Herbal Medicine in India

Saikat Sen • Raja Chakraborty
Editors

Herbal Medicine in India

Indigenous Knowledge, Practice, Innovation and its Value

Springer

Editors
Saikat Sen
Faculty of Pharmaceutical Science
Assam Down Town University
Guwahati, Assam
India

Raja Chakraborty
NEF College of Pharmacy
Lokhra Lalganesh Road, Lokhra
Guwahati, Assam
India

ISBN 978-981-13-7247-6 ISBN 978-981-13-7248-3 (eBook)
https://doi.org/10.1007/978-981-13-7248-3

This Springer imprint is published by the registered company Springer Nature Singapore Pte Ltd.
The registered company address is: 152 Beach Road, #21-01/04 Gateway East, Singapore 189721, Singapore

To our parents, teachers and students.

Preface

Plant-based medicine has a strong tradition in India, with more than 5000 years of practice leading up to the twenty-first century. Codified medicinal system of India, like Ayurveda, Siddha, Unani, and Amchi, has very strong evidences of their effectiveness, and plants are the key component in such systems. It is estimated that Ayurveda, Siddha, and Unani use more than 1200, 900 and 700 species of plant, respectively, in their medicinal preparations. Non-codified or folk medicine in India are playing a key role mainly in remote and rural areas, and it was estimated that about 8000 plants species are in use in folk medicine and about 25,000 effective plant-based formulations are used by local folk medicine practitioners.

Plants are always in the centre of drug discovery and development. In recent years, an enormous resurgence of the use of herbal product is due to the lesser side effect, failure or side effect caused by modern medicine and microbial resistance. The World Health Organization acknowledged the importance of herbal medicine. The goal of "Health for All" cannot be accomplished without herbal medicines. In the twenty-first century, demand for medicinal plants, herbal medicines and pharmaceuticals, food supplements, health products, cosmetics, etc. is growing in, which demand for more research, enhanced regulation and to address quality control issues.

The book *Herbal Medicine in India: Indigenous Knowledge, Practice, Innovation and Its Value* is a vast compendium of information on herbal medicine written by eminent academia and researchers. The book is divided into five major divisions in view of the current need and research on herbal medicine. *Part I: Traditional Medicinal Systems and Herbal Medicine in India* contains chapters devoted to the current situation, importance and role of traditional Indian medicines. *Part II: Plants for Better Future (Therapeutic and Pharmaceutical Consideration)* relates to the research and role of plants considering their therapeutic and pharmaceutical uses. Chapters on plant-based drug discovery, phytochemicals and analytical techniques are included in *Part III: Phytochemicals and Drug Discovery*. *Part IV: Herbal Nutraceuticals and Today's Life* includes the chapters on herbal nutraceuticals and plant-based food which are key aspects in recent time. *Part V: Herbal Medicine—Validation, Quality Control and IPR Issues* discusses on the quality control issues, validation of herbal medicine and IRP issue.

We are very sure this book will have long-lasting effect, and we hope that a wide audience will find this book useful as a database and repository of knowledge, ideas and research on herbal medicine to build on in further research.

Guwahati, Assam, India Saikat Sen
Guwahati, Assam, India Raja Chakraborty

Acknowledgements

Academicians and researchers from diverse fields working on the herbal medicine have shared their ideas/thought and made this book an important repository of information in the field of herbal medicine. We express our gratitude to all the contributing authors who accepted our invitation to give their valuable time and effort and share the expertise they have attained through their extensive research and hard work.

We are greatly indebted to our parents and teachers who played an instrumental role in our life. We are also thankful to our friends, colleagues and well-wishers who were all the time with us during the journey of our education and professional life. We want to express our thanks to our students who are one of the important sources of motivation.

We want to express our sincere thanks to the authorities/managements of Assam Down Town University, Guwahati and NEF College of Pharmacy, Guwahati for providing professional backbone while writing the book.

Most importantly, we are personally indebted to our family members for their motivation, support and tolerance, without which this book would have never been finished.

Finally, we would like to thank Springer Publishers and their staff members, specifically Dr. Naren Aggarwal, Ms. Jagjeet Kaur Saini, Ms. Abha Krishnan and Ms. Vinodhini S, for their help and patience during the preparation of this work.

However, for any errors that remain, despite our best efforts to catch them, we take responsibility. The authors would welcome suggestions from the readers through electronic mail (saikat.pharm@rediffmail.com/dr_rchakraborty@rediffmail.com).

Contents

Part V Herbal Medicine—Validation, Quality Control & IPR Issues

About the Editors

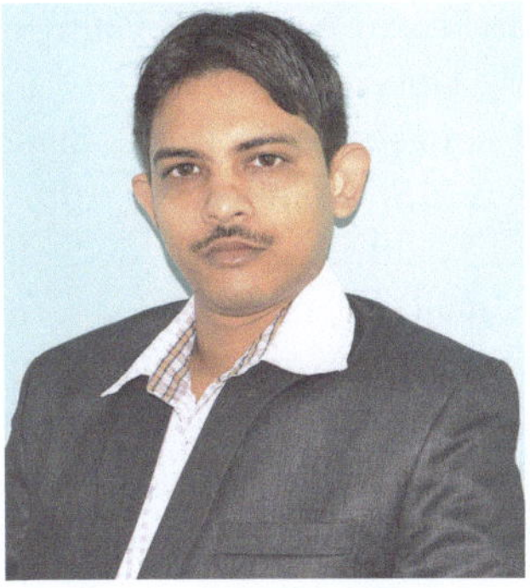

Saikat Sen, M.Pharm., Ph.D., F.I.C.S. is a Professor, Assam Down Town University, Guwahati, India. He received his B.Pharm. degree from JSS College of Pharmacy, Ooty; his M. Pharm (Pharmacology) degree from the College of Pharmacy, Sri Ramakrishna Institute of Paramedical Sciences, Coimbatore; and his Ph.D. in Pharmaceutical Sciences from Jawaharlal Nehru Technological University Anantapur, Andhra Pradesh. He has authored two books and contributed different peer-reviewed edited books published by American Chemical Society (USA), Springer Publishing, Studium Press LLC, Academic Press, etc. More than 60 research and review articles in reputed national/international journals were added to his credit. He presented several scientific papers, attended a number of national and international conferences and delivered invitee lecture in different scientific forums. He is associated with different professional bodies and journals as Life Member, Fellow Member, Scientific Advisor, Editorial Board Member, Advisor Board Member, and Reviewer. His bibliography is published by Marquis Who's Who in the World 2016. He has devoted many years of research into traditional medicine, mainly focusing on herbal medicine. In recognition of his contributions, he received the "Dr. APJ Abdul Kalam Award for Young Scientists 2018" from Marina Labs, Chennai, and the "Best Faculty Award" from The Science & Technology Awards (STA-18) in 2018, as well as an award from the *Journal of Forestry Research* in collaboration with the Government of China to continue his research in herbal medicine. Currently, he is also working as PI in a DBT-sponsored mega networking project on herbal medicine. He is involved enthusiastically in scientific research on traditional/folk medicinal system and to develop active research culture.

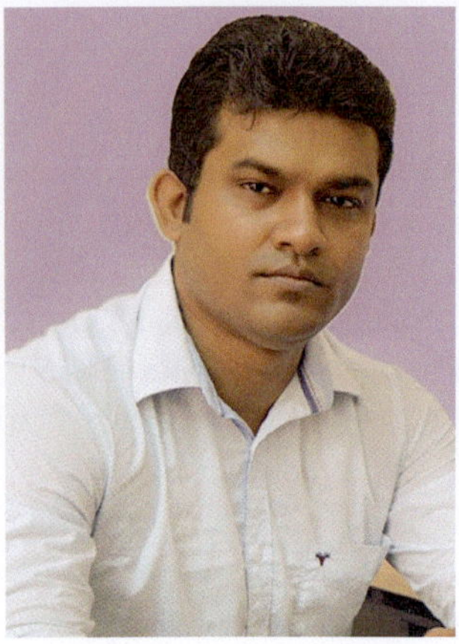

Raja Chakraborty, M.Pharm., Ph.D., F.I.C.S. is Professor and Principal of NEF College of Pharmacy, Guwahati, India. He has received his B.Pharm. from JSS College of Pharmacy, Ooty; M.Pharm. in Pharmaceutical Chemistry from the College of Pharmacy, SRIPMS, Coimbatore, affiliated to The Tamil Nadu Dr. MGR Medical University, Chennai; and Ph.D. in Pharmaceutical Sciences from Jawaharlal Nehru Technological University Anantapur, India, in 2014. With 11 years of academic and research experience, he has published more than 60 research and review articles in reputed national and international journals. He authored two books and also contributed nine book chapters published by ACS Publication, Studium Press, Academic Press, Abhijeet Publications, IGI Global, Write and Print Publications, and Springer Publishing. He serves as a Reviewer for several reputed journals and works as Editorial Board Member for different international journals. Recently, he received "Dr. APJ Abdul Kalam Award for Teaching Excellence 2018". He is guiding a number of Ph.D. students and serving as Co-PI in a DBT-funded megaproject. He wants to contribute his research hand in the field of natural chemistry in respect to traditional knowledge aimed to serve a beneficiary and economic health care.

Part I

Traditional Medicinal Systems and Herbal Medicine in India

Globalisation of Ayurveda: Importance of Scientific Evidence Base

1

Kaushik Chattopadhyay

Contents

1.1 Introduction

This chapter is written from an evidence-based perspective, which is needed for the globalisation of Ayurveda. The author is a qualified Ayurveda practitioner and an evidence-based healthcare academic in a world-class university. This chapter is divided into sections like Ayurveda and its popularity, problems associated with Ayurveda, scientific evidence base of Ayurveda—the way forward, pathways to impact and communication plans and beneficiaries and impacts.

1.2 Ayurveda and its Popularity

Ayurveda is one of the world's oldest medical systems, which originated in the Indian subcontinent more than 5000 years ago. Ayurveda can be considered as a complex intervention, which includes maintaining a healthy lifestyle and using Ayurvedic therapies and medicines (such as herbal and herbo-mineral formulations). Ayurvedic interventions are written in Sanskrit, in the form of classical texts, such as Charaka Samhita (400–200 BC), Sushruta Samhita (400–200 BC) and Astanga Hridaya (around 200 AD) (Sharma 1981; Bhishagratna 1991; Murthy 1991).

K. Chattopadhyay (✉)
Division of Epidemiology and Public Health, School of Medicine, The University of Nottingham, Nottingham, UK
e-mail: kaushik.chattopadhyay@nottingham.ac.uk

S. Sen, R. Chakraborty (eds.), *Herbal Medicine in India*,
https://doi.org/10.1007/978-981-13-7248-3_1

Ayurvedic interventions are particularly used for the prevention and management of chronic diseases (Sharma et al. 2007a, b; Rudra et al. 2017). In India, the Ministry of AYUSH is dedicated exclusively towards traditional therapies, including Ayurveda (Katoch et al. 2017). Globally, different rules and regulations are in place, which may change over time. Many countries had less stringent laws but have now implemented well-defined and well-enforced laws. Some countries consider Ayurvedic medicines as conventional pharmaceuticals and some as dietary supplements (Barnes et al. 2016; Job et al. 2016; Sammons et al. 2016; Teng et al. 2016).

In general, the acceptability of and faith in Ayurveda are high among South Asians, especially among older, women, rural, poor and tribal populations. Ayurveda fits their health beliefs and is compatible with their social and cultural expectations. Many of them do not prefer Western medicines—to avoid the associated side effects and costs (Roy et al. 2015; Rudra et al. 2017; Srinivasan and Sugumar 2017). In fact, Western medicine is facing new challenges arising from its limitations when applied to chronic diseases and ageing (Warrell et al. 2010). Globally, Ayurveda is gaining popularity due to its holistic approach (Patwardhan 2014). Ayurvedic therapies like Panchakarma (i.e. detoxification of the body) are popular among people, especially among foreign tourists who travel to Indian states like Kerala (Ramesh et al. 2010).

1.3 Problems Associated with Ayurveda

Many times, Ayurvedic medicines are either prescribed by an unqualified practitioner or used as self-medication. One of the major reasons behind self-medication is the easy availability of these medicines over-the-counter (which includes online shopping). Many people blindly follow the claims made by others or use a 'trial and error' approach in deciding the medication (Bhamra et al. 2017; Rao et al. 2016; Rudra et al. 2017; Srinivasan and Sugumar 2017). A wide range of non-evidence-based Ayurvedic medicines are used by people, which can have serious negative health and socio-economic consequences. Globally, many cases of heavy metal poisoning (such as lead and mercury) have been reported among people using Ayurvedic medicines (Ernst 2002; Lynch and Braithwaite 2005; Karri et al. 2008; Kales and Saper 2009). Although many Ayurveda practitioners claim that heavy metal poisoning occurs due to the inadequate processing of heavy metals before they are used in Ayurvedic medicines (i.e. if the exact processing methods, as mentioned in Ayurvedic classical texts, are not followed), but robustly designed scientific studies are still lacking on this issue. In addition, many people simultaneously use multiple Western and/or traditional medicines (i.e. polypharmacy)—many times without any evidence of effectiveness and safety and can lead to harmful drug-drug interactions (Aslam and Shaw 1995; Bhamra et al. 2017; Bush et al. 2007; Sarkar et al. 2013). Thus, strong concerns remain about the suboptimal management and care of many people, arising from the unacceptable usage of non-evidence-based Ayurvedic interventions. It is important to use only effective and safe Ayurvedic interventions and minimise the use of interventions that are of no, minimal, or questionable value.

One of the major hurdles in the globalisation of Ayurveda is its poor scientific evidence base. Unfortunately, the interest of commercial pharmaceutical companies in conducting research studies is not always strong, as it is not possible to patent prior published knowledge (Chaudhary and Singh 2012). In most cases, the scientific evidence base does not exist. Even if it does, it is of poor quality. Most of them are short-term studies and are often associated with considerable methodological limitations, such as small sample sizes in treatment groups, resulting in lack of statistical power for outcome assessment and poor concealment of treatment allocation, leading to potential analysis bias. In addition, most of them have evaluated Ayurvedic medicines but not Ayurveda as a system of care or complex intervention (Patwardhan 2014).

1.4 Scientific Evidence Base of Ayurveda: The Way Forward

In the case of Ayurveda, there is a strong need for robustly designed pragmatic studies. One of the major research areas should be the evaluation of effectiveness and safety of Ayurvedic interventions through randomised controlled trials. The World Health Organization says that a traditional therapy (including Ayurveda) with an established history of use can proceed directly from basic animal toxicity studies to a phase III clinical trial (Chaudhury 1992). The UK Medical Research Council's guideline for developing and evaluating complex interventions can be used for designing such studies (MRC 2006). Many internationally recognised checklists for reporting research studies are available, which should be used to design such studies, such as the Consolidated Standards of Reporting Trials (CONSORT) 2010 (includes a specific checklist for herbal medicines) (Gagnier et al. 2006a, b, c; Moher et al. 2010; Schulz et al. 2010). However, research studies on Ayurvedic interventions should not be restricted to randomised controlled trials and should also include basic pharmacological studies, observational (epidemiological) studies, qualitative studies, economic evaluations and systematic reviews (and meta-analysis). Some other important research topics are Ayurveda related education, health services and systems and diagnostic methodologies. These studies will provide a complete picture of the situation and have the potential to make the scientific evidence base of Ayurveda strong.

1.5 Pathways to Impact and Communication Plans

User involvement (patient and public involvement) in research studies is a major pathway to impact (Staley 2009; Bagley et al. 2016). It should also be the backbone of research studies on Ayurvedic interventions. Such studies need to be carried out with patients and the public, to meet their needs and preferences. Research topics should be identified and discussed with users and user groups. They should agree and acknowledge the importance of the research topic. The issues identified during these discussions should be taken into consideration while designing and developing such studies. These users and user groups should regularly take part in discussions and give feedback on different aspects of the project, including research tools, data analyses and interpretation, research updates and reports and different mediums for communicating results. These collaborations should build relationships within the research community and should extend beyond the life of such projects. It is highly recommended to produce reports on user involvement and disseminate such reports.

In order to ensure the translation of research outputs into actions, key stakeholders should be continuously engaged from the beginning of any study. A range of key stakeholders, representing health policymakers and managers (of public and private healthcare providers), healthcare professionals (including Ayurveda practitioners), patient and public groups, non-profit organisations, non-governmental organisations and international organisations, should be involved. Public-friendly research updates and brief final reports should be produced and disseminated through various avenues, including meetings, study and institutional websites and online forums (e.g. Facebook, Twitter). The press offices of host institutions should also advise on how best to present and disseminate the findings. They usually have good contacts with the media. Press releases should be sent to the media in advance of newsworthy publications. The host institutions can release MP3 podcasts of topical research, an additional medium for dissemination.

The findings of research studies should be widely disseminated in the scientific community through publications in high-impact peer-reviewed open-access journals and presentations at national and international conferences. Both general and specialist conferences should be targeted for a wider coverage. The data (anonymised) on which a journal paper is based should be made available to the readers as an additional supporting file. Publications and additional supporting files should also be made available on the study and institutional websites. These dissemination strategies also have the potential to attract researchers for further collaborative research studies.

1.6 Beneficiaries and Impacts

Research studies on Ayurvedic interventions have the potential to directly benefit people (patients and the public), health policymakers and managers (of public and private healthcare providers), Ayurveda practitioners and academics.

If Ayurvedic interventions are found to be clinically and cost effective, the clinical, personal and economic burden of diseases on people and their families/carers will be prevented or reduced. They will be provided with more evidence-based choices to prevent and manage diseases. These interventions may simultaneously empower people to manage their health. These interventions may reduce health inequalities and be beneficial to all of the society.

Health policymakers and managers will benefit from the availability of low-cost and acceptable evidence-based solutions to prevent and manage diseases, since more expensive disease prevention and management models are in use. The economic burden of diseases on the health systems and the economies will be prevented or reduced.

Ayurveda practitioners will have access to evidence-based Ayurvedic interventions. They may potentially get a boost due to greater interest in their services, which may also enhance their job opportunities. These interventions may close the gap between what they do for preventing and managing diseases and what scientific evidence supports. These interventions may reinforce their position in prevention and management of diseases and offer them medico-legal protection.

The scientific research on Ayurvedic interventions has the potential to directly benefit academics working in at least two research disciplines—specific diseases and traditional therapies (including Ayurveda). Such projects can bring together Western medicine and Ayurveda experts. There will be mutual academic benefit and capacity building by cross-sharing of expertise and experience within the groups. A good-quality cross-country project should be a collaboration between academics with complementary strengths, such as the UK's methodological expertise and India's large clinical networks. Such projects have the potential to improve scientific links between countries and more broadly through wider collaborative links and networking. Greater use of these interventions has the potential to highlight the gaps in evidence, which may stimulate further research activities. Funding opportunities for research on Ayurvedic interventions are growing but are still limited. Conclusive evidence of the beneficial effects and safety of some of these interventions may lead to greater funding opportunities and conduct of robust studies. All these may greatly enhance the acceptance of Ayurveda by the scientific and wider communities.

Given that chronic diseases and ageing are global concerns and the cost is a concern everywhere, low-cost Ayurvedic interventions will be of interest to many countries, particularly South Asian countries and in countries with South Asian ethnic minorities. Such projects will involve collaborative research work to evaluate and implement these interventions in a range of settings and populations. Thus, research studies on Ayurvedic interventions have the potential to impact the world.

1.7 Conclusion

Globally, the scope of Ayurveda is huge and has the potential to benefit a range of beneficiaries. In order to achieve this, the scientific evidence base of Ayurveda must be made strong.

References

Aslam M, Shaw J. A case study: dangers of transcultural medicine in the U.K. J Clin Pharm Ther. 1995;20(6):345–7.

Bagley HJ, Short H, Harman NL, Hickey HR, Gamble CL, Woolfall K, et al. A patient and public involvement (PPI) toolkit for meaningful and flexible involvement in clinical trials: a work in progress. Res Involv Engagem. 2016;2:15.

Barnes J, McLachlan AJ, Sherwin CM, Enioutina EY. Herbal medicines: challenges in the modern world. Part 1. Australia and New Zealand. Expert Rev Clin Pharmacol. 2016;9(7):905–15.

Bhamra SK, Slater A, Howard C, Johnson M, Heinrich M. The use of traditional herbal medicines amongst South Asian diasporic communities in the UK. Phytother Res. 2017;31(11):1786–94.

Bhishagratna KL. English translation of Sushruta Samhita. Varanasi, India: Choukhamba Orientalia; 1991.

Bush TM, Rayburn KS, Holloway SW, Sanchez-Yamamoto DS, Allen BL, Lam T, et al. Adverse interactions between herbal and dietary substances and prescription medications: a clinical survey. Altern Ther Health Med. 2007;13(2):30–5.

Chaudhary A, Singh N. Intellectual property rights and patents in perspective of Ayurveda. Ayu. 2012;33(1):20–6.

Chaudhury RR. Herbal medicine for human health. New Delhi, India: World Health Organization, Regional Office for Southeast Asia; 1992.

Ernst E. Heavy metals in traditional Indian remedies. Eur J Clin Pharmacol. 2002;57(12):891–6.

Gagnier JJ, Boon H, Rochon P, Moher D, Barnes J, Bombardier C, et al. Reporting randomised, controlled trials of herbal interventions: an elaborated CONSORT statement. Ann Intern Med. 2006a;144(5):364–7.

Gagnier J, Boon H, Rochon P, Barnes J, Moher D, Bombardier C, et al. Improving the quality of reporting of randomised controlled trials evaluating herbal interventions: implementing the CONSORT statement [corrected]. Explore (NY). 2006b;2(2):143–9.

Gagnier JJ, Boon H, Rochon P, Moher D, Barnes J, Bombardier C, et al. Recommendations for reporting randomised controlled trials of herbal interventions: explanation and elaboration. J Clin Epidemiol. 2006c;59(11):1134–49.

Job KM, Kiang TK, Constance JE, Sherwin CM, Enioutina EY. Herbal medicines: challenges in the modern world. Part 4. Canada and United States. Expert Rev Clin Pharmacol. 2016;9(12):1597–609.

Kales SN, Saper RB. Ayurvedic lead poisoning: an under-recognized, international problem. Indian J Med Sci. 2009;63(9):379–81.

Karri SK, Saper RB, Kales SN. Lead encephalopathy due to traditional medicines. Curr Drug Saf. 2008;3(1):54–9.

Katoch D, Sharma JS, Banerjee S, Biswas R, Das B, Goswami D, et al. Government policies and initiatives for development of Ayurveda. J Ethnopharmacol. 2017;197:25–31.

Lynch E, Braithwaite R. A review of the clinical and toxicological aspects of 'traditional' (herbal) medicines adulterated with heavy metals. Expert Opin Drug Saf. 2005;4:769–78.

MRC. Developing and evaluating complex interventions: new guidance. London, UK: MRC; 2006.

Moher D, Hopewell S, Schulz KF, Montori V, Gøtzsche PC, Devereaux PJ, et al. CONSORT 2010 explanation and elaboration: updated guidelines for reporting parallel group randomised trials. BMJ. 2010;340:c869.

Murthy S. English translation of Astanga Hridaya. Varanasi, India: Choukhamba Orientalia; 1991.

Patwardhan B. Bridging Ayurveda with evidence-based scientific approaches in medicine. EPMA J. 2014;5(1):19.

Ramesh U, Joseph K, Renganathan R. Ayurvedic health tourism in Kerala: a study on the market potential catering to customer perceptions. i-manager's Journal on Management. 2010;4(4):55–62.

Rao KD, Shahrawat R, Bhatnagar A. Composition and distribution of the health workforce in India: estimates based on data from the National Sample Survey. WHO South East Asia J Public Health. 2016;5(2):133–40.

Roy V, Gupta M, Ghosh RK. Perception, attitude and usage of complementary and alternative medicine among doctors and patients in a tertiary care hospital in India. Indian J Pharmacol. 2015;47(2):137–42.

Rudra S, Kalra A, Kumar A, Joe W. Utilization of alternative systems of medicine as health care services in India: evidence on AYUSH care from NSS 2014. PLoS One. 2017;12(5):e0176916.

Sammons HM, Gubarev MI, Krepkova LV, Bortnikova VV, Corrick F, Job KM, et al. Herbal medicines: challenges in the modern world. Part 2. European Union and Russia. Expert Rev Clin Pharmacol. 2016;9(8):1117–27.

Sarkar PK, Chaudhari S, Chattopadhyay A. Concept of interactions between consumable substances in Ayurveda with special reference to foods and drugs. Drug Metabol Drug Interact. 2013;28(3):147–52.

Schulz KF, Altman DG, Moher D, CONSORT Group. CONSORT 2010 statement: updated guidelines for reporting parallel group randomised trials. BMJ. 2010;340:c332.

Sharma H, Chandola HM, Singh G, Basisht G. Utilization of Ayurveda in health care: an approach for prevention, health promotion, and treatment of disease. Part 1: Ayurveda, the science of life. J Altern Complement Med. 2007a;13(9):1011–9.

Sharma H, Chandola HM, Singh G, Basisht G. Utilization of Ayurveda in health care: an approach for prevention, health promotion, and treatment of disease. Part 2: Ayurveda in primary health care. J Altern Complement Med. 2007b;13(10):1135–50.

Sharma PV. English translation of Charaka Samhita. Varanasi, India: Choukhamba Orientalia; 1981.

Srinivasan R, Sugumar VR. Spread of traditional medicines in India: results of National Sample Survey Organization's perception survey on use of AYUSH. J Evid Based Complementary Altern Med. 2017;22(2):194–204.

Staley K. Exploring impact: public involvement in NHS, public health and social care research. Eastleigh, UK: INVOLVE; 2009.

Teng L, Zu Q, Li G, Yu T, Job KM, Yang X, et al. Herbal medicines: challenges in the modern world. Part 3. China and Japan. Expert Rev Clin Pharmacol. 2016;9(9):1225–33.

Warrell DA, Cox TM, Firth JD. Oxford textbook of medicine. 5th ed. New York, USA: Oxford University Press; 2010.

Siddha, an Indigenous Medical System of Peninsular India

2

Subramani Parasuraman
and Pandurangan Perumal

Contents

S. Parasuraman (✉) · P. Perumal
Faculty of Pharmacy, AIMST University,
Bedong, Malaysia
e-mail: Parasuraman@aimst.edu.my

S. Sen, R. Chakraborty (eds.), *Herbal Medicine in India*,
https://doi.org/10.1007/978-981-13-7248-3_2

2.1 History

Globally, the usage of traditional system of medicine/complementary and alternative medicine has increased over the past few eras. Southern part of India has rich cultural heritage of civilisation, education, devotional, medicine, etc. and the traditional medicinal system followed in southern states of India has vibrant and equally important *Ayurvedic* medicine which is practised throughout the country. South India is also known as Peninsular India encompassing the states of Andhra Pradesh, Karnataka, Kerala, Tamil Nadu and Telangana as well as the union territories of Andaman and Nicobar, Lakshadweep and Puducherry. India is known for its traditional system of medicines including *Ayurveda*, *Siddha* and *Unani*. In traditional medicine, plants are most commonly used for the treatment, and part of minerals is also used. *Siddha* system primarily uses herbal products along with animal and mineral substances. *Siddha* system of medicine is one of the prehistoric medical systems in greater India and considered as the mother of the medicine of ancient Tamil peoples in India. *Siddha* medical system is established by Siddhars dating back to 12,000 years B.C. (Shukla et al. 2011). The father of *Siddha* medicine and *Siddha* system of medicine is Maha Rishi Sri Agathiyar (Agastya), a first Siddhar (Fig. 2.1) (Raghunathan 1979).

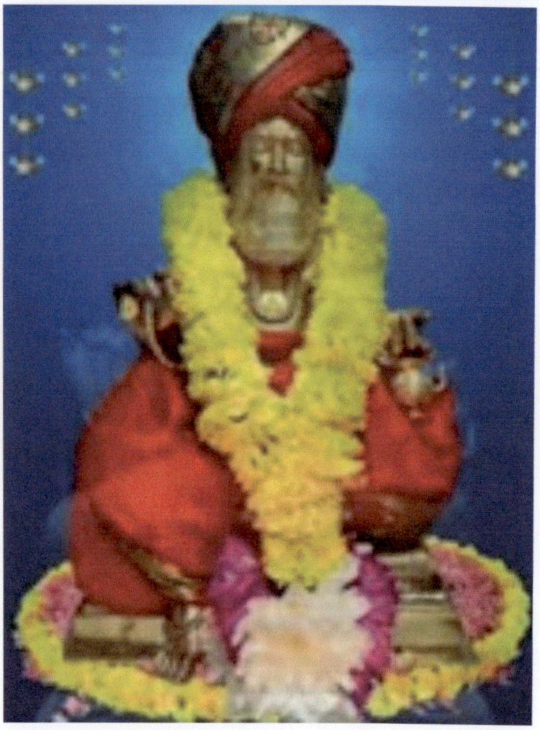

Fig. 2.1 Maha Rishi Sri Agathiyar

Siddha word denotes one who has achieved some extraordinary powers or supernatural powers (*siddhi*) and realisation of soul-superiority of mind over body. This is a state when one can feel the infinite power within oneself. *Siddha* medicine is to make the positive health, and imperishable and harmonious blending of physical, mental, social and spiritual welfare of an individual to promote longevity. Origin is traced to mythological or divine sources belonging to Shaiva tradition. According to the tradition, knowledge of *Siddha* system of medicine is the speech of the Lord Shiva to his concert Goddess Parvati who handed it down to Nandi Deva and from him to the Siddhars (Arunachalam et al. 2009). Another claim is that the *Siddha* system of medicine evolved and developed as an adjuvant to a system of philosophy termed as the *Saiva Siddhanta* which itself is depicted as a product of Tamil culture (Krishnamurthy and Chandra Mouli 1984).

The term *Siddha* is derived from Siddhar (perfected or holy immortals) where saintly persons who achieved results in medicine. Eighteen Siddhars (Agasthiyar, Bogar, Dhanvandri, Idaikkadar, Karuvurar, Kamalamuni, Konganar, Korakkar, Kudhambai, Machamuni, Paambatti, Padhanjali, Ramadevar, Sattainathar, Sivavaakiyar, Sundaranandar, Thirumular and Vanmeegar) are contributed towards the development of *Siddha* system of medicine. *Siddha* literature is in Tamil, a Dravidian language predominantly spoken by the Tamil people, and it is practised largely in Tamil-speaking part of India. Significance of *Siddha* medicine is 'conquest of death' and this statement is attributed to *Thirumoolar*. *Thirumoolar* is the author of *Tirumantiram* and he wrote 3000 stanzas regarding classic text on the basic philosophy of *Siddha* medicine (Wilson et al. 2007). In *Siddha* medical system, drugs are classified into herbs (*Thavaram or Mooligai*), inorganic substance (*Thathu*) and animal products (*Jeevavaguppu*). The theory and concepts of *Siddha* medicines are written in Tamil and largest share of the palm manuscript collection is found in southern part of India. The Oriental Manuscript Library, U. Ve. Swaminatha Iyer Library, Institute of Asian Studies, International Institute of Tamil Studies, *Siddha* Central Research Institute, a Literary division of the Directorate on Indian Medicine and Homeopathy, Govt. of Tamil Nadu, the Saraswathi Mahal Library and Manuscriptology Department of Tamil University at Thanjavur archived a large number of *Siddha* manuscripts and Govt. Oriental Manuscript Library has digitised 1085 *Siddha* manuscripts in the year 2005 (Rajkumar et al. 2012).

In *Siddha* medicine, treatment is based on human body (*Tattva*) or constituent principles. As per *Siddha* literature, the human body is composed of 96 *Tattvas* (principles) under 14 categories. They include ten vital airs and five cases of the sheaths of the soul and nine doors or vents of the body; ten nerves; eight predominant passions; seven constituent elements of the body; six stations of the soul; five basic elements, objects of senses, organs of action, organs of perception and stages of soul; four intellectual faculties; three principles of moral evil; three regions; and imbalances in three humours such as *Vatham*, *Pottham* and *Khapam* causing 4448 diseases (Anonymous 2017).

2.2 Principles of *Siddha*

The universe entails matter and energy. It coexists with inseparable and primordial elements such as *Butas*. The *Panchabutas* (five elements) are said to be *Munn* (solid or earth), *Neer* (fluid or water), *Thee* (radiance or fire), *Vayu* (gas or air) and *Akasam* (space-ether) or earth, water, fire, air and space (Parasuraman et al. 2014). Earth gives fine shape to body. Water represents blood, hormones and vigorous fluid. Fire gives gesture, potency and energy to the body. Air helps in digestion and circulation. Space helps in human's mental and spiritual abilities.

Human body is considered to be made of these five elements in different combinations (*Panchamahabutas*) the universe coexists and functions harmoniously. Physiological functions can be mediated by three humours called as *Tridosha* (three humours) that are *Vatham*, *Pitham* and *Kapham*. *Vatham* consists of *Akasa* and *Vayu* which are responsible for nervous actions such as movement, activity and sensation. *Pitham* consists of *Thee* (fire) which is responsible for the metabolic activity of the body, digestion, assimilation, warmth, etc. *Kapham* consists of *Munn* and *Neer* which are responsible for stability in the body (chest, throat, head and joints). Tissues are called as *dhatus* and there are seven *dathus* (Saptadathus) named as *Rasa* (lymph), *Kurudhi* (blood), *Tasai* (muscle), *Kozhuppu* (adipose tissue), *Elumbu* (bone), *Majjai* (marrow), *Sukkilam* and *Artavam* (male and female hormones).

Vatham is found in the form of five bodily winds which are *Pranam* (inhaled breath), *Apanam* (exhaled breath), *Samanam* (digestion), *Vyanam* (circulation of blood and nutrients) and *Udanam* (upper respiratory functions). There are also five secondary winds which are *Nagam*, *Kurmam*, *Kirukaram*, *Devadhattham* and *Dhananjayam* (Kumar et al. 2012).

The principles of *Siddha* are closely similar to *Ayurveda* with specialisation in iatrochemistry (Chaudhury and Rafei 2001). The *Siddha* system of medicine extensively describes the use of herbomineral products like arsenic, copper, gold, iron, mercury and sulphur (Yadav et al. 2012). Fundamental principles of *Siddha* system of medicine include theories of five elements (*Aimpootham*), three forces/faults (*Mukkuttram*) and eight methods of examination (*Envakai Thervukal*) (Thas 2008).

According to the *Siddha* system, the individual is a microcosm of the universe. The human body is made up of five basic elements such as earth, water, fire, air and space; the three *Uyir Thathukkal, Trithodam* or *Mukkutram* (humours), *viz.*, *vatham*, *pittam* and *kapham*; and seven *Udal Thathukkal* (physical constituents), *viz.*, *Saaram*,

Senneer, *Oon*, *Kozhuppu*, *Elumbu*, *Moolai* and *Sukkilam*. Food is the basic material of the human body and gets processed into humours and imbalances of these humours lead to disease. This was stated by Saint Thiruvalluvar in his *Thirukural* (மிகினும் குறையினும் நோய்செய்யும் நூலோர் வளி முதலா எண்ணிய மூன்று in Tamil. Meaning: As per medical writers imbalance of *vatham*, *pitham* and *kapham* will cause disease.-*Kural* 941) (Kandaswamy 1979; Sowrirajan 1992).

2.3 Tridoshas and Its Characteristics

***Vatham*:** Its characteristics are dryness, lightness, coldness and motility. It regulates the central and the sympathetic nervous system. It can be formed by ether and air (*Akasam* and *Vayu*) and controls the nervous action that constitutes sensation and movement. It predominates in the bone in first 1/3 of life when activity, growth and senses are greater. It pervades in every part of the body.

***Pitham*:** It regulates the functions of thermogenesis and metabolism. It can be formed by fire (*Thee*) and controls the metabolic activity, digestion, warmth, intellect and assimilation. It predominates in the blood in second 1/3 of life. It is located in the alimentary canal from the cardiac end of the stomach to the end of the small intestine.

Kapham: It acts as a thermostat to the body and characteristics are smoothness, firmness, heaviness and viscidity. It regulates the heat and the formation of the various preservative glands. It can be formed by earth and water (*Munn* and *Neer*) and controls the stability, strength, potency and smooth working of joints. It predominates in other tissues in last 1/3 of life with diminishing activity of various organs and limbs. It is located in chest, throat, head and joints (Stephen 2005; Uthamaroyan 1992; Anandan and Thulasimani 2008).

***Tridosha* theory:** The ratio of three humours (*Vatham:Pitham:Kapham*) is 1:1/2:¼ (Shukla et al. 2011). When the equilibrium of these three humours upsets then disease sets in. The characteristics and predominance of *tridoshas* are based on the age of the person and season. The deviation of humours from normal ratio can be found out by pulse diagnosis and there are three types of *nadi vignanam* (*nadi pariksha*) which are index, middle and ring fingers. Index finger may feel the windy humour (movement of cock, or peacock), middle finger may feel bilious humour (movement of tortoise or a leech) and ring finger may feel phlegmatic humour (movement of a frog or a snake). There are eight kinds of diagnostic methods which are *Nadi* (pulse reading), *Sparisam* (sensation of touch), *Naa* (tongue and mouth examination), *Niram* (complexation), *Mozhi* (speech analysis), *Vizhi* (eye examination), *Malam* (examination of stools) and *Moothiram* (urine analysis).

2.4 The Fundamentals of *Siddha* Methodology

According to *Siddha* system, 4448 diseases are treatable based on diagnosis. A physician must be knowledgeable in alchemy, astrology and philosophy and must apply intuition and imagination. The aim of *Siddha* is to give medicine right to the root where the disease is originated (Uthamaroyan 1992; Anandan and Thulasimani 2008).

There are three groups of drugs in *Siddha* medicine which are *mulavargam* (plant products) *thatuvargam* (inorganic substances) and *jivavargam* (animal products) and these are categorised by *rasam* (taste), *gunam* (quality), *viryam* (potency), *vipakam* (post digestive taste) and *prabhavam* (specific action). The fundamental of Siddha medicine can be classified into four types as follows:

(a) Vadham (*alchemy*)
(b) Aithiyam (*medicine*)
(c) Yogam (*yoga*)
(d) Gnanam or thathuvam (*philosophy*)

2.4.1 Vadham *(Alchemy)*

Alchemy was known as the *spagyric art.* Latin: *Solve Et Coagula—Separate, and Join Together*

Table 2.1 The characteristics and properties of inorganic substances

Inorganic substances	Characteristics and properties
Uppu (salts)	Salts are alkaline in nature and soluble in water. More than 25 varieties of salts are used in *Siddha* preparations.
Pashanam (poison)	Pashanam is insoluble in water and emits vapour when heated.
Uparasam	Uparasam is insoluble in water and includes antimony, asafoetida, ferrous sulphate, magnetic, mica, iron, iron pyrites, sulphate and zinc.
Loham (metals)	Six varieties of metals are used in *Siddha* preparations including gold, silver, copper, iron, tin and lead. They are insoluble in water.
Rasam	Rasam contains five chemicals, *viz.*, pure mercury (rasa), red sulphide of mercury (lingam), mercuric chloride (viram), mercurous chloride (puram) and red oxide of mercury (rasachenduram) which are called Panchastutha.
Gandhakam	Gandhakam (English—sulphur) is insoluble in water and burns off when heated. Gandhakam and Rasam combine to make *kattu*.

(or *dissolve and coagulate*). The aim of the alchemists was the transmutation of common metals into gold (called chrysopoeia) or silver and the creation of the elixir of life, which is used to cure all diseases and prolong longevity of life, and the discovery of a universal solvent. Texts of alchemy are *Rasahrdaya*, *Rasaratnakara*, *Rasarnava* and *Rasaratnasamuccya*. The alchemy has many types of substances which include inorganic substances; gems and minerals; mud and siliceous earth; and animals and rocks (Subbarayappa 1971). Inorganic substances are further classified into six types, *viz.*, *uppu*, *pashanam*, *uparasam*, *loham*, *rasam* and *gandhakam*. The characteristics and properties of inorganic substances are summarised in Table 2.1.

2.4.2 Aithiyam (medicine)

Siddha system of medicine is impeccable and a physician should be spiritual and have a thorough knowledge on human physiology, *Siddha* preparations and its characteristics. According to Theraiyar (a *Siddha*) in his '*Theriyar Thylavargachurrukam*', the physician should have pure thought and action, love for all human beings, a detailed knowledge about geographical seasonal variations, correct physical and mental state, and dietary habits. Theraiyar in his '*Thylavarkachurukkam*' insists that a physician should clean his hands many times and have bath after examining a patient (Walter Thomas et al. 2009). According to Maha rishi Agathiyar, the qualities of a physician are kindness, patience, untiring hard work, capability of overcoming hunger and irritation, and knowledge about astrology and numerology. The objective of the medicine is disease prevention. *Siddha* medicine has five branches of Aithiyam, *viz.*, general medicine, paediatrics, surgery, toxicology and mental disorders.

2.4.3 Yogam *(Yoga)*

The yoga philosophy exists beyond the mind and its consciousness, which is the only ultimate reality. It is a system of exercises that encourage the union of mind, body and spirit. The objective of yoga is to evacuate misconceptions from the minds of human being. It believes that it is possible through regular practice of certain yoga practices that bring a complete detachment from all false sources of knowledge and maintain inner sense of balanced calm and tranquillity (Patanjali Yoga Sutras 1953; Parasuraman et al. 2016).

Depending on the degree of distraction, yoga philosophy categorises the mind under five stages are as follows, *viz.*, *Kshipta* or disturbed, *Mudha* or stupefied, *Vikshipta* or distracted, *Ekagra* or concentrated and *Niruddha* or the absolutely balanced state of mind (Aravinda Prabhu and Bhat 2013).

In general, yoga is divided into ten types, *viz.*, *Karma* yoga, *Bhakthi* yoga, *Mantra* yoga, *Tantric* yoga, *Kundalini* yoga, *Hastha* yoga, *Swara* yoga, *Kriya* yoga, *Raja* yoga and *Jnana* yoga (Table 2.2) (Aravinda Prabhu and Bhat 2013; Patanjali Yoga Sutras 1953; Balaramaiah and Vadavaidyattukki 1980).

Table 2.2 Types of yoga

Type of yoga	Description
Karma yoga	It is a way of right action, without the physical motivation (form of prayer) and non-attachment with the work.
Bhakthi yoga	It is a devotion or complete faith to supreme power (God) through Guru (guide) who has a very strong attachment with supreme power.
Mantra yoga	Any person who can chant the *vedas* or *mantras* to achieve the supreme power.
Tantric yoga	Pray the supreme power through statue in temple.
Kundalini yoga	This is concerned with awakening of the psychic chakras, which exists in every individual and there are seven in numbers. The aim of this yoga is to awaken the kundalini and send it to the crown of the head.
Hastha yoga	This is concerned with proper practice of various asana includes pranayama (pranic awakening practices), yogasana (yoga positions), six shatkarmas (physical and mental detox techniques), mudras and bandhas (psychophysiological energy release techniques).
Swara yoga	This is the realisation of cosmic consciousness through control of breath.
Kriya yoga	Kriya yoga is a meditation technique of controlling energy through *pranayama* and meditation, which speeds up the spiritual process of the aspirant. This is a meditation technique to control the internal and external energy by using *pranayama*, which is used to increase our spiritual growth and lead to realisation of our soul.
Raja yoga	This is the state of peace and calm through proper practices of yogasanams by suitable guru (guide). This is divided into eight parts which are *Yama* (non-violence and truthfulness), *Niyama* (purity), *Asana* (yoga postures), *Pranayama* (breathing techniques), *Pratyahara* (detachment of senses), *Dharana* (single-minded concentration), *Dhyana* (meditation) and *Samadhi* (superconscious state).
Gnana yoga	The way of knowledge through insight, proper practice by Guru and knowledge. Gnana Yoga has four principles which are Viveka (discrimination), Vairagya (renunciation), Shatsampatti and Mumukshtva (constant striving for god)

2.4.4 Gnanam or Thathuvam (*Philosophy*)

The philosophy or *thathuvam* describes briefly about God, human body and soul. Our body is the temple and seat of the soul, the mouth is the entrance, soul is the god and five senses are five lamps in the temple. Human body and disease are set by chakras. These chakras can be classified into seven types which are *muladhara*, *swadhisthana*, *manipuraga*, *anahatha*, *vishuthi*, *ajna* and *sahasrara* (Fig. 2.2). Location of chakras and their functions are summarised in Table 2.3.

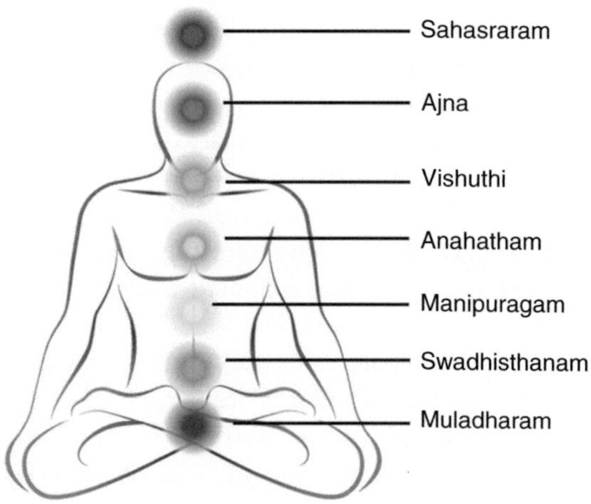

Fig. 2.2 Location of chakras

2.5 Siddhic Process

The process of *siddhic* can be classified into eight forms which are grouped into *Octomiracle* or *Attama* siddhi. *Octomiracle* could keep the body perfect and strong for external life (Anonymous 2018a).The eight primary siddhis are *anima*, *mahima*, *karima*, *laghima*, *prapti*, *prakamya*, *esathwam* and *vashita* (Venkataraman 1990; White 1996).

Table 2.3 Location of chakras and their functions

Chakra name	Location	Function
Sahasraram (Crown Centre)	Top of the head towards the back	Connection to divinity, spirit and bliss
Ajna (Third Eye)	Slightly above the midpoint between eyes	Intuition, metaphysical wisdom and stillness
Vishuthi (Throat Chakra)	Centre of throat	Self-expression and speaking the truth
Anahatham (Heart Chakra)	Centre of the chest at the breastbone	Love, compassion, beauty, joy and balance
Manipuragam (Navel Chakra)	Just below navel	Personal power, self-definition and boundaries
Swadhisthanam (Sacral Chakra)	Internal reproductive organs	Sexuality, creativity, abundance and passion
Muladharam (Root Chakra)	Tailbone	Connection to earth, nature and physicality

2.6 Diagnosis

The proper diagnosis can be possible with those who are having knowledge about *Siddha* medicine and astrology, and experience in the sense of a long period of practice (Narayanaswamy 1975). The diagnosis through *Siddha* medicine is classified into eight categories which are *nadivignanam* (pulse reading), *sparisam* (sensation of touch), *naa* (tongue examination), *niram* (colour of the skin, face), *mozhi* (speech examination), *vizhi* (eye examination), *malam* (tools examination) and *moothiram* (urine examination) (Kandaswamy 1979; Sharma 1992; Walter et al. 2009).

2.6.1 *Nadi Vignanam* (Pulse Reading)

Nadi in *Siddha* means two things, one is the pulse and the other is the nerves. The diagnosis and prognosis are done by the reading of the pulse. In yoga philosophy, there are 72,000 *nadis* or meridians. They take root from the main *sushuma*, intertwined by the *idagalai* (MOON) and the *pingalai* (SUN). These are the three most important nerves in the body along the spinal cord. The *sushuma* resides inside the spinal cord, and *ida* and *pingala* cross at the chakra points along spine and science not yet located these nerves. They are part of the sympathetic nervous system. Certain rules are compulsory to follow before taking pulse as follows: the patients should not have oil on his/her head and the body should not be wet; the pulse should not be taken after a meal, while running, during any physical exercise or when having emotional disturbances (anger and joy); right-hand pulse is taken for male and left-hand for female. Pulse can be taken from ankle joint and ear lobes also but it must be taken at different times based on the season.

The pulse rate may be different in different seasons due to the imbalance of tridhosas such as *vadham, pitham* and *kapham*.

The index, middle and ring fingers are used to feel the *vatham*, *pitham* and *kapham* nadis and it can be read by a *Siddha* practitioner by touching the radial artery of the patient. The internal pressure of the radial artery may be different from finger to finger. *Vatha* nadi imbalance will indicate flatulence of the abdomen, pain and ache all over the body, difficulty in urination, fever, change in voice, constipation, dry cough, discolouration of skin. *Pitha* nadi imbalance will indicate yellowness of eyes, urine and faeces, burning sensation in the stomach, headache, thirst, dryness of mouth, confusion and diarrhoea. *Kapha* nadi imbalance will indicate heaviness of the body and head, sweet taste of tongue, cold to touch, loss of appetite, flatulence, cough with phlegm and difficulty breathing (Nawaz et al. 2010).

2.6.2 Touch

One can feel cold, hot and moist when *vatham, pitham and kapham nadi* are imbalanced.

2.6.3 Colour

Vatham vitiated body of person becomes rough, and skin and hair appear broken. He/she cannot tolerate cold. Memory and self-confidence are affected. *Pitham* in excess can cause excess thirst, hunger and burning sensation. The lips, palms, feet and eyes will be red. Body with excess *kapham* is soft and oily, and symptoms are loss of appetite and thirst.

2.6.4 Tongue

In *vatha* derangement, tongue will be cold, rough and furrowed. In *pitham*, it will be red or yellow. In *kapham*, it will be pale and sticky. In depletion of tridoshas tongue will be dark, with the papillae raised and dry.

2.6.5 Voice

In *kapham* vitiation voice is heavy. In *pitham* vitiation voice will be short. *Vatha* will be different from the other two. Voice also indicates strength.

2.6.6 The Eyes

The eyes are windows to the soul and internal health. If *Vatham* is imbalanced the eyes will be shifty and dry. In *Pitham* imbalance eyes will be yellow and sensitive to light. If *kapham* is in excess, the eyes will have watery secretion, oiliness and lack of luster. In disturbance of all three *doshas*, eyes will be inflamed and red.

2.6.7 Faeces

Undigested food—the stool will sink. Digested food—stool floats. Provoked *vatham*—faeces is hard and dry. *Pitham* vitiation—it is yellow. *Kapham* disturbance—it is pale. Lack of digestion fire—the faeces is watery. Foul smelling of varied colour and shining means the disease is incurable.

2.6.8 Urine Analysis (Moothiram)

Theraiyar was one of the Siddhars in the first 18 Siddhars in *Siddha* medicine who wrote on urine examination. Ramachandiran, explains the colour of the urine in *tridoshas* variance and also explains about the spreading of a single drop of oil on the surface of the urine indicates an imbalance of specific *dosha*. Urine analysis is more important than an examination of *malam* or faeces. Urine is the waste product excreted from the body after metabolism which is carried and transferred from blood to the kidneys which removes the excessive salts and suspensions. Urine analysis can be done early in the morning. Normal urine is thin straw colour and odourless. The colour of the urine comes under five divisions, yellow, red, green, dark and white. The time of day and meals eaten will affect the colour of the urine. The details are further divided as illustrated in Table 2.4 (Ramachandiran 2000; Shanmugavelan 2005; Janani et al. 2016).

2.7 Siddha Preparations

Siddha preparations or medicines can be classified into six categories or six types of formulations as listed below (Subbarayappa 1997):

(a) *Bhasma* (calcined metals and mineral formations)
(b) *Churna* (powder formations)
(c) *Kashaya* (decoction)
(d) *Lehya* (confections)
(e) *Ghrita* (ghee preparation)
(f) Taila (oil preparation)

2.7.1 *Bhasma* (Calcined Metals and Mineral Formations)

Bhasma is a calcined preparation in which the metal or gem is converted into ash. Metals or gems are purified and treated by triturating and macerating in herbal extracts. The dough so obtained is calcinated to obtain the ashes. *Bhasmikaran* is a process by which a substance is made biocompatible by certain *samskaras* or processes (Thottam 2000). The objectives of *samskara* are (1) elimination of toxic matters from the drug; (2) modification of undesirable physical properties of the drug; (3) conversion of some of the characteristics of the drug; and (4) enhancement of the therapeutic value.

Table 2.4 Colour of the urine in tridoshas variance

Colour of the urine		Sign
Yellow	Colour of urine similar to water	Indigestion
	Lemon colour	Good digestion
	Reddish yellow	Heat in body
	Colour similar to forest red or flame	Extreme heat
	Colour of saffron	Heat in body at highest level
Red	Red colour with slight dark red	The blood has become hot
	Bright red colour	More hot than above
	Dark red	Blood in urine
Green	Green with slight dark colour	Cold in the body
	Green with sky blue	Cold and poison in body
	Green with blue	Vatham imbalance
	Blue colour and slimy urine	Early vatham disease
	Leaf green	Late vatham disease
Dark	Dark red	Jaundice or serious pitham disease
	Reddish dark	Destruction of blood cells (haemolysis)
	Greenish dark	Impurities in the blood
	Pale white and dark	Vatham and kapham disease, feverish with kapham diminishing
White	Pale white	Reduction of warmth in body, indicates incurable nature of illness
	Mucous discharge	Kapham dosha due to excessive heat
	Milky white	Indicates destruction of marrow and the possibility of wasting disease
	Pale white with mucous and bad odour	Inflammation and ulcer in the urinary passage from kidney to bladder or renal or urethral calculus
	Semen-like urine	Highly depleted kapham dosha and disturbance of all doshas
	Urine with no sediment	Incurable disease
	Urine like milk or buttermilk	Incurable disease
	Urine resembling washings of spoiled meat	Bad functioning of kidneys and depletion of blood and kapham
	Urine like melted ghee or dense	Indication of impending death

2.7.2 *Churna* (Powders)

Churnas are formulations comprising fine powders of drugs. *Churnas* may be simple or compound. Simple *churnas* consists of only one ingredient while a compound one consists of more than one ingredient. *Churnas* are prepared from powdered roots and herbs after they have been completely dried. The efficacy of *churnas* depends on the use of fresh and genuine herbs and their careful compounding. Examples are *ashwagandhadichurna* and *Triphalachurna*.

2.7.3 *Kashaya* (Decoctions)

Kashaya means 'herbal decoction' or herbal extract and there are more than 1000 kinds of *Kashayas*. In *Kashaya*, herbs are cut into small pieces and boiled in water in an earthen vessel till the liquid is reduced to a quarter of its original volume. The decoction is then strained through fine cloth or muslin. The purpose of *Kashaya* is to remove accumulated digestive wastes and to nourish and strengthen the *dhatus*. *Kashaya* also enhances the immune system of human body by strengthening the body tissues. Diseases caused due to the action of *vata* prakriti are treated this way.

2.7.4 *Lehya* or *Lehyam* (Jam)

Lehya or *Lehyam* is a semisolid jam or thickened herbal extract prepared in a medium of sugar or jaggery in *Siddha*. It is prepared by using powdered drugs and pulp of fruits in the sugar medium of jaggery, sugar, sugar candy or honey in an aqueous medium of water. This can be used for the cure of digestive and respiratory problems and as a general body tonic. The components of *lehya* are easily absorbed to the body, starting from the mouth.

2.7.5 *Ghrita* (Ghee)

Ghritas are made with combination of medicinal herbs or extracts with *ghritas* (ghee) as a base. It is prepared strictly according to *Siddha* system of medicine. These cure diseases and give strength and vigor to the body. They are taken by mixing with hot milk or as directed by a physician. The dose of ghritas should be determined according to the digestive power of the patient. Medicated *Ghritas* are also used as an external application. They act as an emollient.

2.7.6 *Taila* (Oil)

Tailas are medicinal oils meant for application to the skin. They are prepared from the crude drugs and medicines with oil base in accordance with the methods and processes laid down in the traditional system of medicine. They not only cure diseases but also impart strength and vigour to the body. The quantity of the oils depends upon the freshness and fineness of *kalka* (paste) which is specially supervised. Oils are to be massaged gently but briskly so as to be completely absorbed in the skin. Oils can be warmed before the massage and can be used internally also if and when directed by physician.

According to the mode of application, the *Siddha* medicines could be categorised into two classes, *viz.*, internal (internal medicines are further classified into 32 categories based on their form, methods of preparation, shelf life, etc.) and external medicine (Wilson et al. 2007).

2.8 Herbs in Traditional Medical System of India

Medicinal plants/herbs are generally used as substances to treat or prevent diseases. According to the World Health Organisation (WHO), medicinal herbs contribute 80% of the raw materials in the traditional system of medicine and about 80% of world population is dependent on plant-based systems of medicine for their primary healthcare needs (Mishra et al. 2016). People living in developing countries are especially using herbal drugs for the treatment of any diseases and disorders as they are considered as part of the culture in those communities (Ekor 2014). There are numerous types of drugs that are derived from plants such as analgesics, cardiotonic, antimalarial, antihypertensive, memory enhancing, muscle relaxant, anti-inflammatory, anthelmintic, antitussive, central nervous system (CNS) stimulant, anti-parkinsonism, anticholinergic, anti-cancerous and antitumour. Table 2.5 shows the few drugs that are derived from plants and its origin. In India, commonly 573 medicinal plants are used in *Ayurveda*, *Unani* and *Siddha* systems of medicine for the treatment of various illnesses (Anonymous 2018b). Few commonly used medicinal plants in *Siddha* system are listed in Table 2.6 (Ram et al. 2009; Malviya et al. 2010; Mutheeswaran et al. 2011).

Herbal drugs have appeared to exhibit new clinical effects as an alternative choice for the treatment of diseases. A further and deep research had been carried out by targeting at few chronic diseases such as bronchial asthma and diabetes which could lead to the new discovery of drugs for those diseases with improved efficacy. The various medicinal values of plants are daunting for an entrant to the field. The multidisciplinary research approach has provided a motivation in order to identify new pharmacophores which may help to discover new targets as the site of action other than expanding the preventive armamentarium and herbal therapeutic. Different approaches to herbal drugs lead to further drug development efforts in both herbal and single molecule of drug (Vaidya and Devasagayam 2007).

Table 2.5 Drugs that are derived from plants and its origin

Drug action(s)	Drug(s) and its origin
Analgesics	• Codeine and morphine obtained from *Papaver somniferum* • Salicin obtained from *Salix alba* • Tetrahydropalmatine obtained from *Corydalis ambigua*
Cardiotonic	• Acetyldigoxin obtained from *Digitalis lanata* • Adoniside obtained from *Adonis vernalis* • Convallatoxin obtained from *Convallaria majalis* • Deslanoside and Lanatosides A, B, C obtained from *Digitalis lanata* • Digitalin, digitoxin, digoxin, gitalin obtained from *Digitalis purpura* • Ouabain obtained from *Strophanthus gratus* • Scillarin A obtained from *Urginea maritima*
Antimalarial	• Artemsinin obtained from *Artemisia annua* • Quinine obtained from *Cinchona ledgeriana*
Antihypertensive	• Deserpidine obtained from *Rauwolfia canescens* • Protoveratrines A, B obtained from *Veratrum album* • Rescinnamine and reserpine obtained from *Rauwolfia serpentina* • Rhomitoxin obtained from *Rhododendron molle* • Tetrandrine obtained from *Stephania tetrandra*
Memory enhancing	• Physostigmine obtained from *Physostigma venenosum*
Muscle relaxant	• Anabesine obtained from *Anabasis sphylla* • Cissampeline obtained from *Cissampelos pareira* • Papaverine obtained from *Papaver somniferum* • Tubocurarine obtained from *Chondodendron tomentosum*
Anti-inflammatory	• Aescin obtained from *Aesculus hippocastanum* • Bromelain obtained from *Ananas comosus*
Anthelmintic	• Agrimophol obtained from *Agrimonia eupatoria* • Arecoline obtained from *Areca catechu* • Quisqualic acid obtained from *Quisqualis indica*
Antitussive	• Bergenin obtained from *Ardisia japonica* • Codeine and noscapine obtained from *Papaver somniferum* • Glaucine obtained from *Glaucium flavum* • Rorifone obtained from *Rorippa indica*
CNS stimulant	• Caffeine obtained from *Camellia sinensis* • Lobeline obtained from *Lobelia inflate* • Strychnine obtained from *Strychnos nux-vomica* • Vasicine obtained from *Vinca minor*
Anti-parkinsonism	• Levo-dopa obtained from *Mucuna* species
Anticholinergic	• Anisodamine and anisodine obtained from *Anisodus tanguticus* • Atropine obtained from *Atropa belladonna* • Hyoscyamine obtained from *Hyoscyamus niger*
Anti-cancerous	• Betulinic acid obtained from *Betula alba* • Camptothecin, Irinotecan and Topotecan obtained from *Camptotheca acuminate* • Lapachol obtained from *Tabebuia* species • Podophyllotoxin obtained from *Podophyllum peltatum*
Antitumour	• Colchicine and demecolcine obtained from *Colchicum autumnale* • Etoposide and Teniposide obtained from *Podophyllum peltatum* • Monocrotaline obtained from *Crotalaria sessiliflora* • Taxol obtained from *Taxus brevifolia* • Vinblastine and vincristine obtained from *Catharanthus roseus*

Table 2.6 Medicinal plants from *Siddha* system of medicine used for treating various diseases

Disease	Herbal plant
Respiratory diseases	*Acalypha indica* L. (Euphorbiaceae); *Adhatoda vasica* Nees (Acanthaceae); *Apium graveolens* L. (Umbelliferae); *Boerhavia diffusa* L. (Nyctaginaceae); *Borassus flabellifer* L. (Arecaceae); *Caesalpinia bonduc* L. (Caesalpiniaceae); *Calotropis gigantea* L. (Asclepiadaceae); *Crocus sativus* L. (Iridaceae); *Euphorbia hirta* L. (Euphorbiaceae); *Ocimum sanctum* L. (Lamiaceae); *Piper longum* L. (Piperaceae); *Piper nigrum* L. (Piperaceae); *Solanum nigrum* L. (Solanaceae); *Solanum trilobatum* L. (Solanaceae); *Solanum xanthocarpum* (Solanaceae); *Strychnos potatorum* L. (Loganiaceae); *Terminalia bellirica* Roxb. (Combretaceae); *Tylophora indica* Merrill (Asclepiadaceae); etc.
Antidiabetics	*Cassia kleinii* Wight &Arn. (Caesalpiniaceae); *Coscinium fenestratum* Colebr. (Menispermaceae), *Annona squamosa* L. (Annonaceae); *Centella asiatica* L. (Asteraceae); *Gymnema sylvestre* (R.Br.) Schult. (Asclepiadaceae); *Senna auriculata* L. (Fabaceae); *Salacia reticulata* W. (Celastraceae); etc.
Hypercholesterolaemia	*Uvaria narum* Wall (Annonaceae); etc.,
Jaundice	*Viola canescens* Wall. (Violaceae); *Piper longum* L. (Piperaceae); etc.
Anti-allergic	*Hibiscus surattensis* (Malvaceae); etc.
Anti-inflammatory	*Hugonia mystax* L. (Linaceae); *Dodonaea viscosa* (Sapindaceae); *Ruta graveolens* L. (Rutaceae); *Moringa oleifera* Lam. (Moringaceae); *Cassia mimosoides* L. (Fabaceae); *Indigofera heterantha* Wall. (Fabaceae); *Pyrus pashia* Buch.Ham. (Rosaceae); *Rosa brunonii* Lindl. (Rosaceae); *Momordica foetida* L. (Cucurbitaceae); *Centaurea iberica* Trev. (Asteraceae); *Nerium oleander* L. (Apocynaceae); *Lamium amplexicaule* Linn. (Lamiaceae); *Jatropha curcas* L. (Euphorbiaceae); etc.
Male fertility	*Cajanus cajan* (L.) Millsp. (Fabaceae); etc.
UTI	*Medicago polymorpha* L. (Fabaceae); *Morus nigra* L. (Moraceae); etc.
Menstrual cycle	*Rubus pinnatus* Willd. (Rosaceae); etc.
Stomach ache	*Citrus limon* (L.) Burm.F. (Rutaceae); *Woodfordia fruticosa* L. (Lythraceae); *Momordica foetida* L. (Cucurbitaceae)
Dandruff	*Garcinia indica* Choisy (Rubiaceae); etc.
Snake and scorpion bites	*Jasminum malabaricum* W. (Oleaceae), *Cyperus rotundus* L. (Cyperaceae); etc.
Kidney stones	*Centaurea iberica* Trev. (Asteraceae); etc.

2.9 Limitations of *Siddha* Medicine

Siddha medicine is a one of the oldest traditional medicinal system, commonly used by Tamil people. *Siddha* system of medicine mainly concentrates on whole person healing rather than treating symptoms of illnesses. This system of medicine is documented in Tamil, a language predominantly spoken by the Tamil people of India and Sri Lanka. The available document should be made available in multiple languages to reach the global platform. Currently, many pharmaceutical and analytical methods are available to standardise the herbal medicine, which can be extended to *Siddha* medical system to increase the global acceptance rate.

References

Anandan AR, Thulasimani M (Eds). *Siddha* Materia Medica (minerals and animal section) 1st ed. Chennai: Dept of Indian Medicine and Homeopathy. 2008. p. 1–5.

Anonymous. Basic principles of human body 96, Siddhas. 2017. https://ramanan50.wordpress.com/2015/02/05/basic-principles-of-human-body-96-Siddhas/. Accessed 31 Dec 2017.

Anonymous. Glossary—Siddhi. Himalayan academy. 2018a. https://www.himalayanacademy.com/media/books/dancing-with-siva/web/glossary_c.html. Accessed 16 May 2018.

Anonymous. Traditional treatment health center. 2018b. http://www.indiahomeclub.com/botanical_garden/medicinal_plants_uesd_in_ays.htm. Accessed 11 May 2018.

Aravinda Prabhu HR, Bhat PS. Mind and consciousness in yoga—Vedanta: a comparative analysis with western psychological concepts. Indian J Psychiatry. 2013;55:182–6.

Arunachalam G, Karunanithi M, Subramanian N, Ravichandran V, Selvamuthukumar S. Ethno medicines of Kolli hills at Namakkal district in Tamil Nadu and its significance in Indian systems of medicine. J Pharm Sci Res. 2009;1:1–15.

Balaramaiah V, Vadavaidyattukki A. (In Tamil). Part I. Madras: Arul Jyoti Printers. 1980.

Chaudhury RR, Rafei UM. Traditional medicine in Asia. SEARO Regional Publications No. 39. 2001. http://apps.searo.who.int/pds_docs/b0104.pdf. Accessed 2 Jan 2018.

Ekor M. The growing use of herbal medicines: issues relating to adverse reactions and challenges in monitoring safety. Front Pharmacol. 2014;4:177.

Janani L, Anusha S, Elansekaran S, Ramamurthy M, Srinivasan V, Christian GJ. Neerkuri by sage Theraiyar-a review on *Siddha* way of urine examination in the light of contemporary clinical methods. Int J Ayur Pharma Res. 2016;4:80–2.

Kandaswamy PN. History of *Siddha* medicine. Madras: 1979.

Krishnamurthy KH, Chandra Mouli G. *Siddha* system of medicine: a historical appraisal. Indian J Hist Sci. 1984;19:43–53.

Kumar PA, Pankaj G, Abichal C. A comparative study of Siddha & Ayurveda medication system of India. Global J Res Med Plants Indigen Med. 2012;1:470–6.

Malviya N, Jain S, Malviya S. Antidiabetic potential of medicinal plants. Acta Pol Pharm. 2010;67:113–8.

Mishra P, Kumar A, Nagireddy A, Mani DN, Shukla AK, Tiwari R, et al. DNA barcoding: an efficient tool to overcome authentication challenges in the herbal market. Plant Biotechnol J. 2016;14:8–21.

Mutheeswaran S, Pandikumar P, Chellappandian M, Ignacimuthu S. Documentation and quantitative analysis of the local knowledge on medicinal plants among traditional *Siddha* healers in Virudhunagar district of Tamil Nadu, India. J Ethnopharmacol. 2011;137:523–33.

Narayanaswamy V. Introduction to the *Siddha* system of medicine. Director, Pandit S. S. Anandam Research Institute of *Siddha* Medicine, T. Nagar, Madras (Chennai). 1975.

Nawaz GK, Lakshmi MS, JayaSudha M. E-health analysis element for supporting therapeutic through ancient Indian medical science. Int J Comput Appl. 2010;1:92–8.

Parasuraman S, Thing GS, Dhanaraj SA. Polyherbal formulation: concept of Ayurveda. Phcog Rev. 2014;8:73–80.

Parasuraman S, Wen LE, Zhen KM, Hean CK, Sam AT. Exploring the pharmacological and pharmacotherapeutic effects of yoga. PTB Rep. 2016;2(1):6–10.

Patanjali Yoga Sutras. Translated into English with notes by Swarmi Prabhavananda. Madras: Shri Ramakrishna Mission; 1953.

Raghunathan K. Indigenous systems of medicine in India—early history, literature and special features. Bull Ind Inst Hist Med. 1979;XIV:1–13.

Rajkumar S, Srinivasan N, Thirunarayanan T, Sangeetha R. Survey of Tamil *Siddha* manuscripts in possession of traditional healers in Northern Tamil Nadu. Int J Pharmacol Clin Sci. 2012;1(3):68–73.

Ram A, Joseph DA, Balachandar S, Singh VP. Medicinal plants from *Siddha* system of medicine useful for treating respiratory diseases. Int J Pharm Anal. 2009;1:20–30.

Ramachandiran SP. Theraiyar Neerkuri Vaithyam. Chennai: Thamarai Noolagam; 2000.

Shanmugavelan R. Theran Aruliseitha Siru Neerkuri Sodhanai. 3rd ed. Thanjavur: Sarasvati Mahal Library; 2005.

Sharma PV. *Siddha* medicine. In: Sharma PV, editor. History of medicine in India. New Delhi: The Indian National Science Academy; 1992. p. 445–50.

Shukla SS, Saraf S, Saraf S. Fundamental aspect and basic concept of *Siddha* medicines. Systematic Rev Pharm. 2011;2:48–54.

Sowrirajan M. Pathartha Gunapadam. Thanjavur: Saraswathi Mahal Library; 1992.

Stephen ES. Complementary and alternative medicine. In: Dennis LK, Eugene B, Anthony SF, Stephen LH, Llarry JL, editors. Harrisons principles of internal medicine. 16th ed. New York, NY: McGraw-Hill Medical Publishing Division; 2005. p. 67.

Subbarayappa BV. Chemical practices and alchemy. In: Bose DM, Sen SN, Subbarayappa BV, editors. A concise history of science in India. New Delhi: Indian National Science Academy; 1971. p. 315–35.

Subbarayappa BV. *Siddha* medicine: an overview. Lancet. 1997;350:1841–4.

Thas JJ. *Siddha* medicine-background and principles and the application for skin diseases. Clin Dermatol. 2008;26(1):62–78.

Thottam PJ. *Siddha* medicine: a handbook of traditional remedies. New Delhi: Penguin Books; 2000.

Uthamaroyan CS. Thotra Kirama Araiachium *Siddha* Maruthuva Varalarum. Chennai: Tamil Nadu Govt. Siddha Medical Board; 1992.

Vaidya ADB, Devasagayam TPA. Current status of herbal drugs in India: an overview. Recent advances in Indian herbal drug research. J Clin Biochem Nutr. 2007;41:1–11.

Venkataraman R. A history of the Tamil *Siddha* Cult. Madurai: Ennes Publications; 1990.

Walter Thomas M, Rubia G, Sathiya E. Review of ethics in traditional *Siddha* medicine as defined by Siddhar Theraiyar, *Siddha* papers. 2009. https://www.researchgate.net/profile/DrThomas_M_Walter/publication/36448333_Review_of_ethics_in_traditional_Siddha_Medicine_as_defined_by_Siddhar_Theraiyar/links/0e668eccd76d4a5dd1422953/Review-of-ethics-in-traditional-Siddha-Medicine-as-defined-by-Siddhar-Theraiyar.pdf. Accessed 16 May 2018.

Walter TM, Rubia G, Sathiya E. Review of ethics in traditional *Siddha* Medicine as defined by r Theraiyar, *Siddha* Papers. 2009.

White DG. The alchemical body: *Siddha* traditions in medieval India. 1st ed. Chicago: University of Chicago Press; 1996.

Wilson E, Rajamanickam GV, Vyas N, Agarwal A, Dubey GP. Herbs used in *Siddha* medicine for arthritis—a review. Indian J Tradit Know. 2007;6:678–86.

Yadav V, Jayalakshmi S, Singla RK. Traditional systems of medicine - now & forever. WebmedCentral Pharma Sci. 2012;3(4):WMC003299.

Rejuvenation of Interests in Herbal Remedies as Elixir of Life

3

Ambarish Mukherjee and Mousumi Banerjee

Contents

A. Mukherjee (✉)
Centre for Advanced Study, Department of Botany, Burdwan University, Burdwan, West Bengal, India

M. Banerjee
Faculty of Post Graduate Studies, Department of Botany, Scottish Church College, Kolkata, India

S. Sen, R. Chakraborty (eds.), *Herbal Medicine in India*,
https://doi.org/10.1007/978-981-13-7248-3_3

3.1 A General Résumé

Interest in herbal medicines has been growing fast all over the world mainly for their safe remedial virtues especially against refractory diseases, antioxidant properties and efficacy in palliation, immuno-modulation and prophylaction. Contemporary advancement in biochemical and molecular pharmacology has done much to popularize use of herbal remedies. People all over the world are getting acquainted with the benefits obtainable from plants in health care, longevity and improvement of quality of life. They are aware of the fact that stronger new antibiotics are perpetually getting formulated to encounter pathogens that have already become resistant to most of the available antibiotics for their frequent and irrational use. Their usage at the cost of side effects on health has been deteriorating health and vigor, thus leading to growth of aversion towards modern medicines. The herbal medicines for being much economical have been enabling even the low-income group of people to use them.

Recent advancement in molecular and biochemical pharmacology and nutrition science has done much to popularize the use of medicines and food cuisines of plant origin. Presently people in every society are acquainted with the benefits obtainable from plants especially for sustaining health and improving the quality of life. From the reports of WHO (World Health Organization 1983, 1998, 1999a, b, 2002, 2005) it is evident that in developing countries people mostly use plant-based medicines for their primary health care. No less than 30% of world's plant species have been getting used for medicinal purposes. For medicines and cosmetics, nearly 20,000 species of plants are marketed. About 90% of the herbal drugs marketed presently are from natural sources and over 120 important active principles used in modern medicine presently are derived from plants. Approximately half of the drugs currently used clinically are of natural origin. Many more traditionally used herbal medicines have potential to create opportunities for the development of newer therapeutics for several dreadful diseases from natural sources. Diabetes is one of such diseases, the herbal remedies against which are explored (Zhang and Tan 2000; Kavishankar et al. 2011).

The present article is in conformity with the earlier work (Mukherjee 2012) that dealt with various aspects of herbal remedies traditionally used in India with emphasis on ethnobotany, ethnomedicine and the codified systems of traditional medicines and the advent and plant-based progress of modern medicines. It also covers rejuvenation of interest and concern in 'enzyme-inhibition therapy', a newly emerging concept based on traditional food plants all over the world. The future prospect of these systems in the days to come has also been discussed.

3.2 Ethnobotany, Traditional and Modern Medicines

3.2.1 Ethnobotany

People of ethnic communities in different countries of the world have developed in their own ways knowledge about plants in their surroundings so as to integrate them with their life, necessities and sociocultural activities with commitments to develop mutually sustainable relationships. Studies on all aspects of direct man-plant relationship have been given great importance in composing a subject known as ethnobotany. An urgent need has been realized to document with scientific inputs all ethnobotanical information from among the diverse ethnic communities dispersed in our country before the traditional cultures get evolved further. Ethnobotanists have to shoulder the responsibility in stocktaking the traditionally used phyto-resources especially medicinal plants and conserving and revitalizing the traditional beliefs so that the age old cultures win in safeguarding the appropriate use of traditional knowledge. Ethnobotanists also have a responsibility to decide who should, on behalf of the tribals, share the benefits of new discoveries such as medicines or food from plants (Boom 1990; Balick 1996; Balick and Cox 1996) and at what cost (Lalramnghinglova and Jha 1999). Often, ethnobotanists being a part of modern society can also forge closer ties with government and private sector research groups working to develop new food, drug, and energy resources (Balick 1996). There is an urgent need to document and preserve as wide a range as possible of genetic resources region wise on war footing for prevention of genetic erosion, especially of such biotic entities that have evolutionary flexibility. Conservation has to be ensured even of such plants the economic potential and ecological services of which are yet to be fully known (Mukherjee 1997).

The thrust areas in contemporary researches in ethnobotany have been concerning ethnomedicines and edible wild plants need to be more and more explored so as to address in the near future such critical issues as health and food security that are getting progressively intensified by an overgrowth of the population.

3.2.1.1 Ethnomedicine

Ethnomedicine is the study of traditional medical practices, cultural interpretation of health, diseases, and illness as well as the healthcare system and healing practices (Krippner 2003). Ethnomedicine that has been rendering the services of healing for people for millennia (Lowe et al. 2000) is a complex multidisciplinary system based mainly on therapeutic use of plants, spirituality as also the natural environment.

The ethnomedicine, an age-old therapeutic system which is traditionally practiced among folk- and different tribal communities, has always been in India the matrix of codified traditional systems as Ayurveda, Unani, Siddha, etc. that are mostly based on plants and emanate conceptually from folk- or ethnomedicine although they have texts and literature of classical antiquity wherein are documented their unique principles, theory, pharmacy, and pharmacology. Unlike these texted and codified systems, the knowledge in ethnomedicines is transmitted through generations orally in view of which, its documentation collaterally with stocktaking of the phytotherapeutic resources and validation has been currently prioritized. Ayurveda, among different traditional systems of medicines, has been regaining its age-old reputation and gaining popularity abroad. The traditional knowledge about medicinal potential of plants, pharmacy, and therapeutic applications of such plants are well documented in the Ayurvedic literature. The Ayurvedic medicines have been positively responding to scientific evaluations for validation. WHO and UNESCO (United Nations Educational, Scientific and Cultural Organization) have taken a keen interest in promoting use of Indian traditional system of medicine on worldwide basis. Many important medicines of modem age are getting discovered and developed based on the knowledge and wisdom of Great sage Charak (Uniyal et al. 2002). Ethnomedicine has been receiving presently appreciation of modern scientists. Collaterally there has been a tremendous rejuvenation of interest in herbal ethnomedicines all over the world especially among health conscious people in modern societies for their patient-friendly nature and palliative, prophylactic and immunomodulatory functions, efficacy in curing the refractory diseases, and antioxidant properties (Mukherjee 2012). Ethnobotanical investigations have also been revealing edible species capable of preventing and curing various diseases and disorders with the restoration of health. The nutritional and medicinal importance of wild edible plants started subsequently getting realized (Jain et al. 1977; Arora and Pandey 1996; Arjariya and Rawat 2005; Devi and Salam 2016). Efficacy of ethnomedicines, especially of Indian origin, has been attracting most of the corporate world in getting involved in profitable acquisition of the crude drugs along with the traditional knowledge about their use. The situation has eventually given a jolt to Indians to be conscious about their own wealth of medicinal plants and relevant traditional knowledge.

3.2.1.2 A Glimpse of Ethnobotanical Studies in India

In a brief review on the evolution of ethnobotany in India during the last 60 years, Jain and Jain (2015) have regarded E.K. Janaki Ammal as the pioneer scientist to have emphasized on the need for organized ethnobotanical studies in India. Janaki Ammal (1956) for the first time documented over 1500 different plants utilized for food, fodder, medicine, fiber, musical instruments, and sociocultural purposes. Since then scientists have been utilizing the potential of the country so that about 100 books and over 3000 research papers have appeared on the subject. The subject developed progressively in India under the guidance of Dr. S.K. Jain whose publications (Jain 1982, 1987, 1989, 1990, 1991, 1994, 1997, 1999, 2000, 2001a, b, 2002, 2004, 2009, 2010, 2012; Jain et al. 1984; Jain and Borthakur 1980, 1986; Jain and Mitra 1997; Pal and Jain 1989, 1998; Saklani and Jain 1994; Jain and Srivastava 1999; Jain and Jain 2015, 2016a, b) at regular intervals are valued by leading authorities on Ethnobotany as milestones in evolution of Ethnobotany. The ethnobotanical research led by S.K. Jain, the 'Father of Indian Ethnobotany', has made a worldwide impact as a consequence of which India's leadership in this subject has been appreciated in no ambiguous terms by many subject specialists in Europe and America.

There has to be an increasing trend in India to document indigenous traditional knowledge, especially on medicinal plants on war footing since the orally transmitted traditional knowledge has been getting much eroded. In the last few decades emphasis has been laid on stocktaking of medicinal plants of different areas and preparations of written texts on traditional knowledge about their uses as a strategy to safeguard the Intellectual Property Right.

There have been overwhelming important publications in the past few decades on ethnomedicinal plants and herbal remedies used traditionally in India (Ahirwar et al. 2010; Anonymous 1976, 2001; Bhattacharya 2004; Biswas and Mukherjee 2017; Borgohain et al. 2016; Borthakur 1976a, b, 1981, 1992, 1996a, b Borthakur and Goswami 1995; Borthakur and Sharma 1996; Borthakur and Nath 2007; Borthakur et al. 2004; Chopra and Simon 2002; Das and Pandey 2007; Das et al. 2010; Gautam et al. 1998; Jain 1991, 1994, 2004; Jain and De 1966; Jain and Jain 2015, 2016a, b; Jain and Srivastava 1999; Kapoor 1990; Kaushik and Dhiman 1999; Kumar 2014; Lalramnghinghlova 2001; Lalramnghinghlova and Jha 1997; Nadkarni 1992; Nath 2015; Naik 2004; Nair and Mohanan 1998; Rana 2003; Sahu et al. 2015; Satyavati and Gupta 1987; Shah 1992; Swami Brahmananda 2002; Zafar 1999).

Documentation of ethnobotanical knowledge from diverse ethnic communities must be treated as urgent before it gets totally eroded which is not unlikely to happen. Moreover, after the Rio Convention in 1992 and the implementation of the GATT to save the intellectual property and the traditional knowledge of the indigenous communities of a country, it is essential to prioritize such a task on war footing; lest there would be unethical and illegal appropriation of the unattended knowledge and commercial exploitation of the concerned crude drugs. In view of this India has started taking care to establish the claim on traditional cures and encounter biopiracy especially after a long battle to revoke patents received by an antifungal product prepared from the Indian neem plant (*Azadirachta indica*) in Europe in 1994, and a turmeric-based (*Curcuma longa*) product in the United States in 1995.

3.2.2 Health and Traditional Medicines

According to the constitution of the WHO (2006), "Health is a state of complete physical, mental and social well-being and not merely the absence of disease or infirmity."

According to WHO traditional medicine (TM) is defined as health practices, approaches, knowledge, and beliefs incorporating plant, animal and mineral based medicines, spiritual therapies, manual techniques and exercises, applied singularly or in combination to treat, diagnose and prevent illness or maintain well-being. Traditional medicine got included in primary health care systems in all countries subsequent to Alma-Ata declaration: "Health for All" of 1978 as a consequence of which practitioners of Traditional medical systems started getting official recognition. In course of time traditional medicines was given welcome in developed countries for fulfillment of issues related to of primary health care as complementary and alternative medicine (CAM).

3.2.2.1 Traditional Medicines in India

In India, Ayurveda, Yoga, Naturopathy, Unani, Siddha and Homoeopathy happen to be the officially recognized traditional systems, i.e., codified. In March 1995 the Government of India initiated the Department of Indian Systems of Medicine and Homoeopathy (ISM&H) under the Ministry of Health and Family Welfare which in November 2003 was renamed as the Department of Ayurveda, Yoga & Naturopathy, Unani, Siddha and Homoeopathy (AYUSH). A national policy was formulated in 2002 for augmenting growth and development of traditional systems. Attention was focused on promotion and development of education and research in these traditional systems of medicine. The department also included *Amchi or Tibetan medicine* (Sowa-Rigpa/Gso-Rig-pa) which is one of the oldest, well-documented traditional medical systems of the world popularly practiced among Buddhist in Bhutan, Mongolia, Tibet, China and some parts of Nepal, Himalayan regions of India and the former Soviet Union etc.

Restoration of health to the patient is the highest mission of the traditional medical systems of India considering health as the optimal state of physical, psychological, social and spiritual constitutions of a human. Even today no less than 65% of the Indian population depend on the traditional systems of medicine. While giving a brief idea about the Codified Traditional Medicines in India, Mukherjee (2012) mentioned about the Ayurvedic Pharmacopeia which was published by the Pharmacopeia committees of Ayurveda, Siddha and Unani in 3 volumes, and contained as many as 326 Ayurvedic drugs. The Unani pharmacopoeia included no less than 45 drugs. Ayurvedic Formulary of India brought out by the Government of India contained 636 formulations in its 2 volumes. 3 volumes of Unani formulary included no less than 746 formulations. The Ayurvedic, Siddha (single volume used mostly in South India, and Sri Lanka) and Unani Formulary collectively dealt with a total of 1000 medicinal plants, 60 minerals and metals, 60 materials of marine and animal origin. The Tibetan medicine, familiar as Amchi (Sowa-Rigpa), had its reformation and revival in India mainly due to the efforts of Dalai Lama. The Tibetan Medical and Astrological Institute at Dharamsala (Himachal Pradesh) was set up by him after he took refuge in India. This institution has been training the 'would-be-practitioners' in Sowa-Rigpa, so that the people receive quality health service. The practice of Sowa-Rigpa is regulated in India by the Central Council for Tibetan Medicine. Registration is granted to the practitioners by the Council so that proper health care services get catered mainly in places with Buddhist inhabitants like Lahul and Spiti of Himachal Pradesh and Ladakh region of Jammu & Kashmir, Sikkim, Darjeeling of West Bengal, Arunachal Pradeshand and others.

The Department of AYUSH has been giving emphasis on up gradation of educational standards of Ayurveda, Unani, Yoga and Naturopathy, Siddha and Homoeopathy, quality control and standardization of drugs, improving the availability of genuine medicinal plant material, promoting research and development and growth of awareness about the efficacy of the traditional systems at home and abroad. WHO has been collaborating with the Government of India in use of TM, in discovery of novel drugs collaterally with their standardization for quality control for prevention of adulteration of drugs. The World Health Organization is in collaboration with the CDSCO (Central Drugs Standard Control Organization), The Department of AYUSH, Government of India, different Research Councils, National Medicinal Plant Board (NMPB), organizations concerned with Essential Drugs and Medicines (EDM) and Pharmaceuticals to ensure access, quality, safety and rational use of both modern (allopathic) and traditional medicines. Programmes on traditional medicine for promoting safe, rational health services and on capacity building and authentic documentation are given much importance in this regard.

3.2.2.2 Database of Indian Traditional Medicines

The Council of Scientific and Industrial Research (CSIR) and the Ministry of Health and Family Welfare, Govt. of India jointly own a database that has been put in vogue to prevent patenting of traditional medicines by foreign agencies. The database covers formulations numbering no less than 230,000 after screening of ancient texts dealing with Ayurveda, Unani, Siddha and Yoga – in Sanskrit, Hindi, Urdu, Arabic and Persian. The database is also available in English, French, Spanish, German and Japanese. India's massive database on traditional remedies can now be accessed by any country in order to be sure that patents do not granted for remedies and treatments included in Indian systems of medicine. The relevant websites include those of the Department of AYUSH http://www.indianmedicine.nic.in; Ayurvedic foundations http://www.ayur.com; Naturopathy, Herbal, Accu-pressure and Ayurvedic Services -dir. Indiamart. comlindianservicesl buds. Html; Alternative Medicine: Naturopathy, Herbal, Accu-pressure and Ayurvedic Services dir. indiamart.comlindianserviceslbuds.html; Sanjeevani -Asia's largest Yoga and Naturopathy Institution http://www.sanjeevaniindia.org/; Unani medicine http://www.unanLcornlresearch.htm; Siddha Medicine http://www.siddhaquest.com; Central Council for Research in Homoeopathy: http: //www.ccrhindia.org; Phytochemical and Ethnobotanical database: http://www.ars-grin.gov/ and Phytopharmaceuticals: http://www.escop.comlphytonet; Herbal Remedies Information: www.herbalremediesinfo.com; Herbal Remedies: www.herbalremedies.com; National Research Centre for Medicinal and Aromatic Plants: http://nrcap@wilneton/ine.com; Herb Research Foundation: http://www.sunsite.unc.edu/herbs; Herb Society (UK): http://www.sunsite.unc.edu/herbmed/herbSociety; Herb Society of America: http://www.herbsociety.org; Chopra Herbal Centre: http://www.mypotentia1.comlhttp:/I www.chopra.com; Medicinal Plants Global Network: http://www.bellanet/medplants; Medicinal Plants Network: http://www.medplant.net; Medicinal Plants Information Centre: http://www.medicinal-plantinfo.com; Medicinal Plant Database: http://www.Ejb.org/content/voI2/issue2/full/2/duke; International Council for Medicinal and Aromatic Plants: http://www.icmap.org and others.

The Institute of Ayurveda and Integrative Medicine & Foundation for Revitalization of Local Health Traditions (IAIM-FRLHT) took initiatives in 1995 to apply Information Technology so as to process the enormous and valuable data pertinent to Materia Medica of Indian traditional systems of medicines. This innovative work aimed to provide easy access to Indian systems of medicine for augmenting research and development. IAIM-FRLHT has developed multi-disciplinary databases on flora, fauna, metals and minerals of use in Indian traditional medicines. Data from primary sources, i.e., literature and texts covering the period from 1500 BC to 1900 AD have been systematically computerized for easy storage and retrieval of necessary information regarding scientific and Indian names, distribution, medicinal use, trade, pharmacognosy and pharmacology. The database in 32 languages provides pertinent information about 68,000 plants and images of 16,000 plants.

3.2.3 Modern Medicines

Certain epoch making discoveries of natural products from plants used in ethnomedicine in the nineteenth century laid the foundation of modern system of medicine or the so called 'allopathy'. The contribution of Sertürner and Magendie in the nineteenth century deserve special mention in this regard. Friedrich Wilhelm Adam Sertürner (1806), a young German pharmacist, isolated a pure substance from opium that he named morphine, after Morpheus, the Greek God of dreams. It was Sertürner (1817) who was able to isolate morphine in pure from *Papaver sominifer* which without any doubt initiated the development of alkaloid chemistry (Winterstein and Trier 1910). Subsequently, strychnine, a CNS stimulating alkaloid, was discovered from seeds of *Strychnos nuxvomica* by Pelletier and Caventou (1819). The antimalarial quinine was isolated by these authors from *Cinchona* bark (Pelletier and Caventou 1820). The narcotic substance nicotine was then discovered by the German chemists, Wilhelm Heinrich Posselt and Karl Ludwig Reimann from leaves of *Nicotiana tabacum* (tobacco) in 1828 and the anaesthetic compound cocaine was isolated from cocoa leaves by Niemann (1860). It was François Magendie, a French physiologist who in collaboration with Pelletier in 1817, discovered emetine, the active principle of *Caephalis ipecacuanha* (ipecac) (Magendie and Pelletier 1817). Through these outstanding pioneering efforts, experimental pharmacology got established in course of time.

With further progress of medical science, there was refinement of herbal medicines involving isolation, purification and characterization of active principles (secondary metabolites, the non-vital or non-universally vital compounds synthesized by plants), pharmacological screening, clinical evaluation, therapeutic proving and validation. Pharmacognosy proved essential for setting the morpho-anatomical chemical and even molecular standards essential for drug identification to prevent adulteration and ensure quality control of drugs. For their faster curative efficacy, allopathic medicines earned enormous global acceptance and appreciation. A good number of compounds of plant origin are getting used in modern medicine (Table 3.1).

Table 3.1 Some important plants contributing active principles to modern medicines

Name of the Plant	Medicinal Principles	Medicinal Property
Artemisia annua	Artimisinine	Antimalarial
Atropa belladonna	Atropin	Anticholinegic
Camellia sinensis	Theobromine	Diuretic, myocardial activator
Campotheca acuminata	Campothecin	Antitumour
Cassia angustifolia	Rutin	Decreases capillary fragility
Catharanthus roseus	Vinblastine	Antineoplastic
Catharanthus roseus	Vincristine	Antineoplastic
Cephaelis ipecacuanha	Emetine	Emetic, antiamoebic, in dyspepsia
Cephaelis ipecacuanha	Cephaeline	Emetic, antiamoebic, expectorant
Colchicum luteum	Colchicine	Gout amelioration
Coleus forskolli	Forskolin	Antispasmodic and cardiotonic
Curcuma longa	Curcumin	Wound healing, Prevention of Alzheimer's disease
Digitalis purpurea, D. lanata	Digitoxin	Cardiac tonic
Dysosma pleiantha	Podophyllotoxin	Anticancer
Ephedra vulgaris	Ephedrine	Anti- cardiac-asthmatic
Ginkgo biloba	Ginkgolides	Antihistaminic, antitussive
Glycyrrhiza glabra	Glycyrrhizin	Expectorant, demulcent, laxative
Gossypium herbaceum	Gossypol	Male contraceptive
Hypericum perforatum	Hypericin	Prevents capillary fragility
Justicia adhatoda	Vasicine	Bronchodialator
Marsilea minuta	Marsilin	Sedative, anticonvulsive
Mucuna pruriens	L-Dopa	Anti Parkinson
Murraya paniculata	Yuchchulene	Antifertility
Podophyllum emodi	Podophyllotoxin	Antineoplastic
Rauvolfia serpentine	Ajmalcine	Treats insomnia, hypnotic, reduces blood pressure, induces contraction of uterus during child- birth
Taxus brevifolia	Taxol	Prevents cancer

3.3 Enzyme- Inhibition Therapy, A Newly Emerging Concept Based on Traditional Food Plants

One of the important areas of medicines is the application of natural enzyme inhibitors in treatment of many dreadful diseases and disorders resulting from the detrimental activities of specific enzymes, e.g. diabetes from hyperactivity of α-amylase, μ-glucosidase, hepatotoxicity from the activity of β-glucoruinadase, Alzheimer's disease from acetylcholinesterase and hypertension from Angiotensin converting Enzyme (ACE) etc.

Enzyme inhibitors are molecules that can decrease activity of specific enzymes by binding with them. Enzyme inhibition assays are frequently used in drug discovery for toxicity and drug candidate screening (Garcia et al. 2007). The chemical enzyme inhibitors used presently in modern medicine are likely to show side effects in patients for their toxicity. As such presently investigations target discovery of enzyme inhibitors of natural origin, especially those present in food-plants. With the establishment of 'enzyme inhibition therapy' interests have been piling up in discovery of phyto-molecules that can bind with harmfully hyperactive enzymes and step down their actions for giving relief to a patient.

Some of the enzymes the hyperactivity of which results into disorders and disease in man are discussed in the following.

3.3.1 α-Amylase and α-Glucosidase

Interestingly α-Amylase and α-glucosidase inhibitors from food- plants have been known to offer an attractive therapeutic solution to address the issues of post-prandial hyperglycaemia. These natural inhibitors decrease glucose release from starch and delay carbohydrate absorption in the small intestine for which they are likely to be prescribed for the treatment of diabetes mellitus and obesity (Murai et al. 2002). Since the phenolic α-amylase inhibitors extracted from dietary plant sources are potentially safer, they are likely to be a better alternative for modulation of carbohydrate digestion and regulation of glycaemic index of food products (McCue et al. 2005).

3.3.2 β-Glucuronidases

These are enzymes capable of hydrolyzing the glycosidic bond between the glucuronic acid and other molecules of endogenous and exogenous compounds in living organisms. In mammals, glucuronidation, i.e. binding of glucuronic acid with a known or unknown compound, is an essential detoxification process since they form a water soluble product that can be excreted from the body if not hydrolyzed by intestinal β-glucuronidase enzymes (Fior et al. 2009). β-glucuronidase enzymes when hyperactive causes massive deglucuronidation through hydrolysis of the glucuronide moiety from the potentially damaging compounds that consequently get retained in tissues of different organs especially of liver, kidney, spleen, intestinal epithelium, endocrine and reproductive organs (Dutton 1980). Lampe et al. (2002) were successful in showing Serum β-glucuronidase activity to be inversely related to certain plant food intakes in humans.

Certain known hepatoprotective plant extracts and phytoconstituents are proven to inhibit β-glucuronidase. β-Glucuronidase inhibitors reduce the carcinogenic potential of certain xenobiotic compounds compounds that normally get excreted by body after glucuronidation along with bile (Walaszek et al. 1997). Due to this correlation, edible plants with β-glucuronidase inhibitors are suggested as potential hepatoprotective agents (Shim et al. 2000).

3.3.3 Angiotensin Converting Enzyme (ACE)

This enzyme plays an important role in the regulation of blood pressure as well as fluid and salt balance in mammals. The enzyme converts inactive decapeptide, angiotensin I, into vasoconstrictor octapeptide, angiotensin II. ACE also inactivates bradykinin, a vasodilator peptide and raises blood pressure. Naturally hyperactivity of this enzymes leads to hypertension and its related disorders. Under such circumstances, activity of ACE must be therapeutically inhibited to reduce morbidity and mortality in patients with hypertension (Miguel et al. 2009). Food plants that are rich in protein hydrolysates capable of inhibiting angiotensin converting enzyme (ACE) can be ear-marked as novel remedy for prevention of hypertension (Vishkaei et al. 2016). Inclusion of such edible plants in the diet of hypertension-patients can keep them healthy.

3.3.4 Acetylcholinesterase

It catalyzes the hydrolysis of acetylcholine in cholinergic synapses which leads to a deficiency in cholinergic function in the brain causing impairment of memory in the patients of Alzheimer's Disease (AD) (Groner et al. 2007). Approaches to enhance cholinergic function in AD include simulation of cholinergic receptors or prolonging the availability of acetylcholine (ACh) released into the neuronal synaptic cleft by inhibiting hydrolysis of Acetylcholine by acetylcholinesterase (AChE); which may be achieved through the use of AChE inhibitors (Howes and Houghton 2003). Presently the herbal formulations with minimum side effects in AD patients are being evaluated for the discovery of their AChE inhibitory potential. Howes and Houghton (2003) have documented the plants used in traditional medicine of China and India for improving memory and cognitive functions. Curcumin is a good inhibitor of acetylcholine esterase which can be obtained from the rhizomes of *Curcuma longa*.

Since these diseases have presently become very dreadful challenging the global life sustenance it is the enzyme inhibition therapy that has emerged to prove remedial efficacy. As such scientists all over the world have started documenting from the ethnic communities the medicinal properties especially of the wild edible plants to address such issues. Many of the vegetables including the leafy ones, flowers, fruits, seeds and other plant parts have been identified by the scientists as candidates for use in enzyme inhibition therapy (Acharya and De 2015, 2016; Acharya et al. 2016; Begum et al. 2015; Das et al. 2017).

3.4 Immunomodulatory Role of Traditional Plant Medicines

Advancement in the discipline of basic immunology during last 3–4 decades has turned out to be one of the thrust areas of biomedical research, especially in prevention and treatment of a wide range of disorders and diseases (Plaeger 2003). The use of herbal formulations either as immunostimulants or immunosuppresants has a traditional history that corroborates with the use of herbal products for prevention and cure. Considering use of plants for their prophylactic properties as an age long practice, especially in India, it is felt necessary to contemplate immunomodulators which are biological or synthetic substances that can stimulate, suppress or modulate any aspect of the immune system. Clinically, immunomodulators are classified into 3 categories, viz. immunoadjuvants, immunosuppressants and immunostimulants. Immunoadjuvants are used to enhance the efficacy of vaccines and therefore could be considered specific immune stimulants. Immunosuppressants are a structurally and functionally heterogeneous group of drugs, which are often concomitantly administered in combination regimens to treat various types of organ transplant rejection and autoimmune diseases (El-Sheikh 2008). Immunostimulants enhance body's resistance to infection and they are nonspecific. They can act through innate as well as adaptive immune responses in healthy person. Immunostimulants are expected to serve as prophylactic and promoter agents. In a patient who does not have the ability to respond normally to an infection due to an impaired or weakened immune system Immunostimulants act as immunotherapeutic agents. These agents are used to treat immunodeficiency and cancer (Lake et al. 2012).

Many Indian medicinal plants possess immunostimulant properties and they can serve as a potential source for drugs for various immunocompromised states including cancer and other serious infections. *Asparagus racemosus* is a potent immunostimulant (Thatte and Dahanukar 1988). In animal models of intraperitoneal adhesions, *A. racemosus* prevent postoperative adhesions (Rege et al. 1989). Dhuley reported that *A. racemosus* treatment significantly inhibited carcinogen ochratoxin-A induced suppression of chemotactic activity and production of IL-1 and TNF-α by mouse macrophages. *A. racemosus* induced excess production of TNF when compared with control (Dhuley 1997).

Organosulfur compounds of *Allium sativum* extracts have been shown to inhibit growth of tumors in animals probably by activation of natural killer cells, stimulation of T lymphocytes and enhanced production of IL-2 (Tang et al. 1997). Garlic extract enhance cytotoxicity of human peripheral blood lymphocytes against both natural killer cell sensitive (K562) and resistant (M14) cell lines (Morioka et al. 1993). Garlic extract prevented from ultraviolet induced suppression of contact hypersensitivity (Reeve et al. 1993).

Scientists have isolated a lipopolysaccharide from the root of ***Curcuma longa*** which is immunostimulant (Inagawa et al. 1992). NO is an important cellular signaling molecule. It helps modulate vascular tone, insulin secretion, airway tone, and peristalsis, and is involved in angiogenesis and neural development. Curcumin inhibits NO production in activated macrophages (Brouet and Ohshima 1995). The anticancer properties of curcumin may be mediated by inhibition of inducible form of NO-synthase.

Acemannan from gel of *Aloe vera* also induces release of nitric oxide (NO), expression of surface molecules and morphologic changes in mouse macrophage cell line (RAW 264.7) (Zhang Tizard 1996). Acemannan may be responsible for regression of tumors in experimental animals. Oligosaccharides from *A. vera* may prevent ultraviolet induced suppression of delayed type hypersensitivity by reducing keratinocyte derived immunosuppressive cytokines (Byeon et al. 1998).

Some of the plants used in Indian traditional medicine that have been tested to show prospect as immunomodulators include the names of *Emblica officinalis* (Euphorbiaceae), *Evolvulus alsinoides* (Convolvulaceae) (Ganju et al. 2003); *Acorus calamus* (Mehrotra et al. 2003); *Tinospora cordifolia* (Desai et al. 2007; Singh et al. 2004); *Boerhaavia diffusa* (Mungantiwar et al. 1999; Mehrotra et al. 2002); *Nyctanthes arbor-tristis* (Puri et al. 1992); *Eclipta alba* and *Centella asiatica* (Jayathirtha and Mishra 2004).

3.5 Traditional Herbal Remedies for Prevention and Treatment of Viral Diseases

Viral diseases especially influenza viruses have been posing considerable threat to the communities. According to an estimate of the World Health Organization on epidemic influenza, a total of 25–50 million cases each year could be recorded resulting in 150,000 hospitalizations and 30,000–40,000 deaths in the United States alone. During pandemics, the mortality and morbidity may be much higher, imposing tremendous pressure on health system (Fleming et al. 2005; Weber 2009). Due to frequent alterations in the antigenic structures of respiratory viruses, particularly in case of RNA viruses, production of effective vaccines gets much impaired. The inadequacy of effective vaccines and lack of proper medication urge upon discovery of alternative natural therapies based on screening of traditional knowledge documented regarding the herbal medicines used for prevention and treatment viral respiratory diseases. A variety of such herbal remedies are in wide traditional use in different parts of the world for getting rid of viral infections respiratory system. From the very informative publications of Haider Abdul-Lateef Mousa (2015, 2017), on the herbal complementary and natural therapies for prevention and treatment of influenza and influenza-like illness, it is evident that the therapeutic success depends to a great on chemical or biochemical agents that are isolated from plants. These agents include different types of polyphenols, flavonoids, saponins, glucosides, and alkaloids (Wang et al. 2006). The herbal medicine, maoto, a Japanese traditional herbal medicine (Kampo) has been in long traditional use against influenza in Japan. From literature (Anonymous

2006) it is evident that 'maoto' is, composed of *Ephedrae Herba* (stem of *E. sinica* Stapf), *Cinnamomi Cortex* (bark of *Cinnamomum cassia* Blume), *Armeniacae Semen* (kernel of Prunus armeniaca Linne´) and *Glycyrrhizae Radix* (the root of *Glycyrrhiza uralensis* Fisher). Among others with activity against respiratory viruses mention may be made of licorice roots, antiwei, North American ginseng, elderberry, Echinacea, pomegranate, guava tea, and Bai Shao. These were found useful in curing upper respiratory tract infections. There are several mechanisms of action by which herbal extracts encounter respiratory viruses. Future studies are felt necessary for revealing the possible role of alkaline diets or drinks for prevention and treatment of respiratory viral infections.

Many of the traditionally used herbal remedies against viral illness since time immemorial in India can certainly contribute enormously towards contemporary medical science. All such prophylactic and curative herbal remedies need to be documented, collected, authenticated and therapeutically proved for human benevolence.

3.6 Cytoprotective Role of Traditional Plant Medicines in Oxidative Stress and Redox Signaling

Most of the herbal medicines in traditional use owe their origin to antioxidant-rich dietary plants or are rich in certain phytochemicals that can alter the activity of several cell signalling pathways, which can lead to modulation of inflammatory processes, regulation of cytoprotective mechanism, cell growth and differentiation (Surh 2003; Aggarwal and Shishodia 2006). The herbs which show high antioxidant activity play vital role in antioxidant defence and redox signaling. Different dietary antioxidants have different functions and are produced by plants to protect plant cells against oxidative damage. There are many different reactive oxygen species (ROS) that have separate and essential roles in normal physiology and are required for a variety of normal processes. Although flavouring herbs and spices used in the diet for their aroma are with no or low nutritional value are likely to be associated with antioxidant defense and redox signaling (Paur et al. 2008). Different ROS are strongly in correspondence with the etiology of such diseases as infections, chronic inflammatory diseases, cancers, atherosclerosis, autoimmune diseases, neurodegenerative diseases and diabetes (Gutteridge and Halliwell 2000; McCord 2000). Different antioxidants produced by the body (endogenous), e.g. glutathione, thioredoxins, glutaredoxin, and different antioxidant enzymes have specific chemical and physiological characteristics to ensure eventual protection to all parts of the cells, the tissues and organs against oxidative damage.

Based on the complex nature of antioxidants and ROS it is unwise to think that a high dose of one or a few particular antioxidants such as vitamin C or β-carotene can protect all components of the cells, organs, and tissues against oxidative damage and oxidative stress collaterally without impairing any of the numerous normal and beneficial functions of ROS. Recently, several reviews and meta-analyses have concluded that there is no beneficial effect for supplemental vitamin C, vitamin E or β-carotene (Vivekananthan et al. 2003; Eidelman et al. 2004; Bjelakovic et al. 2007). Testing the potential beneficial effects of antioxidant-rich herbs, which contain a large combination of different antioxidants acquired through eventful evolution, to protect every part of the plant cells against oxidative damage is a better option than supplemental use of strong antioxidants like vitamin C, vitamin E or β-carotene . Some herbal medicines that are extremely rich in antioxidants include *Triphala*, an Indian Ayurvedic herbal formulation, that shows anti-inflammatory activity (Rasool and Sabina 2007), antibacterial and wound-healing properties (Srikumar et al. 2007), and cancer chemopreventive potential (Deep et al. 2005). *Arjuna*, another Ayurvedic formula, has been shown to give health benefits (Devi et al. 2007), whereas goshuyu-tou, a traditional kampo medicine, could significantly lower the extracellular concentration of NO in lipopolysaccharide (LPS)-stimulated RAW 264.7 cells (Okayasu et al. 2003). Turmeric, ginger, Clove, thyme and oregano are found to be with the highest total antioxidant capacity when compared with those of other commercially available drugs. Several phytochemicals have been identified as inhibitors of NF-κB, a transcription factor which is crucial in the orchestration of immune and inflammatory responses, such as rosmarinic acid (Lee et al. 2006) in thyme and oregano (Shan et al. 2005), eugenol in clove and allspice (Chainy et al. 2000) and gallic acid in clove. Interestingly thyme and oregano essential oils in combination was seen by Bukovska et al. (2007) to decrease the levels of IL-1β and IL-6 collaterally with subduing inflammation related tissue damage in a model of colitis both of which may also be related to NF-κB. Clove, oregano and thyme are extracted together with walnuts and coffee to produce an inhibitor of NF-κB activation in a synergistic manner *in vitro*, and also *in vivo* in transgenic mice (Paur et al. 2010). Sasaki et al. (2005) were able to observe induction or maintenance of levels of cyto-protective proteins endogenously in the liver by thyme. *In vitro* induction of phase I- and/or phase II-related transcription (through the CYP3A4 promoter, and pregnane X receptor [PXR] and electrophile response element [EpRE]-dependent transcription could be recorded by Kluth et al. (2007) with extracts of thyme, allspice and clove. There are many phytochemical which have been shown by Takada et al. (2004) and Paur et al. (2008) to be equally or even more efficiently inhibiting NF-κB in comparison with classical anti-inflammatory drugs like ibuprofen and dexamethasone.

Traditional herbal remedies and also antioxidant-rich foods prove beneficial by providing a balanced combination of different types of antioxidants so as to impart protection against redundancy of oxidative stress and damage without affecting the reactive oxygen species to perform their normal functions.

3.7 Summing Up

Ethnobotanical studies have been proving their worth in resolving materials and methods ideal for providing good health to all collaterally with improvement of life standards. Traditional medical system prevalent in India since time immemorial deserves acceptance by the contemporary medical science in formulation of remedies for putting forth resilience against worldwide health hazards resulting from environmental pollution and global climatic change.

India certainly has the potential both in terms of traditional knowledge and biodiversity to contribute enormously to medical science. It has immensely rich and complex indigenous medical heritage of its own with strong foundations in biomedical sciences. The Govt. has deep concern for augmentation of traditional medicine for which the Department of AYUSH in the Ministry of Health and other Science and Technology agencies of the Govt. of India like CSIR, ICMR, DBT & DST are collaborating. The National Knowledge Commission (NKC) has resolved important recommendations for promoting rationality of the knowledge systems of traditional medicines. Presently, health systems all over the world have to cope with the changing environment: epidemiologically, in terms of changing age structures, pollution, mutated pathogenic threats and outbreak of diseases over a wide geographic area i.e. the pandemics affecting exceptionally high proportion of the population. Reliance on the traditional systems in health care can reciprocate benevolence to man by ensuring complete physical, mental and social well-being.

References

Acharya J, De B. Evaluation of antidiabetic, neuroprotective, antihypertensive and hepatoprotective potential of flowers of *Cucurbita maxima* Duchesne. Indian J Sci Res. 2015;11(1):17–23.

Acharya J, De B. Bioactivity guided fractionation to identify beta-glucuronidase inhibitors in *Nymphaea pubescens* flower extracts. Cogent Food Agric. 2016;2:1134379.

Acharya J, Karak S, De B. Metabolite profile and bioactivity of Musa X paradisiaca flower extracts. J Food Biochem. 2016;40:724–30.

Aggarwal BB, Shishodia S. Molecular targets of dietary agents for prevention and therapy of cancer. Biochem Pharmacol. 2006;71(10):1397–421.

Ahirwar R, Khan A, Mishra A, Parna SK, Shrivastava IN, Singh G. Ethnomedicinal plants of district Anuppur used in treatment of renal caliculi (kidney stones). Indian J Appl Pure Biol. 2010;25(2):251–5.

Anonymous. Medicinal plants of India, vol. 1. New Delhi: ICMR; 1976.

Anonymous. Herbal products, current status, vision and action plan. New Delhi: TIFAC; 2001.

Anonymous. Appendix—composition and indications of 148 prescriptions. J Kampo Acupuncture Integr Med. 2006;1:85–101.

Arjariya A, Rawat A. An ethnobotanical survey of certain wild edible plants of Chhatarpur district (M.P.). Flora Fauna. 2005;11(1):97–100.

Arora RK, Pandey A. Wild edible plants of India: diversity, conservation and use. New Delhi: National Bureau of Plant Genetic Resources; 1996.

Balick MJ. Transforming ethnobotany for the new Millenium. Ann Mo Bot Gard. 1996;83:58–66.

Balick MJ, Cox PA. Plants, people and culture: the science of ethnobotany. New York: HPHLP; 1996.

Begum S, Acharya J, Banerjee A, De B. Chemical composition and in-vitro study for analysis of potential neuroprotective and antidiabetic activity in *Mimusops elengi* L. Int J Pharmacogn Phytochem Res. 2015;7(4):701–6.

Bhattacharya SK. Handbook of aromatic plants. Jaipur: Pointer Publications; 2004.

Biswas S, Mukherjee A. A census of ethnomedicinal plants used in Bankura District, West Bengal. Res J Pharma Biol Chem Sci. 2017;8(1):424–31.

Bjelakovic G, Nikolova D, Gluud LL, Simonetti RG, Gluud C. Mortality in randomized trials of antioxidant supplements for primary and secondary prevention: systematic review and meta-analysis. JAMA. 2007;297(8):842–57.

Boom BM. Giving native people a share of the profits. Garden. 1990;14:28–41.

Borgohain MP, Teron R, Tamuli AK. Ethnomedicinal plants of the Tai Phake tribe of Upper Brahmaputra Valley in Assam, India. Pleione. 2016;10(1):123–33.

Borthakur SK. Less known medicinal uses of plants among the tribes of Karbi Anglong (Mikir Hills), Assam. Bull Bot Survey India. 1976a;18(1–4):166–71.

Borthakur SK. Traditional weaving implements among the Mikirs (the Karbis) of Assam. Bull Bot Survey India. 1976b;11:46–50.

Borthakur SK. Plants in folklore and folktales of the Karbis (Mikirs) of Assam. In: Jain SK, editor. Glimpses of Indian ethnobotany. New Delhi: Oxford and IBH Publishing Co; 1981. p. 170–81.

Borthakur SK. Native phytotherapy of child and women diseases from Assam. Fitoterapia. 1992;63:483–8.

Borthakur SK. Wild edible plants in markets of Assam, India-an ethnobotanical investigation. In: Jain SK, editor. Ethnobiology in human welfare. New Delhi: Deep Publications; 1996a. p. 31–4.

Borthakur SK. Postnatal care of women in traditional system in Assam. Ethnobotany. 1996b;8:51–5.

Borthakur SK, Goswami N. Herbal remedies from Dimoria of Kamrup district of Assam in Northeastern India. Fitoterapia. 1995;66(4):333–40.

Borthakur SK, Nath KK. Ethnobotanical aspects of weeds from Darrang district of Assam. Ethnobotany. 2007;19:82–7.

Borthakur SK, Sarma UK. Ethnoveterinary medicine with special reference to cattle prevalent among the Nepalis of Assam, India. In: Jain SK, editor. Ethnobiology in human welfare. New Delhi: Deep Publications; 1996. p. 197–9.

Borthakur SK, Choudhury BT, Gogoi R. Folklore hepatoprotective herbal recipes from Assam in Northeast India. Ethnobotany. 2004;16:76–82.

Brouet I, Ohshima H. Curcumin, an anti-tumour promoter and anti-inflammatory agent, inhibits induction of nitric oxide synthase in activated macrophages. Biochem Biophys Res Commun. 1995;206:533–40.

Bukovska A, Cikos S, Juhas S. Effects of a combination of thyme and oregano essential oils on TNBS-induced colitis in mice. Mediat Inflamm. 2007;2007:23296.

Byeon SW, Pelley RP, Ullrich SE, Waller TA, Bucana CD, Strickland FM. *Aloe barbadensis* extracts reduce the production of interleukin-10 after exposure to ultraviolet radiation. J Invest Dermatol. 1998;110:811–7.

Chainy GB, Manna SK, Chaturvedi MM, Aggarwal BB. Anethole blocks both early and late cellular responses transduced by tumor necrosis factor: effect on NF-kappaB, AP-1, JNK, MAPKK and apoptosis. Oncogene. 2000;25(19):2943–50.

Chopra D, Simon D. The Chopra Centre herbal hand book. London: Rider; 2002.

Das AP, Pandey AK (Eds). Advances in ethnobotany. Dehra Dun: Bishen Singh Mahendra Pal Singh; 2007.

Das AP, Ghosh C, Sarker A, Biswas R, Biswas K, Choudhury D, et al. Preliminary report on the medicinal plants from three MPCAs in Terai and Duars of West Bengal, India. Pleione. 2010;4(1):90–101.

Das S, Acharya J, De B. Metabolite profiling, antioxidant activity, and glycosidase inhibition property of the mesocarp tissue extracts of sugar date palm [*Phoenix sylvestris* (L.) Roxb.] fruits. Int J Food Prop. 2017;20:2982–93.

Deep G, Dhiman M, Rao AR, Kale RK. Chemopreventive potential of Triphala (a composite Indian drug) on benzo(a)pyrene induced forestomach tumorigenesis in murine tumor model system. J Exp Clin Cancer Res. 2005;24:555–63.

Desai VR, Ramkrishnan R, Chintalwar GJ, Sainis KB. G1-4A, an immunomodulatory polysaccharide from *Tinospora cordifolia*, modulates macrophage responses and protects mice against lipopolysaccharide induced endotoxic shock. Int Immunopharmacol. 2007;7:1375–86.

Devi MR, Salam S. Wild edible plants used by the Monsang Nagatribe of Manipur, India. Pleione. 2016;10(1):90–6.

Devi RS, Narayan S, Vani G, Shyamala Devi CS. Gastroprotective effect of Terminalia arjuna bark on diclofenac sodium induced gastric ulcer. Chem Biol Interact. 2007;167:71–83.

Dhuley JN. Effect of some Indian herbs on macrophage functions in ochratoxin A treated mice. J Ethnopharmacol. 1997;58:15–20.

Dutton GJ. Acceptor substrates of UDP glucuronosyltransferase and their assay. In: Dutton GJ, editor. Glucuronidation of drugs and other compounds. Boca Raton, FL: CRC Press; 1980. p. 69–78.

Eidelman RS, Hollar D, Hebert PR, Lamas GA, Hennekens CH. Randomized trials of vitamin E in the treatment and prevention of cardiovascular disease. Arch Intern Med. 2004;164:1552–6.

El-Sheikh ALK. Renal transport and drug interactions of immunosuppressants [thesis]. Nijmegen, Netherlands: Radbound University; 2008. p. 62.

Fior S, Vianelli A, Gerola PD. A novel method for fluorometric continuous measurement of β-glucuronidase (GUS) activity using 4-methyl-umbelliferyl-β-D- glucuronide (MUG) as substrate. Plant Sci. 2009;176:130–5.

Fleming DM, Elliot AJ, Nguyen-van Tam JS, Watson JM, Wise R. A winter's tale: coming to terms with winter respiratory illnesses. London: Health Protection Agency; 2005.

Ganju L, Karan D, Chanda S, Srivastava KK, Sawhney RC, Selvamurthy W. Immunomodulatory effects of agents of plant origin. Biomed Pharmacother. 2003;57:296–300.

Garcia E, Hasenbank MS, Finlayson B, Yager P. High-throughput screening of enzyme inhibition using an inhibitor gradient generated in a microchannel. Lab Chip. 2007;7:249–55.

Gautam AL, Rana R, Srivastava V, Ray Choudhuri SP, Singh BR. Prospects of medicinal plants. New Delhi: Indian Society Plant Genetic Resources; 1998.

Groner E, Ashani Y, Apelbaum DS, Sterling J, Herzig Y, Weinstock M. The kinetics of inhibition of human acetylcholinesterase and butyrylcholinesterase by two series of novel carbamates. Mol Pharm. 2007;71(6):1610–7.

Gutteridge JM, Halliwell B. Free radicals and antioxidants in the year 2000. A historical look to the future. Ann N Y Acad Sci. 2000;899:136–47.

Howes MR, Houghton PJ. Plants used in Chinese and Indian traditional medicine for improvement of memory and cognitive function. Pharmacol Biochem Behav. 2003;75(3):513–27.

Inagawa H, Nishizawa T, Tsukioka D, Suda T, Chiba Y, Okutomi T, et al. Homeostasis as regulated by activated macrophage. II. LPS of plant origin other than wheat flour and their concomitant bacteria. Chem Pharm Bull (Tokyo). 1992;40:994–7.

Jain SK. Glimpses of Indian Ethnobotany. New Delhi: Oxford & IBH; 1982.

Jain SK. A manual of ethnobotany. Jodhpur: Scientific Publishers; 1987.

Jain SK. Methods and approaches in ethnobotany. Lucknow: Society of Ethnobotanists; 1989.

Jain SK. Contributions to ethnobotany of India. Jodhpur: Scientific Publishers; 1990.

Jain SK. Dictionary of Indian folk medicine and ethnobotany. New Delhi: Deep Publications; 1991.

Jain SK. Ethnobotany and research on medicinal plants in India. In: Derek J, Chadwick JM, editors. Ethnobotany and the search of new drugs, CIBA Foundation Symposium, 185. Chichester, UK: John Wiley and Sons; 1994. p. 153–68.

Jain SK. Contribution to Indian ethnobotany. 3rd ed. Jodhpur: Scientific Publishers; 1997.

Jain SK. Medicinal plants. New Delhi: National Book Trust; 1999.

Jain SK. Global resurgence of ethnomedicobotany- the Indian scene. Trop Med Plant. 2000;1:75–81.

Jain SK. Ethnobiology in human welfare: index to plant and animal names. New Delhi: Deep Publications; 2001a.

Jain SK. Ethnobotany in modern India. Phytomorphol. 2001b;51(4):39–54.

Jain SK. Bibliography of Indian ethnobotany. Jodhpur: Scientific Publishers; 2002.

Jain SK. Manual of ethnobotany. Jodhpur: Scientific Publishers; 2004.

Jain SK. Plants affecting human mind (psychoactive plants). New Delhi: Deep Publications; 2009.

Jain SK. Ethnobotany in India: some thoughts on future work. Ethnobotany. 2010;22:1–4.

Jain SK. Dictionary of Indian folk medicine and ethnobotany. New Delhi: Deep Publications; 2012. (Reprinted edn.)

Jain SK, Borthakur SK. Ethnobotany of the Mikirs of India. Econ Bot. 1980;34(3):264–72.

Jain SK, Borthakur SK. Solanaceae in India tradition, folklore and medicine. In: D'arehy WG, editor. Solanaceae: biology and systematic. New York: Columbia University Press; 1986. p. 577–83.

Jain SK, De JN. Observations on ethnobotany of Purulia. Bull Bot Surv India. 1966;8:237–51.

Jain SK, Jain V. Evolution of ethnobotany in India during last sixty years: a brief overview. Ethnobotany. 2015;27:1–6.

Jain A, Jain SK. Indian ethnobotany: bibliography of 21st century (2001–2015). Jodhpur: Scientific Publisher; 2016a.

Jain V, Jain SK. Compendium of Indian folk medicine and ethnobotany (1991–2015). New Delhi: Deep Publications; 2016b.

Jain SK, Mitra R. Ethnobotany in India: retrospect and prospect. In: Jain SK, editor. Contribution to Indian ethnobotany. 3rd ed. New Delhi: Scientific Publishers; 1997. p. 1–15.

Jain SK, Srivastava S. Dictionary of ethnoveterinary plants of India. New Delhi: Deep Publications; 1999.

Jain SK, Hajra P, Shanpru R. A survey of wild edible plants in bazaars of Meghalaya. Bull Meghalaya Sci Soc. 1977;2:29–34.

Jain SK, Mudgal V, Banerjee DK, Guha A, Pal DC, Das D. Bibliography of ethnobotany. Calcutta: Botanical Survey of India; 1984.

Janaki-Ammal EK. Introduction to the subsistence economy of India. In: William Jr LT, editor. Man's role in changing face of the earth. Chicago: University of Chicago Press; 1956.

Jayathirtha MG, Mishra SH. Preliminary immunomodulatory activities of methanol extracts of *Eclipta alba* and *Centella asiatica*. Phytomedicine. 2004;11:361–5.

Kapoor LD. Handbook of Ayurvedic medicinal plants. Boca Raton: CRC Press; 1990.

Kaushik P, Dhiman AK. Medicinal plants and raw drugs of India. Dehradun: Bishen Singh Mahenderpal Singh; 1999.

Kavishankar GB, Lakshmidevi N, Murthy SM, Prakash HS, Niranjana SR. Diabetes and medicinal plants: a review. Int J Pharm Biomed Sci. 2011;2:65–80.

Kluth D, Banning A, Paur I, Blomhoff R, Brigelius-Flohe R. Modulation of pregnane X receptor- and electrophile responsive element-mediated gene expression by dietary polyphenolic compounds. Free Radic Biol Med. 2007;42(3):315–25.

Krippner S. Models of ethnomedicinal healing. In: Ethnomedicine Conferences, Munich, 26–27 April and 11–12 October, 2003.

Kumar S. Ethnobotanical studies in India. New Delhi: Deep Publications; 2014.

Lake DF, Briggs AD, Akporiaye ET. Immunopharmacology. In: Katzung BG, Masters SB, Trevor AJ, editors. Basic and clinical pharmacology. 12th ed. New Delhi/New York: Tata/McGraw Hill; 2012. p. 977–1000.

Lalramnghinghlova H. Ethnobotanical interpretations and future prospects of ethnobotany in the North-East India. Sci Vision. 2001;1:24–31.

Lalramnghinghlova H, Jha LK. Forest resources: an overview. In: Jha LK, Nangia SB, editors. Natural resource management, vol. vol. 1. New Delhi: A.P.H. Publishing Corporation; 1997. p. 203–55.

Lalramnghinglova H, Jha LK. Ethnobotany: a review. J Econ Taxon Bot. 1999;23(1):1–27.

Lampe JW, Li SS, Potter JD, King IB. Serum beta-glucuronidase activity is inversely associated with plant –food intakes in humans. J Nutr. 2002;132:1341–4.

Lee J, Jung E, Kim Y. Rosmarinic acid as a downstream inhibitor of IKK-beta in TNF-alpha-induced upregulation of CCL11 and CCR3. Br J Pharmacol. 2006;3(148):366–75.

Lowe H, Payne-Jackson A, Beckstrom-Sternberg SM, Duke JA. Jamaica's ethnomedicine: its potential in the healthcare system. Kingston: Canoe Press, University of West Indies; 2000.

Magendie F, Pelletier J. Recherches chimiques et physiologiques sur l' lpecacuanha. J Pharm. 1817;3:145–64.

McCord JM. The evolution of free radicals and oxidative stress. Am J Med. 2000;108:652–9.

McCue P, Kwon Y-I, Shetty K. Anti-diabetic and anti-hypertensive potential of sprouted and solid-state bioprocessed soybean. Asia Pac J Clin Nutr. 2005;14(2):145–52.

Mehrotra S, Mishra KP, Maurya R, Srimal RC, Singh VK. Immunomodulation by ethanolic extract of *Boerhaavia diffusa* roots. Int Immunopharmacol. 2002;2:987–96.

Mehrotra S, Mishra KP, Maurya R, Srimal RC, Yadav VS, Pandey R, Singh VK. Anticellular and immunosuppressive properties of ethanolic extract of *Acorus calamus* rhizome. Int Immunopharmacol. 2003;3:53–61.

Miguel M, Contreras MM, Recio I, Aleixandre A. ACE-inhibitory and antihypertensive properties of bovine casein hydrolysates. Food Chem. 2009;112(1):211–4.

Morioka N, Sze LL, Mortan DL, Irie RF. A protein fraction from aged garlic extracts enhances cytotoxicity and proliferation of human lymphocytes mediated by interleukin-2 and concanavalin A. Cancer Immunol Immunother. 1993;37:316–22.

Mousa HA. Herbal therapies for prevention and treatment of influenza and influenza-like illness. J Infect Dis Ther. 2015;3:215.

Mousa HA. Prevention and treatment of influenza, influenza-like illness, and common cold by herbal, complementary, and natural therapies. J Evid Based Complementary Altern Med. 2017;22(1):166–74.

Mukherjee A. Biodiversity conservation. J Asiatic Soc. 1997;39:1–6.

Mukherjee A. Herbal remedies: aspects and prospects with special refrence to India. In: Maiti G, Mukherjee SK, editors. Multidisciplinary approaches in angiosperm systematics, vol. 2. Kalyani, West Bengal: University of Kalyani; 2012. p. 576–88.

Mungantiwar AA, Nair AM, Shinde UA, Dikshit VJ, Saraf MN, Thakur VS, Sainis KB. Studies on the immunomodulatory effects of *Boerhaavia diffusa* alkaloidal fraction. J Ethnopharmacol. 1999;65:125–31.

Murai A, Iwamura K, Takada M, Ogawa K, Usui T, Okumura J. Control of postprandial hyperglycaemia by galactosyl maltobionolactone and its novel anti-amylase effect in mice. Life Sci. 2002;71:1405–15.

Nadkarni P. Indian medicinal plants. Hyderabad: Orient Longman; 1992.

Naik VN. Identification of common Indian medicinal plants. Jodhpur: Scientific Publishers; 2004.

Nair CKN, Mohanan N. Medicinal plants in India. Delhi: Nag Publications; 1998.

Nath M. Some less known medicinal uses of plants among Dimsa tribe of Barak valley, Assam (North-east India). Ethnobotany. 2015;27:49–52.

Niemann A. Ueber eine neue organische base in den Cocablättern. Arch Pharm. 1860;153(2):129–256.

Okayasu H, Suzuki F, Satoh K, et al. Comparison of cytotoxicity and radical scavenging activity between tea extracts and Chinese medicines. In Vivo. 2003;17:577–81.

Pal DC, Jain S. Notes on Lodha medicine in Midnapur District, West Bengal. Econ Bot. 1989;43(4):464–70.

Pal DC, Jain SK. Tribal medicine. Calcutta: Naya Prakash; 1998.

Paur I, Austenaa LM, Blomhoff R. Extracts of dietary plants are efficient modulators of nuclear factor kappa B. Food Chem Toxicol. 2008;46(4):1288–97.

Paur I, Balstad TR, Kolberg M, et al. Extract of oregano, coffee, thyme, clove, and walnuts inhibits NF-kappaB in monocytes and in transgenic reporter mice. Cancer Prev Res (Phila). 2010;3(5):653–63.

Pelletier PJ, Caventou JB. Suite: Des recherché chimiques sur les quiquinas. Annales de Chimie et de Physique. 1820;15:337–65.

Plaeger FS. Clinical immunology and traditional herbal medicines. Clin Diagn Lab Immunol. 2003;10:337–8.

Posselt W, Reimann L. Chemisce untersuchng des tabaks und darstellung eines eigengthümlich Wirksamen Prinzips dieser Pflanzen. Magazin für Pharmacie. 1828;6(24):138–61.

Puri A, Saxena RP, Sumati, Guru PY, Kulshreshtha DK, Saxena KC, Dhawan BN. Immunostimulant activity of picroliv, the iridoid glycoside fraction of *Picrorrhiza kurroa* and its protective action against *Leishmania donovani* infection in hamsters. Planta Med. 1992;58:528–32.

Rana AK. Indian medicinal and aromatic plants 1 & 2. Indian Forester. 2003;129:1–297.

Rasool M, Sabina EP. Anti-inflammatory effect of the Indian Ayurvedic herbal formulation Triphala on adjuvant-induced arthritis in mice. Phytother Res. 2007;21:889–94.

Reeve VE, Bosnic M, Rozinova E, Boehm-Wilcox C. A garlic extract protects from ultraviolet B (280-320 nm) radiation-induced suppression of contact hypersensitivity. Photochem Photobiol. 1993;58:813–7.

Rege NN, Nazareth HM, Isaac A, Karandikar SM, Dahanukar SA. Immunotherapeutic modulation of intraperitoneal adhesions by Asparagus racemosus. J Postgrad Med. 1989;35:199–203.

Sahu V, Bajpai R, Upreti DK. Traditional use of lichens of Rudrabhishek (spiritually ceremony): a Hindu practice to worship Lord Shiva in India. Ethnobotany. 2015;27:92–6.

Saklani A, Jain SK. Cross cultural ethnobotany of North East India. New Delhi: Deep Publications; 1994.

Sasaki K, Wada K, Tanaka Y, Yoshimura T, Matuoka K, Anno T. Thyme (Thymus vulgaris L.) leaves and its constituents increase the activities of xenobiotic-metabolizing enzymes in mouse liver. J Med Food. 2005;8(2):184–9.

Satyavati GV, Gupta KA. Medicinal plants of India, vols 1&2. New Delhi: ICMR; 1987.

Sertürner F. Ueber das Morphium, eine neue salzfähige Grundlage, und die Mekonsäure, als Hauptbestandtheile des Opiums. Ann Phys. 1817;55:56–89.

Sertürner F. Darstellung der reinen Mohnsäure (Opiumsäure) nebst einer Chemischen Untersuchung des Opiums mit vorzüglicher Hinsicht auf einen darin neu entdeckten Stoff und die dahin gehörigen Bemerkungen. J der Pharmacie fuer Aerzte und Apotheke. 1806;14:47–93.

Shah S. The selected Indian medicinal plants. Madras: Chemixil; 1992.

Shan B, Cai YZ, Sun M, Corke H. Antioxidant capacity of 26 spice extracts and characterization of their phenolic constituents. J Agric Food Chem. 2005;53(20):7749–59.

Shim SB, Kim NJ, Kim DH. Beta-glucuronidase inhibitory activity and hepatoprotective effect of 18 beta-glycyrrhetinic acid from the rhizomes of *Glycyrrhiza uralensis*. Planta Med. 2000;66(1):40–3.

Singh N, Singh SM, Shrivastava P. Immunomodulatory and antitumor actions of medicinal plant *Tinospora cordifolia* are mediated through activation of tumor-associated macrophages. Immunopharmacol Immunotoxicol. 2004;26:145–62.

Srikumar R, Parthasarathy NJ, Shankar EM, Manikandan S, Vijayakumar R, Thangaraj R, et al. Evaluation of the growth inhibitory activities of Triphala against common bacterial isolates from HIV infected patients. Phytother Res. 2007;21:476–80.

Surh YJ. Cancer chemoprevention with dietary phytochemicals. Nat Rev Cancer. 2003;3(10):768–80.

Swami Brahmananda. Common medicinal plants of India. New Delhi: Dominent Publishers; 2002.

Takada Y, Bhardwaj A, Potdar P, Aggarwal BB. Nonsteroidal anti-inflammatory agents differ in their abilityto suppress NF-kappaB activation, inhibition of expression of cyclooxygenase-2 and cyclin D1, and abrogation of tumor cell proliferation. Oncogene. 2004;23(57):9247–58.

Tang Z, Sheng Z, Liu S, Jian X, Sun K, Yan M. The preventing function of garlic on experimental oral precancer and its effect on natural killer cells, T-lymphocytes and interleukin-2. Hunan Yi Ke Da Xue Xue Bao. 1997;22:246–8.

Thatte UM, Dahanukar SA. Comparative study of immunomodulating activity of Indian medicinal plants, lithium carbonate and glucan. Methods Find Exp Clin Pharmacol. 1988;10:639–44.

Uniyal SK, Awasthi A, Rawat GS. Current status and distribution of commercially exploited medicinal and aromatic plants in upper Gori valley, Kumaun Himalaya, Uttaranchal. Curr Sci. 2002;82(10):1246–52.

Vishkaei MS, Ebrahimpour A, Abdul-Hamid A, Ismail A, Saari N. Angiotensin-I converting enzyme (ACE) inhibitory and anti-hypertensive effect of protein hydrolysate from *Actinopyga lecanora* (sea cucumber) in rats. Mar Drugs. 2016;176:E176.

Vivekananthan DP, Penn MS, Sapp SK, Hsu A, Topol EJ. Use of antioxidant vitamins for the prevention of cardiovascular disease: meta-analysis of randomised trials. Lancet. 2003;361:2017–23.

Walaszek Z, Szemraj J, Narog M, Adams AK, Kilgore J, Sherman U, Hanausek M. Metabolism, uptake, and excretion of a D-glucaric acid salt and its potential use in cancer prevention. Cancer Detect Prev. 1997;21(2):178–90.

Wang X, Jia W, Zhao A, Wang X. Anti-influenza agents from plants and traditional Chinese medicine. Phytother Res. 2006;20:335–41.

Weber O. The role of viruses in the etiology and pathogenesis of common cold. In: Eccles RWO, editor. Common cold. Basel: Birkha¨user Verlag; 2009. p. 132–3.

Winterstein E, Trier G. Die Alkaloide. Berlin: Borntraeger Press; 1910.

World Health Organization. Traditional medicine and health care coverage. Geneva: WHO; 1983.

World Health Organization. Report: technical briefing on traditional medicine. Forty-ninth Regional Committee Meeting. Manila: WHO; 1998.

World Health Organization. Consultation meeting on traditional medicine and modern medicine: harmonizing the two approaches. Geneva: WHO; 1999a.

World Health Organization. Traditional, complementary and alternative medicines and therapies. Washington DC: WHO Regional Office for the Americas/Pan American Health Organization; 1999b.

World Health Organization. Traditional medicine strategy 2002–2005. Geneva: WHO; 2002.

World Health Organization. National policy on traditional medicine and regulation of herbal medicines—report of a WHO global survey. Geneva: WHO; 2005.

World Health Organization. Constitution of the World Health Organization. In Basic Documents, forty-fifth Edition, supplement. 2006.

Zafar R. Medicinal plants in India. New Delhi: CBS Publications; 1999.

Zhang XF, Tan BK. Anti-diabetic property of ethanolic extract of *Andrographis paniculata* in streptozotocin-diabetic rats. Acta Pharma. 2000;21:157–64.

Zhang L, Tizard IR. Activation of a mouse macrophage cell line by acemannan: the major carbohydrate fraction from *Aloe vera* gel. Immunopharmacology. 1996;35:119–28.

An Ethnobotanical Survey of Medicinal Plants Used by Ethnic People of Thoubal and Kakching District, Manipur, India

4

Raja Chakraborty, Saikat Sen, Nongmaithem Randhoni Chanu, Akoijam Bishaljit Singh, and Pratap Kalita

Contents

4.1 Introduction

The infliction of herbs and herbal preparations particularly those based on a traditional system of medicine are increasing in the daily life of people, as a global community is in the search of effective, comparatively safer and better medicine (Sen et al. 2011). According to the World Health Organization (WHO), about 80% of the world's population, especially those who live in rural areas, still depends on herbal medicine for their primary healthcare needs (Ahmad et al. 2006). Traditional local healers abundantly used the natural sources and they conserved the relationship between human society and environments (Sajem and Gosai 2006). Herbal remedies are very popular all over the world as they contain plenty of bioactive molecules to cure the diverse diseases and also considered as safe compared to allopathic medicine (Thirumalai et al. 2009; Verma and Singh 2008; Sannomiya et al. 2007). Ethnic peoples possess immerse knowledge on the usage of biotic resources of traditional medicinal plants (Halim et al. 2007; Uniyal et al. 2006), which helps researchers for better investigation and to find more potent drug formulation based on such information's (Rana et al. 2010).

Manipur is a state situated in the North East part of India. The total area covered by the state is 22,347 km^2 of hill territory. The small state forms a part of the Himalayan mountain system

R. Chakraborty (✉)
Department of Pharmacy, Assam Down Town University, Guwahati, Assam, India

NEF College of Pharmacy, Lokhra, Guwahati, Assam, India

S. Sen · N. R. Chanu · A. B. Singh · P. Kalita
Department of Pharmacy, Assam Down Town University, Guwahati, Assam, India

S. Sen, R. Chakraborty (eds.), *Herbal Medicine in India*,
https://doi.org/10.1007/978-981-13-7248-3_4

which carries this cup-shaped wonderland inside its series of hill ranges (Singha 2014).The climate of Manipur is largely influenced by the topography of this hilly region. Lying 790 m above sea level, Manipur is wedged among hills on all sides. This northeastern corner of India enjoys a generally amiable climate, though the winters can be chilly. The maximum temperature in summer is 32 °C, while it often falls below 0 °C in winter (Singha 2014; Shankar et al. 2009).

Manipur was chosen after the survey because it is blessed with rich flora and fauna which in turn is used in medicines since ancient times by the native people as well as the people inhibited in this hilly region of the state. In this present study, attempts are being made to document such ethnomedicinal information commonly used for various health problems by the people of Thoubal and Kakching district of Manipur, India.

4.2 Methodology

4.2.1 Study Location and Duration

Thoubal district of Manipur lies between latitude 23°45′N and 24°45′N and longitude 93°45′E and 94°15′E, it occupies the larger part of the eastern half of the Manipur Valley, takes the shape of an irregular and triangular with its base facing north. In December 2016, Kakching district came into existence when Government bifurcate Thoubal district. These areas of the state are largely inhibited by a number of communities like *Meitei, Meitei-Muslim, Loi, Taithibi, Chiru, Hmar, Gangte, Kabui, Kom, Lamkang, Maring, Paite, Tangkhul, Vaiphei, Zou, Maring, Kukis, and Thadou*etc (Khan and Yadava 2010). The present study was conducted in different out in different tribal inhabited localities of Thoubal and Kakching district of Manipur during August 2015–June 2016.

4.2.2 Investigating Methods

Ethno-medico-botanical information practised by the different communities of these two districts was collected through field survey. Each locality was visited several times and information was collected through interviewing the local informants. The person we are communicated are above 60 years old and have usually been practicing such knowledge in their locality for more than two decades. Briefly, group discussion prior to the survey was made with the local herbal medicine practitioner at each locality to get their consent and to explain the importance of such study. Methods like a semi-structured interview, face-to-face dialogue, group discussion and field observation were made to collect the data on medicinal plants. Information was collected from both tribal and non-tribal medicine men and medicine women of different castes and religions in the study area. Information on the knowledge and practice of those people were collected and documented. Information on the plant species like their local name, parts of the plant used, medicinal importance, mode of preparation and use were collected. All plant specimens were collected during different seasons. Plants were identified using standard manual, available literature and with the help of traditional medical practitioner followed by confirming with expert plant taxonomists.

4.3 Results and Discussion

Among the 16 districts of Manipur, Thoubal and Kakching districts were surveyed. Traditional healers from Meitei community, as well as other communities, possess rich knowledge on plants which are used in the preparation of traditional medicine. However, a large number of plant species and such knowledge have not been scientifically proven and documented. The plants and herbs are being used for promotion and preservation of health, prevention, and treatment of diseases. A total of 40 ethnomedicinal plants belonging to 35 families were documented in the present study. Informants are generally practised in different section of society by using different parts of plants such as roots, stems, leaves, flowers, fruits in the form of infusion, decoction, paste

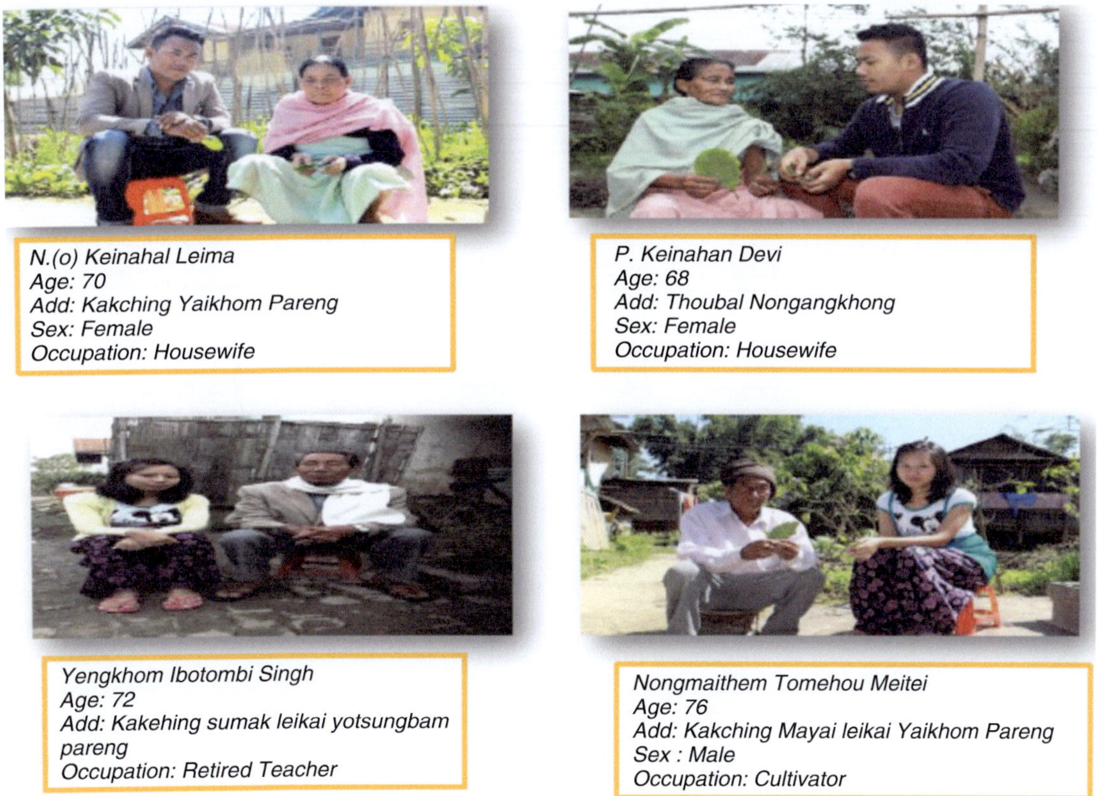
N.(o) Keinahal Leima
Age: 70
Add: Kakching Yaikhom Pareng
Sex: Female
Occupation: Housewife
P. Keinahan Devi
Age: 68
Add: Thoubal Nongangkhong
Sex: Female
Occupation: Housewife
Yengkhom Ibotombi Singh
Age: 72
Add: Kakehing sumak leikai yotsungbam pareng
Occupation: Retired Teacher
Nongmaithem Tomehou Meitei
Age: 76
Add: Kakching Mayai leikai Yaikhom Pareng
Sex : Male
Occupation: Cultivator

Fig. 4.1 Photograph with traditional healers during the survey

Fig. 4.2 Percentage distribution of aboveground, underground and whole plant parts

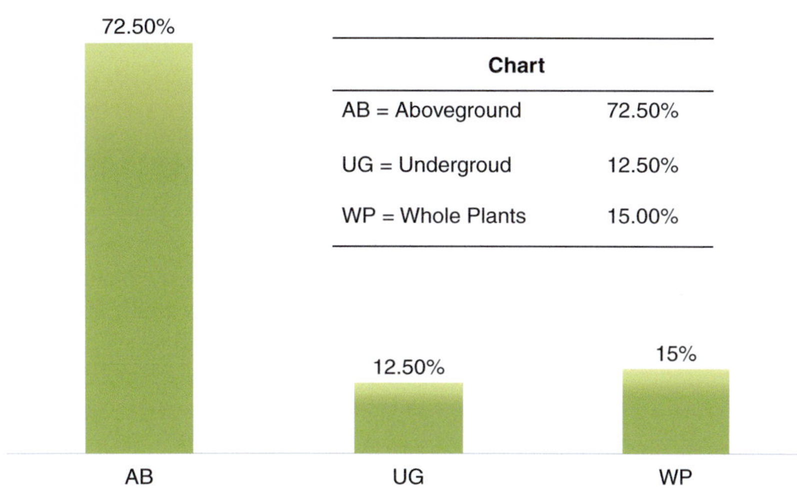

etc. Figure 4.1 shows some clicks captured during the survey with folk medicine practitioners.

Among 40 medicinal plants, the usage of above-ground parts of medicinal plant species consistently higher (72.5%) than the underground plant parts (12.5%) followed by whole plants (15.0%) (Fig. 4.2). All these medicinal plants were used by people of the different community

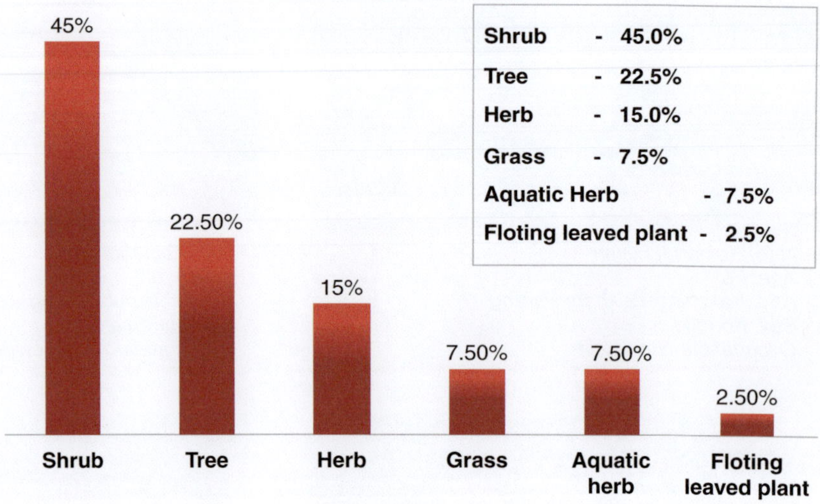

Fig. 4.3 Graphical representation of life forms investigated ethno-medicinal plants

of tribes like *Maitei, Meitei-Muslim, Maring, Kukis, and Thadou* of Thoubal and Kakching district of Manipur for curing of different ailments. The results showed that the shrub was prevalent (45%), followed by tree (22%), herbs (15%), grass (7.5%), aquatic herb (7.5%) and floating winged plant (2.5%) (Fig. 4.3).

The eminent families of the medicinal plant used by ethnic people were presented in Table 4.1 with plant name, habit, common name, parts used and diseases. The percentage of various plant parts used as drug revealed in Fig. 4.4 as leaves (40%), whole plants (15%), seeds (10%), barks (5%), shoots (5%), roots (5%), rhizomes (5%), aerial parts (5%), fruits (2.5%), stems (2.5%), flowers (2.5%) and petioles (2.5%).

In Thoubal and Kakching, as in other parts of the state, herbs or plants have all along been used for promotion of health and prevention and treatment of diseases. They were used in most cases as an infusion, decoction, juice, powder, extract and paste from the parts of plants such as roots, stems, leaves, flowers, fruits, whole plants, barks, seeds, aerial parts, rhizomes, shoots, petioles. Most of the plants are intended as medicine by orally and externally and some of the medicinal plants were intended by both orally and externally. The method of preparation and mode of usage of ethnobotanical medicinal plants were exhibited in Table 4.2.

It was observed that local informants were from the different socio-economic background and a large number of informants were women. The informants were practising folk medicine more than 20 years in their localities. They were from the diverse field like some are housewife, farmer, a retired teacher, daily worker etc. During the discussion, it was observed that they learned such knowledge from their ancestor and also based on their experiences for years. The survey indicated that the people of the study area largely depend on folk practitioners for daily healthcare need. The study area has plenty of plants to treat a wide spectrum of human diseases. It was evident during the survey that knowledge of medicinal plants was mostly limited to traditional healers and elderly persons who are living in rural/remote areas. This study observed that even though the accessibility of modern medicine is easy, many people still continue to depend on medicinal plants, at least for the treatment of some common and daily life diseases such as cold, cough, fever, pain, dysentery, poison bites, skin problem, toothache, diabetes etc.

Table 4.1 List of medicinal plants used by different tribes in Manipur, India

Sl. no.	Plant name	Family	Habit	Common name	Parts used	Diseases claim to cure/manage
1	*Acacia arabica*	Leguminosia	Tree	Babul	Seed, Bark, leaf	Diarrhea, tonsillitis, piles, joint pain
2	*Antidesma acidum*	Phyllanthacae	Shrub	Rohitaka	Leaf	Dyspepsia, diabetes
3	*Alpinia galangal*	Zingeberaceae	Shrub	Blue ginger	Rhizome	Fever, diabetes, irregular menstruation
4	*Ageratum conyzoides*	Asteraceae	Herb	Goat weld	Leaf, shoot	Cut, injury, flatulence, and as hair lotion
5	*Amomum aromaticum* Roxb.	Zingiberaceae	Herb	Bengal cardamom	Seed	High blood pressure, mumps
6	*Alternanthera philoxeroides*	Amaranthaceae	Herb	Alligator weld	Shoot	Dysentery
7	*Arundo donax* L	Poaceae	Shrub	Giant seed	Shoot	Intestinal worm, typhoid, pneumonia
8	*Artocarpus lakoocha* Roxb.	Moraceae	Tree	Monkey jerk	Bark, fruit	Diabetes, bacterial and worm infection, skin rash
9	*Maesa indica* Roxb	Myrsinaceae	Shrub	Ar- ngeng	Leaf	Diabetes, stomach pain
10	*Azadirachta indica*	Meliaceae	Shrub	Neem	Leaf, bark, flower, fruit	Rheumatoid arthritis, diabetes, eye infection, microbial infection
11	*Adhatoda vasica*	Acanthaceae	Shrub	Vasaka	Leaf, flower	Cough, bacterial infection, diabetes
12	*Allium hookeri*	Amaryllidaceae	Shrub	Hooker chives	Whole plant	Diabetes, hypertension, vomiting
13	*Blumea balsamifera*	Compositae	Shrub	Sambung	Whole plant	Fever common cold, stomach pain
14	*Colocasia esculenta* (L) Schott	Araceae	Herb	Green tard,Taro	Petiole, leaf	Injury, body pain, hemorrhage
15	*Cynodon dactylon*	Poaceae	Grass	Bermuda grass	Arial part	Strangury, dysmenorrheal, urogenital disorders, week vision
16	*Cyperus haspan* L.	Cyperaceae	Shrub	Dwarf papyrus	Rhizome	Bronchitis, fever
17	*Celtis timorensis*	Celmaceae	Tree	Stink wood	Bark, leaf	Kidney stone, liver disease, diabetes, respiratory problems
18	*Hibiscus cannabinus*	Malvaceae	Shrub	Kenat	Leaf	Diabetes, cancer, throat diseases
19	*Ipomoea aquatica*	Convolvulaceae	Shrub	Water morning glory	Leaf	Diarrhea and retinitis, Stress, liver problem
20	*Lysimachia obovata*	Primulaceae	Shrub	Manipur loosestrife	Leaf	Dyspepsia, and as diuretic
21	*Magnolia champaca*	Magnoliaceae	Tree	Champak	Seed, bud	Tonsillitis, diabetes
22	*Marsilea minuta* L.	Mareiliaceae	Grass	Dwarf water clover	Whole plants	Strangury, sleep diseases, oral infection
23	*Musa acuminate*	Musaceae	Tree	Banana	Flower, stem	Asthma, diabetes
24	*Nasturtium indicum* L.	Brassicaceae	Grass	Water cress	Whole plant	Diabetes, fungal infection

(continued)

Table 4.1 (continued)

Sl. no.	Plant name	Family	Habit	Common name	Parts used	Diseases claim to cure/manage
25	*Nymphoides indica*	Gentianaceae	Herb	Water snowflak, floating	Stem, rhizome	Cut and injury, headache
26	*Nymphaea stellata* Willd	Nymphaeaceae	Aquatic Herb	Blue water- lily	Whole plants	Erysipelas, and as anti-aphrodisiac and diuretic
27	*Oenanthe javanica*	Apiaceae	Herb	Water dropwort	Arial part	Influenza, jaundice
28	*Parkia javanica*	Fabaceae	Tree	Bitter bean	Leaf, root,	Bacterial infection, diabetes, bleeding
29	*Persicaria sagittata*	Polygonaceae	Shrub	Arrow leaftear thumb	Leaf	Antidote of insect bite, abdominal pain, muscle spasm
30	*Polygonum barbatum*	Polygonaceae	Shrub	Dense flower natured	Leaf, seed	Constipation, stomach problem, cutaneous infection, colic
31	*Punica granatum*	Punicaceae	Shrub	Pramangras	Leaf, fruit	Dysentery, diabetes
32	*Psidium guajava*	Myrtaceae	Tree	Guana	Leaf	Dysentery, diabetes
33	*Pistia stratiotes*	Araceae	Aquatic herb	Water lettuce	Leaf, Stem	Burnt, boil
34	*Ranunculus sceleratus*	Ranunculaceae	Shrub	Cursed buttercup	Leaf	Gout, fever, abdominal problem
35	*Rhuschinensis*	Anacardiaceae	Tree	Chinese gall	Fruit, leaf	Diarrhoea, cough, cancer, diabetes
36	*Salvia officinalis*	Labiateae	Shrub	Sage	Leaf	Tonsillitis, diabetes
37	*Sagittaria sagittifolia*	Alismataceae	Aquatic herb	Gauai-gauai	Root	Cough, scurvy
38	*Syzygium cumini*	Myrtaceae	Tree	Jamun	Seed	Asthma, diabetes, gum infection, ulcer
39	*Solanum xanthocarpum*	Solanaceae	Shrub	Kantakari	Whole parts	Asthma, bronchitis, diabetes, dental pain
40	*Trapa natanas*	Trapaceae	Floating leaved plant	Water chestnut	Roots, fruits	Fungal and bacterial infection, diabetes, sores

Chart	
Leaf	40.00%
Whole plants	15.00%
Seed	10%
Bark	5%
Root	5%
Shoot	5%
Rhizome	5%
Arial part	5%
Fruits	2.50%
Stem	2.50%
Petiole	2.50%
Flower	2.50%

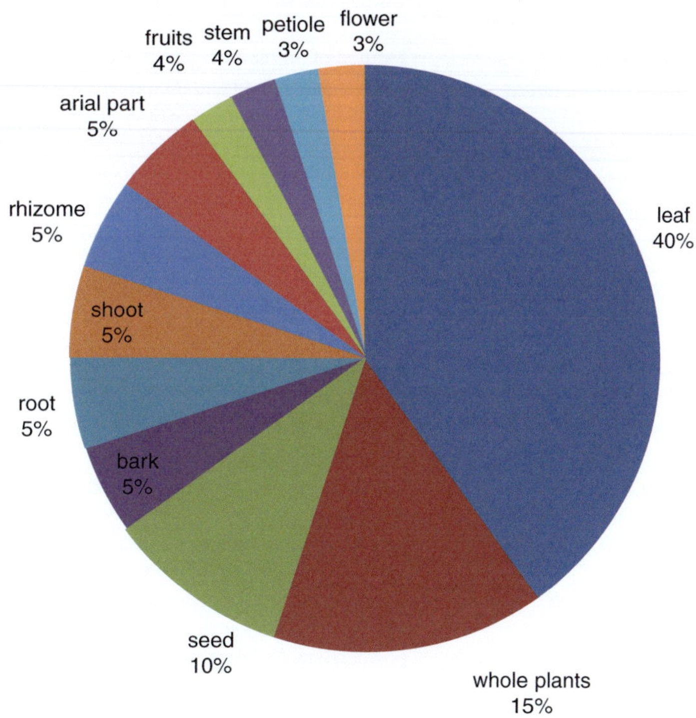

Fig. 4.4 Percentage distribution of medicinal plant parts used as medicine by different tribes for curing ailments

Table 4.2 Mode of application of ethno-botanical medicinal plants (selected uses)

Plant name	Method of preparation and mode of usage
Acacia-arabica	Fruits of the plant were boiled with water and consumed for diarrhoea. A decoction of the bark mixed with salt and used for tonsillitis.
Antidesma acidum	Leaf was boiled with water and mixed with salt and then taken for dyspepsia and diabetes.
Alpinia galangal	Fresh rhizomes were crushed and filtered and mixed with water and taken for dysmenorrheal. Also, the decoction of the leaf used to reduce fever and diabetes.
Ageratum conyzoides	Aqueous extract of leaves or whole plants has been used to treat cold and fevers. Leaf juice also applies for the cut and injury.
Amomum aromaticum	Seed powder boiled with water for blood pressure, root extract with water used for mumps.
Alternanthera philoxeroides	Shoot extract with a little salt is used for dysentery.
Arundo donax	Fresh shoot paste mixes with a spoon of honey and taken for the intestinal worm, boiled leave bud with water is used for typhoid & pneumonia.
Artocarpus lakoocha	Seeds and barks of the plant were boiled with water use for the treatment of antibacterial and anthelmintic, fruit is used for diabetes.
Maesa indica	Leaf was boiled with water and mixed with salt and then taken for diabetes.
Azadirachta indica	Raw neem leaf is used for diabetes; Neem leaves paste also apply for relief of pain for arthritis
Adhatoda vasica	Leaves are crushed and mixed with water and filtered, then the filtrate mixed with honey and utilize a cough and diabetes.
Allium hookeri	The plant is taken as raw to reduce blood pressure. The pasted of leaf used for diabetes.

(continued)

Table 4.2 (continued)

Plant name	Method of preparation and mode of usage
Blumea balsamifera	Leaves are crushed and mixed with water and taken for stomach pain, the leafis crushed and mix with mustard oil and applied on the top of the skull for fever and cold.
Colocasia esculenta	Petiole juice is applied in fresh cut and injury as antiseptic.
Cynodon dactylon	About 20 gm of stolon boiled or soaked in half litre of drinking water and a spoon of honey is added and taken in the empty stomach twice a day for seven days for urination problem. The mixture also used for dysmenorrheal.
Cyperus haspan	Fresh rhizomes paste along with honey is used for bronchitis and fever.
Celtis timorensis	Leaves are boiled with water which is used for kidney stone. Bark used to crushed and soaked for overnight and the filtrate is taken for diabetes as well as liver disease.
Hibiscus cannabinus	Leaves are boiled with water and taken the liquid part with a little salt for diabetes and cancer.
Ipomoea aquatica	Shoot decoction is used as droplet for eye and ear infections. Leaf decoction also used for diarrhoea.
Lysimachia obovata	Leaves are boiled with water and liquid part is taken with salt to treat dyspepsia and diuretics.
Magnolia champaca	Seed is boiled with water and taken as a gargle for tonsillitis. Bud is crushed and make a semisolid paste and used for diabetes.
Marsilea minuta	The fresh plant is boiled with water and taken twice a day for strangury.
Musa acuminate	The flower is boiled with water and taken the liquid portion of diabetes. Stem part powdered and soaked for overnight to use for asthma.
Nasturtium indicum	Leaf is boiled with water for diabetes.
Nymphoides indicum	A paste of the stem applied as a bandage for wound healing. Rhizome paste along with little honey is taken as a diuretic
Nymphaea stellata	Fresh petiole paste mixed with Cuminum cyminum L. seed powder, salt, honey and use for dysmenorrheal. Also, leaf and stem part used for the diuretic purpose.
Oenanthe javanica	Fresh ariel part is boiled with water and use for influenza, jaundice.
Parkia javanica	The leaf is boil with water and takes the liquid extract for diabetes, roots are boiled with water and expose the anus on the liquid for bleeding pile. And also applied as antibacterial purposes.
Persicaria sagittata	Leaves are boiled with water and taken the liquid for stomach pain, the leaf is heated and paste is applied for muscle spasm, the seed is crushed and applied as an antidote for snake bite
Polygonum barbatum	Leaf is boiled with water and use for stomach problem and constipation, leaf paste is applied for cutaneous infection.
Punica granatum	Leave is crush and mixed with water and drink the liquid portion of dysentery and diabetes.
Psidium guajava	Raw leaves are crush and mixed with water and taken for diabetes and dysentery
Pistia stratiotes	Plant paste is applied in burn to reduce the damage of nearby tissue
Ranunculus sceleratus	Leaf is wrapped by banana leaf and slightly burnt in the charcoal then applied internally for gout, leave is boil with water for antipyretic.
Rhus chinensis	Fruit is boil/soak in the water and drinks the liquid parts for diarrhoea and diabetes. Decoction part is also used for the treatment of cough and cancer.
Salvia officinalis	A decoction of the leave is used as a gargle for tonsillitis. Dried leaves were soaked for around 12 hours and the liquid part is consumed for management of diabetes.
Sagittaria sagittifolia	Fresh root paste is mixed with honey and uses for a cough.
Syzygium cumini	Seed is crushed and mixed with water and taken the liquid fractions for diabetes and asthma.
Solanum xanthocarpum	Fruit is boiled or soaked in the water and taken for bronchitis. The leaf part also used for diabetes by preparing the paste solution of leaf in salty water. Stem part is used for the dental analgesic.
Trapa natanas	Fruit peel and root boiled with water and taken for diabetes antibacterial. Dry roots of this plant also used for the antifungal purpose by making the solution of overnight soaked roots.

4.4 Conclusion

Results from the survey revealed that plenty of medicinal plants are available in the area of the study and the local tribal healers used them as a medicine for their common ailments since ancient time. A number of phytochemical moieties like anthocyanins, alkaloids, glycosides, flavonoids, tannin, saponins, carbohydrates etc. present in such plant species may responsible for their curative effect. This study may help towards the conservation of various valuable medicinal plants within the region. Phytochemical and biological screening of different medicinal plants based on such information is a very essential aspect for authors in future. It was also observed during post-study literature survey that a number of plant species were not scientifically investigated and documented, despite the fact that the study area abundantly rich in the medicinal plant and their traditional uses. It thus becomes essential to acquire and preserve such traditional knowledge and diversity of medicinal plant by way of proper documentation and conservation process.

Acknowledgement Authors are thankful to the Assam down town University, Guwahati and traditional practitioners of Thoubal and Kakching district.

References

Ahmad I, Aqil F, Ahmad F, Owais M. Herbal medicines: prospects and constraints, modern phytomedicineturning medicinal plants into drugs. Weinheim: WILEY-VCH Verlag GmbH & Co; 2006.

Halim MA, Chowdhury MSH, Wadud AI, Uddin MS, Sarker SK, Uddin MB. The use of plants in traditional health care practice of the *Shaiji* community in South-Western Bangladesh. J Trop For Sci. 2007;19(3):168–75.

Khan MH, Yadava PS. Antidiabetic plants used in Thoubal district of Manipur, Northeast India. Indian J Trad Knowl. 2010;9(3):510–4.

Rana MP, Sohel MSI, Akhter S, Islam MJ. Ethno-medicinal plants use by the *Manipuri* tribal community in Bangladesh. J For Res. 2010;21:85–92.

Sajem AL, Gosai K. Traditional use of medicinal plants by the Jaintia tribes in North Cachar Hills district of Assam, northeast India. J Ethnobiol Ethnomed. 2006;2:33. https://doi.org/10.1186/1746-4269-2-33.

Sannomiya M, Cardoso CRP, Figueiredo ME, Rodrigues CM, dos Santos LC, dos Santos FV, et al. Mutagenic evaluation and chemical investigation of *Byrsonimaintermedia*A. Juss. leaf extracts. J Ethnopharmacol. 2007;112:319–26.

Sen S, Chakraborty R, De B, Devanna N. An ethnobotanical survey of medicinal plants used by ethnic people in West and South district of Tripura, India. J For Res. 2011;22(3):417–26.

Shankar S, Deb S, Sharma BK (Eds). 2009. Traditional healing practices in North East India. In: Proceeding on traditional healing practices in North East India. Pasighat, Arunachal Pradesh: North Eastern Institute of Folk Medicine.

Singha MN. Manipuri language movement 1924–1992, (PhD Thesis, Assam University, Assam). 2014.

Thirumalai T, Kelumalai E, Senthilkumar B, David E. Ethnobotanical study of medicinal plants used by the local people in Vellore District, Tamil Nadu, India. Ethnobotanical Leaflets. 2009;13:1302–11.

Uniyal SK, Singh KN, Jamwal P, Lal B. Traditional use of medicinal plants among the tribal communities of Chhota Bhangal, Western Himalaya. J Ethnobiol Ethnomed. 2006;2:1–8.

Verma S, Singh SP. Current and future status of herbal medicines. Vet World. 2008;1:347–50.

Scientific Basis for Ayurvedic Medicinal Plants Against Alzheimer's Disease

5

Atanu Bhattacharjee, Raja Chakraborty, and Saikat Sen

Contents

A. Bhattacharjee (✉) · R. Chakraborty · S. Sen
Department of Pharmacy, Assam Down Town University, Guwahati, Assam, India

S. Sen, R. Chakraborty (eds.), *Herbal Medicine in India*,
https://doi.org/10.1007/978-981-13-7248-3_5

5.1 Introduction

Ayurveda (Traditional Indian system of medicine) emphasizes about the root cause of many diseases. According to Ayurveda there are three different bio-energies (Dosha), viz. Vata (all type of movement), Pitta (digestive and metabolic activities), and Kapha (growth, union, stability, and composition), seven different body tissues (Dhatu), and three wastes (Mala) which are very significant for maintaining a healthy life of human beings. Among all Dhatus, the Majja Dhatu (nervous tissue or bone marrow) is responsible for communication, intelligence, and movement. When there is an imbalance between Dosha and Majja Dhatu neurological disorder occurs. Predominance of VATA which is dry and cold in nature, when combines with Majja Dhatu in cerebral cortex, makes cortical shrinkage, shrinkage in hippocampus, and formation of amyloid β plaques, which gradually confronted to various neurological disorders like Alzheimer's disease (Adewusi and Steenkamp 2011). Alzheimer's disease (AD) is a progressive neurodegenerative disorder characterized by a low level of neurotransmitter acetylcholine (ACh) in the cerebrum. It is an irreversible age-related type of dementia that gradually dissolves the mind and burglarizes the individual memory and psychological abilities and causes changes in personality and conduct (Amod et al. 2005; Colucci et al. 2012). AD was first described in 1906 by German neuropsychiatrist Prof. Alois Alzheimer. It is a complex, multifactoral, progressive disorder associated with a diminished level of Ach in brain (Dwivedi and Singh 1978). Normally, ACh is stored in the nerve terminals, in structures called vesicles and released from the nerve endings upon depolarization of nerve terminal and thereby entering the synapse and binding to the receptor. However, in patients with AD, the ACh which is released has a very short half-life due to the presence of large amounts of the enzymes, viz. acetylcholinesterase (AChE) and butyrylcholinesterase (BChE), which are both present in the brain and are detected among neurofibrillary tangles and neuritic plaques. These enzymes hydrolyze the ester bond of ACh molecule to choline and acetate, leading to loss of stimulatory activity (Zhang and Jiang 2015; Anderson 2002). Further, two major pathological hallmarks of AD are characterized by deposition of abnormal amyloid β protein plaques and formation of neurofibrillary tangles of tau protein resulting in diminished impulse transmission from the end of one neuron to the beginning of another neuron (Doraiswamy 2002; Lemstra et al. 2003; Gupta and Bala 2013).

AD is the reason for dementia in the elderly, with a length of around 9 years between the beginning of clinical side effects and demise and has been risen as one of the deadliest issues in developed countries. The World Health Organization (WHO) evaluated that by 2040 around 71% of the dementia cases will happen in developing nations (Atanu et al. 2015). There are considerable financial, social, and emotional burdens associated with the caring for patients with this disease. In fact, in advanced robotic life style, where life expectancy is long, this disease is a major cause of morbidity and it imposes severe strains on the social welfare systems. It is estimated that in the USA alone, more than five million people are affected by AD whereas in Indian scenario the disease has already emerged as one of the deadliest progressive threat of mankind after diabetes, cancer, and cardiac disease (Berrino 2002).

One of the major clinical advances in the treatment of AD have been the utilization of acetylcholinesterase (AChE) and butyrylcholinesterase (BChE) inhibitors to increase ACh level in cerebrum although cholinergic agents with nicotinic and muscarinic agonist properties additionally have pulled in some intrigue (Orhan et al. 2007; Rammohan et al. 2012). BChE, primarily associated with glial cells and specific neuronal pathways cleaves ACh in a similar manner to AChE to terminate its physiological action. Such studies, statistically slower decline in the cognitive performance of dementia patients possessing specific BChE polymorphisms that naturally lower BChE activity, have targeted BChE as a new approach to intercede in the progression of AD (Vinutha et al. 2007; Adewusi and Steenkamp 2011). At present, there are extremely constrained drugs accessible to treat AD and the greater part of the treatment is accessible just to postpone the movement of indications and symptomatic alleviation for a brief time frame. Restorative plants speak to a lot of undiscovered store of characteristic prescriptions and potential wellspring of common AChE inhibitors. The basic assorted variety of their phytoconstituents makes them an important wellspring of novel lead mixes for the mission of medications to treat AD. Consequently, methodical ethnopharmacological screening of these plants may give valuable leads in the disclosure of new medications for AD treatment.

Approaches to enhance cholinergic function in AD have included stimulation of cholinergic receptors or prolonging the availability of ACh released into the neuronal synaptic cleft by use of agents which restore the level of acetylcholine through inhibition of both AChE and BChE (Harvey 2008; Dahanukar et al. 2000). Recent studies indicated that cholinesterase inhibitors hold a key role not only to enhance cholinergic transmission in the brain but also might play a modulatory role on Aβ plaque deposition and neurotoxic fibrils formation via suppressing amyloid precursor protein (APP) expression (Rinne et al. 2003; Mahesh and Tasneem 2014). Therefore, AChE and BChE inhibitors have become remarkable alternatives in the treatment of AD. Existing anticholinesterase drugs, viz. tacrine, donepezil, physostigmine, galantamine, and heptylphysostigmine for the treatment of dementia are reported to have several dangerous adverse effects such as hepatotoxicity, short duration of biological action, low bioavailability, adverse cholinergic side effects in the periphery, and a narrow therapeutic window (Chatellier and Lacomblez 1990; Spiegel 2002; Clegg et al. 2002).

Medicinal plants and their concentrates are assuming an indispensable part in the present treatment of psychological issue either as standard or integral drug with specific reference to their ethnopharmacological perspectives (Philomena 2011). The history of drug discovery has shown that plants contain active compounds that have become new sources to investigate for the pharmaceutical industry. Plant constituents may not only act synergistically with other constituents from the same plant but may also enhance the activity of compounds or counteract toxic effects of compounds from other plant species. In traditional practices, numerous plants have been used to treat cognitive disorders, including neurodegenerative diseases and different neuropharmacological disorders (Perry et al. 1999; Vaidya 1997). Basically, in Ayurveda (traditional Indian medicinal system), these restorative plants were named "medharasayanas" (Sanskrit: "medha" implies intellect/cognition and "rasayana" implies revival). Medharasayanas incorporate a gathering of four therapeutic plants with multifold benefits, particularly to enhance memory and acumen by Prabhava (specific action), viz. Mandukaparni (*Centella asiatica*; Family: Umbelliferae), Yastimadhu (*Glycirrhiza glabra*; Family: Leguminosae), Guduchi (*Tinospora cordifolia*; Family: Menispermaceae), and Shankhapushpi (*Convolvulus pleuricaulis*; Family: Convolvulaceae) (Rammohan et al. 2012; Manyam 1999). Traditional Indian medicinal plants like Ashwagandha (*Withania somnifera*; Family: Solanaceae), Brahmi (*Bacopa monnieri*; Family: Scophulariaceae), Jyothishmati (*Celastrus panniculata*; Family: Celastraceae), Kushmanda (*Benincasa hispida*; Family: Cucurbitaceae), Vacha (Acorus calamus; Family: Araceae), and Jatamamsi (*Nardostachys jatamamsi*; Family: Valerianaceae) are very much archived in Ayurveda and other traditional texts as brain tonics and memory enhancers (Anil et al. 2009). Indian turmeric (*Curcuma longa*; Family: Zingiberaceae) contains curcumin, a demonstrated cell reinforcement and anticholinesterase activity, which is observed to be exceptionally compelling to defer the movement of AD (Rammohan et al. 2012; Ahmed and Gilani 2009). Yokukansan, a Chinese herbal remedy which is used to treat various neurological states, has been reported as being effective to improve overall health status with no adverse effects (Howes and Houghton 2003). Also, galanthamine, an alkaloid from snowdrop, has been approved by the Food and Drug Administration in the United States for use in the treatment of AD (Rhee et al. 2001). Since AD has become a public health burden, and the commonly available synthetic drugs have undesirable side effects, new treatment strategies based on medicinal plants have been the subject of current focus. With this scientific background the chapter has been prepared to bring an up-to-date information about the role of alternative medicine, to encounter AD.

5.2 Etiology and Pathogenesis

In patients with AD, the neurons become disabled. Early stage of AD interferes with the neuron's ability to produce the energy for efficient coordination between them, a process known as metabolism. They also mislay the ability to repair them which ultimately leads to death of neuron cells. Exactly what interferes with the normal functioning of neuron is still a mystery but with recent progression of medical sciences, three pathological hallmarks are being postulated.

5.2.1 β- Amyloid Plaques

Tucked in the spaces between neurons, thick and sticky deposits of plaques made up of a protein called β-amyloid. These plaques also surrounded by other amino acid fragments, neuro- remnants, immune cells, viz. microglia which in turn digests the damaged neurons and causes neuro-inflammation. β-amyloid, a spontaneously aggregating peptide of 39–43 amino acids, is a snipped fragment of larger protein called amyloid precursor protein. APP is an essential component of neuron growth which rests in part inside and outside the cell. β-amyloid is derived from sequential proteolytic cleavage of the amyloid precursor protein (APP) by β- and γ-secretases (Roberts 2002). Initial cleavage by β-secretase (BACE; β-site of APP cleaving enzyme), a membrane-anchored aspartic protease, generates a soluble N-terminal fragment and a membrane-associated C-terminal fragment. The C-terminal fragment then undergoes proteolysis by γ-secretase to give the Aβ peptide which progressively attaches with each other and converted into insoluble plaques (Ghosh and Osswald 2014; Kar et al. 2004). According to the "β-amyloid cascade", deposition of β-amyloid plaques triggers the neurotoxic cascade and promotes neuro-inflammation which ultimately resulted in neurodegeneration (Mahesh and Tasneem 2014).

5.2.2 Neurofibrillary Tangles

One of the pathological hallmarks of AD is the formation of intracellular neurofibrillary tangles which consists of hyperphosphorylated tau protein (Prerna et al. 2010). Tau is an axonal protein which binds to microtubules and promotes their assembly and stability. Phosphorylation of tau protein is regulated by the balance between multiple kinases (e.g. glycogen synthetase kinase-3 (GSK3) and cyclin-dependent kinase-5 (CDK5)) and phosphatases (e.g. PP-1 and PP-2A). Hyperphosphorylation of tau protein leads to destruction of microtubule-associated proteins and thereby prevent microtubule assembly and impair axonal transport resulting in neuronal death (Zhang and Jiang 2015; Gelb 2000; Vladimir and Sophia 2018).

5.2.3 Loss of Cholinergic Neurons

The cholinergic hypothesis claims that decrease in cognitive function in dementia is predominantly related to a decrease in cholinergic neurotransmission. AD leads to selective degeneration of cholinergic neurons of basal forebrain and results in the decline of cholinergic markers, viz. ChAT, Ach level and increase in AChE (Talic et al. 2014; Jemima et al. 2011) (Fig. 5.1).

Moreover, it has been postulated that ACh acts as protein kinase inhibitor and thereby reduces tau phosphorylation. This inhibits intracellular neurofibrillary tangles formation and delays the progression of AD (Prerna et al. 2010).

Formation of extracellular β-amyloid plaques with drastic neuronal and synaptic reduction in cholinergic system of the brain is considered as a major pathological hallmark of AD. Therefore,

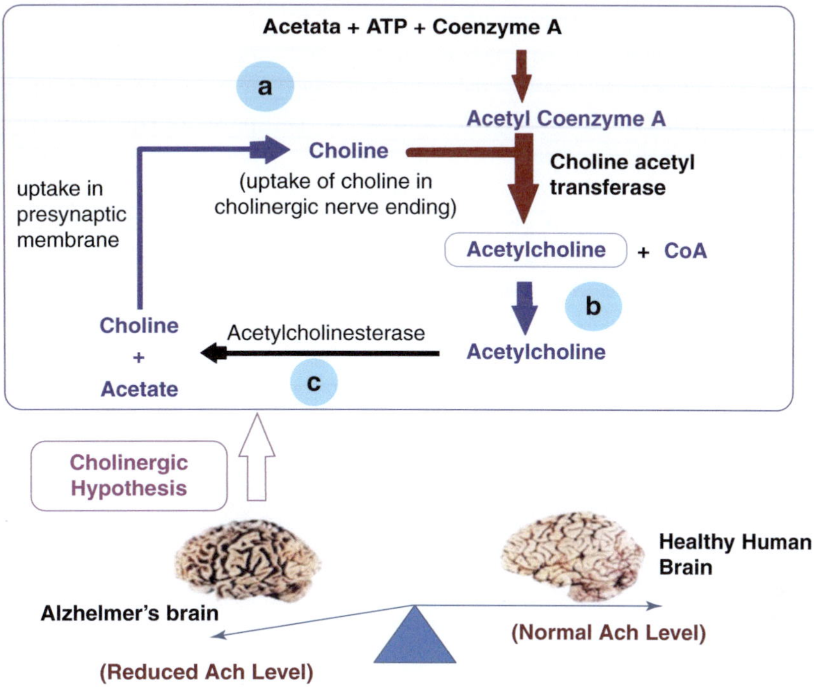

Fig. 5.1 Possible therapeutic approaches in the modulation of cholinergic transmission. (**a**) Increase in ChAT activity. (**b**) Inhibition of Ach release. (**c**) Inhibition of AchE 4. Promotes choline transport (Adapted and modified from Jian-zhi and Ze-fen 2006)

restoration of the central cholinergic function plays a significant role to improve cognitive impairment in patients with AD. There are three principal approaches by which the cholinergic deficit can be addressed: (1) nicotinic receptor stimulation, (2) muscarinic receptor stimulation, and (3) cholinesterase (AChE and BChE) inhibition (Vinutha et al. 2007; Puchchakayala et al. 2012; Jivad and Rabiei 2014).

5.3 Ayurvedic Perspective of AD

There is no condition as described in Ayurveda which can be clinically equated to AD. But in Ayurvedic classics Smṛtināsha (loss of memory) is mentioned among the prodromal symptom of jarā (ageing). In Jarāvasthā (old age; ≥ 60 years), as per Caraka, Smṛti, and other mental coordination gradually deteriorate naturally. As per Vagbhaṭa (As.Sam.Sha 8/25) and Sharṅgadhara (Prathama Khaṇḍa 6/20), the functions of mind and Buddhi decline start declining from the ninth decade of life. Mental function declines at 11th decade of life as per Sharṅgadhara. Further, Smṛtibhramsha (disturbed memory) is described as a symptom where Smṛti (memory) is vitiated by rajas (passion) and tamas (obscurity). Thus, senile dementia can be interpreted as Jarājanya Smṛtibhramsha according to Ayurvedic principles (Singh et al. 1979; Abhang 1987).

AD can be termed as "Smrti Nasha" in Ayurveda and is caused by the depletion of dhatus (tissues) and impairment of Satva Guna (the attribute of mind which represents purity and consciousness) by rajas (the attribute of mind which usually represents energy and dynamism) and tamas (the attribute of mind representing passivity and ignorance). When the Manovaha srotas (channels carrying cyclic impulses principally responsible for memory) are afflicted with Vata dosha, the person is affected and there is malfunctioning of the mental activities (Singh et al. 1979).

This condition is not met as a disease entity in separate chapters of Ayurvedic classics and considered as a natural phenomenon, but sign and symptoms of dementia can be understood in terms of Ayurvedic concepts. In order to understand the etiopathogenesis of dementia in the light of Ayurvedic literature, it is necessary to review the general physiology of *Manas* and *Buddhi*. Before discussing the etiology and psychopathology of *Smritibuddhihrass*, it is worth considering the relation of *Mana*, *Buddhi*, *Medha*, *Dhriti*, and *Smriti* with each other (Akhlaq et al. 2018). In the process of knowledge, mental faculty that determines the nature, merits, and demerits of an object of knowledge is *Buddhi*. *Buddhi* and *Mana* are related with *Karya Karana Sambandh* as in the process of evolution; *Buddhi* is the first entity (*Tatva*), which is responsible for further development of *Indriyas* and *Manas* (Rammohan et al. 2012).

Conventional drug therapy is based on various theories to locate a viable treatment and relief for AD manifestations. These therapies include amyloid cascade and cholinergic hypothesis. Certain other important aspects like inflammatory, oxidative cascade, and hormonal pathways also contribute a vital role in AD (Vaidya 1997; Bush 2003). Some other life style associated possible cause may include lack of routine movement, intake of fast foods with high glycemic index, saturated fats, and less intake of plant-based nutrition, antioxidant substances [e.g., phytoestrogens]), and seafood with rich in ω-3 fatty acids. These may lead to insulin resistance, increased oxidative stress, homocysteine, and estrogen deficiency (Fernando 2008; Huang et al. 2016).

In a planned investigation of hazard factors, expanding age, absence of instruction, and the apolipoprotein E epsilon4 allele were observed to be altogether connected with expanded danger of AD (Huang and Mucke 2012). Then again, utilization of non-steroidal anti-inflammatory drugs, wine, and routine daily activity were observed to be altogether connected with diminished danger of AD (Aisen 2002a, b; Nillert et al. 2017). Some confirmation proposes that oxidative harm of mind tissue might be engaged with pathogenesis, which goes before the event of side effects and the arrangement of amyloid-containing plaques and neurofibrillary tangles (Lindsay et al. 2002). Hereditary variables may likewise be included; however the dilemma associated with the genetic factors responsible for AD has not been clarified in full yet. The disclosure of pathogenic transformations in the β-amyloid peptide (β-APP) and the presenilin qualities provides sound findings to the hereditary theory on the grounds that amyloid β generation and statement add to the causes of AD (Schneider 1996). Certain scientific investigations reported that modifications in the lysosomal framework may play a significant role in the progression of neurodegeneration associated with AD. Lysosomal abnormality perhaps deals with the generation of free radicals in cerebrum and increased oxidative stress prompts steady loss of metabolic movement resulting in diminished life expectancy of a person (Bahr and Bendiske 2002).

5.4 Clinical Examination and Diagnosis

Ayurveda, the Indian system of medicine had developed certain dietary and therapeutic measures to delay ageing and rejuvenating the whole functional dynamics of the body organs. This revitalization and rejuvenation is known as the "Rasayana chikitsa" (rejuvenation therapy).

AD can be considered as advanced form of dementia which in Ayurveda is termed as "Smrti Nasha" (loss of memory). This occurs as a result of depletion of dhatus (tissues) and impairment of Satva Guna (the attribute of mind which represents purity and perception) by rajas (a state mind representing energy and vigor) and tamas (the attribute of mind representing tameness and unawareness). Affliction of Manovaha srotas (retention of sequential events of learning responsible for memory) with Vata dosha may lead to deterioration of mental status of the person suffering from AD. Ayurvedic system of medicine had developed certain dietary and therapeutic measures to delay ageing and rejuvenating the whole functional dynamics of the body organs which is known as "Rasayana chikitsa" (rejuvenation therapy).

AD is a life-changing disease for both the patient and care giver. At present, treatments are available to provide a symptomatic relief from the disease for a short period of time if diagnosed in early stages. According to Ayurveda, the physician must elaborate a concept about the progression and treatment of AD. In the early stages Rookshana and Amapachana medicines are prescribed along with Shadangam kashaya and Saddharanam churna. Rookshana and Amapachana help Srotas prepared for Snehana and Shodhana procedure. Sometimes, Langhana (lightening therapy) is advised even before going for Brihana (nourishing) to induce clarity of senses, expulsion of wastes, and lightness in body. But care must be taken to prevent aggravation of Vata dosha. Snehana therapy is another effective type of treatment where Pranaavruta Samana and Chatushprakara snehana (four types of unctuous substances that are Ghee, oil, fat and bone marrow) are being induced. Medicines which are Brimhana (nourishingh) and Vatanulomana (downward movement of Vata) should be selected like Kshirabala, Vatasini, Dhanwantaram, Narayana, or Lakshaditaila. Murdhatailam with Balalakshadi, Kshirabala or Vatasini can be also done for Snehana. After proper Snehana (oilation), Swedana (Sudation), Shodhana should be done in the form of Vasti or Virechana, while the latter is found to be more effective in Pittanubandha condition.

5.5 Management

Ayurvedic system of medicine utilizes remedy from natural sources (extracts of plant, animal, and mineral) for the treatment of various mental disorders, including impaired memory condition. There are two methodologies of treatment: first one is general or aggregate prosperity of health, including mental activities (memory amusements, perusing, card recreations) and reflection; second methodology specifically targets intellect (medha) and memory (smriti) (Jagdeep et al. 2009; Patel et al. 2014). The patient should be given proper counseling and mental support, i.e., nothing but the Satvavajaya Chikitsa as it is the best in management of Manovikara (psychological disturbances). This will be very helpful to manage the behavioural symptoms of patient of Alzheimer's disease like agitation, wandering, anxiety, anger, and depression. Rasayana therapy including Medhya Rasayan and Achara Rasayana must be planned for the AD because it helps us in strengthening the host defence mechanisms. A regulated lifestyle, wholesome diet, appropriate behaviour, and following ideal code of conduct as quoted in Ayurveda are best to prevent and manage the neurodegenerative diseases in general and AD in particular (Frawley 1989). Some important medications routinely used to treat cognitive dysfunctions are depicted in the following sections.

5.5.1 Brain Tonics (Medhya Rasayana)

Amid vedic time the training framework was conferred by oral guidance and the understudies held and reviewed this information by rehashed recitation. In this way, insight was viewed as identical with memory, and medications that diminished the time of remembering the exercises were produced from regular sources. Several Ayurvedic medicines have been exploited for the treatment and management of acute and chronic neurological diseases associated with cognitive dysfunctions. These medicines from natural sources believed to modulate neuroendocrine-immune systems via antioxidants and anti-inflammatory properties and thereby enhance memory and rejuvenate cognitive functions. Some of the traditionally reputed medhya rasayana drugs are mentioned below:

1. Decoction of Mandhukparni (*Centella asiatica*).
2. Powder of Jastimadhu (*Glycyrrhiza glabra*) with milk.
3. Juice of Guduchi (*Tinospora cordifolia*).
4. Paste of Shankhpushpi (*Convolvulus pluricaulis*) leaves.

A significant integer of medicinal plants of Indian origin is described with brian tonic and memory boosting impacts. Generally, these plants are prescribed in combination as it is believed to provide synergistic effects and provide substantial relief of the symptoms. Sometimes, the formulations are incorporated with mineral originated drugs (Satyavati et al. 1987; Khare 2007). A list of medicinal plants used as brain tonics is enlisted in Table 5.1.

In conventional practice, the main medications at present affirmed for the treatment of AD are cholinomimetics. Infact, tacrine was the first clinically established synthetic AchE inhibitor intro-

Table 5.1 Indian medicinal plant with nootropic effect

Sl. No.	Common name	Scientific name	Family
1	Adrakh	*Zingiber officinalis*	Zingiberaceae
2	Amla	*Emblica officinalis*	Phyllanthaceae
3	Ashwagandha	*Withania somnifera*	Solanaceae
4	Bada Ilaichi	*Amomum subulatum*	Zingiberaceae
5	Badam	*Prunus amygdalis*	Rosaceae
6	Bahera	*Terminalia belerica*	Umbelliferae
7	Bari Saunf	*Foeniculum vulgare*	Umbelliferae
8	Brahmi	*Bacopa monniera*	Plantaginaceae
9	Choti Elaichi	*Elettaria cardamomum*	Zingiberaceae
10	Dalchini	*Cinnamomum zeylanicum*	Lauraaceae
11	Dhak, Palash	*Butea frondosa*	Fabaceae
12	Giloe	*Tinospora cardifolia*	Menispermaceae
13	Ginko	*Ginkgo biloba*	Ginkoceae
14	Guggulu	*Commiphora wightii*	Burseraceae
15	Gulab	*Rosa damascene*	Rosaceae
16	Harar, Hareetaki	*Terminalia chebula*	Combretaceae
17	Heal-all	*Prunella vulgaris*	Lamiaceae
18	Hypericum	*Hypericum perforatum*	Hypericaceae
19	Jadwar Shireen	*Delphinium denudatum*	Ranunculaceae
20	Jatamansi	*Nardostachys jatamansi*	Caprifoliaceae
21	Kava	*Piper methysticum*	Piperaceae
22	Keora	*Pandanus odoratissimus*	Pandanaceae
23	Khas	*Vetiverica zizinoides*	Caprifoliaceae
24	Kuth	*Sassurea lappa*	Compositae
25	Laung	*Eugenia caryophyllus*	Myrtaceae
26	Lavander	*Lavandula officinalis*	Lamiaceae
27	Maca	*Lepidium meyenii*	Brassicaceae
28	Nishoth	*Operculum tarpethum*	Convolvulacea
29	Peepal, Pippali	*Piper longum*	Piperaceae
30	Renuka	*Piper aurantiacum*	Piperaceae
31	Sankha Holi	*Canscora decussate*	Gentianaceae
32	Saunf	*Pimpinella anisum*	Apiaceae
33	Sedge	*Cyperus rotundus*	Cyperaceae
34	Shankhpushpi	*Convolvulus pluricaulis*	Convolvulaceae
35	Shatawar	*Asparagus racemosus*	Asparagaceae
36	Tagar	*Valerian wallachia*	Caprifoliaceae
37	Uood Saleeb	*Paenia emodi*	Paeoniaceae
38	Vacha	*Acorus calamus*	Acoraceae
39	Vayu Vidang	*Embelia ribes*	Phyllanthaceae
40	Vidari Kand	*Ipomea paniculata*	Convolvulaceae

Refs.: Keyvan et al. 2007; Wang et al. 2009; Divya and Lakshmi 2007; Urbain et al. 2004

duced to improve Ach level at the nerve ending. Later, second generation inhibitors are introduced but resulting side effects and cost factor made their utilization limited. Although tacrine provides positive influence on few proportions of memory execution, the size of change was extremely unassuming. Further, long-term use has severe side effects including stomachache, sickness, spewing, and looseness of the bowels, which might be huge and economic constraining (Gupta and Bala 2013). Significant research is being led in different territories, for example, utilizing particular mitigating drugs (specific cyclooxgenase-2 [COX-2] inhibitors) to decrease fiery movement in the mind and cancer prevention agents (Aisen 2002a, b). Other current therapeutic interventions are antiamyloid procedures (e.g., vaccination, collection inhibitors, β-secretase inhibitors), modification of metal chelators (e.g., clioquinol), lipid-bringing down operators, anti-hypertensive, vitamins, and synapse receptors (Dash et al. 1983; Huang and Mucke 2012). Phytoextracts on locally available plant materials with AchE inhibitory properties have demonstrated some promise. Ayurveda has numerous definitions and herbo-mineral drugs talked about underneath that are utilized to enhance intellectual capacities. The exact biochemical system of activity of these herbs is not clear. It is likely that cell reinforcement and mitigating properties of these herbs might be in charge of their gainful impact in the treatment of AD.

5.6 Scientific Basis

5.6.1 Nootropic Plants

Below we describe the various Ayurvedic medicinal nervine herbs that are recommended for AD and their actions on the brain.

5.6.1.1 Pharmacological Studies on Single Herbs

Bacopa monniera (Brahmi)

Central Drug Research Institute (CDRI), Lucknow, and other premiere scientific organizations of Govt. of India, has been conducted a systematic study regarding nootropic effects of *B. monniera*, and based on the outcome a polyherbal preparation "Mentat" is successfully marketed. It has been observed that ethanolic extract of *B. monniera* facilitated acquisition, consolidation, and retention of memory *in vivo* with passive avoidance paradigm and maze tests.

The principal constituents of *B. monnieri* are saponins and triterpenoid bacosaponins that include bacopasides III–V, bacosides A and B, bacosaponins A, B, and C, and jujubogenin bisdesmosides bacopasaponins D, E, and F. Other phytoconstituents include alkaloids, phytosterols, betulic acid, polyphenols, and sulfhydryl compounds that confer strong antioxidant activity. In the hippocampus, *B. monnieri* enhances protein kinase activity that may contribute to its nootropic action. *B. monnieri* also inhibited cholinergic degeneration and thereby displayed a nootropic effect in a rat model of AD. A study with standardized extract of *B. monnieri* inverted cognitive deficits induced by intracerebroventricularly administered colchicines and ibotenic acid into the nucleus basalis magnocellularis. Further, it also inverted the (1) diminution of acetylcholine, (2) reduction in choline acetyltransferase activity, and (3) decrease in muscarinic cholinergic receptor binding in the frontal cortex and hippocampus. The extracts protected neurons from β-amyloid-induced cell death by suppressing cellular acetylcholinesterase activity (Gohil and Patel 2010; Ahirwar et al. 2012).

Centella asiatica (Mandookparni)

C. asiatica (Family: Umbelliferae) aqueous extract showed improved learning and memory potential *in vivo*. Its extract significantly alleviated oxidative stress by decreasing malonaldehyde (MDA) level and increasing glutathione level. Further it also showed AchE inhibitory activity which combinedly may be associated with cognition-enhancing efficacy (Anil et al. 2009).

Convolvulus pluricaulis Chois (Shankhpushpi)

C. pluricaulis (Family: Convulvolaceae) was significantly increased ACh, catechol amine, and

5- hydroxy tryptamine (5-HT) level in brain (Patel et al. 2014). *In-vitro* assay showed its anticholinesterase activity of *Convolvulus pluricaulis* extract at IC_{50} 234 ± 38 μg/mL (Maya and Sarada 2014).

Eugenia caryophyllus spl. (Laung)

The aqueous extract of *E. caryophyllus* (Family: Myrtaceae) significant AchE activity may be due to the presence of water-soluble phytoconstituents present in the extract. Further, another research report with Chavanprash containing *E. caryophyllus* showed significant anticholinesterase and antioxidant potential *in vivo* against scopolamine induce amnesia (Akinrimisi and Ainwannde 1975).

Glycyrrhiza glabra Linn. (Yastimadhu)

The alcoholic extract of *G. glabra* and glabridin, an isolated bioactive component of *G. glabra*, showed both AchE and BuChE inhibitory activities in dose-dependent manner. Further, liquiritin and isoliquirin, isolated flavanoid constituents of the plant, showed significant antioxidant profile against scopolamine induced amnesia *in vivo* (Muralidharan et al. 2009).

Lawsonia intermis Linn. (Mehndi)

Acetone soluble fraction (100 mg/kg body weight) of petroleum ether extract of *L.* intermis leaves showed significant ($p \leq 0.001$) nootropic effect *in-vivo* in dose dependant manner. Further, it affected 5-Hydroxy tryptamine and noradrenaline-mediated behavior in experimental animals (Iyer et al. 1998).

Nardostachys jatamansi DC. (Jatamansi)

Jatamamsi is a safe and highly reputed Ayurvedic medicinal plant used as sedative. The sedative activity is due to the presence of valeranone, a sesquiterpenes, and coumarins. Other terpenoids include spirojatamol, nardostachysin, jatamols A and B, and calarenol.

An alcoholic extract of this plant administered to both young and aged mice significantly improved learning and memory and also reversed the amnesia induced by diazepam and scopolamine. Furthermore, it reversed aging-induced amnesia due to the natural aging of mice, suggesting that the compounds in this plant may prove to be useful in restoring memory in older individuals as well as in patients with age-associated dementia (Habibur et al. 2011).

Pongamia pinnata (Karanj)

Petroleum ether extract of the seed of *P. pinnata* was tested for nootropic activity in an experimental model of Alzheimer's disease (created by ibotenic acid-induced lesioning of nuclear basalis magnocellularis). It reversed both, the cognitive deficits and the reduction in cholinergic markers after 2 weeks of treatment. Reversal of perturbed cholinergic function was considered as the possible mechanism (Prachi et al. 2017).

Tinospora cordifolia F.Vill (Guduchi)

n-butanolic fraction of ethanolic extract of *T. cordifolia* stem which contain saponin showed significant nootropic reduction in cholinergic markers *in vivo* in dose-dependent manner. Further, the extract also showed anti-inflammatory activity against lipopolysaccharide-induced neuro-inflammation. Ethanolic extract of this plant diminish ACh content in rat whole brain but increased it in the cortex. These may be correlated with its nootropic potentiality as anti-Alzheimer's drug (Prakash et al. 2017).

Withania somnifera Dunal (Ashwagandha)

Ashwagandha, a Solanaceous drug is used extensively in Ayurveda as a nervine tonic, aphrodisiac, and "adaptogen" and helps the body adapt to stress. It is categorized as a rasayana (rejuvenative) and is believed to possess antioxidant activity, free radical scavenging activity, and an ability to support a healthy immune system. Ashwagandha has a calming effect and thus may be particularly indicated in people with AD. A total alkaloid extract of Ashwagandha root exhibited CNS depressant activity which is correlated with its relaxation and antidepressant property. Aqueous extracts of this herb have been found to increase cholinergic activity, including increases in the acetylcholine content and cholineacetyl transferase activity in rats and this might partly explain the cognition-enhancing and memory-improving effects. Moreover, recent reports suggested methanol extract of Ashwagandha caused neurite outgrowth in a dose- and time-dependent manner in human neuroblastoma cells. The levels of two dendritic markers, viz. MAP2 and PSD-95, were found to be markedly increased in cells treated with Ashwagandha, suggesting that it stimulates dendrite formation (Bhattacharya and Kumar 1995; Schiloers et al. 1997; Mishra et al. 2000).

5.6.1.2 Clinical Studies of Nootropic Plants

The data on clinical examinations on Indian therapeutic plants possessing nootropic nootropic is displayed underneath.

Bacopa monniera Linn. (Brahmi)

A significant increase in intelligent quotient (IQ) scores was seen after treatment of 110 guys aged 10–13 years for 9 months with a suksma (miniaturized scale) medication got from *B. monniera*. Memory (direct) and arithmatic tests were utilized. The medication was all around endured in single (20–300 mg) and different (100 and 200 mg for 4 weeks) measurements in a twofold visually impaired fake treatment controlled and non-hybrid stage I preliminary clinical trails were done in human volunteers (Carlo et al. 2008).

Centella asiatica Linn. (Mandookparni)

C. asiatica (Family: Umbelliferae) aqueous extract showed improved learning and memory potential *in vivo*. Its extract significantly alleviated oxidative stress by decreasing malonaldehyde level and increasing glutathione level. Further it also showed AchE inhibitory activity which combinedly may be associated with cognition-enhancing efficacy (Anil et al. 2009). In recent randomized clinical trials, 28 participants (>61 years of age) were administered of *C. asiatica* extracts (250, 500, and 750 mg/daily; p.o.) for 2 months. After 2 months, patients with 750 mg dose extract showed significant improvement in cognitive function (as assessed by event-related potential and the computerized assessment battery test) and mood (using BondLader visual analogue) (Kashmira et al. 2010; Soumyanath et al. 2012).

5.7 Pharmacological and Clinical Studies on Polyherbal Formulation with Nootropic Activity

5.7.1 Indian Noni

Noni, a polyherbal formulation of *Morinda citrifolia* extract and *Garcinia cambogi* was tested *in vivo* for its nootropic potential against scopolamine induce amnesia. The formulation (dose: twice/day for 14 days) showed significant ($p < 0.01$) decline in transfer latency against scopolamine induced group. Further, it significantly inhibited acetylcholinesterase enzyme in rat brain homogenate and showed antioxidant property. These results suggested that formulation Noni might offer a useful therapeutic choice in either the prevention or the treatment of AD (Uma and Uma Maheswari 2014).

5.7.2 Memorin (Phytopharma)

Memorin is a dietary supplement designed to enhance brain functions. The formulation consists of aqueous juice of seven well-known Ayurvedic medicinal plant, viz. *C. aiatica* (150 mg), *C. alsonoids* (150 mg), *G. glabra* (100 mg), *A. calamus* (100 mg), *R. serpentina* (30 mg), *W. sominifera* (100 mg), and *S. lappa* (50 mg). Pretreatment with the formulation (200 mg/kg/day for 21 days) attenuated electroconvulsive shock (ECS)-induced retrograde amnesia in rats. The method used was a passive-avoidance test in a shuttle box (Dahanukar et al. 2000).

5.7.3 Mentat (Himalaya Healthcare)

Mentat, a polyherbal formulation containing extracts of *C. asiatica, B. monneri*, and *W. somnifera* is marketed by Himalaya Pvt. Ltd. *B.*

monneri is well known for its nootropic effect. *In vivo* experimentation revealed that the herb enhances memory and learning process and also calms restlessness in several mental disorders. *C. asiatica* possesses antiepileptic properties and is commonly used as an adjuvant to epileptic drugs. It balances amino acid levels, which is beneficial in treating depression. It also prevents cognitive impairment. Ashvagandha is used as a mood stabilizer in clinical conditions of anxiety and depression. Withanolides, the chemical constituents present in Winter Cherry, possess rejuvenating properties. The herb also reduces oxidative stress, which can cause mental fatigue (Kulkarni and Verma 1994; Handa and Bhargava 1997).

5.7.4 Shankhpushpi Syrup (Baidyanath)

Shankhpushpi Syrup is an Ayurvedic remedy for memory and intellect. It is beneficial in mental weakness, forgetfulness, memory loss, low retention power, etc. The formulation consists of C. alsinoids (200 mg), Brahmi (50 mg), Sugar (8000 mg), and Citric Acid (6 mg). Shankhpushpi is traditionally being used as brain tonic. Brahmi calms the mind and reduces anxiety, mental stress, work-related stress, and depression. The formulation showed excellent nootropic activity *in vivo* in normal and scopolamine-amnesic models. It (dose>40 mL/kg p.o.) also showed significant anticholinesterase activity but showed moderate effects on other neurotransmitter contents of whole brain tissue (Sharma et al. 2005).

5.7.5 Trasina (Dey's Pharmaceuticals)

Trasima is a polyherbal capsule containing *O. sanctum* (190 mg) and *W. somnifera* (80 mg). Trasina (1 cap/day for 21 days) showed a beneficial effect in mental activity in two *in vivo* models, viz. intracerebroventricular injection of colchicine (15 mg/rat) and ibotenic acid induced neurotoxicity (10 mg/rat). The drug caused significant reduction in time spent on maze apparatus transfer and augmented cholinergic markers and M1 receptor binding of rat brain. Further, it also showed significant anticholinesterase activity in dose-dependent manner (Kulkarni and Verma 1994; Handa and Bhargava 1997).

5.7.6 Saraswatarishta (Baidyanath)

Saraswatarishta, a polyherbal Ayurvedic liquid formulation containing juice of *C. asiatica* (960 mg), *A. racemosus* (240 mg), *P. tuberose* (240 mg), *T. chebula* (240 mg), *F. vulgare* (240 mg), *Z. officinale* (240 mg), *V. zizanioidis* (240 mg), *W. fruticosa* (240 mg), *V. negundo* (240 mg), *O. turpethum* (240 mg), and Honey. Saraswatarishta contains 5–10% of self-generated alcohol in it. This self-generated alcohol and the water present in the product acts as a media to deliver water and alcohol soluble active herbal components to the body. A clinical study in 25 patients with the formulation (20 mL two times/day for 1 year) showed prominent antiepileptic activity. The drug showed nootropic effects against various experimental models *in vivo* via anticholinesterase activity (Kulkarni and Verma 1994; Handa and Bhargava 1997).

5.7.7 Vidyarthi Amrit (Maharishi Ayurveda)

Vidyarthi amrit, a polyherbal Ayurvedic liquid formulation containing juice of *C. alsinoids*, *C. asiatica*, *V. wallichii*, *E. ribes*, *A. racemosus*, *W. somnifera*, *E. cardamomum*, *P. anisum*, and *A. calamus*. The formulation exhibited significant anticholinesterase and antiglutamate activity and increase in L-aspartate and GABA levels of whole brain tissue *in vivo* which may be associated with nootropic potentiality of the formulation (Kulkarni and Verma 1994; Handa and Bhargava 1997).

5.7.8 Dimagh Pushtak Rasayan (Baidyanath)

Dimagh Pushtak Rasayan is an Ayurvedic Rasayana formulation composed of *C. alsinoids*, *W. somnifera*, *C. asiatica*, *B. monnerie*, Makaradhwaj (Sulphide of Mercury), and *N. jatamansi*. This drug exhibited nootropic effects *in vivo* experimental models. The memory-enhancing effects of the formulation were attributed to cholinergic mechanisms (Kulkarni and Verma 1994; Handa and Bhargava 1997).

5.7.9 Geriforte (Himalaya)

Geriforte is an Ayurvedic formulation. Each Geriforte tablet contains: Chyavanprash concentrate (100 mg), Himsra (*C. spinosa*) (13.8 mg), Kasani (*C. intybus*) (13.8 mg), Daruharidra (*B. aristata*) (10 mg), Vasaka (*A.vasica*) (10 mg), Kakamachi (*S. nigrum*) (6.4 mg), Arjuna (*T. arjuna*) (6.4 mg), Biranjasipha (*A. millefolium*) (3.2 mg), Kasamarda (*C. occidentalis*) (3.2 mg). Jhavuka (*T. gallica*) (3.2 mg), Ashvagandha (*W. somnifera*) (30 mg), Shatavari (*A. racemosus*) (20 mg), Yashtimadhu (*G. glabra*) (20 mg), Mandukaparni (*C. asiatic*) (20 mg), Shilajeet (purified) (20 mg), Haritaki (*T. chebula*) (15 mg), Makardhwaj (10 mg), Musali (*A. adscendens*) 910 mg), Udakiryaka (*C. digyna*) (10 mg), Kapikachchu (*M. pruriens*) (10 mg), Jatiphalam (*M. fragrans*) (10 mg), Pippali (*P. longum*) (10 mg), Jaatipatree [*M. fragrans* (Mace)] (10 mg), Bhringaraja (*E. alba*) (10 mg), Vriddadaru (*A. speciosa*) (10 mg), Abhrak bhasma (10 mg), Jasad bhasma (10 mg), Kumkuma (*C. sativus*) (7 mg), Mandur bhasma (5 mg), Lavanga (*S. aromaticum*) (5 mg), Ela (*E. cardamomum*) (5 mg), Yawani (*C. copticum*) (5 mg), Haridra (*C. longa*) (5 mg), Jyothishmati (*C. paniculatus*) (5 mg), and Loh bhasma (5 mg). The natural ingredients in Geriforte work synergistically to prevent free radical-induced oxidative damage to various organs. The ingredients are natural rejuvenators and cardioprotective agents. As an immunomodulator, Geriforte stimulates the immune system to respond against disease-causing microorganisms. Geriforte is adaptogenic which effectively combats stress and fatigue. It also increases stamina and improves overall performance. Clinical psychobiological thinks about on obviously typical matured subjects 45–50 years were treated for 3 months with the test definition. Results demonstrated an expanding feeling of prosperity, physical effectiveness, and enhancement in mental capacities. The treatment diminished uneasiness and aided in better nitrogen maintenance. The medication has all the earmarks of being a normal blend of natural parts for capturing fast beginning of mental and physical handicap in matured people (Singh et al. 1979; Boral et al. 1989).

5.8 Nootropic Mineral Preparations

In Ayurveda minerals are used as therapeutic agents in their calcinated forms. Ayurvedic preparations like Bhasmas of metal is therapeutically effective and safe for internal use. Few such mineral preparations associated with learning and memory are mentioned below.

5.8.1 Siddh Makardhwaja (Mercury)

This medicine is traditionally administered along with milk. The preparation helped in the overall progress of the overall status of experimental animals. It revealed growth-promoting, memory-improving, and carbohydrate-sparing properties without affecting other central nervous system (CNS) parameters in rodents (Vohora et al. 1995).

5.8.2 Swarna Bhasma (Gold)

Swarna Bhasma showed potent antioxidant and free radical scavenging activity. The preparation (25 mg/kg orally for 7–10 days) exhibited a nootropic effect *in vivo* compared with *P. ginseng* tea

(350 mg/kg orally for 10 days). The preparation showed significant anticholinesterase activity which may be associated with a beneficiary effect on cognitive function (Bajaj et al. 1999; Bajaj and Vohora 2000).

5.9 Summary and Conclusion

At present, restricted solutions accessible to treat AD and the greater part of them are used either to postpone the movement of indications or symptomatic alleviation for a brief timeframe. Yet, the subsequent adverse reactions with economic factors related to these medications have made their utility constrained. In this manner, it is beneficial to shift the paradigm from synthetic to natural medicine as the latter is considered to be more safe and economical by the WHO (Perry et al. 2000). In the field of AD therapy, several interventions on the possible role of natural products have already been supported by the experimental outcomes. Till date, the greatest successes have resulted from plant-based AchE inhibitors and antioxidant discovery programs, which have provided substantial progress in the treatment of AD (Perry et al. 2001). Other approaches include anti-amyloid agents, β-secretase inhibitors, anti-inflammatory drugs, nicotinic and muscarinic receptor agonists, tau proteins inhibitors (Ingkaninan et al. 2006). Currently, the investigation of natural products that can act as functional foods is of utmost interest to delay the progression and symptomatic relief from AD and promote other associated health benefits. A significant shift from a single-target to a multi-target drug approach, especially for chronic and complex disease syndromes, is being witnessed for the management of AD. However, cellular level assay to find out mechanism is indeed very much essential to establish their therapeutic claim as anti-Alzheimer's drug. In a recent study, life style modification like stress-free life, vacation, spending quality and happy moments with family members, etc. are found to be beneficial to reduce risk of dementia. Moreover, yoga and meditation also exert preverol dementia and AD progression (Mukherjee et al. 2007; Atanu et al. 2015). If the research is progressed in a successful manner, the drugs derived from natural sources could be a good substitute for conventional medicine, as they are easily and economically available these days.

References

Abhang RY. Medhya rasayana: past, present and future. Deerghayu Int. 1987;4:8–18.

Adewusi EA, Steenkamp V. *In vitro* screening for acetylcholinesterase inhibition and antioxidant activity of medicinal plants from Southern Africa. Asian Pac J Trop Med. 2011;5(2):829–35.

Ahirwar S, Tembhre M, Gour S, Namdeo A. Anticholinesterase efficacy of *Bacopa monnieri* against the brain regions of rat—a novel approach to therapy for Alzheimer's disease. Asian J Exp Sci. 2012;26(1):65–70.

Ahmed T, Gilani AH. Inhibitory effect of curcuminoids on acetylcholinesterase activity and attenuation of scopolamine-induced amnesia may explain medicinal use of turmeric in Alzheimer's disease. Pharmacol Biochem Behav. 2009;91:554–9.

Aisen PS. Anti-inflammatory agents in Alzheimer's disease. Curr Neurol Neurosci Rep. 2002a;2:405–52.

Aisen PS. Evaluation of selective COX-2 inhibitors for the treatment of Alzheimer's disease. J Pain Symptom Manag. 2002b;23:S35–42.

Akhlaq AF, Tahira F, Anil M, Jolin Hwee-Jing O, Wei-Yi O. Ayurvedic medicine for the treatment of dementia: mechanistic aspects. Evid Based Complement Alternat Med. 2018;40(2):1–11.

Akinrimisi ED, Ainwannde AI. Effect of aqueous extract of *Eugenia caryolphyllus* on brain acetylcholinesterase in rats. West Afr J Pharmacol Drug Res. 1975;2:127–33.

Amod PK, Laurie AK, Girish JK. Herbal complement inhibitors in the treatment of neuroinflammation. Ann N Y Acad Sci. 2005;1056:413–29.

Anderson RN. Deaths: leading causes for 2000. Natl Vital Stat Rep. 2002;50:1.

Anil K, Samrita D, Atish P. Neuroprotective effects of *Centella asiatica* against intracerebroventricular colchicine-induced cognitive impairment and oxidative stress. Int J Alzheimer's Dis. 2009;9:1–8.

Atanu B, Shastry CS, Saha S. Nootropic activity of *Crataeva nurvala* Buch-ham against scopolamine induced cognitive impairment. EXCLI J. 2015;14:335–45.

Bahr BA, Bendiske J. The neuropathogenic contributions of lysosomal dysfunction. J Neurochem. 2002;83:481–92.

Bajaj S, Vohora SB. Anticataleptic, anti-anxiety and anti-depressant activity of gold preparation used in Indian systems of medicine. Indian J Pharmacol. 2000;32:339.

Bajaj S, Ahamad I, Fatima M, Raisuddin S, Vohora SB. Immunomadulatory activity of a Unani gold preparation used in Indian system of medicine. Immunopharmacol Immunotoxicol. 1999;21:151.

Berrino F. Western diet and Alzheimer's disease. Epidemiol Prev. 2002;26:107.

Bhattacharya SK, Kumar A. Effect of glycowithanolides from Withania somnifera on an animal model of Alzheimer's disease and perturbed central cholinergic markers of cognition in rats. Phytother Res. 1995;9:110–6.

Boral GC, Gautam B, Anjan B, Das NN, Nandi PS. Geriforte in anxiety neurosis. Indian J Psychiatry. 1989;31(3):258–60.

Bush AI. The metallobiology of Alzheimer's disease. Trends Neurosci. 2003;26(4):207–14.

Carlo C, William LG, Michael L, Dale K, Kerry B, Barry O. Effects of a standardized *Bacopa monnieri* extract on cognitive performance, anxiety, and depression in the elderly: a randomized, double-blind, placebo-controlled trial. J Altern Complement Med. 2008;14(6):707–13.

Chatellier G, Lacomblez L. Tacrine (teterahydroaminoacridine; THA) and lecithine in senile dementia of the Alzheimer type: a multicenter trial. Br Med J. 1990;300:495.

Clegg BJ, Nicholson T, McIntyre L, De Broe S, Gerard K, Waugh N. Clinical and cost effectiveness of donepezil, rivastigmine, and galantamine for Alzheimer's disease: a systematic review. Int J Technol Assess Health Care. 2002;18:497.

Colucci L, Bosco M, Ziello AR, et al. Effectiveness of nootropic drugs with cholinergic activity in treatment of cognitive deficit: a review. J Exp Pharmacol. 2012;4:163–72.

Dahanukar SA, Kulkarni RA, Rege NN. Pharmacology of medicinal plants and natural products. Indian J Pharmacol. 2000;32:S81–S118.

Dash SC, Tripathi SN, Singh RH. Clinical assessment of medhya drugs in the management of psychosis (unmada). Ancient Sci Life. 1983;3:77–83.

Divya SV, Lakshmi CM. Alzheimer's disease. Scientific basis for Ayurvedic medicines. New York: CRC Publishers; 2007.

Doraiswamy PM. Non-cholinergic strategies for treating and preventing Alzheimer's disease. CNS Drugs. 2002;16:24.

Dwivedi KK, Singh RH. A clinical study of medhya rasayana therapy in the management of convulsive disorder. J Res Ayurveda Siddha. 1978;13:97.

Fernando GP. Brain foods: the effects of nutrients on brain function. Nat Rev Neurosci. 2008;9(7):568–78.

Frawley D. Ayurvedic Healing. Delhi, India: Motilal Banarsidass Publishers; 1989.

Gelb DJ. Measurement of progression in Alzheimer's disease: a clinician perspective. Stat Med. 2000;19:1390–8.

Ghosh AK, Osswald HL. BACE1 (β-Secretase) inhibitors for the treatment of Alzheimer's disease. Chem Soc Rev. 2014;43(19):6765–813. https://doi.org/10.1039/c3cs60460h.

Gohil KJ, Patel JA. A review on *Bacopa monniera*: current research and future prospects. Int J Green Pharma. 2010;2:1–9.

Gupta BM, Bala A. Alzheimer's disease research in India: a scientometric analysis of publications output during 2002–11. Res Neurol Int J. 2013;2013:11. https://doi.org/10.5171/2013.204542.

Habibur R, Muralidharan P, Anand M. Inhibition of AChE and antioxidant activities are probable mechanism of Nardostacys Jatamansi DC in sleep deprived Alzheimer's mice model. Int J Pharma Tech Res. 2011;3(3):1807–16.

Handa SS, Bhargava VK. Effect of BR 16-A (Mentat) on cognitive deficits in aluminum treated and aged rats. Indian J Pharmacol. 1997;28:258–64.

Harvey AL. Natural products in drug discovery. Drug Discov Today. 2008;13:894–901.

Howes MJ, Houghton PJ. Plants used in Chinese and Indian traditional medicine for improvement of memory and cognitive function. Pharmacol Biochem Behav. 2003;75:513–27.

Huang Y, Mucke L. Alzheimer mechanisms and therapeutic strategies. Cell. 2012;148(6):1204–22.

Huang W, Zhang X, Chen W. Role of oxidative stress in Alzheimer's disease. Biomed Rep. 2016;4(5):519–22.

Ingkaninan K, Phengpa P, Yuenyongsawad S, Khorana N. Acetylcholinesterase inhibitors from *Stephania venosa* tuber. J Pharm Pharmacol. 2006;58:695–700.

Iyer MR, Pal SC, Kasture VS, Kasture SB. Effect of *Lawsonia inermis* on memory and behaviour mediated via monoamine neurotransmitters. Ind J Pharmacol. 1998;30:181–5.

Jagdeep SD, Prasad DN, Avinash CT, Rajiv G. Role of traditional medicine in neuropsychopharmacology. Asian J Pharm Clin Res. 2009;2(2):72–6.

Jemima J, Bhattacharjee P, Singhal RS. Melatonin—a review on the lesser known potential nutraceutical. Int J Pharm Sci Res. 2011;2(8):1975–87.

Jian-zhi W, Ze-fen W. Role of melatonin in Alzheimer-like neurodegeneration. Acta Pharmacol Sinica. 2006;27(1):41–9.

Jivad N, Rabiei Z. A review study on medicinal plants used in the treatment of learning and memory impairments. Asian Pac J Trop Biomed. 2014;4:780–9.

Kar S, Slowikowski SPM, Westaway D, Mount HTJ. Interactions between β-amyloid and central cholinergic neurons: implications for Alzheimer's disease. J Psychiatry Neurosci. 2004;29(6):427–41.

Kashmira JG, Jagruti P, Anuradha KG. Pharmacological review on *Centella asiatica*: a potential herbal cure-all. Ind J Pharma Sci. 2010;72(5):546–56.

Keyvan D, Damien Dorman HJ, Heikki V, Raimo H. Plants as potential sources for drug development against Alzheimer's disease. Int J Biomed Pharm Sci. 2007;1(2):83–104.

Khare CP. Indian medicinal plants an illustrated dictionary. Berlin: Springer; 2007.

Kulkarni SK, Verma A. BR 16-A (Mentat): a herbal preparation improves learning and memory performance in mice. PRO. 1994;3(222):28.

Lemstra AW, Eikelenboom P, Van Gool WA. The cholinergic deficiency syndrome and its therapeutic implications. Gerontology. 2003;49:55.

Lindsay J, Laurin D, Verreault R, Hebert R, Helliwell B, Hill GB, McDowell I. Risk factors for Alzheimer's disease: a prospective analysis from the Canadian study of health and aging. Am J Epidemiol. 2002;156:445–52.

Mahesh G, Tasneem S. Biomarker controversies and diagnostic difficulties in Alzheimer's disease. Am J Phytomed Clin Therap. 2014;2(4):463–8.

Manyam BV. Dementia in Ayurveda. J Altern Complement Med. 1999;5:81–8.

Maya M, Sarada S. *In vitro* screening for anticholinesterase and antioxidant activity of methanolic extracts of Ayurvedic medicinal plants used for cognitive disorders. PLoS One. 2014;9(1):e86804.

Mishra LC, Singh BB, Dagenais S. Scientific basis for the therapeutic use of *Withania somnifera* (ashwagandha): a review. Altern Med Rev. 2000;5:334–46.

Mukherjee PK, Kumar V, Mal M, Houghton PJ. Acetylcholinesterase inhibitors from plants. Phytomedicine. 2007;14:289–300.

Muralidharan P, Balamurugan G, Venu B. Cerebroprotective effect of *Glycyrrhiza glabra* Linn. root extract on hypoxic rats. Bangladesh J Pharmacol. 2009;4:60–4.

Nillert W, Pannangrong W, Welbat JU. Neuroprotective effects of aged garlic extract on cognitive dysfunction and neuroinflammation induced by β-amyloid in rats. Nutrients. 2017;9:24–36.

Orhan I, Kartal M, Naz Q, Ejaz A, Yilmaz G, Kan Y, et al. Antioxidant and anticholinesterase evaluation of selected Turkish Salvia species. Food Chem. 2007;103:1247–54.

Patel VS, Jivani NP, Patel SB. Medicinal plants with potential nootropic activity: a review. Res J Pharm Bio Chem Sci. 2014;5(1):1–11.

Perry EK, Pickering AT, Wang WW, Houghton PJ, Perry NS. Medicinal plants and Alzheimer's disease: from ethnobotany to phytotherapy. J Pharm Pharmacol. 1999;51:527–33.

Perry NSL, Houghton PJ, Theolad AE, Jenner P, Perry EK. *In vitro* inhibition of human erythrocyte acetylcholinesterase by *Salvia lavandulaefolia* essential oil and constituent terpenes. J Pharm Pharmacol. 2000;52:895–902.

Perry NSL, Houghton PJ, Sampson J, Theolad AE, Hart S, Lis-balchin M. *In vitro* activities of *Salvia lavandulaefolia* (Spanish Sage) relevant to treatment of Alzheimer's disease. J Pharm Pharmacol. 2001;53:1347–56.

Philomena G. Concerns regarding the safety and toxicity of medicinal plants—an overview. J Appl Pharma Sci. 2011;1(6):40–4.

Prachi S, Lakshmayya L, Vinod SB. Anti-Alzheimer activity of isolated karanjin from *Pongamia pinnata* (L.) pierre and embelin from Embelia ribes Burm.f. Int Quarterly J Res Ayurveda. 2017;38(1):76–81.

Prakash R, Sandhya E, Ramya N, Dhivya R, Priyadarshini M, Sakthi Priya B. Neuroprotective activity of ethanolic extract of Tinospora cordifolia on LPS induced neuroinflammation. Transl Biomed. 2017;8(4):135–42.

Prerna U, Vikas S, Mushtaq A. Therapy of Alzheimer's disease: an update. Afr J Pharm Pharmacol. 2010;4(6):408–21.

Puchchakayala G, Akina S, Thati M. Neuroprotective effects of meloxicam and selegiline in scopolamine-induced cognitive impairment and oxidative stress. Int J Alzheimers Dis. 2012;12:1–8.

Rammohan VR, Olivier D, Varghese J, Dale EB. Ayurvedic medicinal plants for Alzheimer's disease: a review. Alzheimers Res Ther. 2012;4(22):1–12.

Rhee IK, Meent MV, Ingkaninan K, Verpoorte R. Screening for acetylcholinesterase inhibitors from Amaryllidaceae using silica gel thin-layer chromatography in combination with bioactivity staining. J Chromatogr. 2001;915:217–23.

Rinne JO, Kaasinen V, Jarvenpaa T, Någren K, Roivainen A, Yu M, et al. Brain acetylcholinesterase activity in mild cognitive impairment and early Alzheimer's disease. Neurol Neurosurg Psychiatry. 2003;74:113–5.

Roberts SB. Gamma-secretase inhibitors and Alzheimer's disease. Adv Drug Deliv Rev. 2002;54:1579–82.

Satyavati GV, Gupta AK, Tandon N, Seth SD. Medicinal plants of India, Vol. 2. New Delhi, India: Indian Council of Medical Research; 1987.

Schiloers R, Liermann A, Bhattacharya SK, Kumar A, Ghoshal S, Rich V. Systemic administration of defined extracts from Withania Somnifera (Indian ginseng) and shilajit differentially affects cholinergic but not glutaminergic and gabaergic markers in rat brain. Neurochem Int. 1997;30:181.

Schneider LS. New therapeutic approaches to Alzheimer's disease. Psychiatry. 1996;57:30–6.

Sharma PC, Yelne MB, Dennis TJ. Database on medicinal plants used in Ayurveda and Sidha. 1st ed. New Delhi: CCRAS, Dept. of AYUSH, Ministry of Health and Family Welfare, Govt. of India; 2005.

Singh RH, Sinha BN, Sarkar FH, Udupa KN. Comparative biochemical studies on the effect of four Medhya Rasayana drugs described by Caraka on some central neurotransmitters in normal and stressed rats. J Indian Med Yoga Homeopathy. 1979;14:7–14.

Soumyanath S, Zhong Y, Henson E, et al. *Centella asiatica* extract improves behavioral deficits in a mouse model of Alzheimer's disease: investigation of a possible mechanism of action. Int J Alzheimers Dis. 2012;12:381–94.

Spiegel R. Rivastigmine: a review of its clinical effectiveness. Rev Neurol. 2002;35:859.

Talic S, Dragicevic I, Corajevic L, Martinovic BA. Acetylcholinesterase and butyrylcholinesterase inhibitory activity of extracts from medicinal plants. Bulletin Chemists Technol Bosnia Herzegovania. 2014;43:11–4.

Uma G, Uma Maheswari S. Neuroprotective effects of polyherbal formulation (Indian Noni) on scopolamine-induced memory impairment in mice. Int J Pharm Pharm Sci. 2014;6(1):354–7.

Urbain A, Marston A, Queiroz EF, Ndjoko K, Hostettmann K. Xanthones from *Gentiana campestris* as new acetylcholinesterase inhibitors. Planta Med. 2004;70:1011–4.

Vaidya AB. The status and scope of Indian medicinal plants acting on the central nervous system. Indian J Pharmacol. 1997;29(S340):228–34.

Vinutha B, Prashanth D, Salma K, Sreeja SL, Pratiti D, Padmaja R, et al. Screening of selected Indian medicinal plants for acetylcholinesterase inhibitory activity. J Ethnopharmacol. 2007;109:359–63.

Vladimir V, Sophia R. Results of beta secretase-inhibitor clinical trials support amyloid precursor protein-independent generation of beta amyloid in sporadic Alzheimer's disease. Med Sci (Basel). 2018;6(2):45–58.

Vohora SB, Kim HS, Shah SA, Khanna T, Dandiya PC. CNS and adaptogenic effects of Siddh Makardhwaja: an Ayurvedic mercury preparation, in trace elements in nutrition and health. New Delhi, India: Jamia Hamdard and Wiley Eastern Ltd.; 1995.

Wang BS, Wang H, Wei ZH, Song YY, Zhang L, Chen HZ. Efficacy and safety of natural acetylcholinesterase inhibitor huperzine A in the treatment of Alzheimer's disease: an updated meta-analysis. J Neural Transm. 2009;116(4):457–65.

Zhang F, Jiang L. Neuroinflammation in Alzheimer's disease. Neuropsychiatr Dis Treat. 2015;11:243–56.

Integrating Indigenous Systems of Medicines in the Healthcare System in India: Need and Way Forward

6

Vandana Roy

Contents

V. Roy (✉)
Department of Pharmacology, Maulana Azad Medical College and Associated Hospitals, University of Delhi, New Delhi, India

S. Sen, R. Chakraborty (eds.), *Herbal Medicine in India*,
https://doi.org/10.1007/978-981-13-7248-3_6

6.1 Introduction

The purpose of Universal Health Coverage (UHC) is to ensure that all people have access to promotive, preventive, curative and rehabilitative health services, of sufficient quality to be effective, while also ensuring that they do not suffer financial hardship when paying for these services (World Health Organization 2018). The Alma Ata declaration in 1978 recommended primary healthcare as a way to achieve the goals of universal health. It called for integration of preventive, promotive, curative and rehabilitative health services (United Nations 1978). These had to be made accessible to people, guided by principles of universality, comprehensiveness and equity (Nundy 2005). The Declaration called for a balanced distribution of available resources.

Since there are multiple ways of understanding health and disease, it is imperative that all available choices for healthcare be available for fulfillment of the above goal. This implies that medical pluralism involving multiple healing options be offered to patients. The choices need to be offered to the patients in a well-defined, transparent, accountable, affordable, accessible, balanced and stand-alone way. The patients also need to be informed about the choices. At all times the efficacy, safety, affordability and patient acceptability of the treatments offered should be kept prime while making or giving choices.

The healthcare needs of people in India have been taken care of by a multitude of persons, some practicing conventional western medicine, others indigenous or traditional systems. *"Traditional medicine has been defined as the sum total of the knowledge, skill and practices based on the theories, beliefs and experiences indigenous to different cultures, whether explicable or not, used in the maintenance of health as well as in the prevention, diagnosis, improvement or treatment of physical and mental illness. Traditional medicines of proven quality, safety and efficacy contribute to the goal of ensuring that all people have access to care."* For many people around the world, traditional systems of medicines are the main and many times the only source of health care. The reasons in favor of traditional systems of medicines include their ready acceptability, availability, accessibility and affordability. There is also a perception that these systems are safe. Most of these are offered by healers who live in proximity to the people (World Health Organization 2013).

India has a rich heritage of indigenous systems of medicines. Some of which have been in existence for thousands of years. Others were brought by travellers, invaders and rulers who came from outside and settled here. These assimilated into the local culture and healthcare practices. After independence, India adopted a health policy that integrated principles of universality and equity. The indigenous systems were incorporated as part of the National health policy. Both the Western allopathic and indigenous, traditional systems of medicines coexist in India and have Government recognition. Yet in spite of this, access to affordable healthcare eludes the majority of the population.

The present article aims to explore the situation regarding the coexistence of indigenous, traditional systems of medicines in India with the allopathic system and reasons for the same. Ways to optimize utilization of indigenous systems in India will be explored.

6.2 Medical Systems in India

India has a rich heritage of traditional medical systems dating back to antiquity. These include Ayurveda, Siddha, Naturopathy and Yoga which originated in India itself. In addition, the Unani system which came from Greece and Homeopathy which came from Germany have also been incorporated in the Indian systems of medicines more commonly referred to as AYUSH (Ayurveda, Yoga, Unani, Siddha and Homeopathy). Ayurveda originated around 5000–1000 BC, Siddha developed in South India in Tamil culture. It has been suggested that it could have originated during the time of the Harappan civilization. The medical literature of the Siddha system was scientifically codified in the eighteenth century. Unani medicine came to India around the eleventh century and Homeopathy came to India from Germany in the eighteenth century (Subbbarayappa 2001).

These systems were officially recognized as Indian Systems of Medicine and Homoepathy (ISM & H) systems of medicines in the year 1959. In 2011 Sowa Rigpa was included in the official lists of ISM. In addition, there are many folk medicines other than the codified traditional medicine in existence in India.

In 1970 the Central Council of Indian Medicine was constituted which was involved in framing and implementation of different regulations including curriculum and syllabus in ISM & H. A separate Department of ISM & H was set up in 1995. This was renamed in 2003 as the Department of Ayurveda, Yoga, Unani, Siddha, Homeopathy (AYUSH). In 2014, a separate ministry on AYUSH was formed. These official changes were associated with many developments which have led to each system being regulated by an official body, specific education and training programs, research, and manufacture of healthcare products required (AYUSH Ministry 2015).

These systems are characterized by their own individual philosophy, ways of defining disease and treatment modalities. All AYUSH medical systems use naturally available parts and products of plants, animals and minerals to promote health, prevent and cure disease. Ayurveda and Unani involve the use of herbal products as part of their therapy to a great extent.

6.3 Existing Status: Some Observations

India has a large network of AYUSH dispensaries, hospitals and colleges, largely government supported (AYUSH Ministry 2018). Surveys done over various periods to find out the extent of utilization of AYUSH systems by the people for healthcare problems showed that it ranged from 4% to 70% (FOD (NSSO)—Ministry of Statistics and PI 2016; Sundar 1995; Singh et al. 2005). The stand-alone AYUSH facilities were better utilized than those co-located in existing healthcare facilities where the modern system was being practiced. The utilization in some states like Tamil Nadu, Kerela and Delhi was high (Priya and Shweta 2010). These are also states where the public health system is better organized. Studies for assessing the feasibility of integrating AYUSH, specifically Ayurveda with allopathy system of medicine have shown that sustained effort, communication and sensitization is required for integration (Bhatt et al. 2007). Surveys on folk medicine have shown that about 2% of the population during the survey period was using folk medicine (some places the use was high as 14%) (Central Council for Research in Ayurveda and Siddha 1999). About 5000 folklore/ethnomedical claims used by tribal people have been documented by Central Council for Research in Ayurvedic Sciences (Anonymous 2002). Household remedies are commonly used by people and over 3000 such remedies have been documented in the publications of Ayurveda and Unani Medicine. A study done has shown that people use Ayurveda for chronic ailments such as skin diseases, gastrointestinal disorders, liver diseases, arthritis, gynecological problems and some acute ailments (Sujatha 2011; Chandra 2011).

Current Status of the Infrastructure Available in Indian Systems of Medicines in India (2015) (AYUSH Ministry 2018)

- Total number of AYUSH Hospitals is 3632. Among these, 2833, 265, 279, 212 and 43 are Ayurveda, Unani, Siddha, Homoeopathy and other (Yoga, Naturopathy) hospitals, respectively.

- Total bed strength is 58,020; of these, 43,454, 3623, 2440, 7182, 85 and 1236 numbers of beds are of Ayurveda, Unani, Siddha, Homoeopathy, Yoga, Naturopathy respectively.
- Out of total 26,325 dispensaries 15,555, 1491, 835, 8117, 327, 34 are of Ayurveda, Unani, Siddha, Homoeopathy, Yoga and Naturopathy, and Sowa Rigpa, respectively.
- Total number of registered practitioners are 744,563. Out of this, 402,079, 48,213, 8388, 283,840, 2043 are Ayurveda, Unani, Siddha, Homoeopathy and Naturopathy practitioners, respectively.
- Among 525,663 institutional qualified registered practitioners 267,998, 734,619, 74,733 and 215,327 are from Ayurveda, Unani, Siddha and Homoeopathy, respectively.
- Total number of colleges (undergraduate) is 544. Numbers of Ayurveda, Unani, Siddha, Homoeopathy and Sowa Rigpa undergraduate colleges are 279, 43, 8, 195 and 19, respectively.
- In these colleges total number of students is 32,256: Ayurveda (15,117), Unani (2131), Siddha (410), Homoepathy(13,658) and Sowa Rigpa (940).
- Total number of colleges with post-graduation is 170. The numbers of Ayurvedic, Unani, Siddha, and Homoeopathy colleges with post-graduates are 112, 9, 3 and 43, respectively.
- In these colleges total number of students is 4339: Ayurveda (3029), Unani (147), Siddha (140) and Homoeopathy (918).
- Total Drug Manufacturing Units are 9282. Among this 7995, 505, 379 and 403 are from Ayurveda, Unani, Siddha, and Homoeopathy, respectively.

6.4 Status of AYUSH as Independent Medical Systems: Ground Reality

Despite the existence of these systems in the country for such a long time, these systems have not been optimally utilized as well as the allopathic system. As a result, the contribution of these systems to the healthcare system in the country is below par and not what it should be. There are many reasons for this.

6.4.1 Historical

Prior to British colonization, the ISM had an independent identity and was the mainstay of medical and healthcare in India. During British colonization, a deliberate and conscious effort to suppress the practitioners of ISM was made. Government policies and actions aimed at marginalizing ISM and its practitioners. The Bombay Medical Registration Act in 1912, requiring registration of Western medical practitioners with no recognition to the Vaidyas and Hakims was one such Act. The Indian Medical Association was formed in 1928 and concentrated exclusively on practitioners of Western medicine. The Sub Committee of the National Planning Commission (1938) drawing up a plan for healthcare services for independent India also recommended integration of Vaidyas and Hakims after "training". During this time support for integrated colleges decreased while that for pure colleges of ISM increased (Chandra 2011). Thus the practitioners and believers in ISM were sidelined and did not receive the political and official patronage that the Western medicine system did.

6.4.1.1 Towards Utilization of Indigenous Medical Systems. Committee Recommendations, Policy Changes, Plans

Many committees were formed around independence and after to recommend steps to bring the ISM & H at par with the Western medicine system in India. These include the Bhore committee (1946), Sokhey Committee (1946), Chopra Committee (1948), Pandit Committee (1951), Dave Committee (1956), Uduppa committee (1958), Mudaliar Committee (1962), Vyas report (1963) and Sampurnananda Committee (1964). All of them looked at the ISM and ways to establish them in the country through education, training and assimilation in the healthcare system. The government wanted research in Ayurveda and Unani medicine along scientific lines. The thrust was on having a single medicine system and teaching of modern medicine was considered essential for the betterment of Indian medicine (Chandra 2011).

The third Five Year Plan (1961–1966) was the first plan where a specific section was devoted to strategies to promote Indian Medicine. Between 1970 and 2014, the Indian Medicine Central Council Act was enacted, a Department of ISM & H was notified, the name was changed to AYUSH and subsequently, a Ministry of AYUSH was created. The first ISM & H policy was announced only in 2002. It was only in the ninth Five Year Plan (1997–2002) that separate chapter was devoted to the ISM & H. It is obvious that recognition of ISM & H within the country has been a relatively recent phenomenon.

6.4.2 Government Policies

Various National Health Policies of the Government included specific mention of ISM & H for the delivery of healthcare services. These include National Health Policy 1983, 2002 and 2017. In 2002 a separate National Health policy for ISM & H was formulated. Each policy has built upon the previous one. However, while expanding and achieving some extent of acceptance in the public healthcare system, it has not achieved widespread utilization. The reason is that there are problems and lacunae in the way the policies have been implemented (Ministry of Health & Family Welfare 1983, 2002, 2017; Department of AYUSH 2002; Ministry of Health & Family Welfare 2012).

6.4.3 Education and Training: Not Optimum

Initially, these systems and their philosophy were propagated through the Guru shishya tradition. During British rule, strategies were used to see that the ISM did not flourish. The English language was also chosen as the language for training in allopathy medicine. Efforts to keep the ISM alive were made by individuals, who wrote on the subjects, made institutions and colleges (Chandra 2011). But these did not get as much patronage from the rulers that allopathy medicine did. Thus the institutions of learning and training in ISM had structural weaknesses in content and process.

Efforts to start the integrated system of medicine, wherein both the ISM and allopathy systems would be taught and would complement each other, were made after independence unsuccessfully, as this was opposed by both the Allopathic and Ayurvedic practitioners.

While many colleges and institutes have opened up in ISM & H, the quality of education and training requires improvement. The curriculum requires changes to make it relevant and interesting for the students. Learning objectives have to be defined in various subjects. Some amount of understanding of subjects of modern medicine is also required. There is a need of infrastructure in terms of audio-visual aids and laboratories for learning. More practical training for the learners with experienced teachers is the need of the hour (Chandra 2011, Vaidya 2005).

6.4.4 Research and Development: Lack of Evidence

Evidence-based medicine is the foundation of modern medicine. Scientific research methodology has laid down principles of how all therapies must be investigated, evaluated for efficacy and safety. Lack of data about the research outcomes related to AYUSH (henceforth ISM & H will be referred to as AYUSH) is a major reason why these therapies have not been adopted for development by the drug industry as well as not been accepted by modern medicine doctors.

While a lot of research work has been initiated by Government bodies such as Indian Council of Medical Research (ICMR), Council of Scientific and Industrial Research (CSIR), Department of Biotechnology (DBT), Department of Science and Technology (DST), Universities, individual Councils of Ayurveda, Unani and Siddha, since the 1960s, the outcome has not been satisfactory.

Either the research was not directed properly or was of poor quality. Where promising evidence was generated, there the drug industry did not show an interest to take the formulation forward (Chandra 2011). This has not helped in increasing confidence in the indigenous systems of medicines among practitioners of allopathy medicine who are taught to make decisions based on scientific evidence.

6.4.5 Western (Allopathy) Medicine and AYUSH: Existence in Silos

Both allopathy system and AYUSH have grown in individual silos in the country. Although many attempts to integrate the learning of modern system of medicine with the AYUSH were made even before independence, the idea could not develop. Some examples include the establishment of Ashtanga Ayurveda College and Hospital by Kaviraja Jaminibhushan Ray in 1916 and the Vishwanta Ayurveda Mahavidyalaya in 1932 by Kaviraja Gananath Sen. There was opposition from both allopathy and Ayurveda practitioners (Chandra 2011).

Thus complete separation in the education of AYUSH and allopathy system and no integration at all in the public health system has been the norm. The medical curriculum of students pursuing allopathy medicine also finds no mention of even sensitizing students to AYUSH systems of medicine. The closest the Government has reached is having clinics of AYUSH in health facilities which primarily are allopathy hospitals. Some hospitals have attempted centers for integrative medicine for specific diseases, but these are a rarity and not the norm.

6.4.6 Language as a Barrier

The original manuscripts and texts of AYUSH are written in languages which are not easily understood by the common people. These are Sanskrit, Urdu, Tamil and Homeopathy in German, whereas modern medicine is taught in English. There is no way to bridge this gap either in AYUSH systems or in allopathy medicine. The texts are not easily comprehensible, even by students of AYUSH. For modern medicine doctors and lay people, it is even more difficult.

6.4.7 Practice

Confusion and opposition prevail in India regarding prescribing of medicines by practitioners of different systems of medicines, that is, allopathic medicines by AYUSH practitioners and AYUSH medicines by allopathic doctors, the so called "Cross pathy". The use of allopathic medicines by AYUSH practitioners and increasing demands that they be allowed to prescribe allopathic medicines have not been considered appropriate by the Indian Medical Association. The term quackery is used and this further results in widening the divide between the two systems. This has added to the conflicting perception regarding the AYUSH systems in some quarters (IMA 2013).

6.4.8 Administrative and Court Orders

Legally also in India, confusion prevails regarding prescribing of medicines by practitioners of different systems of medicines. Some State Governments have allowed practitioners of AYUSH to prescribe drugs of modern system (Maharashtra, Punjab, Haryana, Assam, Himachal Pradesh, Karnataka, Tamil Nadu, Goa). These have been contested in courts. The courts have given contradictory judgments: some allowing and others not allowing.

The "Supreme Court judgement in the case of Poonam Verma Vs. Ashwin Patel and Others (1996) 4 SCC 332 where a doctor holding Diploma in Homeopathic Medicine and Surgery (DHMS) and registered under Bombay Homeopathic Practitioners Act, caused the death of a patient due to administration of allopathic medicine, held the doctor as not qualified to practice allopathy, and hence guilty of negligence per se. The court said *"the doctor must not only be qualified, but he must also be registered with the appropriate Medical Council in order to practice as a doctor. A homeopath would not have knowledge about allopathic medicines and its drug actions, so administration of allopathic treatment by a homeopath would be proof enough to establish negligence"* As per this judgment, homeopathic doctors are not legally permitted to prescribe allopathic medicines (Supreme Court of India 1996).

According to Sect. 2(ee) of the Drugs and Cosmetics Act Rules, allopathic medicines can be prescribed only by a Registered Medical Practitioner (RMP). Three categories of RMPs are defined in three sub-clauses of this Rule. *Subclause (I) and (ii) are practitioners holding a qualification and registration for practicing modern medicine. Subclause (iii) however allows practitioners who are registered in a medical register (other sthan a register of Homeopathic practitioners) of a State, who although not falling within subclause (I) or subclause (ii) is declared by a general or special order made by the State Government in this behalf, as a person practicing the modern scientific system of medicine.* Thus according to this subclause (iii) of Rule 2(ee) of the Drugs and Cosmetics Act Rules, practitioners of AYUSH so declared by the respective State Government are legally permitted to prescribe allopathic medicines (Government of India 2014).

Based on this many State Governments have issued orders and thereby permitted practitioners of AYUSH to prescribe allopathic medicines. Such State Government orders have been upheld by the Hon'ble Supreme Court in the case of Mukhtiar Chand versus the State of Punjab and Others 1998, where the apex court gave a ruling that a practitioner of one system of medicine has to adhere to his own system or by registered medical practitioners in the State Medical Register. This ruling has been quoted whenever this debate surfaces (Supreme Court of India 1998). A judgment by the Tamil Nadu High Court has permitted the use of modern drugs by ASU practitioners on the ground that the state has approved the same.

The subclause(iii) of Rule 2(ee) of Drugs and Cosmetic Act, which gives the State Governments power to declare who can prescribe allopathic medicine, on a criteria other than that based on the requisite educational qualification and training to practice, is itself fraught with contradictions and is a major reason for the court cases.

Such administered orders, court cases and judgments indicate the problems in the practice of these systems in the country.

6.4.9 Quality Issues

Quality assurance in AYUSH practice as well as in products has not been as stringent as for allopathy medicine.

6.4.9.1 Practitioners

Many practitioners of AYUSH have learned their skills from generational transfer. Thus while there are many ISM practitioners who have received their qualification from regulated institutes, there are many who have not. Even in regulated colleges, many issues concerning the curriculum, lack of exposure to sufficient clinical material, teaching modern system by AYUSH practitioners, insufficient regulation of quality control of the colleges are there which may impact the quality of the practitioners (Ministry of Health & Family Welfare 2012).

6.4.9.2 Quality Issues in Medicinal Products

Many products used in AYUSH are of herbal origin, some are of animal and mineral origin. Originally, all AYUSH medicines were prepared by the vaidyas or hakims themselves. In the late nineteenth century large scale, mechanized production of Ayurvedic medicines began. The traditional procedures were preserved until modern dosage forms were made available. This process of large-scale manufacturing of AYUSH products has replaced classical medicine, wherein the practitioner gave individualized therapies.

Issues concerning regulation of manufacture and marketing of AYUSH products and quality of raw material are of paramount importance. The Drugs and Cosmetics Act of 1940 was amended in 1964 and Chap. IV A was introduced with regulations for the manufacture and sale of AYUSH products. Standards have been issued and Good

Manufacturing Practice (GMP) introduced. Despite notifying of these regulations, there is laxity in there adoption by the manufacturers in the States. Lack of technically qualified resource people to inspect the manufacturer's facilities and claims of manufacturers have led to many GMP non-compliant manufacturers in the market. The total number of GMP compliant units in India was 62% in 2010. Some states with more than 50% non-compliant GMP manufacturers are Madhya Pradesh, Gujarat, Tamil Nadu, Bihar and Uttarakhand (Chandra 2011).

Thus products of questionable quality are available in the market. As a result, quality of AYUSH products is questioned by consumers and it erodes confidence in the system.

6.4.9.3 Herbal Products

Most AYUSH medicinal products are of herbal origin, some are of animal and mineral origin.

Herbal medicines: Herbs or herbal products are used by a large number of populations for basic healthcare needs. Herbal medicines include herbs, herbal materials or plant parts, herbal health products, pharmaceuticals, nutraceuticals, food supplements and cosmeceuticals. Herbal medicines are an integral part of the indigenous and folk medicine. A large number of plants are used. It has been estimated that Ayurveda uses 1200–1800 plants, Siddha medicine uses 500–900 plants, Unani utilizes 300 plants while folk healers use more than 7500 (Sen and Chakraborty 2015, 2017; Galor and Benzie 2011). Many of the plants and therapies have been documented in classical texts. But there are many others which are being passed on down generations and are not documented.

Herbal medicines are preferred by some because of the perception that they are safer, being natural and less costly (Sahoo and Manchikanti 2013). However, there are many quality issues related to herbal medicines. These pertain to their identification, collection of appropriate plants, storage of raw material, processing of raw material, metallic content, standardization, packaging, labeling information, use, research, ethical advertising (Sen and Chakraborty 2017; Sahoo and Manchikanti 2013; Anonymous 2018).

To take care of all the above regulations are required. These are there for most issues mentioned above in India but the problem is lack of implementation. Standards for medicines have been specified in Pharmacopoeias (Ayurveda, Unani and Siddha), all manufacturing units must be GMP compliant. Most important evidence and scientific information about them must be available in a way that is comprehensible to all especially practitioners of modern medicine. Quality as an integral aspect has as yet not got institutionalized in the AYUSH medical systems and its drug manufacturing processes.

6.5 Integration of AYUSH with Allopathy (Modern Medicine) in India

Integrative medicine (IM), recently advocated in the West, has been defined as *"the practice of medicine that reaffirms the importance of the relationship between practitioner and patient, focuses on the whole person, is informed by evidence, and makes use of all appropriate therapeutic approaches, healthcare professionals, and disciplines to achieve optimal health and healing"* (Academic Consortium of Academic Health Centers for Integrative Medicine and Health 2018). According to the Consortium of Academic Health Centers for Integrative Medicine, over 50 universities and institutions, including Harvard University, Stanford University, and the University of Maryland, have established integrative medicine centers in North America.

Integrative medicine values all aspects of a person's health, mind, body and spirit, and considers a patient's overall satisfaction with life. It lays emphasizes on preventing disease and living well with chronic diseases.

Appropriate integration has been addressed by Dr. Margaret Chan, Director General, World Health Organization (WHO), who stated that *"the two systems of traditional and Western medicine need not clash. Within the context of primary health care, they can blend together in a beneficial harmony, using the best features of each system and compensating for certain weaknesses in each. This is not something that will happen all by itself. Deliberate policy decisions have to be taken. But it can be done successfully*" (World Health Organization 2013).

6.5.1 Reasons for Integrating Allopathy and AYUSH Systems

There are many reasons why AYUSH and Allopathy systems must be integrated into the public health system in India. Some reasons are included below.

6.5.1.1 Improve Access to Health Care

At present, India has a ratio of 0.7 doctors per 1000 patients. This is much lower than the WHO average of 2.5 doctors per 1000 people. The situation is aggravated by the concentration of medical professionals in urban areas which have only 30% of India's population.

The registered practitioners on Medical Council of India are 10.2 lakhs. Assuming there is 8.18 lakh active allopathic doctors across private and public sectors, then the doctor-patient ratio comes to 1:1612. This translates into a shortage of about 5 lakh doctors, which is going to increase as the population grows.

If the AYUSH practitioners are added to this number, the ratio will come to 1:800. This is much better than the 1:1000 recommended by WHO. The AYUSH doctors are also available in remote, rural areas, where there is an acute shortage of healthcare facilities.

Integration of AYUSH into the healthcare system has the potential to improve access to health care for the population. It will enable consumers to have a wider choice when they wish to use such services (Dua 2005; Albert and Porter 2015).

6.5.1.2 Take Care of Public Healthcare Needs in India

The prevalence and incidence of non-communicable diseases (diabetes, cardiovascular disorders, degenerative disorders, e.g., osteoarthritis) in India is increasing. For many, there are no treatments to prevent in allopathy medicine. The cost of healthcare is also skyrocketing.

Studies have shown that people use traditional and complementary medicines for chronic conditions, e.g., musculoskeletal complaints, ischemic heart disease, hypertension, hemorrhoids, for the promotion of health and some cases for treatment of acute diseases. Some of the areas where therapies of AYUSH are showing promise include bronchial asthma, rheumatoid arthritis, sinusitis, diabetes and osteoarthritis. Some therapies could be used as adjuvants and complementary to the modern medicine, for example, yoga and naturopathy for stress and hypertension (World Health Organization 2013, Chandra 2011; Bhatt et al. 2007; Buch 2014; Chopra et al. 2010).

Under the various research activities initiated by Government of India, many herbal formulations are showing promise and undergoing Phases 2, 3 of clinical trials. These include diabetes, arthritis, psoriasis and hepatocellular protection. The Central Council for Research in Unani Medicine has investigated formulations for vitiligo, sinusitis, infective hepatitis, rheumatoid arthritis and bronchial asthma. There are innumerable other therapies being offered by AYUSH systems for many conditions. The only drawback for some therapies may be lack of evidence for effectiveness as per standard criteria (Chandra 2011; Aggarwal et al. 2011; Mandhare et al. 2015; Payyappallimana 2010).

6.5.1.3 Pluralistic Medicine: Offer True Choices to Patients

With the increased availability of information on the internet, people are increasingly turning to self-health care involving the use of traditional and complementary medicine (TCM) all over the world. The acceptability of systems of medicines other than allopathy is increasing (World Health Organization 2012).

The reasons why individuals chose TCM includes their belief that it is more affordable, more closely corresponds to the patients ideology, allays concerns about adverse effects of chemical medicines, increasing demand for healthcare services, increased awareness of available options, an increased dissatisfaction with existing healthcare services, a desire for holistic care, health promotive and preventive services, desire for healthy lifestyle, failure with conventional treatments and side effects (Sahoo and Manchikanti 2013; World Health Organization 2013). In the Indian context, TCM would imply the use of AYUSH.

6.5.1.4 Promote Assimilation of Different Medical Systems

Integration of AYUSH will result in assimilation. These systems focus more on promotive and preventive healthcare. They involve a change in thinking, meditation, physical exercises, cleaning of the body and diet control. The allopathy system of medicine focuses more on the treatment of diseases and medicines form the bulk of the treatments. The best in each science will have the opportunity of getting assimilated with the other. There will be a better understanding and strengthening of the healthcare systems. History is witness to the fact that modern medicine has evolved over the centuries by the intermingling of ideas, thoughts, practices in existence all over the world. The ancient and medieval civilizations have been the building blocks on which modern medicine has been built upon.

6.5.1.5 Affordability

Out-of-pocket expenditure accounts for nearly 60% of healthcare spending (Planning Commission 2011). Many families incur debts and bankruptcy because of the same. About 3.9 million Indians are pushed to poverty because of ill health every year. Around 30% of rural India did not go for any treatment due to financial constraints in 2004. In urban areas, 20% of ailments were not treated for financial reasons in the same year. About 47% and 31% of hospital admissions respectively in rural and urban India were financed by loans and sales of assets (Kooreman and Baars 2012).

The use of AYUSH may actually bring down the healthcare costs. A study indicated that patients, whose General Practitioner (GP) has additional training in complementary and alternative systems of medicines (CAM), have lower healthcare costs and mortality rates than those who do not. This was due to fewer hospital stays and fewer prescription drugs (World Health Organization 2002).

Costs of allopathic medicine are increasing. With pharmaceutical companies filing patents for minor changes made to medicine formulations, tested AYUSH products may help offset the increased costs due to evergreening of patents.

6.5.1.6 Economic Development

Traditional medicine is being used globally. In developed countries like Australia, Canada and the United Kingdom, the annual expenditure on traditional medicine is in billions of dollars (Sahoo and Manchikanti 2013). In 1995 the total commercial value of ethnobotanicals market in 1995 was estimated to be US$ 5.1 billion. It was estimated that the annual worldwide market for these products approached US$ 60 billion around 2005 (Anonymous 2014).

In India, use of herbal medicine is a common practice. It has been estimated that approximately 25,000 plant-based formulations are available in AYUSH. Also, more than 2000 tons of medicinal plant raw materials are required annually. More than 1500 herbals are also sold as dietary supplements or ethnic traditional medicines (Sen and Chakraborty 2017; Galor and Benzie 2011). About 960 plant species are used by Indian herbal industry of which 178 are high volume, exceeding 100 metric tons per year (Sahoo and Manchikanti 2013). During 2014–2015 the export of AYUSH products was 13,620.57 cores. During the same period (2014–2015) the share of AYUSH products in the total trade of India was 0.32% (Anonymous 2014; Gangadharan and Shankar 2009).

Proper integration of AYUSH with allopathic medicine will in all likelihood increase its use. Since proper integration will require quality assurance of AYUSH products, the market for AYUSH products is likely to increase.

6.5.1.7 Promote Quality Research

Presently there is insufficient research in the area of AYUSH especially about outcomes: efficacy and the safety of the AYUSH products. This lack of evidence is a major reason why some AYUSH therapies may be looked at doubtfully. On the other hand, allopathic medicine works on evidence, created through research.

The AYUSH are traditional systems of medicines that work on different philosophies and theories. These cannot be tested or validated using the same parameters and research methodology as for allopathic medicine. A different model for evaluating therapies in AYUSH needs to be formed (Gangadharan and Shankar 2009).

AYUSH is being used by people, in many cases concomitantly along with allopathic medicines (Roy et al. 2015). There are insufficient data on the possible interactions that can occur when medicines of both systems are given. There is a possibility that adverse drug reactions may occur which may not be accounted for in the specific system of medicine since the doctor is not aware that the patient is using other traditional medicines. Most doctors do not ask and most patients do not think it is required to tell their doctor that they are taking other medicines also (Zaman et al. 2007). Many consumers think that medicines of AYUSH or other traditional medicines are safe and harmless and self-medicate (Cohen and Ernst 2010).

Integration will promote research in this area. Practitioners of both the systems, allopathy and AYUSH, will get to learn about the principles and philosophy of treatment in each system. Formulation of research methodology suitable for evaluating outcomes with AYUSH systems will evolve. AYUSH practitioners stand to gain in learning research methodology which will improve the quality of research. Research is likely to get an impetus in the area of outcomes of concomitant use of allopathic and AYUSH medicines.

6.5.1.8 Widen Global Outreach

Traditional and complementary medicines (TCM) are being used globally along with the allopathic system, in some countries to the extent of 70%–80%. It is imperative that the AYUSH products and practices be understood by healthcare providers of different streams within the country. Proper integration within the healthcare system will help in better understanding. Once the awareness and acceptance of AYUSH within the country are increased, this in itself will give an impetus to widening the global outreach of AYUSH. Chinese medicine especially acupuncture has a global acceptance because of the way in which it is established within its country of origin and the way it has been promoted (World Health Organization 2013).

6.5.1.9 Enrichment of Knowledge

As different systems grow together, one modern and others ancient and traditional, there is bound to be the enrichment of knowledge of the practitioners and users both. As they try to understand the philosophy of the other systems, new paradigms of understanding of health and the human body may emerge.

6.5.1.10 Increased Acceptance by Practitioners of Allopathy Medicine

A public health program where different medicine systems are integrated keeping in mind the advantages and disadvantages of different systems of medicines for the public in a well-informed way, where all stakeholders are aware of their roles, with regulations in place which are implemented and where quality is assured will increase its acceptance.

6.5.1.11 Holistic Healthcare

Most important integration of modern medicine and AYUSH systems will result in the provision of holistic healthcare to the people of India.

6.6 Efforts to Integrate AYUSH with Allopathy Medicine in India

There is no doubt that integration of AYUSH with the modern system is the way to go ahead. The Government of India is committed to providing pluralistic healthcare to the people of India. Various National health policy plans, Planning Commission documents all point to the intention of the Government. A brief overview (extracts) of how various National policies, Plans and Missions have tried to incorporate utilization of AYUSH over the years in the public healthcare system in India is given below. This has been done to show how the relevance of indigenous traditional systems in healthcare in India evolved. It began with only a brief mention about the ISM & H or AYUSH as they later came to be known, to gradually a complete section about them and then as the relevance of the systems to provide healthcare to the people was realized, a separate National policy for AYUSH came into being.

6.6.1 The National Health Policy 1983 (Ministry of Health & Family Welfare 1983)

Visualized a role for the ISM & H practitioners in the delivery of healthcare service.

"The policy realized that India has a large number of health manpower comprising of practitioners in various systems including AYUSH. These doctors are accepted and respected by the communities. Therefore it was necessary to utilize the services of these practitioners and integrate their services in the health care delivery system."

6.6.2 National Health Policy 2002 (Ministry of Health & Family Welfare 2002)

In the National Health Policy 2002 more emphasis was given. These, however, were mentioned as alternative systems of medicines.

"The policy stated that the alternative systems of medicine (Ayurveda, Unani, Sidha and Homeopathy) have a substantial role in healthcare delivery in the country, as they have inherent advantages such as diversity, modest cost, and growing popularity of natural plant-based products. Developing these systems would help serve the remote, underserved areas. At the same time enable India to become a global center for plant diversity in medicinal and aromatic plants. The policy aimed to encourage research in alternative systems to determine their efficacy, safety and dosage. Certification and quality assurance of products with consolidation of documentary knowledge contained in these systems to protect it against commercial exploitation by other countries was also emphasized. ".

"The policy further stated that all the main components of the NHP-2002 apply equally to the alternative systems of medicines. However, the Policy features specific to the alternative systems of medicines will be presented as a separate document."

6.6.3 National Rural Health Mission 2006–2012 (Ministry of Health & Family Welfare 2012)

The mission talked about mainstreaming and utilizing AYUSH practitioners in the National healthcare delivery systems in India, under "National Rural Health Mission (NRHM)". Yoga and Naturopathy also came to be considered under the umbrella term of AYUSH.

"The Mission document said that the AYUSH doctors shall work in the same health infrastructure available for modern practitioners. They would work according to the terms laid down by the appropriate Regulatory Authorities. AYUSH medicines would be made available and cross referrals between allopathic and AYUSH doctors will be encouraged."AYUSH health workers will work in primary health centres, Community health centres and district hospitals".

6.6.4 National Health Policy 2017 (Ministry of Health & Family Welfare 2017)

The recent National Health Policy 2017 has elaborated in detail about the role of AYUSH in the healthcare system (under different subheadings). It talks about mainstreaming all healthcare systems. For the first time the policy talks of bridge courses between AYUSH and allopathy, as well as integrated courses for Indian Systems of Medicines.

6.6.4.1 Mainstreaming the Potential of AYUSH

The policy aimed to do so by increasing access by co-location in public health facilities, introducing Yoga in schools, standardizing and validating Ayurvedic medicines and establishing quality assurance systems for AYUSH medicines. The Policy recognized the need for development of teaching institutions and capacity building of professionals. It also aimed to give a bridge course to AYUSH doctors in 15 competencies of allopathic remedies. Sensitization of practitioners of each system to the strengths of others, development of sustainable livelihoods of local communities in processing of medicinal plants, strengthening farming of herbal plants, engaging traditional community healthcare providers in conservation and generation of raw materials required, enhancing their skills and developing mechanisms for certification of "prior knowledge" of traditional community were all aspects of the policy".

A complete National Policy on Indian Systems of Medicine and Homeopathy evolved in 2002.

6.6.5 National Policy on Indian Systems of Medicine and Homeopathy-2002 (Department of AYUSH 2002)

"*Objectives: The basic objectives of this Policy are:*

(a) *To promote good health and expand the outreach of health care to our people, particularly those not provided health cover, through preventive, promotive, mitigating and curative intervention through ISM & H.*
(b) *To improve the quality of teachers and clinicians by revising curriculum to contemporary relevance and researchers by creating model institutions and Centers of Excellence and extending assistance for creating infrastructural facilities.*
(c) *To ensure affordable ISM & H services and drugs which are safe and efficacious.*
(d) *To facilitate the availability of raw drugs which are authentic and contain essential components as required under pharmacopoeial standards to help improve the quality of drugs, for domestic consumption and export.*
(e) *Integrate ISM & H in the healthcare delivery system and National Programs and ensure optimal use of the vast infrastructure of hospitals, dispensaries and physicians.*
(f) *Re-orient and prioritize research in ISM & H to gradually validate therapy and drugs to address in particular the chronic and new lifestyle related to emerging diseases.*
(g) *Create awareness about the strengths of these systems in India and abroad and sensitize other stakeholders and providers of health.*
(h) *To provide full opportunity for the growth and development of these systems and utilization of the potentiality, strength and revival of their glory."*

Various strategies for fulfilling the above have been put forth in the policy. These include for education, research, medicinal plants, intellectual property rights and patents, integration of ISM & H and National healthcare programs and delivery systems, drug standardization, and quality control, ISM industry, revitalization of local health traditions, home remedy kits, veterinary medicine, medical tourism, exposing foreign students and Indian modern graduates and increasing awareness etc."

6.6.6 The 11th Plan (2007–2012)

Recommended mainstreaming of AYUSH systems to actively supplement the efforts of the allopathic system (Planning Commission 2007).

6.6.7 The 12th Five-Year Plan

Some recommendations of the Steering Committee on Health for the 12th Five-Year Plan, pertaining to the integration of medicine systems in India are presented below. It included aspects related to research, human resource development and practice and promotion of AYUSH (Planning Commission, 2012).

6.6.7.1 Research

Standardization of terminologies and of classical therapies and development of standard treatment guidelines must be taken up as priority.

Classical drugs listed in formularies and therapies should be validated for their safety and efficacy.

All five Research Councils of AYUSH need to pool resources, human, clinical facilities and information.

6.6.7.2 Human Resource Development

1. *Doctors and nursing staff of the allopathic system need to be introduced to the positive aspects of the AYUSH systems through "short orientation modules" on AYUSH.*
2. *Development for cross-referral understanding between all systems, based on the strengths of respective systems.*
3. *At the postgraduate levels, cross-disciplinary learning between allopathy and AYUSH systems ought to be promoted. For this purpose, coordinated efforts need to be made. Suggestions given included.*
   (a) *Modifications in syllabi at undergraduate level.*
   (b) *AYUSH chairs to be established in medical colleges to provide necessary technical expertise to jointly take up research, teaching and patient care.*

6.6.7.3 On Practice and Promotion of AYUSH

Standards need to be established and tertiary level AYUSH facilities similar to Indian Public Health Standard (IPHS)

- *Standard treatment guidelines and Model Drug Lists need to be developed for community health workers.*
- *AYUSH services of an appropriate standard should be provided at all primary, secondary and tertiary care institutions under the MOHFW, State Health Departments and other Ministries like Railways, Labor and Home Affairs.*
- *Roles and responsibilities of AYUSH colleges should be defined for contributing towards National Health Outcomes.*
- *AYUSH-based lifestyles guidelines should be considered for RCH, adolescent health, geriatric care, mental health, non-communicable diseases, anemia, nutrition and health promotion by establishing "Joint behavioural change plans".*
- *"Bridge courses" and appropriate modifications in regulations "should be considered so as to facilitate the prescription of essential allopathic medicines by AYUSH practitioners.*

Table 6.1 Level of integration of AYUSH in the public healthcare facilities

Facility	Total units	Number (%) of co-located AYUSH facilities
Primary Health Centers	23,391	8366 (35.77)
Community Health Centers	4510	2945 (65.3)
District Hospitals	602	404 (70.2)

The Government is committed to the integration of healthcare systems. Prior to 2005, the working of AYUSH systems was completely separate from the existing medical and public health systems. A physical integration was introduced as a part of National Rural Health Mission. Despite plans and policy changes the level of integration at different levels of health care as per the Steering Committee's report is shown in Table 6.1. (This may have improved in the last few years).

It is obvious that there is a gap between the state of modern medicine and AYUSH in the country. This gap needs to be bridged.

6.7 Way Forward

A lot has been achieved as regards development of the different AYUSH systems in the country. But true integration is still far off. Even utilization of AYUSH systems is not optimum due to many reasons which have been highlighted above.

What is needed is for a quality assured AYUSH system to get established within the country, where the purity, philosophy and approach to healthcare of each system are maintained. No dilution of AYUSH with allopathy should be attempted. The orders and demands that AYUSH practitioners be allowed to prescribe allopathic medicines, using the justification that they are needed to meet the public healthcare needs of rural India are far-fetched. Such actions will result in dilution of AYUSH systems and at the same time not achieve public health goals (Chandra and Parwardhan 2018). It will only result in further eroding the essence and strength of the AYUSH systems of medicines.

Basically, two approaches are needed Top down and Bottom up.

6.7.1 Top Down

This means working from policy downwards, as is what is happening at the moment. These include:

- *Policy:* Various National Health Policies have been incorporating and defining the role of AYUSH. With each new policy, the role of AYUSH in public health care has expanded.
- *Planning:* Different plan documents have already written about the need to integrate AYUSH with the modern system in the public health system.
- *Implementation:* This is a problem area. An important policy initiative has been the utilization of AYUSH practitioners in public health facilities under NRHM. AYUSH practitioners have been posted along with allopathic doctors. There are many gaps in the way this has been done. The AYUSH doctors sent through NHRM are working in isolation from AYUSH doctors posted through the non-NHRM system. The roles of AYUSH doctors, especially in emergency duties have not been clearly defined. Thus there is a lack of communication even among the AYUSH practitioners posted in health facilities. Confusion prevails as regards prescribing of allopathic medicines by AYUSH doctors (this aspect, in any case, will not be looked upon favorably by allopathic doctors). There is a lack of infrastructure in many AYUSH facilities. Lack of availability of AYUSH medicines has also been a problem (Chandra 2011; Vaidya 2005).

  There must be a planned coordination between the Central Government and State Governments. Further, there should not be any division between doctors of AYUSH posted through State postings and NRHM. The hierarchy within the HF must be established, so the AYUSH doctor knows who to report to.

  The role of AYUSH practitioners must be clearly defined. This includes the medical problems that they will handle. The infrastructure and medicines needed by the AYUSH practitioners must be made available.
- *Education and Training:* This is an extremely relevant area. The quality of training being imparted to AYUSH graduates needs to improve significantly. In a way that the philosophy, science and art of the system are retained. The different Central Councils making the curriculum must be trained on planning curriculum, based on what are the objectives of teaching in that subject. In the same way that the Medical Council of India does for allopathy courses. Curriculum changes, skills to be imparted and resources required for the same must be identified. Most importantly Government support to provide infrastructure, training and hand holding of the institutes is a must. These institutes of learning must be monitored to assess outcomes. The graduates and postgraduates coming out of these institutes must be confident of their knowledge and learning. Most important they must feel pride in their achievement and their qualification.

To begin with, a few centers already imparting quality AYUSH education in the country must be identified. These should be developed as Centers of Excellence. The graduates and postgraduates from these institutes must be absorbed in the public health system. Their roles and work well identified.

Having established their quality, these centers could then work with allopathic institutes. Again these institutes would also have to be identified.

A program for continuous monitoring of these AYUSH centers for learning will have to be established.

6.7.2 Bottom Up Approach

In addition to the above, what is also needed in addition is a bottom up approach. Here the immediate providers of healthcare to the public need to be trained in the best practices of each other's medicine system. More important allopathic doctors need to be sensitized to the philosophy and basic fundamentals of AYUSH. Educational intervention needs to be planned and implemented for both doctors of allopathy and AYUSH. This has to be both short term and long term. In short-term bridge courses, continuous medical education workshops, development of modules and standard operating procedures along with research must be done. In long term starting of courses in integrative medicine must be done.

6.7.2.1 Short-Term Educational Intervention

- *Bridge Courses*: These should be started for both practitioners of allopathy medicine in AYUSH medicine and for practitioners of AYUSH in allopathy medicine. A group of doctors from both systems who are interested in integrated medicine, need to be brought together to help formulate the course content for such a course. A dialogue must be started between doctors from different systems. Like-minded people should be brought together to begin the process.

  There are practitioners of allopathic medicine who are open to the idea of utilizing AYUSH and would be willing to give their time and thoughts to develop such a course module. They should be invited for the same.

  The purpose of these bridge courses must be defined right in the beginning. These must be for sensitizing and increasing awareness of doctors about each other's system of medicine. *Undergoing the Bridge course will not, in any case, give them a licentiate to practice that system. This must be told before in no uncertain terms and legal repercussions of doing the same must also be told beforehand.*
- *Continuous Medical Education Workshops*: On the best practices in AYUSH must be organized. Wherever there is sufficient evidence those therapies must be told and shown to the allopathic doctors. There are some therapies and procedures in AYUSH for which evidence of their efficacy is there. These need to be highlighted. A healthy discussion between doctors from allopathy and AYUSH must be encouraged.
- *Modules:* Modules for treatment of a limited number of medical conditions where there are proven therapies in AYUSH need to be made. These must also be based on evidence made available in the best possible way. These modules must be highlighted and discussed in CMEs with allopathy doctors.
- *Research*: In AYUSH therapies, as well as on outcomes when both allopathy and AYUSH is used concomitantly must be conducted.

6.7.3 Starting Departments of Integrative Medicine

Once the above actions are done, it is expected that a minimum number of human resource personnel, aware and trained in both allopathy and AYUSH systems would be available. These practitioners could be then asked to plan and implement a course in integrative medicine.

- *Course in integrative medicine*: The course must be developed by doctors interested and aware about AYUSH from allopathy. A multidisciplinary team including AYUSH and allopathy doctors should be given the task. The course must undergo rigorous scrutiny by experts from all branches from both AYUSH and allopathy systems. The course could be brought under the ambit of Medical Council of India or any other authority regulating medical education in India. It could be a diploma or degree course.

- *Patient services in integrative medicine*: At the same time, with this minimum resource material ready, departments of integrative medicine should be started. To begin with, a few medical colleges need to be identified where the department of integrative medicine could be started. The educational environment of those institutions must be assessed first. Medical colleges where there are already outpatients departments (OPDs) or departments of AYUSH functioning and where some allopathic faculty is interested should be selected.

  This idea must not be imposed from the top, rather the enthusiasm of the institute to take the idea ahead must be assessed. These could be Medical colleges or institutes under Government of India.

  All help in terms of planning, financial support, human resources required must be given to these centers by the Government.

  These centers must be nurtured. The progress and problems in the implementation of the program must be monitored.

- *Research in integrative medicine*: Simultaneously research in specific areas must be encouraged. The findings of which should be publicized. All protocols for research must be made by investigators from both allopathic and AYUSH streams.

  Slowly these centers of integrative medicine, as they are nurtured, will expand. The confidence of policymakers, administrators, doctors and the public will increase. These can then be expanded to more medical colleges in the country. This can only happen when there is sufficient faculty from both the allopathic and AYUSH trained in the other system of medicine and integrative medicine.

  While integrative courses are the future, right now it is too early to think of degree or even a diploma course in integrative medicine as is there in other countries like China and USA. A critical mass of professionals who are aware of what integrative medicine entails is required before India can start degree courses in integrative medicine.

  In the meantime, it is of paramount importance that the Government ensures quality in the practice and products of AYUSH. This is required not only for increasing its acceptance nationally but also globally.

6.8 Conclusion

India has a rich heritage of indigenous medical systems. Realization of their value along with their nurturing is the need of the hour. AYUSH should be allowed to grow and develop independently with inbuilt quality assurance measures. True integration of indigenous medicine systems will happen only when AYUSH has established its own true identity. It is the right of the people of India to be offered true choices, which include integrated medicine in healthcare.

References

Academic Consortium of Academic Health Centers for Integrative Medicine and Health. Definition of integrative medicine. 2018. https://imconsortium.org/about/introduction/. Accessed 20 Jul 2018.

Aggarwal BB, Prasad S, Reuter S, et al. Identification of novel anti-inflammatory agents from ayurvedic medicine for prevention of chronic diseases: "reverse pharmacology" and "bedside to branch" approach. Curr Drug Target. 2011;12:1595–653.

Albert S, Porter J. Is mainstreaming AYUSH the right policy for Meghalaya, north east India? BMC Complement Altern Med. 2015;15:288.

Anonymous. CCRAS research an overview, Central Council for Research in Ayurveda and Sciences. New Delhi: Department of AYUSH, Ministry of Health & Family Welfare, Government of India; 2002. p. 63–8.

Anonymous. Section 9: AYUSH related Foreign Trade 2014. AYUSH. http://www.indianmedicine.nic.in/writercaddata/linkimages/0145351269-AYUSH-related-foreign-trade.pdf. 2014. Accessed 12 Jul 2018.

Anonymous. The basics: defining integrative medicine. 2018. http://www.thenewmedicine.org/about_integrative_medicine/defining.html. Accessed 25 Jun 2018.

AYUSH Ministry. Government of India. Summary of All India AYUSH infrastructure facility. 2018. http://www.ayush.gov.in/sites/default/files/summary.pdf. Accessed 18 Jul 2018.

AYUSH Ministry. Government of India. AYUSH. 2015. http://www.nhp.gov.in/ayush_ms. Accessed 18 Jul 2018.

Bhatt S, Gupta V, Srikanth N. Feasibility of integrating Ayurveda with modern system of medicine in a Tertiary Care Hospital for management of osteoarthritis (knee)- an observational study. Technical report Central Council for Research in Ayurveda and Siddha. 2007.

Buch ZM. Role of Ayurveda integrated cancer rehabilitation: Ayurvaids integrated cancer rehabilitation program (ICRP)—a role model. Int Ayurvedic Med J. 2014;2:233–8.

Central Council for Research in Ayurveda and Siddha. An appraisal of tribal- folk medicines. New Delhi: Department of AYUSH, Ministry of Health and family Welfare, Government of India; 1999.

Chandra S, Parwardhan K. Allopathic, AYUSH and informal medical practitioners in rural India- a prescription for change. J Ayurveda Integr Med. 2018;9:143–50.

Chandra S. Status of Indian medicine & folk healing: with a focus on benefits that the systems have given to the public. Under the aegis of Department of AYUSH, Ministry of Health & Family Welfare, Government of India. 2011. http://www.over2shailja.wordpress.com/2011/10/13status-of-indian-medicine-and-folk-healing/.

Chopra A, Saluja M, Tillu G. Ayurveda- modern medicine interface- a critical appraisal of studies of ayurvedic medicines to treat osteoarthritis and rheumatoid arthritis. J Ayurveda Integr Med. 2010;1:190–8.

Cohen PA, Ernst E. Safety of herbal supplements a guide for cardiologists. Cardiovasc Ther. 2010;28:246–53.

Department of AYUSH. Ministry of health & family welfare, Government of India. National policy on Indian systems of medicine and homeopathy 2002. http://ayush.gov.in/sites/default/files/7870046089-Ayush%20%20n%20policy%20ISM%20and%20H%20Homeopathy_0.pdf (2002). Accessed 12 Jul 2018.

Dua AS. Human resources for health. In: Lal PG, Byword Editorial Consultants, editors. In financing & delivery of health care services in India. New Delhi: Cirrus Graphics Pvt. Ltd. National Commission on Macroeconomics and Health, Ministry of Health & Family Welfare, Government of India; 2005. p. 153–71.

FOD(NSSO)—Ministry of Statistics and PI. Government of India. Utilization of medical services (42nd Round), New Delhi 1986–1987. 2016. http://www.icssrdataservice.in/datarepository/index.php/catalog/17/access-policy. Accessed 5 Aug 2018.

Galor SW, Benzie IFF. Herbal medicine: an introduction to its history, usage, regulation, current trends and research needs. In: Benzie IFF, Wachtel-Galor S, editors. Herbal medicine: biomolecular and clinical aspects. 2nd ed. Boca Raton (FL): CRC Press Taylor & Francis; 2011. https://www.ncbi.nlm.nih.gov/books/NBBK92773.

Gangadharan GG, Shankar D. Medical Pluralism-the challenges ahead. Indian J Tradit Knowl. 2009;8:181–4.

Government of India. Ministry of Health & Family Welfare. Drugs & Cosmetics Act (1940) and Rules (1945). 2014. http://www.cdsco.nic.in/writereaddata/Drugs&CosmeticAct.pdf. Accessed 29 Oct 2014.

IMA. IMA against AYUSH practitioners prescribing allopathy. 2013. https://www.homeobook.com/ima-against-ayush-practitioners-prescribing-allopathy/. Accessed 5 Aug 2018.

Kooreman P, Baars EW. Patients whose GP knows complementary medicine tend to have lower costs and live longer. Eur J Health Econ. 2012;13(6):769–77.

Mandhare PM, Garje BH, Khade AA. Importance of herbal remedies in the treatment of HIV and TB infection. Int J Sci Res Methodol. 2015;1:1–17.

Ministry of Health & Family Welfare. Government of India. National RURAL Health Mission—Meeting people's health needs in rural areas (Framework for Implementation 2005–2012). 2012. http://nhm.gov.in/images/pdf/about-nrhm/nrhm-framework-implementation/nrhm-framework-latest.pdf. Accessed 9 Jul 2018.

Ministry of Health & Family Welfare. Government of India. National Health Policy. 1983. http://www.communityhealth.in/~commun26/wiki/images/6/64/Nhp_1983.pdf. Accessed 10 Jun 2018.

Ministry of Health & Family Welfare. Government of India. National Health Policy 2017. https://www.nhp.gov.in/nhpfiles/national_health_policy_2017.pdf. Accessed Jun 2018.

Ministry of Health & Family Welfare. Govt. of India. National Health Policy-2002. 2002. https://www.india.gov.in/national-health-policy-2002-0. Accessed 10 Jun 2018.

Nundy M. Primary health care in India: review of policy, plan and committee reports. In: Lal PG, Byword Editorial Consultants, editors. Financing & delivery of health care services in India. New Delhi: Cirrus Graphics Pvt. Ltd. National Commission on Macroeconomics and Health, Ministry of Health & Family Welfare, Government of India; 2005. p. 39–42.

Payyappallimana U. Role of traditional medicine in primary health care: an overview of perspectives and challenges. Yokohama J Soc Sci. 2010;14:57–77.

Planning Commission. Government of India. Report of the Steering Committee on Health for the 12th 11th Five-Year Plan 2007-12. 2007. http://planningcommission.nic.in/aboutus/committee/wrkgrp11/wg11_hayush.pdf. Accessed 9 Jul 2018.

Planning Commission. Government of India. High level expert group report on universal health coverage for India 2011. 2011. http://planningcommission.nic.in/reports/genrep/rep_uhc0812.pdf. Accessed 12 Jul 2018.

Planning Commission. Government of India. Steering Committee on Health. 12th Five Year Plan 2012. http://planningcommission.nic.in/aboutus/committee/strgrp12/st_health0203.pdf. Accessed 5 Aug 2018.

Priya R, Shweta AS. Status and role of AYUSH and local health traditions under the National Rural Health Mission-Report of a study. New Delhi: National Health Systems Resource Centre (NHSRC), National Rural Health Mission, Ministry of Health and Family Welfare, Government of India; 2010.

Roy V, Gupta M, Ghosh RK. Perception, attitude & usage of complimentary & alternative medicines among doctors and patients in a tertiary care hospital in India. Indian J Pharmacol. 2015;47:137–42.

Sahoo N, Manchikanti P. Herbal drug regulation and commercialization: an Indian industry perspective. J Altern Complement Med. 2013;19:957–63.

Sen S, Chakraborty R. Toward the integration and advancement of herbal medicine: a focus on traditional Indian medicine. Bot Target Ther. 2015;5:33–44.

Sen S, Chakraborty R. Revival, modernization and integration of Indian traditional herbal medicine in clinical practice: importance, challenges and future. J Trad Complent Med. 2017;7:234–44.

Singh P, Yadav RJ, Pandey A. Utilization of indigenous systems of medicines and homeopathy in India. Ind J Med Res. 2005;122:137–42.

Subbbarayappa BV. The roots of ancient medicine: a historical outline. J Biosci. 2001;26:135–43.

Sujatha V. What could integrative medicine mean? Social science perspectives on contemporary Ayurveda. J Ayurveda Integr Med. 2011;2:115–23.

Sundar R. Household survey of Health Care utilization and expenditure. National Council of Applied Economic Research, New Delhi 1995. http://www.ncaer.org/publication_details.php?pID=142. Accessed 5 Aug 2018.

Supreme Court of India. Judgement in the case of Dr. Mukhtiar Chand and others vs State of Punjab and Others, 08/10/1998. 1998. https://www.indiankanron.org/doc/484509/. Accessed 29 Oct 2014.

Supreme Court of India. Judgment in the case of Poonam Verma Vs Ashwin Patel and others. 1996. http:// indiankanoon.org/doc/611474/. Accessed 5 Aug 2018.

United Nations. The Declaration of Alma Ata. 1978. http://www.who.int/publications/almaata_declaration_en.pdf. Accessed 14 Jul 2018.

Vaidya ADB. Effective integration of Indian Systems of Medicine in health care delivery: people's participation, access and choice in a pluralistic democracy. In: Lal PG, Byword Editorial Consultants, editors. Financing & delivery of Health Care Services in India. New Delhi: National Commission on Macroeconomics and Health, Ministry of Health & Family Welfare, Government of India; 2005. p. 39–42.

World Health Organization. Traditional Medicine Strategy 2014–23. 2013. http://www.who.int/medicines/publications/traditional/trm_strategy14_23/en/. Accessed 12 Jul 2018.

World Health Organization. Global Health Statistics 2012. 2012. http://www.who.int/gho/publications/world_health_statistics/2012/en. Accessed 12 Jul 2018.

World Health Organization. Universal Health Coverage. 2018. https://www.paho.org/hq/index.php?option=com_content&view=article&id=9392%3Auniversal-health-coverage&Itemid=40244&lang=en. Accessed June 2018.

World Health Organization. WHO Traditional medicine strategy 2002–2005. 2002 Geneva: World Health Organization; http://apps.who.int/iris/bitstream/handle/10665/92455/9789241506090_eng.pdf;jsessionid=C198C0977291DEBCE60D69D7DC8B329B?sequence=1/.

Zaman T, Agarwal S, Handa R. Complimentary and alternative medicine use in rheumatoid arthritis: an audit of patients visiting a tertiary care center. Natl Med J India. 2007;20:236–9.

Home Herbal Garden for Promotion of Herbal Health Care System in Tripura

7

Pawan K. Kaushik and Poulami Saha

Contents

7.1 Background

Ayurveda, which literally means the science of life, is an ancient Indian system of natural and holistic medicine. The Atharvaveda, one of the four Vedas in Indian civilization, is the origin of Ayurvedic practices which includes the use of herbal medicines along with mineral or metal supplementation, surgical techniques, opium, and application of oil by massages. A herb can be broadly defined as a plant used for a specific purpose other than nourishment (Hemadri 1981; Kumar 2002). It includes a wide diversity of forms including trees, shrubs, Sub-shrubs, herbaceous perennials, ground covers, and vines. In many developing countries, a large proportion of the population relies on traditional practitioners and their armamentarium of medicinal plants in order to meet health care needs and where the herbal plants are one of them on treated as traditional practitionaries. Ayurveda is a medical system primarily practiced in India that has been known for nearly 5000 years; it includes herbal plants to made traditional diagnosis. Ayurveda is gaining prominence as the natural system of health care all over the world. Today this system of medicine is being practiced in countries like Nepal, Bhutan, Sri Lanka, Bangladesh, and Pakistan, while the traditional system of medicine in the other countries like Tibet, Mongolia, and Thailand appear to be derived from Ayurveda,

P. K. Kaushik (✉) · P. Saha
Forest Research Centre for Livelihood Extension (FRC-LE), Agartala, India

Indian Council of Forestry Research and Education, Dehradun, India

S. Sen, R. Chakraborty (eds.), *Herbal Medicine in India*,
https://doi.org/10.1007/978-981-13-7248-3_7

but this Ayurveda is a system of herbal medicine used and practice in India with its medicinal value to diagnosis different diseases (Billore et al. 1998; Rao and Jamir 1982; Kumar 2002).

7.2 Concept of Home Herbal Garden

In the medicinal world, herbs have been used for centuries to help with a variety of ailments. "Old fashioned remedies" are for the most part herb based and have been used for generations to help with conditions from upset stomachs to anxiety and even strengthening the immune system. The first apothecaries (pharmacies) were stocked with botanical ingredients. Garlic is considered to be good for the heart and cholesterol conditions and has been shown in studies to possess anti-bacterial an anti-viral properties effective in boosting the immune system and fighting all types of infections. Lemon balm, lavender, and marjoram can calm nerves and reduce anxiety. And peppermint is soothing and settling to a "sour stomach."' In studies, it has shown that "The wise, old herbs" such as sage and rosemary enhance the brain function and may help to ward away Alzheimer's disease. Planting a herb garden is a wonderful way to enjoy the sights, smells, and tastes of a wide variety of plants. Fresh herbs are often easy to cultivate and can grow in a small garden in the back yard, in pots on an outdoor patio or sunroom, or even in a window box inside a kitchen. It is a great activity that can be shared with others like grandchildren, with friends in a club as a social activity, or even alone. Not only is gardening relaxing but it also improves hand-eye coordination, motor skills, and self-esteem. Herbs have an important role in human life; they are beneficial for getting a fruitful healthy body and they also have lots of medicinal benefits. Herbs have the capacity of treating dreaded diseases. Many users go for herbs supplements for overcoming their shortcomings related to health. Today varied types of herbs are used as a medicinal plant with different qualities like flavour, scent, and other things. Also herbs are used in the preparation of herbal foods and for spiritual activities in social life. Herbs have an important role in providing effective healthy life. Also it is found that herbs show its importance in varied forms such as culinary, spiritual, and medicinal. Different parts of the herbs such as leaves, roots, flowers, seeds, resin, stems, root barks, or essential oils are used in several activities especially for spiritual activities. The idea behind the herbal garden besides preservation is to get access to various herbs at one spot as and when necessary or required.

7.3 Traditional Healing Practices in Tripura

Vadyaraj Herbal Grower's Society (VHGS) operates in Kanchanpur. The traditional healers (Kaviraj) at Netaji Nagar and Dupatachara area of Kanchanpur have established herbal gardens (400–2000 m^2) on their homesteads and about 100 species of medicinal herbs have been planted and well maintained in the gardens. A participatory plan to study their performance under domestication and thereby livelihood development and promotion of medicinal plants is under finalization. The practitioners of Vaidyaraj Herbal Growers Society (VHGS) have created ten such herbal gardens across Kanchanpur sub-division in North Tripura district. The members of the society, who belong to different tribes like Tripuri, Reang, Jamatia, Noatia, Chakma, gather regularly in the garden to nurture the herbal medicinal plant and share their traditional knowledge. The group is also preserving their ancestral knowledge and compiling and documenting experiences on Ayurveda in the form of a book to pass it on to the future generations. The garden is one among the many herbal gardens started in the area by some 55 traditional Ayurveda practitioners.

7.4 Species Composition in Home Herbal Garden

7.4.1 Initiatives and Preferences of Traditional Healers

The members of the society, with some financial and technical help from the "Forest Research Centre for Livelihood Extension (FRCLE), Agartala" have collected hundreds of rare species of herbs useful in preparing Ayurvedic medicines from far-flung areas and are growing them in these gardens to study the *Ex-situ* conservation of medicinal plants on promotion of traditional healing practices under Vadyaraj Herbal Grower's Society. It creats a self-help healers group with 55 traditional healers from different tribes to collect, grow, and market over 200 varieties of rare and endangered medicinal plants. The sampling, survey, and interviews are held individually as well as collectively, for the further information gathered in the future. The data/information thus gathered is taken back to the community not only for verification but also to ensure that the community gets the benefit that data offer.

7.4.2 Participatory Appraisal on Common Diseases and Preferred Plants

7.4.2.1 Aspects of Healing Practices

A survey among the folk medicine practitioners carried out to understand their treatment strategy and to know about available folk medicine to treat different diseases or conditions like bone fracture, skin disease, heart disease, stomach disorder, arthritis, fever, cold and cough, general weakness, fistula and piles, and gynaecological disorders. Server results are tabulated in Table 7.2 and Figs. 7.1, 7.2, 7.3, 7.4, 7.5, 7.6, 7.7, 7.8, 7.9, 7.10, and 7.11.

7.4.2.2 Issue of Traditional Healers

During the survey questions also asked on few issues like sustainability of the practices and availability of medicinal plants.

Out of the 30 respondent traditional healers 12 claimed that the practices of herbal medicine are sustainable whereas the rest respondents think that practices of herbal medicine as "Vaidyaraj" are sustainable for their life (Fig. 7.12).

Out of the 30 respondent traditional healers 25 claimed that the herbal gardens and herbs are available for preparing medicine whereas the rest respondents said that it is difficult for them to collect herbal medicines from the forest (Fig. 7.13). Figure 7.14 includes picture of herbal medicine, herbal garden and its plantation design. Figure 7.15 includes picture of training workshop conducted. Table 7.3 includes list of medicinal plants and their uses.

Table 7.1 List of Herbal garden established by Kanchanpur Herbal group, North Tripura

Sl No	Name	Location in Tripura		Date of establishment	No of species
		Village	Area		
1	Harendra Reang	Kanchanpur	Mitrojoy Para	17/09/2014	22
2	Puronjoy and Suronjoy	Kanchanpur	Company para	19/09/2014	07
3	Arun Kumar Chakma, Nandalal Chakma and Premnlal Chakma	Kanchanpur	Dopatacherra	08/04/2014	18
4	Agni Kumar Chakma	Kanchanpur	Chandra Mohan para	02/09/2012	100
5	Harendra Reang	Urichara	Subhash Nagar	05/11/2014	07
6	Ananda Goswami	Joysree Gram	Subhash Nagar	16/12/2014	75
7	Amiya Chowdhury	Kanchanpur	Netaji Nagar	16/12/2014	150
8	Sukanta Choudhury	Kanchanpur	Netaji Nagar	16/12/2014	100
9	Bikash Ch. Reang Parendra Reang Khajaram Reong	Kanchanpur	PurbaSatnala (Dangasara)	02/01/2015	21
10	Sri Ratenshar Chakma	Kanchanpur	PurbaSatnala (Dangasara)	02/01/2015	35
11	Barana Ram Reang	Kanchanpur	Purba Satnala (Dangasara)	02/01/2015	33
12	Purnamani Chakma	Kanchanpur	Netaji Nagar	02/01/2015	50
13	Karnamoy Chakma	Kanchanpur	Netaji Nagar	02/01/2015	50
14	Shri Bir Bahadur Reang	Kanchanpur	Gobinda para	2014	100

Table 7.2 Response of traditional healers in respect to cure different diseases/conditions

Sl No	Name of disease	Response of traditional healers	Figure
1	Bone fracture	Out of the 30 respondent traditional healers 24 claimed they have the ailments for bone fracture	Fig. 7.1
2	Jaundice	Out of the 30 respondent traditional healers 24 claimed they have the ailments for the disease	Fig. 7.2
3	Skin disease	Out of the 30 respondent traditional healers 26 claimed they have the ailments for the disease	Fig. 7.3
4	Heart disease	Out of the 30 respondent traditional healers 14 claimed they have the ailments for the disease	Fig. 7.4
5	Stomach disorder	Out of the 30 respondent traditional healers 27 claimed they have the ailments for the disease	Fig. 7.5
6	Arthritis	Out of the 30 respondent traditional healers 23 claimed they have the ailments for the disease	Fig. 7.6
7	Fever	Out of the 30 respondent traditional healers 27 claimed they have the ailments for the disease	Fig. 7.7
8	Cold and cough	Out of the 30 respondent traditional healers 26 claimed they have the ailments for the disease	Fig. 7.8
9	General weakness	Out of the 30 respondent traditional healers 27 claimed they have the ailments for the disease	Fig. 7.9
10	Fistula and piles	Out of the 30 respondent traditional healers 18 claimed they have the ailments for the disease	Fig. 7.10
11	Gynecological disorders	Out of the 30 respondent traditional healers 21 claimed they have the ailments for the disease	Fig. 7.11

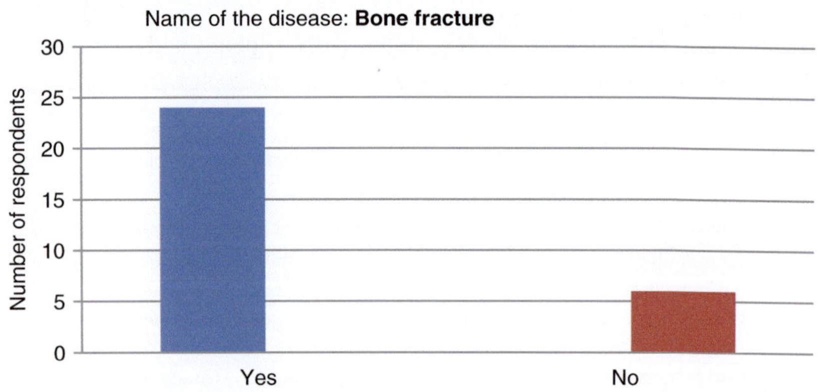

Fig. 7.1 Response of traditional healers about healing of bone fracture by folk medicine

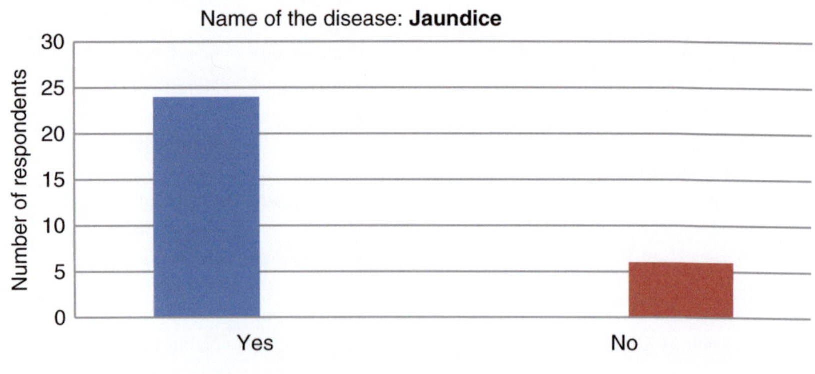

Fig. 7.2 Response of traditional healers about the treatment of jaundice by folk medicine

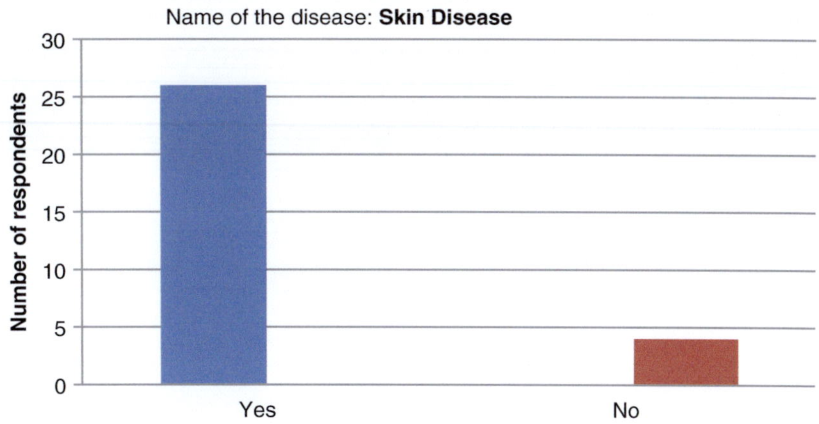

Fig. 7.3 Response of traditional healers about the treatment of skin disease by folk medicine

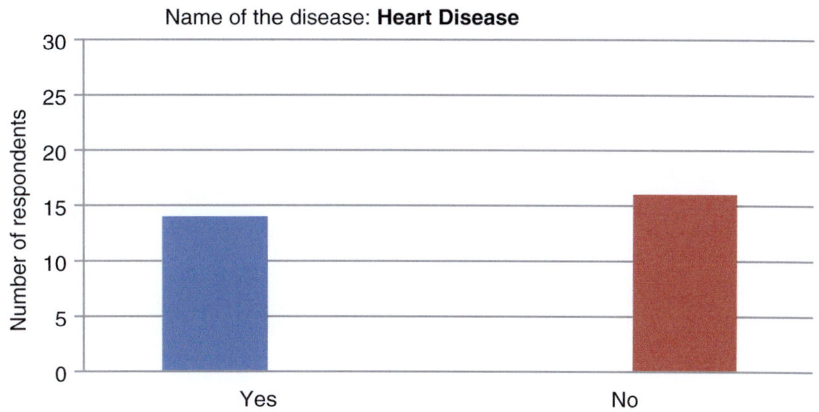

Fig. 7.4 Response of traditional healers about the treatment of heart disease by folk medicine

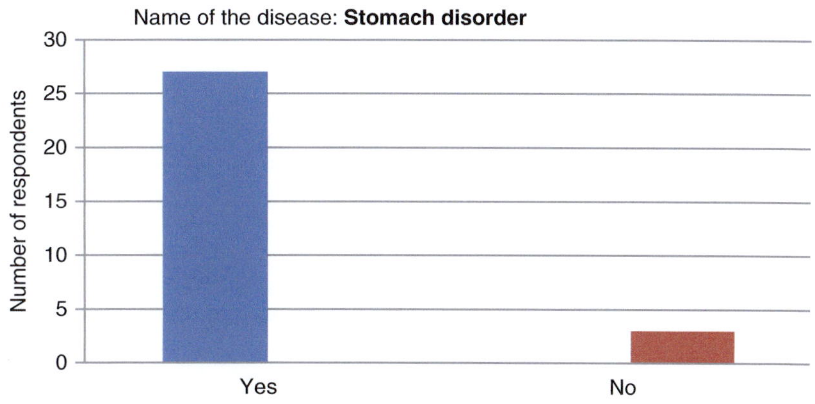

Fig. 7.5 Response of traditional healers about the treatment of stomach disorders by folk medicine

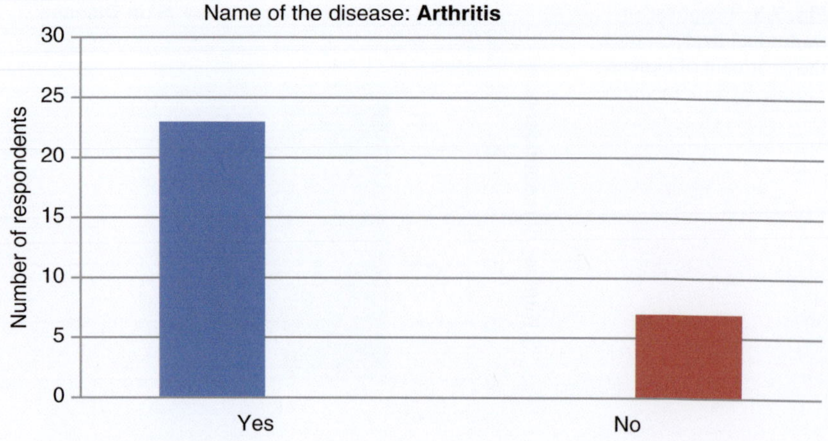

Fig. 7.6 Response of traditional healers about the treatment of arthritis by folk medicine

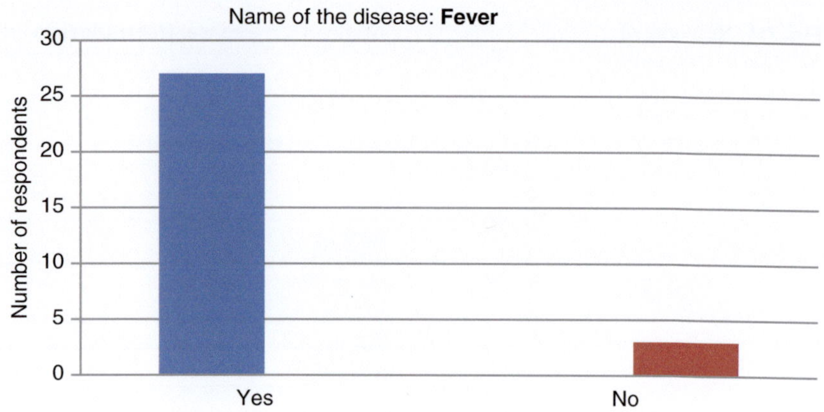

Fig. 7.7 Response of traditional healers about the treatment of fever by folk medicine

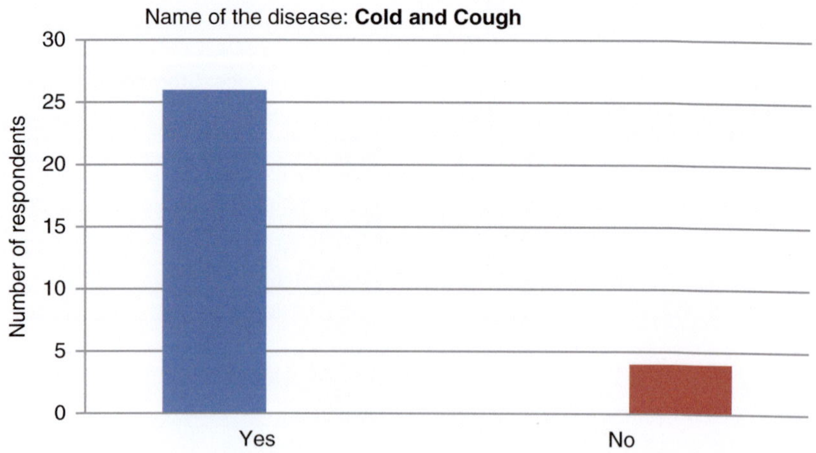

Fig. 7.8 Response of traditional healers about the treatment of cold and cough by folk medicine

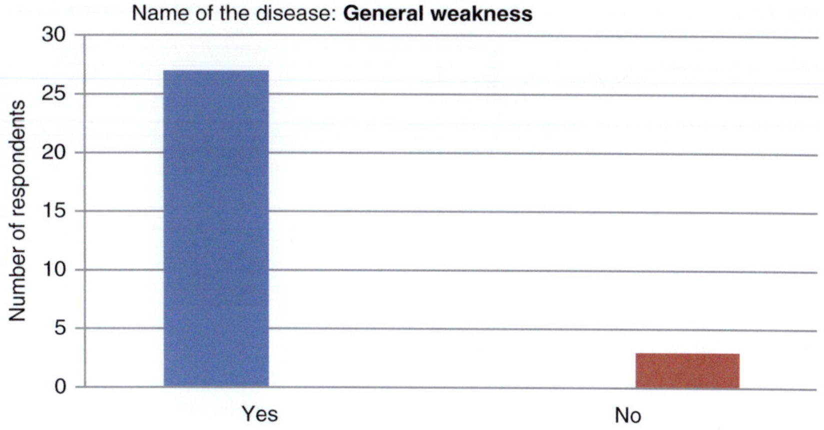

Fig. 7.9 Response of traditional healers about the treatment of general weakness by folk medicine

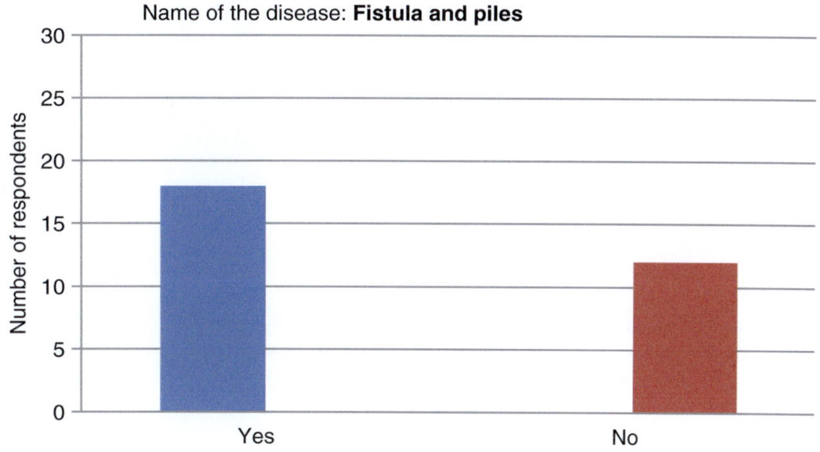

Fig. 7.10 Response of traditional healers about the treatment of fistula and piles by folk medicine

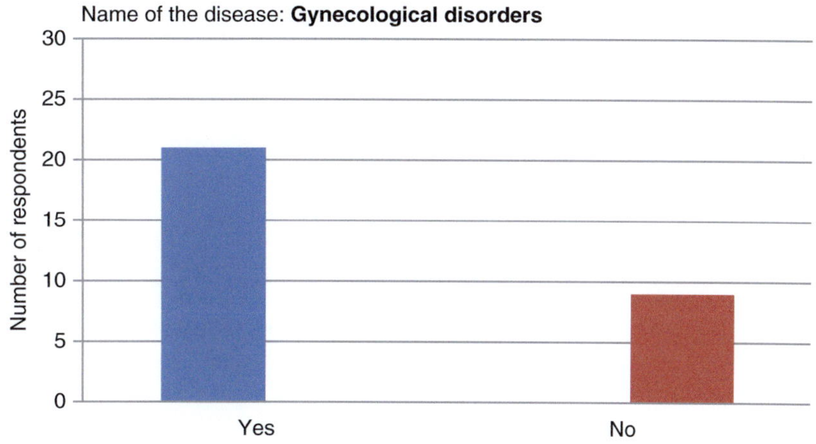

Fig. 7.11 Response of traditional healers about the treatment of fistula and piles by folk medicine

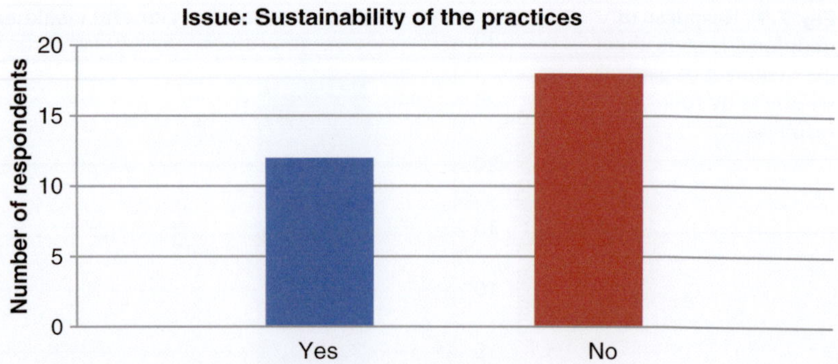

Fig. 7.12 Response of traditional healers on the issue sustainability of the practices

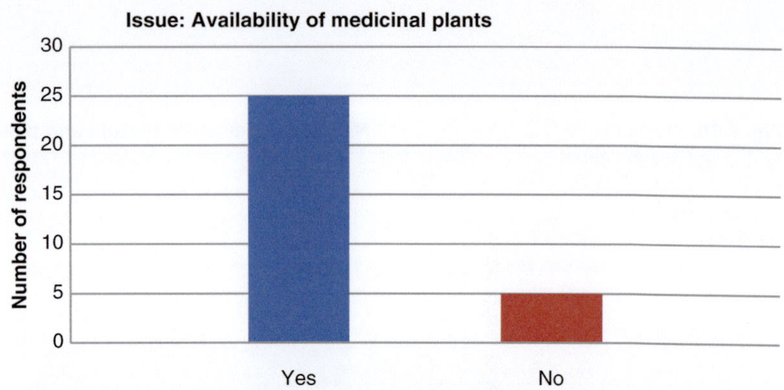

Fig. 7.13 Response of traditional healers on the availability of medicinal plants

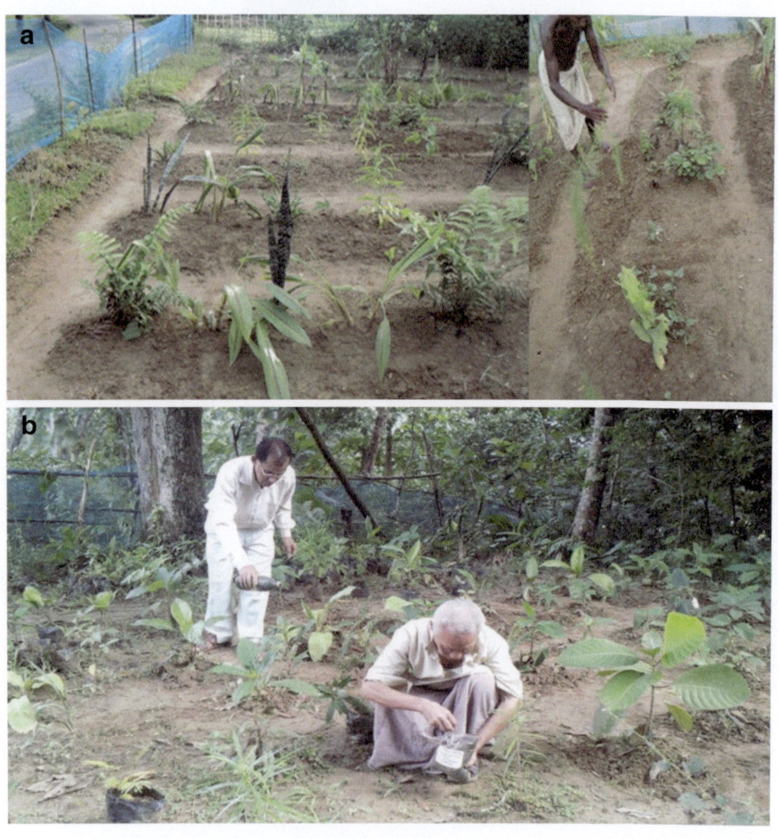

Fig. 7.14 (**a**) and (**b**) Plantation design for home herbal garden and (**c**) a folk medicinal practitioner with his medicine

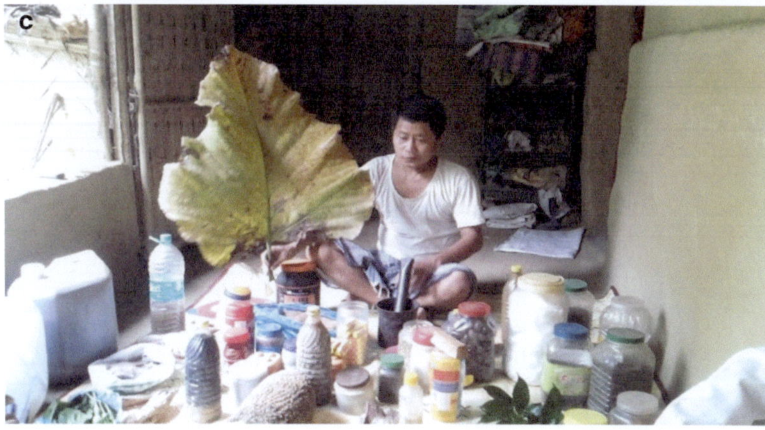

Fig. 7.14 (continued)

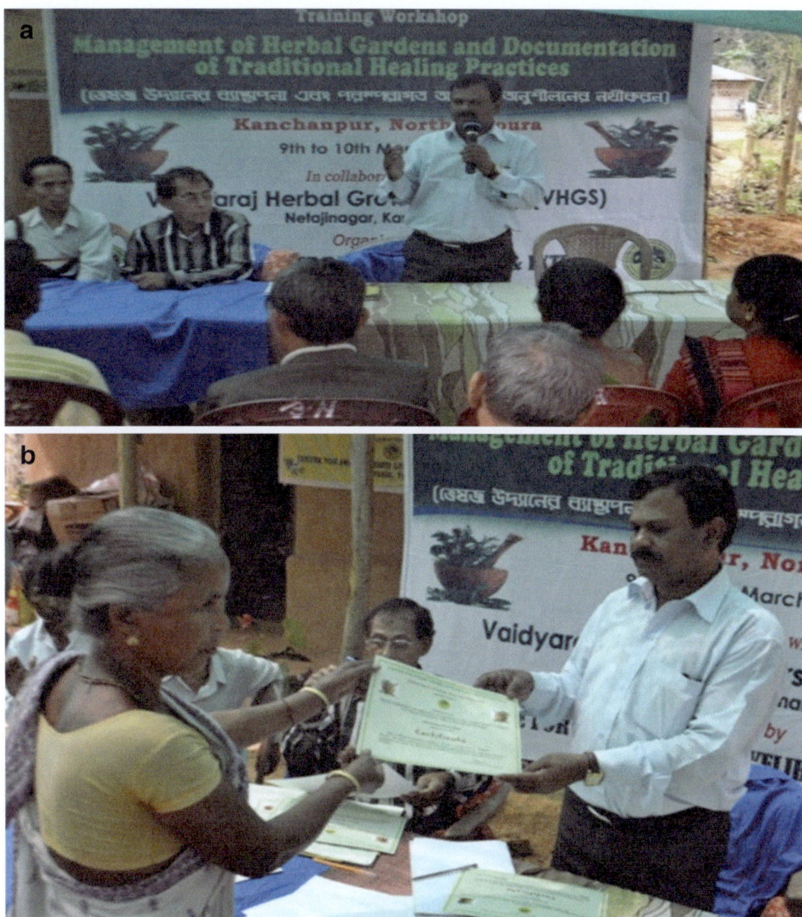

Fig. 7.15 (**a**) and (**b**) Training workshop held at Kanchanpur and handing over the certificate by Regional Director to the traditional healers

Table 7.3 Participatory appraisal on preferred plants and their parts

Sl. No.	Common diseases	Name of plants used		Family	Parts used
		Local name	Scientific name		
1	Stomach disorder	Ginger	*Zingiber officinale*	Zingiberaceae	Rhizome
		Golmorich	*Piper nigrum*	Piperaceae	Fruits
		Loung/Cloves	*Syzygium aromaticum*	Myrtaceae	Flower bud
		Hetranga	*Hydrangea macrophylla*	Hydrangeaceae	Roots
		Amla	*Phyllanthus emblica*	Phyllanthaceae	Fruits
		Hartaki	*Terminalia chebula*	Combretaceae	Fruits
		Bahera	*Terminalia bellirica*	Combretaceae	Fruits
		Pipul	*Ficus religiosa*	Moraceae	Fruits
		Boroi	*Ziziphus mauritiana*	Rhamnaceae	Seed
		Mango	*Mangifera indica*	Anacardiaceae	Seed
2	Diabetes	Surchang/Thyme	*Thymus vulgaris*	Lamiaceae	Roots and leaf
		Hiumbetya/Comfrey	*Symphytum officinale*	Boraginaceae	Leaf
		Telakuchi	*Coccinia grandis*	Cucurbits	Leaf
3	Jaundice	Chirata	*Swertia perennis*	Gentianaceae	Leaf
		Arhar	*Cajanus cajan*	Legumes	Leaf
		Amla	*Phyllanthus emblica*	Phyllanthaceae	Fruit
		Bahera	*Terminalia bellirica*	Combretaceae	Fruit
		Balsakow	*Viburnum prunifolium*	Adoxaceae	Root
		Gandhari	*Fagonia cretica*	Zygophyllaceae	Root
		Jongolerkejpata	*Neolamarckia cadamba*	Rubiaceae	Root
		Bakormo	*Brugmansia suaveolens*	Solanaceae	Root
		Hartaki	*Terminalia chebula*	Combretaceae	Fruit
		Arjun	*Terminalia arjuna*	Combretaceae	Tuber
		Alkoshi	*Mucuna pruriens*	Fabaceae	Bark
		Ashwagandha	*Withania somnifera*	Solanaceae	Fruit
		Guruchi	*Tinospora cordifolia*	Menispermaceae	Root
		Gukhur	*Tribulus terrestris*	Zygophyllaceae	Stem
5	Bone fracture	Harjora	*Cissus quadrangularis*	Vitaceae	Whole plant
		Ginger	*Zingiber officinale*	Zingiberaceae	Rhizome
		Bati	*Cissus quadrangularis*	Vitaceae	Leaf
		Neem	*Azadirachta indica*	Meliaceae	Leaf
		Basaka	*Adhatoda vasica*	Acanthaceae	Leaf
6	Gynecological disorder	Golmorich	*Piper nigrum*	Piperaceae	Fruits
		Loung/Cloves	*Syzygium aromaticum*	Myrtaceae	Flower bud
		Hetranga	*Hydrangea macrophylla*	Hydrangeaceae	Roots
7	General weakness	Bashak	*Adhatodavasica*	Acanthaceae	Leaf
		Tulsi	*Ocimum tenuiflorum*	Acanthaceae	Leaf
		Kalmegh	*Andrographis paniculata*	Acanthaceae	Leaf
		Kobabchini	*Piper cubeba*	Piperaceae	Fruits
		Ginger	*Zingiber officinale*	Zingiberaceae	Rhizome
8	Paralysis	Kolathur, chainohula	*Musa* spp.	Musaceae	Whole plant
		Dhenuaatpho	*Cannabis sativa*	Cannabaceae	Hemp
		Elaichi	*Elettaria cardamomum*	Zingiberaceae	Fruit
		Pora, Panipuri	*Tephrosia hookeriana*	Fabaceae	Whole plant
		Thankuni	*Centella asiatica*	Umbellifers	Leaf
		Jaba	*Hibiscus rosasinensis*	Malvaceae	Leaf

Table 7.3 (continued)

Sl. No.	Common diseases	Name of plants used		Family	Parts used
		Local name	Scientific name		
9	Skin disease	Neem	*Azadirachta indica*	Meliaceae	Leaf
		Aakon	*Auguste ferrier*	Cannaceae	Extract
		Turmeric	*Curcuma longa*	Zingiberaceae	Whole
		Cassia	*Cassia fistula*	Fabaceae	Leaf
10	Eczema	Aakon	*Auguste ferrier*	Cannaceae	Extract
		Cusmilka	*Brassica napus*	Brassicaceae	Extract
		Neem	*Azadirachta indica*	Meliaceae	Leaf
		Turmeric	*Curcuma longa*	Zingiberaceae	Whole
11	Fistula and piles	Lotichoria	*Arum* spp.	Araceae	Rhizome
		Muli Bamboo	*Melocanna baccifera*	Poaceae	Choung/
		Tulsi(black)	*Ocimum tenuiflorum*	Lamiaceae	Leaf
		Chalmugra	*Hydrocarpus wightiana*	Achariaceae	Fruit
		Jam	*Sizygium cuminii*	Myrtaceae	Leaf
		Genda	*Tagetes patula*	Asteraceae	Leaf
		Durba	*Cynoton daetylon*	Poaceae	Whole plant
		Jungle Hartaki	*Terminalia chebula*	Combretaceae	Fruit
12	Worm infestation	Bati	*Cissus quadrangularis*	Vitaceae	Leaf
		Neem	*Azadirachta indica*	Meliaceae	Leaf
		Basaka	*Adhatoda vasica*	Acanthaceae	Leaf
		Shepalika	*Nyctanthes arbor*	Oleaceae	Leaf
		Chirata	*Swertia chirayaita*	Gentianaceae	Leaf
		Ginger	*Zingiber officinale*	Zingiberaceae	Rhizome
		Manjistha	*Rubia cordifolia*	Rubiaceae	Root

7.5 Conclusion

Herbal medicines have been widely utilized as effective remedies for the prevention and treatment of multiple health conditions for centuries by almost every known culture. It has been recorded that nowadays it is estimated that 80% of the population uses herbs as in daily basis of work in different purposes, the culture plays an important role in the manner in which people use herbs. Herbs can serve as a major way of treating certain conditions or diseases or even more cost effectively, especially if the herb can be grown locally or regionally. The reason for the use of herbal plants is that it is part of the culture and belief of some people for the maintenance of health with its aromatic, medicinal, or cosmetic properties and for the increased use of herbals is the relatively cheaper cost of herbal products and hence affordability to the lower income group that the practitioners can grow their economic prospects from the healing traditional practices. Traditional medicines used to be extremely popular across India and steps are now being taken to revive the old practices. Besides helping in conserving the local biodiversity, this will also go a long way in generating employment. And this kind of activity also enriches the participatory mechanism to ensure the conservation of endangered, threatened, and rare species of herbal plants in a sustainable manner. It evolves the importance of Biological Diversity of Herbal Medicinal plants in Traditional Health Care Management System. The goal is to promote traditional medicines and preserve traditional knowledge as well as provide forest-based livelihood to growers and practitioners for the conservation of bio-diversity and preservation of certain endangered plants of traditional importance for the promotion of local healthcare practices by the use of medicinal plant parts.

References

Billore KV, Joseph TG, Dave SK. Interesting folk remedies by the local vaidyas of Rajasthan for SwasRoga. Ethnobotany. 1998;10:42–5.

Hemadri K. Rheumatism: tribal medicine. Anc Sci Life. 1981;1:117–20.

Kumar S. The medicinal plants of Northeast India. Jodhpur; 2002.

Rao RR, Jamir NS. Ethnobotanical studies in Nagaland-I medicinal plants. J Econ Taxon Bot. 1982;36:176.

Cultivation of Medicinal Plants: Special Reference to Important Medicinal Plants of India

8

Tridip Bhattacharjee, Saikat Sen,
Raja Chakraborty, Praveen Kumar Maurya,
and Arup Chattopadhyay

Contents

T. Bhattacharjee (✉)
College of Agriculture, Lembucherra, Tripura, India

S. Sen · R. Chakraborty
Department of Pharmacy, Assam Down Town University, Guwahati, Assam, India

P. K. Maurya · A. Chattopadhyay
Department of Vegetable Science, Faculty of Horticulture, BCKV, Nadia, West Bengal, India

S. Sen, R. Chakraborty (eds.), *Herbal Medicine in India*,
https://doi.org/10.1007/978-981-13-7248-3_8

8.1 Introduction

Herbal medicine and medicinal plants are playing an integral role in the modern healthcare system. Acceptance and utilization of herbal medicine are increasing day by day for their better compatibility, lesser side effect, and economic health management. Herbal sources are mainly used as medicine, cosmetic and supplement (Sen and Chakraborty 2017; Sen et al. 2011). The growing interest towards the herbal medicines made this a prime area of research and development. India is a rich repository of codified and folk knowledge of medicinal plants as well as differences in climatic condition, attitude, and rainfall makes this land a gold mine of medicinal plants. The word "herb" taken from the Latin word, *"herba"* and an old French word *"herbe"* (Rajak and Singh 2017). The market of traditional medicinal plants and herbal formulations are also lucrative and increasing day by day. Indian traditional medicine is well-established traditional medicinal system and received global acceptance particularly Ayurveda. The demand for Ayurvedic and other herbal medicine is increasing day by day. A number of herbal formulations are presently available in market equally competing allopathic medicines. Codified medicinal texts like Ayurveda, Unani, Siddha are the main sources of information for the preparations of marketed herbal products. World Health Organization (WHO) estimated that about 80% world population rely on herbal medicines mainly in their primary healthcare needs. It is estimated that 300,000 plant species exist globally and only 15% have been screened to find their possible therapeutic potential (De Luca et al. 2012). Ministry of Environment and Forests, Government of India, documented more than 9500 plant species based on their importance in the pharmaceutical industry. Medicinal and aromatic plants MAP species are collected from wild sources and comparatively a few are grown in farmland (Maiti and Geetha 2007). Maximum herbal industries are collection the medicinal plants/plant parts from the forest source. The excessive or irrational collection may also result in threat to the availability of medicinal plants. Loss of biodiversity, industrializations are became a big threat to medicinal plants species (Kala et al. 2006; Sen and Chakraborty 2017). Therefore, conservation of medicinal plants and commercial harvesting of medicinal plants could be useful for sustainable availability of medicinal plants. Collection of forest source in different season and different area may vary the phytochemical content which may ultimately effect in the biological activity of the plant. Commercial herbal garden is one of the very effective solutions to overcome these problems. Scientific research and science tools developed a number of isolated phytochemicals with prominent biological activity. A number of drugs are inspired from the isolated phytochemicals and successfully used in the management of modern healthcare. Recent era, the growing market of herbal medicine has an important aspect of economic growth of the country. This article deals with majorly deals cultivation with some very common and commercially important medicinal plants of India.

8.2 Important Medicinal Plants of India

8.2.1 Yam

Botanical Name: *Dioscorea spp.*
Family: Dioscoreaceae.
The chemical present in the yam is diosgenin, which is obtained from tubers root of dioscorea and important chemical for several steroid hormones including sex hormones, cortisone, and various corticosteroids and is the major ingredient in the oral birth control pill. The growing necessity for steroidal drugs and the high expenditure of obtaining them from animal sources led to an extensive search for plant sources of steroidal sapogenins; which eventually led to the identification of the Genus *Dioscorea* as the most promising one. This genus *Dioscorea* with more than 600 species is broadly distributed in the tropical world. The species like *Dioscorea alata* and *Dioscorea esculenta* are also cultivated for their edible tuber and time of cultivation time is longer. About 15 *Dioscorea* species contain

diosgenin. Among them, *Dioscorea floribunda, Dioscorea villosa, Dioscorea composita* etc. are extensively grown for diosgenin production. The diosgenin content ranges from 2% to 7% based on the age of the tuber (Das et al. 2013; Bhattacharjee et al. 2015).

Cultivation details of *Dioscorea* spp.:

Climate and soil	Varieties	Propagation	Planting	Harvesting and yield
Subtropical warm humid weather and light soil; pH 5.5–6.5	FB(c)-1, Arka Upkar	Tubers 250–300 gm/ piece/pit	60 cm × 30 cm (R-R × P-P) for 1 year crop 60 cm × 45 cm (R-R × P-P) for 2 year crop	February-March 50–60 tonnes/ha

8.2.2 Sarpagandha

Botanical Name: *Rauvolfia serpentina.*
Family: Apocynaceae.
Rauvolfia (Sarpagandha) or Serpentine root is one of the vital crude drugs used in present medicine and known since 3000 years (Dey and De 2010). Roots are prominent, tuberous, usually branched, 0.5–2.6 cm girth, 40–60 cm long into soil. The bark of root, which constitutes 40–60% of total root volume, is rich in alkaloids known for their usefulness in lowering high blood pressure and as a sedative or tranquillizing agent. The fresh roots give a unique acrid aroma and are very astringent in taste. The root contains high alkaloid concentration. In allopathic means of medicine, reserpine is the most active principle used for hypertension for life-saving drug.

Cultivation details of Sarpagandha:

Climate and soil	Variety	Propagation	Planting	Harvesting, processing and yield
Well suited at 10–30 °C and sandy alluvial loam to red lateritic loam and pH –4.6 to 6.5.	Wild and R.S-1	Seed and also by vegetative means like root stumps, and stem cutting.	Seedlings of 40–50 days and 30 cm × 30 cm spacing, 80,000–1, 00,000/ha	After 30 months of planting (during winter months), the roots are cleaned, washed and cut into 12–15 cm pieces for drying and storage. Dry root 2000–2500 kg/ ha.

8.2.3 Opium

Botanical Name: *Papaver somniferum* L.
Family: Papaveraceae.
Papaver somniferum is an outstanding medicinal plant. Opium and codeine are the products of opium that used for their analgesic and hypnotic property (Dhakad et al. 2017). A semi-synthetic morphine known as heroin has led to worldwide social problem. But morphine and another opium alkaloid still have important and non-replaceable role in the healthcare sector. Poppy is a strait, rarely branched, annual, growing to a length of 0.60–1.20 m. With operation of lancing on fruits (capsular) latex known as opium is obtained. In nature, all parts of the poppy plant have milky white latex, but large amount contains on unripe capsules.

Cultivation details of Sarpagandha:

Climate and soil	Variety	Propagation	Planting	Harvesting and yield
Cool climate favors high yield and light black or loam soil with highly fertility, pH around 7.0.	Ranghatak, Talia, Dhola Chota, Sujatha, NBRI-3 and Shubhra	Seed rate is 4–5 kg/ ha for line and 7–8 kg/ha for broadcast.	broadcast or in lines, 30 cm × 30 cm	95–115 days after sowing and 50–60 kg/ha.

8.2.4 Periwinkle

Botanical Name: *Catharanthus roseus* (L) G. Don.
Family: Apocynaceae.
It is one of the important medicinal plant's mentions in the literature of folks medicinal. The plant has been extensively used as a purgative, abortifacient, antidiabetic, hemorrhagic antimalarial, diuretic, antidysenteric and against skin diseases by the antique people (Devi et al. 2017). Modern studies have shown that periwinkle contains more than 100 alkaloids found in various parts of the plant. Periwinkle gained additional importance after the separation of vinblastine and vincristine alkaloids which having importance in cancer (Moudi et al. 2013). Other alkaloids like rovidine, leurosovine and leurosidine isolated from the plant and acquired medicinal importance for their preclinical anticancer properties.

Cultivation details of Periwinkle:

Climate and soil	Variety	Propagation	Planting	Harvesting and Yield
Tropical and subtropical and deep sandy loam to loam soils	No improved variety	Periwinkle or Vinca is propagated by seeds	45 × 30 cm	After 6, 9 and 12 months of sowing. Yield- 4 t/ha of leaves, 1.5 t/ha of stem, and 1.5 t/ha of roots.

8.2.5 Aloe/Gheekumari

Botanical Name: *Aloe spp* (L) G. Don.
Family: Liliaceae.
It is commonly called as healing plant, miracle plant, fountain of youth and plant of immortality. Out of the 275 species, only three species are commercially vital which are the majorly used in pharmaceutical industries or medicinal purpose. They are: *A. barbadensis,* Mill. (*A. vera* Linn) which yields Indian aloe or Curacao aloe or Barbados aloe or Jaffarabad aloe, and *A. ferox* and yield Cape aloe, and *A. perryi* (socotrine aloe). Other aloe species (*A. africana* and *A.* spicata) yield aloes of lesser importance. Aloe gel or *A. vera* gel derived from the leaves, and the yellow, bitter juice present in specific cells underneath the bulky epidermis yields the drug aloe and the parenchymatous tissue in the leaf center found to contains a mucilaginous gel; at present it is obtained from *A. barbadensis.* Aloe contains cathartic anthraglycosides as its lively principles; are mostly C-glucosides, notably barbaloin (glucoside of aloe emodin) (Patel et al. 2012). The concentrations glucosides may differ with the types of aloe varying from 4.5% to 25% of aloin. Aloe gel is well known for domestic medicinal importance. For this cause, *Aloe vera* is also called first-aid for burn or medicine plant. When newly obtained, the gel has the property of relieving sunburn and thermal burns, also wound healing; it has moisturizing and emollient properties. As a food, aloe extracts are used as a flavor ingredient mainly in non-alcoholic and alcoholic beverages.

Cultivation details of Aloe:

Climate and soil	Variety	Propagation	Planting	Harvesting and yield
Warm, humid or dry climate and sandy coastal to loamy soils of the plains with a pH of up to 8.5	Non	By root-suckers or rhizome cuttings	60 cm × 30 cm or 60 cm × 45 cm	Harvested eight months after planting and around 10,000–12,000 kg/ha

8.2.6 Guggal

Botanical Name: *Commiphora wightii (Arn.) Bhandari syn. Commiphora mukul.*
Family: Burseraceae.
The gum is acrid, bitter, thermogenic, astringent, expectorant, aromatic, anthelmintic, digestive, anti-inflammatory, antiseptic, anodyne, nervine tonic, alterative, aphrodisiac, stimulant, antispasmodic, liver tonic, hemostatic, emmenagogue,

rejuvenating, diuretic, general tonic (Joy et al. 1998), and is useful in scrofula, gout, sciatica, facial paralysis cough, diplegia, asthma, pectoral, bronchitis and hepatic, otorrhoea, disorders, fever, epilepsy, stangury, dysmenorrhoea, hemorrhoids, wounds, amenorrhea and ulcers.

Cultivation details of Guggal:

Climate and soil	Variety	Propagation	Planting	Harvesting and yield
Warm, humid or dry climate and sandy to silt-loam or rocky soils	No	Semi-wood stem cuttings	Rainy season	After 8–10 years ready for tapping of the gum by shallow incision on bark during December and March and 500–800 g gums per plant.

8.2.7 Belladona

Botanical Name: *Atropa belladonna L.*
Family: Solanaceae.
Atrops is commonly called as 'Deadly night Shade'. The commercial drug is obtained from the roots, leaves and flowering tops of *A.belladonna*. Belladonna leaves are extensively used for the produce of tinctures and plasters. The drug serves as a sedative, anodyne, stimulant, antiasthmatic, antidiuretic, antispasmodic and anti-inflammatory. It is found beneficial in treatment of stomach, renal disorders, bilary colic, and to stop sweating. The roots are mainly used in the external treatment of rheumatism, gout and other affiliations.

Cultivation details of Belladonna:

Climate and soil	Variety	Propagation	Planting	Harvesting and Yield
Perennial in temperate climates and deep fertile soils of medium texture.	Gurguva	Seeds and May to the end of autumn	March–April or October–November	3 months after planting and average of 1000 kg of dry herb, 1500 kg per hectare during second and third years and dry roots will vary from 170 to 335 kg/ha.

8.2.8 Nux Vomica

Botanical Name: *Strychnosnux-vomica* Linn.
Family: Strychnaceae (Loganiaceae).
Dried seeds or beans, and occasionally its bark (called *nux vomica*) are used in herbal remedies (Akbar et al. 2010). The seeds contain organic substances, brucine, and strychnine. Dried seeds of kuchila are stomachic, nervine, and aphrodisiac, cardio-tonic, and respiratory stimulant. It is used as a remedy in paralytic, chronic dysentery and neuralgic disorders, rheumatic arthritis, epilepsy, and hydrophobia. It is an important drug in all systems of medicine. *Strychnos* species is a deciduous tree, medium-sized, with fairly long and cylindrical bole and dark-grey or yellowish-grey bark with minute tubercles.

Cultivation details of Nux vomica:

Climate and soil	Variety	Propagation	Planting	Harvesting & Yield
Dry or humid tropical and laterite, sandy, and alluvial soil.	no	Seeds, also through cuttings	Onset of South-west monsoon in May or early June and 5 m × 5 m.	50–75 kg of dry seeds per tree per year.

8.2.9 Medicinal Solanum

Botanical: *Solanum spp,*
Family: Solanaceae.
Species include *S. indicum, Solanum anguivi* Lam. (Poison berry), *Solanum nigrum* Linn. (Black night shade), *Solanum torvum* (West Indian turkey berry), *Solanum surattense* Burm, *Solanum khasianum* C.B. Clarke. It is source of low cost steroidal drugs, due to its quick growth and low first investment in its commercial cultivation. It yields a solasodine, glyco-alkaloid, a

nitrogen analogue of diosgenine. Solasodine through 16-dehydro-pregnenolone (16 DPA) is converted of compounds like methyl testosterone and testosterone and corticosteroids like hydrocortisone and predinisolone (Sunitha and Swapna 2014). These steroidal compounds have anabolic, anti-inflammatory and antifertility properties, due to which they find huge-scale use in family and health planning programs through the world.

Cultivation details of Medicinal Solanum:

Climate and soil	Variety	Propagation	Planting	Harvesting and Yield
Moderate climate red lateritic soil with a moderate quantity of organic matter.	Arka Sanjeevini, Arka Mahima, Pusa-1, RRL 20-2	Seed	June to September or October, 50 cm × 50 cm, 75 cm × 75 cm and 90 cm × 120 cm.	6 months to be ready for harvesting and 2500 kg/ha of dried.

8.2.10 Aonla/Amla

Botanical Name: *Emblica officinalis* Gaertn., Syn. *Phyllanthus emblica*,
Family: Euphorbiaceae.
Amla is an antioxidant with the free radical scavenging quality, which may be presence of high levels of super oxide dismutase (Hazra et al. 2010). It is efficient in the treatment of dyspepsia, peptic ulcer and diabetes. Further reported are antioxidant, hepatoprotective, cytoprotective, antimutagenic, antimicrobial and anti-tumor (Deori et al. 2017).

Cultivation details of Medicinal Amla:

Climate and soil	Variety	Propagation	Planting	Harvesting and Yield
Tropical plant and medium heavy soil except purely sandy	NA-7, NA-6, NA-10 and Chakaiya	Generally propagated by shield budding.	May–June and 4.5 m × 4.5 m.	After 4–5 years, harvested during February and 50–70 kg of fruit.

8.2.11 Senna

Botanical Name: *Cassia angustifolia* Vahl.
Family: Leguminaesae.
Senna is used in medicine as a cathartic and habitual constipation. It increases the peristaltic movement of the colon (Balasankar et al. 2013). Senna on storage, lose biological action faster than revealed by chemical estimation. The leaves/pods as such or in powder form do not lose potency easily (Sreeramu 2004).

Cultivation details of Medicinal Senna:

Climate and soil	Variety	Propagation	Planting	Harvesting and Yield
Sun-loving crop and tropical climate. Red loam, alluvial loam and the rich clayey rice-fields.	Thenkalam local type, 'ALFT –2' Sona and KKM 1	Seeds	Seeds are broadcast or 30 cm × 30 cm.	50–70 days, 90–100 days and 130–150 days after sowing. 15 q/ha of dry leaves and 7 q/ha of pods.

8.2.12 Isubgol

Botanical Name: *Plantago ovata* Forsk.
Family: Plantaginaceae.
Isabgol (*Plantago ovata* Forsk.) is key medicinal plants used widely that have originated from arid and semi-arid zones and widely used by traditional medicinal industries. It is an annual herb and cultivated in Gujarat, Rajasthan, Madhya Pradesh and Haryana (Meena et al. 2015).

Cultivation details of Isabgol:

Climate and soil	Variety	Propagation	Planting	Harvesting and yield
Cool and dry weather, that is, from November–December to March–April and sandy loam to rich loamy soil with a pH of 7–8 is ideal	Gujarat Isabgol-1 Gujarat Isabgol-2, Gujarat Isabgol-3, Jawahar Isabgol-4, Hariyana Isabgol-5 and Niharika	Seed (4–6 kg/ha)	November–December	110–130 days after sowing and 800–1000 kg/ha.

8.2.13 Stevia

Botanical Name: *Stevia rebaudiana.*
Family: Asteraceae.
Stevia is a subtropical perennial that produces sweet steviol glycosides in the leaves for which it is also known as 'Mou Tulsi' or 'Cheeni Tulsi'. Plants grown-up at higher latitudes generally has a higher percentage of sweet glycosides (Mathur et al. 2017). Origin of Stevia is North Eastern Paraguay. Stevia uses include regulating blood sugar, treatment of skin disorders, preventing hypertension and prevention decay of tooth. The compound obtains from stevia is consider to be the best alternate source of sugar for diabetic patient.

Cultivation details of Stevia:

Climate and soil	Variety	Propagation	Planting	Harvesting and Yield
Semi-humid subtropical plant and well-drained fertile sandy loam or loam soil and prefers acidic to neutral (pH 6–7) soil	S.R.B-123, S.R.B-512 and S.R.B-128	Stem cuttings @ 75,000/ha	March to mid- May and distance of 40 cm × 30 cm	4 months after planting during mid to late September. About 15,000 kg/ha of green herb is obtained which on drying gives about 4166 kg/ha.

8.2.14 Coleus

Botanical Name: *Coleus forskohlii* Syn: *Coleus barbatus* Brig.
Family: Lamiaceae
Coleus is used as an emmenagogue, expectorant and diuretic. Interestingly its foliage is employed for intestinal disorders treating, and it has been utilized as a condiment for a long time before in India. The tuberous roots of the plant similar to a carrot in shape and brown in color are the economical parts.

Cultivation details of Coleus:

Climate and soil	Variety	Propagation	Planting	Harvesting and Yield
Crop of the tropics, 10–25 °C and 100–160 cm rainfall and porous and well-drained soils pH from 5.5 to 7.	Garmai, Manganiper, Maimul and Selection K-8	Terminal cuttings (10 cm) or rooted cuttings..	June–July, 60 cm × 45 cm spacing (37,030 plants/ha).	4.5–5 months after planting. Fresh tubers: 15–20 t/ha Dry tubers: 2000–2200 kg/ha.

8.2.15 Acorus

Botanical Name: *Acorus calamus.*
Family: Acoraceae (Araceae).
Acorus calamus is a semi-aquatic, perennial and smelly plant, habituated in both sub-temperate and temperate zones (Meena et al. 2010). It is very well known for the remedies of cold and cough and also like bronchitis. It is considered as a useful aid to the digestive system as it helps against colic, flatulent, dyspepsia and vomiting. It is composed in the formulation for psychosomatic disorders like epilepsy and it roots having insect repellent characters.

Cultivation details of Acorus:

Climate and soil	Variety	Propagation	Planting	Harvesting and Yield
Sub tropical climate and shallow water or in a very moist loamy soil and pH 5.5–7.5	No	Roots/rhizomes and seeds.	–	Early spring before new growth, or late autumn and 1–1.5 tons of dry rhizome per acre

8.2.16 Ocimum (Holy Basil/Tulsi)

Botanical Name: *Ocimum sanctum* Linn.
Family: Lamiaceae/Labiatae.
Tulsi is one of the important medicinal plants of India, which has its medicinal and religious importance since ancient time. Essential oil of tulasi has various medicinal importance. It is extensively used as an herbal tea, commonly used in Ayurveda. It is widely used in various aspects drugs, flavouring insecticide, culinary purposes and perfumery. The plant possesses mainly phenols, tannins, aldehydes, saponin, and fats (Ansari 2015).

Cultivation details of Ocimum:

Climate and soil	Variety	Propagation	Planting	Harvesting and Yield
Fairly high rainfall and humid conditions, Rich loam to poor laterite, saline and alkaline to moderately acidic soils.	Sri Tulsi (green type) and Krishna Tulsi (second type)	Seed (200–300 g/ha)	Nursery- third week of February and transplanting-middle of April. 40 cm × 40 cm, 40 cm × 50 cm, 50 cm × 30 cm.	First harvest at full bloom i.e. 90–95 days after planting and harvested at every 65–75 days. About 5 tonnes/ha of fresh harvest can be obtained twice or thrice a year.

Yam, sarpagandha, opium, periwinkle, aloe, guggal, belladonna, nux vomica, medicinal solanum, aonla/amla, senna, isubgol, stevia, coleus, acorus, and ocimum are medicinally important plants. Researches on these plants isolated different important phytomolecule and investigated for their therapeutic potential. Table 8.1 included the major phytochemicals and pharmacological activity of these plants.

Table 8.1 Major phytoconstituents and pharmacological activity of selected medicinal plants of India

Name	Major bioactive phytomolecules	Pharmacological properties
Yam (*Dioscorea spp;* Family: Dioscoreaceae)	Diosgenin, dioscorin, dioscoreanoside A-K, dioscin, diosbulbisin, diosbulbisides, bafoudiosbulbin, quercetin and its derivatives, kaempferol and its derivatives, hyperoside, neoxanthin, auroxanthin, violaxanthin, cryptoxanthin, daucosterol, β-sitosterol, 3-o-β-d-glucopyranosyl-b-sitosterol, stigmasterol, catechin, protocatechuic acid, (+) epicatechin, (−) epicatechin, vanillic acid, isovanillin acid, protodioscin, protoneodioscin (Galani and Patel 2017; Sautour et al. 2007)	Anti hypertensive, antioxidant, anticancer, antimicrobial, immunomodulatory, antidiabetic, hypolipidemic and hypocholesterolemic, analgesic and anti-inflammatory, anti-HIV activity, diuretic, gastro protective, cardioprotective Activity (Kanu et al. 2018; Galani and Patel 2017)
Sarpagandha (*Rauvolfia serpentine;* Family: Apocynaceae)	Reserpine, serpentinine, ajmalicine, ajmaline, ajmalimine, reserpiline, deserpidine, indobidine, rescinnamidine, rescinnamine, serpentine, yohimbine, indobinine, serpentinine etc. (Chauhan et al. 2017; Kumari et al. 2013).	Antihypertension activity, inhibition of ACE, antivenom activity, antioxidant activity, antimicrobial activity, hypolipidemic activity, hepatoprotective activity, hyperglycemic activity, antivenom activity, anti-diarrheal activity (Chauhan et al. 2017; Kumari et al. 2013).

Table 8.1 (continued)

Name	Major bioactive phytomolecules	Pharmacological properties
Opium (*Papaver somniferum;* Family: Papaveraceae)	Morphine, codeine, narcotine, thebaine, papaverine, narceine, cryptopine, pseudomorphine, protopine, hydrocatarnine, laudanosine, meconidine, laudanine, rhoeadine, codamine, meconidine, nascopine, xanthaline, lanthopine, apocodeine, apomorphine, thebamine, desoxycodeine, catarnine, prophyroxine (Mani and Dhawan 2014; Chalise 2015)	Poppy latex and poppy alkaloids exerted number of activities like hypnotic and sedative, expectorant, astringent, diaphoretic, antispasmodic, antitussive, antispasmodic, analgesic, sedative, narcotic, antiperistaltic, anticonvulsant etc. (Mani and Dhawan 2014).
Periwinkle (*Catharanthus roseus*; Family: Apocynaceae)	Vindoline, vinblastine, vincristine, vindolidine, vindolicine, vindolinine, ibogaine, lochnerine, yohimbine, raubasine, leurosine, catharanthine, leurosine, lochnerine, catharanthine, vindoline, ajmalacine, serpentine, reserpine, lochnerine, alstonine, tabersonine, horhammericine, echitovenine, tricin, vingramine, methylvingramine (Renjini et al. 2017). Zeatin ribosyl, zeatin, zeatin-9-riboside, vinaphamine vinaspine, vincaline, vincathicine, vinosidine, vinsedicine, vinsedine, yohimbine, vanillic acid, syringic acid, quercetin, isovincoside, kaempferol, catharine, catharosine, cathenamine, cathindine (Nisar et al. 2016)	Antioxidant, antimicrobial, antiulcer, antidiabetic, hypotensive, wound healing, anticancer, memory enhancing activity, anti-diarrheal, anthelmintic, biopesticidal (Das and Sharangi 2017; Renjini et al. 2017).
Aloe (*Aloe vera,* Family: Liliaceae)	It contain high levelof water (99%–99.5%) and small amount of solid contents (0.5%–1%). Aloin; Barbaloin; Isobarbaloin; Emodin; Anthracene; Anthranol; Emodin; Aloetic acid, Resistannol (Minwuyelet et al. 2017; Maan et al. 2018).	Anti-microbial activity (antibacterial, antifungal, antiviral), anti-inflammatory, antioxidant, wound healing, antidiabetic, antiulcer, immunomodulatory, antitumor, hepatoprotective, antihyperlipidemic, laxative, anthelmintic, antiseptic, detoxifying effect, moisturizing and anti-aging effect. Aloe or its component can enhance drug absorption. Lactobacillus brevis were observed in naturally fermented *A. vera.* Juice of *A. vera* used in skin care and tooth and gum protective products. It also used in infection caused by genital herpes, asthma, HIV infection (Minwuyelet et al. 2017; Radha and Laxmipriya 2015; Sharma et al. 2014a, b; Maan et al. 2018). Aloin is a major component of *A. vera* that possesses antidiabetic, antimicrobial, antioxidant, hypotensive, anti-inflammatory and anticancer activity (Patel and Patel 2013)

(continued)

Table 8.1 (continued)

Name	Major bioactive phytomolecules	Pharmacological properties
Guggal (*Commiphora wightii syn. Commiphora mukul;* Family: Burseraceae)	Guggulsterol I-VI; *E* and *Z*-guggulsterone; Z-guggulsterol; guggulsterone M and Y; *α*-camphorene; cembrene-A; cembrene; mukulol; isocembrol; 4-epiisocembrol; dimyrcene; oleic acid; linoleic acid; palmitic acid; stearic acids, sitosterol; eugenol; ellagic acid; (8R)-3α,8-dihydroxy-polypoda-13E, 17E, 21 triene, 20S-acetyloxy-4-pregnene-3,16-dione; 4,17(20)-(*trans*)-pregnadiene-3,16-dione; 16β-acetyloxy-pregn- 4,17(20)-*trans*-dien-3-one; 4,17(20)-(*cis*)- pregnadiene-3,16-dione; (1*E*, 4*E*, 8*E*)-4,8,14-Trimethyl-11-(1-methylethyl)4-methoxycyclotertradeca-1,4,8-triene; 3α-acetyloxy-5α- pregnan-16-one; (2*E*, 12*E*)-2,7,13-trimethyl-9-(1-methylethyl)-15-oxabicyclo [12.1.0] pentadeca-2,12-diene-7-ol; (4*Z*, 6*E*)-4,7,12,15,15-pentamethylbicylco [9.3.1] pentadeca-4,6-diene-12-ol; myrrhanone A; myrrhanone B; myrrhanone A acetate; commipherol; commipherin; pelargonidin-3,5,di-*O*-glucoside; quercetin-3-*O*-β-L-arabinose; quercetin 3-*O*-β-D-glucuronide; quercetin-3-*O*-β-D-galactoside; quercetin-3-*O*-β-L-rhamnoside, (Kalshetti et al. 2014; Sarup et al. 2015)	Hypolipidemic activity, antiatherosclerotic activity, platelet aggregation and fibrinolytic activity, thyroid stimulatory activity, anti-inflammatory activity, antiarthritic activity, cardioprotective activity, antioxidant activity, antutumor and anticancer activity, antifertility activity, antihyperglycemic activity, antimicrobial activity (Kalshetti et al. 2014; Sarup et al. 2015)
Belladonna (*Atropa belladonna;* Family: Solanaceae)	Atropine, scopalamine, norhyoscyamine, δ-N-methylornithrine, atroposide (A,B,C,D,E,F, G and H), 3-O-α-D-galactopyramoside, 3-O-β-D-glucopyranosyl (1-- > 4)-β-D-galactopyramoside (Paul and Dutta 2011)	Treatment of colitis, irritable bowel syndrome, diverticulitis, colic, peptic ulcer, diarrhea, asthama, extreme sweating, nighttime incontinence, headaches, migraines, muscle pains and spasms, motion sickness and vertigo, Parkinson's disease, Biliary colic, colic of liver or gallbladder (Long 2005)
Nux vomica (*Strychnosnux-vomica;* Family: Strychnaceae)	Strychnine; brucine; vomicine; α & β- colubrine; *n*-methyl pseudostrychnine; 7-hydroxy coumarin; kaempferol-7-glucoside; kaempferol 3-rutinoside; quercetin-3-rhamnoside; rutinbrucine; mavacurine; strychnochrysine; vomicine; strychnoflavine; icajine; salidroaide; stryvomicine; stryvomitine; α-colubrine-chloromethochloride; igasuric acid; pseudostrychnine; pseudobrucine; lupeol; loganin; β-colubrine; icajine; 16-hydroxy-α-colubrine; vomicine; novacine; pseudostrychnine; isostrychnine; isobrucine; 3-methoxy icajine; 15-hydroxy strychnine (Behera et al. 2017; Patel et al. 2017).	Amticancer activity, antitumor activity, antimicrobial activity, antidiarrhoeal activity, anti HIV effect, neuropharmacological activity; antiamnesic activity; antiallergic and immunomodulatory property; analgesic and anti-inflammatory activity, antipyretic effect, hepatoprotective and anticholestatic activity, antisnake venom activity (Behera et al. 2017; Patel et al. 2017).

Table 8.1 (continued)

Name	Major bioactive phytomolecules	Pharmacological properties
Medicinal Solanum (*Solanum spp,;* Family: Solanaceae)	***S. indicum:*** Indiosides (A to F), protodioscin, carpesterol, isoanguivine, solanidine, solasodine, solamargine, solavetivone, isofraxidin, fraxetin, trilinolein, arteminorin a, indicumin (Sharma et al. 2017) ***S. virginianum (*Syn. *S. xanthocarpum*):** Solasonine, solasonine, solanocarpidine solamargine, sitosterol, solanocarpine, β–solamargine, isochlorogenic acid, neochronogenic acid, chronogenic acid, caffeic acids, cycloartanol, sitosterol, cycloartenol, stigmasterol, stigmasterol glucoside, solamargine, beta-solamargine, khasianine (Rane et al. 2014). ***S nigrum:*** Solamargine, Solasonine, α and β- solanigrine, degalactotigonin, nigrumnins I and II. Tigogenin, spirosestanol glycoside, furostanol glycoside, ascorbic acid, ethyl b-D-thevetopyranosyl-(1-4) b-D-oleandropyranoside, ethylb-D-thevetopyranosyl-(1-4)-a-D-oleandropyranoside (Saleem et al. 2009; Nyeem et al. 2017).	***S. indicum:*** Antibacterial, antioxidant, anthelmintic, antiplasmodial, hepatoprotective, anticancer, laxative, cardiotonic activity, CNS depressant and anti hypertensive activity (Sharma et al. 2017). ***S. virginianum (*Syn. *S. xanthocarpum*):** Anthelmintic, antipyretic, anti-inflammatory, anti-asthmatic, laxative, aphrodisiac effect, hypoglycemic, antiasthmatic, hepatoprotective antibacterial, anticancer and insect repellent properties. Treatment of epilepsy, pain, migraine, head ache, hair fall, bronchial asthma, skin problems, cough, cough, asthma, rheumatism and chest pain and as tonic (Rane et al. 2014; Subharani 2016). ***S nigrum:*** Antimicrobial, antioxidant, hepatoprotective, anticancer, antidiabetic, antiulcer, cardiotonic activity, CNS depressant and anti hypertensive activity, immunostimulant, anti-HCV, anti gastritis, antihyperlipidemic, antidiarrhoeal, cytotoxic, antioxigenic, anti-inflammatory (Saleem et al. 2009; Nyeem et al. 2017).
Aonla/Amla (*Emblica officinalis* Syn. *Phyllanthus emblica*, Family: Euphorbiaceae)	Apigenin, ellagic acid, gallic acid, quercetin, chebulagic acid, chebulinic acid, corilagin, isostrictiniin, methyl gallate, luteolin, emblicanin A, emblicanin B, phyllaemblicin B, phyllantine, phyllantidine, punigluconin, pedunculagin (Hasan et al. 2016).	Antibacterial, antifungal, antiviral, insecticidal, larvicidal and mosquitocidal, radioprotective, hypolipidemic, immunomodulatory activity, antimutagenic and wound healing, antidepressant activity, anticancer, HIV-reverse transcriptase inhibitory, hepatoprotective, anti ulcerogenic activity. It also use in piles, jaundice, gout, respiratory disorders, migraine, urinary problems, (Hasan et al. 2016; Kulkarni and Ghurghure 2018; Gaire and Subedi 2014).
Senna (*Cassia angustifolia*; Family: Leguminaesae)	sennoside A, sennoside B, sennoside C, sennoside D, rhein-anthrone- 8-diglucose, rhein-8-glucoside, rhein-8-diglucoside, aloe-emodine-8-glucoside, aloe-emodine-anthrone diglucoside, rhein, aloe emodine, palmidine A, kaempferol, isorhamnetin, sennacrol, sennapicrin, cathartomannite, mannitol, sodium potassium tertarate, myricyl alcohol, salicylic acid, phytosterolin, mucilage, resin, chrysophanic acid, calcium oxalate, beta sitosterol (Tripathi 1999; Ganapaty et al. 2002).	Laxative, anticancer, purgative, anthchiiintic, antipyretic, cathartic, antimicrobial, anti-inflammatory activity, body detoxing, vermifuge, diuretic (Tripathi 1999; Balasankar et al. 2013).

(continued)

Table 8.1 (continued)

Name	Major bioactive phytomolecules	Pharmacological properties
Isubgol (*Plantago ovate*; Family: Plantaginaceae)	Psyllium husk contains hemicelluloses, a xylan backbone attached with arabinose, rhamnose, and galacturonic acid units (arabinoxylans); iridoids; phenols; fatty acids; luteolin-7-O-β-glycoside; polysaccharides; sterols. Among two poly saccharine fractions one fraction soluble in clod another one in hot water. Cold water soluble fraction on hydrolysis produces xylose, aldobiouronic acid, arabinose. Hot water soluble fraction on hydrolysis yields xylose, arabinose, aldobiouronic acid, galactose (Sarfraz et al. 2017; Haddadian et al. 2014; Deokar et al. 2016).	Laxative activity, wound healing activity, anti-diarrheal and anti-constipation activity, anti-inflammatory activity, hypocholestrolemic activity, hypoglycemic activity, hypolipidemic activity, hypocholestrolemic activity, antibacterial activity, anticancer activity (Sarfraz et al. 2017; Deokar et al. 2016; Haddadian et al. 2014).
Stevia (*Stevia rebaudiana;* Family: Asteraceae)	Stevioside, steviolbioside, steviolmonoside, rebaudioside (A to F), dulcoside A, austroinullin, β-carotene, dulcoside, nilacin, rebaudi oxides, riboflavin, steviol, stevioside, thiamine, isosteviol, 4-methoxybenzoic acid, p-coumaric acid, 4-methylcatechol, caffeoylquinic acid, dicaffeoylquinic acid, 4-caffeoyl-5-feruloylquinic acid, 4-methoxybenzoic acid, 4-coumaric acid, 4-methylcatechol, sinapic acid, caryophyllene, β-caryophyllene, β-pinene (Momtazi-Borojeni et al. 2017; Wolwer-Rieck 2012)	Anti-diabetic, antihypertensive, antimicrobial, antiviral, antifungal, antitumor, anti-inflammatory, hepatoprotective, immune stimulating activity. It is also used as natural sweetener (Momtazi-Borojeni et al. 2017).
Coleus (*Coleus forskohlii* Syn: *Coleus barbatus;* Family: Lamiaceae)	Forskolin (E, F, G, H, I, J, L); 6-acetyl-1,9-dideoxy forskolin; 6-acetyl-1-deoxyforskolin; deactylforskolin; 1, 9-deoxyforskolin; 9-deoxyforskolin; 1,9-dideoxy-7-deacetylforskolin; 1,6-diacetoxy-9-deoxyforskolin; 1-acetyl forskolin; isoforskolin;1,6-di-O-acetylforskolin; forskoditerpenoside A and B; forskoditerpenoside C, D and E; forskoditerpene A; coleonol E and coleonol F; coleol; coleosol; 3-hydroxy forskolin; 3-hydroxyisoforskolin (Bhowal and Mehta 2017).	Antiasthmatic, antiglaucoma, antidiabetic, antiobesity, antiplatelet, antimicrobial, anti-inflammatory, hypotensive, anticancer and antiproliferative, antidepressant, antidyspeptic, antioxidant, antiulcer, antimycotic, hepatoprotective activity. It also possesses relaxative, immune system enhancement and vasculogenic property, and found useful in UTI, psoriasis, thyroidism (Bhowal and Mehta 2017).
Acorus (*Acorus calamus;* Family: Acoraceae/ Araceae)	β-asarone, α- asarone, caryophyllene, eugenol, methyl isoeugenol, pinenes, myrcene, cymene, cisisoelemicine, calamen, calameon, clamenol, camphene, α-selinene, elemicine, *cis* and *trans* isoeugenol, camphor, calarene, P-cymene, bgurjunene, β-cadinene, camphor, terpinen-4-ol, aterpineol, calacorene, acrenone, acorone, acoragermacrone, linalool, shyobunones, preisocalamendiol, acoradin, galangin, calamendiol, sitosterol, spathulenol, (E)-β-ocimene, α-selinene, s-cadinol, isoshyobunone, bsesquiphellandrene, preiso calamendiol, acorone (Sharma et al. 2014a, b; Imam et al. 2013).	Antibacterial activity, antifungal activity, anti-inflammatory activity, analgesic activity, antioxidant activity, antidiabetic activity, anticancer activity, antimutagenic activity, Radioprotection and DNA Repair Activity, Wound-healing Activity, Immunosuppressive Activity, antidiarrhoeal activity, antiulcer activity, antispasmodic activity, anti-asthmatic activity, anti-convulsant activity, Antidepressant activity, Anti HIV Activity, Antihypertensive activity, as tranquiliser (Imam et al. 2013; Sharma et al. 2014a, b).

Table 8.1 (continued)

Name	Major bioactive phytomolecules	Pharmacological properties
Ocimum (*Ocimum sanctum*; Family: Lamiaceae/ Labiatae)	Eugenol, euginal, urosolic acid, carvacrol, linalool, limatrol, caryophyllene, methyl carvicol, fatty acids, sitosterol; rosmarinic acid, apigenin, vallinin, vitexin, cirsimaritin, isothymusin, isothymonin, orientin, stigmsterol, vicenin, camphor, *cis*-α-terpineol, cubenol, D-limonene, cardinene, eucalyptol, eicosane, eugenol, farnesol, farnesene, limonene, *n*-butylbenzoate, oleic acid, sabinene, veridifloro, selinene, α-camphene, αmyrcene, α-pinene, α-thujene, β-pinene, β-gurjunene, β-guaiene, caffeic acid, chlorgenic acid, gallic acid, galuteolin, isovitexin, luteolin, isorientin, procatechuic acid, urosolic acid, (Pattanayak et al. 2010; Kulkarni and Adavirao 2018).	Antibacterial activity, antifungal activity, antiviral activity, antimalarial activity, antiprotozoal activity, anthelmintic activity, antidiarrheal activity, as mosquito repellent, anti-oxidant activity, anti-inflammatory activity, anti-cataract potency, chemopreventive and radioprotective effect, anticancer activity, hepatoprotective effect, neuroprotective activity, cardioprotective effect, hypoglycaemic effect, anti-hypercholesterolemic and hypolipidemic activity, anti-hypertensive activity, analgesic effect, anti-pyretic activity, anti-allergic activity, immunomodulatory activity, anti-fertility, Anti-psychotic, CNS depressant activity, memory enhancement effect, antiasthmatic activity, anti-tussive potency, diaphoretic activity, antiulcer activity, anti-thyroid activity, anti-fertility activity, anti-emetic activity, anti-spasmodic activity, stress reducing activity, anti-arthritic activity, adaptogenic activity, as anti-coagulant effect (Cohen 2014; Kulkarni and Adavirao 2018).

8.3 Conclusion

Our lifestyle is becoming modernized as we are becoming more dependent on technology, adopting unhealthy lifestyle and moving away from nature. Herbs are important to maintain our health and discover of new medicine. Traditionally, we are gifted by our ancestors with medicinal knowledge and nature since its existence providing lot of herbs used for the ailments related to different seasons. Loss of biodiversity is huge problem or unscientific collection of medicinal plants from wild source will create a problem in future related to the sustainable availability of plant sources. Cultivation outside their natural habitat will be useful for sustainable availability of medicinal plants, preservation of medicinal plants and to promote economic development.

References

Akbar S, Khan SA, Masood A, Iqbal M. Use of *Strychnos Nux-Vomica* (Azraqi) seeds in Unani system of medicine: role of detoxification. Afr J Tradit Complement Altern Med. 2010;7(4):286–90.

Ansari AK. Study of Plant Tulsi and its benefits for human beings. Int J Appl Res. 2015;1(3):148–51.

Balasankar D, Vanilarasu K, Preetha PS, et al. Senna—a medical miracle plant. J Med Plants Stud. 2013;1(3):41–7.

Behera MC, Mohanty TL, Paramanik BK. Silvics, phytochemistry and ethnopharmacy of endangered poison nut tree (*Strychnos nux-vomica* L.): a review. J Pharmacog Phytochem. 2017;6(5):1207–16.

Bhattacharjee T, Sen D, Das SP, Datta M. Underutilized tuber crops for food, feed and nutritional security in Tripura. Int J Biores Sci. 2015;2(3):241–9.

Bhowal M, Mehta DM. *Coleus forskholii*: phytochemical and pharmacological profile. Int J Pharm Sci Res. 2017;8(9):3599–18.

Chalise U. The poppy plant: phytochemistry & pharmacology. Indo Global J Pharma Sci. 2015;5(1):58–65.

Chauhan S, Kaur A, Pareek RK. Pharmacobotanical and pharmacological evaluation of Ayurvedic crude drug: *Rauwolfia serpentina* (Apocynaceae). Int J Green Pharm. 2017;11(4):S686–93.

Cohen MM. Tulsi—*Ocimum sanctum*: a herb for all reasons. J Ayur Integr Med. 2014;5(4):4251–9.

Das S, Sharangi AB. Madagascar periwinkle (*Catharanthus roseus* L.): diverse medicinal and therapeutic benefits to humankind. J Pharmacog Phytochem. 2017;6(5):1695–701.

Das S, Dutta Choudhury M, Mazumder PB. In vitro propagation of genus Dioscorea—a critical review. Asian J Pharm Clin Res. 2013;6:26–30.

De Luca V, Salim V, Atsumi SM, Yu F. Mining the biodiversity of plants: a revolution in the making. Science. 2012;336:1658–61.

Deokar G, Kshirsagar S, Deore P, Kakulte H. Pharmaceutical benefits of *Plantago ovate* (Isabgol seed): a review. Pharm Biol Eval. 2016;3:32–41.

Deori C, Das S, Bordoloi SK. Study of hepatoprotective activity of *Emblica officinalis* (AMLA) in Albino rats. J Evid Based Med Healthc. 2017;4(54):3298–301.

Devi N, Gupta AK, Prajapati SK. Indian tribe's and villager's health and habits: popularity of apocynaceae plants as medicine. Int J Green Pharm. 2017;11:256.

Dey A, DE JN. *Rauvolfia serpentina* (L). Benth. ex Kurz.-a review. Asian J Plant Sci. 2010;9:285–98.

Dhakad D, Choudhary S, Wankhede A, Swarnakar VK. Knowledge and adoption level of improved production technology among opium poppy growers in Mandsaur District (M.P.). Int J Appl Agric Res. 2017;12(3):325–31.

Gaire BP, Subedi L. Phytochemistry, pharmacology and medicinal properties of *Phyllanthus emblica* Linn. Chin J Integr Med. 2014; https://doi.org/10.1007/s11655-014-1984-2.

Galani VJ, Patel DM. A comprehensive phytopharmacological review of *Dioscorea bulbifera* Linn. Int J Environ Sci Nat Res. 2017;4(5):1–11.

Ganapaty S, Thomas PS, Ramana KV, Vidyadhar K, Chakradhar V. A review of phytochemical studies of *Cassia* species. J Nat Remid. 2002;2:102–20.

Haddadian K, Haddadian K, Zahmatkash M. A review of plantago plant. Indian J Tradit Knowl. 2014;13:681–5.

Hasan MR, Islam MN, Islam MR. Phytochemistry, pharmacological activities and traditional uses of *Emblica officinalis*: a review. Int Curr Pharma J. 2016;5(2):14–21.

Hazra B, Sarkar R, Biswas S, Mandal N. Comparative study of the antioxidant and reactive oxygen species scavenging properties in the extracts of the fruits of Terminalia chebula, Terminalia belerica and Emblica officinalis. BMC Complemen Altern Med. 2010;10(20):1–15.

Imam H, Riaz Z, Azhar M, Sofi G, Hussain A. Sweet flag (*Acorus calamus* Linn.): an incredible medicinal herb. Int J Green Pharm. 2013;7:288–96.

Joy PP, Thomas J, Mathew S, Skaria BP. Medicinal plants. Kerala Agricultural University. Aromatic and Medicinal Plants Research Station. 1998. pp. 1–211.

Kala CP, Dhyani PP, Sajwan BS. Developing the medicinal plants sector in northern India: challenges and opportunities. J Ethnobiol Ethnomed. 2006;2:32.

Kalshetti P, Thakurdesai P, Alluri R. A review on bioactive phytoconstituents and pharmacological uses of *Commiphora mukul*. J Curr Pharma Res. 2014;5:1392–405.

Kanu AN, Ezeocha CV, Ogunka NP. A review on bioactive compounds of yam varieties for human disease management. Asian Food Sci J. 2018;1(4):1–10.

Kulkarni KV, Adavirao BV. A review on: Indian traditional shrub Tulsi (*Ocimum sanctum*): the unique medicinal plant. J Med Plants Studies. 2018;6(2):106–10.

Kulkarni KV, Ghurghure SM. Indian gooseberry (*Emblica officinalis*): complete pharmacognosy review. Int J Chem Studies. 2018;2:5–11.

Kumari R, Rathib B, Ranic A, Bhatnagar S. *Rauvolfia serpentina* L. Benth. ex Kurz.: phytochemical, pharmacological and therapeutic aspects. Int J Pharm Sci Rev Res. 2013;23(2):348–55.

Long JL. The gale encyclopedia of alternative medicine, vil I. 2nd ed. Detroit: Thomson; 2005.

Maan AA, Nazir A, Khan MKI, et al. The therapeutic properties and applications of *aloe vera*: a review. J Herb Med. 2018;12:1–10. https://doi.org/10.1016/j.hermed.2018.01.002.

Maiti S, Geetha KA. Medicinal and aromatic plants in India. 2007. http://nsdl.niscair.res.in/jspui/bitstream/123456789/742/4/Medicinal%20and%20Aromatic%20plants.pdf.

Mani D, Dhawan SS. Scientific basis of therapeutic uses of opium poppy (*Papaver somniferum*) in Ayurveda. Actahorticulturae. 2014;1036:175–80.

Mathur SI, Bulchandani N, Parihar S, Shekhawat GS. Critical review on steviol glycosides: pharmacological, toxicological and therapeutic aspects of high potency zero caloric sweetener. Int J Pharmacol. 2017;13(7):916–28.

Meena AK, Rao MM, Singh A, Kumari S. Physicochemical and preliminary phytochemical studies on the rhizome of *Acorus calamus* Linn. Int J Pharma Pharm Sci. 2010;2(2):130–1.

Meena VD, Dotania ML, Meena BP, Das H. Beena. Isabgol (*Plantago ovata* Forsk.)—a medicinal herb: good source of income generation in water scarcity regions. Popular Kheti. 2015;3(4):2–5.

Minwuyelet T, MogesSewalem M, Gashe M. Review on therapeutic uses of *Aloe vera*. Global J Pharmacol. 2017;11(2):14–20.

Momtazi-Borojeni AA, Esmaeili SA, Abdollahi E, Sahebkar A. A review on the pharmacology and toxicology of steviol glycosides extracted from *Stevia rebaudiana*. Curr Pharm Des. 2017;23(11):1616–22.

Moudi M, Go R, Yien CYS, Nazre M. Vinca alkaloids. Int J Preventive Med. 2013;4(11):1231–5.

Nisar A, Mamat AS, Hatim MI, Aslam MS, Ahmad MS. An updated review on *catharanthusroseus*: phytochemical and pharmacological analysis. Ind Res J Pharm Sci. 2016;3(2):631–53.

Nyeem MAB, Rashid AKMMU, Nowrose M, Hossain MA. *Solanum nigrum* (Maku): a review of pharmacological activities and clinical effects. Int J Appl Res. 2017;3(1):12–7.

Patel K, Patel DK. Medicinal importance, pharmacological activities, and analytical aspects of aloin: a concise report. J Acute Dis. 2013;2:262–9.

Patel DK, Patel K, Tahilyani V. Barbaloin: a concise report of its pharmacological and analytical aspects. Asian Pac Trop Biomed. 2012;2(10):835–8.

Patel K, Laloo D, Singh GK, Gadewar M, Patel DK. A review on medicinal uses, analytical techniques and pharmacological activities of Strychnos nux-vomica Linn.: a concise report. Chin J Integr Med. 2017; https://doi.org/10.1007/s11655-016-2514-1.

Pattanayak P, Behera P, Das D, Panda SK. *Ocimum sanctum* Linn. A reservoir plant for therapeutic applications: an overview. Pharmacog Rev. 2010;4(7):95–105.

Paul R, Dutta KA. An updated overview on *Atropa belladonna* L. Int Res J Pharm. 2011;2:11–7.

Radha MH, Laxmipriya NP. Evaluation of biological properties and clinical effectiveness of Aloe vera: a systematic review. J Tradit Complemen Med. 2015;5:21–6.

Rajak AR, Singh R. Contribution of medicinal plants in economic growth. World J Pharma Pharma Sci. 2017;6:367–72.

Rane MH, Sahu NK, Ajgoankar SS, Teli NC, Verma DR. A holistic approach on review of *Solanumvirginianum*. L. J Pharm Pharma Sci. 2014;3(3):1–4.

Renjini KR, Gopakumar G, Latha MS. The medicinal properties of phytochemicals in catharanthusroseus—a review. Eur J Pharma Med Res. 2017;4(11):545–51.

Saleem TSM, Chetty CM, Ramkanth S. *Solanum nigrum* Linn.—a review. Phcog Rev. 2009;3:342–5.

Sarfraz RM, Khan H, Maheen S, et al. *Plantago ovata:* a comprehensive review on cultivation, biochemical, pharmaceutical and pharmacological aspects. Acta Pol Pharm. 2017;74:739–46.

Sarup P, Bala S, Kamboj S. Pharmacology and phytochemistry of oleo-gum resin of *Commiphora wightii* (Guggulu). Scientifica (Cairo). 2015;2015:138039. https://doi.org/10.1155/2015/138039.

Sautour M, Mitaine-Offer A, Lacaille-Dubois M. The Dioscorea genus: a review of bioactive steroid saponins. J Nat Med. 2007;61:91–101.

Sen S, Chakraborty R. Revival, Modernization and integration of Indian traditional herbal medicine in clinical practice: importance, challenges and future. J Trad Complemen Med. 2017;7:234–44.

Sen S, Chakraborty R, De B. Challenges and opportunities in the advancement of herbal medicine: India's position and role in global context. J Herb Med. 2011;1(3–4):67–75.

Sharma P, Kharkwal AC, Kharkwal H, Abdin MZ, Varma A. A review on pharmacological properties of *Aloe vera*. Int J Pharm Sci Rev Res. 2014a;29(2): 31–7.

Sharma V, Singh S, Chaudhary P. *Acorus calamus* (the healing plant): a review on its medicinal potential, micropropagation and conservation. Nat Prod Res. 2014b;28(18):1454–66.

Sharma V, Hem K, Seth A, Maurya SK. *Solanum indicum* Linn.: an ethnopharmacological, phytochemical and pharmacological review. Curr Res J Pharma Allied Sci. 2017;1:1–9.

Sreeramu BB. Cultivation of medicinal and aromatic crops. Hyderabad, India: University Press Pvt. Ltd; 2004.

Subharani K. Chemical constituents and medicinal properties of *Solanum xanthocarpum*. A review. Int J Sci Res. 2016;5(10):824–6.

Sunitha K, Swapna D. Preliminary evaluation of antioxidant and antimicrobial activity of *Solanum khasianum* berries. Int J Pharmacog Phytochem Res. 2014;6(1):104–6.

Tripathi YC. Cassia Angustifolia, a versatile medicinal crop. Int Tree Crops J. 1999;10:121–9.

Wolwer-Rieck U. The leaves of *Stevia rebaudiana* (Bertoni), their constituents and the analyses thereof: a review. J Agric Food Chem. 2012;60:886–95.

Part II

Plants for Better Future (Therapeutic & Pharmaceutical Consideration)

Preclinical and Clinical Trials of Indian Medicinal Plants in Disease Control

9

Md. Harun Al Rashid, Anindita Kundu, Vivekananda Mandal, Phurpa Wangchuk, and Subhash C. Mandal

Contents

The original version of this chapter was revised. A correction to this chapter can be found at https://doi.org/10.1007/978-981-13-7248-3_39

Md. H. Al Rashid (✉) · A. Kundu · S. C. Mandal
Pharmacognosy and Phytotherapy Research Laboratory, Division of Pharmacognosy, Department of Pharmaceutical Technology, Jadavpur University, Kolkata, West Bengal, India

V. Mandal
Institute of Pharmacy, Guru Ghasidas Central University, Bilaspur, India

P. Wangchuk
Centre for Molecular Therapeutics, Australian Institute of Tropical Health and Medicine, James Cook University, Townsville, QLD, Australia

S. Sen, R. Chakraborty (eds.), *Herbal Medicine in India*,
https://doi.org/10.1007/978-981-13-7248-3_9

9.1 Introduction

At the beginning of human civilization, herbs have been an integral part of the society, valued for both their culinary and medicinal properties. Herbal medicine plays a great role to fulfil the needs and has been used for curing ailments for many centuries. Broadly, medicinal plants are used as major compounds or as a crude substance. Just a small number of plant species has been methodically investigated for their therapeutic effect (Heinrich and Gibbons 2001). India is one of the large countries in the world, which has distinctive assets of medicinal herbs and enormous traditional awareness of the use of herbal medicine for treating diverse ailments. Traditionally some medicinal plants such as 'Rasayana' has been used for over 1000 years in the Indian traditional health care systems (Scartezzini and Sproni 2000; Majumder et al. 2016). Nearly all Indian practitioners formulate and dispense their own regimens. However, there many formulations that are manufactured in large industrial scale and marketed worldwide. According to the World Health Organization (WHO), 21,000 plants are used for medicinal purposes worldwide and 3000 species are reported from India alone (Wangchuk et al. 2016) out of which 150 species are used commercially in large scale. India is the largest producer of herbs and it is often known as botanical garden of the world (Seth and Sharma 2004).

This chapter focuses on medicinal plants used in the treatment of a major chronic disease, which are associated with huge socio-economic losses. It highlights the preclinical and clinical trials outcomes, and discusses the role of WHO and Government policies on medicinal herbs.

9.2 Biological Background of Herbs

Chemical compounds (also commonly known as phytochemicals) are manufactured by all herbs as part of their normal metabolic activities or as part of their defensive mechanism. These phytochemicals are divided into (1) primary metabolites (examples are sugars and fats), which are found in all herbs; and (2) secondary metabolites (examples are alkaloids and terpenoids), which are found in a smaller range of herbs, serving a more specific function (Vaidya 1997). A number of chemical constituents are toxins used to deter-predation and others are pheromones utilized to magnetize insects used for pollination. Medicinal herbs produce a baffling array of phytochemicals (Vaidya et al. 1996) and few of them including quinine, morphine, codeine, digoxin and artemisinin have been developed into drugs for treating many human diseases (Vaidya 1997).

9.3 Herbs Used in Disease Control

9.3.1 CNS Active Herbs

According to Vaidya, the span of CNS dynamic Indian Medicinal Plants in therapeutics has been exemplifying in an assessment commentary. The subsequent clause center on the supplementary effort conceded (Singh et al. 1997).

9.3.1.1 Nootropics

Different seeds extracts of *Pongamia pinnata* (Karanj) lessen pentobarbitone sleeping time, by stimulation of the hepatic microsomal enzyme method and also roots having the same activity (Kumar and Singh 1996). However, the petroleum ether extract (PEE) of the roots enhanced pentobarbitone sleeping time, probably due to CNS depression (Singh and Dhawan 1997). Additionally, the PEE of the seed obtained from *Pongomia pinnata* was screened for nootropic action in an experimental model of Alzheimer's disease (created by ibotenic acid-induced lesioning of nucleus basalis magnocellularis). It invested equally, the cognitive shortages and the decrease in cholinergic markers after 2 weeks of cure (Bhattacharya and Kumar 1997).

The alcoholic *Bacopa monniera* extract assisted the attainment, consolidation and maintenance of memory as observed in albino rats, viz. foot shock provoked intensity bias, dynamic conditioned avoidance and Sidman continuous avoidance responses (Jaiswal et al. 1994).

A polyherbal formulation, Trasina was seen to exert important nootropic effect subsequently 21 days treatment in two experimental models of Alzheimer's ailment. These types of models used either injecting colchicine (15 μg/rat) intracerebroventricular (i.c.v.) or injuring nucleus basalis magnocellularis by ibotenic acid (10 μg/rat). This polyherbal agent enhanced equally memory and levels of various cholinergic markers resembling acetylcholine concentration, choline acetyltransferase action and muscarinic cholinergic receptor binding in frontal cortex and hippocampus of rat brain. Consequently, its nootropic result might be recognized to modification of cholinergic dysfunction (Makwana et al. 1994).

9.3.1.2 Psychoactives

Azadirachta indica (Neem) leaf extract showed anxiolytic activities comparable to diazepam at small doses (10–200 mg/kg) in rats. High doses (>400 mg/kg), did not illustrate anxiolytic action (Mukherjee et al. 1996).

Vitex leucoxylon (Nirnochi in Tamil) leaf extract and cold aqueous infusion down spontaneous motor activity, provoked d-amphetamine-induced sterotypy and oxotremorine-induced vibrations and reduced the time of calmness in the behavioral 'despair' examination in mice (Mitra et al. 1996).

Nelumbo nucifera rhizomes extract created a major diminution in impulsive action, reduced in the investigative behavioral model by the head dip and Y maze tests, muscle relaxant function and potentiation of pentobarbitone-induced sleeping time (Kulkarni and Ninan 1997).

The entire leaf extracts of *Abies pindrow* Royle (Silver fir) [petroleum ether (PEE), benzene (BE), chloroform (CE), acetone (AE), and ethanol (EE)] demonstrated potentiation of pentobarbitone sleeping time i.e. CNS depressant effect. The PEE, BE, CE and AE (highest efficacy) proved important anti-depressant action. On the other hand, EE was found to potentiate immobility, signifying that this fraction is absent of anti-depressant action (Manocha et al. 1996).

9.3.1.3 Agents Attenuating Dependence

Withania somnifera (Ashwagandha) root extract has been used in the treatment of chronic disease and attenuated the improvement of tolerance and also the improvement of dependence to morphine in mice. By itself, *Withania somnifera* has no analgesic effect (Manocha et al. 1997).

9.3.1.4 Anticonvulsants

According to Vaz et al. 1998, *Ginkgo biloba* reduced the defensive result of sodium valproate and carbamazepine against picrotoxin as well as strychnine-induced convulsions in mice (Vaz et al. 1998). More studies demonstrated that pretreatment by *Ginkgo biloba* extract potentiated the convulsions produced by picrotoxin and strychnine, representing the connection of GABAergic system and chloride channels (for picrotoxin) and modulation of activity of the glycine neurotransmitter (for strychnine) by *Ginkgo biloba* (Johri et al. 1995).

Caffeine intake has been shown to increase the plasma half-life (two-fold) and reduce the bio availability by 32% of carbamazepine in normal human volunteers. No interaction was seen with sodium valproate. These results indicate the need for restriction of xanthine/caffeine consumption in patients on carbamazepine therapy (Ramaswamy and Viswanathan 1997).

9.3.1.5 Sedatives

Vernonia lasiopus and *Vernonia galamensis* leaf fractions have been revealed to have sedative properties using *in vitro* model (Makwana et al. 1994).

9.3.1.6 Analgesics

Gossypin (a bioflavonoid compound) isolated from the yellow petals of *Hibiscus vitifolius* (Bhasadwaji) has demonstrated the anti-nociceptive activity, which was similar to morphine. The cholinergic and GABAergic neurotransmitter pathways of gossypin pre-treatment extensively diminished the progress of acute tolerance to morphine-induced anti-nociception (acetic acid-induced writhing assay). As an analgesic, gossypin is a possible contestant for clinical trials with the advantages of lack of tolerance and dependence liability (Mitra et al. 1996). Inhibition of acetic acid writhing was observed with both the ethanol extract and cold aqueous infusion of *Vitex leucoxylon* (Narayanan et al. 1999).

A novel furopyridine alkaloid is Cerpegin obtained from *Ceropegia juncea* Roxb. (Bhutumbi) showed an analgesic activity (not involving the opioid pathway) against acetic acid induced writhing in mice. Important analgesic effect was noticed in leaf and seed of *Vernonia lasiopus* and *Vernonia galamensis* (Makwana et al. 1994) and alcoholic extract of *Ochna obtusata* (Kanakchampak) stem bark using the above model in rats. *Panax ginseng* revealed anti-nociceptive action and potentiated the anti-nociceptive effect of both pentazocine and aspirin (Makwana et al. 1994).

An important analgesic effect in mice was noticed in alcoholic extract of the roots of *Clerodendron serratum* (Bharanji) (Kumar and Basu 1994).

9.3.1.7 Anti-inflammatory Agents

Vitex leucoxylon leaf extract demonstrated important inhibition of carrageenan paw oedema and granulation tissue formation *in vivo* (Mengi and Deshpande 1995). Leaf extract obtained from the plant *Ficus racemosa* demonstrated anti-inflammatory activity on carrageenan, serotonin, histamine and dextran-induced rat hind paw oedema models (Mandal et al. 2000a, b).

Suspension of *Calotropis procera* (Arka) latex showed anti-inflammatory action when examined in the carrageenan and formalin induced rat paw oedema models (Vimala et al. 1997). Aspirin transdermal patch is one type of formulation which is basically used as anti-inflammatory activity (Banerjee et al. 2012). Ocular anti-inflammatory activity of roots and leaves extract obtained from *Butea frondosa* (Palash) was screened in rabbits. The gel formulation of leaves reduced the intra-ocular pressure, declined leucocytosis and miosis and was similar to flubiproten gel (Rao and Mishra 1997).

Michelia champaca Linn. (Champaka) flowers extracts, *Ixora brachiata* Roxb (Rasna) and *Rhynchosia cana* Willd have shown noteworthy anti-inflammatory action against cotton pellet-induced subacute inflammation in rats (Suresh et al. 1995).

Sida rhombifolia (Atibala) extract proved important oedema suppressant effect in the carrageenan -induced paw oedema model in rats. Possible mechanism of action might be due to its inhibitory property on release of mediators of inflammation such as histamine, 5-hydroxytryptamine, bradykinin etc. (Subramoniam et al. 1995).

9.3.1.8 Antipyretics

The ethanolic extracts of *Ailanthus excels* (Mahanimba), *Toddalia asiatica* (Kanchana) and *Araucaria bidwilli* (Monkey puzzle) extracts demonstrated reasonable to a significant degree of antipyretic effect in an experimental rat model of 20% yeast suspension induced hyperthermia (Narayanan et al. 1999).

Andrographis elongate has shown more potent antipyretic action when compared to *Andrographis paniculata* (Kalmegh). *Nelumbo nucifera* rhizome extract produced a momentous dose-dependent lowering of body temperature in normal rats and antipyretic effect in pyretic rats (Ganguli et al. 1996).

Rhynchosia cana showed significant antipyretic activity in rats (Andrade et al. 1994). Alcoholic extract of the roots of *Clerodendron serratum* showed significant antipyretic activity following typhoid TAB vaccination in rabbits (Kayath and Goel 1995).

As against these antipyretic plants, *Panax ginsengs* showed hyperthermic effect and attenuated the hypothermic response of reserpine and 5-HTP induced hyperthermia in animals (Makwana et al. 1994).

9.3.1.9 Neurotransmitter Modulation

Analysis of the neurochemical results of diverse fusarial toxins isolated from *Fusarium moniliform* and *Fusarium orysporum* demonstrated that *Fusarium moniliform* had irreversible and nonspecific Mono amino oxidase inhibitory action comparable to nialamide (Bhattacharya et al. 1994). Studies on the effect of BR-16A on adrenergic and dopaminergic function in rats showed that it did not interfere with α2-adrenergic and dopamine auto-receptor functioning. However, its effects on mobility in the open field test following challenge with clonidine or apomorphine showed that it enhanced dopamine post-synaptic receptor activity (Dhanasekaran et al. 1994).

9.3.2 Plants Modulating Autonomic and Autacoids Activity

The development to estimate agents modulating autonomic and autacoid action are declining. Though, the consequence of using certain methodologies such as isolated tissue tests to assemble preliminary data about the relations of a herbal product with host receptor methods remains conclusive. Some of the attempts in this way are discussed below. The outcome of *Cuscuta reflexa* (Amarvalli) extract resembled those of acetylcholine when examined on isolated rabbit ileum, frog rectus abdominis and heart and these actions were blocked by atropine. The action of this extract on isolated frog rectus abdominis muscle was blocked by pancuronium and potentiated by neostigmine (Dalvi et al. 1994).

Beta-adrenoceptor mediated tracheal rest or the diminished sensitivity of the tracheal smooth muscle induced by down-regulation of receptors with terbutaline in guinea pigs was unchanged by Abana, a herbomineral formulation. This is perhaps due to need of Abana's effects on ß-receptors of the airway. Though, pretreatment with Abana improved potassium chloride-induced contractions and improved the compassion to the relaxant properties of isoprenaline, terbutaline and aminophylline following such contractions, possibly by increasing membrane permeability to calcium ions (Srinivasan and Srinivasan 1995).

9.3.3 CVS Active Herbs

Last few years cardiovascular pharmacology mainly aimed on agents with hypolipidaemic properties and plant drugs are no exemption. This part describes diverse agents that have been calculated for their outcome on the cardiovascular system.

9.3.3.1 Anticoagulant

The methanolic extracts and petroleum ether obtained from *Araucaria bidwillii* leaf and oleo resin confirmed slight delaying effect on bleeding and clotting times at 1 h interval in rabbits when experienced using Wright's and Dukes capillary tube method (Sharma et al. 1995).

9.3.3.2 Hypolipidaemic

Vitex leucoxylon leaf extract and cold aqueous infusion mainly decreased serum total cholesterol levels in mice (Mengi and Deshpande 1995).

Gugulipid is a main constituent obtained from *Commiphera mukul* that has been widely examined for its hypolipidaemic action. Administration of gugulipid with propranolol or diltiazem in normal volunteers was found to reduce the bioavailability of both drugs (Shaila et al. 1995).

When *Adenocalymma alliaceum* flowers was administered at 2% level for 6 weeks to hypercholesterolaemic rats, it extensively decreased serum cholesterol levels and lowered the absorption of dietary cholesterol from the intestines (Srividya and Periwal 1995).

Alcoholic extract of *Semecarpus anacardium* (Bhallatak, nut shell) also showed hypocholesterolemic activity and prevented cholesterol-induced atheroma in hypercholesterolaemic rabbits (Chattopadhyay 1997).

Correspondingly, *Terminalia belerica* (Bibhitak) extract decreased the levels of lipids in experimentally induced hypercholesterolaemia in rabbits. There was also a major decrease in liver and heart lipids (Singh et al. 1998).

9.3.3.3 Anti-Hypertensives

Preparation of the whole plant of *Phyllanthus amarus* (Bhuiamalaki) was administered to nine mild hypertensive subjects for 10 days. The results suggest that it is a potential diuretic, hypotensive and hypoglycemic drug for humans (Bhatt et al. 1998).

Hydroalcoholic extract obtained from *Azadirachta indica* leaf caused a dose-dependent hypotensive result. It did not alter the force of contraction or heart rate at low doses in isolated frog heart, but caused a temporary cardiac arrest in diastolic at high doses (Nyman et al. 1998). The petroleum ether extract of *Abies pindrow* leaf explained an important hypotensive effect in anaesthetized dogs (Chopra and Singh 1994).

Treatment with a polyherbal formulation is Abana having normotensive rats produced significant lowering of blood pressure, improvement of vaso-pressor reactions to low dose of noradrenaline (with no effect on dopamine β hydroxylase activity) and no activity on the vaso-depressor responses of acetylcholine and isoprenaline. Abana mainly confined against ethinyl oestradiol induced hypertension and increased dopamine β hydroxylase action in these hypertensive animals. It recommends to makes activities against ethinyl oestradiol induced hypertension by its sympatholytic property (Vaidya 1994).

9.3.3.4 ACE (Angiotensin Converting Enzyme) Inhibitors

Approximately 72 species of traditional medicinal plants belonging to 42 families have been explored for their capacity to inhibit the angiotensin converting enzyme. 4 species out of 72 were found to have a high ACE inhibiting capability and were low in their tannin content (Mukherjee et al. 1997).

9.3.3.5 Cardio Protectives

The plant *Sophora japonica* contain a flavonoid called rutin clearly reduced the infarct size and prohibited the loss of the 'R' wave in anaesthetized rats subjected to coronary artery ligation. Rutin had no activity on heart rate and systolic blood pressure. This constitute reduced the ligation-induced enhance in serum malonyldialdehyde levels and prevented the loss of glutathione peroxidase effect. It inhibited *in vitro*, luminol-induced chemiluminescence of rat PMN's. Consequently rutin has beneficial action is possibly due to its ability to harm the generation of reactive oxygen species (Saha et al. 1997).

9.3.3.6 Positive Ionotropics

Ionotropic actions of *Terminalia arjuna* (Arjuna) is controversial according to Vaidya. Some studies proved the positive ionotropic effects of Arjuna but some scientists have observed negative ionotropic and chronotropic effects as well. Hence, he had recommended more detailed experimental and clinical studies on the plant and its active principle. Statistics of placebo-controlled clinical studies carried out consequently with this herb is presented below. It was observed in phase II clinical trial after compared to placebo in 12 patients with refractory CCF that treatment with *Terminalia arjuna* was associated with an improvement in symptoms and signs of heart failure, improvement in the NYHA class (from IV & III), decrease in echo-left ventricular end-diastolic and end-systolic volumes indices, increase in the left ventricular stroke volume index and increase in left ventricular ejection fraction at the end of 2 weeks. Long-term treatment (i.e. 24 months) also proved sustained development in the signs and symptoms, effort tolerance and NYHA class among the patients (Nair et al. 1994).

9.3.4 Herbs Acting on Respiratory System

Drymaria cordata willd and *Leucas lavandulaefolia* (Dronapushpi) extracts were explored for their effects on a cough model induced by sulfur dioxide gas in mice. These two herbs showed major antitussive activity, comparable to that of codeine phosphate and increasing concentrations explained better inhibition of cough (Nair and Saraf 1995; Gupta et al. 1995a, b).

Solanum xanthocarpum (Kantakari) and *Solanum trilobatum* (Alarka), the plants mentioned in Siddha, have been shown to improve various parameters of pulmonary function (FVC, FEV1, PEFR & FEF25–75%) in asthmatic subjects with mild-moderate asthma (Gupta et al. 1997).

9.3.5 Anti-allergic Herbs

Alcoholic extract of *Vitex negundo* (Nirgundi) has demonstrated anti-allergic activity against immunologically induced degranulation of mast cells superior than that with compound 40/80. This plant extract can inhibit in oedema during active paw anaphylaxis using *in vitro* model in mice (Gupta et al. 1997).

Nair and Saraf (Barua et al. 1997) additionally examined their activities on mediator release and smooth muscle contractions of sensitized and non-sensitized guinea pig trachea using antigen and compound 48/80 correspondingly. This fraction mainly inhibited both the initial and later continued phases of tracheal contractions. The first phase was principally due to histamine release which was blocked by the extract (confirmed in guinea pig ileal studies). The final phase was due to the release of lipid mediators from arachidonic acid. Inhibition of the final phase may be secondary to inhibition of arachidonic acid by the ethanolic extract. Arbortristoside A & C are two chemical constituent obtained from the seeds of *Nyctanthus arbortristis* (Srividya and Periwal 1995) alcoholic extract, two diterpenes, andrographolide and neoadrographolide, derived from *Andrographis paniculata* (Rizvi et al. 1995), and Himachalol, a sesquiterpene alcohol, isolated from the hexane soluble extract of the wood of *Cedrus deodara*. These were found to have momentous anti-allergic effect comparable to disodium cromoglycate when tested in the experimental models of passive cutaneous anaphylaxis and mast cell degranulation in rats. Correspondingly, the bark of *Albizzia lebbeck* (Shirish) aqueous extract was found to have anti-allergic effects in an experimental model of passive cutaneous anaphylaxis and mast cell stabilization property (Manickam et al. 1997).

9.3.6 Hypoglycemic Herbs

A formulation of *Phyllanthus amarus* was found to have hypoglycemic activities in nine human subjects, four of whom were diabetics (Tripathi and Chaturvedi 1995).

Rizvi et al., have confirmed that *Pterocarpus marsupium* (Vijaysar) contain principal constituent epicatechin that demonstrated a defensive action on erythrocyte osmotic fragility, similar to insulin, but by a different mechanism of action using *in vitro* model (Gomes et al. 1995). Out of three important phenolic constituents of the heartwood of *Pterocarpus marsupium* (pterosupin, marsupin and pterostilbene) tested, marsupin and pterostilbene considerably lowered the blood glucose levels and the results were analogous to metformin (Chattopadhyay 1996).

The hypoglycemic efficacy of *Pterocarpus marsupium* has been further evaluated in a multicentric (4 centres) flexible-dose open trial in newly-diagnosed patients of non-insulin-dependent diabetes mellitus (Sheel et al. 1995).

The alcoholic extract of *Inula racemosa* (Pushkarmula) lowered blood glucose and enhanced liver glycogen in rats. However, there was no increase in plasma insulin levels or an increase in the degree of degranulation of beta cells of the pancreas. Its action may be at the peripheral level by potentiating insulin sensitivity (Talwar et al. 1995).

Camellia sinensis (Black tea leaf) extract extensively reduced the blood glucose level and was found to have both preventive and healing activity in streptozotocin induced diabetic rats (Joshi et al. 1996).

Azadirachta indica leaf extract had no activity on the peripheral utilization of glucose (determined by intravenous glucose tolerance tests) and on hepatic glycogen in normal and streptozotocin induced diabetic rats. Though, it blocked the action of epinephrine on glucose metabolism and decrease in peripheral glucose exploitation in diabetic rats and to several extents in normal rats, investigative of an anti-hyperglycemic prospective of the herb (Deka et al. 1994).

9.3.7 Anti- and Pro-Fertility Herbs

Bupleurum marginatum extract was found to have vital oestrogenic effect as seen by the improved uterine weight and early opening and cornification of vagina in embryonic rats and histological features of the uterus (Sarkar 1994).

Azadirachta indica seed contain oil known as Praneem vilci which was found to be safe when taken as a single intra-uterine instillation in 18 healthy tubectomised female. No problematic actions were seen. The menstrual pattern and ovulatory condition did not alter and the endometrial biopsy was average. 10 female had taken the HSD-hCG vaccine, co-administration of Praneem vilci did not prevent the antibody reaction to HSD-hCG vaccine (Rasik et al. 1996). *Azadirachta indica* leaves were found to have reversible, anti-androgenic properties in male rats (Prasad et al. 1994).

9.3.8 Herbs Promoting Skin and Bone Healing

Cissus quadrangularis (Asthishunkala) methanolic extract healed the experimentally cracked radius-ulna of dogs as visually demonstrated in radiological and histopathological assessments (Anand et al. 1995). It also exhibited a decrease in serum calcium levels as balanced to saline control animals after treatment. Essential oils obtained from the leaves of *Eucalyptus hybrid* and seeds of *Seseli indicum* when administered intradermal route improved cutaneous capillary permeability against Evan's blue treated rabbits test. This action may be advantageous in their possible wound curing effect (Mukherjee et al. 1995). Aqueous extract of latex obtained from *Euphorbia neriifolia* (Nivadung) assisted the curing of surgically produced cutaneous wounds inguinea pigs as proofed by an increase in tensile strength, DNA content, epithelialisation and angiogenesis in topical route (Dahanukar et al. 1998).

9.3.9 Herbs Acting on Genito-Urinary System

Ammannia baccifera (Bhatjambol) extract was found to be efficient in reducing the development of urinary stones (mostly of magnesium ammonium phosphate with traces of calcium oxalate) as well as liquefying preformed ones (curative) that were provoked by instillation of zinc discs in the urinary bladders of rats. Management with *Ammannia baccifera* also extensively reduced calcium and magnesium levels (Dalvi et al. 1994).

Crateva nurvala (Varun) contain Lupeol and a number of its derivatives those were found to have major anti-hyperoxaluric and anti-hypercalciuric effect when tested in rats against hydroxyproline induced hyperoxaluria and calciurial (Johri et al. 1995).

9.3.10 Gastro-Intestinal Pro- and Anti-Kinetic Herbs

Alcoholic extract of rhizomes obtained from *Nelumbo nucifera* demonstrated important inhibitory effect against castor oil induced diarrhea and PGE2 induced entero-pooling in rats. It also demonstrated major diminution of gastro-intestinal motility in rats, thus signifying its usefulness as an anti-diarrhoeal substance (De et al. 1997).

Aqueous extract, dry powder and incinerated powder are dosage formulation obtained from *Emblica officinalis* (Amalki). These formulations were tested for the action on gastro-intestinal motility at various dose levels (210,420 and 840 mg/kg) in mice. Out of three formulation, the dry powder and the aqueous extract proved pro-kinetic action at all the three dose levels. The incinerated powder formulation at lower doses, proved pro-kinetic action, where at higher doses, it reduced gastro-intestinal motility (Vaidya et al. 1996).

9.3.11 Cytoprotective Herbs

9.3.11.1 Ulcero- Protectives

Gastric and Duodenal Ulcers

The alcoholic, oleoresin and petroleum ether extracts of leaf obtained from *Araucaria bidwillii* showed moderate degree of ulcero-protective effect in pylorus ligated rat model of gastric ulceration (Bhatt and Bhatt 1996). *Vernonia lasiopus* and *Vernonia galamensis* leaf and seed extracts were responsible for antiulcerogenic activities when examined using either hydrochloric acid or ethanol as the necrotizing agent in rats (Nagarkatti et al. 1994).

The protective action of hot water extract obtained from *Camellia sinensis* (black tea) demonstrated positive effects against ulcers induced in rats by various ulcerogens (NSAIDs, ethanol, reserpine, 5-HT, histamine) and by cold limit stress 5-HT and histamine. It distorted the acid and peptic action of gastric secretion. The four sitavirya plants viz. Satavari (*Asparagus racemosus*: fresh root juice, 1250 mg/kg), Yastimadhu (*Glycerrhiza glabra*: water decoction of root, 600 mg/kg), Kutaja (*Holorrhena antidysentrica*: water decoctions of bark, 400 mg/kg) and Aswattha (water decoctions of bark, 500 mg/kg) were derive to have ulceroprotective properties against 2 h cold restraint stress ulcers, pylorus ligation-induced gastric and cysteamine-induced duodenal ulcers in rats. However, they were uncreative against acute aspirin-induced gastric ulcers (Thorat et al. 1995).

Ulcerative Colitis

Boswellia serrata has defensive effect in patients suffering from (grade II and III) ulcerative colitis. The stool distinctiveness along with histopathological, scan microscopical alters in rectal biopsies and blood parameters (hemoglobin, serum iron, calcium, phosphorus, proteins, total leukocytes and eosinophils) improved subsequent treatment with *Boswellia serrata* gum resin preparation; the results being similar to sulfasalazine.

9.3.11.2 Hepato-Protectives

According to Vaidya et al., the experimental and clinical research work linked to hepato-protective effects of different formulations available in the Indian market (Ziauddin et al. 1996). Bhatt and Bhatt have not only assembled the information available regarding the studies on different potential plant drugs from India but also have talked about the troubles and drawbacks pertaining to this research (Kumar et al. 1996). A number of the agents value mentioning are as follows.

Tinospora cordifolia has been shown to reduce fibrosis in rats, induced by CCl_4, was to significantly develop the suppressed Kupffer cell function in another rat model of chronic liver injure induced by heterologous serum. This raises the possibility that anti-fibrotic effect of *Tinospora cordifolia* is mediated through activation of kupffer cells (Kuttan 1996).

9.3.11.3 Pancreato-Protectives

Experimentally the defensive action of *Emblica officinalis* mainly induced acute necrotizing pancreatitis in dogs. This plant inhibited the increase in serum amylase caused by pancreatitis (Sharma et al. 1998). Microscopical experiment proved that the acinar cell injury and the entire inflammatory score were extensively fewer in dogs pretreated with *Emblica officinalis*.

9.3.11.4 Myelo-Protectives

Withania somnifera contains three compounds, cyclophosphamide, azathioprine or prednisolone and one or more of these mainly prevented mylosuppression, as seen by a major increase in hemoglobin concentration, RBC and WBC count, platelet count and body weight and hemolytic antibody responses to human erythrocytes (Johri et al. 1995).

9.3.11.5 Radio-Protectives

It was found to significantly increase total WBC count, bone marrow cellularity, natural killer cell and antibody-dependent cellular cytotoxicity after oral administration of Rasayana group of drugs (from Ayurveda) in gamma radiation exposed mice. Rasayanas mainly decrease radiation induced lipid peroxidation in liver (Mohanan et al. 1997).

9.3.11.6 Oculo-Protectives

Ocimum sanctum leaves delayed the beginning as well as the successive maturation of cataract extensively in two models of cataract i.e. galactosamic cataract in rats and naphthalene cataract in rabbits (Chaurasia et al. 1995).

9.3.11.7 Membrane Stabilizers

The plant part leaf and root extracts of *Vernonia lasiopus* and *Vernonia galamensis* confirmed outstanding *in vitro* membrane soothing action as determined by the percentage inhibition of RBC lysis (Tripathi et al. 1996).

9.3.12 Herbs Protecting Against Oxidative Stress

9.3.12.1 UV Light-Induced

The chemical constituent sobatum basically obtained from *Solanum trilobatum* (Alarka) after purification revealed important protection *in vitro* against UV light induced injury by free radicals on the bacteria *Salmonella typhimurium*. Equally, this herb also confined against superoxide production that was generated by the reaction of photo reduced riboflavin andoxygen (Tripathi et al. 1997).

9.3.12.2 Cumene Hydroperoxide Induced

An organomineral compound is Tamrabhasma obtained from Ayurveda, revealed important protection against cumene hydroperoxide induced lipid peroxidation and lesser reduced glutathione and superoxide dismutase levels in rat liver homogenate. This constitutes also extensively reduced malondealdehyde (MDA) levels. No modification in biochemical and histopathological factors were recorded. After experimenting it was proven that tamrabhasma is a powerful antioxidant drug and can be utilized in the treatment of lipid peroxidation (Chakraborty et al. 1995).

Correspondingly, an Ayurvedic drug Sandhika was estimated *in vitro* using the same model (cumene hydroperoxide) and demonstrated important antioxidant activity (Padmaja et al. 1995).

9.3.12.3 Iron Induced

The plant Jatamanasi known as *Nardostachys jatamanasi* was evaluated *in vitro* on the basis of iron-induced lipid peroxidation in rat liver homogenate for antioxidant property. Thiobarbituric acid reactive substance (TBARS) content is the process for determination of peroxidation method. Two fractions viz., one is hexane more potent and another one alcoholic extracts afforded protection against lipid peroxidation signifying that the plant having antioxidant property (Suresh et al. 1994).

A dihydroxy anthraquinone is rubiadin obtained from *Rubia cordifolia* (manjistha) extract, which showed significant antioxidant activity as it prevented lipid peroxidation induced by $FeSO_4$ and t-butylhydroperoxide (t-BHP) in a dose dependent manner. The case of Fe^{2+} induced lipid peroxidation was more percent inhibition. Comparatively, anti-oxidant activity of the formulation was better than EDTA, mannitol, Vitamin E and p-benzoquinone (Thyagaran et al. 1988).

9.3.13 Chemotherapeutic Herbal Products

Antimicrobial, antifungal, antiviral, antiprotozoal, and antihelminthic activity of herbs has been described in this section. Standard assays have been used by various investigators and most of the work was carried out *in vitro*.

9.3.13.1 Antimicrobial Agents

A carbazole alkaloidis clausenol obtained from the stem bark of *Clausena anisata* alcoholic extract was seen to be active against gram positive and gram negative bacteria and fungi (Doshi et al. 1994). Leaf extract obtained from the plant *Ficus racemosa* demonstrated potential antibacterial activity against different microorganisms (Mandal et al. 2000a, b).

The hexane fraction obtained from the stem bark of *Amona glabra* demonstrated antimicrobial, antifungal and moderate insecticidal, sporicidal and cytotoxic activities. Biological activities observed of the stem led to the isolation of kaur-16-en-19-oic acid after chromatographic fractionation (Jayaram and Thyagarajan 1996).

9.3.13.2 Antifungal Agents

Azadirachta indica leaves extract confirmed that antidermatophytic activity is more significant when compared to the aqueous extract against 88 clinical isolates of dermatophytes using the agar dilution techniquein an *in vitro* model. The MIC90 of ethanolic extract was 100 μg/mL whereas that of aqueous extract was 500 μg/mL 166. Four Siddha drugs viz. Nandhi mezhugh, Parangipattai choornam, Erasa kenthimezhugu and Vaan mezhugu (in order of efficacy) were found to have significant anti-fungal activity when tested against 14 strains of *Candida albicans* (Nagpal et al. 1995).

9.3.13.3 Antiviral Agents

However, at first *Phyllanthus amarus* showed positive results in Hepatitis B carriers (Dua et al. 1995) but additional studies found that the plant has no effect on hepatitis B surface antigen (HbsAg) in asymptomatic carriers of the antigen (Ray et al. 1996). Though, newly, *Phyllanthus amarus* extract was incubated with the Alexandar cell line in an *in vitro* model, a human hepatocellular carcinoma derived cell line which has the property of hidingthe Hepatitis B surface antigen (HbsAg) in the supernatant. The outcome established that *Phyllanthus amarus* was efficient in reducing the secretion of HbsAg for 48 h thus showing its anti-hepatitis B virus property at the cellular level (Talakal et al. 1995).

9.3.13.4 Antiprotozoal Agents

Antimalarial

In vivo and *in vitro* assay were screened for antimalarial activity against ethanolic and petroleum extracts of *Artemisia japonica*, *Artemisia maritimia* and *Artemisia nilegarica*. *In vivo* tests were done in Balb/c mice using the Rane test wherein all the constituents extended the survival time of the mice. *In vitro*, all three compounds inhibited schizont maturation in chloroquine sensitive strains of *Plasmodium falciparum* (Kumar et al. 1995).

Ball formed wood scrapings soaked in 5% Neem oil obtained from *Azadirachta indica* diluted in acetone and positioned in water storage overhead tanks elicited the breeding of *Anopheles stephensi* and Aedes aegypti in 45 days (Singh et al. 1996).

Likewise, application of a cream obtained from the herb *Azadirachta indica* on exposed body parts at the rate of 2.0 g/person considerably protected against Aedes, Culex and Anopheles musquitoe bites (Roy and Tandon 1996).

Antileishmanial

The herb *Swertia chirata* extract was found to reduce the catalytic effect of topoisomerase I enzyme of *Leishmania donovani*. After fractionation of the extract with suitable solvent, it yielded three secoiridoid glycosides, amarogentin, amaroswerin and sweroside. The compound amacogentin was found to be a strong inhibitor of topoisomerase I and exerted its activity by cooperating with the enzyme and therefore preventing binary complex formation (Singh et al. 2012).

Antitrypanosomial

Crude 50% ethanolic extract of flowers obtained from the herb *Parthenium hysterophorus* showed trypanocidal effect against *Trypanosoma evansi* both *in vitro* and *in vivo*. Toxicity was noticed only at a dose of 1 g/kg (Ghaisas and Bhide 1994).

9.3.13.5 Anthelmintic Agents

Antinematodes

The mechanism of action of the active principle palasoninis described on *Ascaridia galli*. This constituent is obtained from *Butea frondosa* seeds. Palasonin inhibited glucose uptake and depleted the glycogen content (Hastak et al. 1997) and thus the promising mechanism of its anthelminthic action may be connected to inhibition of energy metabolism. Two extract aqueous and alcoholic obtained from the leaves of herb *Senecio nudicaulis* Buch Ham were found to exert antifilarial effect when examined against *Setariacervi* (*Nematoda Filarioidea*). The useful concentrations varied for the aqueous and alcoholic extracts signifying the existence of a cuticular permeability barrier. These two fractions also revealed micro-filaricidal effect *in vitro*. Their anti-filarial reactions were parallel to diethylcarbamazine. They did not block the stimulant action of acetylcholine on the worm (Elangovan et al. 1994).

Antitrematode (Fluke)

A local medicinal plant in Meghalaya, *Flemingia vestita* root extract revealed antihelminthic function *in vitro* causing paralysis against two species of flukes, *Artyfechinostomum sufrartyfex* and *Fasciolopsis buski*. Stereo-scanning clarification on the tegument surfaces exposed sloughing off of most of the spines or their deformation and wrinkling and rupture of the common tegument (Upadhyay 1997).

9.3.14 Antimutagenic Herbs

Punark, a mixture of solvent extracts of herbs, namely turmeric (*Curcuma longa*), betel leaf (*Piper betel*) and catechu (*Acacia catechu*) is call punark protected against benzo (a) pyrene induced chromosomal spoil in human lymphocytes *in vitro* (Dahanukar et al. 1997). Alcoholic extracts of tumeric oil (TD) and tumeric oleoresin (TOR) proved antimutagenic action *in vitro*.

They also revealed chemoprotective activity in lymphocytes of standard healthy subjects *in vitro* when examined against benzo (a) pyrene induced DNA damage. The extracts reduced DNA spoilage (cytogenetic damage) in oral mucosal cells of patients with oral submucous fibrosis *in vivo* (Srinivasan 2005).

9.3.15 Anticancer Herbs

The important function of different herbs in cancer therapy as a direct anticancer agent, chemo preventive agent, radio sensitizer or immunity improver is offered in the following paragraphs. Estimation of the *in vitro* anticancer activities of bioflavonoids, viz. quercelon, catechin, luteolin and rutin against human carcinoma of larynx (Hep-2) and sarcoma 180 (S-180) cell lines revealed that only luteolin and quercetin inhibited the proliferation of the cells. Luteolin is responsible for depletion of glutathione in the cells and a decline in DNA synthesis, as seen by thymidine uptake studies, thus demonstrating its anticancer potential (Pittler et al. 2000). Different solvent fractions and its formulation showed anticancer activity. The pentacyclic triterpenoid ursolic acid obtained from the herb *Diospyros melanoxylon* Roxb. leaves used in the treatment of cancer therapy (Rashid et al. 2017a, b, c). The fractions and its nanoparticle of methanolic extract obtained from *Diospyros melanoxylon* Roxb. leaves demonstrated significant anticancer activity against different cancerous cell line (Rashid et al. 2017a, b, c; Rashid et al. 2018).

9.3.16 Immune Active Herbs

Immunomodulatory extracts and compounds can initiate immune responses through stimulation or inhibition and can help patients to attain healthy immune system. Some agents generate host resistance mechanisms in the occurrence of a damaged immune responsiveness can afford encouraging treatment to conventional chemotherapy. Upadhyay has focused the beneficial prospective of immunomodulatory substances from herbs. They have estimated Indian medicinal herbs for immunomodulatory activity (Cravotto et al. 2010). The authors have also evaluated the Ayurvedic perceptions of precautionary health need. A list of Ayurvedic medicinal herbs including *Withania somnifera, Allium sativum, Azadirachta indica, Piper longum, Asparagus racemosus, Glycyrrhiza glabra, Aloe vera, Gmelina arborea and Tinospora cordifolia* shown potent immunoregulatoy properties.

9.3.17 Adaptogens

Adaptogen is substances that enhance the nonspecific conflict of micorganisms against an array of stressors. A modern appraisal explains the growth taking place in this ground and the troubles connected in the estimation of adaptogens. The aqueous fractions of *Tinospora cordifolia, Asparagus racemosus, Emblica officinalis, Withania somnifera, Piper longum* and *Terminalia chebula* all showed adaptive responses against chemical stressors. In empty stomach these herbs upturnedthe effects of cisplatin, while *Tinospora cordifolia* and *Asparagus racemosus* also controlled cisplatin-induced intestinal hypermotility, fulfilling to the explanation of an adaptogen. These types of plants are secure in both acute and subacutetoxicity studies. The methanolic fraction obtained from the herb *Withania somnifera* (as more active) was observed the best effects after pretreatment administration. The herb *Emblica officinalis* reinforced the protection mechanisms against free radical injury marked through stress. The outcome of *Emblica officinalis* showed to depend on the capability of target tissues to produce prostaglandins. On the other hand, gastroprotective activity of *Tinospora cordifolia* was possibly mediated during a principally immune stimulant mechanism as the protection was found to vanish by blocking the macrophage role (Fabricant and Farnsworth 2001) (Table 9.1).

Table 9.1 Different activity of herbal medicine

Sl. No.	Drugs	Plant	Part used	Mechanism of action	Traditional uses	Models available	References
1	Glipizide, Metformin, Miglitol, Acarbose	*Inula racemosa*		Lowered blood glucose and enhanced liver glycogen, potentiating insulin sensitivity in rats.	Antidiabetic	Pancreatic α-amylase, α-Glucosidase	Talwar et al. (1995)
2	Loperamide, Bismuth subsalicylate, **Co-phenotrope, Racecadotril**	*Nelumbo nucifera*	Rhizomes	Reduce gastric motility	Antidiarrhoeal	Prostaglandin E2 (PGE 2) induced enteropooling, Magnesium sulphate induced diarrhoea	Fabricant and Farnsworth (2001)
3	Nizatidine, famotidine, lanzoprazole, esomeprazole.	*Araucaria bidwillii*	Leaf	Moderate degree of ulcero-protective activity in pylorus ligated rat model of gastric ulceration.	Gastric and duodenal ulcer	Rabbit acetic acid-induced gastric ulcer modeling (AAU model), Rabbit endoscopic mucosal resection (EMR)-related ulcer model (MRU model)	Vaidya et al. (1996)
4	Tamoxifen, Pirfenidone, Riociguat, BMS-986020	*Tinospora cordifolia*		Significantly improve the suppressed Kupffer cell function.	Anti-fibrotic effect.	Bleomycin-induced pulmonary fibrosis, Transplant-induced pulmonary fibrosis, Allergen-induced airway remodelling	Kuttan (1996)
5	Latanoprost, Timolol, apraclonidine, dorzolamide.	*Ocimum sanctum*	Leaves	Delayed the onset as well as the subsequent maturation of cataract.	Oculo-protective	galactosamic cataract in rats and naphthalene cataract in rabbits.	Chaurasia et al. (1995)
6	Doxycycline, Erythromycin, Bacitricin.	Clausena anisata	Stem bark	Inhibits cell wall synthesis, DNA and RNA synthesis,protein synthesis.	Anti-microbial, anti-fungal and moderate insecticidal, sporicidal.	Monte Carlo stimulations for static and dynamic *in vitro* infection models, monoparametric models.	Jayaram and Thyagarajan (1996)
7	Miconazole, Nystatin, Echinocandin, Terbinafine.	*Azadirachta indica*	Leaves	Impaired biosynthesis of ergosterol,allowing leakage of a variety of intracellular channels such as potassium,magnesium etc.	Antifungal	The C. elegans model of microbial pathogenesis, C. elegans bioassays as a screen for novel antimicrobial compounds	Nagpal et al. (1995)

(continued)

Table 9.1 (continued)

Sl. No.	Drugs	Plant	Part used	Mechanism of action	Traditional uses	Models available	References
8	Amphotericin B, Miltefosine, Pentamidine, Sitamaquine.	*Swertia chirata*		The catalytic activity of topoisomerase I enzyme of *Leishmania donovani.*	Anti-leishmanial		Singh et al. (2012)
9	Nitrogen- and oxygen-containing heterocyclic compounds, Pyrrolidine-2,5-dione derivatives, Aminoalkanolic derivatives of xanthones.	*Curcumin longa*	Oleoresin	Reduced DNA damage (cytogenetic damage) in oral mucosal cells.	Anti-mutagenic	Mouse heritable translocation assay, *In vitro* comet assay.	Srinivasan (2005)
10	Alprazolam, Meprobamate,Buspirone, Eszopiclone.	*Azadirachta indica*(Neem)		Exert their action by producing the GABA ergic, serotonergic and dopaminergic transmission	Anxiolytics	Elevated plus maze test	Mukherjee et al. (1996)
11	Lanotrigine, Topiramate, Gabapentine, Denzimol.	*Ginkgo biloba*		Blocks sodium channels and NMDA receptors, having action on GABAergic receptors and calcium, potassium ion concentration	Anti-convulsant	TBPS binding assay, Kindled rat seizure model	Johri et al. (1995)
12	Fentanyl, Hydrocodon, Hydromorphone.	*Hibiscus vitifolius* (Bhasadwaji)	Petals	Acts on cholinergic and GABAergic neurotransmitter pathways	Anti-nociceptive	Formalin-induced hind paw-licking test, Acetic acid-induced writhing test	Mitra et al. (1996)
13	Paracetamol, Diclofenac, Nambutone, Nimesulide.	*Calotropis procera* (Arka)	Dried latex	inhibitory effects on release of mediators of inflammation such as histamine, 5-hydroxytryptamine, bradykinin etc	Anti-inflammatory	Carrageenin and formalin induced rat paw oedema models, Cotton pellet induced granuloma	Vimala et al. 1997; Andrade et al. (1994)
14	Paracetamol, Ibuprofen, Nimesulide.	*Nelumbo nucifera*	Rhizome	Inhibits the cyclo-oxygenase enzyme and stops release of prostaglandin.	Antipyretic		Ganguli et al. (1996)
15	Dicoumarol, Fondaparinux, Ximelagatran, Warfarin.	*Araucaria bidwillii*	Leaf and oleoresin	Interacts with KO reductase enzyme and blocking the formation of prothrombin.	Anticoagulant	Regional citrate anticoagulation.	Sharma et al. (1995)

16	Etofibrate, Ezetimibe, Clofibrate, Lovastatin.	*Commiphoramukul*	Gugulipid	Acts as a HMG CO-A reductase inhibitor, increase VLDL clearance,fatty acid oxidation and lipoprotein lipase activity.	Hypo-lipidaemic activity.	Cholesterol rich HFD induced hepatic steatosis, triton induced hyperlipidemia model.	Shaila et al. (1995)
17	Ouabain, Deslanoside,Digoxine.	*Terminalia arjuna*	Bark	Increased cardiac contractility, Prolongation of action potential and thereby increased cardiac output.	Positive inotropic	Chronic nitric oxide inhibition-induced hypertension, Hypertension induced by external compression of renal parenchyma	Nair et al. (1994)
18	Labetalol, Nifedipine, Losartan, Irbesartan, Eprosartan	*Agathosma betulina*	Leaves	Decrease the calcium influx, inhibits the angiotensin converting enzyme and β-adrenergic receptive regions.	antihypertensive	Transgenic rat (TGR) models, Hypertension induced by cholinomimetic agents	Badyal et al. (2003)
19	Mebendazole, Oxamniquine, Praziquantel, Eflornithine.	*Butea frondosa*	Seeds	Palasonin inhibited energy metabolism such as glucose uptake and depleted the glycogen content.	Anthelmintic	Heligmosomoides bakeri. Model, Ancylostoma ceylanicum model.	Hastak et al. (1997)
20	Vinblastine, Cisplatin, Methotrexate, Pemetrexed.	*Catharanthus reseus*	Leaves	Inhibits DHFR, uridylic acid, the disassembly of the key cytoskeleton and thereby preventing the biosynthesis of DNA and RNA.	Anticancer	SRB assay, MTT assay	Sahpazidoua et al. (2014)

9.4 Clinical Tests of Herbs

Many herbs have shown positive results *in vitro, in vivo* animal model or small-scale clinical tests, while studies on some herbal treatments have found negative results (Eric et al. 2002).

In 2002, the U.S. National Center for Complementary and Alternative Medicine of the National Institutes of Health began funding clinical trials into the effectiveness of herbal medicine (Brater and Daly 2000). In a 2010 survey of 1000 plants, 356 had clinical trials published evaluating their "pharmacological activities and therapeutic applications" while 12% of the plants, although available in the Western market, had "no substantial studies" of their properties (Lind 1754).

Presently, there is no strong proof from experiments in public that herbal remedies can treat, prevent or cure cancer according to Cancer Research UK (Patwardhan et al. 2004).

Herbalists criticize the manner in which many scientific studies make insufficient use of historical knowledge, which has been shown useful in drug discovery and development in the past and present (Ammon et al. 1993). They maintain that this traditional knowledge can guide the selection of factors such as optimal dose, species, time of harvesting and target population (Jayaprakasam and Muraleedharan 2003).

9.5 Research of Medicinal Herbs

Although the basis of clinical research was first advanced in Avicenna's The Canon of Medicine (Dwivedi et al. 1992), and had been applied in James Lind's famous clinical trials of citrus fruits in the cure scurvy (Visen et al. 1993); a somewhat modified, viewpoint on "clinical trial" has emerged lately:

India has world-class expertise and facilities for organic synthesis, isolation and structure elucidation, biological screening, toxicological testing and pharmacokinetics. The expertise has supplemented for the progress of agro-technology for the cultivation of medicinal plants. Industry contribution to ensure successful upscaling and completion of technology is rising. Production of leads among structural varieties through the construction of natural product libraries, detection of suitable objectives and their appropriate validation and optimization is of paramount significance (Johri and Zutshi 2000). India has progressive research institutes like Central Drug Research Institute (CDRI), Central Institute of Medicinal and Aromatic Plants and National Botanical Research Institute at Lucknow, Regional Research Laboratories (RRL), at Jammu, Bhubaneswar and Jorhat, National Chemical Laboratory at Pune, which regularly accepts research on medicinal plants. Most of the mare involved in standardizing the herbal medicines and isolating active compounds. Fews selected medicinal crops have been taken for improvement there is a need for research on quality planting materials for farmers, conservation of end angered species and to prevent exploitation of the natural resources. Antihypertensive agent is reserpine obtained from Rauwolfia is a tremendously expensive contribution from Ayurvedic systems. Curcumin is an anti-inflammatory agent obtained from turmeric (Bhatt 2001), Withaferin A (Sekhar et al. 2003) (anti-inflammatory from ashwagandha), kutkoside (Gupta et al. 1998) (hepatoprotective from kutki), andrographolide (Chopra et al. 2000) (hepatoprotective from andrographis) and vasicine (Gupta et al. 2000) (bronchodilator and expectorant from vasaka) are chemical entities with beautiful gallows for drug discovery.

Controlled clinical trials are important to develop evidence for safety and efficacy. Clinical trials have shown encouraging results (Kumar et al. 1999), but lot more clinical research is required to establish validity of the system. Ayurvedic preparations have been successfully evaluated for treatment of bronchial asthma (Majeed et al. 1999; Atal et al. 1985), rheumatoid arthritis, ischaemic heart disease (Gautam et al. 2004). Piperine from pipali has come out as a bioenhancer in recent clinical evaluation (Kumar 2000). Botanicals like *Withania somnifera* (Barbara and Ginger 1997); *Asparagus racemosus* (Ganguli 2004) have exhibited significant vaccine adjuvant activity in experimental systems, which have valuable applications in immunobiological industry. An IND application of Lupin Ltd. is in process and US patent has been granted for development of herbal-based antipsoriatic composition containing *Argemone mexicana* (Ganguli 2004). Standardized fraction of gugulipid from *Commiphora wightii* developed by CDRI has been marketed (Guglip, Cipla Ltd) for treating hyperlipidemia and atherosclerosis (Prashant et al. 2012). RRL Jammu has commercialized *Boswellia serrata* gumresinas NSAID (Non-SteroidalAnti-Inflammatory Drug) (Sallaki Gufic). It is also hypolipidemic. A multicentric study by the Indian Council of Medical Research (ICMR) showed promising results that a preparation from *Pterocarpus marsupium* was effective in reducing levels of blood glucose and glycosylated haemoglobin in patients with non-insulin-dependent diabetes mellitus (Maeng et al. 2013). Beside the crude extract traditional formulations, Indian medicinal herbs have huge potential to contribute to modern drug discovery programs. Most of the Indian universities have rich research facilities that can be used for modern drug discoveries. Small molecule drug lead identification from the diverse range of Indian medicinal plants can be carried out using the natural products techniques and technologies (Wangchuk et al. 2018; Rashid et al. 2015, 2017a, b, c).

9.6 Role of WHO in Herbal Medicine

Two decades ago, WHO referred to traditional health systems (including herbal medicine) as 'holistic'—'that of viewing man in his totality within a wide ecological spectrum, and of emphasizing the view that ill health or disease is brought about by an imbalance or disequilibrium of man in his total ecological system and not only by the causative agent and pathogenic evolution' (WHO), probably implying that the indigenous system drugs (including herbal medicine) restore the imbalance or disequilibrium leading to the cure of ill health or disease. Such an attitude sent signals that WHO as an organization has failed to provide leadership to establish traditional systems of medicine which provide health care to about 80% of the world population. However, it helped the inclusion of proven traditional remedies in national drug policies and regulatory approvals by developing countries. The World Health Assembly continued the debate and adopted a resolution (WHA 42.43) in 1989 that herbal medicine is of great importance to the health of individuals and communities. The redefined definition of traditional medicine thus issued in the early nineties is given vide supra (see herbal medicine). Consequently, in 1991 WHO developed guidelines for the assessment of herbal medicine 7, and the same were ratified by the sixth International Conference of Drug Regulatory Authorities held at Ottawa in the same year. The salient features of WHO guidelines are: (1) Quality assessment: Crude plant material; Plant preparation; and Finished product. (2) Stability: Shelf life. (3) Safety assessment: Documentation of safety based on experience or/and; Toxicology studies. (4) Assessment of efficacy: Documented evidence of traditional use or/and; Activity determination (animals, human).

9.7 Government Policies

In China and India, formal training is an integral part of the national health program, which helps in ensuring quality standards in healthcare delivery. In Bhutan traditional herbal medicine was integrated with allopathic medicine since 1967, long before the WHO traditional medicine integration policy was put in place (Wangchuk et al. 2016). Government of India also has expressed support and encouragement for the TIM. A separate department for Indian Systems of Medicine and Homeopathy (ISM & H) known as AYUSH (Ayurveda, Yoga, Unani, Siddha, Homoeopathy) was established in March 1995 to promote indigenous systems. Priorities include education, standardization of drugs, enhancement of availability of raw materials, research and development, information, communication and larger involvement in the national system for delivering healthcare. The Central Council of Indian Medicine over sees teaching and training institutes while Central Council for Research in Ayurveda and Siddha deals with interdisciplinary research. Some TIM products are being added into family welfare programs of the Government under the World Bank project. These medicines are mainly for common diseases like anemia, edema during pregnancy, postpartum problems such as pain, uterine and abdominal complications, difficulties with lactation, nutritional deficiencies and childhood diarrhoea (Walters and Kleeberger 2008). The Government has also established 10 new drug testing laboratories for TIM and is upgrading existing laboratories to provide documented high-quality evidence to licensing authorities for the safety and quality of herbal medicines. This replaces the earlier ad-hoc system of testing that was considered unreliable.

In 2002, the Council for Scientific and Industrial Research has launched are research program under New Millennium Indian Technology Leadership Initiatives scheme in Ayurveda. Identifying the disease are as such as arthritis, diabetes and hepatic disorders, which afflict large numbers of the Indian population. Many additional concerns need to be addressed. The quality of education in many colleges needs to be improved. Under the pretext of integration, attempts to make hybrid curricula producing inadequately trained graduates remain unacceptable for either modern or traditional systems (Ji et al. 2015). A paucity of funds is noticeable; ISM & H gets only 2% of the total health budget of the nation. A corrective and promotive policy needs to be initiated for TIM to fully realize its potential and contribute more meaningfully to integrative health services. The industry has not been able to grow and develop optimally during the last few decades. Largely, the achieved grow this owing to industry's own initiatives, in-house research and development. A national organization, Ayurvedic Drugs Manufacturers' Association is taking a proactive role to improve quality and research that needs to be nurtured, stimulated and sustained by providing special funding or incentives. Preparations of formularies and pharmacopoeial standards have been attempted but a lot remains to be done. Indian botanical resources and their medicinal utilization such as in case of turmeric have been patented .Essential actions to defend such intellectual assets are vital as there trivial and contesting of patents is extremely expensive and time-consuming issue (Jacobs et al. 2016). For this purpose, the Government of India has established a Traditional Knowledge Digital Library on traditional medicinal plants, which will also lead to a Traditional Knowledge Resource Classification (Walf and Frye 2007). Connecting this to globally accepted International Patent Classifications structure will establish a link among the information on Indian old Sanskrit extend .This may control the problem of mistakingly granting patents since the examiner will know the Indian rights to that knowledge. It could integrate widely scattered and distributed references on TIM in retrievable for mand will be a major impetus to modern research in the developing world.

9.8 Conclusion

It is strongly considered that the traditional herbal drugs have a vital responsibility to participate in primary health care as well as serving to discover promising medicinal herb remedies and to assist their development to clinical trial stages both as crude formulations or in isolated compound-based regimens. Traditional medicines plays significant role in modern drug discoveries. However, it requires collaborations because the small numbers of pharmaceutical firms that are present in these countries have little or no R&D base. It seems that the underlying issue in herbal clinical trials is not so much about whether traditional herbal remedies work but how much is suitable for the condition for which the remedy in question is traditionally prescribed. With compared to conventional drugs or single entity drugs; the herbal medicines are more intricate and mostly act holistically or synergistically. Consequently, most of their mechanisms of action in molecular/systems levels are still unexplored. Empirically, the medicinal herbs have been successfully used all around the world to improve health, energy, and vitality by extensive clinical experience and observation. The systems pharmacology model might facilitate to understand the mechanisms of action of the medicinal herbs, which brings about new development for complementary and alternative medicine. Some significant scientific evidences suggest that a large number of herbal medicines exert their effect on different body systems which supports and confirms the extensive empirical testimony gained over the years. These scientific evidences reinforce the case for including herbal medicines in the mainstream therapy of a number of chronic disorders, either alone, or as part of a programme of integrative medicine (Fig. 9.1).

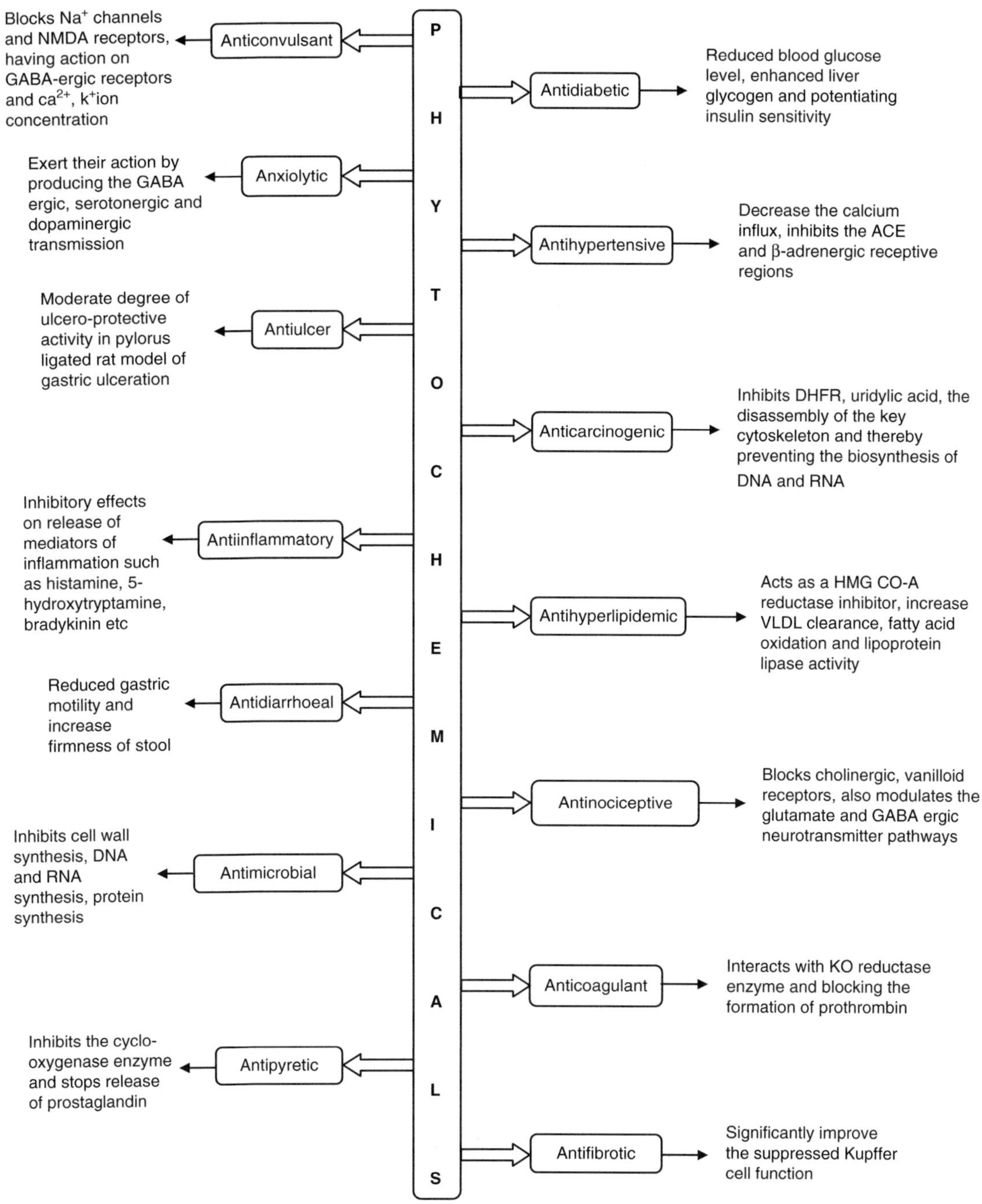

Fig. 9.1 Mechanism of action of some important diseases

Acknowledgments The authors are thankful to the Department of Biotechnology, New Delhi for financial assistance to Prof. (Dr.) Subhash C Mandal under DBT's Twinning Program (DBT-NER/AGRI/29/2015 (Group 2), Dated: 19/10/2016) for the North East, India.

References

Ammon HP, Safayhi H, Mack T, Sabieraj J. Mechanism of anti-inflammatory actions of curcumin and boswellic acids. J Ethnopharmacol. 1993;38:113–9.

Anand R, Patnaik GK, Roy K, Bhaduri AP. Antioxaluric and anticalciuric activity of lupeol derivatives. Indian J Pharmacol. 1995;27:265–8.

Andrade C, Raj T, Udaya HB, Suresh JC. Effect of BR-16A on alpha-2 adrenergic, dopamine autoreceptor and dopamine postsynaptic receptor functioning. Indian J Pharmacol. 1994;26:292–5.

Atal CK, Dubey RK, Singh J. Biochemical basis of enhanced drug availability by piperine: evidence that piperine is a potent inhibitor of drug metabolism. J Pharmacol Exp Ther. 1985;232:258–62.

Badyal DK, Lata H, Dadhich AP. Animal models of hypertension and effect of drugs. Indian journal of pharmacology 2003; 35: 349–62.

Banerjee A, Rashid Md. HA, Chakraverty R, Dey S, Basak D, Biswas C. Preparation and evaluation of aspirin transdermal patch using HPMC. Int J Pharma Sci Rev Res. 2012;15(1):45–6.

Barbara AJ, Ginger W. Turmeric patent over turned in legal victory. HerbalGram. 1997;41:11.

Barua CC, Gupta PP, Patnaik GK, et al. Studies on anti-anaphylactic activity of fractions of *Albizzia lebbeck*. Cur Sci. 1997;72:397–9.

Bhatt AD. Clinical trials of Ayurvedic medicine: myths, realities and challenges. J Assoc Physicians India. 2001;49:558–62.

Bhatt AD, Bhatt NS. Indigenous drugs and liver disease. Indian J Gastroenterol. 1996;15:63–7.

Bhatt JD, Panchakshari UD, Hemavati KG, Gulati OD. Effect of Abana, an Ayurvedic preparation of ethinyl estradiol-induced hypertension in rats. Indian J Pharmacol. 1998;30:399–403.

Bhattacharya SK, Kumar A. Effect of Trasina, an Ayurvedic herbal formulation, on experimental models of Alzheimer's disease and central cholinergic markers in rats. J Altern Complement Med. 1997;3: 327–36.

Bhattacharya P, Bhatt JD, Hemavathi KG, Gulati OD. Effects of chronic terbutaline and Abana pretreatments on beta-adrenoceptor mediated relaxant responses of guineapig isolated trachea. Indian J Pharmacol. 1994;26:270–6.

Brater DC, Daly WJ. Clinical pharmacology in the middle ages: principles that presage the 21st century. Clin Pharmacol Ther. 2000;67(5):447–50.

Chakraborty A, Chowdhury BK, Bhattacharya P. Clausenol and clausenine-two carbazole alkaloids from Clausena anisata. Phytochemistry. 1995;40:295–8.

Chattopadhyay RR. Possible mechanism of antihyperglycemic effect of *Azadirachta indica* leaf extract. Part IV. Gen Pharmacol. 1996;27:431–4.

Chattopadhyay RR. Effect of *Azadirachta indica* hydroalcoholic leaf extract on the cardiovascular system. Gen Pharmacol. 1997;28:449–51.

Chaurasia S, Tripathi P, Tripathi YB. Antioxidant and antiinflammatory property of Sandhika: a compound herbal drug. Indian J Exp Biol. 1995;33:428–32.

Chopra K, Singh M. Involvement of oxygen free radicals in cardioprotective effect of rutin-A naturally occurring flavonoid. Indian J Pharmacol. 1994;26:13–8.

Chopra A, Lavin P, Patwardhan B, Chitre D. Randomized double blind trial of an Ayurvedic plant derived formulation for treatment of rheumatoid arthritis. J Rheumatol. 2000;27:1365–72.

Cravotto G, Boffa L, Genzini L, Garella D. Phytotherapeutics: an evaluation of the potential of 1000 plants. J Clin Pharm Ther. 2010;35(1):11–48.

Dahanukar SA, Rege NN, Thatte UM. Adaptogens. In: Ed. Medicinal plants, their bioactivity, screening and evaluation - Proceedings of the International Workshop, CDRI, Lucknow (India), December 2–5, 1997;143–63.

Dahanukar SA, Rege NN, Thatte UM. Omnipotent officinale. Amruth. 1998;2:21–3.

Dalvi SS, Nayak VK, Pohujani SM, et al. Effect of gugulipid on bioavailability of diltiazem and propranolol. J Assoc Phys India. 1994;42:454–5.

De B, Maiti RN, Joshi VK, Agrawal VK, Goel RK. Effect of some Sitavirya drugs on gastric secretion and ulceration. Indian J Exp Biol. 1997;35:1084–7.

Deka DK, Lahon LC, Saikia J, Mukit A. Effect of *Cissus quadrangularis* in accelerating healing process of experimentally fractured radius-ulna of dog: a preliminary study. Indian J Pharmacol. 1994;26:44–5.

Despina Sahpazidou, George D. Geromichalos, Dimitrios Stagos, Anna Apostolou, Serkos A. Haroutounian, Aristidis M. Tsatsakis, George N. Tzanakakis, A. Wallace Hayes, Dimitrios Kouretas, (2014) Anticarcinogenic activity of polyphenolic extracts from grape stems against breast, colon, renal and thyroid cancer cells. Toxicology Letters 230 (2):218–24

Dhanasekaran S, Ravishankar R, Sumitra Devi K, et al. Pharmacological studies of *Araucaria Bidwillii* hook. Geobios New Rep. 1994;13:49–52.

Doshi JC, Vaidya AB, Antarkar DS, et al. A two-stage clinical trial of *Phyllanthus amarus* in Hepatitis B carriers: failure to eradicate the surface antigen. Indian J Gastroenterol. 1994;13:7–8.

Dua VK, Nagpal BN, Sharma VP. Repellent action of neem cream against mosquitoes. Indian J Malariol. 1995;32:47–53.

Dwivedi Y, Rastogi R, Garg NK, Dhawan BN. Picrolivandits components kutkoside and picroside I protect liver against galactosamine-induced damage in rats. Pharmacol Toxicol. 1992;71:383–7.

Elangovan V, Ramamoorthy N, Balasubramanian S, et al. Studies on the antiproliferative effect of some naturally occurring bioflavonoidal compounds against human carcinoma of larynx and sarcoma-180 cell lines. Indian J Pharmacol. 1994;26:266–9.

Eric Y, ND RH, Kathy AJD. Dilemmas of traditional botanical research. Herbal Gram. 2002;55:46–54.

Fabricant DS, Farnsworth NR. The value of plants used in traditional medicine for drug discovery. Environ Health Perspect. 2001;109(1):69–75.

Ganguli P. Patents and patent information in 1979 and 2004: a perspective from India. World Patent Inf. 2004;26:61–2.

Ganguli S, Hota D, Goel RK, et al. Neuropharmacological studies on Fusarium toxins-III: Neurochemical investigations on total toxin extracts from *F. moniliforme* and *F. oxysporum*. Indian J Exp Biol. 1996;34:531–4.

Gautam M, Diwanay SS, Gairola S, Shinde YS, Jadhav SS, Patwardhan BK. Immune response modulation to DPT vaccine by aqueous extract of *Withania somnifera* in experimental system. Int Immunopharmacol. 2004;4:841–9.

Ghaisas SD, Bhide SV. *In vitro* studies on chemoprotective effect of Purnark against Benzo (A) pyrene-induced chromosomal damage in human lymphocytes. Cell Biol Int. 1994;18:21–7.

Gomes A, Vedasiromoni JR, Das M, et al. Anti-hyperglycemic effect of black tea (Camellia sinensis) in rat. J Ethnopharmacol. 1995;45:223–6.

Gupta PP, Srimal RC, Srivastava M, et al. Antiallergic activity of arbortristosides from *Nyctanthusarbortristis*. Int J Pharmacog. 1995a;33:70–2.

Gupta PP, Tandon JS, Patnaik GK. Antiallergic activity of andrographolides isolated from *Andrographis paniculata* (Burm.F) Wall. Int J Pharma Biol. 1995b;36:1–3.

Gupta PP, Kulshrestha DK, Patnaik GK. Antiallergic activity of *Cedrusde odara*. J Med Aromatic Plant Sci. 1997;19:1007–8.

Gupta I, Gupta V, Parihar A, Gupta S, Ludtke R, Safayhi H. Effects of *Boswellia serrata* gum resin in patients with bronchial asthma: results of adouble-blind, placebo-controlled, 6-week clinical study. Eur J Med Res. 1998;3:511–4.

Gupta R, Singhal S, Goyle A, Sharma VN. Antioxidant and hypocholesterolaemic effects of *Terminaliaarjuna* tree-bark powder: a randomized placebo-controlled trial. J Assoc Physicians India. 2000;49:231–5.

Hastak K, Lubri N, Jakhi SD, et al. Effect of turmeric oil and turmeric oleoresin on cytogenetic damage in patients suffering from oral submucous fibrosis. Cancer Lett. 1997;116:265–9.

Heinrich M, Gibbons S. Ethnopharmacology in drug discovery: an analysis of its role and potential contribution. J Pharm Pharmacol. 2001;53:425–32.

Jacobs M, Grégoire N, Couet W, Bulitta JB. Distinguishing antimicrobial models with different resistance mechanisms via population pharmacodynamic modeling. PLoS Comput Biol. 2016;12(3):1004782.

Jaiswal AK, Bhattacharya SK, Acharya SB. Anxiolytic activity of *Azadirachta indica* leaf extract in rats. Indian J Exp Biol. 1994;32:489–91.

Jayaprakasam B, Muraleedharan GN. Cyclooxygenase-2enzyme inhibitory withanolides from *Withania somnifera* leaves. Tetrahydron. 2003;59:841–9.

Jayaram S, Thyagarajan SP. Inhibition of HBsAg secretion from Alexander cell line by *Phyllanthus amarus*. Indian J Pathol Microbiol. 1996;39:211–5.

Ji L, Li C, Shen N, Huan Y, Liu Q, Liu S, Shen Z. A simple and stable galactosemic cataract model for rats. Int J Clin Exp Med. 2015;8(8):12874–81.

Johri RK, Zutshi U. Mechanism of action of 6,7,8,9,10,12-hexahydro-azepino-[2,1-b]quinazolin-12-one-(RLX)-a novel bronchodilator. Indian J Physiol Pharmacol. 2000;44:75–81.

Johri RK, Singh C, Kaul BL. *Vernonialasiopus* and *Vernoniagalamensis*: a medicinal perspective. Res Ind. 1995;40:327–8.

Joshi AR, Ahamed RN, Pathan KM, Manivannan B. Effect of *Azadirachta indica* leaves on testis and its recovery in albino rats. Indian J Exp Biol. 1996;34:1091–4.

Kayath HP, Goel NK. Effects of cuscuta stem extract on various animal tissues. Indian J Pharmacol. 1995;27:227–9.

Kulkarni SK, Ninan I. Inhibition of morphine tolerance and dependence by *Withania somnifera* in mice. J Ethnopharmacol. 1997;57:213–7.

Kumar S. India's government promotes traditional healing practices. Lancet. 2000;335:1252.

Kumar VL, Basu N. Anti-inflammatory activity of the latex of *Calotropis procera*. J Ethnopharmacol. 1994;44:123–5.

Kumar A, Singh RK. Effect of Pongamia pinnata on perturbed central cholinergic markers of cognition in experimentally demented rats. J Basic Appl Biomed. 1996;4:43–8.

Kumar D, Mishra SK, Tandan SK, Tripathi HC. Possible mechanism of anthelmintic action of palasonin on Ascaridia galli. Indian J Pharmacol. 1995;27:161–8.

Kumar P, Kuttan R, Kuttan G. Radioprotective effects of Rasayanas. Indian J Exp Biol. 1996;34:848–50.

Kumar PU, Adhikari P, Pereira P, Bhat P. Safety and efficacy of Hartone instable angina pectoris-an open comparative trial. J Assoc Physicians India. 1999;47:685–9.

Kuttan G. Use of Withania somnifera Dunal as an adjuvant during radiation therapy. Indian J Exp Biol. 1996;34:854–6.

Lind J. James Lind biography. 1754: pp. 1716–1794.

Maeng JH, Lee E, Lee DH, Yang SG. Rabbit gastric ulcer models: comparison and evaluation of acetic acid-induced ulcer and mucosectomy-induced ulcer. Lab Anim Res. 2013;29(2):96–102.

Majeed M, Badmaev V, Rajendran R. Use of piperineasa bioavailability enhancer. US Patent 5972382, Sabinsa Corporation USA, 1999.

Majumder S, Rashid Md. HA, Chowdhury S, Gupta BK, Mandal SC. Physicochemical and antioxidant assay of Ayurvedic formulations of Alternanthera philoxeroides. Int Res J Pharma. 2016;7(5):20–3.

Makwana HG, Ravishankar B, Shukla VJ, et al. General pharmacology of *Vitex leucoxylon* Linn leaves. Indian J Physiol Pharmacol. 1994;38:95–100.

Mandal SC, Maity TK, Das J, Saba BP, Pal M. Anti-inflammatory evaluation of *Ficus racemosa* Linn. leaf extract. J Ethnopharmacol. 2000a;72(1–2):87–92.

Mandal SC, Saha BP, Pal M. Studies on antibacterial activity of *Ficus racemosa* Linn. leaf extract. Phytother Res. 2000b;14(4):278–80.

Manickam M, Ramanathan M, Jahromi MA, et al. Antihyperglycemic activity of phenolics from *Pterocarpus marsupium*. J Nat Prod. 1997;60:609–10.

Manocha A, Pillai KK, Husain Z. Influence of *Ginkgo biloba* on the effect of anticonvulsants. Indian J Pharmacol. 1996;28:84–7.

Manocha A, Pillai KK, Husain Z. Effect of *Ginkgo biloba* in chemo shock in mice. Indian J Pharmacol. 1997;29:198–200.

Mengi SA, Deshpande SG. Evaluation of ocular anti-inflammatory activity of *Butea frondosa*. Indian J Pharmacol. 1995;27:116–9.

Mitra SK, Chakraborti A, Bhattacharya SK. Neuropharmacological studies on Panax ginseng. Indian J Exp Biol. 1996;34:41–7.

Mohanan PV, Rathinam K, Devi KS. Effect of Sobatum on ultra violet-induced damage and superoxide production. Indian J Pharmacol. 1997;29:129–31.

Mukherjee PK, Das J, Balasubramanian R, et al. Antidiarrhoeal evaluation of *Nelumbo nucifera* rhizome extract. Indian J Pharmacol. 1995;27:262–4.

Mukherjee PK, Saha K, Balasubramanian R, et al. Studies on pyschopharmacological effects of *Nelumbo nucifera* Gaertn. rhizome extract. J Ethnopharmacol. 1996;54:63–7.

Mukherjee PK, Saha K, Bhattacharya S, et al. Studies on antitussive activity of *Drymaria cordata* Willd. J Ethnopharmacol. 1997;56:77–80.

Nagarkatti DS, Rege NN, Desai NK, Dahanukar SA. Modulation of Kupffer cell activity by *Tinospora cordifolia* in liver damage. J Postgrad Med. 1994;40:65–7.

Nagpal BN, Srivastava A, Sharma VP. Control of mosquito breeding using wood scrapings treated with neem oil. Indian J Malariol. 1995;32:64–9.

Nair AM, Saraf MN. Inhibition of antigen and compound 48/80 induced contractions of Guinea pig trachea by the ethanolic extract of the leaves of Vitex negundo Linn. Indian J Pharmacol. 1995;27:230–3.

Nair AM, Tamhankar CP, Saraf MN. Studies on the mast cell stabilising activity of *Vitex negundo* Linn. Indian Drug. 1994;32:277–82.

Narayanan N, Thirugnanasambantham P, Viswanathan S, et al. Antinociceptive antiinflammatory and antipyretic effects of ethanol extract of *Clerodendron serratum* roots in experimental animals. J Ethnopharmacol. 1999;65(3):237–41.

Nyman U, Joshi P, Madsen LB, et al. Ethnomedical information and in vitro screening for angiotensin-converting enzyme inhibition of plants utilized as traditional medicines in Gujarat, Rajasthan and Kerala (India). J Ethnopharmacol. 1998;60:247–63.

Padmaja V, Thankamany V, Hara N, et al. Biological activities of *Amonaglabra*. J Ethnopharmacol. 1995;48:21–4.

Patwardhan B, Vaidya ADB, Chorghade M. Ayurveda and natural product drug discovery. Curr Sci. 2004;86:789–99.

Pittler M, Abbot NC, Harkness EF, Ernst E. Location bias in controlled clinical trials of complementary/alternative therapies. Int J Epidemiol. 2000;53(5):485–9.

Prasad KV, Bharathi K, Srinivasan KK. Evaluation of *Ammannia baccifera* Linn. For antiurolithic activity in albino rats. Indian J Exp Biol. 1994;32:311–3.

Prashant B, Shamkuwar S, Shahi R. Evaluation of antidiarrhoeal activity of mebarid: an ayurvedic formulation. Int J Pharm Pharm Sci. 2012;4(2):714–6.

Ramaswamy S, Viswanathan S. Influence of gossypin on the development of acute tolerance to morphine induced antinociception. Indian J Expt Biol. 1997;35:413–4.

Rao KS, Mishra SH. Anti-inflammatory and hepatoprotective activities of *Sidarhombifolia* Linn. Indian J Pharmacol. 1997;29:110–6.

Rashid Md. HA, Mandal V, Choudhury SR, Mandal SC. Herbal nanotechnology: an emerging tool in cancer therapy. Biology, biotechnology and sustainable development. New Delhi: Research India Publications (RIP); 2015. p. 86–108.

Rashid Md. HA, Deepak Bharadwaj PVP, Mandal V, Pal M, Mandal SC, Rajarajan AT. Preparation and characterization of PLGA loaded nanoparticles obtained from *D. melanoxylon Roxb. leaves for their* antiproliferative and antidiabetic activity. Int J Green Pharma. 2017a;11(3):S438–47.

Rashid Md. HA, Majumder S, Mandal V, Mandal SC, Rajarajan AT. Regulatory and trading issues in traditional medicine: an overview. Natural products chemistry. New Delhi: Write & Print Publications; 2017b. p. 177–89.

Rashid Md. HA, Mandal V, Mandal SC, Rajarajan AT. *Diospyros melanoxylon* Roxb. in cancer prevention: pharmacological screening, pharmacokinetics and clinical studies. Int J Pharmacogn. 2017c;4(7): 217–23.

Rashid Md. HA, Deepak Bharadwaj PVP, Majumder S, Mandal V, Pal M, Mandal SC, Rajarajan AT. Antioxidant and anticancer activity of extract and fractions obtained from *Diospyros melanoxylon* Roxb. Leaves and correlation with their polyphenolic Profiles. Int J Pharm Pharm Sci. 2018;10(11):6–16.

Rasik AM, Shukla A, Patnaik GK, et al. Wound healing activity of latex of *Euphorbia neriifolia* Linn. Indian J Pharmacol. 1996;28:107–9.

Ray S, Majumder HK, Chakravarty AK, et al. Amarogentin, a naturally occurring secoiridoid glycoside and a newly recognized inhibitor of topoisomerase I from *Leishmania donovani*. J Nat Prod. 1996;59:27–9.

Rizvi SI, Abu ZM, Suhail M. Insulin-mimetic effect of (−) epicatechin on osmotic fragility of human erythrocytes. Indian J Exp Biol. 1995;33:791–2.

Roy B, Tandon V. Effect of root-tuber extract of *Flemingiavestita*, a leguminous plant, on *Artyfechinostomumsufrartyfex* and *Fasciolopsisbuski*: a scanning electron microscopy study. Parasitol Res. 1996;82:248–52.

Saha K, Mukherjee PK, Murugesan T, et al. Studies on in vivo antitussive activity of *Leucaslavandulaefolia* using a cough model induced by sulfur dioxide gas in mice. J Ethnopharmacol. 1997;57:89–92.

Sarkar SN. Capillary permeability-increasing effect of Eucalyptus hybrid leaf and *Seseli indicum* seed oils in rabbit. Indian J Pharmacol. 1994;26:55–6.

Scartezzini P, Sproni E. Review on some plants of Indian traditional medicine with antioxidant activity. J Ethnopharmacol. 2000;71:23–43.

Sekhar AV, Gandhi DN, Rao NM, Rawal UD. An experimental and clinical evaluation of anti-asthmatic potentialities of Devadaru compound (DC). Indian J Physiol Pharmacol. 2003;47:101–7.

Seth SD, Sharma B. Medicinal plants of India. Indian J Med Res. 2004;120:9–11.

Shaila HP, Udupa AL, Udupa SL. Preventive actions of *Terminalia belerica* in experimentally induced atherosclerosis. Int J Cardiol. 1995;49:101–6.

Sharma A, Mathur R, Dixit VP. Hypocholesterolemic activity of nut shell extract of *Semecarpusana cardium* (Bhilawa) in cholesterol fed rabbits. Indian J Exp Biol. 1995;33:444–8.

Sharma P, Kulshreshtha DK, Sharma AL. Anti-cataract activity of *Ocimum sanctum* on experimental cataract. Indian J Pharmacol. 1998;30:16–20.

Sheel J, Dehadrai S, Prakash AO. Estrogenic activity in the ethanolic extract of *Bupleurum marginatum*. Indian J Pharmacol. 1995;27:258–61.

Singh HK, Dhawan BN. Neuro psycho pharmacological effects of the ayurvedic nootropic *Bacopamonniera* Linn. (Brahmi). Indian J Pharmacol. 1997;29: S359–65.

Singh K, Singh A, Singh DK. Molluscicidal activity of neem (*Azadirachta indica* A. Juss). J Ethnopharmacol. 1996;52:35–40.

Singh RK, Nath G, Acharya SB, et al. Pharmacological actions of *Pongamia pinnata* roots in albino rats. Indian J Exp Biol. 1997;35:831–6.

Singh RK, Nath G, Goel RK, Bhattacharya SK. Pharmacological actions of *Abiespindrow*Royle leaf. Indian J Expt Biol. 1998;36:187–91.

Singh RL, Singh P, Agarwal A. Chemical constituents and bio-pharmacological activities of *Swertia chirata*: a review. Nat Pro Indian J. 2012;8:238–47.

Srinivasan K. Spices as influencers of body metabolism: an overview of three decades of research. Food Res Int. 2005;38(1):77–86.

Srinivasan MR, Srinivasan K. Hypocholesterolemic efficacy of garlic-smelling flower *Adenocalymma alliaceum* Miers. in experimental rats. Indian J Exp Biol. 1995;33:64–6.

Srividya N, Periwal S. Diuretic, hypotensive and hypoglycaemic effect of *Phyllanthusamarus*. Indian J Exp Biol. 1995;33:861–4.

Subramoniam A, Pushpangadan P, Rajasekharan S, Latha PG. Antipyretic activity of TBR-002, a herbal formulation. Ancient Sci Life. 1995;15:7–14.

Suresh B, Kalyanaraman VR, Dhanasekaran S, et al. Evaluation of certain Siddha drugs in the treatment of candidiasis. Ancient Sci Life. 1994;14:16–20.

Suresh B, Dhanasekaran S, Elango K, et al. Anti-pyretic activity of some plants in female albino rats: a preliminary report. Ancient Sci Life. 1995;14:253–7.

Talakal TS, Dwivedi SK, Sharma SR. In vitro and in vivo therapeutic activity of *Parthenium hysterophorus* against *Trypanosoma evansi*. Indian J Exp Biol. 1995;33:894–6.

Talwar GP, Pal R, Singh OM, et al. Safety of intra-uterine administration of purified neem seed oil (Praneem vilci) in women and effect of its co-administration with the hetero species driver birth control vaccine on antibody response to human chorionic gonadotropin. Indian J Med Res. 1995;102:66–70.

Thorat SP, Rege NN, Naik AS, et al. *Emblica officinalis*: a novel therapy for acute pancreatitis—an experimental study. HPB Surg. 1995;9:25–30.

Thyagaran SP, Subramanian S, Thirunalasunder T, Venkateswaran PS, Blumberg BS. Effects of *Phyllanthusamarus* on chronic carriers of hepatitis B virus. Lancet. 1988;2:764–6.

Tripathi YB, Chaturvedi P. Assessment of endocrine response to *Inula racemosa* in relation to glucose homeostasis in rats. Indian J Exp Biol. 1995;33: 686–9.

Tripathi YB, Tripathi E, Upadhyay A. Antilipid peroxidative property of *Nardostachys jatamanasi*. Indian J Exp Biol. 1996;34:1150–1.

Tripathi YB, Sharma M, Manickam M. Rubiadin, a new antioxidant from *Rubia cordifolia*. Indian J Biochem Biophys. 1997;34:302–6.

Upadhyay SN. Therapeutic potential of Immunomodulatory agents from plant products. In: Upadhyay SN, editor. Immunomodulation. New Delhi: Narosa Publishing House; 1997. p. 149–54.

Vaidya AB. *Terminalia chebula* in cardiovascular therapy. J Assoc Phys India. 1994;42:281–2.

Vaidya AB. The status and scope of Indian medicinal plants acting on central nervous system. Indian J Pharmacol. 1997;29:S340–3.

Vaidya AB, Sirsat SM, Doshi JC, Antarkar DS. Selected medicinal plants and formulations as hepato-biliary drugs–an overview. Indian J Clin Pharmacol Ther. 1996;17:7–11.

Vaz J, Kulkarni C, David J, Joseph T. Influence of caffeine on pharmacokinetic profile of sodium valproate and carbamazepine in normal human volunteers. Indian J Exp Biol. 1998;36:112–4.

Vimala R, Nagarajan S, Alam M, Susan T, Joy S. Anti-inflammatory and antipyretic activity of *Micheliachampaca* Linn, (white variety), *Ixorabra chiata* Roxb. and *Rhynchosia cana* (Willd.) D.C. flower extract. Indian J Exp Biol. 1997;35:1310–4.

Visen PK, Shukla B, Patnaik GK, Dhawan BN. Andrographolide protects rat hepatocytes against paracetamol-induced damage. J Ethnopharmacol. 1993;40:131–6.

Walf AA, Frye CA. The use of the elevated plus maze as an assay of anxiety-related behavior in rodents. Nat Protoc. 2007;2(2):322–8.

Walters DM, Kleeberger SR. Mouse models of bleomycin-induced pulmonary fibrosis. Curr Protoc Pharmacol. 2008;5:5.46.1–5.46.17.

Wangchuk P, Namgay K, Gayleg K, Dorji Y. Medicinal plants of Dagala region in Bhutan: their diversity, distribution, uses and economic potential. J Ethnobiol Ethnomed. 2016;12:28.

Wangchuk P, Apte SH, Smout MJ, Groves PL, Loukas A, Doolan DL. Defined small molecules produced by Himalayan medicinal plants display immunomodulatory properties. Int J Mol Sci. 2018;19(11):E3490.

Ziauddin M, Phansalkar N, Patki P, Diwanay S, Patwardhan B. Studies on the immunomodulatory effects of Ashwagandha. J Ethnopharmacol. 1996;50:69–76.

Plant Latex: A Rich Source of Haemostatic Proteases

10

Maheshwari Kumari Singh and O. S. Bindhu

Contents

10.1 Introduction

Traditional medicine is emerging as one of the increasingly popular therapeutic systems globally. In one of its surveys WHO reported that over 80% of the world's population is still dependent on traditional medicine for various health problems. Even in developed countries, 25% of medicinal products are obtained from plants and their derivatives (Kasarla et al. 2012; Priya et al. 2002; Stanley et al. 2010; Steenkamp et al. 2004). Use of medicinal plants is popular among the indigenous people in rural regions of most of the third world countries. In addition to the modern medical practices, over 65% of the Indian population relies upon traditional system of medicine for their primary treatments especially in the management of skin injury (Kumar et al. 2007; Samuel and Andrews 2010). Description of classical role of plant-based medicine as remedy for wounds and cuts can even be found in various Indian epics. A great number of these plants are vital in modern pharmaceutical industries either as therapeutic agents or as starting materials for the manufacture of classical and modern medicines (Ramproshad et al. 2012). 70% of wound healing Ayurvedic medicines are plant-based and remaining 20% and 10% are mineral and animal product based respectively. In most cases, scientific validation to support efficacies of these plants are not performed (Kumar et al. 2007;

M. K. Singh · O. S. Bindhu (✉)
Department of Biochemistry, School of Sciences, Jain (Deemed- to- be) University, Bangalore, Karnataka, India
e-mail: os.bindhu@jainuniversity.ac.in

S. Sen, R. Chakraborty (eds.), *Herbal Medicine in India*, https://doi.org/10.1007/978-981-13-7248-3_10

Sathya and Kokilavani 2013; Verpoorte 2000). Studies that attempted to understand the scientific basis behind the therapeutic efficacy of many traditionally used medicinal plants revealed the protagonist role by their proteases. Even though there is vast information on plant protease being used in ancient times as illustrated in Homeric writings such as the Íliad, the number of industrially used plant proteases is sparse (de Roos et al. 2004).

Among herbal medicines, latex and its constituents provide a major basis for wound care and management. Use of plant latex from several medicinal plants to stop bleeding from minor injuries, and to enhance wound healing has been in tribal/rural practice for thousands of years in India and other countries. Latex producing plants were reported to be the primary constituents of traditional medicine employed in the management of wounds and burns (Biswas and Mukherjee 2003; Kumar et al. 2007). Latex is a plant-derived natural milky fluid secreted by specialized laticifers. Local tribal communities and traditional healers have extensively explored the medicinal values associated with this plant exudates from various angiospermic families for treating diverse ailments including various skin injuries (common wounds, cuts, burns, boils, blisters, bruises, thorn wounds, cracks, ulcers and warts) (Priyanka Uday et al. 2015). The search for novel protease/s from medicinal plants continues to be of extreme importance in recent research programs around the world primarily due to high incidence of multidrug resistance and toxicity of some antibiotics already in use for the management of wounds (Subramanian and Saratha 2010). The interference of proteases in biofilm eradication of gram-positive bacteria via hydrolyzing the matrix proteins and adhesins which are crucial proteins favoring the cell attachment have been reported. Biofilm eradication role by these protease also involves cleavage of signaling peptides associated with the intercellular communication (Lequette et al. 2010; Park et al. 2012; Pavlukhina et al. 2012; Powers et al. 2011). The effectiveness of selected wound healing latex proteases such as ficin as the antibiofilm agent has been reported recently by few studies (Baidamshina et al. 2017). The escalating demand for herbal products in recent time for various purposes has led to booming of scientific investigations in latex biochemistry.

Latex from several plant families has been reported to be a mixture of several hydrolytic enzymes and secondary metabolites (Domsalla and Melzig 2008; Guimaraes-Ferreira et al. 2007). Of these hydrolytic enzymes, proteases are known to be the key molecules responsible for many of the observed pharmacological effects of latex *in vivo* and *in vitro*. Research in latex Biochemistry till date has demonstrated their suitability as agents in numerous processes associated with pharmaceuticals, food, detergent, leather industries etc. (Anusha et al. 2014; Li et al. 2013). Interestingly, protease obtained from certain plant species has even shown compound functions and hence multifaceted utility (Badgujar and Mahajan 2013; Bindhu and Singh 2014; Lopez-Otin and Bond 2008; Sawant and Nagendran 2014).

10.2 Plant Latex and Its Physiological Role

Latex is a natural plant polymer with molecular composition of carbon, hydrogen and nitrogen (C_3H_3N). It is a complex blend of chemicals (terpenoids, alkaloids, rubber, cardenolides etc.) and proteins. It generally exudes from highly specialized laticifers/ducts of laticiferous tissue of plant parts due to injury. Laticifers, the latex-bearing structures, vary in origin, anatomy, and distribution (Domsalla and Melzig 2008; Lewinsohn 1991; Yagami et al. 1998). Color of latex is generally white with some exceptions of yellow, orange, or scarlet (Upadhyay 2011). Approximately 10% of all angiosperm plants produce latex. Nearly 35,000 species, with the inclusion of conifers and resin-exuding plants, exude latex (Agrawal and Konno 2009; Farrell et al. 1991; Lewinsohn 1991; Metcalfe 1967). Latex production is a typical trait of plants belonging to the families like Asteraceae, Caricaceae, Moraceae,

Asclepiadaceae, Apocynaceae and Euphorbiaceae (Metcalfe 1967). Furthermore, latex has also been documented to be present in mushrooms and pteridophytes.

The term "latex" was first coined by an English physician in 1600 AD and its function was found to be analogous to lymphatic vessels of animals (Mahlberg 1993). There have been several hypotheses regarding its function in plants which include expulsion of waste metabolites, coverage of affected tissue and protection against herbivores/pathogens etc. James in 1887 proposed the first defensive hypothesis describing North American milkweeds (James 1887). Kniep, a German Scientist in the early twentieth century, noted that slugs could damage only the leaves of plants without latex (Kniep 1905). In the following years, a couple of findings supported the presence of diverse biologically active compounds such as secondary metabolites and latex proteins to be the reason for this characteristic defensive property (Agrawal and Konno 2009; Konno 2011; Upadhyay 2011). Many of biologically active compounds in latex provide resistance to herbivores via toxicity or antinutritive effects whereas others are involved in the stickiness that can mire insect herbivores.

The presence of proteases in latex of several plant families is known from many years. Initial report on the presence of proteolytic enzymes in plant latex was from Winnick et al. (1940). One or more proteolytic enzymes are found in over 110 latex producing plants from various angiospermic families (Domsalla and Melzig 2008). Attempts have been made to study the role of these proteases in various physiological processes *in vitro* and *in vivo*. These enzymes play an important role in plant physiology. In addition to maintaining the cellular protein pool, they are also involved in processes such as leaf senescence, defence against pathogens, fruit ripening, germination etc. (Domsalla and Melzig 2008; Ramos et al. 2010). Over 90 latex proteases have been reported to be purified from plants belonging to various families (Domsalla and Melzig 2008; Li et al. 2013; Mahajan and Badgujar 2010).

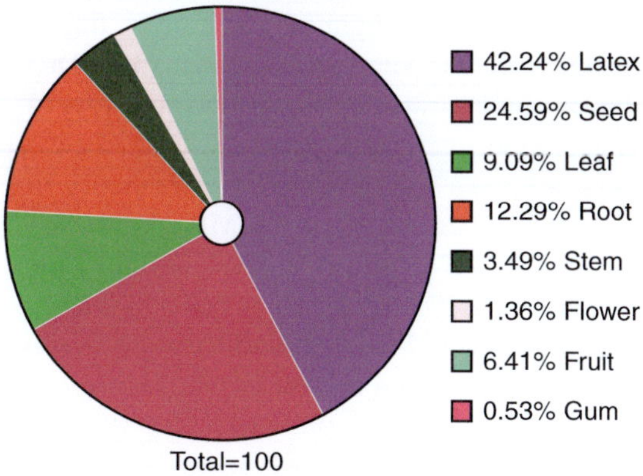

Fig. 10.1 Distribution of proteases in different plant parts

10.3 Distribution of Latex Proteases

Proteases are abundant in nature, extensively spread among all animals, plants and microorganisms. Plants form the major source of proteases, followed by bacteria, fungi, animals, algae and viruses. Plant proteases are prevalent literally in all parts of plants i.e. root, stem, leaf, flower, fruit, seed, gum, and latex. Among the plant parts, latex has been considered as the richest protease source. Figure 10.1 summarizes the distribution of proteases in different plant parts. Cysteine proteases abundantly occur in plants (34.92%) with a minor contribution of serine (13.21%) aspartic (8.81%) and asparaginyl proteases (0.53%). Nearly 43% of plant proteases are yet to be characterized (Domsalla and Melzig 2008; Mahajan and Badgujar 2010). Proteases identified from latex producing plants so far are either cysteine or serine proteases and rarely aspartic proteases family (Rawlings et al. 2009).

10.3.1 Serine Proteases

Serine proteases possess over forty peptidases family grouped into six clans. Their catalytic mechanism is based on transfer of acyl group of the substrate to enzyme's functional group (Barrett et al. 2012). They are irreversibly inhibited by phenylmethylsulfonyl fluoride (PMSF), 3, 4-dichloroisocoumarin (3, 4-DCI), diisopropylfluorophosphate (DFP) and tosyl-L-lysine chloromethyl ketone (TLCK). Few of them are even inhibited by thiol reagents like p-chloromercuribenzoate (PCMB) because of the presence of a cysteine residue in the vicinity of active site. The optimum pH of serine proteases is between 7 and 11, and they are usually functional at neutral and basic pH. The isoelectric points of serine proteases are generally between pH 4 and 6. They possess wide substrate preference in addition to esterolytic and amidase activities. Their molecular weights vary between 18 and 35 kDa and seldom the molecular weight is found to be more than 100 kDa (Barrett 1994). Ficinsare serine protease purified from genus *Ficus* (Devaraj et al. 2008).

10.3.2 Cysteine Protease

Majority of latex cysteine proteases belong to the Papain family (C1). Their molecular weight ranges from 21 to 49 kDa with a few exceptions. These are stable over pH range of 3–12 and up to 80 °C temperature and are comparable to serine proteases (Mahajan and Badgujar 2010). Typically utilized inhibitors are iodoacetamide (IAA), sodium tetrathionate, mercuric chloride, trans epoxysuccinyl-L-leucylamido-(4-guanidino) butane (E-64) and p-chloromercury benzoate (PCMB). Cysteine proteases derived from plants are known to perform a significant role in intracellular and extracellular activities such as growth and ripening of fruits, degradation of storage protein in germinating seeds, activation of proenzymes, degradation of defective proteins etc. (Salas et al. 2008; Taylor and Cuming 1993; Gomes et al. 2011). Apart from their crucial physiological roles, plant cysteine proteases have attracted attention in the food and biotech industries. They are also useful in the pharmaceutical industry for managing wounds, infections, burns etc. (Yegin and Dekker 2013). Papain is the best-known cysteine protease which has been explored for its profound industrial applications.

10.3.3 Aspartic Proteases (EC 3.4.23)

Aspartic proteasesutilize aspartic acid residues for catalytic function and are commonly known as acidic proteases. Contrary to the case of serine or cysteine proteases, these proteases do not generate a covalent intermediate during cleavage. Hence proteolysis takes place in a single step. Acidic proteases are categorized into three families namely pepsin (AP1), retropepsin (AP2) and enzymes from para retroviruses (AP3) (Barrett 1995). Majority of aspartic proteases exhibit high activity between pH 3 and 4 and their isoelectric points fall between pH 3 and 4.5. Their molecular masses range from 30 to 45 kDa, with a few exceptions (Labarère 1980). Aspartic proteases are generally inhibited by pepstatin. They are also sensitive to diazoketone compounds like diazoacetyl-DL-norleucine methyl ester (DAN) and 1, 2-epoxy-3-(p-nitrophenoxy) propane (EPNP) when copper ions are present (Mahajan and Badgujar 2010). An unusual thermostable aspartic protease from the latex of *Ficus racemosa*is known to be only aspartic protease from latex so far (Devaraj et al. 2008).

10.4 Latex Proteases as Hemostatic Agents in Wound Healing

Research on wound healing agents is one of the developing areas in modern biomedical sciences. Plant based natural agents were shown to induce healing and regeneration of lost tissue by multiple mechanisms. In spite of tremendous advances in pharmaceutical industry, the availability of drugs capable of stimulating the process of wound repair particularly chronic wounds is still limited (Porras-Reyes et al. 1993; Suh et al. 1998). Ankaferd and haemocer/starcil are a few examples of plant based therapeutic haemostats operating via different mechanisms leading to arrest bleeding (Uday et al. 2017). Biochemical and pharmacological characterization of plant latex in the past has revealed involvement of latex proteases in wound healing. Extensive characterization studies are carried out for a few of them while others are yet to be explored (Agrawal and Konno 2009; Ashwani 1999; Begum and Nath 2000; Osoniyi and Onajobi 2003; Prusti and Behera 2007; Ramachandra Reddy et al. 2003).

Wounds are defined as physical injuries that result in breaking or opening of the tissue due to either the external environment (external injury) or the internal environment of the body (internal injury) (Sharma et al. 2013). Wound healing is a complicated and intricate phenomenon that restores the function and integrity of damaged tissues (Clark 1996; Glynn 1981; Kumar et al. 2007; Martin 1996; Martin 1997). The process of healing of wound or cicatrisation involves repairing of skin post injury by itself within a defined period of time involving four phases–hemostasis phase (within minutes), inflammatory phase (24–48 h may be up to 2 week), proliferative phase (2 days to 3 weeks) and remodeling phase (3 weeks to 2 years) (Arun et al. 2013; Priyanka Uday et al. 2015). Hemostasis and fibrinolysis, being major steps in this process, have drawn much attention in the present research world. They involve the collaborative action of various cellular entities and clotting factors. Reports supporting the role of latex constituents in wound healing include their role in the formation and dissolution of clot which are two vital events of healing (Fig. 10.2). Research directed towards solving the puzzle of healing mechanism by latex has led to new emphasis and drive in latex based plant research in wound management (Kumar et al. 2007).

Hemostasis, the initial event of wound healing, is a proteolytically regulated system which involves platelet and blood coagulation cascade activation. The key enzymes that play a role in the cascades of blood clotting and fibrinolysis are thrombin and plasmin respectively (Shivaprasad et al. 2009; Shivaprasad et al. 2010a, b). Many proteolytic enzymes are involved in these processes *in vivo* (Sherry et al. 1959). Thrombin, a specific fibrinogenolytic enzyme, breaks down Aα and Bβ chains of fibrinogen and forms fibrin clot by releasing fibrinopeptide A and B with partially maintaining the γ band intact (Gowda et al. 2011; Magalhães et al. 2007; Rajesh et al. 2006). Proteases found in plant latex have been shown to influence blood coagulation. Thrombin-like enzymes present in latex represent group of proteases that have similar fibrinogen hydrolytic pattern as mediated by thrombin and involve in the formation of fibrin clots. The procoagulant effects of some of these proteases (serine/cysteine) are due to their hydrolytic effect on a few of the intermediates in the coagulation cascade.

Fibrinolysis is the immediate second significant proteolytic event after fibrin clot formation which favors the process of wound healing. This process involves plasmin as main enzyme that breaks both fibrin clot and haemostatic plug to facilitate wound healing (Lijnen 2002).

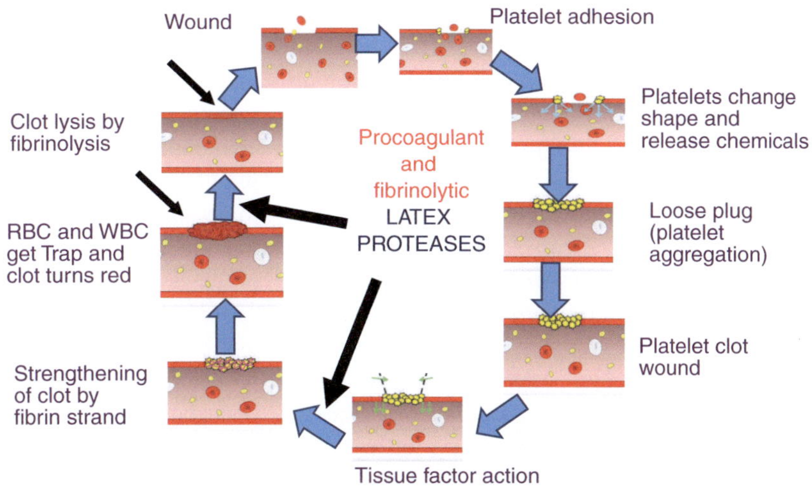

Fig. 10.2 Procoagulant and fibrinolytic involvement of proteolytic enzymes from latex

Interestingly, most of the plant latex proteases that have procoagulant activity also possess fibrinolytic/ plasmin-like activity (Fig. 10.2).

Until 1930s, no scientific study was conducted on the involvement of latex in the context of hemostasis and wound healing. Year 1937 witnessed procoagulant (fibrinogen to fibrin conversion) effect of a cysteine protease (papain) isolated from *C. papaya* (Eagle and Harris 1937). Two latex based studies in 1979 and 1984 showed presence of several hydrolytic enzymes in aqueous extracts of *Calotropis gigantea* latex (Abraham and Joshi 1979; Sengupta et al. 1984). Latex from several plant species, principally members of Asclepidiaceae, Apocyanaceae, Euphorbiaceae and Moraceae family, has been shown to involve in pain-relieving and wound healing (Bolay 1979; Richter et al. 2002; Thankamma 2003). As early as 1991, Nath and Dutta isolated curcain, a serine protease from latex of *Jatropha curcus*, and proved its wound healing activity in mice (Nath and Dutta 1992). Proteases derived from *Ficus carica* (common fig) were known to involve in the activation and deactivation of human factor X suggesting their hemostatic potency (Richter et al. 2002). Cysteine proteases from crude latex extract of *C. gigantea* exhibited strong proteolytic activity accompanied with hydrolysis of purified fibrinogen (human) and fibrin clot in a dose dependent manner suggesting potent procoagulant and thrombolytic activity (Rajesh et al. 2005). Mechanism of action of *Jatropha gossypifolia* stem latex belonging to the family Euphorbiaceae as a haemostatic agent was investigated (Oduola et al. 2005). A unique fibrinogen and fibrin hydrolytic pattern, unlike thrombin and plasmin, was exhibited by purified 34 kDa latex glycoprotein (serine protease) from *Synandenium grantii,* a Euphorbiaceae member (Rajesh et al. 2006). Rajesh et al. (2007), carried out a comparative study on latex proteases from *C. gigantea* R. Br., *S. grantii Hook.* f. and *Wrightia tinctoria* R. Br. latex extracts and provided a foundation for the likely action of plant latex proteases to arrest bleeding and augment wound healing (Rajesh et al. 2007). A similar observation on cysteine proteases from the latex of *Asclepias curassavica* L., *C. gigantea* R. Br, *Pergularia extensa* R. Br. and *Cynanchum puciflorum* R. Br. of family Asclepiadaceae substantiated their pharmacological significance in wound healing (Shivaprasad et al. 2009).

Ficin from *Ficus carica* and pergularine I from *P. extensa* latex were other potent haemostatic agents reported (Devaraj et al. 2008; Shivaprasad et al. 2010a, b). Protective effect of latex proteases from *C. procera* in sepsis model and their efficacy in maintaining coagulation homeostasis via thrombin- and plasmin-like activities was investigated (Ramos et al. 2012). Similar to Asclepediaciae, Moraceae, Euphorbiaceae and Apocynaceae family members also have received much attention regarding the characterization of biochemical properties of their proteolytic enzymes (Mekkriengkrai et al. 2004). A 79.5 kDa serine protease (artocarpin) has been isolated from *Artocarpus heterophyllus* (jackfruit) latex. A novel serine protease, AMP48, from *A. heterophyllus* latex exhibited both fibrinogenolytic and fibrinolytic activity suggesting its potential utility towards thromboembolic disorder treatment as anti-thrombotic agent (Siritapetawee et al. 2012).

Purified 34 kDa serine protease (hirtin) from *Euphorbia hirta*, was studied for its fibrinolytic activity and its industrial and therapeutic applications were suggested (Patel et al. 2012). New perspectives about the pharmacological potential of latex cysteine proteases from *C. grandiflora* and *P. rubra* in blood homeostasis reinforced their fibrinogenolytic (thrombin like) activity (Viana et al. 2013). Latex from selected Euphorbiaceae members was found responsible for arresting wound bleeding and accelerating whole blood coagulation process. Latex augmented the healing of experimentally induced excision wound in mice showing its direct involvement in wound healing process (Yariswamy et al. 2013). Multiple proteases (Cysteine and serine) from *Maclura spinosa* (Roxb. ex Willd.) latex exhibited synergistic caseinolytic and differential fibrinogenolytic action with serine proteases as the exclusive contributor for hemostatic activity (Venkatesh et al. 2015). Heynein, a cysteine protease purified from *Ervatamia heyneana* showed strong thrombin like action with mild fibrinolytic activity (Uday et al. 2017).

Tables 10.1 and 10.2 compile the details of partially purified and purified plant latex proteases respectively with proteolytic activity that are shown to interfere with hemostasis and their target coagulation factors and action (ND: not determined).

Table 10.1 Partially purified plant latex proteases and their wound healing contribution

Latex extract	Type	Action	Target	References
Calotropis gigantea	Cysteine	Thrombin and plasmin-like	Fibrinogen and Fibrin	Rajesh et al. (2005)
Synadenium grantii	Serine	Procoagulant	Fibrinogen and Fibrin	Rajesh et al. (2006)
Wrightia tinctoria	Serine	Procoagulant	Fibrinogen and Fibrin	Rajesh et al. (2007)
Asclepias curassavica	Cysteine	Thrombin- and plasmin-like	Fibrinogen and Fibrin	Shivaprasad et al. (2009)
Euphorbia caducifolia	ND	Effect on clotting and angiogenesis .	Excision and incision wounds model	Goyal et al. (2012)
Plumeria rubra	Cysteine	Thrombin- and plasmin-like	Fibrinogen and Fibrin	Viana et al. (2013)
Cryptostegia grandiflora	Cysteine	Thrombin- and plasmin-like	Fibrinogen and Fibrin	Viana et al. (2013)
Wrightia tinctoria	Serine	Healing of excision wound in mice models	Topical wound	Yariswamy et al. (2013)
Euphorbia nivulia	Cysteine	Procoagulant	Whole Blood	Badgujar (2014)
Pedilanthus tithymaloides	ND	Procoagulant	Whole Blood	Badgujar (2014)
Maclura spinosa	Serine Proteases	Procoagulant	Fibrinogen	Venkatesh et al. (2015)
Tabernaemontana divaricata	Cysteine	Thrombin- and plasmin-like	Fibrinogen and Fibrin	Singh et al. (2015)
Artocarpus altilis	Cysteine	Thrombin- and plasmin-like	Fibrinogen and Fibrin	Singh et al. (2015)

Table 10.2 Purified plant latex proteases and their wound healing contribution

Purified protease	Type	Action	Target	References
Ficin (Cysteine)	*Ficus Carica*	Factor X activator	Factor X	Richter et al. (2002)
LGP (Serine)	*Synadenium grantii*	Procoagulant	Fibrinogen and Fibrin	Rajesh et al. (2006)
Eumiilin (Cysteine)	*Euphorbia milii var. hislopii*	ND	Fibrinogen	Fonseca et al. (2010)
Pergularain e I (Cysteine)	*Pergularia extensa*	Thrombin- and plasmin-like	Fibrinogen and Fibrin	Shivaprasad et al. (2010a, b)
Crinumin (Serine)	*Crinum asiaticum*	Plasmin-like and platelet aggregation inhibition	Fibrin	Singh et al. (2010)
Hirtin (Serine)	*Euphorbia hirta*	Thrombin- and plasmin-like	Fibrinogen and Fibrin	Patel et al. (2012)
LPPII and LPPIII (Cysteine)	*Calotropis procera*	Thrombin- and plasmin-like	Fibrinogen and Fibrin	Ramos et al. (2012)
AMP48 (Serine)	*Artocarpus heterophylus*	Fibrino(geno)lytic	Fibrinogen and Fibrin	Ramos et al. (2012)
Heynein	*Ervatamia heyneana*	Strong thrombin like action with mild fibrinolytic	Fibrinogen and Fibrin	Uday et al. (2017)

Apart from its usage to stop bleeding, plant latex has been used since time immemorial in folk medicine as remedy for wound healing (Rajesh et al. 2005). Although fibrin clot supports initial events of wound healing, subsequent breakdown leading to removal of clot is a pre-requisite for the events of repair phase that involve tissue repair and its remodeling (Clark 1996; Green et al. 2008). Clot dissolution process *in vivo* is mediated by the serine protease, plasmin. Proteases from plant lattices have been shown to exhibit blood clot dissolving properties indicating their plasmin like behavior. The dual activities by some latex proteases have projected them as good alternatives in the management of fresh cuts/wounds (Siritapetawee et al. 2012).

Plant latex proteases have distinct action on blood coagulation pathways. This property makes them suitable candidates to serve as potential research tools and as topical agents at therapeutic level. Studies till date strongly support latex proteases' dual role as an inducer (blood clot formation/thrombin like action) and dissolver of fibrin clot (plasmin like action). Detailed characterization along with understanding of structure-activity relationships and the diversity of these latex proteases may allow them to be explored for practical applications of these enzymes in therapeutics.

10.5 Summary and Path Forward

Advancements in research focusing on latex proteases have led to the understanding from their physiological role as primary plant defence providers to other multiple biological functions (Shivaprasad et al. 2016). Even much before their nature and properties were known, plant latex has been an active ingredient in traditional medicine for centuries. Treatment of wounds, burns, infections, pain etc. were some such latex facilitated applications. Their contribution is now obvious even in cheese making, leather processing, meat tenderization, detergent industries, water treatment etc. (Badgujar and Mahajan 2013; Baidamshina et al. 2017; Headon and Walsh 1994; Li et al. 2013; Walsh 2002). A lot of plant latex derived proteases are still at the level of academia research. Even with this much progress, very few have come to the industrial level. Papain and ficin are a few of those kinds that have arrived at the level of commercialization. Papain has evolved asan industrial enzyme since decades in various fields such as meat tenderization, detergent, food, water treatment, pharmaceutical etc. (Fernández-Lucas et al. 2017). Accuzyme®, Penafil® are the only papain based commercial enzymatic debriding ointments that are currently available in market (Miner et al. 2006; Whitley 2005).

Lack of complete understanding of precise mechanism behind wound healing process is one of the major concerns in the pharmacological validation of many identified potential hemostatic agents. Hence most of the wound healing studies restrict the validation to the initial phases of wound healing without going into much detail of biochemical changes, epithelization, antioxidant defense etc. Extended assessments on the basis of dosage, toxicity, mode of administration, efficacy etc. at molecular level along with addressing the issues associated with cost, quality control, sustainable availability etc. may facilitate the promotion of at least a few of those proteases which are in pipeline/academic research to make it to level of commercialization.

References

Abraham KI, Joshi PN. Studies on proteinases from *Calotropis gigantea* latex: purification and some properties of two proteinases containing carbohydrate. Biochim Biophys Acta. 1979;568:111–9.

Agrawal AA, Konno K. Latex: a model for understanding mechanisms, ecology, and evolution of plant defense against herbivory. Annu Rev Ecol Evol Syst. 2009;40(1):311–31.

Anusha R, Singh MK, Bindhu O. Characterisation of potential milk coagulants from *Calotropis gigantea* plant parts and their hydrolytic pattern of bovine casein. Eur Food Res Technol. 2014;238(6):997–1006.

Arun M, Satish S, Anima P. Herbal boon for wounds. Wounds. 2013;6(7):8.

Ashwani K, editor. Ayurvedic medicines: some potential plants for medicine from India. a meeting of the international forum on traditional medicines.

Toyama, Japan: Toyama Medical and Pharmaceutical University; 1999.

Badgujar SB. Evaluation of hemostatic activity of latex from three Euphorbiaceae species. J Ethnopharmacol. 2014;151(1):733–9.

Badgujar SB, Mahajan RT. Characterization of thermo- and detergent stable antigenic glycosylated cysteine protease of *Euphorbia nivulia* Buch.-Ham. and evaluation of its ecofriendly applications. Sci World J. 2013;2013:716545.

Baidamshina DR, Trizna EY, Holyavka MG, Bogachev MI, Artyukhov VG, Akhatova FS, et al. Targeting microbial biofilms using Ficin, a nonspecific plant protease. Sci Rep. 2017;7:46068.

Barrett AJ. Classification of peptidases: proteolytic enzymes: serine and cysteine peptidases. Methods Enzymol. 1994;244:1–15.

Barrett AJ. Proteolytic enzymes: aspartic and metallo peptidases. Cambridge, MA: Academic Press; 1995.

Barrett AJ, Woessner JF, Rawlings ND. Handbook of proteolytic enzymes. Amsterdam: Elsevier; 2012.

Begum D, Nath SC. Ethnobotanical review of medicinal plants used for skin diseases and related problems in Northeastern India. J Herbs Spices Med Plants. 2000;7(3):55–93.

Bindhu OS, Singh MK. Hemostatic, milk clotting and blood stain removal potential of cysteine proteases from Calotropis gigantea (L.) R. Br. Latex. Pharmacogn Mag. 2014;10(Suppl 2):S350.

Biswas TK, Mukherjee B. Plant medicines of Indian origin for wound healing activity: a review. Int J Low Extrem Wounds. 2003;2(1):25–39.

Bolay E. Feigenund wurgefeigen. Pharm Unserer Zeit. 1979;4:97–112.

Clark R. Wound repair: overview and general con- 17. Becker, DL, McGonnell, I, Makarenkova, H, Patel, K, Tickle, sideration In The Molecular and Cellular Biology of Wound Re- C, Lorimer, J, and Green, CR (1999) Roles for alpha. 1996;1:3–50.

Devaraj KB, Gowda LR, Prakash V. An unusual thermostable aspartic protease from the latex of *Ficus racemosa* (L.). Phytochemistry. 2008;69(3):647–55.

Domsalla A, Melzig MF. Occurrence and properties of proteases in plant latices. Planta Med. 2008;74(7):699–711.

Eagle H, Harris TN. Studies in blood coagulation: V. The coagulation of blood by proteolytic enzymes (trypsin, papain). J Gen Physiol. 1937;20(4):543.

Farrell BD, Dussourd DE, Mitter C. Escalation of plant defense: do latex and resin canals spur plant diversification? Am Nat. 1991;138(4):881–900.

Fernández-Lucas J, Castañeda D, Hormigo D. New trends for a classical enzyme: papain, a biotechnological success story in the food industry. Trends Food Sci Technol. 2017;68:91–101.

Fonseca KC, Morais NC, Queiroz MR, Silva MC, Gomes MS, Costa JO, et al. Purification and biochemical characterization of Eumiliin from *Euphorbia milii* var. hislopii latex. Phytochemistry. 2010;71(7): 708–15.

Glynn L. The pathology of scar tissue formation. Handbook of inflammation. 1981;3:120–128.

Gomes MT, Oliva ML, Lopes MT, Salas CE. Plant proteinases and inhibitors: an overview of biological function and pharmacological activity. Curr Protein Pept Sci. 2011;12(5):417–36.

Gowda CD, Shivaprasad HV, Kumar RV, Rajesh R, Saikumari YK, Frey BM, et al. Characterization of major zinc containing myonecrotic and procoagulant metalloprotease 'malabarin'from non lethal *Trimeresurus malabaricus* snake venom with thrombin like activity: its neutralization by chelating agents. Curr Top Med Chem. 2011;11(20):2578–88.

Goyal M, Nagori B, Sasmal D. Wound healing activity of latex of *Euphorbia caducifolia*. J Ethnopharmacol. 2012;144(3):786–90.

Green KA, Almholt K, Ploug M, Rønø B, Castellino FJ, Johnsen M, et al. Profibrinolytic effects of metalloproteinases during skin wound healing in the absence of plasminogen. J Investig Dermatol. 2008;128(8):2092–101.

Guimaraes-Ferreira CA, Rodrigues EG, Mortara RA, Cabral H, Serrano FA, Ribeiro-dos-Santos R, et al. Antitumor effects in vitro and in vivo and mechanisms of protection against melanoma B16F10-Nex2 cells by fastuosain, a cysteine proteinase from *Bromelia fastuosa*. Neoplasia. 2007;9(9):723–33.

Headon D, Walsh G. The industrial production of enzymes. Biotechnol Adv. 1994;12(4):635–46.

James JF. The milkweeds. Am Nat. 1887;21(7):605–15.

Kasarla R, Elumalai A, Chinna Eswaraiah M, Ravi P, Naresh V. An annual review on wound-healing medicinal plants (Jan–Dec 2011). Scholars Res Library. 2012;2:182–5.

Kniep H. Über die Bedeutung des Milchsafls der Pflanzen. Flora oder Allgemeine Botanische Zeitung. 1905;94:129–205.

Konno K. Plant latex and other exudates as plant defense systems: roles of various defense chemicals and proteins contained therein. Phytochemistry. 2011;72(13):1510–30.

Kumar B, Vijayakumar M, Govindarajan R, Pushpangadan P. Ethnopharmacological approaches to wound healing exploring medicinal plants of India. J Ethnopharmacol. 2007;114(2):103–13.

Labarère J. Proteolytic activities during growth and aging in the fungus *Podospora anserina*: effect of specific mutations. Arch Microbiol. 1980;124(2):269–74.

Lequette Y, Boels G, Clarisse M, Faille C. Using enzymes to remove biofilms of bacterial isolates sampled in the food-industry. Biofouling. 2010;26(4):421–31.

Lewinsohn TM. The geographical distribution of plant latex. Chemoecology. 1991;2(1):64–8.

Li Q, Yi L, Marek P, Iverson BL. Commercial proteases: present and future. FEBS Lett. 2013;587(8):1155–63.

Lijnen H. Matrix metalloproteinases and cellular fibrinolytic activity. Biochem Mosc. 2002;67(1):92–8.

Lopez-Otin C, Bond JS. Proteases: multifunctional enzymes in life and disease. J Biol Chem. 2008;283(45):30433–7.

Magalhães A, Magalhães HP, Richardson M, Gontijo S, Ferreira RN, Almeida AP, et al. Purification and properties of a coagulant thrombin-like enzyme from the venom of *Bothrops leucurus*. Comp Biochem Physiol A Mol Integr Physiol. 2007;146(4):565–75.

Mahajan RT, Badgujar SB. Biological aspects of proteolytic enzymes: a review. J Pharm Res. 2010;3(9):2048–68.

Mahlberg PG. Laticifers: an historical perspective. Bot Rev. 1993;59(1):1–23.

Martin A. The use of antioxidants in healing. Dermatol Surg. 1996;22(2):156–60.

Martin P. Wound healing-aiming for perfect skin regeneration. Science. 1997;276(5309):75–81.

Mekkriengkrai D, Ute K, Swiezewska E, Chojnacki T, Tanaka Y, Sakdapipanich JT. Structural characterization of rubber from jackfruit and euphorbia as a model of natural rubber. Biomacromolecules. 2004;5(5):2013–9.

Metcalfe C. Distribution of latex in the plant kingdom. Econ Bot. 1967;21(2):115–27.

Miner KJ, CWCN F, Agbim SN, editors. Papain-urea-chlorophyllin copper complex sodium ointment (PUC) and trypsin, balsam peru, and castor oil (TBC) in the treatment and healing of recurrent Stage II and Stage III pressure ulcers. In: The 38th Annual WOCN Society Conference; 2006.

Nath L, Dutta S. Wound healing response of the proteolytic enzyme curcain. Indian J Pharmacol. 1992;24(2):114.

Oduola T, Adeosun GO, Oduola TA, Avwioro GO, Oyeniyi MA. Mechanism of action of *Jatropha gossypifolia* stem latex as a haemostatic agent. Eur J Gen Med. 2005;2(4):140–3.

Osoniyi O, Onajobi F. Coagulant and anticoagulant activities in *Jatropha curcas* latex. J Ethnopharmacol. 2003;89(1):101–5.

Park J-H, Lee J-H, Cho MH, Herzberg M, Lee J. Acceleration of protease effect on *Staphylococcus aureus* biofilm dispersal. FEMS Microbiol Lett. 2012;335(1):31–8.

Patel GK, Kawale AA, Sharma AK. Purification and physicochemical characterization of a serine protease with fibrinolytic activity from latex of a medicinal herb *Euphorbia hirta*. Plant Physiol Biochem. 2012;52:104–11.

Pavlukhina SV, Kaplan JB, Xu L, Chang W, Yu X, Madhyastha S, et al. Noneluting enzymatic antibiofilm coatings. ACS Appl Mater Interfaces. 2012;4(9):4708–16.

Porras-Reyes BH, Lewis WH, Roman J, Simchowitz L, Mustoe TA. Enhancement of wound healing by the alkaloid taspine defining mechanism of action. Proc Soc Exp Biol Med. 1993;203(1):18–25.

Powers ME, Smith PA, Roberts TC, Fowler BJ, King CC, Trauger SA, et al. Type I signal peptidase and protein secretion in *Staphylococcus epidermidis*. J Bacteriol. 2011;193(2):340–8.

Priya KS, Gnanamani A, Radhakrishnan N, Babu M. Healing potential of *Datura alba* on burn wounds in albino rats. J Ethnopharmacol. 2002;83(3):193–9.

Priyanka Uday RRA, Bhat PR, Rinimol VR, Bindu J, Nafeesa Z, Swamy SN. Laticiferous plant proteases in wound care. Int J Pharm Pharm Sci. 2015;7(1):44–9.

Prusti A, Behera K. Ethnobotanical exploration of Malkangiri district of Orissa, India. Int J Ethnobot Res Ethnobot Leaflets. 2007;2007(1):14.

Rajesh R, Gowda CR, Nataraju A, Dhananjaya B, Kemparaju K, Vishwanath B. Procoagulant activity of *Calotropis gigantea* latex associated with fibrin (ogen) olytic activity. Toxicon. 2005;46(1):84–92.

Rajesh R, Nataraju A, Gowda C, Frey B, Frey F, Vishwanath B. Purification and characterization of a 34-kDa, heat stable glycoprotein from *Synadenium grantii* latex: action on human fibrinogen and fibrin clot. Biochimie. 2006;88(10):1313–22.

Rajesh R, Shivaprasad HV, Gowda CDR, Nataraju A, Dhananjaya BL, Vishwanath BS. Comparative study on plant latex proteases and their involvement in hemostasis: a special emphasis on clot inducing and dissolving properties. Planta Med. 2007;73(10):1061–7.

Ramachandra Reddy P, Rao PP, Prabhakar M. Ethnomedicinal practices amongst Chenchus of Nagarjunasagar Srisailam Tiger Reserve (NSTR), Andhra Pradesh: plant remedies for cuts, wounds and boils. Ethnobot. 2003;15:67–71.

Ramos MV, Grangeiro TB, Freire EA, Sales MP, Souza DP, Araújo ES, et al. The defensive role of latex in plants: detrimental effects on insects. Arthropod Plant Interact. 2010;4(1):57–67.

Ramos MV, Viana CA, Silva AF, Freitas CD, Figueiredo IS, Oliveira RS, et al. Proteins derived from latex of *C. procera* maintain coagulation homeostasis in septic mice and exhibit thrombin-and plasmin-like activities. Naunyn Schmiedeberg's Arch Pharmacol. 2012;385(5):455–63.

Ramproshad S, Afroz T, Mondal B, Khan R, Ahmed S. Screening of phytochemical and pharmacological activities of leaves of medicinal plant *Plumeria rubra*. Int J Res Pharma Chem. 2012;2(4):1001–7.

Rawlings ND, Barrett AJ, Bateman A. MEROPS: the peptidase database. Nucleic Acids Res. 2009;38(suppl 1):D227–D33.

Richter G, Schwarz HP, Dorner F, Turecek PL. Activation and inactivation of human factor X by proteases derived from *Ficus carica*. Br J Haematol. 2002;119(4):1042–51.

de Roos A, Grassin C, Herweijer M, Kragh KM, Poulsen CH, Soe JB, et al. Industrial enzymes: enzymes in food applications. In: Enzymes in industry: production and applications. 2nd ed; 2004. p. 101–55.

Salas CE, Gomes MT, Hernandez M, Lopes MT. Plant cysteine proteinases: evaluation of the pharmacological activity. Phytochemistry. 2008;69(12):2263–9.

Samuel JK, Andrews B. Traditional medicinal plant wealth of Pachalur and Periyur hamlets Dindigul district, Tamil Nadu. Indian J Trad Knowl. 2010;9(2):264–70.

Sathya M, Kokilavani R. Phytochemical screening and *in vitro* antioxidant activity of *Saccharum spontaneum* Linn. Int J Pharm Sci Rev Res. 2013;18(1):75–9.

Sawant R, Nagendran S. Protease: an enzyme with multiple industrial applications. World J Pharm Sci. 2014;3:568–79.

Sengupta A, Bhattacharya D, Pal G, Sinha N. Comparative studies on calotropins DI and DII from the latex of *Calotropis gigantea*. Arch Biochem Biophys. 1984;232(1):17–25.

Sharma Y, Jeyabalan G, Singh R, Semwal A. Current aspects of wound healing agents from medicinal plants: a review. J Med Plants Studies. 2013;1:2320–3862.

Sherry S, Fletcher AP, Alkjaersig N. Fibrinolysis and fibrinolytic activity in man. Physiol Rev. 1959;39(2):343–82.

Shivaprasad H, Rajesh R, Nanda B, Dharmappa K, Vishwanath B. Thrombin like activity of *Asclepias curassavica* L. latex: action of cysteine proteases. J Ethnopharmacol. 2009;123(1):106–9.

Shivaprasad HV, Rajaiah R, Frey BM, Frey FJ, Vishwanath BS. Pergularain e I'–a plant cysteine protease with thrombin-like activity from *Pergularia extensa* latex. Thrombosis Res. 2010a;125(3):e100–e5.

Shivaprasad HV, Rajesh R, Yariswamy M, Vishwanath BS. Procoagulant properties of plant latex proteases. Toxin Hemost. 2010b:591–603.

Shivaprasad H, Rajesh R, Vishwanath B. Hemostatic interference of plant latex proteases. SM J Clin Pathol. 2016;1(1):1–7.

Singh KA, Kumar R, Rao GRK, Jagannadham MV. Crinumin, a chymotrypsin-like but glycosylated serine protease from *Crinum asiaticum*: purification and physicochemical characterisation. Food Chem. 2010;119(4):1352–8.

Singh MK, Usha R, Hithayshree K, Bindhu O. Hemostatic potential of latex proteases from *Tabernaemontana divaricata* (L.) R. Br. ex. Roem. and Schult. and *Artocarpus altilis* (Parkinson ex. FA Zorn) Forsberg. J Thromb Thrombolysis. 2015;39(1):43–9.

Siritapetawee J, Thumanu K, Sojikul P, Thammasirirak S. A novel serine protease with human fibrino(geno) lytic activities from *Artocarpus heterophyllus* latex. Biochim Biophys Acta. 2012;1824(7):907–12.

Stanley LR, Vinay K, Abul K, Ramzi S, Nelson F. Robbins & cotran pathologic basis of disease-8th Edition. 8th ed. Philadelphia, PA: Saunders/Elsevier; 2010.

Steenkamp V, Mathivha E, Gouws M, Van Rensburg C. Studies on antibacterial, antioxidant and fibroblast growth stimulation of wound healing remedies from South Africa. J Ethnopharmacol. 2004;95(2):353–7.

Subramanian SP, Saratha V. Evaluation of antibacterial activity of *Calotropis gigantea* latex extract on selected pathogenic bacteria. J Pharm Res. 2010;3(3):517–21.

Suh DD, Schwartz IP, Canning DA, Snyder HM, Zderic SA, Kirsch AJ. Comparison of dermal and epithelial approaches to laser tissue soldering for skin flap closure. Lasers Surg Med. 1998;22(5):268–74.

Taylor RM, Cuming AC. Purification of an endoproteinase that digests the wheat 'Em'protein in vitro, and determination of its cleavage sites. FEBS Lett. 1993;331(1–2):76–80.

Thankamma L. Hevea latex as a wound healer and pain killer. Curr Sci. 2003;84(8):971–2.

Uday P, Maheshwari M, Sharanappa P, Nafeesa Z, Kameshwar VH, Priya B, et al. Exploring hemostatic and thrombolytic potential of heynein-A cysteine protease from *Ervatamia heyneana* latex. J Ethnopharmacol. 2017;199:316–22.

Upadhyay R. Plant latex: a natural source of pharmaceuticals and pesticides. Int J Green Pharm. 2011;5(3):169.

Venkatesh B, Achar RR, Sharanappa P, Priya B, Swamy SN. Synergistic caseinolytic activity and differential fibrinogenolytic action of multiple proteases of *Maclura spinosa* (Roxb. ex Willd.) latex. Pharmacogn Mag. 2015;11(Suppl 3):S457.

Verpoorte R. Pharmacognosy in the new millennium: leadfinding and biotechnology. J Pharm Pharmacol. 2000;52(3):253–62.

Viana CA, Oliveira JS, Freitas CD, Alencar NM, Carvalho CP, Nishi BC, et al. Thrombin and plasmin-like activities in the latices of *Cryptostegia grandiflora* and *Plumeria rubra*. Blood Coagul Fibrinolysis. 2013;24(4):386–92.

Walsh G. Proteins: biochemistry and biotechnology. Hoboken, NJ: John Wiley & Sons; 2002.

Whitley P. Papain-urea-chlorophyllin copper complex sodium debriding ointment to assist with resolution of traumatic leg wound: 634. J Wound Ostomy Cont Nurs. 2005;32(3S):S13.

Winnick T, Davis AR, Greenberg DM. Physicochemical properties of the proteolytic enzyme from the latex of the milkweed, *Asclepias speciosa* Torr. some comparisons with other proteases. J Gen Physiol. 1940;23(3):275–88.

Yagami T, Sato M, Nakamura A, Komiyama T, Kitagawa K, Akasawa A, et al. Plant defense–related enzymes as latex antigens. J Allergy Clin Immunol. 1998;101(3):379–85.

Yariswamy M, Shivaprasad H, Joshi V, Urs AN, Nataraju A, Vishwanath B. Topical application of serine proteases from *Wrightia tinctoria* R. Br.(Apocyanaceae) latex augments healing of experimentally induced excision wound in mice. J Ethnopharmacol. 2013;149(1):377–83.

Yegin S, Dekker P. Progress in the field of aspartic proteinases in cheese manufacturing: structures, functions, catalytic mechanism, inhibition, and engineering. Dairy Sci Technol. 2013;93(6):565–94.

Antidiabetic Activity of Indian Medicinal Plants

11

Vibha Rani, Anubhuti Gupta, Megha, Sakshi Awasthi, Tanya Suneja, Mohini Yadav, and Shanya Verma

Contents

V. Rani (✉) · A. Gupta · Megha · S. Awasthi
T. Suneja · M. Yadav · S. Verma
Department of Biotechnology, Jaypee Institute of Information Technology, Noida, Uttar Pradesh, India
e-mail: vibha.rani@jiit.ac.in

S. Sen, R. Chakraborty (eds.), *Herbal Medicine in India*,
https://doi.org/10.1007/978-981-13-7248-3_11

11.1 Introduction

Plants are an intrinsic part of our lives and have been an important source of food, fodder, medicine, and fuel since old times. Non-being non-toxic, having typically fewer side effects, better compatibility with physiological flora, and inexpensive prices are the reasons for the fondness for plant based medicines. Ayurveda and the various Indian literatures describe the usefulness of plants in treating numerous human ailments. India is graced with a rich wealth of medicinal plants therefore making it the botanical garden of the world and the largest producer. Diabetes mellitus is a metabolic, non-communicable diseases and the fourth largest killer in many developing and industrialized nations globally, posing a serious threat in the twenty-first century (Wild et al. 2004) diagnosed.

11.1.1 Diabetes and Significance

Diabetes is termed as a group of chronic metabolic diseases characterized by hyperglycemia \\ resulting from the defects in insulin secretion, its action, or both. It is diagnosed by high blood glucose level and subsequent insulin deficiency. Diabetes is a major threat and co-morbidity for heart diseases, such as ischemic heart disease and diabetic cardiomyopathy. The cases of diabetes are estimated to increase from 4% in 1995 to 5.4% by the year 2025 globally (American Diabetes Association 2010).

11.1.2 Classification of Diabetes Mellitus

Depending upon the circumstances at the time of diagnosis, an individual is assigned a type of diabetes. An individual may not fit into the single class and maybe assigned multiple classes.

- **Type I Diabetes**: Also termed as insulin-dependent diabetes or juvenile onset diabetes is an absolute insulin deficiency occurs because of β-cell destruction. It accounts for only 5–10% of the total number of people suffering with diabetes (Atkinson et al. 2014).
- **Type II Diabetes**: Previously referred to as non-insulin dependent diabetes, occurring due to insulin resistance leading to a predominantly insulin secretory defect. It accounts for 90–95% of a total number of people with diabetes (American Diabetes Association 2010).
- **Gestational Diabetes**: It marked by glucose intolerance with its onset or first recognition during pregnancy. Studies shows that most cases of gestational diabetes resolve with delivery, stating whether or not the condition stays after pregnancy and did not exclude the chances that unrecognized glucose intolerance may have initiated concomitantly with the pregnancy (Atkinson et al. 2014).

There are various ways in which the antidiabetic drugs act could be stimulation of beta-cell of pancreatic islet releasing insulin, restricting the hormones that increase blood glucose, increasing the glycogen content, increasing the number and sensitivity of insulin receptors, free radical scavenging, correcting the metabolic disorder of lipid and protein, enhancing the use of organ glucose in the tissue, resisting lipid peroxidation, and promoting microcirculation in the body (Bösenberg and van Zyl 2008).

11.1.3 Indian Medicinal Plants with Antidiabetic Potential

Natural plants are used as major sources of medicine since ancient times. A major portion of population, say about 80–85%, both in developed and developing countries depends on traditional medicine made from medicinal plants for their primary health care needs. It is estimated that a major part of traditional therapy includes the use of plant extracts or their active components (Ignacimuthu and Ayyanar 2006; Elujoba et al. 2006). Before the discovery of insulin, the only options for the treatment of diabetes were the traditional practices based on the usage of medicinal plants (Ribnicky et al. 2006). Metformin, derived from a medicinal plant *Galega officinalis*

Table 11.1 Some important traditional antidiabetic plants of India

S. no.	Plant botanical name	Common name	Family	Major phytoconstituents
1	*Ficusreligiosa*	Peepal	Moraceae	Lanosterol, Bergaptol, Stigmasterol, Fucosterol
2	*Eugenia jambolana*	Jamun	Myrtaceae	Isoquercetin, Kaempferol, Myricetin, Petunidin
3	*Momordicacharantia*	Karela	Cucurbitaceae	Momordicin, Charantin, Galacturonic acid, Linoleic acid
4	*Aloe barbadensis*	Gritkumari	Aloeaceae	Aloin A and B, Aloe-Emodin, Anthranol, Aloetic-Acid
5	*Brassica juncea*	Rai	Brassica	Quercetin, Kaempferol, Isorhamnetin and Cyaniding
6	*Allium cepa*	Onion	Liliaceae	Allin, Ajoene, Di-Allyl-Tri-Sulphide and S-Allyl Cysteine
7	*Acacia Arabica*	Babul	Fabaceae	Catechin, Epicatechin, Gallate, Procatechinic Acid and Tannins
8	*Azadirachtaindica*	Neem	Malaceae	Nimocin, Nimbin and Quercetin
9	*Tinosporacordifolia*	Giloy	Menispermaceae	Berberin, Palmative, Columbin
10	*Allium sativum*	Garlic	Amaryllidaceae	Alliin, Allicin, Allyl sulfide,1,2-Vinyldithin
11	*Ocimum sanctum*	Tulsi	Lamiaceae	Orientin, vicenin, eugenol, urosolic acid

is the major orthodox drug approved, till today, for the treatment of non-insulin dependent diabetes mellitus. (Hussain 2002; Oubre et al. 1997).

Herbal mixtures contains various active ingredients that targets multiple mechanisms, unlike western medicine which generally contains a single active ingredient targeting a specific mechanism. Herbal medicines are based on the holistic theory, putting an emphasis on the body as a whole (Rawat and Namita 2013).

11.1.4 Phytoconstituents Present in Medicinal Plants

Plants show antidiabetic properties due to the various types of phytoconstituents present in them. These phytoconstituents present in medicinal plants can be described as (Sen et al. 2016):

- Imidazoline alkaloids triggers insulin secretion in a glucose-dependent manner.
- The blood glucose level is reduced by polysaccharides increasing the serum insulin level.
- Flavanoids are antidiabetic agents that act by suppressing the glucose level, by lowering plasma cholesterol and triglycerides remarkably, and by increasing hepatic glucokinase activity, may be by enhancing the insulin release from the beta pancreatic islets (Chauhan et al. 2010).
- Dietary fibers can help in lowering the rate of glucose absorption and concentration of postprandial serum glucose.
- Ferulic acid stimulates insulin secretion and saponins trigger the release of insulin blocking the formation of glucose in the bloodstream (Mishra et al. 2010).

According to the ethnobotanical information reports, several plants possess antidiabetic potential. The active components of many plant can be used directly as drugs, lead compounds or pharmacological agents (Table 11.1).

11.2 Important Medicinal Plants Explored as Anti-Diabetic

11.2.1 *Ficus religiosa*

Ficus religiosa: common name peepal, comes from the Moraceae family. *F. religiosa* has many important compounds which are beneficial in the treatment of diseases such as skin diseases, diabetes, central nervous system disorder, respiratory disorders (Gautam et al. 2014) (Table 11.2).

Table 11.2 *Ficus religiosa*—classification

Ficus religiosa			
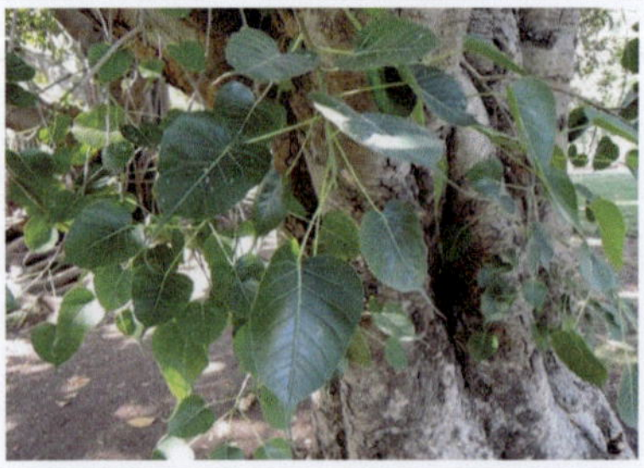		Kingdom:	Plantae
		Division:	Magnoliophyta
		Class:	Magnoliopsida
		Order:	Rosales
		Family:	Moraceae
		Genus:	*Ficus*

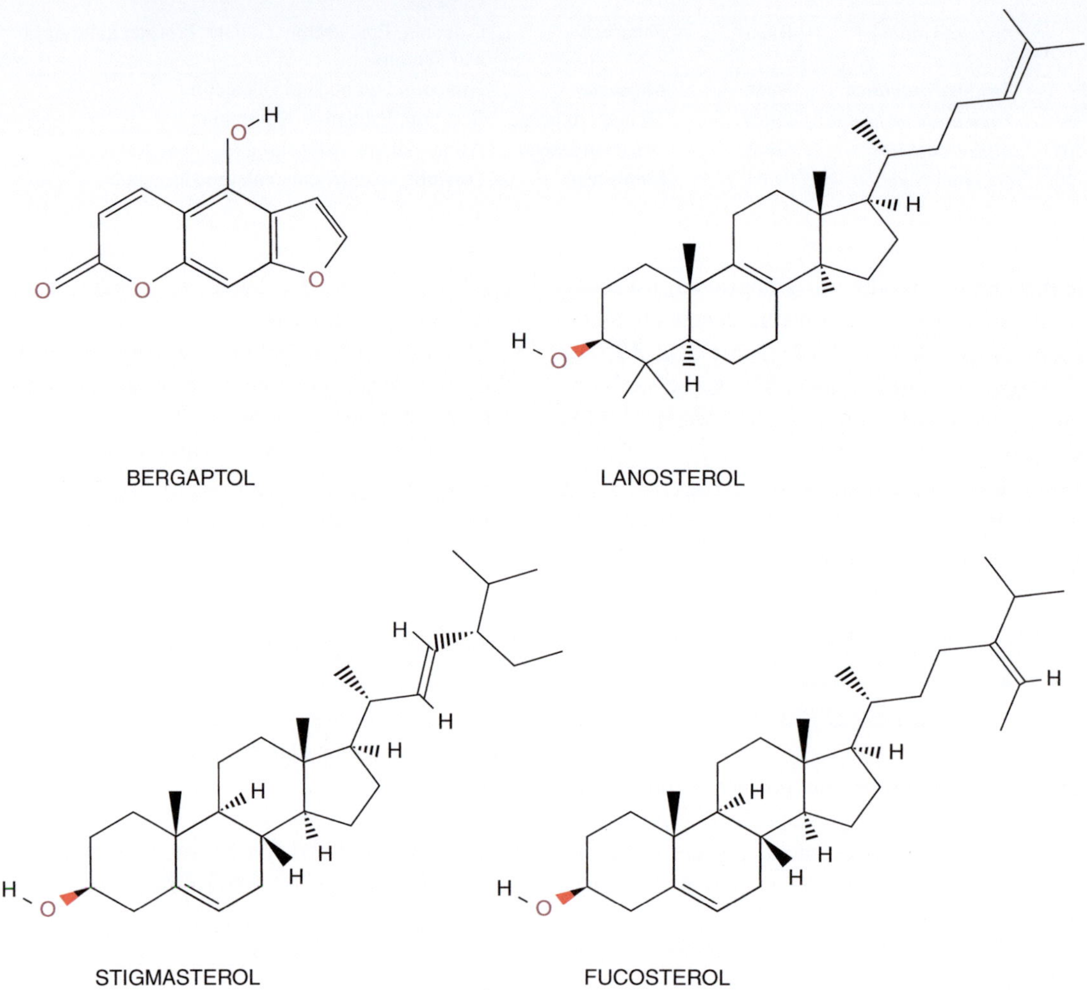

Fig. 11.1 Bioactive compounds in *Ficus religiosa*

11.2.1.1 Bioactive Compounds in *Ficus religiosa*

These are several bioactive compounds present in *Ficus* that can provide a major antidiabetic effect. The documented phytoconstituents of stem bark of *F. religiosa* are steroids, phenols, alkaloids, flavonoid, tannins, β-sitosteryl-d-glucoside, noctacosanol, methyl oleanolate, vitamin K, lanosterol, lupen-3-one, stigmasterol which are shown in Fig. 11.1 (Manorenjitha et al. 2013).

11.2.1.2 Anti-Diabetic Activity

Aqueous extract of *F. religiosa* in doses of 50 and 100 mg/kg has been studied to significantly reduce blood glucose levels. Glibenclamide, a well-known hypoglycemic drug was used as a control for comparison. Thereafter the aqueous extract of *F. religiosa* showed a gradual rise in serum insulin levels, liver glycogen content, body weight, and skeletal muscle of experimental diabetic rats (Pandit et al. 2010).

- The bark root showed highest decrease of the blood sugar level.
- Aqueous extract of *F. religiosa* orally decreases the fasting blood glucose.
- *F. religiosa* regulates the enzymes of an antioxidant defense system to fight against oxidative stress. Therefore, glutathione levels went up and it helped in blocking the formation of malondialdehyde, proving its antidiabetic activity along with antioxidant potential.
- An experiment on STZ diabetic rats showed reduction in serum triglycerides and total cholesterol levels significantly.

11.2.2 *Eugenia jambolana*

Eugenia jambolana, or black plum or jamun, belongs to the family Myrtaceae. This species is popularly found in the Indian subcontinent and in regions of South Asia such as Pakistan, Sri Lanka, Nepal, Burma, Bangladesh and Indonesia from ancient time (Ravi et al. 2004) (Table 11.3).

11.2.2.1 Bioactive Compounds in *Eugenia jambolana*

The plant is rich in bioactive compounds such as anthocyanins, isoquercetin, glucoside, ellagic acid, myricetin, kaempferol, and hydrolysable tannins (1-0-galloyl castalagin and casuarinin) are shown in Fig. 11.2 (Faria et al. 2011).

11.2.2.2 Anti-Diabetic Activity

The jambul fruit has a direct effect on pancreas so it is a major medication for diabetic sufferers. The major anti-diabetic effects include (Faria et al. 2011):

- Jambul seeds include jamboline, a glycoside that blocks the transformation of starch into sugar in cases of elevated blood sugar levels.
- It increases the secretion of insulin from the pancreas or by inhibition of insulin degradation.
- Ethanolic extract of seeds and seed powder of *Eugenia jambolana* when supplemented in alloxan-induced diabetic rats showed a remarkable decrease in blood sugar level and increase in the histopathology of pancreatic islets.
- The ash of dried bark of jambul tree is helpful to deal with diabetic effects.

11.2.3 *Momordica charantia*

Momordica charantia (bitter gourd or karela) belonging to the family Cucurbitaceae is a popular fruit helpful for the treatment of diabetes, cardiovascular diseases, and related ail-

Table 11.3 *Eugenia jambolana*—classification

Eugenia jambolana	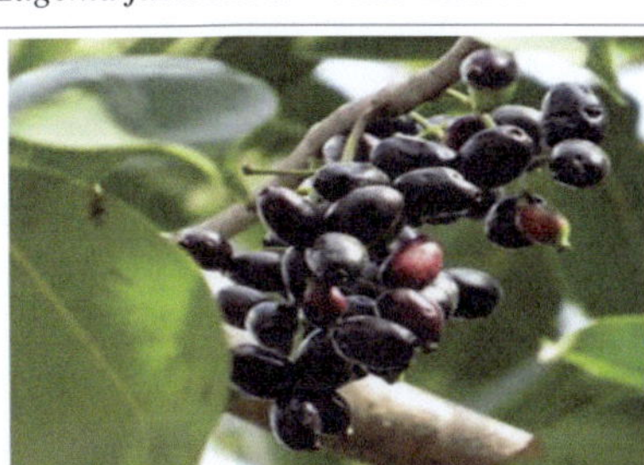	Kingdom:	Plantae
		Division:	Magnoliophyta
		Class:	Magnoliopsida
		Order:	Myrtales
		Family:	Myrtaceae
		Genus:	*Eugenia*

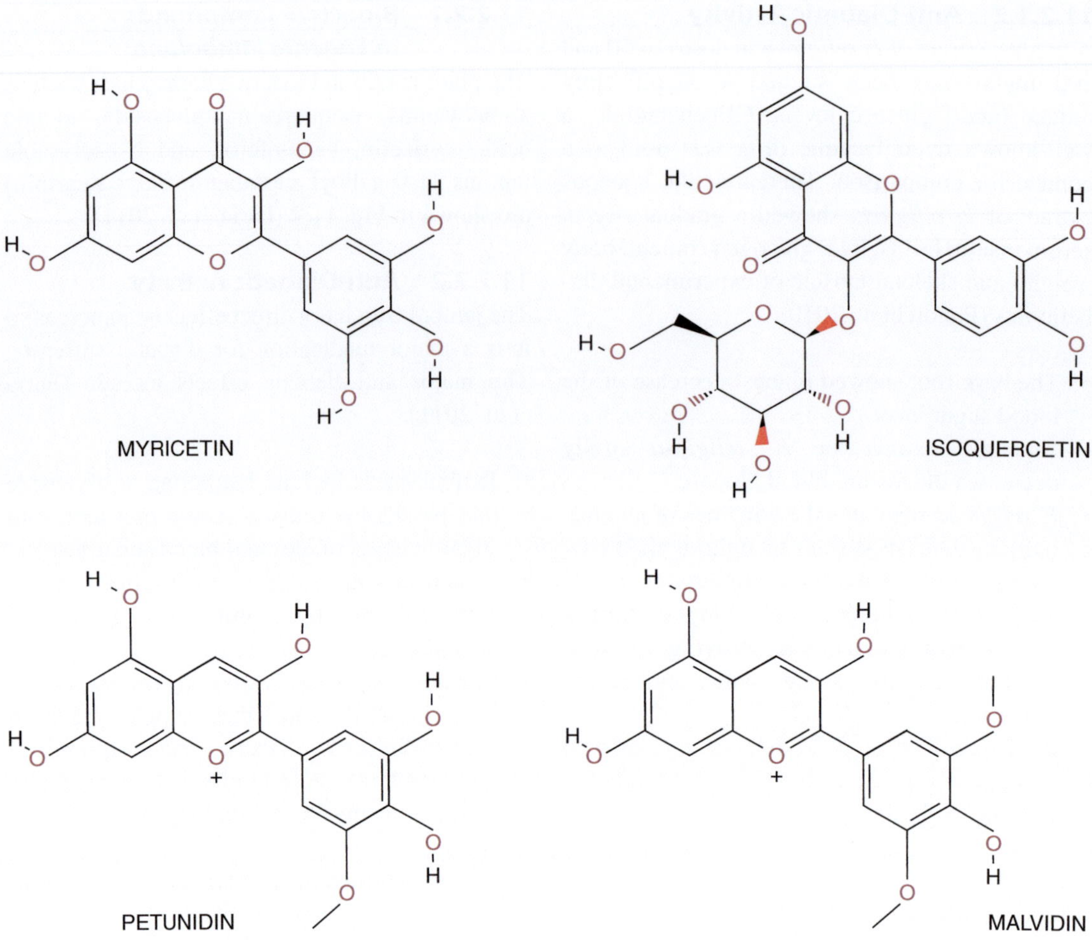

Fig. 11.2 Bioactive compounds in *Eugenia jambolana*

Table 11.4 *Momordic acharantia*—classification

Momordica charantia	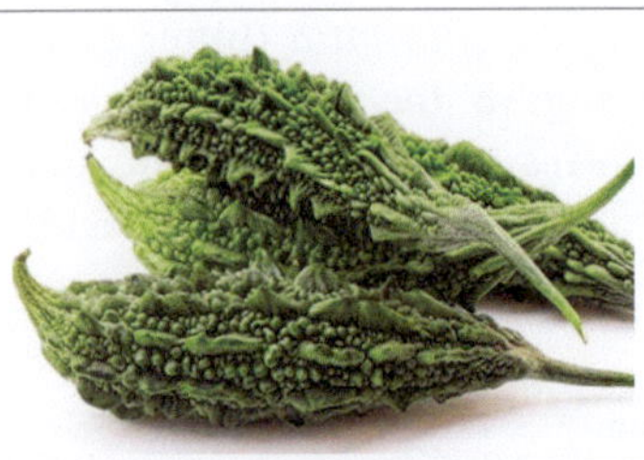	Kingdom:	Plantae
		Division:	Tracheophyta
		Class:	Magnoliopsida
		Order:	Cucurbitales
		Family:	Cucurbitaceae
		Genus:	*Momordica*

ments in the areas of Asia, East Africa and South America. It has also been demonstrated to show antibacterial, antiviral, anticancer activities; however, the anti-diabetic activity has been widely reviewed (Basch et al. 2003) (Table 11.4).

11.2.3.1 Bioactive Compounds in *Momordica charantia*

The specific chemical constituents of *M. charantia* are momordicin, charantin, galacturonic acid, linoleic acid, spinasterol and nerolidolcitrulin which are shown in Fig. 11.3 (Kumar et al. 2010a, b).

Fig. 11.3 Bioactive compounds in *Momordica charantia*

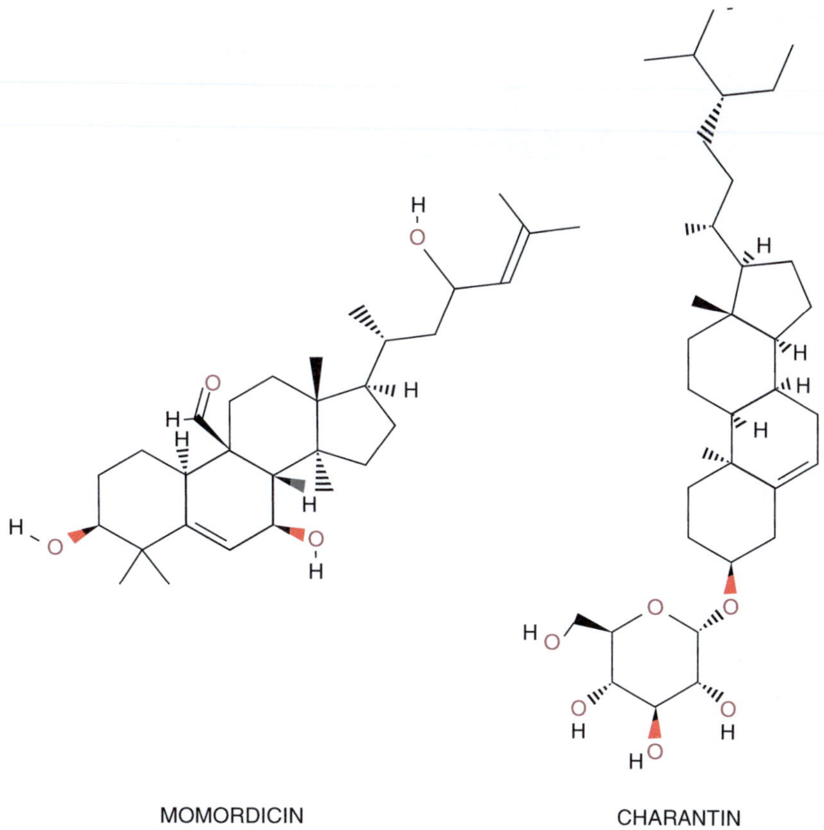

11.2.3.2 Anti-Diabetic Activity

M. charantia shows certain hypoglycemic effects via different pharmacological modes (Perumal et al. 2015).

- It contains bioactive substances such as vicine, along with some antioxidants which are known to have anti-diabetic potential. It obstructs the absorption of glucose by obstructing glucosidase.
- It helps in triggering insulin levels and also improves signaling or sensitivity of insulin by repairing the damaged β-cells.
- It helps in the suppressing glucose-6-phosphatase and also triggering of the activity of hepatic glucose-6-phosphate dehydrogenase.
- It also shows the inhibitory properties on α-glucosidase and α-amylase. Saponins also increase insulin secretion.

11.2.4 *Aloe barbadensis*

Aloe barbadensis is commonly known as Ghritkumari (Aloe Vera). It popularly grows as hedgerows in the drier part of India. It is used as an Ayurvedic medicine for coping up with painful conditions and is also stated in folk medicine of Arabian Peninsula for treatment of diabetes (Ghannam et al. 1986) (Table 11.5).

Table 11.5 *Aloe barbadensis*—classification

Aloe barbadensis

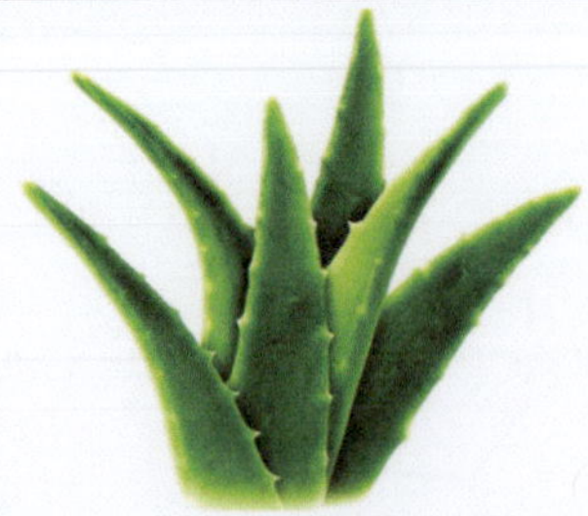

Kingdom:	Plantae
Division:	Magnoliophyta
Class:	Liliopsida
Order:	Liliales
Family:	Aloeaceae
Genus:	*Aloe*

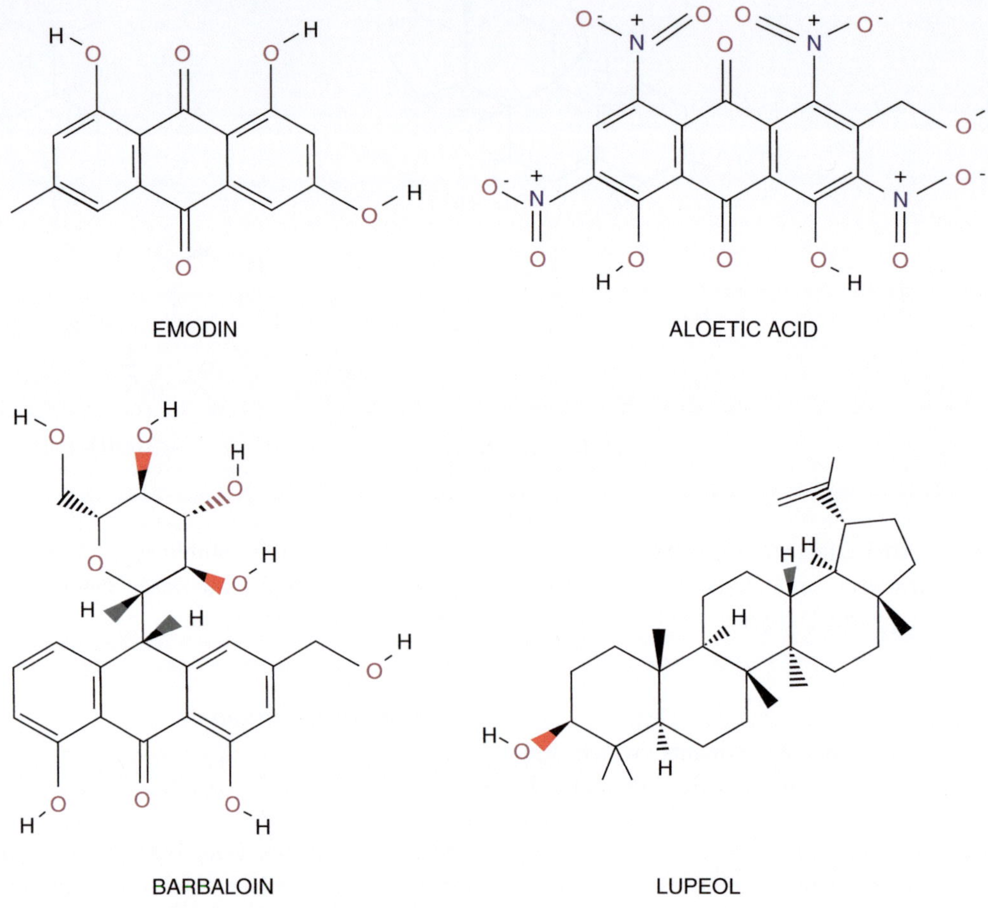

Fig. 11.4 Bioactive compounds in *Aloe barbadensis*

11.2.4.1 Bioactive Compounds in *Aloe barbadensis*

The plant is rich in various active phytoconstituents such as aloetic-acid, aloe-emodin, isobarbaloin, emodin, anthranol, aloin A and B, and ester of cinnamic acid which are shown in Fig. 11.4 (Arunkumar and Muthuselvam 2009).

11.2.4.2 Anti-Diabetic Activity

The Ghritkumari is mainly famous for its antidiabetic and anti-inflammatory activities. It helps to stabilize blood sugar level for a very long time (Saminathan and Kavimani 2015).

- *Aloe vera* gel at 200 mg/kg has magnificent antidiabetic and cardio protective activity retaining the catalase and superoxide dismutase activity up to the normal level and enhancing reduced glutathione by four folds in diabetic rats.
- The effectiveness can be enhanced in type II diabetes rats by using the leaf pulp extract that showed certain hypoglycemic effects.
- Both *Aloe gibberellins* and *Aloe vera* (over a dose range of 2–100 mg/kg) prevents inflammation in a dose-response manner and stimulates wound healing in STZ diabetic mice.
- The hypoglycemic effects could be observed with the help of dried sap of the plant.
- Aloe had a definite role in the prevention and management of atherosclerotic heart disease and the blood sugar level in the diabetic patient.

11.2.5 *Brassica juncea*

Brassica juncea generally known as raiis popularly used as spice in various food items in India. The plant is cultivated throughout in India but mostly in U.P and Bihar. India is the third largest rapeseed-mustard producer in the world. Its effect was attributed to increase glycogen synthetase causing an increasing in hepatic glycogen content and decrease of glycogen phosphorylase and other glyconeogenic enzyme in animal body (Khan et al. 1995) (Table 11.6).

11.2.5.1 Bioactive Compounds in *Brassica juncea*

The main phytoconstituents present in *Brassica* are quercetin, kaempferol, isorhamnetin and cyaniding are shown in Fig. 11.5 (Khan et al. 1995).

11.2.5.2 Anti-Diabetic Activity

It helps to stabilize blood sugar level in the following manner (Chauhan et al. 2010):

- *Brassica juncea* given orally in diet for 60 days to normal rats led to notable hypoglycemic effects.
- Potent hypoglycemic activity is contained in *B. juncea* aqueous seed extract which was investigated in STZ induced diabetic male albino rats.
- The Brassica vegetables contain certain polyphenols which have high antioxidant activities.
- The hypoglycemic effect of the seed extract increases glycogen synthesis causing an increase in hepatic glycogen content and decrease of glycogen phosphorylase, and other gluconeogenic enzymes.

11.2.6 *Allium cepa*

Allium cepa (Onion) is very commonly cultivated in Central Asia. It is grown everywhere India and is one of the significant dietary constituents. Several soluble and insoluble fractions of dried onion powder show anti-hyperglycemic activity in diabetic rabbits. *Allium cepa* is also possesses hypolipidaemic and antioxidant properties (Kumar et al. 2010a, b) (Table 11.7).

Table 11.6 *Brassica juncea*—classification

Brassica juncea

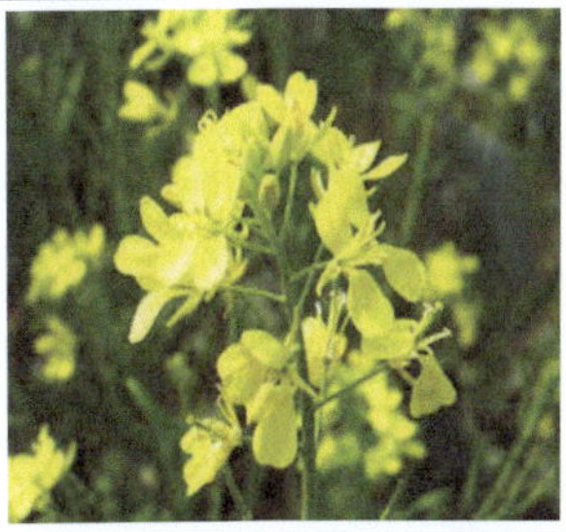

Kingdom:	Plantae
Division:	Magnoliophyta
Class:	Magnoliopsida
Order:	Brassicales
Family:	Brassica
Genus:	*Juncea*

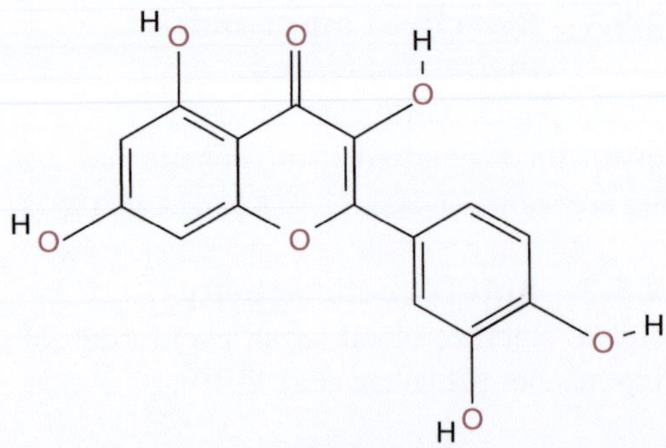

QUERCITIN

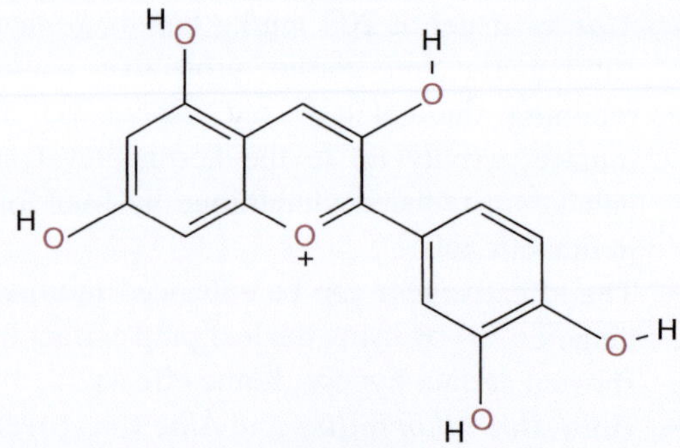

CYANIDIN

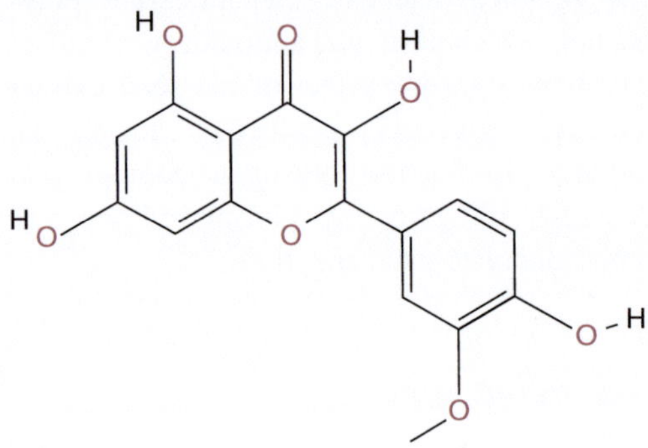

ISORHAMNETIN

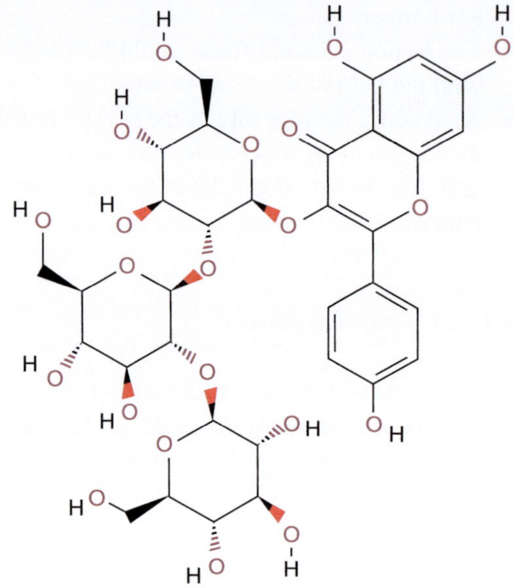

KAEMPFEROL

Fig. 11.5 Bioactive compounds in *Brassica juncea*

Table 11.7 *Allium cepa*—classification

Allium cepa	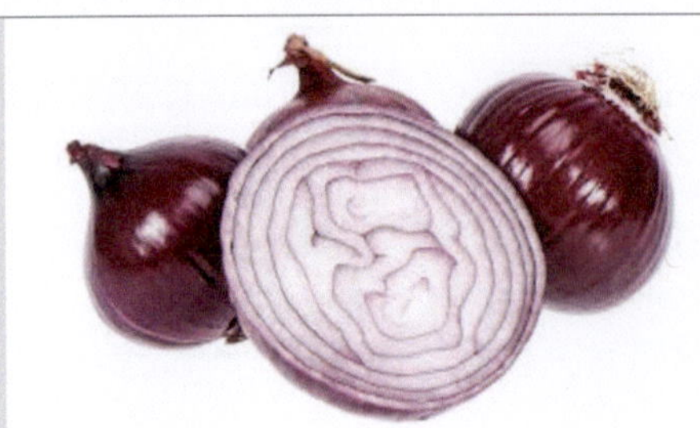	Kingdom:	Plantae
		Division:	Magnoliophyta
		Class:	Liliopsida
		Order:	Liliales
		Family:	Liliaceae
		Genus:	*Allium*

11.2.6.1 Bioactive Compounds in *Allium cepa*

The plant is rich in phytoconstituents such as allin, ajoene, di-allyl-tri-sulphide, S-allyl cysteine and allicin which are shown in Fig. 11.6 (Benítez et al. 2011).

11.2.6.2 Anti-Diabetic Activity

Onion helps in controlling blood glucose levels by (Benítez et al. 2011):

- Onion has hypocholesterolemic and hypoglycemic properties, therefore, feeding onion improves the metabolic status of diabetes patients.
- Decreases blood glucose level and has significant antioxidant activity, which may be the reason for its hypoglycemic potential.
- Onion extract counteracts the concentration of thiobarbituric acid reactive substances and the activity of glutathione S-transferase in plasma, liver, brain and kidney which are normally high for diabetic patients.
- Onion powder supplementation in high-fat diet diabetic rats leads to an increase in insulin secretion.
- The onion extract is helpful in reducing the plasma glucose concentrations and body weight in diabetic patients.

11.2.7 *Acacia arabica*

Commonly known as 'Babool' in India, it has a lot of medicinal significance for the treatment of skin, stomach and tooth problems. The fresh plant's parts of *Acacia arabica* is considered as astringent, antidiarrhoeal, aphrodisiac, antimicrobial, anthelmintic, with good nutritional value in Indian traditional medicine system (Roqaiya et al. 2017) (Table 11.8).

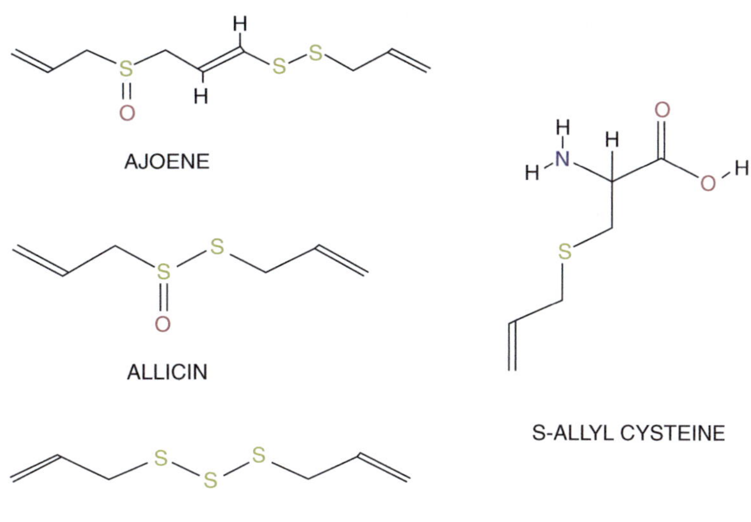

Fig. 11.6 Bioactive compounds in *Allium cepa*

Table 11.8 *Acacia arabica*—classification

Acacia arabica	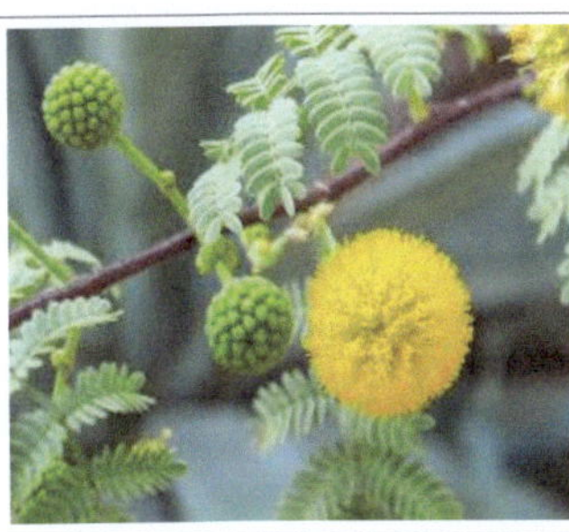	Kingdom:	Plantae
		Division:	Tracheophyta
		Class:	Magnoliopsida
		Order:	Fabales
		Family:	Fabaceae
		Genus:	*Acacia*

11.2.7.1 Bioactive Compounds in *Acacia arabica*

The major phytochemical constituents of *Acacia arabica* are catechin, epicatechin, procatechinic acid, tannins, alkaloids, kaempferol, and glucosides are shown in Fig. 11.7 (Khadem and Marles 2010).

11.2.7.2 Anti-Diabetic Activity

It occurs throughout India and is also cultivated. Significant hypoglycemic effect versus controls were observed when normal rats were feeded with 94% of the seed diets (Shori 2015).

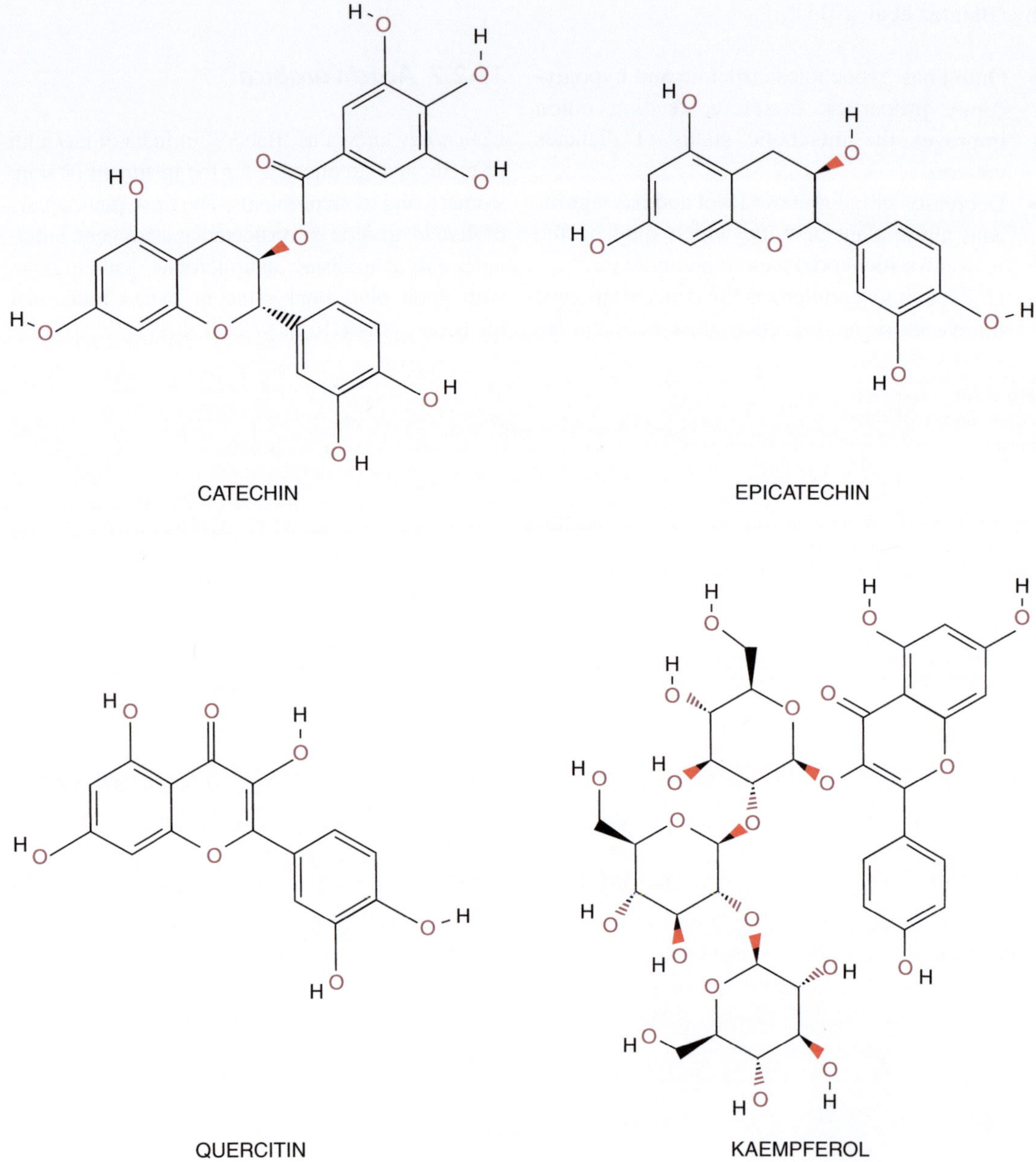

Fig. 11.7 Bioactive compounds in *Acacia arabica*

- Alloxanized rats were observed with no hypoglycemic effect which indicated that plant acts through the release of insulin.
- Also, significant hypoglycemic effect was observed in normal rabbits when release of insulin was initiated from pancreatic beta cells. At these doses, acute toxicity and behavioral changes were not observed.

11.2.8 *Azadirachta indica*

It is commonly known as neem. It is a type of species in the genus *Azadirachta* which is native to the Indian subcontinent. The major areas of its growth are tropical and sub-tropical regions. It is used for many purposes such as its oil is used for healthy hair. Neem improves liver function, detoxify the blood and balance blood sugar level. It is also used to manufacture variety of cosmetics like soaps, shampoo, skin creams, body lotion and toothpastes. It also acts as a nutritive tonic to the skin and treats eczema (López-Pantoja et al. 2007) (Table 11.9).

11.2.8.1 Bioactive Compounds in *Azadirachta indica*

The plant is rich in various bioactive compounds like nimocin, nimbin and quercetin as shown in Fig. 11.8 (Samy et al. 2008).

11.2.8.2 Anti-Diabetic Activity

Neem root bark extract suppresses blood sugar levels and also reduces antihyperglycemic and hypoglycemic activity (Samy et al. 2008).

- Ethanolic extract of *Azadirachta indica* was studied, and significant decrease in elevated blood glucose level was observed.

Table 11.9 *Azadirachta indica*—classification

Azadirachta indica

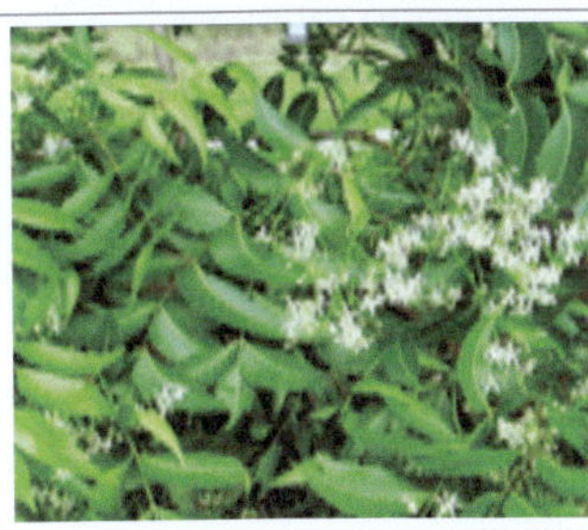

Kingdom:	Plantae
Division:	Tracheophyta
Class:	Magnoliopsida
Order:	Sapindales
Family:	Mellaceae
Genus:	*Azadirachta*

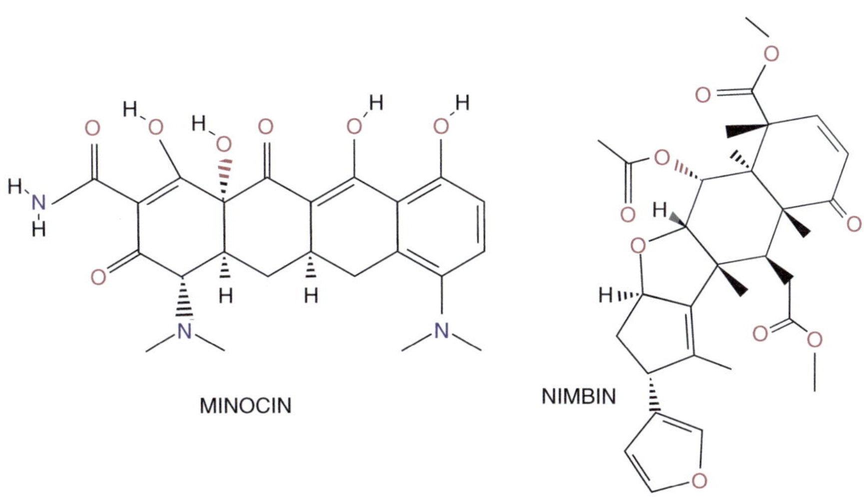

Fig. 11.8 Bioactive compounds in *Azadirachta indica*

- *A. indica* chloroform extract stimulates oral glucose tolerance and suppress the intestinal glucosidase activity. It is also involved in the regeneration of insulin-producing cells.
- Neem oil is beneficial in reducing blood glucose level in short period of time. It also improves glucose tolerance.

11.2.9 *Tinospora cordifolia*

It is generally named as 'guduchi', 'giloy'. It is herbaceous vine found in tropical areas of India, Myanmar, and Sri Lanka. *T. cordifolia* contains many different chemicals which are beneficial for the body. Some of which possess antioxidant properties while others might boost the immune system of the body (Sharma et al. 2010) (Table 11.10).

11.2.9.1 Bioactive Compounds in *Tinospora cordifolia*

The plant is rich in various bioactive compounds like berberin, palmative, columbinas is shown in Fig. 11.9 (Pandey et al. 2012).

11.2.9.2 Anti-Diabetic Activity

Blood and urine glucose and lipids in serum is reduced by oral extracts of *T. cordifolia* (Pandey et al. 2012).

- It also decreases body weight.
- Its aqueous extract reduces blood glucose level.
- And its methanol extract suppress blood glucose level and also helps in decreasing glycosylated hemoglobin level.

11.2.10 *Allium sativum*

Garlic or *Allium sativum* plays an important role throughout the world whether it be a raw material for culinary processes or it be as an important ingredient in traditional as well as modern medicine. It is considered to be one of the plentiful sources of phenolic compounds and is either taken as a raw vegetable or after processing it with different chemical and biological composition such as garlic oil, powder or extracts (Capasso 2013) (Table 11.11).

Table 11.10 *Tinospora cordifolia*—classification

Tinospora cordifolia	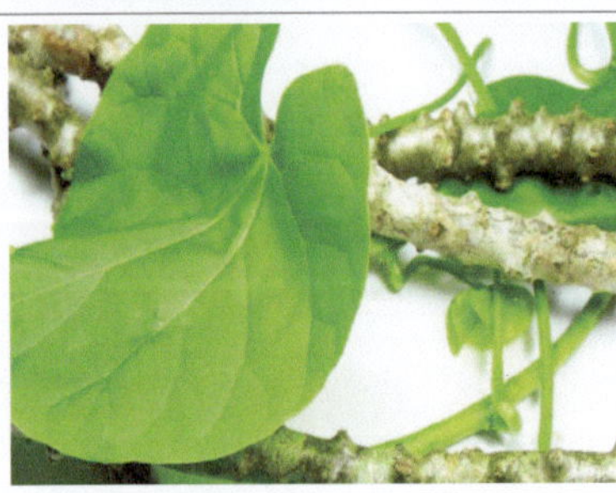	Kingdom:	Plantae
		Division:	Tracheophyta
		Class:	Magnoliopsida
		Order:	Ranunculalas
		Family:	Menispermaceae
		Genus:	*Tenospora*

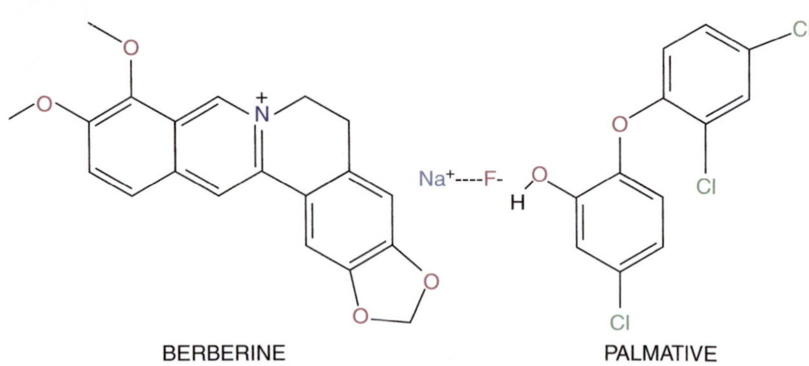

Fig. 11.9 Bioactive compounds in *Tinospora cordifolia*

Table 11.11 *Allium sativum*—classification

Allium sativum

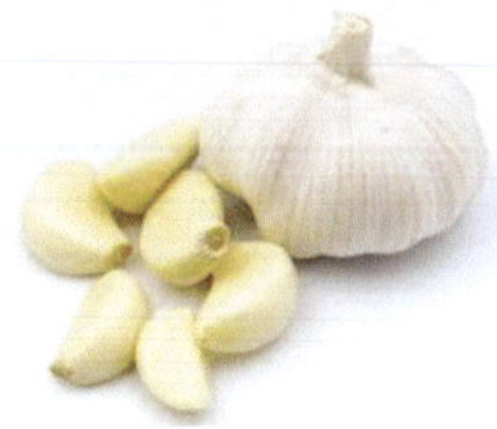

Kingdom:	Plantae
Division:	Angiosperms
Class:	Monocots
Order:	Asparagales
Family:	Amaryllidaceae
Genus:	*Allium*

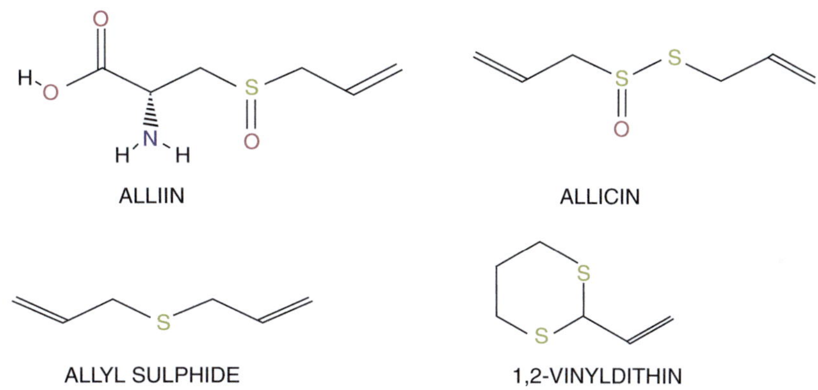

Fig. 11.10 Bioactive Compounds of *Allium sativum*

11.2.10.1 Bioactive Compounds of *Allium sativum*

The peculiar flavor of clove is considered to be the main quality attribute of garlic products and this is obtained as an outcome of various biochemical reactions. The main bioactive compounds are thiosulfinates- sulfur that contains non-volatile amino acids which further includes alliin, allicin, allyl sulfide, 1, 2-vinyldithin are shown in Fig. 11.10 (Martins et al. 2016).

11.2.10.2 Anti-Diabetic Activity

S-allyl-cysteine sulfoxide (alliin) has been reported to show hypoglycemic properties as shown by glyburide, an antidiabetic drug which belongs to the class sulfonylureas and also lowers down the serum glucose levels (Ried and Fakler 2014).

- The mechanism for the hypoglycemic condition is that garlic increases the sensitivity of insulin along with increase in pancreatic secretion of insulin from β cells, the release of bounded or attached insulin.
- It contains a compound called allicin that enhances serum insulin by combining with compounds like cysteine which makes insulin free from S-H group reactions which commonly causes inactivation of insulin.

11.2.11 *Ocimum sanctum*

Known as tulsi and its leaves are considered to be holy and is considered to be part of the Hindu spiritual rituals. It is mainly found in two main varieties black and green, having a same chemical composition and medicinal properties. From prehistoric times, tulsi leaves are being used to reduce inflammation, to cure respiratory tract infections etc. this plant is known for its significant aromatic odor due to the presence of essential volatile oils. This volatile oil is mainly composed of terpenes, phenols, aldehydes and is extracted from the seeds. Other than the oil the plant also contains glycosides, saponins, tannins and alkaloids whereas the leaves contain ascorbic acid and carotene (Singh et al. 2012) (Table 11.12).

Table 11.12 *Ocimum sanctum*—classification

Ocimum sanctum			
	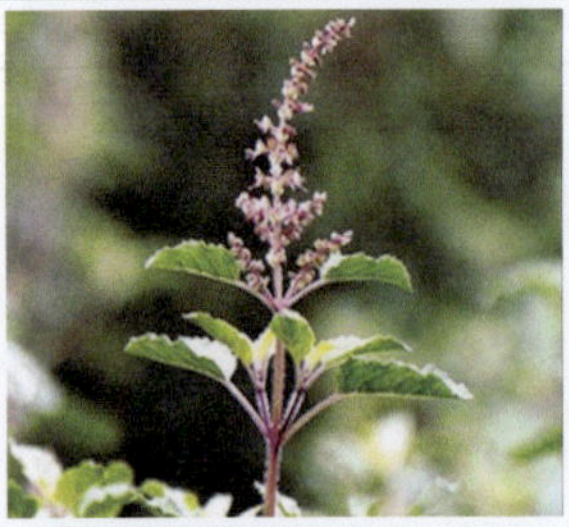	Kingdom:	Plantae
		Division:	Angiosperms
		Class:	Magnoliopsida
		Order:	Lamiales
		Family:	Lamiaceae
		Genus:	*Ocimum*

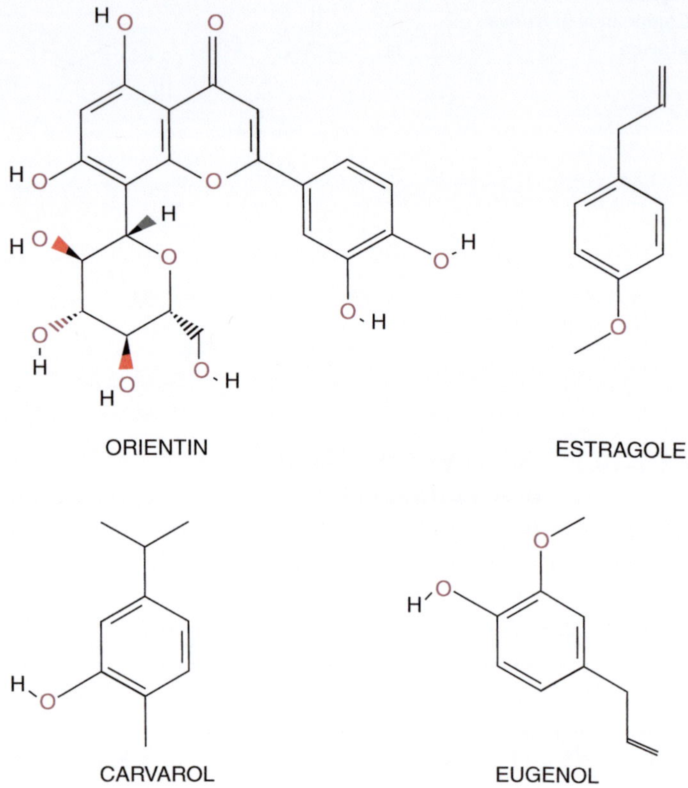

Fig. 11.11 Bioactive compounds in *Ocimum sanctum*

11.2.11.1 Bioactive Compounds in *Ocimum sanctum*

The leaf of this plant contains about 0.7% of volatile oil consisting of 71% eugenol, and 20% methyl eugenol. Various phenolic compounds are also extracted from the fresh leaves and stem of tulsi like orientin, vicenin, eugenol, urosolic acid, and apigenin from aqueous leaf extracts as shown in Fig. 11.11 (Kelm et al. 2000).

11.2.11.2 Anti-Diabetic Activity

Insulin secretion from the pancreas and clonal pancreatic β cells is enhanced due to the alcoholic and various organic solvent extract. (Kelm et al. 2000).

- Tulsi extracts are known for reducing blood sugar levels and it also has aldose reductase activity which further helps in reducing the diabetes related complications.
- The mechanism by which it enhances insulin secretion is that it stimulates adenylatecyclase (cAMP) and also exerts direct effect which leads to mobilization of calcium ions present within the cell as well as promoting the entry of calcium ions.

11.3 Adverse Effects of Indian Medicinal Plants

11.3.1 *Ficus religiosa*

- *Ficus* leaf contains a compound known as psoralens, which may cause photodermatitis when applied on the skin. While using products that contain *ficus* leaf excessive sunlight or ultraviolet light exposure should be avoided (Olaokun et al. 2013).
- Certain cases have been reported about the weeping *ficus* plant that it can cause allergy and side effects may include conjunctivitis, rhinitis, anaphylactic shock or asthma.
- Certain diseases, although rare, such as obstructive ileus (intestinal/bowel obstruction), hemolytic anemia (deficiency of red blood cells), and retinal hemorrhages (bleeding of the retina) have been reported (Olaokun et al. 2013).

11.3.2 *Eugenia jambolana*

- There may be a body-aches if taken in excess amount.
- Symptoms of vomiting may appear.
- According to Ayurveda, it may enhance the Vata-Dosha causing sleep-disorder.
- The Java-plum available in the market may be contaminated with dirty-water and as such it may cause health issues such as diarrhea or dysentery on its consumption if hygienic conditions are not maintained (Chaturvedi et al. 2007).

11.3.3 *Momordica charantia*

- *Momordica charantia* may irritate the digestive tract. For this reason, stomach discomfort, abdominal pain or diarrhea may be observed.
- Reduced blood sugar levels is the primary effect of bitter melon that may be potentially beneficial for people with uncontrolled diabetes, and might be problematic for people taking diabetes drugs or with normal or low blood sugar levels. The plant extracts and certain components have been reported to exert hypoglycemic effects (Baby and Jini 2013).
- Severe toxicity side effects include fever and coma and require prompt medical attention.
- Red arils (covering on bitter melon seeds) is also toxic to children. Improper consumption of these seed coverings may lead to diarrhea, vomiting or, in severe cases, death (Baby and Jini 2013).
- This natural supplement may induce vaginal bleeding, abortion or premature contractions in pregnant women so it must be avoided.
- The seeds of *Momordica charantia* contain vicine, a substance that cannot be digested by people with glucose-6-phosphate dehydrogenase. So the people with G6Pd may have worsened symptoms from this condition (Baby and Jini 2013).

11.3.4 *Aloe barbadensis*

- Topical and oral use of *Aloe vera* can cause skin irritation, hives, cramping, and diarrhoea to those who are allergic to other plants in the lily family, for example, onion (Guo and Mei 2016).
- *The* synthesis of prostaglandin can be reduced by *Aloe vera*, thus inhibiting secondary aggregation of platelets.
- Aloe gel or aloe latex should not be taken in case of ulcer, irritable bowel syndrome.
- Never give aloe gel or aloe latex if one has hemorrhoids (Guo and Mei 2016).

11.3.5 *Brassica juncea*

- It contains certain compounds in large quantities such as glucosenolates, alkaloids, thioglucosides and SMCO (S-methylcysteinesuphoxide), which are linked to a host of conditions including: poor performance, hemolytic anemia, goitre, stasis (paralysis) (Blackman and Rey 2005).
- It also causes embryonic death, poor conception, polioencephalomalacia syndrome, tongue extension, bloat, reduced birth weights, excess salivation, and acute respiratory distress resulting in sudden death, blindness and diarrhea.

11.3.6 *Allium cepa*

- Frequent contact with onion seeds has been reported as an occupational allergen. It contains some compounds (e.g., propanethial-s-oxide) that escape from the onion in the form of vapor and hydrolyze to sulfuric acid when it is cut, causing the eye irritation and lacrimation. Corneal swelling from onion exposure has also been reported (Oyewusi et al. 2017).
- The stomach gets affected, and frequent contact with onion may cause allergic reactions. Onion toxicity is only associated with high intake.
- Other clinical signs observed by *Allium* species in dogs and cats that include depression, haemoglobinuria, and presence of haemosiderin, urinary casts, icterus, tachycardia, tachypnea, weakness and exercise intolerance.

11.3.7 *Acacia arabica*

- *Acacia* inhibits tumor cell growth and selectively toxic to tumor cells at low doses (Pradeep et al. 2012).
- It has also shown to have potent cytotoxicity activity against human T-cell leukaemia.

11.3.8 *Azadirachta indica*

- Neem can help in reducing the blood sugar levels and might cause blood sugar level to go too low (Solanki et al. 2013).
- Neem should not be used at least 2 weeks before a scheduled surgery as there is a concern that it might interfere with blood sugar control during and after surgery.

11.3.9 *Tinospora cordifolia*

- It is safe for short duration of time but the longer duration can cause certain side effects.
- *Tinospora cordifolia* is advised to use cautiously if you have diabetes as it might lower blood sugar levels and one should monitor blood sugar levels. The doses of diabetes medications might need to be adjusted.

11.3.10 *Allium sativum*

- Intake of one or two cloves of raw garlic is considered to be safe for an adult human being. One of the most common side effects is breath and body odor (Tattelman 2005).
- If it is ingested in empty stomach in the excessive amount it can cause various problems like gastrointestinal disturbances, flatulence and can also cause changes in the intestinal flora, allergic dermatitis, burns and blisters.
- Due to the presence of sulfur compounds, it causes different allergic reactions like asthma, rhinitis, conjunctivitis, urticaria, anaphylaxis and angioedema.

11.3.11 *Ocimum sanctum*

- Holy Basil or Tulsi can cause a wide variety of allergic reactions as tulsi acts as a blood thinner so the patients who are taking blood thinners as their medications should not take tulsi (Prakash et al. 2015).
- This herb intensifies the blood thinning properties of the drug due to which there are chances of prolonged bleeding. This herb should also be avoided by pregnant or breastfeeding women as it induces contractions in the uterus (Prakash et al. 2015).
- Eugenol which is one of the most important constituents of tulsi, its concentration can be increased due to an overdose of this herb. Overdose can result in presence of blood while coughing, hyper-breathing and traces of blood in the urine (Prakash et al. 2015).

References

American Diabetes Association. Diagnosis and classification of diabetes mellitus. Diabetes Care. 2010;33(Suppl 1):S62.

Arunkumar S, Muthuselvam M. Analysis of phytochemical constituents and antimicrobial activities of *Aloe vera* L. against clinical pathogens. World J Agri Sci. 2009;5(5):572–6.

Atkinson MA, Eisenbarth GS, Michels AW. Type 1 diabetes. Lancet. 2014;383:69–82.

Baby J, Jini D. Antidiabetic effects of *Momordicacharantia* (bitter melon) and its medicinal potency. Asian Pac J Trop Dis. 2013;3(2):93–102.

Basch E, Gabardi S, Ulbricht C. Bitter melon (*Momordica charantia*): a review of efficacy and safety. Am J Health Syst Pharm. 2003;60(4):356–9.

Benítez V, Mollá E, Martín-Cabrejas MA, Aguilera Y, López-Andréu FJ, Cools K, et al. Characterization of industrial onion wastes (*Allium cepa* L.): dietary fibre and bioactive compounds. Plant Foods Hum Nutr. 2011;66(1):48–57.

Blackman SC, Rey JAG. Hematologic emergencies: acute anemia. Clin Pediatr Emerg Med. 2005;6(3):124–37.

Bösenberg LH, van Zyl DG. The mechanism of action of oral antidiabetic drugs: a review of recent literature. J Endocrinol Metab Diabetes S Afr. 2008;13:80–8.

Capasso A. Antioxidant action and therapeutic efficacy of *Allium sativum* L. Molecules. 2013;18(1):690–700.

Chaturvedi A, Kumar MM, Bhawani G, Chaturvedi H, Kumar M, Goel RK. Effect of ethanolic extract of *Eugenia jambolana* seeds on gastric ulceration and secretion in rats. Indian J Physiol Pharmacol. 2007;51(2):131.

Chauhan A, Sharma PK, Srivastava P, Kumar N, Dudhe R. Plants having potential antidiabetic activity: a review. Der Pharm Lett. 2010;2:369–87.

Elujoba AA, Odeleye OM, Ogunyemi CM. Traditional medicine development for medical and dental primary health care delivery system in Africa. Afr J Tradit Complement Altern Med. 2006;2(1):46–61.

Faria AF, Marcella MC, Mercadante AZ. Identification of bioactive compounds from jambolão (Syzygiumcumini) and antioxidant capacity evaluation in different pH conditions. Food Chem. 2011;126(4):1571–8.

Gautam S, Meshram A, Bhagyawant SS, Srivastava N. Ficus religiosa-potential role in pharmaceuticals. Int J Pharm Sci Res. 2014;5(5):1616–23.

Ghannam N, Kingston M, Al-Meshaal IA, Tariq M, Parman NS, Woodhouse N. The antidiabetic activity of aloes: preliminary clinical and experimental observations. Horm Res. 1986;24(4):288–94.

Guo X, Mei N. *Aloe vera*: a review of toxicity and adverse clinical effects. J Environ Sci Health C Environ Carcinog Ecotoxicol Rev. 2016;34(2):77–96.

Hussain HEMA. Hypoglycemic, hypolipidemic and antioxidant properties of combination of curcumin from *Curcuma longa* Linn, and partially purified product from *Abromaaugusta* Linn. instreptozotocin induced diabetes. Indian J Clin Biochem. 2002;17(2):33–43.

Ignacimuthu S, Ayyanar M. Ethnobotanical investigations among tribes in Madurai district of Tamil Nadu (India). J Ethnobiol Ethnomed. 2006;2:25.

Kelm MA, Nair MG, Strasburg GM, DeWitt DL. Antioxidant and cyclooxygenase inhibitory phenolic compounds from *Ocimum sanctum* Linn. Phytomedicine. 2000;7(1):7–13.

Khadem S, Marles RJ. Monocyclic phenolic acids; hydroxy-and polyhydroxybenzoic acids: occurrence and recent bioactivity studies. Molecules. 2010;15(11):7985–8005.

Khan BA, Abraham A, Leelamma S. Hypoglycemic action of *Murrayakoenigii* (curry leaf) and *Brassica juncea* (mustard): mechanism of action. Indian J Biochem Biophys. 1995;32(2):106–8.

Kumar SKP, Debjit D, Pankaj T. Allium cepa: a traditional medicinal herb and its health benefits. J Chem Pharm Res. 2010a;2(1):283–91.

Kumar DS, Sharathnath KV, Yogeswaran P, Harani A, Sudhakar K, Sudha P, Banji D. A medicinal potency of *Momordica charantia*. Int J Pharm Sci Rev Res. 2010b;1:95–100.

López-Pantoja Y, Angulo-Escalante M, Martínez-Rodríguez C, Soto-Beltrán J, Chaidez-Quiroz C. Antimicrobial effect of crude extracts of neem (*Azadirachtaindica* A. Juss) and venadillo (*Swieteniahumilis* Zucc) against *E. coli, S. aureus* and the bacteriophage P22. Bioquimia. 2007;32(4):117–25.

Manorenjitha MS, Norita AK, Norhisham S, Asmawi MZ. GC-MS analysis of bioactive components of *Ficusreligiosa* (Linn.) stem. Int J Pharm Bio Sci. 2013;4(2):99–103.

Martins N, Petropoulos S, Ferreira IC. Chemical composition and bioactive compounds of garlic (*Allium sativum* L.) as affected by pre-and post-harvest conditions: a review. Food Chem. 2016;211:41–50.

Mishra SB, Rao CV, Ojha SK, Vijayakumar M, Verma A, Alok S. An analytical review of plants for antidiabetic activity with their phytoconstituent and mechanism of action. Int J Pharm Sci Res. 2010;1(1):1647–52.

Olaokun OO, McGaw LJ, Eloff JN, Naidoo V. Evaluation of the inhibition of carbohydrate hydrolysing enzymes, antioxidant activity and polyphenolic content of extracts of ten *African Ficus* species (Moraceae) used traditionally to treat diabetes. BMC Complement Altern Med. 2013;13(1):94.

Oubre AY, Carlson TJ, King SR, Reaven GM. From plant to patient: an ethnomedical approach to the identification of new drugs for the treatment of NIDDM. Diabetologia. 1997;40(5):614–7.

Oyewusi JA, Oridupa OA, Saba AB, Oni O, Oyewusi IK, Mshelbwala MF. Assessment of cardiotoxic potential of methanol extract of red cultivar *Allium cepa.* Sokoto J Vet Sci. 2017;15(3):69–77.

Pandey M, Chikara SK, Vyas MK, Sharma R, Thakur GS, Bisen PS. *Tinosporacordifolia*: a climbing shrub in health care management. Int J Pharm Bio Sci. 2012;3(4):612–28.

Pandit R, Phadke A, Jagtap A. Antidiabetic effect of *Ficusreligiosa* extract in streptozotocin-induced diabetic rats. J Ethnopharmacol. 2010;128(2):462–6.

Perumal V, Khoo WC, Abdul-Hamid A, et al. Evaluation of antidiabetic properties of Momordica charantia in streptozotocin induced diabetic rats using metabolomics approach. Int Food Res J. 2015;22(3):1298–306.

Pradeep AR, Agarwal E, Bajaj P, Naik SB, Shanbhag N, Uma SR. Clinical and microbiologic effects of commercially available gel and powder containing *Acacia arabica* on gingivitis. Aust Dent J. 2012;57(3):312–8.

Prakash O, Kumar R, Srivastava R, Tripathi P, Ajeet MS. Plants explored with anti-diabetic properties: a review. Am J Pharmacol Sci. 2015;3(3):55–66.

Ravi K, Sivagnanam K, Subramanian S. Anti-diabetic activity of *Eugenia jambolana* seed kernels on streptozotocin-induced diabetic rats. J Med Food. 2004;7(2):187–91.

Rawat M, Namita P. Medicinal plants with antidiabetic potential: a review. Am Eurasian J Agric Environ Sci. 2013;13(1):81–94.

Ribnicky DM, Poulev A, Watford M, Cefalu WT, Raskin I. Antihyperglycemic activity of Tarralin, an ethanolic extract of *Artemisia dracunculus* L. Phytomedicine. 2006;13(8):550–7.

Ried K, Fakler P. Potential of garlic (*Allium sativum*) in lowering high blood pressure: mechanisms of action and clinical relevance. Integr Blood Press Control. 2014;7:71–82.

Roqaiya M, Begum W, Jahufer R. *Acacia arabica* (Babool): a review on ethnobotanical and Unani traditional uses as well as phytochemical and pharmacological properties. Int J Pharm Phytopharmacol Res. 2017;4(6):315–21.

Saminathan K, Kavimani S. Current trends of plants having antidiabetic activity: a review. J Bioanalysis Biomed. 2015;7:55.

Samy RR, Pushparaj PN, Gopalakrishnakone P. A compilation of bioactive compounds from Ayurveda. Bioinformation. 2008;3(3):100–10.

Sen P, Sahu K, Prasad P, Chandrakar D, Sahu RK, Roy A. Approach to phytochemistry and mechanism of action of plants having antidiabetic activity. UK J Pharma Biosci. 2016;4:82–120.

Sharma S, Gupta A, Batra SSA. *Tinospora cordifolia* (Willd.) Hook. F. & Thomson-a plant with immense economic potential. J Chem Pharm Res. 2010;2(5):327–33.

Shori AB. Screening of antidiabetic and antioxidant activities of medicinal plants. J Integr Med. 2015;13(5):297–305.

Singh E, Sharma S, Dwivedi J, Sharma S. Diversified potentials of *Ocimum sanctum* Linn (Tulsi): an exhaustive survey. J Nat Prod Plant Resour. 2012;2(1):39–48.

Solanki JD, Makwana AH, Mehta HB, Kamdar P, Desai C, Gandhi P. Comparison of regional variation of body composition in Type 2 Diabetics and matched controls of an urban area of Gujarat, India using bio-electrical impedance method. Int J Basic Appl Physiol. 2013;2(1):94–8.

Tattelman E. Health effects of garlic. Am Fam Physician. 2005;72(1):103–6.

Wild S, Roglic G, Green A, Sicree R, King H. Global prevalence of diabetes: estimates for the year 2000 and projections for 2030. Diabetes Care. 2004;27(5):1047–53.

12 Novel Drug Delivery System in Phytochemicals: Modern Era of Ancient Science

Rinku Baishya, Jyoti L. Hati Boruah, Manob J. Bordoloi, Deepak Kumar, and Pratap Kalita

Contents

12.1 Introduction

Since primeval times, plants and plant-derived extracts containing bio-active molecules (phytochemicals) have been used as a source of medicines for the treatment of ailments. As per a guesstimate, a total of 25–48% of currently approved medicines by FDA (food and drug administration) is derived from the natural products (Russo 2007; Orlikova and Diederich 2012). Natural products derived from plants (Phytochemicals) are a large diversified group of chemical compounds granting color, flavor,

R. Baishya (✉) · J. L. Hati Boruah · M. J. Bordoloi
Pharmacology Laboratory, Natural Products Chemistry Group, Chemical Science and Technology Division, CSIR-North East Institute of Science and Technology, Jorhat, Assam, India
e-mail: rbaishya@neist.res.in

D. Kumar
Organic and Medicinal Chemistry Division, CSIR-Indian Institute of Chemical Biology, Kolkata, India

P. Kalita
Department of Pharmacy, Assam Down Town University, Guwahati, Assam, India

S. Sen, R. Chakraborty (eds.), *Herbal Medicine in India*,
https://doi.org/10.1007/978-981-13-7248-3_12

aroma, and texture along with various medicinal properties. These phytochemicals are widely distributed among the plant kingdom ranging from vegetables, legumes, grains, fruits, flowers, nuts, seeds, herbs and spices into plant-based beverages such as wine and tea. Potential pharmacologically active phytochemicals are time tested and extracted from edible and medicinal plants, which means they are usually safe and exhibit low or no toxicity at a physiologically relevant concentration on normal human organs and cells. The profusion and readily available plants and plant products (fruits, flowers, bark, leaf, etc.) make the derived chemical constituents diverse and economical to use and study for human benefits.

Naturally occurring compounds derived from plants hold a major proportion of prospective therapeutically active agents (Al-Farsi and Ellis 2014; Overby et al. 2014). It is pertinent to mention that, paclitaxel from *Taxus baccata* (Legha et al. 1986; Riondel et al. 1986; Wiernik et al. 1987), vinblastine from *Vinca rosea* (Costa et al. 1963; Frei et al. 1961) and topotecan a synthetic derivative of natural compound (Cheson and Arbuck 1993; Wall et al. 1992), have been successfully developed into clinically used drugs for the treatment of cancer. However, several encumbrances are to be overcome for their extensive use as drugs. These encumbrances range from low solubility, poor penetration into the targeted cells, and high hepatic clearance due to first pass effect, to narrow therapeutic index (Lipinski 2000; Mastropaolo et al. 1995). Additionally, undesired pharmacokinetic profile and emerging drug resistance are also major obstacles for the development of phytochemicals in the clinically used drugs (Lin et al. 2003).

Novel drug delivery system (NDDS) is a novel approach to drug delivery that overcomes the restrictions of the traditional drug delivery systems of phytochemicals. Modern medicine exerts its actions by targeting precisely the affected areas of a patient and delivering the drug to the particular organ or area. The drug targeting with NDDS to individual organs improves selectivity, drug delivery and effectiveness with dose reduction, and safety, and increases compliance. The NDDS as an ideal drug carrier should be capable of extended circulation in the bloodstream, tiny enough to penetrate target cells and tissues, and finally delivering the active constituents in a predetermined manner.

12.2 Novel Drug Delivery Systems

The NDDS are classified by multiple schemes depending on the types and techniques—based on therapeutic group of drug loaded, the physical form of the NDDS, administration route, mode of delivery or action, etc. Therefore, a few most popular and promising NDDS have been discussed in the following sections which are Polymeric Nanoparticles, Liposomes, Ethosomes, Phytosomes, Nanoemulsion/Microemulsion, Microsphere, Micelles, Transferosome, Implants, Cyclodextrins, Niosomes, Transdermal Patches, etc.

12.2.1 Nanoparticles

There has been substantial research interest in the particulate drug delivery systems (submicron particle size ranging 10–1000 nm) as a transporter for small and large molecules of therapeutic interest. Nanoparticles have many advantages, such as solubility enhancement, thereby leading to bioavailability enhancement, reduction in dose, improvement in therapeutic effectiveness, better stability, and improved absorption of herbal medicines or phytochemicals in comparison with the respective crude formulation or preparations. The nanoparticles can be designed with different particle size and surface characteristics for controlled and targeted drug delivery of both hydrophobic and hydrophilic phytochemicals. The phytochemical release from nanoparticles is either through bulk erosion in the matrix or by surface erosion in the polymer depending on the drug characteristics and method adopted for preparation (Chan et al. 2010a, b; Kumari et al. 2010; Rao and Geckeler 2011; Leo et al. 2006). There are various methods employed for the preparation of nanoparticles, viz. salting out method, solvent evaporation method, nanoprecipitation, and dialysis method. Polymeric nanoparticles are extensively used in nanotechnology due to their tiny size and exceptional biocompatibility. Interesting synthetic polymers for research include chitosan (Anitha et al. 2011; Das et al. 2010), poly (D,L-lactide-co-glycolide) (PLGA) and PEG (Anand et al. 2010; Shaikh et al. 2009; Yallapu et al. 2010). Among these, PLGA is considered an efficient material for the formulation of a variety of nano delivery systems.

Curcumin, a natural diarylheptanoid polyphenol is an indispensable curcuminoid present in the turmeric rhizome—*Curcuma longa* (L.) (Family: Zingiberaceae) and is accredited as "Wonder drug of life". Despite its enormous therapeutic potential against a wide variety of physiological disorders, the poor aqueous solubility, resulting poor systemic bioavailability and quick degradation are a few of the major constraints which put a ceiling on the clinical development of curcumin (Gera et al. 2017). To advance clinically applicable parameters of curcumin, the nanoparticle has been prepared using different polymers by many researchers with enhanced aqueous solubility and site-specific delivery of curcumin that prompts to augment the bioavailability, transportation, and quick treatment leading to better clinical applications. Mathew et al. coupled Tet-1 peptide with PLGA coated-curcumin nanoparticles, and reported that this complex of curcumin encapsulated-PLGA nanoparticles is non-cytotoxic and exerted the antioxidant property alongside destroying amyloid aggregates. The PLGA encapsulated curcumin does not hamper its intrinsic therapeutic potential and so, the PLGA encapsulated curcumin nanoparticles provides a hope for its use as a drug with multiple therapeutic potentials in the treatment of Alzheimer's disease (Mathew et al. 2012). Yallapu et al. reported enhanced intracellular uptake of curcumin-PLGA nanoparticles and antibody conjugation attributed in cancer cells (Yallapu et al. 2010). Furthermore, Curcumin loaded PLGA nanoparticles with thiolated chitosan such as bis sulfosuccinimidyl suberate facilitated conjugation of annexin A2 and displayed efficient delivery of curcumin to annexin A2-positive MDA-MB-231 cancer cells (Thamake et al. 2011). Curcumin encapsulated in polycaprolactone nanoparticles (650 nm) showed elevated intracellular levels of curcumin in liver cells upon intravenous administration to male wistar rats. This study demonstrated the therapeutic efficiency of this formulation in liver diseases (Anuradha and Aukunuru 2010).

In another study, a remarkable improvement in A549 cells (human lung adenocarcinoma epithelial cell line) cytotoxicity was reported by the combinations of PLGA encapsulated quercetin (a naturally occurring flavonoid) nanoparticles and etoposide-loaded PLGA nanoparticles, as compared to free quercetin and etoposide (Pimple et al. 2012). Quercetin has been studied extensively as a potential drug candidate for the treatment of cancer but its implementation as a clinically used therapeutic drug are limited because of the poor aqueous solubility and low oral bioavailability. Nanoformulations developed for quercetin have shown promising epithelial system uptake as well as enhanced targeted delivery to the site.

Triptolide, a diterpenoid epoxide, is known for its anti-inflammatory, anti-fertility, anti-neoplastic and immunosuppressive properties. It shows some of the undesirable toxic effects because of the poor aqueous solubility. The anti-inflammatory activity of nanoparticles and microemulsions containing triptolide were evaluated in the rat paw oedema model and the solid lipid nanoparticle (SLN) formulation displayed better activity than the microemulsion (Mei et al. 2003). PLA nanoparticles encapsulating Taxol, produced by emulsion solvent evaporation method, displayed improved bioavailability with sustained release pattern compared to the free drug (Fu et al. 2006). SLN of silibinin showed the hepatoprotective effects and an improved bioavailability due to improved circulation time and enhanced (Zhang et al. 2007).

12.2.2 Liposomes

Liposomes are microscopic, vesicular phospholipids/cholesterol carrier system formulated by one or more concentric lipid bilayers encapsulating small proportion of the solvent in which they unreservedly diffuse into the interior of the liposomes. It is built of polar lipids containing both hydrophilic and lipophilic groups on the same molecule (Lasic 1993). The interaction of polar lipids with water results in self-assembly of the polar lipids to form self-organized colloidal particles. Hydrophilic molecules of interest or drugs are encapsulated in the hydrophilic/aqueous compartment and the lipophiles are inserted into the membrane. Liposomes can be classified based on the size, a number of lamellae, and the surface charge. The liposomes are further classified based on the surface charge into, anionic, cationic, or neutral subcategories (Bonifacio et al. 2014). Liposomes have the property of encapsulating both hydrophilic and lipophilic materials, therefore, as a carrier, it can indiscriminately deliver molecules of interest through the cell membrane by increasing ingredient solubility and enhance intracellular uptake. Liposomal mode of drug delivery can maintain therapeutic concentrations of the drugs or other phytochemicals for prolonged periods of time, thus significantly improves the therapeutic activity, remedial effect and safety profiles. It releases herbal drugs/phytochemicals in a sustained release fashion with reducing peak-valley fluctuations and targeting into the desired area, by improving the solubility and bioavailability (Singh 2015; Abou ElWafa et al. 2003; Barragan-Montero et al. 2005; Weiss and Fintelmann 2000; Ajazuddin and Saraf 2010).

Liposomes were discovered in 1970 as drug delivery vehicles for targeting at the active site into desired concentration. The first successful example of a liposomal drug delivery system is the formulation of doxorubicin (anti-cancer drug) encapsulated in sterically stabilized liposomes (Doxil®). It was approved in 1995 by the FDA for clinical use in the US market (James 1995). Liposomes have been found to be a delivery system for vitamins and enzymes, small cytotoxic molecules as liposomes are biocompatible, nontoxic, and biodegradable in nature (Musthaba et al. 2009; Allen and Cullis 2013). Liposomal drug delivery systems play a vital role owing to easy preparation, and charged liposomes could enhance the percutaneous permeation through the skin, resulting in transdermal drug delivery. The applications of liposomes in herbal formulations have been investigated widely and it's evident from the latest researches that are more focused on enhancing the bioavailability of phytoconstituents (Musthaba et al. 2009; Ajazuddin and Saraf 2010). *Atractylodes macrocephala* Koidz essential oil entrapped into liposomes for the treatment of digestive diseases and tumors has displayed lesser side effects (Wen et al. 2010). *Tripterygium wilfordi* extract displayed better heat stability and lesser side effects on liposomal entrapment (Li et al. 2007).

Quercetin liposomes increased anxiolytic and cognitive effects with a significant reduction in dose when administered through oral and intranasal route (Priprem et al. 2008; Blumenthal et al. 2000). To improve the solubility of Silymarin in the gastrointestinal tract, it has been incorporated into liposomal dosage form which on oral administration improved its bioavailability. Soybean lecithin has been used to incorporate silymarin in liposomal form to improve the bioavailability in a stable buccal dosage form. Silymarin has also been encapsulated as hybrid liposomes (El-Samaligy et al. 2006) to prevent aggregation by maintaining liposomal stability. Commercially available liposome as a delivery system for herbal extracts is Liposomal based powder form Herbasec® by a Swiss-based company Cosmetochem International AG. It is available in the freeze-dried form which is reformed-encapsulating the concentrated plant extract on dispersion in water (Saraf 2010).

12.2.3 Ethosome

Ethosomes are the slightly modified un-shakable drug carrier liposome. It was developed by Touitou et al. (1997), as a non-invasive drug delivery carrier that facilitates drug delivery into the deep skin layers and/or into the systemic circulation through the stratum corneum barrier (Bendas and Tadros 2007). Ethosomes are malleable soft vesicles containing ethanol (20–45%), phospholipids, and water customized for enhanced delivery of desired compounds. These phospholipids are mainly phosphatidylserine, phosphatidylcholine, phosphatidic acid (Merdan et al. 1998). Ethanol is added to make vesicular systems an elastic nanovesicle. The property of ethanol to disturb the skin lipid bilayer organization acts as a competent permeation enhancer and helps in penetration of stratum corneum by interacting with the hydrophilic polar part of the lipid molecules imparting lipid fluidity, and enhances cell membrane permeability as a result of a decrease in the melting point of the stratum corneum lipid. The addition of ethanol imparts high flexibility to the vesicular membrane making elastic enough to squeeze through the pores smaller than their size (Verma and Pathak 2010). Ethosomes can penetrate through the skin at a higher rate than liposomes, rendering them to replace liposomes. Ethosomes entraps phytochemicals and drug molecule with differing physicochemical properties i.e. hydrophilic, lipophilic, and also amphiphilic molecules like proteins and peptides. Herbal ethosome preparations have effectively enhanced the bioavailability of many medicinal plants including *Sophora alopecuroides*, *Cannabis sativa*, *Glycyrrhiza glabra*, etc. for various diseases (Pawar et al. 2015). These ethosomes are suitable for various applications in cosmeticeuticals, phyto-pharmaceuticals, pharmaceuticals, nutraceuticals, veterinary and biotechnology segments. Topical application of Vitamin E, exogenous lipophilic vitamin with antioxidant property reported to enhance the skin protection from exogenous oxidants and used widely in various dermatological preparations. Vit E addition decreases the production of lipid peroxides and protect against UV exposure, destructive chemicals, and physical agents as well. Antioxidants rapidly undergo degradation when exposed to light. Ethosomes have been reported to be an advantage in cosmeceuticals for topical administration of antioxidants to diminish oxidative injury in the skin. Koli and Lin (2009) developed antioxidant ethosomes using the synergistic properties of Vit A palmitate with Vit C for Vit E transport into the deeper layer of stratum corneum. An absolute protection of the ethosome formulations from the oxidation was observed due to the synergistic interaction of Vit C and Vitamin A and E in the aqueous core and lipid bilayer, respectively.

Ethosomes application in transcutaneous immunization of antigen against Hepatitis B showed superior entrapment efficiency when compared to conventional liposomes. *In vitro* assay in murine dendritic cells demonstrated an efficient uptake of HBsAg-loaded ethosomes. It also generated a robust systemic and mucosal humoral immune response on the topical application in mice in comparison with alum-adsorbed HBsAg suspension (i.m.), the topical application plain HBsAg solution, and the hydroethanolic (25%) HBsAg solution. HBsAg-loaded ethosomes were capable to produce a protecting immune response. It was further tested using human cadaver skin, which displayed a superior skin penetration of the antigen than the conventional liposomes and soluble antigen formulation (Mishra et al. 2007). The ethosomes may be used for the development of a Hepatitis B vaccine via a transcutaneous route due to its ability to transverse and target the immunological environment of the skin.

Other applications of ethosome have been reported in the administration of hormones by Ainbinder and Touitou (2005). Paolino et al. (2005) investigated the anti-inflammatory ammonium glycyrrhizinate ethosomes for dermal delivery for various skin diseases. Lodzki et al. (2003) prepared a transdermal cannabidiol ethosomal formulation for the treatment of rheumatoid arthritis.

12.2.4 Phytosome

In most of the cases, biological activities are partially or totally lost during the isolation and purification process of the molecules having therapeutic potential. It has been observed that the bioavailability and biological activities of the active constituents is dependent on the complexity of the different ratios of the constituents present in the crude or partially purified extract. Extracts, when taken orally, may sometimes lead to the destruction of active constituents in the gastric environment due to digestive secretions and gut bacteria. Therefore poor bioavailability hinders their effects. As most of the bioactive water-soluble phytochemicals like flavonoids, tannins, terpenoids, etc. have large molecular weight and this leads to poor absorption by passive diffusion, and possibly their poor lipid solubility also limits their ability to permeate through lipophilic biological membranes, thus results in poor bioavailability of these molecules (Manach et al. 2004; Kumar and Kesari 2011). Therefore, for such herbal extracts to be effectively utilized as herbal drugs is hugely dependent on the delivery to an effective level. Indena S.p.A. of Italy developed the Phytosome® technology which markedly enhanced the bioavailability of select phytomedicines. This technology involves incorporation of water-soluble phytoconstituents or standardized plant extracts or fractions into phospholipids molecular complexes; improves their bioavailability (Bombardelli et al. 1989; Manach et al. 2004).

Phytosomes display structural and functional differences from liposome as phytosomes are a molecular unit of few molecules bound together while the liposomes are made of several phospholipid molecules aggregating together to enclose the phytochemicals or drugs without specifically binding with them. The water-soluble active principles are hosted in the inner cavity of liposomes with limited interaction with surrounding lipid core. On the contrary, the phytosomes accompany their polyphenolic guest at their surface and the guest having polar functionalities via polar interactions with phospholipids bearing charged phosphate groups. The spectroscopic technique can evident these interactions. The topical application of phytosomes enhances the absorption of desired active compounds and oral administration significantly improves the systemic bioavailability and thus phytosomes are superior to liposomes in these modes of administration (Fry et al. 1978; El Maghraby et al. 2000; Jain 2005).

Phytosome being able to cross the lipophilic biological membranes to reach into systemic circulation results in higher plasma concentrations than the individual compounds (Mauri et al. 2001; Kidd and Head 2005; Rossi et al. 2009). The resulting higher plasma concentration ensure that more amount of the desired constituent is available at the site of action (liver, kidney, brain, heart, or another organ) at the same or even low dose. Therefore, the therapeutic action improves, prolongs and becomes detectable. Absorption of phytosome in gastro-intestinal tract can be favorably deployed in the treatment of acute hepatic disorders of metabolic and/or infective origin. Phosphatidylcholine can also be used as a hepatoprotective besides its use as a phytosome carrier, thus it may exert a synergistic effect as hepatoprotective (Saraf and Kaur 2010). The phytosomes can be used for various ailments including cardiovascular, anti-inflammatory, immunomodulatory, anticancer, antidiabetic, etc and also for prophylactic and health benefits as neutraceuticals.

Several therapeutically important phytochemicals developed in this form displayed excellent therapeutic activity in the animal and human models. Meriva®, a patented curcumin-soy phosphatidylcholine complex (Kidd 2009; Marczylo et al. 2007) demonstrated greater bioavailability in rats in comparison with standardized curcumin extract in rats. Indena complexed soyphospholipids exploiting the Phytosome® technology to defeat the poor bioavailability of silybin. Ginkgoselect® Phytosome® have been used in human trials for Raynaud's disease and the study exerted the usefulness of the phytosome in the reduction of Raynaud's attacks, both the frequency (56%) and severity (Muir et al. 2002).

12.2.5 Nanoemulsions/ Microemulsions

Emulsions are thermodynamically unstable formulations of oil and water phase, stabilized by a suitable emulsifying agent. Nano and micro emulsions O/W or W/O type emulsion possess the size range of several microns. These emulsions are widely used in drug delivery formulations to enhance the solubility of inadequately soluble drugs and possess various advantages such as good thermodynamic stability, ease of manufacturing, fewer chances of drug degradation, etc. (Kumar et al. 2012; Mujaffar et al. 2013).

FDA approved surfactants, considered safe for human use, are utilized for the preparation of these emulsions. The higher surface area and lower size enable them to penetrate easily through the skin. Nanoemulsions can be prepared by various methods including the high-pressure homogenization and microfluidisation technique (Lieberman et al. 1998; Lachman et al. 1996) unlike to microemulsions which form spontaneously. The scope of microemulsions and nanoemulsions in herbal drug delivery is wide and has been used clinically as well as commercially (Goyal et al. 2011).

An enhanced anti-inflammatory activity of curcumin in O/W nanoemulsion was reported in 2008 (Wang et al. 2008). It was prepared by an optimized high pressure and high-speed homogenization method to achieve droplet sizes in the 618.6–79.5 nm range. 12-O-tetradecanoyl phorbol-13-acetate-induced edema of mouse ear was used to compare this formulation against 1% curcumin in 10% Tween 20 water solution and it was observed that high-pressure homogenization microemulsion showed improved activity compared to microemulsion prepared with the high-speed method; no activity was observed with 1% curcumin in 10% Tween 20 water solution. The eutectic properties of ubiquinone was utilized to develop a self nanoemulsion (Nazzal et al. 2002). This drug delivery system enhanced the solubility and bioavailability and reduced precipitation of the drug in the vehicle.

12.2.6 Microsphere

Microspheres are spherical particles having a diameter in the range of 1–1000 μm in which drug is dispersed in finely divided form or crystalline form and also referred to as microparticles. They can be prepared from various materials of natural and synthetic origin like albumin, gelatin, chitosan, polypropylene, polylactic acid, polyglycolic acid, modified starch, dextran, etc. The first order kinetics is followed by microsphere for the drug release and controlled by the matrix dissolution and disintegration. The drug release is majorly affected by the matrix type, size and concentration of the polymer (Brahmankar and Jaiswal 1998). Microspheres are having wide commercial applications including sustained drug delivery, they can be ingested or injected, overcome handling issues with potent molecules and improved targeting at the active site in desired concentration to maintain overall effective plasma concentration for a longer duration (Singh 2015; Varde and Pack 2004; Freiberg and Zhu 2004). Mucoadhesive microsphere has been prepared by evaporation technique and ionic cross-linking technique, etc. (Kanan et al. 2009; Das and Senapati 2008). In recent times, microspheres are widely used to enhance the therapeutic potential of various poorly soluble phytoconstituents.

Gastro-retentive floating microspheres of curcumin have been prepared with a prolonged gastric residence time in simulated gastric fluid for at least 20 h, resulting in increased drug bioavailability (Kumar & Rai 2012). Rutin-alginate-chitosan microsphere delivered rutin specifically to cardiovascular and cerebrovascular organelles (Xiao et al. 2008). *Piper sarmentosumn* extract encapsulated with calcium alginate beads used an industrially feasible process of adsorption (Chan et al. 2010a, b). Zedoary turmeric oil was microencapsulated to enhance bioavailability and sustained-release application. This was achieved by emulsion-solvent diffusion method (You et al. 2006). Turmeric oleoresin microspheres were prepared after emulsification of oleoresin followed by spray drying technique. The microspheres displayed an improved therapeutic effect and also protected the oleoresin from degradation when exposed to light, oxygen, heat, and alkali (Kshirsagar et al. 2009). Camptothecin was encapsulated in oxidized cellulose microspheres by spray drying process; enhanced its solubility and cytotoxicity (Chao et al. 2010).

12.2.7 Micelles

Micelles are lipid molecules organize themselves in a spherical shape in aqueous solutions.

Polymeric micelles are usually very small in size and range from 10 to 100 nm (Kataoka et al. 2001). Micelles protect the drug from its surrounding which may inactivate the drug and thus increases the drug bioavailability and retention (Kwon 2002). There are various factors which govern the drug release from micelles, such as micelle stability, drug diffusion rate, the partition coefficient, and the copolymer biodegradation rate (Kwon and Okano 1996). The drug release is also affected by its concentration and location inside the micelles, molecular weight and physicochemical properties (Teng et al. 1998). Targeted delivery of poorly soluble herbal drugs has been achieved by using polymeric micelles. Micelles formulations of poorly soluble drugs like Artemisinin and Curcumin with sodium dodecyl sulphate increased their solubility by 25-folds. The micellar formulation also increased the solubility of paclitaxel and has been used for the treatment of hormone refractory prostate cancer in LN Cap tumor model (Simon et al. 2000).

12.2.8 Transferosome

The transferosome concept was introduced in 1991 by Gregor Cevc. Transferosomes are phospholipid vesicles which can penetrate the stratum corneum to be used as potential transdermal drug delivery carriers (Pandey et al. 2009). Transferosomes exhibit better elasticity than the standard liposomes and thus more suitable for the transdermal drug delivery. Transferosomes squeeze themselves along the intracellular lipids of the stratum corneum and penetrate the skin (Eldhose et al. 2016). Hydration or osmotic force in the skin enhances the penetration through stratum corneum. They can be used as a potential carrier for drugs with a wide range molecular weights and different pharmacological actions including analgesic, sex hormones, anesthetic, anticancer, corticosteroids, and insulin, etc. They are biocompatible, biodegradable and have high entrapment efficiency (near to 90% for the lipophilic drug). They act as a depot for the encapsulated drug protecting from metabolic degradation, and release the drugs slowly and gradually. They are used in both systemic and topical drug delivery. The preparation of transferosomes is simple, short and do not involve pharmaceutically unacceptable additives (Cevc et al. 1998). Transferosomes are prepared using following: (a) phospholipids, a vesicle-forming material, (b) surfactant for providing flexibility, (c) alcohol as a solvent and (d) a buffering agent as a hydrating medium.

Curcumin is largely used as a potent anti-inflammatory herbal drug, but it has low bioavailability due to poor gastrointestinal absorption. Transferosomes encapsulating curcumin gel showed an increase in skin permeation compared with the plain gel containing curcumin, paving the transferosome as potential carriers for the curcumin transdermal delivery (Patel et al. 2009). High shear dispersion technique was used to prepare Capsaicin transferosomes and it showed better topical absorption compared to pure Capsaicin (Xiao-Ying et al. 2006). Colchicine transferosomes for topical delivery were prepared using handshaking method and prevented the GI side effects of oral absorption (Singh et al. 2009). Transferosomes encapsulating Vincristine sulfate were prepared by lecithin and sodium deoxycholate (70/20). The *in vitro* tests through mouse skin showed penetration through the skin at zero order rate (Lu et al. 2005).

12.2.9 Implants

Another approach of controlled drug delivery is to formulate into polymeric implants. Implants are polymeric devices which provide controlled drug delivery of wide variety of drugs. These are prepared using biodegradable polymers and can be directly placed at the site of action by a microsurgery for the insertion of these devices (Brahmankar and Jaiswal 1998). Two types of polymeric matrices are used for the preparation of Implants: Biodegradable and Nondegradable polymeric matrices. Nondegradable bio-matrices are made of either silicone or poly (ethylene-co-vinyl acetate) (Saltzman and Fung 1997). The Norplant system of contraception uses these non-biodegradable biomatrices for this type of drug delivery (Darney 1994). Vadhanam et al. have delivered ellagic acid using this system of delivery in a mammary tumorigenesis model and observed tumor reduction with 130-fold less compound (silastic implants v/s dietary route) (Vadhanam et al. 2011). Although implant delivery system has the potential to deliver for a long duration, it has the risks of mechanical failure of implants that may lead to dose dumping. Another drawback of the system is the likelihood for fibrous growth in the region of the implants, which become difficult to remove after the treatment is over (Aqil et al. 2013). A biodegradable polymeric system can overcome those disadvantages of a nondegradable matrix system. A sustained-release implant containing plant extract has proved to be beneficial. An implant containing the extract of Danshen (*Radix Salvia miltiorrhiza*) using chitosan and gelatin was developed to support anastomosing and healing on muscles and tissues in abdominal cavities. The sustained delivery of the implant was observed for up to 28 days. The repairing of the wounds and tissues were healed better with this implant system and frequent dosing was reduced for the patient (Zhao et al. 2002).

12.2.10 Cyclodextrins

Cyclodextrins (CDs) are cyclic oligosaccharides that contain six to eight dextrose units (α-, β-, and γ-cyclodextrins, respectively) connected through 1–4 bonds. The outer side of CDs is hydrophilic and the inner side is relatively lipophilic, enabling them to interact and entrap molecules forming noncovalent inclusion complexes (Challa et al. 2005). The application of cyclodextrins is also to enhance the drug bioavailability by enhancing the solubility, stability and overcoming the undesirable physiochemical properties of drugs (Le and Rysanek 1987; Szejtli 1982, 1988).

CDs enhance the permeability of hydrophobic drugs by increasing the availability of the drug on the surface of the biological barrier like skin and mucosa, where the drug partitions into the membrane and thus penetrating the lipid layers of these barriers. The optimum CDs should be used to solubilize the drug in the aqueous vehicle increasing the drug availability (Loftsson and Stefansson 1997).

Cyclodextrin scan be used for both oral and intravenous drug delivery and when used as vehicles/carriers for oral delivery they can increase the bioavailability of insoluble drugs by molecular dispersion, shielding it from degradation in different gastro intestinal tract pH, and increasing the availability at the intestinal wall. When it is used as parenteral vehicles, they solubilize the hydrophobic drugs without changing their pharmacokinetic properties (Thompson 1997).

Due to volatile properties, oxidation, photodegradation and/or polymerization, many naturally occurring compounds, like vanillin, cinnamaldehyde, essential oils and flavoring agents such as lemon and orange peel oil, tends to vanish from solid formulations. CDs formulation could overcome those problems up to an adequate level (Vyas et al. 2008).

High hydrophobicity and sensitivity to air, light and oxidative enzymes caused remarkable problem for resveratrol formulation. β-CD and G2 β-CD complexation with resveratrol reduced the oxidation as it is entrapped in the internal cavity of CDs (Lucas-Abellan et al. 2007).

CD complexation can stabilize many famous paramedical foul smelling and volatile products like cinnamon leaf oil and garlic oil (Ayala-Zavala et al. 2008). The glucopyranose rings of β-cyclodextrins are able to form inclusion complexes of small molecular weight with flavor substances. The stable β-cyclodextrin complexes have the advantages of persistent composition, macroscopic and microbiological purity, and reduced sensitivity to external factors (Lindner 2006).

12.2.11 Niosomes

Niosomes are vesicles composed of multiple lamellas and are non-ionic in nature. It consists of non-ionic surfactant and differs from liposomes which have phospholipids. Because of the similarity in structure with a liposome, niosome can be an alternative to liposomal drug carriers.

The properties of the niosomes are influenced by additives, mode of preparation, drug's physicochemical properties, surfactant's amount, structure and type, cholesterol content and resistance to osmotic stress (Rajera et al. 2011). Niosomes can enhance the therapeutic effect of drugs by targeted delivery as they are non-ionic in nature and are less toxic.

They can be prepared by any of the following methods—ether injection, sonication, reverse phase evaporation, extrusion, remote loading, hand shaking, and microfluidization. These vesicles act as a storehouse for the drug and release it in a controlled manner. They improve the stability of the entrapped drug molecule and thus enhance the oral bioavailability of poorly absorbed drugs. They cross the anatomical barrier of GIT via transcytosis of M cells of Peyer's patches in the intestinal lymphatic tissues (Jadon et al. 2009). Such highly contained drug accrual is beneficial in the treatment of diseases like leishmaniasis where parasites attack liver and spleen cells (Sheena et al. 1998; Baillie et al. 1986). Niosomes have been suggested for treatments of various diseases such as cancer and infection (Balasubramaniam et al. 2002), also as immunological adjuvants (Jain et al. 2005), as anti-inflammatory drug carrier (Shahiwala and Misra 2002) and also as a diagnostic imaging agent (Uchegbu and Vyas 1998). Niosomes can be administered through various routes and particular emphasis has been given for transdermal drug delivery systems. The evolution of niosomal drug delivery technology is in its formative years but it has displayed promising potential in cancer chemotherapy and anti-leishmanial therapy.

12.2.12 Transdermal Drug Delivery System (Transdermal Patches)

Delivery of phytochemicals via skin is widely investigated and an increase in interest for drug delivery through transdermal patch has been observed for enhancing permeation and therapeutic efficacy. The major advantages of topical delivery are an evasion of the first-pass metabolism, decrease adverse effects associated with oral and intravenous (IV) doses and improved therapeutic efficacy. Various strategies are used to enhance the transdermal permeation including transdermal patches, ethosomes, transferosomes, and SLNs (Prausnitz and Langer 2008; Benson and Watkinson 2011; Prausnitz et al. 2004). Ethosomes, transferosomes, and SLNs are already discussed in this chapter.

The medication delivery by transdermal patches is done through an adhesive patch which is attached to the patient's skin. The patch is made up of special membrane which can control the rate of drug release. Treatment through such patches is non-invasive and medication delivery is designed to release the active ingredient at a constant rate over a specific period ranging from several hours to days after application to the skin. It involves percolation of the drug from the surface of the skin passing through the layers of dermal tissue and finally into the circulatory system.

Transdermal patches are the novel approach which utilizes permeation enhancers (terpenes, ozones, and surfactants) for topical delivery. Various physical methods are used such as iontophoresis, sonophoresis, microneedles, and skin electroporation for delivery of the drug through a transdermal patch. The main limitation in transdermal patch approach is that it causes skin irritation or skin infection due to the high frequency applied through iontophoresis, which will overcome by the novel vesicular carriers such as transferosomes and ethosomes, which supplies essential nutrients results in maintaining the integrity of the skin.

Some examples of marketed preparations

(a) The virility patch: The RX male virility enhancement patch is an ultra-concentrated formulation infused in discreetly small patch containing a variety of herbs which exist to enhance male vigor. Other nicotine patch and diet patches are similar examples, where these products use advanced physiological technology to feed the formulation into the blood circulation of a patient in a timely manner. The effective mixture of ingredients is right away absorbed into the skin from the patch. The major advantage of this product is that the formulation can bypass the digestive system and working mechanism of the formulation immediately fasten up and provides effective virility enhancement. This transdermal delivery system is approved by the FDA (Bayarski 2010).

(b) Transdermal slimming patch (Levin Health Care): This product is prepared on a soft patch embedded with formulation entirely made of natural herbs with the transdermal delivery system. It reduces the overburden to the vital organs and works for 24 h. Once applied it helps in the acceleration of the fat burning process, alleviating hunger pangs and provides the feeling of fullness, even when one has not eaten (Anonymous 2010).

12.3 Conclusion

Herbal drugs have the potential to treat all diseases with one or more active constituents present in them and they have been extensively used throughout the world since ancient times. With fewer side effects when compared with modern medicines, it's well-recognized between physicians and patients. Plant actives and extracts are now also been recognized for high therapeutic value in the new dimension of novel drug delivery and targeting. This change has been brought by the rising demand of herbal drugs in the market and also with the growth of awareness among people about the safety of plant origin drugs. NDDS for herbal drugs can bring down the repeatable dose administration to overcome non-compliance and elevate the therapeutic value increasing the bioavailability thus reducing toxicity and so on. This technology being an exploratory stage demands some more research, to resolve issues with production and application. The pharmaceutical companies have started focusing on adopting new drug delivery technology for existing drugs, for various reasons, such as reducing the dosing frequency to meet patient compliance, and these developed products are normally filed a new drug application (NDA) to capture the generic market because the development of investigational new drugs (IND) is slow and developing new drugs for specific diseases takes a long time. Several excellent phytochemicals have been successfully delivered using this technology. In years to come, there is definitely a great potential in the field of novel drug delivery systems for active phytochemicals.

References

Abou ElWafa AA, Mursi NM, El-Shaboury KM. A pharmaceutical study on certain ocular drug delivery systems. MS Thesis. Cairo University, Cairo (2003).

Ainbinder D, Touitou E. Testosterone ethosomes for enhanced transdermal delivery. Drug Deliv. 2005;12:297–303.

Ajazuddin, Saraf S. Applications of novel drug delivery system for herbal formulations. Fitoterapia. 2010;81:680–9.

Al-Farsi A, Ellis PM. Treatment paradigms for patients with metastatic non-small cell lung cancer, squamous lung cancer: first, second, and third-line. Front Oncol. 2014;4:157.

Allen TM, Cullis PR. Liposomal drug delivery systems: from concept to clinical applications. Adv Drug Deliv Rev. 2013;65:36–48.

Anand P, Nair HB, Sung B, Kunnumakkara AB, Yadav VR, Tekmal RR, Aggarwal BB. Design of curcumin-loaded PLGA nanoparticles formulation with enhanced cellular uptake, and increased bioactivity in vitro and superior bioavailability in vivo. Biochem Pharmacol. 2010;79:330–8.

Anitha A, Maya S, Deepa N, Chennazhia KP, Naira SV, Tamurab H, Jayakumara R. Efficient water soluble O-carboxymethyl chitosan nanocarrier for the delivery of curcumin to cancer cells. Carbohydr Polym. 2011;83:452–61.

Anonymous. Transdermal patch. http://www.levinhealthcare.com. 2010.

Anuradha CA, Aukunuru J. Preparation, characterisation and in vivo evaluation of bis-demethoxy curcumin analogue (BDMCA) nanoparticles. Trop J Pharm Res. 2010;9:51–8.

Aqil F, Munagala R, Jeyabalan J, Vadhanam MV. Bioavailability of phytochemicals and its enhancement by drug delivery systems. Cancer Lett. 2013;334:133–41.

Ayala-Zavala JF, Soto-Valdez H, Gonzalez-Leon A, Alvarez-Parrilla E, Martın-Belloso O, Gonzalez-Aguilar GA. Microencapsulation of cinnamon leaf (cinnamomumzeylanicum) and garlic (Allium sativum) oils in β -cyclodextrin. J Incl Phenom Macrocycl Chem. 2008;60:359–68.

Baillie AJ, Coombs GH, Dolan TF, Laurie J. Non-ionic surfactant vesicles, niosomes, as delivery system for the anti-leishmanial drug, sodium stibogluconate. J Pharm Pharmacol. 1986;38:502–5.

Balasubramaniam A, Kumar VA, Pillai KS. Formulation and *in-vivo* evaluation of niosome encapsulated daunorubicin hydrochloride. Drug Dev Ind Pharm. 2002;28:1181–93.

Barragan-Montero V, Winum J, Moles J, Juan E, Clavel C, Montero J. Eur J Med Chem. 2005;40:1022–9.

Bayarski Y.. http://www.google.com/Transdermalpatches/NDDS/Herbal drugs.in. 2010.

Bendas ER, Tadros MI. Enhanced transdermal delivery of sulbutamolsulfate via ethosomes. AAPS Pharm Sci Tech. 2007;8:1–7.

Benson HE, Watkinson AC. Topical and transdermal drug delivery: principles and practice. New Jersey: Wiley Online Library; 2011.

Blumenthal M, Goldberg A, Brinkmann J. Herbal medicine. Newton: Integrative Medicine Communications; 2000.

Bombardelli E, Curri SB, Loggia DR, Del NP, Tubaro A, Gariboldi P. Fitoterapia. 1989;60:1–9.

Bonifacio BV, Silva PB, Ramos MA, Negri KMS, Bauab TM, Chorilli M. Nanotechnology-based drug delivery systems and herbal medicines: a review. Int J Nanomedicine. 2014;9:1–5.

Brahmankar DM, Jaiswal SB. Biopharmaceutics and pharmacokinetics—a treatise. 1st ed. New Delhi: Vallabh Prakashan; 1998.. (reprint 2008):61:359–362

Cevc G, Gebauer D, Steiber J, Schatzlein A, Blume G. Ultraflexible vesicles, transfersomes, have an extremely low pore penetration resistance and transport therapeutic amounts of insulin across the intact mammalian skin. Biochem Biophys Acta. 1998;1368:201–15.

Challa R, Ahuja A, Ali J, Khar RK. Cyclodextrins in drug delivery: an updated review. AAPS Pharm Sci Tech. 2005;6:E329–57.

Chan ES, Yim ZH, Phan SH, Mansa RF, Ravindra P. Encapsulation of herbal aqueous extract throughabsorption with ca-alginate hydrogel beads. Food Bioprod Process. 2010a;88(40239):195–201.

Chan JM, Valencia PM, Zhang L, Langer R, Farokhzad OC. Polymeric nanoparticles for drug delivery. Methods Mol Biol. 2010b;624:163–75.

Chao P, Deshmukh M, Kutscher HL, Gao D, Rajan SS, Hu P, Laskin DL, Stein S, Sinko PJ. Pulmonary targeting microparticulate campothecin delivery system: anticancer evaluation in a rat orthotopic lung cancer model. Anticancer Drugs. 2010;21:65–76.

Cheson BD, Arbuck SG. Clinical trials referral resource. Clinical trials with topotecan. Oncology. 1993;7:49–51.

Costa G, Carbone PP, Gold GL, Owens AH Jr, Miller SP, Krant MJ, Bono VH Jr. Clinical trial of vinblastine in multiple myeloma. Cancer Chemother Rep 1. 1963;27:87–9.

Darney PD. Hormonal implants: contraception for a new century. Am J Obstet Gynecol. 1994;170:1536–43.

Das MK, Senapati PC. Furosemide loaded alginate microspheres prepared by ionic cross linking technique: morphology and release characteristics. Indian J Pharm Sci. 2008;70:77–84.

Das RK, Kasoju N, Bora U. Encapsulation of curcumin in alginate-chitosan-pluronic composite nanoparticles for delivery to cancer cells. Nanomedicine. 2010;6:153–60.

El Maghraby GM, Williams AC, Barry BW. Skin delivery of oestradiol from deformable and traditional liposomes: mechanistic studies. J Pharm Pharmacol. 1999;51:1123–34.

El Maghraby GM, Williams AC, Barry BW. Oestradiol skin delivery from ultradeformable liposomes: refinement of surfactant concentration. Int J Pharm. 2000;196:63–74.

Eldhose MP, Mathew F, Mathew NJ. Transfersomes – A Review. Int J Pharma Pharma Res. 2016;6:436–52.

El-Samaligy MS, Afifi NN, Mahmoud EA. Int J Pharm. 2006;319:121–9.

Frei E, Franzino A, Shnider BI, Costa G, Colsky J, Brindley CO, Hosley JF, Gold GL, Jonsson U. Clinical studies of vinblastine. Cancer Chemother Rep 1. 1961;12:125–9.

Freiberg S, Zhu XX. Polymer microspheres for controlled drug release. Int J Pharm. 2004;282:1–18.

Fry DW, White JC, Goldman ID. Rapid secretion of low molecular weight solutes from liposomes without dilution. Anal Biochem. 1978;90:809–15.

Fu RQ, He FC, Meng DS, Chen L. Taxol PLA nanoparticles. ACTA Academiae Medicinae Militaris Tertiae. 2006;28:1573–4.

Gera M, Sharma N, Ghosh M, Huynh DL, Lee SJ, Min T, Kwon T, Jeong DK. Nanoformulations of curcumin: an emerging paradigm for improved remedial application. Oncotarget. 2017;8:66680–98.

Goyal A, Kumar S, Nagpal M, Singh I, Arora S. Potential of novel drug delivery system for herbal drugs. Ind J Pharm Edu Res. 2011;45:3.

Jadon PS, Gajbhiye V, Jadon RS, Gajbhiye KR, Ganesh N. Enhanced oral bioavailability of griseofulvin via niosomes. AAPS Pharm Sci Tech. 2009;10:1186–92.

Jain NK. Liposomes as drug carriers, controlled and novel drug delivery. 1st ed: CBS Publisher; 2005. p. 321–6.

Jain S, Singh P, Mishra V, Vyas SP. Mannosylated niosomes as adjuvant carrier system for oral genetic immunization against Hepatitis B. Immunol Lett. 2005;101:41–9.

James JS. DOXIL approved for KS. AIDS Treat News. 1995;236:6.

Kanan K, Karar PK, Manavalan R. Formulation and evaluation of sustained release microspheres ofacetazolamide by solvent evaporation technique. J Pharm Sci Res. 2009;1:36–9.

Kataoka K, Harada A, Nagasaki Y. Block copolymer micelles for drug delivery: design, characterization and biological significance. Adv Drug Deliv Rev. 2001;47:113–31.

Kidd PM. Bioavailability and activity of phytosome complexes from botanical polyphenols: the silymarin, curcumin, green tea, and grape seed extracts. Altern Med Rev. 2009;14:226–46.

Kidd P, Head K. A review of the bioavailability and clinical efficacy of milk thistle phytosome: a silybin-phosphatidylchoiine complex (Siliphos'). Altern Med Rev. 2005;10(3):193–203.

Koli JR, Lin S. Development of anti oxidantethosomes for topical delivery utilizing the synergistic properties of Vit A palmitate, Vit E and Vit C. AAPS Pharm Sci Tec. 2009;11:1–8.

Kshirsagar AC, Yenge VB, Sarkar A, Singhal RS. Efficacy of pullulan in emulsification of turmeric oleoresin and its subsequent microencapsulation. Food Chem. 2009;113:1139–45.

Kumar VS, Kesari A. Herbosome—a novel carrier for herbal delivery. Int J Curr Pharm Res. 2011;3:36–41.

Kumar K, Rai AK. Development and evaluation of floating microspheres of curcumin. Trop J Pharm Res. 2012;11:713–9.

Kumar R, Kumar MS, Mahadevan N. Multipleemulsions: a review. Int J Adv Pharm Res. 2012;2:9–19.

Kumari A, Yadav SK, Yadav SC. Biodegradable polymeric nanoparticles based drug delivery systems. Colloids Surf B Biointerfaces. 2010;75:1–18.

Kwon GS. Block copolymer micelles as drug delivery systems. Adv Drug Deliv Rev. 2002;54:167.

Kwon GS, Okano T. Polymeric micelles as new drug carriers. Adv Drug Deliv Rev. 1996;21:107–16.

Lachman L, Lieberman HA, Kanig JL. The Theory and practice of Industrial Pharmacy. 3rd ed. Philadelphia: Lea & Febiger; 1996. p. 510–1.

Lasic DD. Liposomes: from physics to applications. Amsterdam/London, New York, Tokyo: Elsevier; 1993.

Le BG, Rysanek N. Cyclodextrins and their industrial uses. Duchene D Ed.; Editions de Santé. 1987.p.107–30.

Legha SS, Tenney DM, Krakoff IR. Phase I study of taxol using a 5-day intermittent schedule. J Clin Oncol. 1986;4:762–6.

Leo E, Scatturin A, Vighi E, Dalpiaz A. Polymeric nanoparticles as drug controlled release systems: anew formulation strategy for drugs with small or largemolecular weight. J Nanosci Nanotechnol. 2006;6:3070–9.

Li HR, Li SF, Dua HQ. Preparation of liposomes containing extracts of Tripterygium wilfordii and evaluation of its stability. Zhongguo Zhong Yao Za Zhi. 2007;32:2128–31.

Lieberman HA, Rieger MM, Banker GS. Pharmaceutical dosage forms: disperse systems. 2nd ed. New York: Marcel Dekker Inc.; 1998. p. 339–44.

Lin J, Sahakian DC, de Morais SM, Xu JJ, Polzer RJ, Winter SM. The role of absorption, distribution, metabolism, excretion and toxicity in drug discovery. Curr Top Med Chem. 2003;3:1125–54.

Lindner K. Using cyclodextrin aroma complexes in the catering. Food Nahrung. 2006;26:675–80.

Lipinski CA. Drug-like properties and the causes of poor solubility and poor permeability. J Pharmacol Toxicol Methods. 2000;44:235–49.

Lodzki M, Godin B, Rakou L, Mechoulam R, Gallily R, Touitou E. Cannabidiol-transdermal delivery and anti-inflammatory effect in a murine model. J Control Release. 2003;93(3):377–87.

Loftsson T, Stefansson E. Effect of cyclodextrins on topical drug delivery tothe eye. Drug Dev Ind Pharm. 1997;23:473–81.

Lu Y, Hou SX, Chen T, Sun YY, Yang BX, Yuan ZY. Preparation of transferosomes of vicristine sulfate and study on its precutaneous penetration. Zhongguo Zhong Yao Za Zhi. 2005;30:900–3.

Lucas-Abellan C, Fortea I, Lopez-Nicolas JM, Nunez-Delicado E. Cyclodextrins as resveratrol carrier system. Food Chem. 2007;104:39–44.

Manach C, Scalbert A, Morand C, Rémésy C, Jiménez L. Polyphenols: food sources and bioavailability. Am J Clin Nutr. 2004;79:727–47.

Marczylo TH, Verschoyle RD, Cooke DN, Morazzoni P, Steward WP, Gescher AJ. Comparison of systemic availability of curcumin with that of curcumin formulated with phosphatidylcholine. Cancer Chemother Pharmacol. 2007;60:171–7.

Mastropaolo D, Camerman A, Luo Y, Brayer GD, Camerman N. Crystal and molecular structure of paclitaxel (taxol). Proc Natl Acad Sci U S A. 1995;92:6920–4.

Mathew A, Fukuda T, Nagaoka Y, Hasumura T, Morimoto H, Yoshida Y, Maekawa T, Venugopal K, Kumar DS. Curcumin Loaded-PLGA nanoparticles conjugated withTet-1 peptide for potential use in Alzheimer's disease. PLoS One. 2012;7(3):e32616.

Mauri P, Simonetti P, Gardana C. Liquid chromatography/atmospheric pressure chemical ionization mass spectrometry of terpene lactones in plasma of volunteers dosed with Ginkgo biloba L. extracts. Rapid Commun Mass Spectrom. 2001;15:929–34.

Mei Z, Chen H, Weng T, Yang Y, Yang X. Solid lipid nanoparticle and microemulsion for topical delivery of triptolide. Eur J Pharm Biopharm. 2003;56:189–96.

Merdan VM, Alhaique F, Touitou E. Vesicular carriers for topical delivery. Acta Techno Legis Medicament. 1998;12:1–6.

Mishra D, Mishra PK, Dubey V, Nahar M, Jain NK. Systemic and mucosal immune response induced by transcutaneous immunization using Hepatitis B surface antigen-loaded modified liposomes. J Control Release. 2007;33:424–33.

Muir AH, Robb R, McLaren M, Daly F, Belch JJ. The use of *Ginkgo biloba* in Raynaud's disease: a double-blind placebo-controlled trial. J Vasc Med. 2002;7:265–7.

Mujaffar F, Singh UK, Chauhan L. Review of micro-emulsion as futuristic drug delivery. Int J Pharm Sci. 2013;5:39–51.

Musthaba SM, Baboota S, Ahmed S, Ahuja A, Ali J. Status of novel drug delivery technology for phytotherapeutics. Expert Opin Drug Deliv. 2009;6:625–37.

Nazzal S, Smalyukh II, Lavrentovich OD, Khan MA. Preparation and in vitro characterization of a eutectic based semisolid self nanoemulsified drug delivery system of ubiquinone: mechanism and progress of emulsion formation. Int J Pharm. 2002;235:247–65.

Orlikova B, Diederich M. Power from the garden: plant compounds as inhibitors of the hallmarks of cancer. Curr Med Chem. 2012;19:2061–87.

Overby A, Zhao CM, Chen D. Plant phytochemicals: potential anticancer agents against gastric cancer. Curr Opin Pharmacol. 2014;19C:6–10.

Pandey S, Goyani M, Devmurari V, Fakir J. Transferosomes: a Novel approach for transdermal drug delivery. Pharm Lett. 2009;1:143–50.

Paolino D, Lucania G, Mardente D, Alhaique F, Fresta M. Ethosomes for skin delivery of ammonium glycyrrhizinate: in vitro percutaneous permeation through human skin and in vivo anti-inflammatory activity on human volunteers. J Control Release. 2005;106:99–110.

Patel R, Singh SK, Singh S, Sheth NR, Gendle R. Development and characterization of curcumin loaded transferosomes for transdermal delivery. J Pharm Sci. 2009;1:71–80.

Pawar P, Kalamkar R, Jain A, Aberkar S. Ethosomes: a novel tool for herbal drug delivery. IJPPR Human. 2015;3:191–202.

Pimple S, Manjappa AS, Ukawala M, Murthy RS. PLGA nanoparticles loaded with etoposide and quercetin dihydrate individually: in vitro cell line study to ensure advantage of combination therapy. Cancer Nanotechnol. 2012;3:25–36.

Prausnitz MR, Langer R. Transdermal drug delivery. Nat Biotechnol. 2008;26:1261–8.

Prausnitz MR, Langer R, Mitragotri S. Current status and future potential of transdermal drug delivery. Nat Rev Drug Discov. 2004;3:115–24.

Priprem A, Watanatorn J, Sutthiparinyanont S, Phachonpai W, Muchimapura S. Anxiety and cognitive effects of Quercetin liposomes in rats. Nanomedicine. 2008;4:70–8.

Rajera R, Nagpal K, Singh SK, Mishra DN. Niosomes: a controlled and novel drug delivery system. Biol Pharm Bull. 2011;34:945–53.

Rao JP, Geckeler KE. Polymer nanoparticles: preparation techniques and size-control parameters. Prog Polym Sci. 2011;36:887–913.

Riondel J, Jacrot M, Picot F, Beriel H, Mouriquand C, Potier P. Therapeutic response to taxol of six human tumors xenografted into nude mice. Cancer Chemother Pharmacol. 1986;17:137–42.

Rossi R, Basilico F, Rossoni G, Riva A, Morazzoni P, Mauri PL. J Pharm Biomed Anal. 2009;50:224–7.

Russo GL. Ins and outs of dietary phytochemicals in cancer chemoprevention. Biochem Pharmacol. 2007;74:533–44.

Saltzman WM, Fung LK. Polymeric implants for cancer chemotherapy. Adv Drug Deliv Rev. 1997;26:209–30.

Saraf S, Kaur CD. Phytoconstituents as photoprotective novel cosmetic formulations. Pharmacogn Rev. 2010;4:1–11.

Shahiwala A, Misra A. Studies in topical application of niosomally entrapped Nimesulide. J Pharm Pharm Sci. 2002;5:220–5.

Shaikh J, Ankola DD, Beniwal V, Singh D, Kumar MN. Nanoparticle encapsulation improves oral bioavailability of curcumin by at least 9-fold when compared to curcumin administered with piperine as absorption enhancer. Eur J Pharm Sci. 2009;37:223–30.

Sheena IP, Singh UV, Kamath R, Uma Devi P, Udupa N. Niosomal with a ferin A, with better tumor efficiency. Indian J Pharm Sci. 1998;60:45–8.

Simon YL, Jackson J, Miyake H, Burt H, Gleave ME. Polymeric micellar paclitaxel phosphorylates Bcl-2 and induces apoptotic regression of androgen-independent LNCaP prostate tumors. Prostate. 2000;44:156–63.

Singh D. Application of novel drug delivery system in enhancing the therapeutic potential of phytoconstituents. Asian J Pharm. 2015;9(4):S1–S12.

Singh HP, Utreja P, Tiwari AK, Jain S. Elastic liposomal formulation for sustained delivery of colchicine: in vitro characterization and in vivo evaluation of anti-gout activity. AAPS J. 2009;11:54–64.

Szejtli J. Cyclodextrins and their inclusion complexes. Budapest: AkadémiaiKiadó; 1982. p. 296.

Szejtli J. Cyclodextrin technology. Dordrecht: Kluwer Academic; 1988. p. 450.

Teng Y, Morrison ME, Munk P, Webber SE, Prochazka K. Release kinetics studies of aromatic molecules into water from block polymer micelles. Macromolecules. 1998;31:3578–87.

Thamake SI, Raut SL, Ranjan AP, Gryczynski Z, Vishwanatha JK. Surface functionalization of PLGA nanoparticles by non-covalent insertion of a homo-bifunctional spacer for active targeting in cancer therapy. Nanotechnology. 2011;22(3):035101.

Thompson DO. Cyclodextrins—enabling excipients: their present and future use in pharmaceuticals. Crit Rev Ther Drug. 1997;14:1–104.

Touitou E, Alkabes M, Dayan N, Eliaz M. Ethosomes: the novel vesicular carriers for enhanced skin delivery. Pharm Res. 1997;14:305–6.

Uchegbu IF, Vyas SP. Non-ionic surfactant based vesicles (niosomes) in drug delivery. Int J Pharm. 1998;33:172–6.

Vadhanam MV, Ravoori S, Aqil F, Gupta RC. Chemoprevention of mammary carcinogenesis by sustained systemic delivery of ellagic acid. Eur J Cancer Prev. 2011;20:484–91.

Varde NK, Pack DW. Microspheres for controlled release drug delivery. Expert Opin Biol Ther. 2004;4:35–51.

Verma P, Pathak K. Therapeutic and cosmeceutical potential of ethosomes: an overview. J Adv Pharm Technol Res. 2010;1:274–82.

Vyas A, Saraf S, Saraf S. Cyclodextrin based novel drug delivery system. J Incl Phenom Macrocycl Chem. 2008;62:23–42.

Wall JG, Burris HA, Von Hoff DD, Rodriguez G, Kneuper-Hall R, Shaffer D, et al. A phase I clinical and pharmacokinetic study of the topoisomerase I inhibitor topotecan (SK&F 104864) given as an intravenous bolus every 21 days. Anticancer Drugs. 1992;3:337–45.

Wang X, Jiang Y, Wang YW, et al. Enhancing anti-inflammation activity of curcumin through O/W nanoemulsions. Food Chem. 2008;108:419–24.

Weiss R, Fintelmann V. Herbal medicine. 2nd ed. Stuttgart, New York: Thieme; 2000.

Wen Z, Liu B, Zheng Z, You X, Pu Y, Li Q. Preparation of liposomes entrapping essential oil from Atractylodes macrocephala Koidz by modified RESS technique. Chem Eng Res Design. 2010;88:1102–7.

Wiernik PH, Schwartz EL, Strauman JJ, Dutcher JP, Lipton RB, Paietta E. Phase I clinical and pharmacokinetic study of taxol. Cancer Res. 1987;47:2486–93.

Xiao L, Zhang YH, Xu JC, Jin XH. Preparation of floating rutin-alginate-chitosan microcapsule. Chin Trad Herb Drugs. 2008;2:209–12.

Xiao-Ying L, Luo JB, Yan ZH, Rong HS, Huang WM. Preparation and in vitro-in vivo evaluations of topically applied capsaicin transferosomes. Yao Xue Xue Bao. 2006;41:461–6.

Yallapu MM, Gupta BK, Jaggi M, Chauhan SC. Fabrication of curcumin encapsulated PLGA nanoparticles for improved therapeutic effects in metastatic cancer cells. J Colloid Interface Sci. 2010;351:19–29.

You J, Cui FD, Han X, Wang YS, Yang L, Yu YW, Li OP. Study of the preparation of sustained releasemicrospheres containing zedoary turmeric oil by the emulsion solvent diffusion method and evaluation of theself emulsification and bioavailability of the oil. Colloids Surf B Biointerfaces. 2006;48:35–41.

Zhang J, Jasti B, Li X. Formulation and characterization of silibinin-loaded sterically stabilized solid lipid nanoparticles. Drug Deliv. 2007;15:381–7.

Zhao HR, Wang K, Zhao Y, Pan LQ. Novel sustained release implant of herbal extract using chitosan. Biomaterials. 2002;23:4459–62.

Plant Derived Polysaccharides as Pharmaceutical Excipients: An Overview

13

Rajendra Awasthi, Bhupesh Sharma, and Giriraj T. Kulkarni

Contents

13.1 Introduction

Polysaccharide hydrogels possess high adhesive and cohesive properties due to their branched and complex polymeric structure. This makes them highly useful in pharmaceutical preparations. Polysaccharide hydrogels resemble the extracellular matrices of tissues comprised of various glycosaminoglycans. Hence, polysaccharide hydrogels find diverse applications in the pharmaceutical industry. The biotechnological applications of polysaccharide hydrogels are due to their gelling properties and entrapment capabilities. They are used for separation of gene and chromosome fragments and in the entrapment of living microorganisms, plant and

R. Awasthi · B. Sharma · G. T. Kulkarni (✉)
Amity Institute of Pharmacy, Amity University Uttar Pradesh, Noida, Uttar Pradesh, India

S. Sen, R. Chakraborty (eds.), *Herbal Medicine in India*,
https://doi.org/10.1007/978-981-13-7248-3_13

animal cells, and enzymes. This is called immobilization. The immobilized cells and enzymes can be used for carrying out bioconversions, which are difficult to achieve by chemical methods. This chapter describes early investigations carried out on pharmaceutical, biotechnological and biomedical (tissue engineering) applications of polysaccharide hydrogels. Extremely large number of polysaccharide hydrogels has been investigated for the preparation of drug products.

13.2 Pharmaceutical Applications of Polysaccharide Hydrogels

The polysaccharide hydrogels have been widely used as adhesive and laxative. These hydrophilic polymers are used as disintegrant, binder and sustaining agent in tablet formulation, emulsifier, gelling and stabilizing agent, thickening agent, and suspending and protective colloid in suspensions. Pharmaceutical applications of some polysaccharide hydrogels are summarized in Table 13.1.

Table 13.1 Pharmaceutical applications of polysaccharide hydrogels

Name	Source	Family	Pharmaceutical applications	Reference
Guar gum	*Cyamompsis tetraganolobus*	Leguminosae	Disintegrant, binder, emulsifier, thickening agent, laxative	Tharanathan (1995)
Locust bean gum	*Ceratania siliqua*	Leguminosae	Stabilizer, thickening agent	Tharanathan (1995)
Xanthan gum	*Xanthomonas lempestris*		Suspending agent, emulsifier, stabilizer in tooth paste and ointments	Tharanathan (1995)
Pectin	*Citrus aurantium*	Rutaceae	Thickening agent, suspending agent	Tharanathan (1995)
Karaya gum	*Sterculia urens*	Sterculiaceae	Suspending agent, emulsifier, dental adhesive, bulk laxative	Tharanathan (1995), Kokate et al. (2002), Evans (1996)
Sodium alginate	*Macrocytis pyrifera*	Lessoniaceae	Suspending agent, gelation for dental films, stabilizer	Bruneton (1995)
Agar	*Gelidium amansii*	Gelidaceae	Suspending agent, emulsifier, gelling agent in suppositories, surgical lubricant, disintegrant, base for bacterial culture, laxative	Bruneton (1995)
Carrageenan	*Chondrus crispus*	Gliganrtinaceae	Gelling agent, stabilizer in emulsions and suspensions, demulcent and laxative	Bruneton (1995)
Ispagol mucilage	*Plantago psyllium, Plantago ovata*	Plantaginaceae	Cathartic, lubricant, laxative, demulcent, tablet disintegrant	Kokate et al. (2002), Evans (1996), Bruneton (1995)
Fenugreek mucilage	*Trigonellafoenum graecum*	Leguminosae	Sustaining agent, emollient and demulcent, gelling agent	Kokate et al. (2002), Evans (1996), Bruneton (1995), Baveja et al. (1988), Sarasija and Hota (2000)
Gum ghatti	*Anogeissus latifolia*	Combretaceae	Binder, emulsifier, suspending agent, sustaining agent	Tharanathan (1995), Baveja et al. (1988)
Linseed mucilage	*Linium usitatissiumum*	Linaceae	Sustaining agent in tablets	Tharanathan (1995), Baveja et al. (1988)
Abelmoschus mucilage	*Abelmoschus esculentus*	Malvaceae	Binder in tablets, matrix material for sustaining the drug release	Ofoefule et al. (2001), Ofoefule and Chukwu (2001)

Table 13.1 (continued)

Name	Source	Family	Pharmaceutical applications	Reference
Tamarind seed polysaccharide	*Tamarindus indica*	Leguminosae	Sustaining agent	Kulkarni et al. (1997)
Mesquite gum	*Prosopis tulifora*	Leguminosae	Binding agent	Khanna et al. (1997)
Bavchi mucilage	*Ocimum canum*	Labiatae	Suspending agent, emulsifying agent	Patel et al. (1987), Patel and Chauhan (1987)
Asario mucilage	*Lepidum sativum*	Cruciferae	Suspending agent, emulsifying agent	Patel et al. (1987), Patel and Chauhan (1987)
Shatavari mucilage	*Asparagus racemosus*	Apocynaceae	Sustaining agent, binding agent	Kulkarni et al. (2002a), Tharanathan (1995), Baveja et al. (1988)
Drumstick mucilage	*Moringa pterygosperma*	Moringaceae	Suspending agent, emulsifier, film forming agent	Rao and Mishra (1993)
Hibiscus mucilage	*Hibiscus esculentus*	Malvaceae	Emulsifying agent	Wahi et al. (1985)
Cashew gum	*Anacardium occidentale*	Anacardiaceae	Suspending agent	Ibezim et al. 2000
Aloe mucilage	*Aloe species*	Liliaceae	Sustaining agent in tablets	Tharanathan (1995), Baveja et al. (1988)
Neem gum	*Azadirachta indica*	Meliaceae	Sustaining agent	Tharanathan (1995), Baveja et al. (1988)
Coco yam mucilage	*Colocasia esculenta*	Araceae	Sustaining agent	Tharanathan (1995), Baveja et al. (1988)
Ocimum mucilage	*Ocimum canum*	Labiatae	Sustaining agent	Tharanathan (1995), Baveja et al. (1988)

13.2.1 Application of Polysaccharide Hydrogels in Tablet Formulation

Polysaccharide hydrogels are widely used as a binding agent in tablet formulation because of their adhesive nature. They impart cohesiveness to the powdered material and convert it into a granular mass with improved flow properties. A polysaccharide gum from the pods of *Abelmoschus esculentus* was used as a binder for a poorly water soluble drug sulfaguanidine, and it has been reported that the solubility of the drug improved when the gum was used at 4% concentration (Ofoefule et al. 2001). A gum from *Prosopis juliflora* has been used as a binder and a comparison was made between the isolated gum and standard binders acacia and tragacanth in lactose tablets. The gum had equivalent binding property as that of acacia and tragacanth (Khanna et al. 1997). Locust bean gum is galactomannan polysaccharide obtained from seeds of *Ceratonia siliqua*. It contains linear α-(1-6)-D-galactopyranosyl and β-(1-4)-D-mannopyranosyl. The hydrophobic nature of Locust bean gum is due to the presence of high content of mannose. High viscosity of Locust bean gum makes it a suitable binding agent, thickening agent and rate controlling agent in the development of controlled release systems (Upadhyay et al. 2018).

Antony and Sanghavi (1997a) have reported the use of gellan gum as binding agent for ibuprofen tablets. The gellan gum tablets exhibited better physical properties than those of other binders, such, as acacia, starch, gelatin, hydroxypropyl methyl cellulose (HPMC), polyvinyl alcohol (PVA) and Polyvinylpyrrolidone (PVP), and the drug release was faster in gellan gum tablets.

Jain and Dixit (1988) evaluated the binding properties of three polysaccharide gums from *Cochlospermum gossypium*, *Anogeissus latifolia* and *Buchanania lanzan* and their carbozymethyl and methoxyl derivatives in sodium bicarbonate tablets. They have reported that the gum from

Cochlospermum gossypium produced harder tablets than acacia, but the disintegration was faster than acacia tablets. Also, the derivatives exhibited less friability than the gums.

Gum karaya and its modified low viscosity form have been mixed with nimodipine using co-grinding technique (Murali et al. 2002). The mixture was then compressed into tablets. The tablets prepared using modified gum exhibited better dissolution profiles. *Cassia fistula* galactomannan has been used as a binder in lactose tablets. The tablets exhibited better physical properties than other gums used for comparison (Tausif et al. 1992).

Kulkarni et al. (2002a) have reported the use of *Asparagus racemosus* and *Cassia sophera* mucilages as binders in paracetamol tablets. The polysaccharide mucilage from *Plantago ovata* and *Trigonellafoenum-graecum* have been used as binders in paracetamol tablets (Kulkarni et al. 2002b). It has been reported that the hardness of tablets increased with binder concentration and the drug release was delayed up to 3 h.

The polysaccharide hydrogels can also be used as disintegrants in tablets. The disintegrant property of polysaccharide hydrogels is due to their ability to absorb water and swell (Deshpande and Panya 1987). This swelling leads to faster disintegration of tablets, which improves the dissolution. Modified USP xanthan gum (Rizk et al. 1997), gellan gum (Antony and Sanghavi 1997b), *Ocimum basilicum* and *Plantago ovate* (Srinivas et al. 2003) mucilages have been studied for their disintegrants properties in tablet formulations.

13.2.2 Polysaccharide Hydrogels as Emulsifying and Suspending Agents

Polysaccharide hydrogels can act as suspending and emulsifying agent. Emulsions can be effectively stabilized by polysaccharide hydrogels via interfacial adsorption and subsequent development of condensed film of high tensile strength, which resist coalescence of droplets. They stabilize oil-in-water emulsions by forming a strong multimolecular film (Martin et al. 2002) around oil globules. This retards coalescence due to the presence of a hydrophilic barrier between the oil-water phase. Filled hydrogels have gained special attention of formulation scientist in emulsification process. This new class of hydrogels consists of (1) an external phase of hydrophilic polymer, and (2) an internal phase of materials, such as oils, natural polymers such as protein and polysaccharide (Choudhary et al. 2018).

When used as suspending agents, the polysaccharide hydrogels increase the strength of hydration layer developed around suspended particles via hydrogen bonding, and molecular interactions. Polysaccharide hydrogels do not reduce the interfacial and surface tension and thus, effective in the presence of wetting agent. Natural polysaccharide hydrogels are hydrophilic colloids, which form dispersion with water and increase the viscosity of continuous phase, so that the solid particles remain suspended in it for a sufficiently long time to measure a uniform dose.

The emulsifying properties of *Hibiscus esculentus* and *Hygrophila spinosa* mucilages have been studied using liquid paraffin and turpentine oil as oily phases (Wahi et al. 1985). The mucilage from *H. spinosa* was found to be a better emulsifying agent. Patel et al. (1987) have studied the emulsifying properties of *Lepidium sativum* and *Ocimum canum* mucilages. Both the mucilages exhibited excellent emulsifying properties at 0.4% w/v, and *Ocimum* mucilage was found to be superior to *Lepidium* mucilage.

A polysaccharide gum from the seeds of *Leucaena leucocephala* was evaluated as an emulsifying agent using liquid paraffin as oily phase, in a concentration range of 1-4% w/v. It has been reported that the isolated gum had better emulsifying properties than gum acacia (Verma and Razdan 2003a).

Lepidium sativum and *Ocimum canum* polysaccharides have been evaluated as suspending agents in ammoniated mercury, bismuth subnitrate, kaolin, sulfur and zinc oxide suspensions and comparison was made with tragacanth (Patel et al. 1987). Among the two polysaccharides, *Ocimum canum* mucilage was the best suspending agent. The suspending properties of *Anacardium occidentale* gum were studied by Ibezim et al. (2000). Chalk suspensions were prepared with different concentrations of the selected gum and veegum, which was used for comparison. The effect of pH, preservatives and electrolytes on the stability was studied. The selected gum was found to be a good suspending agent.

Verma and Razdan (2003b) used *Leucaena leucocephala* seed gum as a suspending agent for sulfadimidine suspensions. Tragacanth was used as standard for comparison. The suspensions prepared with isolated gum had good stability and redispersion properties.

13.2.3 Polysaccharide Hydrogels as Sustaining Agents

Polysaccharide hydrogels can be used for sustaining the drug release. They have been used in tablets, suspensions, or as matrix systems for sustaining the drug release (Subramanian and Vijayakumar 2015). Polysaccharide hydrogels, get hydrated and form gel in presence of water. The drug release from this gel is usually diffusion controlled and hence sustains the drug release (Babu et al. 2002).

Many polysaccharides have been used as matrix materials for sustaining the drug release. *Abelmoschus esculentus* gum was used as matrix material for furosemide and diclofenac sodium tablets (Ofoefule and Chukwu 2001). Sodium carboxymethyl cellulose was used as standard. The selected gum was equally good as standard in prolonging the drug release. Billa and Yuen (2000) studied the effect of thermal treatment on the drug release from diclofenac sodium matrix tablets prepared using wet granulation method. It has been reported that the thermal treatment did not affect the swelling of tablets and release of drug.

Sodium alginate has been used as hydrophilic matrix material for prolonging the release of ketoprofen from tablets prepared by direct compression using sodium alginate, calcium gluconate and HPMC, in different combinations (Giunchedi et al. 2000). The matrix tablets prepared with sodium alginate alone or in combination with 10% or 20% HPMC gave a prolonged drug release at a fairly constant rate. Methylated guar gum has been evaluated as matrix material for chlorpheniramine maleate (CPM) and the release kinetics have been reported (Baweja and Misra 1997). The methylation of guar gum was found to reduce its swelling property, and thus reduced the drug release significantly. Also, wet granulation was found to impart better cohesiveness and retard the release, when compared to direct compression.

Tamarind seed polyose has been evaluated as matrix material for sustaining the release of verapamil hydrochloride (Kulkarni et al. 1997). *In vitro* release was correlated with *in vivo* bioavailability of the drug in rabbits. A good *in vitro-in vivo* correlation has been reported. Xanthan gum, in combination with n-octenyl succinate starch, has been evaluated as matrix material, using ibuprofen as a model drug (Ntawukulilyayo et al. 1996). The matrix tablets were prepared by direct compression. The combination matrix did not erode completely during dissolution, whereas pure xanthan gum matrix eroded completely. Also, the combination matrix was found to avoid the initial slow absorption phase in the bioavailability studies. The swelling and release behaviour of xanthan gum matrix tablets were studied (Talukdar and Kinget 1995) using three different drugs, caffeine (soluble-neutral), indomethacin (insoluble-acidic) and sodium salt of indomethacin (soluble-acidic). The swelling property of tablets was found to be influenced by ionic strength and buffer concentrations and the drug release was influenced by the solubility of the drug.

Sujja-areevath et al. (1996) have studied the release characteristics of diclofenac sodium from encapsulated natural mini-matrix formulations. Carrageenan, karaya locust bean, and xanthan gums were used to produce mini matrices containing gum, drug and other release regulating excipients. The release characteristics showed sustained release of the drug up to 77% from mini-matrices containing locust bean, karaya and xanthan gum. Carrageenan did not produce sufficient sustained release. The drug release process followed swelling and relaxation. The concentration of gum present played a dominant role in determining the drug release rate.

Baveja et al. (1988, 1989) examined natural gums and mucilages for their sustaining properties in tablet dosage forms. Twenty-two natural gums and mucilages were evaluated for their ability to sustain the release of freely soluble drug propranolol hydrochloride from tablets. Comparison was made with synthetic methylcellulose polymers. Tablets produced from plant products had *in vitro* release rates ranging from 4 to 12 h; whereas those prepared using the polymers had release rates from 1 to 7.4 h.

13.2.4 Polysaccharide Hydrogels as Coating Agents

Many polysaccharide hydrogels have been investigated as coating agents to sustain the drug release or to protect active ingredient from degradation in gastric fluid. A patent has been granted to Hingston et al. (2018) for their invention based on adhesive stent coating for anti-migration drugs using polysaccharide. The mucilage from drumstick polysaccharide (*Moringa pterygosperma*) has been documented as a good film-coating polymer, which retarded drug release from granules at 2% w/w concentration (Rao and Mishra 1993). Tamarind seed polysaccharide has also been used as aqueous coating agent for paracetamol granules (Nagarsenkar and Deshpande 1990). The granules were evaluated for flow rate, Hausner ratio, granule strength and drug release. The flow properties and Hausner ratios were not affected by coating. The granule strength and t_{90} of dissolution were found to increase with an increase in the concentration of coating material. In an interesting report, soluble soybean polysaccharide and tragacanth gum polysaccharide have been reported as an effective edible coating material in the presence of calcium chloride and ascorbic acid for fresh cut apple slices (Jafari et al. 2018).

13.2.5 Application of Polysaccharide Hydrogels in Microencapsulation

The polysaccharide hydrogels, because of their coating ability, find application in microencapsulation to sustain the drug release (Anderson and Langer 2018). Microencapsulation properties of *Acacia senegal* gum *and Acacia nilotica* gum have been investigated for their microencapsulating properties using spray-drying technique. *A. nilotica* gum is reported to be a better microcapsulating agent (Chattopadhyay et al. 1997). Polysaccharide hydrogel isolated from *Tamarindus indica* (tamarind) seeds has been reported as release modifier from spheroid formulations. The study reported a reliable correlation between swelling index, surface roughness of the polysaccharide, viscosity, and *in vitro* drug release profile. In bioavailability studies, the spheroids containing polysaccharide hydrogel were able to sustain the drug release over 8 h (Kulkarni et al. 2005). Locust bean gum and sodium alginate based interpenetrating polymeric network containing Capecitabine encapsulated in microbeads have shown promising pharmacokinetic and cytotoxicity results in HT-29 cells (Upadhyay et al. 2018).

13.2.6 Polysaccharide Hydrogels as Gelling Agents

Polysaccharide hydrogels find application in the formulation of pharmaceutical gels. Polysaccharide hydrogels can form gels as a result of inter and intra molecular association and formation of a water entrapped three-dimensional network (Rees et al. 1982). Gel formation is induced by either physical (change in temperature and pH) or chemical (addition of suitable reagents) treatments. In case of acidic polysaccharides such as pectin, the gelatin is due to the formation of junction zones within wide hydrogen bonded chains (Mabeau and Fleurence 1993). In case of alginic acid, the gel formation occurs as a result of formation of calcium alginate due to the interaction with calcium ions. Galactomannans form elastic gel by interacting synergistically with carrageenans or xanthan gum.

Even though a variety of structures are involved with gel networks, most of the pharmaceutical gels are random coil networks, the mechanism of which is rooted in the polymer-polymer and polymer-solvent interactions (Bruneton 1995). The strength of gel network increases with increase in polymer concentration. This reduces the interparticle distance, which subsequently leads to chain entanglement and further development of crosslinks. Polysaccharide hydrogel from the seeds of *Trigonellafoenum graecum* has been reported to possess good gelling property and it has been used as transdermal gel with diclofenac diethylammonium as model drug (Gowthamarajan et al. 2002).

13.2.7 Polysaccharide Hydrogels for Colon Targeting of Drugs

Colon targeted drug delivery is valuable in the treatment of ulcerative colitis and Chron's disease where high local concentration of drug is desired while minimizing premature drug release and side effects. Colon is a desirable site for vaccine delivery due to rich lymphoid tissue of colonic mucosa (Sarasija and Hota 2000). Colon is also attracting interest as a site for improving the bioavailability of poorly absorbed drugs. Many approaches are used for colonic delivery of drugs and one among them is embedding of drug in polymer matrices, which can degrade in colon and liberate the entrapped drug. Polysaccharides are known to retain their structural integrity in gastric and intestinal fluids. These are resistant to the gastrointestinal enzymes. The polysaccharide matrix degrades by colonic bacterial polysaccharidases and allows the drug to release (Chaurasia and Jain 2003). Many polysaccharide hydrogels have been used as matrices for colon targeting of drugs. Some of them include xanthan gum (Sinha et al. 2004), guar gum (Sinha et al. 2004), amylase (Siew et al. 2004) and calcium alginate (Xing et al. 2003). They have been used to deliver anticancer drugs, antibiotics and peptides to the colon.

13.2.8 Applications of Polysaccharide Hydrogels in Ocular Delivery Systems

Ocular drug delivery systems present major challenges for formulation scientists due to the extensive precorneal loss caused by the drainage of tear fluid. Only 10% of the drug crosses the corneal barriers and reach the posterior segment of the eye. Polysaccharide hydrogels have been widely used in the development of ocular drug delivery system to increase the residence time of drugs on the eye and minimize the loss of drug due to the precorneal loss. In situ gelation property of polysaccharide hydrogels makes them a suitable candidate for the development of ocular drug delivery systems. In situ hydrogels undergoes a sol-to-gel transition in the cul-de-sac with change in ions, pH and temperature.

Lin and coworkers reported in situ gelling system of alginate and Pluronic solutions for ocular delivery of Pilocarpine. Effective in situ gel was formed at 2% w/w and 14% w/w for alginate solution and Pluronic solution, respectively. The mixture of alginate solution (0.1% w/w) and Pluronic solution (14% w/w) had highest gel strength with free flow at room temperature (25 °C) and pH 4.0. The solution containing a mixture of alginate/Pluronic retained Pilocarpine for prolonged time than the alginate or Pluronic solutions alone (Lin et al. 2004). Film forming and release modifier properties of *Tamarindus indica* seed polysaccharide have been reported by Kulkarni and co-workers. They reported controlled drug release over a period of 8 h from the polysaccharide containing ocular films. The films were stable and reduced the intraocular pressure for 24 h in a more efficient manner than the eye drops (Kulkarni et al. 2016).

Cyclodextrins are cyclic oligosaccharides with a hydrophobic internal cavity and a hydrophilic outer surface. It has been reported that the drug reached retina and optic nerve and maintained desired concentrations for 8 h after administration of the eye drops containing cyclodextrin (Sigurdsson et al. 2005). Co-polymerization of glycidyl methacrylate with hydrogels of acetazolamide, hydrocortisone has been reported to create poly (hydroxyl ethyl methacrylate) hydrogels for ophthalmic delivery (dos Santos et al. 2008, 2009). Diaz-Tome et al. used cyclodextrin to improve the solubility of econazole for the effective management of fungal keratitis. Econazole-α-cyclodextrin complex was incorporated in two types of ocular hydrogels (a hyaluronic acid hydrogel and a natural polysaccharides ion-sensitive hydrogel). These hydrogels were non-irritating and controlled drug release over

24 h. Ocular bio-permanence studies indicated retention of antifungal drug on eye for prolonged time periods (Diaz-Tome et al. 2018).

Sodium hyaluronate is frequently used polysaccharide due to its extreme water holding capacity and viscoelastic properties. It is used in the formulation of drug products to treat dry eye disease. Vismed® (Horus Pharma, France), Hylo™ (Candorvision, Canada), and Aqualarm® (Bausch + Lomb, Bridgewater, NJ, USA) are the example of Sodium hyaluronate based ophthalmic products available in the example (Lai et al. 2010; Bora et al. 2016; Widjaja et al. 2014). Lei and co-workers (2018) fabricated cross-linked Chitosan hydrogel sheets for the ocular delivery of levofloxacin. These hydrogel sheets were porous (20–150 μm) and allowed diffusion of the encapsulated drug first 30 min, followed by a sustained release up to 24 h. The results of cytocompatibility test with L-929 cells after 24 h of incubation suggested that the formulated hydrogels were noncytotoxic (Lei et al. 2018).

13.3 Applications of Polysaccharide Hydrogels in Tissue Engineering

Synthesis, derivetization, evaluation, and characterization of natural polysaccharide bioactive compounds are an interdisciplinary field of biomedical science. Khan and Ahmad reviewed chemistry and modifications of various polysaccharides for tissue engineering applications (Khan and Ahmad 2013). Polymeric systems are used in tissue engineering due to their sol-to-gel transition ability under physiological conditions (Gutowska et al. 2001). Polysaccharides obtained from the marine eukaryotes and marine prokaryotes could be the alternative to traditional polysaccharides such as glycosaminoglycans present in all animals (Senni et al. 2011). Sulfated polysaccharides, obtained from different marine algae, are receiving growing interest in tissue engineering due to resemble chemical and biological properties of mammalian glycosaminoglycans (Silva et al. 2012). During the past 2–3 decades, polysaccharides have been reported to be useful in the engineering of various body tissues such as articular cartilage, blood vessels, bone, heart valves, intervertebral discs, liver, menisci, myocardium, neural tissue, skeletal muscle, skin, tracheal cartilage, and urinary bladder. Polysaccharides have been used as hydrogels or fibrous or porous scaffolds (Bacakova et al. 2014). Poly(lactide-co-glycolide) is the common scaffold material approved by US FDA for use in the body (Drury and Mooney 2003). Mohan and Nair prepared highly porous 3D scaffolds using alginate for tissue engineering of bone, cartilage and liver (Mohan and Nair 2005).

Chitosan, obtained from crustacean exoskeleton, is the most versatile biopolymer used for tissue engineering and orthopaedic applications (Di Martino et al. 2005; Venkatesan and Kim 2010; Croisier and Jerome 2013). It has been used for the preparation of porous scaffold in tissue-relevant geometries by controlled freezing and lyophilization. The scaffold formed included porous membranes, blocks, tubes and beads. Depending on the freezing conditions, the pore diameter varied from 1 to 250 μm. The pore structure can be retained by treating lyophilized Chitosan scaffold with glycosaminoglycans due to the formation of ionic complex (Madihally and Matthew 1999). Scaffolds composed of the natural hydrophilic polysaccharides (dextran and pullulan) supplemented or not with nanocrystalline hydroxyapatite has been proposed as a material for stimulating bone cell differentiation of host mesenchymal stem cells and bone formation for orthopedic and maxillofacial surgical applications (Fricain et al. 2013).

Many investigators have described the combination of polysaccharides with natural or synthetic polymers. Agar, alginate, cellulose, chitin and chitosan, dextran, gellan, glycosaminoglycans, pectins, pullulan, starch, and xanthan are the most widely used polysaccharides in tissue engineering (Bacakova et al. 2014). Suh and Matthew published an interesting review reporting application of chitosan-based polysaccharide hydrogel in cartilage tissue engineering (Suh and Matthew 2000). Bioartificial blends of poly-(ϵ-caprolactone) with a polysaccharide (dextran, gellan and starch) prepared by a solution-precipitation technique have shown promising outcomes in tissue engineering. The thermal stability of these blends was affected by the type of polysaccharide (Ciardelli et al. 2005). Tan et al. reported application of Chitosan and oxidized hyaluronic acid derived injectable hydrogel in tissue engineering. They synthesized aldehyde hyaluronic acid and *N*-succinyl-chitosan for the preparation of hydrogels. Bovine articular chondrocytes were encapsulated within the hydrogel. The derived hydrogel confirmed cell survival and retention of cellschondrocytic morphology (Tan et al. 2009, 2010). Iwasaki and co-workers tested the hypothesis that alginate-based chitosan hybrid biomaterials could provide excellent supports for chondrocyte adhesion. Alginate-chitosan copolymer fibers showed better adhesion property with chondrocytes than the alginate polymer fiber. The study demonstrated the applicability of alginate-chitosan copolymer fiber as cartilage tissue scaffold biomaterial (Iwasaki et al. 2004).

13.4 Biotechnological Applications of Polysaccharide Hydrogels

Polysaccharides, especially from marine algae, find a vast range of applications in biotechnology due to their gelling properties and entrapment capabilities. Some of the important applications are described below.

13.4.1 Gene Fragment Separation

DNA sequence coding for a specific protein can be cut from a gene using restriction endonucleases, which cleave the DNA between certain defined nucleotide sequences. After cleavage of DNA using restriction enzymes, the required fragments are separated using agarose gel electrophoresis (Alexander et al. 1985; Andrews 1986). In genetic engineering, agarose gel electrophoresis has a major role. Isolation of required gene from genome or a particular chromosome, isolation of 'plasmid' DNA which is used as vector, essentially needs agarose gel electrophoresis. Without this, it would not have been possible to carry out gene manipulation in microorganisms to produce human proteins such as recombinant insulin, interferon, growth hormones and other such proteins (Andrews 1986).

13.4.2 Chromosome Fragment Separation

Small and large chromosomal DNA fragments created by restriction enzyme treatment are separated on agarose gels pulsed field gel electrophoresis (PFGE) technique. In this technique, an electric current is alternately imposed at a predetermined angle to the direction of electrophoretic migration (Schwartz et al. 1983). Modified PFGE techniques have been reported for genetic disorder-specific chromosomal fragment separations.

13.4.3 Artificial Organs

An implant containing insulin or other hormone developing cells produces reverse physiological consequences due to the deficiency of such hormones. The techniques are under investigation to implant the living tissues or cells to keep them isolated to avoid problems like rejection by immune system. Cages of agarose, its low-gelling-temperature hydroxyethyl derivatives and calcium alginate are compatible with this application (Guiseley 1976, 1987, 1989). Encapsulated insulin-producing islets of Langerhans cells have been reported by various researchers (Lim and Sun 1980; Howell et al. 1982; Bouhaddioui et al. 1985; Goosen et al. 1989; Goosen et al. 1985; Gin et al. 1987; Iwata et al. 1988). Immobilized rat hepatocytes in alginate droplets retained enzymatic detoxifying activity (Yarmush et al. 1988). Adaniya reported live pre-implantation mouse embryos encapsulated in calcium alginate womb (Adaniya et al. 1987).

13.4.4 Cell and Enzyme Immobilization

Immobilization (imprisonment) refers to physical or chemical trapping of cell or enzyme into the polymer matrix. Most commonly used techniques of immobilization are 'entrapment' and 'encapsulation' (Trevan 1987; Kierstan and Coughlan 1985) using polysaccharides such as agar, agarose, κ-carrageenan, starch gel, cellulose derivatives or alginates as encapsulating agents (Rees et al. 1982; Madan 1979; Trevan 1987; Guilbault and Neto 1985; Zucca et al. 2016). Mohan et al. (2015) reported a hydrophobically modified biocompatible nanolayer polysaccharide derivative suitable for the immobilization of horseradish peroxidase. They reported formation of water-soluble benzylamide of carboxymethyl cellulose from carbodiimide mediated reaction of benzylamine with carboxymethyl cellulose yields.

13.4.4.1 Immobilization by Entrapment

Entrapment of enzyme/cell within a polymer matrix is easy to perform. For entrapment, two types of polymers, namely, synthetic (like polyacrylamide) or natural (like cellulose derivatives, agar, gelatin, carrageenan) are used. The natural polymers, because of their biocompatible and hydrophilic nature, allow better activity of cells and enzymes entrapped in them (Trevan 1987). The physicochemical properties of seaweed polysaccharides utilized for cell immobilization have been extensively studied by Guiseley (1989). He has reported that sodium alginate was the most suitable and convenient polymer for cell immobilization as they are thermally irreversible. Nehra et al. (1998) studied the alkaline protease production by mycelium of *Aspergillus* species immobilized in agar, sodium alginate and polyacrylamide gel matrices and found that the immobilized mycelia performed better over a wide range of temperatures and pH compared to free mycelia and cells immobilized in sodium alginate proved better and performed well up to seventh cycle of reuse.

Sutar et al. (1986) have studied the alkaline protease secretion by immobilized mycelium of *Conidiobolus* (NCL 82-1-1) entrapped in carrageenan and polyurethane sponge. They found that both immobilized mycelia could be repeatedly used in batch mode under aseptic conditions.

A novel enzyme immobilization method using ascorbic acid on celluloses and polyvinyl alcohol has been developed by Tiller et al. (1999). The enzymes glucose oxidase, glutamase oxidase, lactate oxidase, urate oxidase and peroxidase have been covalently fixed with a high surface loading to ultra-thin and transparent films of selected polymers. They have reported that the immobilized enzymes could be stored for one month's time without becoming detached from the films. The system did not reduce the enzyme activity.

Polymeric alginate films and beads have been used for controlled delivery of bovine serum albumin as model protein (Hermis and Narayani 2002). The films were prepared by moulding technique and the beads were prepared by extrusion-congealing technique. The entrapment of protein into the developed systems was found to be 96–98%. The release of protein was sustained for a period of 18 days.

Orive et al. (2003) have studied the behaviour of hybridoma cells after immobilization in alginate-agarose microcapsules. The results showed that the hybridoma cells exhibited better growing pattern and improved viability. The antibody production also increased within the liquefied beads. However, the beads did not show mechanical strength, when compared to solid beads. In solid beads, the hybridoma cells exhibited prolonged viability for 70 days, in comparison to the 15 days' viability of normal hybridoma cells.

13.4.4.2 Immobilization by Encapsulation

Microencapsulation of enzymes can be done by enclosing a droplet of enzyme solution in a semipermeable membrane capsule (Trevan 1987) The polymers used for this purpose are classified into two groups, namely, permanent (like nylon) or biodegradable (like polylactic acid, phospholipids). The disadvantage of this system is its mechanical instability. Hence, it is not widely used (Trevan 1987).

Polysaccharides find applications in dosage form development and in techniques of biotechnology. Systematic investigation of natural polysaccharide hydrogels can lead to interesting discoveries in the fields of pharmaceutical investigations. Various plant polysaccharide hydrogel materials have not been investigated till date. Hence, it is worthwhile to evaluate the pharmaceutical and biotechnological applications of polysaccharide hydrogels from plant origin.

13.5 Conclusions

Polysaccharides are widely used materials in pharmaceutical, biotechnological and biomedical fields due to their excellent biocompatibility profiles. It is evident that the plant based polysaccharides are much better than synthetic polymers for making hydrogels. The formation to polysaccharide hydrogels is quite easy due to the presence of several chemical groups in linear chain of polysaccharide. Thixotropy of these materials is high due to the presence of large amounts of water. It means polysaccharide hydrogels gets liquid under mechanical stress and return to gel after rest (sol-gel transition). It is expected that the polysaccharide hydrogel-network will extremely useful in drug delivery and tissue engineering.

Acknowledgement *Competing financial interests:* The authors declare no competing financial interests.

References

Adaniya GK, Rawlins RG, Miller IF, Zaneveld LJD. Effect of sodium alginate encapsulation on the development of preimplantation mouse embryos. J In Vitro Fertil Embryo Transf. 1987;4:343–5.

Alexander RR, Griffiths JM, Wilkinson ML. Basic biochemical methods. New York: Wiley; 1985. p. 95–101.

Anderson DG, Langer RS, Dang TT, inventors; Children s Medical Center Corp, Massachusetts Institute of Technology, assignee. Hydrogel encapsulated cells and anti-inflammatory drugs. United States patent application US 15/831,570. 2018 Apr 5.

Andrews AT. Electrophoresis: theory, techniques and biochemical and clinical applications. 2nd ed. Oxford: Clarendon Press; 1986. p. 75–108.

Antony PJ, Sanghavi NM. A new binder for pharmaceutical dosage forms. Drug Dev Ind Pharm. 1997a;23:417–8.

Antony PJ, Sanghavi NM. A new disintegrant for pharmaceutical dosage forms. Drug Dev Ind Pharm. 1997b;23:413–5.

Babu GVMM, Himasankar K, Janaki Ram B, Seshasayana A, Ramana Murthy KV. Studies on preparation and evaluation of modified form of gum karaya. Indian J Pharm Sci. 2002;64:244–9.

Bacakova L, Novotna K, Parizek M. Polysaccharides as cell carriers for tissue engineering: the use of cellulose in vascular wall reconstruction. Physiol Res. 2014;63:S29.

Baveja SK, Rangarao KV, Arora J. Examination of natural gums and mucilages as sustaining materials in tablet dosage forms. Indian J Pharm Sci. 1988;50:89–92.

Baveja SK, Rangarao KV, Arora J. Examination of natural gums and mucilages as sustaining materials in tablet dosage forms-part II. Indian J Pharm Sci. 1989;51:115–8.

Baweja JM, Misra AN. Studies on kinetics of drug release from modified guar gum hydrophilic matrices. Indian J Pharm Sci. 1997;59:316–20.

Billa N, Yuen K. Formulation variables affecting drug release from xanthan gum matrices at laboratory scale up and pilot scale. AAPS Pharm Sci Tech. 2000;1:35–42.. Available from: http//www.pharmscitech.com

Bora M, Mundargi RC, Chee Y, Wong TTL, Venkatraman SS. 5-Flurouracil microencapsulation and impregnation in hyaluronic acid hydrogel as composite drug delivery system for ocular fibrosis. Cogent Med. 2016;3(1):1182108.

Bouhaddioui N, Crespy N, Orsetti A. Functional study of rat islets of Langerhans cultured in agarose cells. CR Soc Biol. 1985;179:21–6.

Bruneton J. Pharmacognosy, phytochemistry, medicinal plants. New York: Lavoisier; 1995.

Chattopadhyay S, Singhal RS, Kulkarni PR. Microencapsulation of vanillin using *Acacia nilotica* gum. J Sci Ind Res (India). 1997;56:109–10.

Chaurasia MK, Jain SK. Pharmaceutical approaches to colon targeted drug delivery systems. J Pharm Pharm Sci. 2003;6:33–66.

Choudhary B, Paul SR, Nayak SK, Qureshi D, Pal K. Synthesis and biomedical applications of filled hydrogels. In: Pal K, Banerjee I, editors. Polymeric gels. Cambridge: Woodhead Publishing; 2018. p. 283–302.

Ciardelli G, Chiono V, Vozzi G, Pracella M, Ahluwalia A, Barbani N, Cristallini C, Giusti P. Blends of poly-(ε-caprolactone) and polysaccharides in tissue engineering applications. Biomacromolecules. 2005;6(4):1961–76.

Croisier F, Jerome C. Chitosan-based biomaterials for tissue engineering. Eur Polym J. 2013;49(4):780–92.

Deshpande AV, Panya LB. Evaluation of sorghum starch as a tablet disintegrants and binder. J Pharm Pharmacol. 1987;39:495–6.

Di Martino A, Sittinger M, Risbud MV. Chitosan: a versatile biopolymer for orthopaedic tissue-engineering. Biomaterials. 2005;26(30):5983–90.

Diaz-Tome V, Luaces-Rodríguez A, Silva-Rodríguez J, Blanco-Dorado S, García-Quintanilla L, Llovo-Taboada J, Blanco-Mendez J, García-Otero X, Varela-Fernández R, Herranz M, Gil-Martinez M. Ophthalmic econazole hydrogels for the treatment of fungal keratitis. J Pharm Sci. 2018;107(5):1342–51.

dos Santos JF, Couceiro R, Concheiro A, Torres-Labandeira JJ, Alvarez-Lorenzo C. Poly (hydroxyethyl methacrylate-co-methacrylated-β-cyclodextrin) hydrogels: synthesis, cytocompatibility, mechanical properties and drug loading/release properties. Acta Biomater. 2008;4(3):745–55.

dos Santos JF, Alvarez-Lorenzo C, Silva M, Balsa L, Couceiro J, Torres-Labandeira JJ, Concheiro A. Soft contact lenses functionalized with pendant cyclodextrins for controlled drug delivery. Biomaterials. 2009;30(7):1348–55.

Drury JL, Mooney DJ. Hydrogels for tissue engineering: scaffold design variables and applications. Biomaterials. 2003;24(24):4337–51.

Evans WC. Trease and Evans' Pharmacognosy. 14th ed. London: W.B. Saunders Company; 1996.

Fricain JC, Schlaubitz S, Le Visage C, Arnault I, Derkaoui SM, Siadous R, Catros S, Lalande C, Bareille R, Renard M, Fabre T. A nano-hydroxyapatite-pullulan/dextran polysaccharide composite macroporous material for bone tissue engineering. Biomaterials. 2013;34(12):2947–59.

Gin H, Dupuy B, Baquey C, Ducassou D, Aubertin J. Agarose encapsulation of islets of Langerhans: reduced toxicity *in vitro*. J Microencapsul. 1987;4:239–42.

Giunchedi P, Gacini E, Moretti MDL, Pirisino G. Evaluation of alginate compressed matrices as prolonged drug delivery systems. AAPS Pharm Sci Tech. 2000;1:E19.. Available from: http//www.pharmscitech.com

Goosen MFA, O'Shea GM, Gharapetian HM, Chou S, Sun AM. Optimization of microencapsulation parameters: semipermeable microcapsules as bioartificial pancreas. Biotechnol Bioeng. 1985;27:146–50.

Goosen MFA, O'Shea GM, Sun AM. Microencapsulation of living tissue and cells, US Patent, No. 4, 806, 355 (1989).

Gowthamarajan K, Kulkarni GT, Muthukumar A, Mahadevan N, Samanta MK, Suresh B. Evaluation of fenugreek mucilage as gelling agent. Int J Pharm Excip. 2002;4(1):16–9.

Guilbault GG, Neto GO. Immobilized enzyme electrodes. In: Woodward J, editor. Immobilized cells and enzymes-a practical approach. Oxford: IRL Press; 1985. p. 55–74.

Guiseley KB. Modified agar and method of making same. US Patent. 3, 956, 273 (1976).

Guiseley KB. Natural and synthetic derivatives of agarose and their use in biochemical separations. In: Yalpani M, editor. Industrial polysaccharides: genetic engineering, structure/property relations and applications. Amsterdam: Elsevier; 1987. p. 139–47.

Guiseley KB. Chemical and physical properties of algal polysaccharides used for cell immobilization. Enzyme Microb Technol. 1989;11:706–16.

Gutowska A, Jeong B, Jasionowski M. Injectable gels for tissue engineering. Anat Rec. 2001;263(4):342–9.

Hermis RS, Narayani R. Polymeric alginate films and beads for the controlled delivery of macromolecules. Trends Biomater Artif Organs. 2002;15(2):54–6.

Hingston J, Jordan G, Bertolino W, Norton PK, Weiner J, inventors; Boston Scientific Scimed Inc, assignee. Adhesive stent coating for anti-migration. United States patent US 9,993,582. 2018 Jun 12.

Howell SL, Ishaq S, Tyhurst M. Possible use of agarose gels as encapsulating media for transplantation of islets of Langerhans. J Physiol. 1982;324:20.

Ibezim EC, Khanna M, Singh S. A study of the suspending properties of *Anacardium occidentale* gum. J Sci Ind Res (India). 2000;59:1038–43.

Iwasaki N, Yamane ST, Majima T, Kasahara Y, Minami A, Harada K, et al. Feasibility of polysaccharide hybrid materials for scaffolds in cartilage tissue engineering: evaluation of chondrocyte adhesion to polyion complex fibers prepared from alginate and chitosan. Biomacromolecules. 2004;5(3):828–33.

Iwata H, Amemiya H, Matsuda T, Takano H, Akutsu T. Microencapsulation of Langerhans islets in agarose microbeads and their application for a bioartificial pancreas. J Bioact Compat Polym. 1988;3:356–69.

Jafari S, Hojjati M, Noshad M. Influence of soluble soybean polysaccharide and tragacanth gum based edible coating to improve the quality of fresh-cut apple slices. J Food Process Preserv. 2018:e13638. https://doi.org/10.1111/jfpp.13638.

Jain JK, Dixit VK. Studies on some gums and their derivatives as binding agents. Indian J Pharm Sci. 1988;50:113–4.

Khan F, Ahmad SR. Polysaccharides and their derivatives for versatile tissue engineering application. Macromol Biosci. 2013;13(4):395–421.

Khanna M, Dwivedi AK, Singh S, Soni PL. Mesquite gum (*Prosopis juliflora*): potential binder in tablet dosage forms. J Sci Ind Res (India). 1997;56:366–8.

Kierstan MPJ, Coughlan MP. Immobilization of cells and enzymes by gel entrapment. In: Woodward J, editor. Immobilized cells and enzymes—a practical approach. Oxford: IRL Press; 1985. p. 39–47.

Kokate CK, Purohit AP, Gokhale SB. Pharmacognosy. 21st ed. Pune: Nirali Prakashan; 2002.

Kulkarni D, Dwedi AK, Sarin JPS, Singh S. Tamarind seed polyose: a potential polysaccharide for sustained release of verapamil hydrochloride as a model drug. Indian J Pharm Sci. 1997;59:1–7.

Kulkarni GT, Gowthamarajan K, Brahmajirao G, Suresh B. Evaluation of binding properties of selected natural mucilages. J Sci Ind Res (India). 2002a;61:529–32.

Kulkarni GT, Gowthamarajan K, Rao BG, Suresh B. Evaluation of binding properties of *Plantago ovata* and *Trigonellafoenum* graecum mucilages. Indian Drugs. 2002b;39:422–5.

Kulkarni GT, Gowthamarajan K, Dhobe RR, Yohanan F, Suresh B. Development of controlled release spheriods using natural polysaccharide as release modifier. Drug Deliv. 2005;12(4):201–6.

Kulkarni GT, Sethi N, Awasthi R, Pawar VK, Pahuja V. Development of ocular delivery system for glaucoma therapy using natural hydrogel as film forming agent and release modifier. Polym Med. 2016;46(1):25–33.

Lai JY, Ma DHK, Cheng HY, Sun CC, Huang SJ, Li YT, Hsiue GH. Ocular biocompatibility of Carbodiimide cross-linked hyaluronic acid hydrogels for cell sheet delivery carriers. J Biomater Sci Polym Ed. 2010;21:359–76.

Lei L, Li X, Xiong T, Yu J, Yu X, Song Z, Li X. Covalently cross-linked chitosan hydrogel sheet for topical ophthalmic delivery of levofloxacin. J Biomed Nanotechnol. 2018;14(2):371–8.

Lim F, Sun AM. Microencapsulated islets as bioartificial endocrine pancreas. Science. 1980;210:908–10.

Lin HR, Sung KC, Vong WJ. *In situ* gelling of alginate/pluronic solutions for ophthalmic delivery of pilocarpine. Biomacromolecules. 2004;5(6):2358–65.

Mabeau S, Fleurence J. Seaweed in food products: biochemical and nutritional aspects. Trends Food Sci Technol. 1993;4:103–7.

Madan PL. Microencapsulation-new techniques and applications. Tokyo: Techno Inc; 1979. p. 11.

Madihally SV, Matthew HW. Porous chitosan scaffolds for tissue engineering. Biomaterials. 1999;20(12):1133–42.

Martin A, Bustamante P, Chun AHC. Physical Pharmacy. 4th ed. New Delhi: B.I. Waverly Pvt. Ltd.; 2002.. p. 423–448, 453–473, 490

Mohan N, Nair PD. Novel porous, polysaccharide scaffolds for tissue engineering applications. Trends Biomater Artif Organs. 2005;18(2):219–24.

Mohan T, Rathner R, Reishofer D, Koller M, Elschner T, Spirk S, Heinze T, Stana-Kleinschek K, Kargl R. Designing hydrophobically modified polysaccharide derivatives for highly efficient enzyme immobilization. Biomacromolecules. 2015;16(8):2403–11.

Murali MBGV, Himasankar K, Kishore Kumar N, Janaki Ram B, Seshasayana A, Ramana Murthy KV. Formulation and evaluation of tablet dosage forms of nimodipine-modified gum karaya co-grinding mixtures. Indian J Pharm Sci. 2002;64:449–54.

Nagarsenkar MS, Deshpande SG. Pan coating of paracetamol granules using tamarind seed polysaccharide. Indian Drugs. 1990;27:48–54.

Nehra KS, Dhillon S, Chaudhary K, Singh R. Production of alkaline protease by immobilized Aspergillus mycelia. Indian J Microbiol. 1998;38:153–6.

Ntawukulilyayo JD, Vervaet C, Remon JP, Gortz JP, Berlo JA. *In vitro* and *in vivo* evaluation of a xanthan gum-n-octenylsuccinate starch matrix tablet containing ibuprofen as a model drug. Int J Pharm. 1996;139:79–85.

Ofoefule SI, Chukwu A. Application of *Abelmoschus esculentus*gum as mini matrix for furosemide and diclofenac sodium tablets. Indian J Pharm Sci. 2001;63:532–5.

Ofoefule SI, Chukwu A, Anyakoha N, Ebebe IM. Application of *Abelmoschus esculentus* in solid dosage formulation 1: Use as a binder for a poorly water soluble drug. Indian J Pharm Sci. 2001;63:234–8.

Orive G, Hernández RM, Gascón AR, Igartua M, Pedraz JL. Survival of different cell lines in alginate-agarose microcapsules. Eur J Pharm Sci. 2003;18:23–30.

Patel NM, Chauhan GM. Suspending properties of the mucilages of *Lepidium sativum* Linn (Asario) and *Ocimumcanum Sims* (Bavchi). East Pharm. 1987;30:137–8.

Patel NM, Chauhan GM, Patel LD. Mucilages of *Lepidium sativum* Linn (Asario) and *Ocimumcanum* Sims (Bavchi) as emulgents. Indian J Hosp Pharm. 1987;24:200–2.

Rao KS, Mishra SH. Drumstick polysaccharide as pharmaceutical adjuvant. Indian J Nat Prod. 1993;9:3–6.

Rees DA, Morris ER, Thom DA, Madden JK. Shapes and interactions of carbohydrate chains. In: Aspinall GO, editor. The polysaccharides, vol. 1. New York: Academic Press; 1982. p. 195.

Rizk S, Barthelemy C, Duru C, Guyot-Hermann AM. Investigation on a new modified USP xanthan with tablet disintegranting properties. Drug Dev Ind Pharm. 1997;23:19–26.

Sarasija S, Hota A. Colon-specific drug delivery systems. Indian J Pharm Sci. 2000;62:1–8.

Schwartz DC, Saffran W, Welsh J, Haas J, Goldenberg MM, Cantor CR. New techniques for purifying large DNAs and studying their properties and packaging. Cold Spring Harb Symp Quant Biol. 1983;47:189–95.

Senni K, Pereira J, Gueniche F, Delbarre-Ladrat C, Sinquin C, Ratiskol J, Godeau G, Fischer AM, Helley D, Colliec-Jouault S. Marine polysaccharides: a source of bioactive molecules for cell therapy and tissue engineering. Mar Drugs. 2011;9(9):1664–81.

Siew LF, Man S, Newton JM, Basit AW. Amylose formulations for drug delivery to colon: a comparison of two fermentation models to assess colonic targeting performance *in vitro*. Int J Pharm. 2004;273:129–34.

Sigurdsson HH, Stefánsson E, Gudmundsdóttir E, Eysteinsson T, Thorsteinsdóttir M, Loftsson T. Cyclodextrin formulation of dorzolamide and its distribution in the eye after topical administration. J Control Release. 2005;102(1):255–62.

Silva TH, Alves A, Popa EG, Reys LL, Gomes ME, Sousa RA, Silva SS, Mano JF, Reis RL. Marine algae sulfated polysaccharides for tissue engineering and drug delivery approaches. Biomatter. 2012;2(4):278–89.

Sinha VR, Mittal BR, Bhutani KK, Kumria R. Colonic drug delivery of 5-fluorouracil: an *in vitro* evaluation. Int J Pharm. 2004;269:101–8.

Srinivas K, Prakash K, Kiran HR, Prasad PM, Rao MEB. Study of *Ocimumbasilicum* and *Plantago ovata* as disintegrants in the formulation of dispersible tablets. Indian J Pharm Sci. 2003;65:180–3.

Subramanian K, Vijayakumar V. *In vitro* release characteristics of 5-fluorouracil from Aloe vera gel/guar gum blend as a carrier matrix. Indian J Chem Technol. 2015;3:120–5.

Suh JK, Matthew HW. Application of chitosan-based polysaccharide biomaterials in cartilage tissue engineering: a review. Biomaterials. 2000;21(24):2589–98.

Sujja-areevath J, Munday DL, Cox PJ, Khan KA. Release characteristics of diclofenac sodium from encapsulated natural gum mini-matrix formulations. Int J Pharm. 1996;139:53–62.

Sutar I, Vartak HG, Srinivasan MC, Sivaraman H. Production of alkaline protease by immobilized mycelium of Conidiobolus. Enzyme Microb Technol. 1986;8:632–4.

Talukdar MM, Kinget R. Swelling and drug release behaviour of xanthan gum matrix tablets. Int J Pharm. 1995;120:63–72.

Tan H, Chu CR, Payne KA, Marra KG. Injectable *in situ* forming biodegradable chitosan–hyaluronic acid based hydrogels for cartilage tissue engineering. Biomaterials. 2009;30(13):2499–506.

Tan H, Rubin JP, Marra KG. Injectable *in situ* forming biodegradable chitosan-hyaluronic acid based hydrogels for adipose tissue regeneration. Organogenesis. 2010;6(3):173–80.

Tausif M, Malhotra AK, Kapoor VP. *Cassia fistula* seed galactomannan: potential binding agent for pharmaceutical formulation. Indian J Pharm Sci. 1992;54:234–40.

Tharanathan RN. Polysaccharide gums of industrial importance: a review. J Sci Ind Res (India). 1995;54:512–23.

Tiller J, Berlin P, Klemm D. A novel efficient enzyme-immobilization reaction on NH_2 polymers by means of L-ascarbic acid. Biotechnol Appl Biochem. 1999;30:155–62.

Trevan MD. Enzyme applications. In: Trevan MD, Boffey S, Goulding KH, Stanbury P, editors. Biotechnology: the biological principles. New Delhi: Tata McGraw-Hill; 1987. p. 178–228.

Upadhyay M, Adena SK, Vardhan H, Yadav SK, Mishra B. Development of biopolymers based interpenetrating polymeric network of capecitabine: a drug delivery vehicle to extend the release of the model drug. Int J Biol Macromol. 2018;115:907–19.

Venkatesan J, Kim SK. Chitosan composites for bone tissue engineering—an overview. Mar Drugs. 2010;8(8):2252–66.

Verma PRP, Razdan B. Studies on *Leucaena leucocephala* seed gum: emulsifying properties. J Sci Ind Res (India). 2003a;62:198–206.

Verma PRP, Razdan B. Evaluation of *Leucaena leucocephala* seed gum as suspending agent in sulphadimidine suspensions. Indian J Pharm Sci. 2003b;65:665–9.

Wahi SP, Sharma VD, Jain VK, Sinha P. Studies on emulsifying property of mucilage of *Hygrophilaspinosa* and *Hibiscus esculentus*. Indian J Nat Prod. 1985; 1:3–6.

Widjaja LK, Bora M, Chan PNPH, Lipik V, Wong TTL, Venkatraman SS. Hyaluronic acid-based nanocomposite hydrogels for ocular drug delivery applications: Ha-based nanocomposite hydrogels. J Biomed Mater Res A. 2014;102:3056–65.

Xing L, Dawei C, Kiping X, Rongqing Z. Oral colon-specific drug delivery for bee venom peptide: development of a coated calcium alginate gel beads-entrapped liposome. J Control Release. 2003;93:293–300.

Yarmush ML, Tomkins RG, Carter EA, Burke JF. Enzymatic function of alginate immobilized rat hepatocytes. FASEB J. 1988;2:A738.

Zucca P, Fernandez-Lafuente R, Sanjust E. Agarose and its derivatives as supports for enzyme immobilization. Molecules. 2016;21(11):1577.

Green Synthesis of Nanoparticles Using Herbal Extract

14

Subhashis Debnath, Dakshinamurthy Swetha, and M. Niranjan Babu

Contents

S. Debnath (✉)
Royal School of Pharmacy, Royal Global University, Guwahati, Assam, India

D. Swetha · M. N. Babu
Seven Hills College of Pharmacy, Tirupati, Andhra Pradesh, India

S. Sen, R. Chakraborty (eds.), *Herbal Medicine in India*,
https://doi.org/10.1007/978-981-13-7248-3_14

14.1 Introduction

Nanotechnology deals with synthesis and manipulation of colloidal particles ranging from 1 to 100 nm in size. Applications of nanoparticles are growing significantly due to their enhanced properties based on size, morphology and their distribution.

Metallic nanoparticles are extensively used in the field of imaging, sensing, catalysis and antimicrobial applications.

Two approaches are used to synthesize metallic nanoparticles, namely (a) top-down and (b) bottom-up (Tyagi 2016). In the top-down approach, lithographic techniques are used to prepare nanoparticles. In this technique, nanoparticles are prepared by size reduction of bulk material. Mechanical techniques are also used to prepare metallic nanoparticles. It is done by machining and grinding. The bottom-up approach is another method to prepare metallic nanoparticles where small building blocks of the metals are assembled into a larger structure. Chemical synthesis and green synthesis of nanoparticles are an example of bottom-up approach (Masarovicova and Kralova 2013) (Figs. 14.1 and 14.2).

However, bottom-up approach is used extensively, as it is the most effective and acceptable approach for the preparation of nanoparticle. Here reaction precursors are grown to prepare nanoparticle. These reaction precursors are simpler molecules (Saha et al. 2017).

Different methods are widely used to prepare metallic nanoparticles of desired characteristics. They are

(a) Physical process
(b) Chemical processes

However, the above methods suffer from various disadvantages like

1. Production methods are expensive,
2. Labour-intensive process and
3. Potentially hazardous to the living organisms and environment. These methods use toxin-reducing agents like sodium hydrazine hydrate and borohydride. These toxic reagents cause hazardous impacts on the plant, environment and animal life (Saif et al. 2016).

Thus, there is a need for an alternative method for the production of metallic nanoparticles. The method should be cost-effective and at the same time environmentally safe method of nanoparticle production. Hence green nanotechnology is the method of choice for the production of nanoparticles, as it does not use toxic chemicals. During the past decade, it has been observed that many biological systems, including plants and algae, bacteria, yeast, fungi, diatoms, and human cells, can be used to prepare metallic nanoparticle. They transform metal ions (inorganic) into metal nanoparticles by reductive capacities of the proteins and metabolites present in them. The

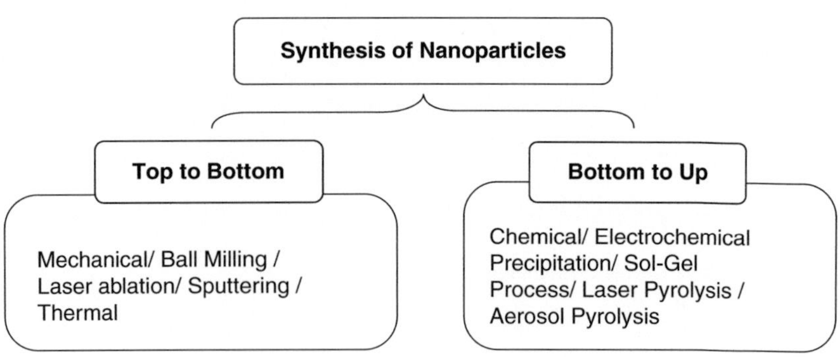

Fig. 14.1 Various synthesis process of nanoparticles

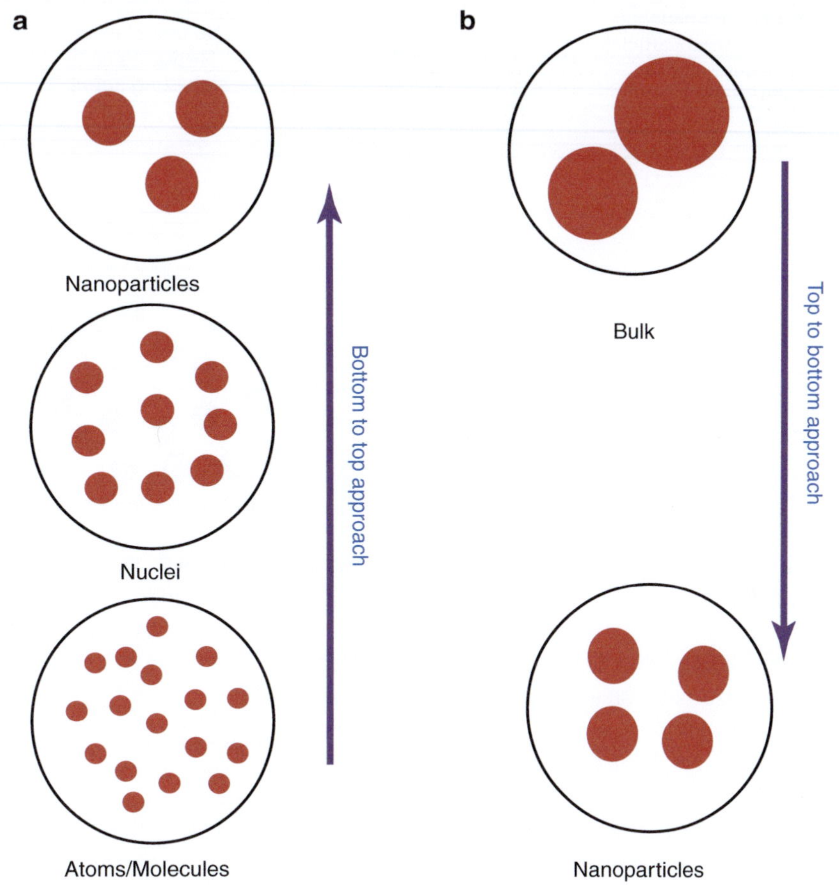

Fig. 14.2 (**a**) Bottom-to-top approaches and (**b**) top-to-bottom approaches

short production time, low cost of cultivation and safety make plants an alternative platform to synthesize metallic nanoparticle.

14.2 Phytomining

Phytomining is the process of production of a metal 'crop' by growing plants that accumulate high concentrations of metal. Mostly high-biomass plants are used for this purpose. Some may be natural hyperaccumulators, and in other plants, it can be induced. Since the ancient time it is known that plants reduce metal ions on their surface and in various tissues and organs far from the ion penetration site. Based on the above facts plants have been used for metal extracting via phytomining. Recovery of the metal accumulated in the plant can be done after harvesting. Extensive studies on bioaccumulation of metal in the plant have revealed that these metals are normally accumulated as nanoparticles (Masarovicova and Kralova 2013) (Table 14.1).

Table 14.1 Metallic nanoparticles accumulated in various plants

Plant	Accumulated metallic nanoparticles
Medicago sativa (alfalfa) and *Brassica juncea* (mustard greens)	Silver nanoparticles of 50 nm when grown on silver nitrate
Medicago sativa	Gold icosahedra of 4 nm in size
Iris pseudacorus (yellow iris)	Semi-spherical copper particles with a size of 2 nm when grown on substrates containing salts of the respective metals

Fig. 14.3 Formulation of metallic nanoparticles using plant extract as reducing agent (*in vitro* process)

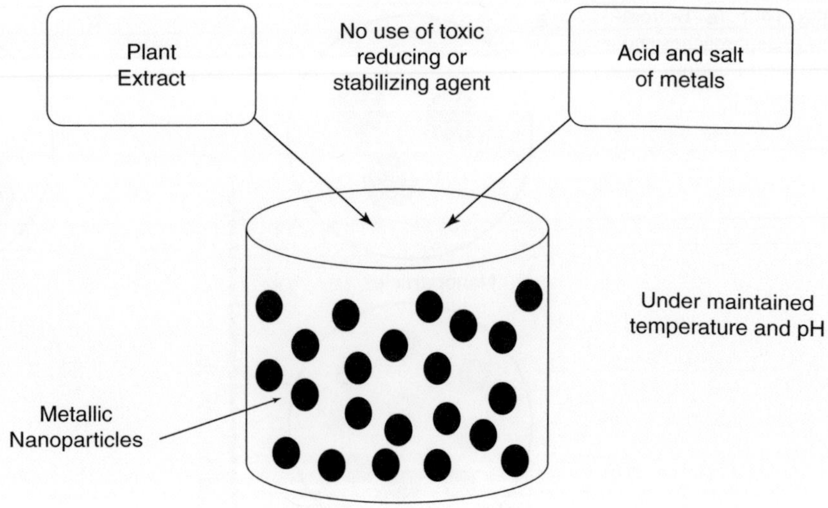

However, this process has the following disadvantages:

1. Depending on their localization in the plant, the size and shape of nanoparticles vary, which may depend on differences in the content of metal ions in various tissues and the subsequent possibility of nanoparticle movement and penetration.
2. In this, the nanoparticles vary in size and in morphology. This may affect their application where there is a need for uniformity in size and shape.
3. Extraction, isolation and purification of the nanoparticles are difficult with limited recovery.

Due to the above disadvantages, *in vitro* approaches were developed, in which bioreduction of metal ions is done using plant extract to formulate nanoparticles (Fig. 14.3).

Control over the size and shape of the nanoparticles by altering the pH of the medium or reaction temperature is possible by these approaches. The purification process is very easy; moreover, this process occurs faster than the whole plant synthesis of nanoparticles. This process takes place instantaneously and there is no delay in the uptake and diffusion of metal ions throughout the plant. In this method, extracts from different plant species are combined with salts and acids of metal, like silver, gold, copper, iron, platinum, etc. (Table 14.2).

Table 14.2 Plant extracts used to prepare metallic nanoparticles

Plants extract used	Nanoparticles produced
Pelargonium graveolens (*Rose geranium*)	Gold nanoparticles (decahedral icosahedral shaped) of 20–40 nm
Cymbopogon flexuosus (lemon grass)	Gold nanospheres and nanotriangles 0.05–18 μm in size
Azadirachta indica (neem, Indian lilac)	Gold nanoparticles of 50–100 nm
Aloe barbadensis (*Aloe vera*)	Cubic In_2O_3 particles 5–50 nm in size
Carica papaya (papaya)	Silver nanoparticles of 25–30 nm
Aloe vera	Spherical, triangular silver nanoparticles of 50–350 nm
Hibiscus cannabinus L. (kenaf)	Silver nanoparticles of 9 nm
Mentha piperita L. (peppermint)	Gold and silver nanoparticles of 90–150 nm
Ocimum sanctum L. (holy basil)	Gold, silver and platinum nanoparticles of 40–30 nm
Zingiber officinale (ginger)	Gold and silver nanoparticles of 10 nm

Terpenoids, phenolic acids, sugars, polyphenols and proteins play an important role in the reduction of metal ions into nanoparticles and its stability. Interaction of these biomolecules with metal ions controls the size and morphology of the nanoparticles formed (Ahmed et al. 2016; Varahalarao et al. 2013)

14.3 Role of Plant Metabolites in the Binding and Reduction of Metal Ions

Various plant metabolites like terpenoids, alkaloids, sugars, proteins, etc. play an important role in the production of metallic nanoparticles by bioreduction of metal ions. Polyhydroxy group is present in secondary metabolites, and this polyhydroxy group is responsible for their antioxidant property. It also plays a curtail role in the production of nanoparticles by reducing metal ions. Examples of the main types of secondary metabolites capable of reducing metal ions are shown in Table 14.3.

14.3.1 Terpenoids

Terpenoids are also called isoprenoids. These are the largest group of natural products and about 60% of known natural products are terpenoids. It is synthesized in plants from five-carbon isoprene units and possesses antioxidant activity. Terpenoids play an important role in the formation of silver ions into nanoparticles. Extracts of geranium leaves are used to reduce silver ions into the silver nanoparticle. It has been observed that eugenol is the main terpenoid of an extract of *Cinnamomum zeylanisum* (cinnamon) and used in the bioreduction of $AgNO_3$ and $HAuCl_4$ to nanoparticles. The first step in this process is an active reduction of metal ions, followed by the formation of the nanoparticle.

14.3.2 Flavonoids

Flavonoids are a class of secondary metabolites of the plant. Chemically, it is having the general structure of a 15-carbon skeleton. It also contains two phenyl rings and a heterocyclic ring. Pure flavonoids: hesperidin, naringin and diosmin are used for the synthesis of silver nanoparticles. A pure aqueous solution of hesperidin, naringin and diosmin are popularly used to prepare silver nanoparticles with a size range of 5–80 nm. Bioreduction of silver ions into AgNPs using pure polyhydroxylated plant secondary metabolite was studied, and it was observed that the reaction involves hydroxyl group. These silver nanoparticles possess mild antimicrobial efficacy and cytotoxicity against HL-60 cells. Hence these nanoparticles can be used as a drug for cancer treatment.

Flavonoids contain a wide verity of functional groups capable of formation of the nanoparticle. These functional groups can actively chelate and reduce metal ions into nanoparticles. A reactive hydrogen atom is released during the tautomeric transformation of flavonoids from enol to keto form. Formation of silver nanoparticles using *Ocimum basilicum* extract is the result of the transformation of the flavonoids from enol to keto form of luteolin and rosmarinic acid. Researchers investigated various characteristics of silver nanoparticles synthesized using plant extract like Tulsi leaf and quercetin and it has been examined for its antibacterial and morphological characteristics. It was observed that silver nanoparticles prepared using several plant extracts exhibit similar characteristics.

14.3.3 Sugars

Various researches showed that sugars present in the extract of the plant can also play a potential role in the formation of nanoparticles. Glucose, a monosaccharide, possesses liner structure with an aldehyde group and acts as a reducing agent. Another monosaccharide fructose contains keto group and undergoes several tautomeric transformations, which convert ketone to an aldehyde, and it acts as an antioxidant. Disaccharides and polysaccharides can also reduce metal ions but their reducing ability depends on the ability to form an aldehyde group from their individual monosaccharide. This monosaccharide should have the ability to adopt an open-chain form within an oligomer and, hence, to provide access to an aldehyde group. Maltose and lactose (disaccharides) show reducing ability as their monomers assume open-chain form. Sucrose, on the

Table 14.3 Various plant metabolites used in the bioreduction of metal ions

Plant metabolites used in the bioreduction of metal ions	Chemical structure
Eugenol (terpenoids)	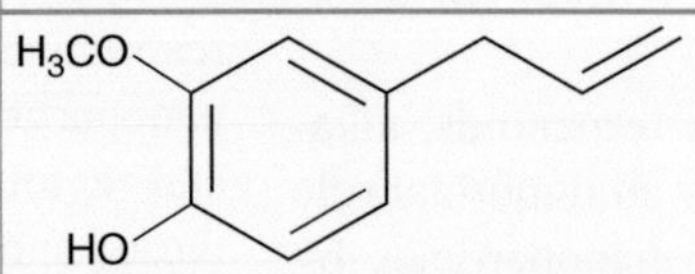
Luteolin (flavonoids)	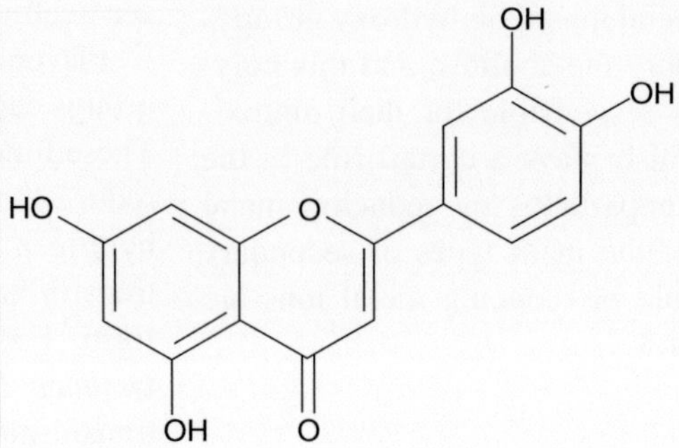
Tryptophan (amino acids)	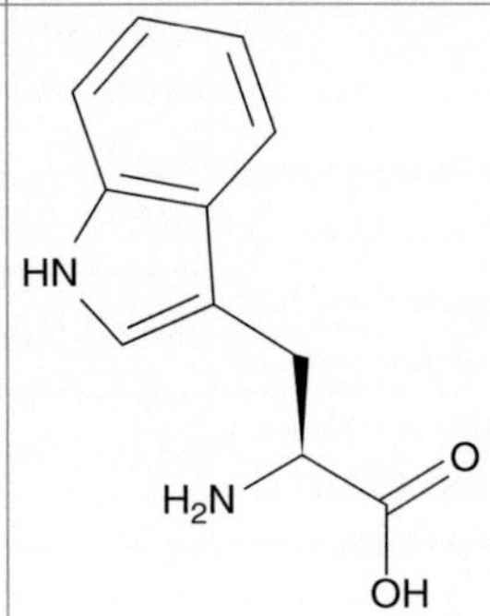
Galangin (flavonoids)	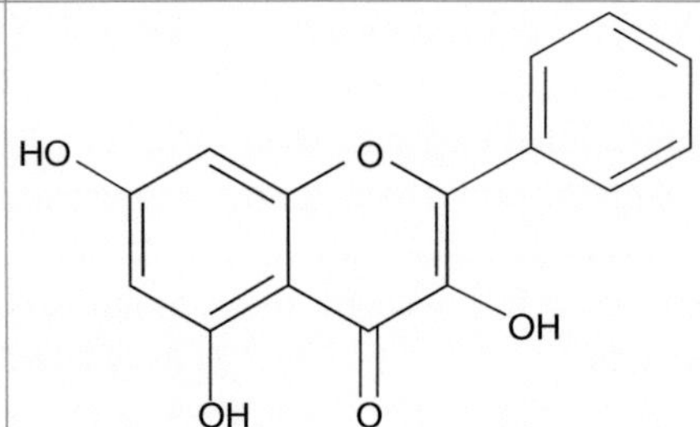
Epicatechin (flavonoids)	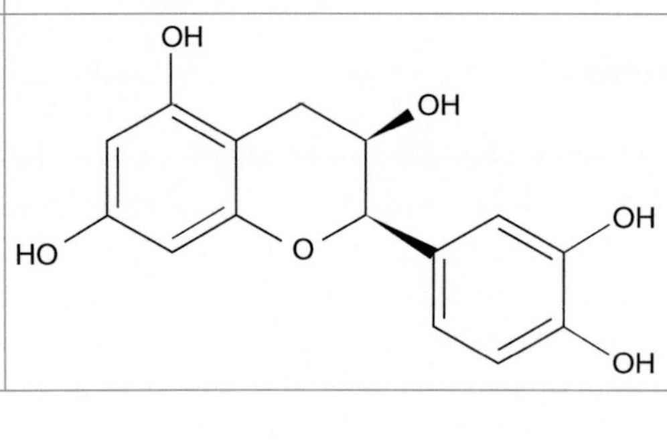

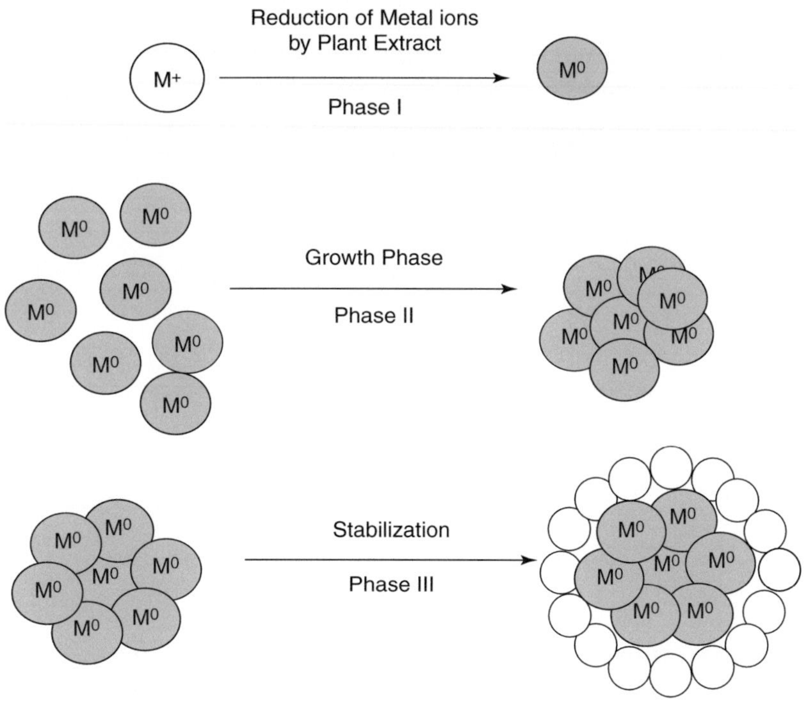

Fig. 14.4 Various phases of synthesis of metallic nanoparticles

other hand, does not reduce metal ions, because monomers of sucrose, that is glucose and fructose, are arranged in such a way that they cannot assume open-chain form. Fructose is a weaker reducing agent than glucose as the potential of antioxidant activity of fructose is limited by its kinetic tautomeric shifts. It is believed that aldehyde group of the sugar is oxidized into a carboxyl group via the nucleophilic addition of OH–, which in turn leads to the reduction of metal ions and to the synthesis of nanoparticles.

14.4 Overall Mechanism of Green Nanoparticle Synthesis

The mechanism involved in the formation of metal nanoparticle using plant extract involves three important phases:

First phase: This phase is called an activation phase. During this phase reduction of metal ions occurs. Nucleation of the reduced metal ions also occurs in this phase.

Second phase: This phase is known as the growth phase. In this phase growth of nanoparticles occurs. Small nanoparticles coalesce into a larger size by a process called Ostwald ripening. This is a phase where thermodynamic stability of nanoparticle increases.

Third phase: Third phase is known as the termination phase. This phase determines the shape of the final nanoparticle. In this phase, nanoparticles are the most stable.

Increase in the second phase that is growth phase corresponding nanoparticles aggregates and form different irregularly shaped nanoparticles like nanoprisms, nanotubes, etc. (Fig. 14.4).

14.5 Bio-Reduction Mechanism

Silver: $AgNO_3$ reacts with plant extract and synthesizes nanoparticle by the following reaction.

$$Ag + NO_3^- + \text{plant extract} \rightarrow Ag^{\circ}\ \text{NPs} + \text{byproducts}.$$

Gold: Au^{+} ions react with different biomolecules like sugars, proteins, enzymes, amino acids and other traces of metals. These metabolites reduce Au^{+} ions into metallic Au° nanoparticles. The reaction proceeds as follows:

$$HAu + Cl_4 \bullet 4H_2O + \text{plant extracts} \rightarrow Au^{\circ}\ \text{NPs} + \text{byproducts}$$

Platinum: Synthesis of platinum nanoparticle involves the following reaction:

$$H_2Pt + Cl_2 \bullet 6H_2O + \text{Plant extracts} \rightarrow Pt^{\circ}\ \text{NPs} + \text{byproducts}$$

Copper: Copper nanoparticles can be synthesized by the following reduction reaction using herbal extract:

$$CuSO_4 \bullet 5H_2O + \text{Plant metabolites} \rightarrow Cu^{\circ}\ \text{NPs} + \text{byproducts}$$

14.6 Factors Affecting Green Synthesis of Nanoparticles Using Plant Extract

Preparation of metallic nanoparticles using herbal extract not only affected by nature of herbal extract and their contents, but also affected by various other factors like (a) reaction mixture pH, (b) incubation temperature, (c) pressure, (d) reaction, (e) time, (f) concentration and (g) metal ion electrochemical potential (Patra and Baek 2014).

14.6.1 pH of the Reaction Mixture

The pH value of the herbal extract influences the formulation of metallic nanoparticle. The charge of the natural phytochemicals present in the extract changes with a change in pH. This may affect their binding ability to the metal ions during the process of synthesis of nanoparticle. Changes in the pH also affect the yield of nanoparticle including its size and shape. It has observed that in *Avena sativa* extract at pH 3.0 and 4.0 more small-sized gold nanoparticles were formed, whereas at pH 2.0 aggregated gold nanoparticles were observed.

14.6.2 Incubation Temperature

Preparation of metallic nanoparticle using plant extract is also affected by incubation temperature. Increase in temperature increases the rate of reaction and production of the nanoparticle. It has observed that formation of silver nanoparticles (triangular shape) using an extract of alfalfa plants initiates at temperatures above 30 °C only. Reduction of silver ion efficacy can also be increased by increasing reaction temperature when extracts of lemon verbena are used to prepare silver nanoparticle. However the formation of crystal particle at room temperature is difficult; this can easily be achieved at high temperature. Nucleation rate increases with increase in temperature and helps in the formation of nanoparticles. It has also observed that temperature can also affect the structural form of the nanoparticle synthesized. For example, though silver nanoparticle formed at room temperature using *Cassia fistula* extracts, production of nanoparticle with spherical shape mostly occurs at a temperature above 60 °C.

14.6.3 Pressure

Synthesis of metallic nanoparticles also affected by the pressure applied to the reaction medium. The rate of reduction of metal ions using plant extract is faster at ambient temperature. The size and shape of the nanoparticles can also vary with changes with pressure.

14.6.4 Time

The time of incubation greatly affects the quantity and type of nanoparticles formed. The characteristics of the metallic nanoparticles synthesized are influenced time, synthesis process, exposure to light, etc. Time of incubation affects the aggregation of particles, particles growth and their potential.

14.7 Conclusions

Though preparation of metallic nanoparticles using plant extracts suffers from several limitations, it is having its own significance and advantages relative to conventional methods of preparation of nanoparticle. Green synthesis of nanoparticles using plant extract has been used only in small-scale production, and it is needed to scale up for large-scale production. The preparation method should be less expensive and easily accepted by the industries. Cost of metal salt and reducing agent governs the cost of nanoparticles prepared by chemical synthesis, whereas cost of the green synthesized nanoparticles depends on the cost of metal salt only. In the green synthesis of nanoparticles, plant waste from the various food industries can serve as a reducing agent. Hence food industries can be encouraged to recycle plant waste and that can be used to produce nanoparticles. This recycling process can also control pollution from the food industries and emphasize the environmental advantages of the synthesis of metallic nanoparticles using herbal extracts.

References

Ahmed S, Ahmad M, Swami BL, Ikram S. A review on plants extract mediated synthesis of silver nanoparticles for antimicrobial applications: a green expertise. J Adv Res. 2016;7:17–28.

Masarovicova E, Kralova K. Metal nanoparticles and plants. Ecol Chem Eng S. 2013;20:9–22.

Patra JK, Baek K. Green nanobiotechnology: factors affecting synthesis and characterization techniques. J Nanomater. 2014;10:1–12.

Saha J, Begum A, Mukherjee A, Kumar S. A novel green synthesis of silver nanoparticles and their catalytic action in reduction of methylene blue dye. Sust Environ Res. 2017;27:245–50.

Saif S, Tahir A, Chen Y. Green synthesis of iron nanoparticles and their environmental applications and implications. Nanomaterials. 2016;6:209–35.

Tyagi PK. Production of metal nanoparticles from biological resources. Int J Curr Microbiol App Sci. 2016;5:548–58.

Varahalarao V, Kaladhar DSVGK, Behara M, Sujatha B, Naidu GK. Synthesis of green metallic nanoparticles (NPs) and applications. Orient J Chem. 2013;29:1589–95.

Sassurea lappa: A Scientific Review 15

Mohammad Kamil

Contents

15.1 Introduction

A large number of studies have been carried out on different aspects of *Sassurea lappa*. Observing the medicinal importance of the plant, studies were carried out in laboratory to find out the quality control studies of the plant material (root) including pharmacognostic, phytochemical, pharmacological and toxicological studies. The physiochemical data such as total ash, water soluble and acid insoluble ash, loss of weight on drying, solubilities in alcohol and water as well as successive extractive values in petrol, chloroform and alcohol were studied. Finger printing pattern of all the successive extractives was carried out using IR, UV, TLC and HPLC. GC–MS and LCMS studies of the extract have also been carried out. These pharmacognostic and

M. Kamil (✉)
TCAM Research, HealthCare Licensing and Medical Education Division (HL&ME), Department of Health, Zayed Complex for Herbal Research & Traditional Medicine, Abu Dhabi, UAE

S. Sen, R. Chakraborty (eds.), *Herbal Medicine in India*,
https://doi.org/10.1007/978-981-13-7248-3_15

phytochemical studies provide a standard data for *S. lappa* root and its method of processing to be included in any pharmacopoeia and monographic references (Kamil et al. 2002a).

The present paper deals with a review on different scientific studies carried out to date globally for such an important plant—*Sassurea lappa* along with some phytochemical, chemical, quality control, and pharmacological studies carried out in our laboratories (Kamil et al. 2002b) (Fig. 15.1).

Plant's Name:	*Sassurea lappa* C.B. Clarke
English Name:	Costos
Arabic Name:	Qust/Qast-Hindi
Family:	Asteraceae
Part Used:	Root

Saussurea lappa is a robust, erect perennial with: a stout stem up to 2 m in height; leaves membranous, basal ones very large, upper ones small, irregularly toothed; flowers bluish purple in axillary and terminal heads; and fruits compressed, curved achenes. The roots are stout, up to 60 cm long having a penetrating characteristic odour. It is brown with longitudinal ridges and a rough reticulated surface having a resinous appearance and dirty white color. The used parts are roots, which are bitter, acrid, sweet, thermogenic, aromatic, aphrodisiac, carminative, digestive, stimulant, diuretic, expectorant, rejuvenating, and tonic (Indian Medicinal Plants 1996).

Falconer was the first to prove that among many species, *S. lappa's* roots only were used by the ancient physicians and recently by Japanese scientists for therapeutic use against cancer as it contains more than one antimutagenic compounds. During its antimutagenic study on *E. coli*, it showed no toxic effects to the cells (Kuroda et al. 1987). The alkaloids also produced a definite relaxation of the bronchioles, similar to adrenaline. The extracts and tinctures of *S. lappa* have been included in different pharmacopoeias.

Saussurea lappa is a traditionally known and potent plant, which is well considered for its medicinal uses in different indigenous Indian systems of medicine. It is popularly known as Kuth root or costus and used in various traditional system of medicine for its anti-ulcer, anti-convulsant, anti-cancer, hepatoprotective, anti-arthritic, and anti-viral activities. Several of its activities are well proved and established through *in vitro*, *in vivo* methods which gave a rationale scientific approach to the traditional claims. Phytochemical compounds isolated from this plant such as costunolide, Isodihydrocostunolide, cynaropicrin, etc. were proven to be bio-active and potential source for developing new molecules. Due to the significant proven activities, *Saussurea lappa* is having a considerable chance for new drug discovery. This review is an effort to explore the different phytoconstituents and the pharmacological activities of *Saussurea lappa* (Madhuri et al. 2012).

Besides diverse pharmaceutical applications, *Saussurea lappa* roots (family: Asteraceae) have been widely recommended in inflammation-related diseases characterized by rheumatoid arthritis, chronic gastritis, asthma, and bronchitis in traditional medicine (Chopra 1982; Ikram and Hussain 1978; Jain 1968). The scientific evi-

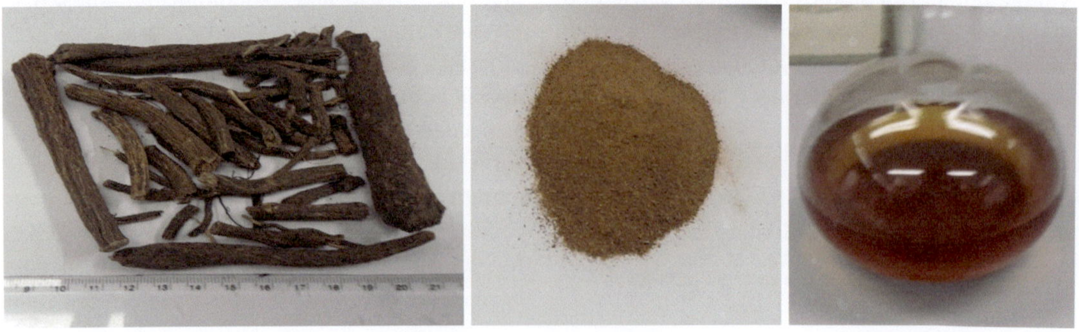

Fig. 15.1 Image of the *Sassurea lappa* root; powder and its cold extraction

dences of their significance are inadequate. Akhtar and Farah (1987) reported chemical contents exerting anthelmintic effects in animals. Recently, a small number of *in vitro* studies have been published describing effects of the methanolic root extracts of *Saussurea lappa* on cell-mediated immunity in rats (Lee et al. 1995; Taniguchi et al. 1995; Cho et al. 1998; Jung et al. 1998; Lee et al. 1999). However, the toxicological effects of these preparations on individual's general health remain yet to be ascertained. Taken as a whole, these findings suggest that inhibition of lymphocyte proliferation and IFN-γ by homeopathic dilutions of *Saussurea lappa* may contribute to suppress immune-mediated inflammatory reactions possibly through a cell-mediated cytokine pathway. On the other hand, enhanced leukocyte phagocytic activity may be helpful to clear the soluble immune complexes produced during a sustained immune response against self-antigens which causes chronic inflammatory injury of tissue. Thus, homeopathic preparations of *Saussurea lappa* may be considered as a possible therapeutic support in autoimmune and chronic inflammatory disorders (Sarwar and Enbergs 2007).

15.2 Phyto-Constituents of *Saussurea lappa*

15.2.1 Thin-Layer Chromatographic (TLC) Finger Printing

A number of standards were chromatographed along with different extracts of the *Sassurea lappa* powder and were identified as Piperazine, D-glucitol, n-valeraldehyde, Xanthosine, Stevioside, Cinnamic acid, Lupeol, Betulin, Alpha terpinenyl acetate, Cholesterol, Ethyl linoleate, etc.

15.2.2 Gas Chromatography–Mass Spectrometric (GC–MS) Studies

Essential oil of *Sassurea lappa* roots was analyzed by gas chromatography (GC) and mass spectrometry. Quite a large number of components of the essential oil of *Sassurea lappa* roots were identified. The essential oil has higher content of (80%) of sesquiterpenoids than monoterpenoids (14%). The principal compounds in *Sassurea lappa* essential oil were dehydrocostus lactone (46.00%), costunolide (10%), 8-cedren-13-ol (5.09%), and α-curcumene (5.33%). Based on bioactivity-directed fractionation, dehydrocostus lactone and costunolide were isolated from *S. lappa* essential oil. The following compounds were detected using GC/MS in other fractions from column chromatography (unpublished data from current research of author).

Sorbitol; Piperazine; Ethyl linoleate; Diethl succinate; Diethyl di maleate; Dehydrosanssure lactone; D-glucitol; n-valeraldehyde; Xanthosine; Stevioside; Cinnamic acid Diazoprogesterone; Andrographolide; Caryophylline oxide; Aromadendrene Pseudosarsasapogenin, 5, 20-dien; Eremanthin; Androstan-17-one3-ethyl-3-hydroxy (5 alpha); 1-Heptatriacotanol; Tetrahydroisovelleral9,19-Cyclolanost-23-ene-3, 25-diol; Glaucyl alcohol; Lupeol; Betulin; Alpha terpinenyl acetate Cholesterol; Alpha terpineol; Pyrrolidine; Thunbergol Doconexent; Cinnamic acid; Diazoprogesterone; Andrographolide; Glycine; 1-beta-hydroxycolartin; 5-alpha-hydroxy-beta-costic acid; 11-alpha, 13-dihydroxy-dehidrocostuslactone; 11, 13-dihydro-7,11-dehydro-13-hydroxy-3-desoxyzaluzanin; 8alpha-hydroxyl-11betaH-11,13-dihydrodehydrocostuslactone; Soulangianolide A; Syringaresinol; Scopoletin; 2,5-Di tert butyl-p-quinone; 3-Angeloyloxy-10-oxy-Furoexmophilan; 8,9-Dehydro-9-formyl-cycloisolongifolene (unpublished data from current research of author).

15.3 Acute Toxicity Evaluation

Two groups of eight TO mice were formed with four males and four females each and average body weight of 30 g; one group was given the sample decoction at a dose of 1 mL/mouse orally and the other group kept as control and given only 1 mL of water per mouse daily for 7 days (unpublished data from current research of author).

The following observations were made 30 min following the acute administration of the *Sassurea lappa* extract and then observed for 7 days.

Autonomic:	No signs
Behavioral:	The treated group showed no restricted movement, drooping head, pitosis, preening, irritability, aggressive behavior, righting reflex, sensitivity to pain, touch, sound and phonation.
Neuromuscular:	No lethargy' tremors, weakness, muscle tone, ataxia, convulsions, prostration, and hind limb weakness.
Gastrointestinal:	No salivation, defecation, diarrhea, urination.
Coetaneous:	No piloerection, alopecia, erythema, edema, swelling, necrosis.

The following tests were also carried out:

Pole and string tests	No animal fail the tests
Motor coordination	The motor impairment was assessed using rotarod and found no difference in a number of falls between treated and control group.
Rectal temperature measurement	The rectal temperature of the mice measured using rectal probe, the treated group showed no change as compared to the control.
Body weight changes	Initial (before drug administration), and after 24 h and 7 days, body weight was recorded. No difference between treated and control groups was detected after 7 days of observation.

Inference: The above results have been given on the basis of 7-day observation period. The acute oral administration of the test sample of *Sassurea lappa* water extract to the mice showed no change in the animals' behavior. No toxic signs and symptoms observed at the dose tested. The treated animals showed normal motor coordination tests. No change in body weight. No animal died after 7 days of drug daily administration. To ensure further safety of the sample, chronic toxicity test should be carried out (unpublished data from current research of author).

15.4 Literature Survey

15.4.1 Medicinal Uses

Costus is regarded as tonic for vital organs but more useful for liver and lungs. As aromatic stimulant and antiseptic, its fumes are considered useful fumigation, as incense or in pestilence when the patient is fumigated with gives pleasurable sensation. Its use confines the bowls and the infusion with some cardamoms is useful in cough, asthma, chronic rheumatism and other nervous disorders, skin diseases, fever and dyspepsia, and in cholera. It is useful antispasmodic serviceable in paralysis, facial paralysis, diphtheria, cholera, gout and sciatica and finds frequent use in preparations administered for the treatment of intermittent fevers, malaria, leprosy, persistent hiccough, bronchitis, and rheumatism. With honey, the powdered root is applied on freckles, leucodermal conditions, and vitiligo as well as in alopecia (Indus Yunic Medicine 1997).

It is the root of *Saussurea lappa* that was narrated in *Sunnah* of Prophet Mohammed (SAW) (PBUH) as a treatment for headaches and upper respiratory tract infections. Root is tonic, stomachic, carminative, stimulant, and aphrodisiac and is used as spasmodic in asthma, cough and cholera and as alterative in chronic skin diseases and rheumatism. Cupping and sea costus are the best of your remedies (Al-Jauziyah 1999).

In the *Sahihain*, it is narrated that Anas (RAA) related from the Prophet (SAW) that he said: "Cupping and marine Castus are the best of your remedies." According to Imam Ali ibn Abi Talib the Prophet (SAW) said, " You have Costus (kust) which contains seven remedies: administered by mouth it is useful against pleurisy and heart pain; administered by nose, it is effective against aludra and headaches; and as an incense it is effective against the cold." Imam Ali allegedly did not remember the two other diseases (Ibn Habib 1992). It is also reported that the Messenger of Allah allowed women to use a little costus (kust) when they did their ritual ablutions after menstruations (Suyuti 1994).

Imam Zahbi said that it is useful in paralysis, an antidote for snake poison and its oil is effective in back pain. According to the authentic books of Al-Hadith, it is described accompanied with the description of cupping. Anas Bin Malik narrates that Prophet stated "Out of those things which are being used by you for treatment, the cupping and Qust Bahri are the best treatment" (Sahih Bukhari 5371). This description might be interpreted to mean that if somebody fails to use to cupping, he may use the *Saussurea lappa* instead of cupping (Al-Jauziyah 1999).

Hadith—Mustadrak-al-Hakim, Narrated Jabir Bin Abdullah narrates that Prophet stated: "If someone's child gets Azra (upper respiratory tract infection) or a headache then she should take Qust and after grinding it in water, apply it to the child" (Mustadrak-Al-Hakim 405 A.H., n.d.). Azra is an ancient term, might be interpreted as tonsillitis, in which tonsils become swollen and painful with or without pus formation. Hence, this drug is especially effective against any type of tonsillitis and might be used in all types of phlegmatic diseases. It is effective in general weakness after diarrhoea and cholera. The water extract of the root was used to wash the females' internal organs after the menstruation. Oil mixture of *Saussurea lappa* and olive oil is effective against alopecia and tones up the body. It is a good insect repellant hence, might be used to keep off the insects from the clothes (Mustadrak-Al-Hakim 405 A.H., n.d.).

In recent years, the anti-cancer property of various sesquiterpene lactones had attracted a great deal of interest and extensive research work has been carried out to characterize the anticancer activity, the molecular mechanisms, and the potential chemotherapeutic application of sesquiterpene lactones. Costunolide, a sesquiterpene lactone isolated from the root of *Saussurea lappa*, is known to have anti-fungal activities (Cho et al. 2000).

15.4.2 Anti-Convulsant Activity

Sasuurea lappa root extracts prepared from different solvents such as petroleum, ether, water were evaluated for the anti-convulsant activity by pentylenetetrazole, picrotoxin-induced convulsions and maximal electroshock tests performed in mice by which it is proved that the petroleum extract of SL roots at a dose of 100 and 300 mg/kg ip showed potent anti-convulsant activity (Shirishkumar et al. 2009).

15.4.3 Anti-Viral Activity

The extract obtained from the root of SL was evaluated for the activity against Hepatitis B virus (HBV). Costunolide and dehydrocostus lactone suppressed the expression of Hepatitis B surface antigen (HBsAg) in human hepatoma Hep3B cells in a dose-dependent manner (IC50 values 1.0 and 2.0 mm), by the method of northern blotting analysis, and the suppression was also observed in the human hepatoma cell line HepA2 derived from the HepG2 cells. By all the observations it was proved that the tested compounds showed significant activity against HBV (Chen et al. 1995).

15.4.4 Gastro-Protective Activity

In healthy volunteers, a decoction of *Sassurea lappa* was found to accelerate gastric emptying and increase endogenous motilin release, an amino acid peptide that regulates upper GI motility (Chen et al. 1994; Matsuda et al. 2000).

15.4.5 Anti-Hepatotoxic Activity

Aqueous and methanolic extracts of SL root was investigated for hepatotoxic activity against D-galactosamine (D-GalN) and lipopolysaccharide (LPS)-induced hepatitis in mice. Pretreatment of mice with different doses of SL led to rising in creatinine plasma levels in a dose-dependent manner and AST, ALT levels as well. Whereas, post-treatment led to the restricted progression of hepatic damage, which was induced by D-GalN and LPS. By the studies, it is revealed that the root extract works against hepatotoxic activity (Yaeesh et al. 2010).

15.4.6 Anti-Microbial Activity

Disk-diffusion assay was used to determine the anti-microbial activity (Bauer et al. 1966). Müller-Hinton Agar (MAST, UK) was prepared by suspending 36 g of the powder in 1 L of distilled water. 20 μL of the microbial suspension was added to 20 mL of sterile Mueller-Hinton agar and poured into sterile petri dishes. Sterile filter paper discs with 6 mm in diameter were impregnated with 20 μL of the extract. The filter papers then were allowed to evaporate before placing them on the surface of the inoculated Mueller-Hinton agar plates. To enable the prediffusion of the extract, plates were incubated for 2 h in refrigerator. Then plates were incubated for 24 h at 37° C for bacteria, whereas for fungus they were incubated for 48 h at 30° C. Filter paper discs impregnated with 20 μL of distilled water were used as negative control. The antimicrobial activity was evaluated according to the size of the inhibition zone around the discs after the incubation period (Chang et al. 2011).

15.4.7 Anti-Ulcer Effects

Plant extract exhibited cholagogic and anti-ulcer effects in mice (Chem. Pharm. Bull. 1985, 33:1285); it inhibited KC1-induced contractions of aorta but the effect was less on nor epinephrine-induced contractions, indicating a possible calcium antagonistic action. Dehydro costus lactone showed similar effects but its specific inhibition of KC1-induced contraction was less than that of costunolide (J. Nat. Prod. 1986, 49:1112).

15.4.8 Treatment of Ischemic Heart Diseases (IHD)

A study of the usefulness of Saussurea lappa on the treatment of Ischaemic Heart Diseases (IHD): This communication described a preliminary clinical trial of (*Saussurea lappa*, Clarke) water extract on the cases of IHD. The drug was used both individually and in combination with Segontin (Upadhyay et al. 1993).

This study induced 45 patients suffering from IHD the cases. The cases were divided into three groups ($n = 15$ in each), group I have treated with *Saussurea lappa* alone, group II was treated with *Saussurea lappa* + Segontin and group III was received Segontin alone. To evaluate the response of the drug *Saussurea lappa*, the clinical features, ECG, and bio chemical parameters were recorded. The responses were graded as significant, moderate, and no response. After the treatment for four months, significant improvement was observed in clinical and biochemical parameters of *Sassurea lappa*, Segontin group. Apart from that more marked improvement in ECG was observed in the group II where ECG comes to normal. It can be interpreted:

- That the combination of *Sassurea lappa* and Segontin is more effective and suitable without the occurrence of any major side effects.
- The dose of Segontin could be reduced in combined drug therapy (group II) in comparison to sengontin group. The side effects were also less in combined group.

15.4.9 Anti-Oxidant Activity

A recent study conducted by the National Botanical Research Institute in India seems to confirm the anti-oxidative activity of *Sassurea costus* and its activity to scavenge DPPH, nitric oxide, and super oxide radicals along with its ability to inhibit lipid peroxidation and GSH oxidation (Pandey et al. 2005; Chang et al. 2012).

15.4.10 Side Effects

When taken in large doses it may produce irritation and a feeling of discomfort in the abdomen, which may last for several hours; the patient at the same time feels somewhat drowsy. Large doses of the extract may: produce giddiness, headache, and drowsiness; also produce a harmful effect on urinary bladder and lungs function (unpublished data from the research of author).

Acknowledgements The author would like to thanks Department of Health in general and Division of HL&ME in particular for providing facilities to complete this review.

References

Akhtar MS, Farah N. Phytochemical screening of the fruit of *Caesalpinia crista* (Kranjwa), Meliaazadarach (Bakain) and roots of *Sausurea lappa* (Qusti-shireen). Pakistan J Agri Sci. 1987;24(4):235–40.

Al-Jauziyah IIQ. Healing with the medicine of the prophet (SAW). Riyad, Saudi Arabia: Darrussalam; 1999.

Bauer AW, Kirby WMM, Sheriss JC, Turck M. Antibiotic susceptibility testing by standardized single method. Am J Clin Pathol. 1966;45:493–6.

Chang K, Choi S, Chung SJ, Kim G. Anti-microbial activity of *Saussurea lappa* C.B. Clarke Roots. Prev Nutr Food Sci. 2011;16(4):376–80.

Chang K, Choi S, Kim G. Anti-oxidant activity of *Saussurea lappa* C.B. Clarke roots. Prev Nutr Food Sci. 2012;17(4):306–9.

Chen SF, Li YQ, Fy H. Effect of *sassurea lappa* on gastric functions. Zhongguo Zhong Xi Yi Jie He Za Zhi. 1994;14(7):406–40-8.

Chen HC, Chou CK, Lee SD, Wang JC, Yeh SF. Active compounds from *Saussurea lappa* Clarke that suppress hepatitis B virus surface antigen gene expression in human hepatoma cells. Antiviral Res. 1995;27(1-2):99–109.

Cho JY, Park J, Yoo ES, Baik KU, Jung JH, Lee J, Park MH. Inhibitory effect of sesquiterpene lactones from *Saussurea lappa* on tumor necrosis factor-alpha production in murine macrophage-like cells. Planta Med. 1998;64:594–7.

Cho JY, Baik KU, Jung JH, Park MH. *In vitro* anti inflammatory effect of cynaropicrin, a sesquiterpene lactone from, *Saussurea lappa*. Eur J Pharmacol. 2000;398:399–407.

Chopra RN. Indiginous Plants of India. Calcutta, India: Academic Publishers; 1982.

Ibn Habib A. Mujtasar fi l-tibb/compendio de medicina. In: Alvarez de Morales C, Giron Irueste F, editors. Madrid: Consejo Superior de Investigations Cientificas; 1992:78/45.

Ikram M, Hussain SF. Compendium of medical plants. Peshawar: Pakistan Council of Scientific and Industrial Research; 1978.

Indian Medicinal Plants, Orient Longman Limited; 1996,Vol 5,p 80.

Indus Yunic Medicine (1997) Khan Usman Ghani, Aftab Saeed, Muhammad Tanweer Alam, Univ. Karachi, Pakistan, pp. 394–95.

Jain SK. Medicinal plants. India: Nation Book Trust; 1968.

Jung JH, Kim Y, Lee CO, Kang SS, Park JH, Im KS. Cytotoxic constituents of *Saussurea lappa*. Arch Pharm Res. 1998;23:153–6.

Kamil M, Ahmad F, Gunasekhar G, Samuel S, Naji MA. Quality control studies for the *Sassurea lappa* roots. In: 2nd Arab Conference of Pharmacology (5–7 September 2002), Fez, Morocco; 2002a.

Kamil M, Ahmad F, Gunasekhar G, Samuel S, Naji MA. 'Quality control studies for the *Saussurea lappa* roots'. In: 50th Annual Congress of the Society for Medicinal Plant Research, Barcelona (Spain), September 8–12; 2002b.

Kuroda M, Yoshida D, Kodama H. Antimutagenic effects of sesquiterpene lactones from costus root oil. Agric Boil Chem. 1987;51:585–7.

Lee GI, Ha JY, Min KR, Nakagawa H, Tsurufuji S, Chang IM, Kim Y. Inhibitory effects of oriental herbal medicines onIL-8 induced in lipopolysaccharide activated rat macrophages. Planta Med. 1995;61:26–30.

Lee HJ, Kim NY, Jang MK, Son HJ, Kim KM, Sohn DH, Lee SH, Ryu JH. A sesquiterpene, dehydrocostus lactone, inhibits the expression of inducible nitric oxide synthesis and TNF-alpha in LPS –activated macrophages. Planta Med. 1999;65:104–8.

Madhuri K, Elango K, Ponnusankar S. *Saussurea lappa* (Kuth root): review of its traditional uses, phytochemistry and pharmacology. Orient Pharma Exp Med. 2012;12:1–9.

Matsuda H, Kageura T, Inoue Y, Morikawa T, Yoshikawa M. Absolute stereo structures and syntheses of Saussure amines A, B, C, D and E, amino acid-sesquiterpene conjugates with gastroprotective effect from the roots of *Saussurea lappa*. Tetrahedron. 2000;56:7763–77.

Mustadrak-Al-Hakim, Abu Abd Allah Muhammad ibn Abd Allah al-Hakim al-Nishapuri (d. 405 A.H). Sahih Al-Bukhari, Hadith on Medicine, 5371, n.d..

Pandey MM, Govindarajan RA, Rawat AK, Pushpangadan PA. Free radical Scavenging potential of Sassurea costus. Acta Pharm. 2005;55(3):297–304.

Sarwar A, Enbergs H. Effects of Saussurea lappa roots extract in ethanol on leukocyte phagocytic activity, lymphocyte proliferation and interferon-gamma (IFN-gamma). Pak J Pharm Sci. 2007;20(3):175–9.

Shirishkumar DA, Nilesh AM, Amol PM, Subhash LB. Pharmacological evaluation of anticonvulsant activity of root extract of *Saussurea lappa* in mice. Eur J Integ Med. 2009;1:131–7.

Suyuti J. As-Suyuti's medicine of the prophet. London: Ta-Ha Publishers; 1994. p. 77.. Thomson A (editor)

Taniguchi M, Kataoka T, Suzuki H, Uramato M, Ando MK, Magae J, Nishimura T, Otake N, Nagai K. Costunolide and dehydrocostus lactone as inhibitors of killing function of cytotoxic T lymphocytes. Biosci Biotechnol Biochem. 1995;59(11):2064–7.

Upadhyay OP, Ojha JK, Bajpai HS, Hathwal AK. Study of (*Saussurea lappa,* Clarke) in ischaemic heart disease. Ancient Sci Life. 1993;XIII(1–2):11–8.

Yaeesh S, Jamal Q, Shah AJ, Gilani AH. Antihepatotoxic activity of *Saussurea lappa* extract on D-galactosamine and lipopolysaccharide-induced hepatitis in mice. Phytother Res. 2010;24:S229–32.

Agarwood: Medicinal Side of the Fragrant Plant

16

Pratap Kalita, Probin Kr. Roy, and Supriyo Sen

Contents

P. Kalita
Faculty of Pharmaceutical Sciences, Assam Down Town University, Guwahati, Assam, India

P. K. Roy
BIRAC BIG Project (Ouija Biosolutions Pvt. Ltd.), Guwahati Biotech Park, Indian Institute of Technology-Guwahati Campus, Guwahati, Assam, India

Division of Pharmaceutical Technology, Defence Research Laboratory (DRL), Tezpur, Assam, India

S. Sen (✉)
BIRAC BIG Project (Ouija Biosolutions Pvt. Ltd.), Guwahati Biotech Park, Indian Institute of Technology-Guwahati Campus, Guwahati, Assam, India

School of Life Sciences, Assam Don Bosco University, Sonapur, Assam, India

S. Sen, R. Chakraborty (eds.), *Herbal Medicine in India*,
https://doi.org/10.1007/978-981-13-7248-3_16

16.1 Agarwood: An Interesting Profile of a Tree

Agarwood is synonymous with flavor and fragrances owing to the rich and ancient traditions in perfumery and religious rituals associated with it. The distinct woody aroma of agarwood has a strong presence in commercial incense and perfumes industry particularly in the Middle East and Europe. However, the equally important medicinal aspect of agarwood has been rather overlooked in terms of popular perception, commercial use and scientific research. Even though the Eastern world, particularly China and Japan, has used agarwood in traditional medicine, the global view continues to be predominantly that of perfumes and aroma. It is not that there has not been scientific studies exploring or validating its medicinal aspects, but the focus has been by and large on its aroma. The reason for this is largely related to economics. The agarwood resin which is traded as its fragrant principle is among the most expensive natural products in the world. The essential oil distilled out of the resinous wood sells at a whopping 70,000–80,000 USD/litre while the raw resinous wood can be sold at up to 8000–10,000 USD/kg depending upon quality in the global market. Most of the agarwood products find their way into the global flavor and fragrance market registering trade estimated at 6–8 billion USD (Akter et al. 2013). The demand is consistently higher than supply which maintains such a high price for agarwood in the market. The reason for the supply shortage is primarily agarwood resin formation itself. The fragrant resin is formed by a complex process of challenge to plants of the genera *Aquilaria* and *Gyrinops* under the family Thymelaeaceae by biotic (insects, microorganisms) and abiotic stressors in the environment where the tree grows. The genetic make-up of the plant is the other contributor to the nature of response to the stresses by the plant. However, this is a matter of chance and hence only 10% of plants in a plantation do actually produce any resin. Moreover, agarwood is confined only to a definite geographical zone of the world comprising parts of South and Southeast Asia which makes it a highly exclusive forest product and a rare commodity.

Aquilaria is the most prominent genus that produces agarwood. However, all the 19 known species of the genus are highly endangered and included under the Convention on International Trade in Endangered Species of Wild Fauna and Flora (CITES 2018) and 9 of them are listed in the Red List of the International Union for Conservation of Nature (IUCN 2018). The commercially exploited species are *A. malaccensis, A. crassna, A. sinensis*, and *A. filaria*. *A. malaccensis* is the most popular species of agarwood which, apart from India, is also found in Bangladesh, Bhutan, Indonesia, Malaysia, Myanmar, the Philippines, Singapore, and Thailand (Oldfield et al. 1998). All *Aquilaria* species can survive in altitudes up to 1000 m with average temperature of 20–22 °C and can grow up to a height of 40 m with 60 cm diameter. Age is a major factor in resin formation, as trees mostly produce resin from the age of 15 years and those aged 50 years and above give the best yields both in quality and quantity of aroma (Chakrabarty et al. 1994; Soehartono and Newton 2001).

Agarwood has a special place of reverence in the religious and aesthetic practices among followers of Islam. Agarwood products have the largest market in the Middle East, where oil (*attar*) and incense are used extensively in religious, decorative, aesthetic, and medicinal purposes. Artistic shapes are used to decorate homes and incense is burnt for relaxation and meditation by affluent sections of the society. In Southeast Asia agarwood is used primarily for medicinal and religious purpose apart from fragrance. In Chinese *Materia medica*, agarwood-derived therapies for abdominal pain, vomiting, diarrhea, and asthma are found. In India, agarwood is used in Ayurvedic formulations as carminative and refrigerant while in Unani as a stimulant, stomachic, laxative, and aphrodisiac.

Scientific studies on agarwood have largely emphasized on elucidation of the mechanisms of fragrant agarwood formation, chemical nature of constituents of wood and oil and techniques for artificial induction of resin for aroma production. There are studies that have attempted at understanding the medicinal value of the plant but compared to other aspects are in fewer number. Therefore, more such studies, a comprehensive cataloguing and critical deliberations on the medical aspect of agarwood are urgently required to highlight this neglected aspect of agarwood.

This chapter is an attempt in this direction and it aspires to be a primer for more research, writings, and discussion on this aspect of the fragrant plant.

16.2 Phytoconstituent Profile of *Aquilaria* Species

An early comprehensive review of the phytochemical constituents of agarwood appeared in 2011 (Naef 2011). Since then there has been a steady continuity on research aimed at elucidating the phytochemical nature of agarwood. Numerous bioactive compounds have been already screened out from the different *Aquilaria* species in order to explore their biological activities. *Aquilaria* species like *A. crassna* and *A. malaccensis* are rich in phytoconstituents. Powder of the *A. crassna* seeds is very rich in the glycerides including triglycerides, diglycerides, and monoglycerides in addition to free fatty acid content (Chen et al. 2010). Four types of bi-2-(2-phenylethyl) chromone moieties have been elucidated from *A. crassna,* and from the same source six uncommon ester-bonded dimeric compounds were isolated with the addition of units of a 5,6,7,8-tetrahydroxy-2-(2-phenylethyl)-5,6,7,8-tetrahydro-4H-chromone (Yang et al. 2017, 2018). *A. sinensis* is a source of artificial agarwood in China, where presence of novel bi-phenylethylchromones has been reported (Xiang et al. 2017). Five new 5,11-epoxyguaiane sesquiterpenes were extracted from the *A. sinensis* found in south China. Qi-Nan is familiar as high-quality agarwood that is abundant source for different active sesquiterpenes. Isolation of guaiane and acorane sesquiterpenes (Yang et al., 2016a), comparison of natural and artificial agarwood through GC-MS (Gao et al. 2014), and identification of sesquiterpenes from the agarwood oil originated from the *A. malaccensis* (Tajuddin et al. 2013) are some new approaches adopted for understanding the phytoconstituent profile of agarwood. Refer to Table 16.1 for the details of research on chemical components of the agarwood and agarwood oil.

16.3 Medicinal Properties of Agarwood: Traditional Therapy and Beliefs

Agarwood has been used since thousands of years and is reported to be part of Ayurveda, Muslim, Tibetan, and traditional East-Asian medical practice and even finds mention in *Sushruta Samhita* (Chakrabarty et al. 1994; Fratkin 1994). The highly valued material from agarwood plant is the scented heartwood produced by different species of *Aquilaria.* It has been a key material for perfumery and many products. It is used as incense in religious and festive celebrations by Arabians, Indians, and Japanese since many centuries. It has also been reported to act as sedative or tranquilizer, detoxifying agent of body, and for maintaining healthy stomach (Jung 2009; http://citeseerx.ist.psu.edu/viewdoc/download?doi=10.1.1.459.1016&rep=rep1&type=pdf). Essential oils have countless benefits. The benefits of agarwood are vast ranging from psychoactive and spiritual to therapeutic and medicinal. Ayurvedic practitioners prescribe the essential oils for spiritual and emotional benefits. Inhaling a few drops of oil at bedtime can help induce sound sleep. It is used in the treatment of insomnia by promoting calm and deep sleep. Tibetan monks used to bring inner peace, positive energy, and self-awareness (http://citeseerx.ist.psu.edu/viewdoc/download?doi=10.1.1.459.1016&rep=rep1&type=pdf).

Agarwood has been established for its medicinal properties in Indian and Chinese medicine. In Tibetan medicine agarwood is used to treat emotional, nervous, and psychological issues. In Chinese medicine agarwood has been reported to treat digestive problems and spasms, regulate the vital organs, and relieve pain. It is also used in treating abdominal pain, vomiting, diarrhea, and asthma. In Ayurveda, agarwood is used as incense, which has beneficial effects on the mind. The powdered heartwood is also used to treat diarrhea, dysentery, vomiting, and anorexia (Radosevic 2018).

16.4 Pharmacological Properties of Agarwood

Agarwood has been used traditionally for curing many diseases in several countries. The different parts of the plant such as leaves, bark, and wood have been used as acrid, anodyne, aphrodisiac, aromatic, astringent, bitter, cardiotonic, carminative, stimulant, and fragrant (Alam et al. 2015).

Table 16.1 Compounds present in agarwood and agar oil originated from *Aquilaria* spp.

Sl No	*Aquilaria* spp.	Plant parts	Variety	Methods	Extract type	Compounds isolated	References
1	*A. crassna*	Seeds	Indonesia	Super-critical CO_2 extraction	n-Hexane, methanol, dichloromethane etc	Triglycerides, diglycerides, monoglycerides, free fatty acids including myristic acid, palmitic acid, palmitoleic acid, strearic acid, linoleic acid	Chen et al. (2010)
2	*A. crassna*	–	Laos	Spectroscopic methods including UV, 1D and 2D NMR, MS, IR, ECD	Ethyl acetate, methanol, ethanol, chloroform fractions	Crassin A, Crassin B, Crassin C, and Crassin D	Yang et al. (2017)
3	*A. crassna*	–	Laos	Spectroscopic methods including UV, NMR, MS, IR, ECD	Ethyl acetate and other fractions	Aquilacrassnins A, B, C, D, E, and F with units of 5,6,7,8-tetrahydroxy-2-(2-phenylethyl)-5,6,7,8-tetrahydro-4H-chromone	Yang et al. (2018)
4	*A. crassna*	–	Laos	Spectroscopic methods including UV, 1D and 2D NMR, MS, IR	Ethyl acetate and other fractions	(7β,8β,9β)-8,9-epoxycalamenen-10-one, 11,13-dihydroxy-9(10)-ene-8β,12-epoxyemophilane, (4S,5R,7R)-11,12-dihydroxy-eremophila-1(10)-ene-2-oxo-11-methyl ester	Wang et al. (2016)
5	*A. sinensis*	–	China	Spectroscopic methods including 1D and 2D NMR ECD, HRESIMS, MS, UV, IR	Ethyl acetate extract, methanol, ethanol, chloroform fractions	Nine new bi-phenylethylchromones	Xiang et al. (2017); Huo et al. (2017)
6	*Gyrinops salicifolia*	–	Papua New Guinea	Spectroscopic methods including UV, 1D and 2D NMR, IR	Different solvent fractions	Six new fragrants of sesquiterpenes isolated, namely 4β,7α-H-eremophil-9(10)-ene-12,13-diol, 4β,7α-H-eremophil-9(10)-ene-11,12,13-triol, 4β,7α-H-eremophil-1(2),9(10)-dien-11,12,13-triol, 4β,7α,8α-H-eremophil-9(10)-ene-8,12-epoxy-11α,13-diol, 4β,7α-H-11,13-dihydroxy-eremophil-1(10)-ene-11-methyl ester, 4β,5α,7α,8α-H-3β-hydroxy-1(10)-ene-8,12-epoxy-guaia-12-one	Shao et al. (2016)
7	*A. sinensis*	–	South China	Spectroscopic methods including 1D and 2D NMR, HRESIMS, IR	Total 11 fractions	Qinanol A, qinanol B, qinanol C, qinanol D, qinanol E, and sinenofuranol	Yang et al. (2016a)
8	*A. sinensis*	–	China	Spectroscopic methods including NMR, ECD, X-ray crystallographic	Different solvent systems like chloroform, ethanol, butanol, methanol, etc.	5,6,7,8-Tetrahydro-2-(2-phenylethyl)chromones include tetrahydrochromone A, B, C, D, E, F, G, H, I, G, K, L, M	Liao et al. (2017)

9	*A. sinensis*	–	South China	Spectroscopic methods including 1D and 2D NMR, HRESIMS, IR	Different solvent fractions	Qinanlactone, Qinan-guaiane-one, 4-epi-10-hydroxyacoronene, −epi-15-hydroxyacorenone	Yang et al. (2016b)
10	*A. sinensis*	–	China	GC-MS	Chloroform fractions	22 metabolites reported including farnesol, β-selinenol, aristolone, ledene oxide-(I), baimuxinal, verrucarol, glaucyl alcohol, velleral, hydrastine, (−)-spathulenol, etc.	Gao et al. (2014)
11	*A. crassna*	–	Vietnam, South China	NMR	Ethyl acetate extract with different fractions	Oxidoagarochromone A, oxidoagarochromone B, oxidoagarochromone C	Yagura et al. (2005)
12	*A. sinensis*	–	China	HPLC	–	5S, 7S, 9S, 10S)-(+)-9-hydroxyselina-3, 11-dien-12-al	Zhu et al. (2016)
13	*A. agallocha*	–	Japan	GC, GC-MS, NMR, IR	Different solvent fractions	(−)-Guaia-l(10),ll-dien-15-al,(−)-selina-3,ll-dien-pane,(+)-selina-3,11-dien-9-01	Ishihara et al. (1991)
14	*A. malaccensis*	–	Malaysia	GC × GC	Agarwood oil	Total 30 components screened out including benzaldehyde, acetophenone, copaene, α-cedrene, caryophyllene, α-guaiene, α, and β-selinene, agarospirol, elemol, α-muurolene, α-bulnesene, etc.	Tajuddin et al. (2013)
15	*A. agallocha, A. malaccensis*	–	Vietnam, Indonesia	GLC, GC/MS	Essential oil from agarwood	β-Agarofuran, α-agarofuran, agarospirol, Jmkohol, Kusunol, Dlhydrokaranone, Jmkohol II, Oxo-agarospirol	Yoneda et al. (1984)
16	*A. malaccencis*	Leaves	Malaysia	HPLC	Leaf extract	4'-Hydroxyacetanilide	Afiffudden et al. (2015)
17	*A. sinensis*	Petiole and leaves	China	Chromatographic techniques	Different solvent fractions including butanol, ethyl acetate, chloroform, methanol, etc.	5-Hydroxy-6-methoxy-2-(2-phenylethyl)chromone, 6-methoxy-2-[2-(3-methoxy-4-hydroxyphenyl)ethyl]chromone, 6-hydroxy-2-[2-(4-hydroxyphenyl)ethyl]chromone, aquilacallane B, aquilacallane A, cucurbitacin L, bryoamaride, 2-O-b-D-glucopyranosylcucurbitacin I, 2-O-b-D-glucopyranosylcucurbitacin J, 2-O-b-D-glucopyranosyl-cucurbitacin K, uridine, cytidine, thymidine, inosine, adenosine, guanosine, iriflophenone 3-C-b-D-glucopyranoside, aquilarisinin	Wang et al. (2015)
18	*A. sinensis*	Leaves	China	Spectroscopic methods including 1D and 2D NMR, HRMS, and chemical analysis	Ethanol extract with other solvent fractions	Five new benzophenone glycosides isolated namely aquilarinenside A aquilarinenside B, aquilarinenside C, aquilarinenside D, aquilarinenside E	Sun et al. (2014)

Use of agarwood in different rituals is also well documented but the therapeutic effects produced by different parts of the plant or compounds present and their mechanisms of action are not well understood. Development of science and technology in the recent years has helped to indentify and study a number of compounds which are mainly responsible for the pharmacological effects.

A summary of the pharmacological activities studied in agarwood is detailed below:

16.4.1 Antidiabetic Activity

Diabetes mellitus is a metabolic disorder where the body is incapable of converting glucose into energy. Health complications associated with diabetes include heart disease, diabetic nephropathy, diabetic retinopathy, immune suppression, delayed wound healing, etc. Nowadays herbal drugs have impressed the worldwide population because of their least side effects, least toxicity, and better safety compared to synthetic or semisynthetic drugs. Studies of antidiabetic activity of plants have been well documented in literature. The antidiabetic activity of agarwood plant was not recognized until the story of a diabetic patient who drank infusion of agarwood leaf to reduce his blood sugar to normal came to light. Methanol and aqueous extracts of the leaf were tested against streptozotocin (STZ)-induced diabetic rats. *In vitro* α-glucosidase and α-amylase inhibitory effects of methanol and aqueous extracts were also determined. The comparative results suggested that agarwood leaf extract can be a potential candidate as a dietary supplement (Zulkifle et al. 2013). In another study antihyperglycemic activity of agarwood leaf extracts in STZ-induced diabetic rats and glucose uptake enhancement activity in rat adipocytes were evaluated. Methanol and water extracts of agarwood leaf had shown potential antihyperglycemic activity in STZ-induced diabetic rats and also increased glucose uptake by adipocytes in normal rats. At 3 and 10 μg/mL, both extracts exhibited slightly high glucose uptake than 1.5 nM of insulin which was used as a control. They concluded that the mechanism of antihyperglycemic activity of both extracts apparently was linked to glucose uptake by adipocyte and can be a potential source for antidiabetic agent (Pranakhon et al. 2011). Ethanol extract of leaves of *A. sinensis* contains mangiferin, iriflophenone 2-O11 α-L-rhamnopyranoside, iriflophenone 3-C-β-D-glucoside, and iriflophenone 3,5-C-β-D-diglucopyranoside. These compounds have been reported to have antidiabetic effect and reduce blood sugar by reducing absorption of carbohydrate in intestine (Feng et al. 2011). Ethanol extract of *A. malaccensis* has the capability to raise the levels of type 4 (GLUT4) transporter, thereby regulating the glucose in whole body. The extract has been reported to have higher antidiabetic activity by increasing GLUT4 levels than pioglitazone (Said and Kamaluddin 2016).

16.4.2 Antioxidant Activity

The effects of free radicals on human beings are strongly linked to toxicity, disease, and aging (Maxwell 1995). Almost all the living species have their own defense system to protect themselves from oxidative stress produced by reactive oxygen species (ROS) (Sato et al. 1996). Antioxidant properties of plants are correlated with oxidative stress defense from different human diseases including cancer, atherosclerosis, and aging process (Stajner et al. 1998; Sanchez-Moreno et al. 1999). They are generated as by-products through the oxidative damage of DNA molecules, lipids and proteins (Farber 1994). Antioxidants can greatly reduce the damage due to oxidants by neutralizing the free radicals before they can attack the cells and preventing damage to lipids, proteins, enzymes, carbohydrates, and DNA. *In -vitro* antioxidant property of ethyl acetate extract of *A. agallocha* was tested on nitrite-induced oxidation of hemoglobin in human blood hemolysate. Strong inhibitory effects on methemoglobin, the oxidation product of hemoglobin, produced by the treatment with sodium nitrite activity was observed at a dose range of 500–3500 μg/mL (Miniyar et al. 2008). In another study antioxidant and antibacterial activities of *A. malaccensis* were reported. The study was conducted to identify the group of compounds which are responsible for the different activities. Old and young leaves of the plants were selected for the purpose. Dried leaves were powdered and then extraction was done in Soxhlet apparatus using three different polarities of solvents such as chloroform, methanol, and water. After fractioning through vacuum liquid chromatography (VLC) antioxidant activity was analyzed using 2,2-diphenyl-1-picrylhydrazyl (DPPH). To identify the bioactive compounds in the potential fraction thin-layer chromatography (TLC) was used. In the result it was reported that the methanol extract of the old leaves was the most potential extract with an IC_{50} value of 19.62 ± 1.49 μg/mL and the combined fraction of 1:3 chloroform:methanol and 100% methanol showed the highest antioxidant activity with IC_{50} 17.39 ± 1.43 μg/mL. The compounds which were responsible for the antioxidant properties were found to be of phenolic and flavonoid group (Hendra et al. 2016). In another study antioxidant activities of flavonoids from *A. sinensis* have been investigated by DPPH and 2,2′-azinobis-(3-ethylbenzothiazoline-6-sulfonate) (ABTS) radical scavenging, and potassium ferricyanide reduction assays. The flavonoids reported to possess strong antioxidant activity to scavenge DPPH and ABTS radicals with median effective concentrations (EC_{50}) of (1.14 ± 0.08) mg/mL and (0.23 ± 0.01) mg/mL, respectively (Duan et al. 2015). *A. crassna* leaves have been used traditionally by people of Thailand without proper scientific analysis to treat numbers of disorders. Extract of *A. crassna* was tested for antioxidative properties using DPPH antioxidant assay. Antioxidative activity of the leaf extract was reported to be with IC_{50} value of 47.18 μg/mL. They had reported that there was surprisingly a significant reduction in body weight from second day to consecutive seven days of administration with a dose of 8000 mg/kg compared to control. They concluded that the antioxidant properties of the extract and the possible ability to inhibit α-glucosidase may be applicable in the treatment and prevention of metabolic disorders (Sattasai et al. 2012). The tradition of drinking herbal tea is well familiar worldwide since past 2000 years (Cabrera et al. 2006). The benefit of herbal tea is often associated with refreshing mood, aroma taste, and also numerous health benefits (Adam et al. 2017). Agarwood tea became popular in China as a health drink and from studies that suggested antioxidant properties the health benefits were confirmed (Han and Li 2012).

16.4.3 Hepatoprotective Activity

Many herbs are traditionally used by different ethnic groups of people for liver disease. Liver is the primary drug-metabolizing organ which performs numerous functions such as synthesis, secretion, and metabolism of xenobiotics. It is revealed that different factors responsible for liver damage and hepatic injury are infectious virus, pollutants, and hepatotoxic chemicals (Singhal and Gupta 2012). Liver transforms many drugs and toxins and converts to inactive form. During transformation liver converts much water-insoluble entity to soluble form, thereby enhancing excretion through kidneys (Strunin 1971). Ethanol extract of *A. agallocha* has been reported to have hepatoprotective activity in CCl4-induced rats. In a histopathological study CCl4-induced rats exhibited necrosis with disappearance of hepatocytes, areas of inflammation, and increased sinusoidal spaces. Liver section of the rat treated with 400 mg/kg of the extract and CCl4 was found to exhibit normalization of cells and reduced sinusoidal dilation along with mild inflammation (Vakati et al. 2013). In another study hepatoprotective potential of ethanol extract of *A. agallocha* leaves was reported against paracetamol-induced hepatotoxicity in Sprague-Dawley rats. Extract at a dose of 400 mg/kg/day was reported to be comparable with 100 mg/kg/day of standard silymarin drugs. Results showed significant decrease in serum alanine transaminase, aspartate aminotransferase, alkaline phosphatase, lactate dehydrogenase, cholesterol, and bilirubin level and increased level of albumin and total protein. It was summarized that agarwood possesses hepatoprotective effect against paracetamol-induced hepatotoxicity (Alam et al. 2017).

16.4.4 Anticancer and Antitumor Activity

Cucurbitacins are tetracyclic triterpenoids which are biologically distributed mostly in

Cucurbitaceae family. *Aquilaria* leaves have been reported to contain cucurbitacin glycosides such as 2-O-β-D-glucopyranosyl cucurbitacin I and bryoamaride (Sun et al. 2015; Adam et al. 2017). Cucurbitacin I found in the different parts of the *Aquilaria* plants has been reported to inhibit cancer cells and cytotoxic effect against MDA-MB-468 human breast cancer cells and inhibit cell motility by indirectly interfering with actin (Knecht et al. 2010). *In -vitro* anti-metastatic activity of agarwood oil (*A. crassna*) had been reported against pancreatic cancer cells. The essential oil is found to possess potential cytotoxic activity against MIA PaCa-2 cells (Dahham et al. 2015). *In vitro* toxicity and antitumor activity of essential oil extract from agarwood (*A. crassna*) showed that it is safe with LD_{50} above 2000 mg/kg and has antitumor activity in HCT 116 subcutaneous tumor model established in NCR nu/nu nude mice (Yang et al. 2016a, 2016b). Anticancer activity of agarwood oil against MCF-7 breast cancer cell has been reported with IC_{50} value of 900 μg/mL. ß-caryophyllene, a sesquiterpene isolated from essential oil of *A. crassna*, was studied for *in- vitro* antitumor-promoting activity using colon cancer cells. The results suggested that β-caryophyllene is the principal compound for the selective anticancer properties and can be a promising chemotherapeutic agent for colorectal cancer (Dahham et al. 2015). Studies have also indicated that the cytotoxic properties of supercritical fluid extract of *A. malaccensis* have potent anticancer activity in human colon cancer cell (Ibrahim et al. 2011).

16.4.5 Analgesics, Anti-arthritic, and Anti-inflammatory Activities

Inflammation involves increased vascular permeability which results in exudation of fluids from interstitial space followed by infiltration of leukocyte into the tissues and granuloma formation (Ritter 2000; Haslett et al. 2002; Vogel et al. 2002). Inflammation and pain are treated by non-steroidal anti-inflammatory drugs (NSAIDs), opioid analgesics, and corticosteroids. However, their serious side effects forced the search for alternative agents of treatment. Herbal sources have been preferred because of the lesser side effects and history of using herbal medicine has been well recognized by different traditional systems of medicine. Ethyl acetate extract of *A. agallocha* has been reported to have analgesic and anti-inflammatory activity (Chitre et al. 2007). Extract of *A. crassna* has also been experimentally reported to have anti-inflammatory (Kumphune et al. 2011), antipyretic, and analgesic activity (Sattasai et al. 2012). Rheumatoid arthritis (RA) is an autoimmune chronic inflammatory disorder which affects the joints of the bone. Ethanolic extracts and the oil from the heartwood of *A. agallocha* have been found with potent anti-arthritic activity *in-vitro* and *in vivo* (Rahman et al. 2012). In the recent studies, many anti-inflammatory 2-(2-phenylethyl) chromone derivatives have been identified from Chinese agarwood (*A. sinensis*) (Chen et al. 2012; Huo et al. 2017).

16.4.6 Antibacterial and Antifungal Activities

Agarwood leaves contain hexadecanoic acid, a saturated fatty acid usually found in both plants and animals, familiar for its antibacterial and antifungal activity (Khalil et al. 2013). Hexadecanoic acid exhibits antibacterial activity against both Gram-negative as well as Gram-positive bacteria which is comparable to ampicillin but in case of *Streptococci* hexadecanoic acid shows better antibacterial activity than ampicillin (Saidana et al. 2008). A sesquiterpene β-caryophyllene from essential oil of *A. crassna* was found to have selective antibacterial activity against *Staphylococcus aureus* with a minimum inhibitory concentration (MIC) of 3 ± 1.0 μM and have more prominent antifungal activity than kanamycin (Dahham et al. 2015). In other studies, plant crude extracts have also been evaluated for antimicrobial activity (Dash et al. 2008; Hendra et al. 2016).

16.4.7 Laxative Effects

Leaves of *A. sinensis* have been found to have intestinal motility activity in small intestines

(Li et al. 2013). Two compounds, mangiferin and genkwanin-5-O-β-premeveroside, found in the ethanol extract of *A. sinensis* and *A. crassna* have been found to be responsible for the laxative effects (Kakino et al. 2010; Kakino and Hara 2016).

16.4.8 Antihistaminic Activities

Allergic reaction is partly mediated by IgE, involving multiple mediators. Histamine is one of the earliest recognized mediators of allergy derived from the mast cells (White 1990). Histamine is one of the potential mediators to be known to cause bronchoconstriction in the pathogenesis of asthma (Liu et al. 1990). Genkwanin and luteolin present in the *Aquilaria* leaves are reported to have cough-relieving and soothing effects in asthma (Wang 2008; Lin et al. 2012). Aqueous extract of the stems of *A. agallocha* has been reported to have anti-hypersensitivity effect by inhibition of histamine release from mast cells (Kim et al. 1997).

16.4.9 Other Effects

Alcoholic heartwood extract of *A. agallocha* has been reported to have anxiolytic and anticonvulsant effect on mice (Alla et al. 2007). A number of compounds such as benzylacetone, gurjunene, and (+)-calarene found in *Aquilaria* species have been reported to have sedative effect (Takemoto et al. 2008). Benzene extracts of *Aquilaria* species have been reported to have central nervous system (CNS) depressant potential (Okugawa et al. 1993). Nutrients present in the leaves of *Aquilaria* make them usable for the farm animals to improve their digestibility and growth (Huang et al. 2016; Suhatri et al. 2017).

16.5 Toxicity and Safety Measurement of *Aquilaria* Species

The toxicological studies still remain unclear due to lack of scientific reports on the consumption of *Aquilaria* spp. But some recent investigations reported the effects on the basis of laboratory assays. Consumption of agarwood leaves (2000 mg/kg) and oil (2000 mg/kg) by the female experimental Wistar rats showed normal behavior without any toxic effect. No sign of depression (tested animals expressed normal motor activity) as well as gland secretion were visible (Rahman et al. 2012). Toxicity studies on Malaysian agarwood leaf extracts exhibited normal observations in case of single-sex animals administered a fixed dose. Normal-behavior profile included parameters like changes in skin, eye, respiration, circulatory, and mucus secretion (Zulkifle et al. 2013). Sattasai et al. (2012) repeated administration of effective doses (800 mg/kg) to 8000 mg/kg in rodents which showed no sign of unusual characters with additional reduction of body weight from the second day of administration up to seventh day. Extract of *A. crassna* was studied for the cell viability test on the rat cardiac myoblast cell line (H9c2) and the outcomes prescribed normal cellular viability (Jermsri and Kumphune 2012; Jermsri et al. 2012). No sign of cytotoxicity was observed against the ethyl acetate extract of *A. crassna* after exposure of extract to lipopolysaccharide-stimulated human peripheral blood mononuclear cell culture (Kumphune et al. 2011). Aquilacrassnin A-F from the *A. crassna* displayed effective cytotoxic potency against the varieties of tumor cell lines including A549, Hela, SGC-7901, BEL-7402, and K562 (Yang et al. 2018). The effect of essential oil from the *A. crassna* stem bark on human pancreatic carcinoma cell lines (MIA PaCa-2) confirmed strong prevention of cell viability at high concentration and moderate cell viability at lower concentration (Dahham et al. b). Long- and short-term effects of inhalation or smoking of agarwood linked with weight loss and adverse metabolic functions and biochemical parameters due to alteration of the group of the cytochrome enzymes in the empirical Wistar albino rats are also reported (Alokail et al. 2011; Hussain et al. 2014; Karimi et al. 2012). Please refer to Table 16.2 for a more detailed catalogue of the studies on toxicity of agarwood phytoconstituents.

Table 16.2 Toxicological studies on *Aquilaria* species

Sl No	*Aquilaria* spp.	Plant parts	Experiment/trial	Variety	Extract/Fractions	Tested dose	Results	References
1	*A. agallocha*	Leaves	Oral toxicity studies	India	Ethanolic extract	2000 mg/kg	Normal behavior	Rahman et al., (2016)
2	*A. agallocha*	Oils	Acute toxic class method	Marketed product, India	Oil	2000 mg/kg	Normal behavior	Rahman et al. (2012)
3	*A. malaccensis, A. hirta, A. beccariana, A. rostrata*	Leaves	Acute toxic—fixed-dose method	Malaysia	Methanol and aqueous extract	250, 500, 1000, 2000 mg/kg	No negative signs	Zulkifle et al. (2013)
4	*A. crassna*	Leaves	Oral toxicity procedure	Thailand	Methanol extract	8000 mg/kg	No abnormal behavior	Sattasai et al. (2012)
5	*A. crassna*	Heartwood	Cell viability assay (based on MTT)	Thailand	Ethyl acetate extract	1–8 mg/mL	Cell viability (%) was found within the range of 96.58 ± 3.129 to 100.4 ± 2.972 when tested on H9c2 cell as compared to control (DMSO) 98.29 ± 5.178	Jermsri and Kumphune (2012)
6	*A. crassna*	Heartwood	Cell viability assay (based on MTT)	Thailand	Ethyl acetate extract	1 mg/mL–10 mg/mL	Findings were significantly different against cell viability on H9c2 cell	Jermsri et al. (2012)
7	*A. crassna*	Heartwood	Trypan blue dye exclusion assay	Thailand	Ethyl acetate extract	0.5–3 mg/mL	No sign of cytotoxicity when tested on LPS-stimulated human peripheral blood mononuclear cell culture	Kumphune et al. (2011)
8	*A. crassna*	Heartwood	MTT assay	Luang Prabang, Laos	Fractions of EtOAc extract (Aquilacrassnin A-F)	Different concentrations of all compounds	Significant cytotoxic potential has been observed for all the tested compounds against the different tumor cell lines	Yang et al. (2018)
9	*A. crassna*	Stem bark	MTT cell proliferation assay	Malaysia	Essential oil extract	3.1–200 μg/mL	Strong and moderate resistance against the proliferation of cancer cell in MIA PaCa-2	Dahham et al. (2016b)
10	*A. crassna*	Leaves	Acute toxicity test in mice	Thailand	Water extract	2000–15,000 mg/kg	No sign of mortality	Kamonwannasit et al. (2013)
11	*A. crassna*	Stem bark	Limit test procedure (fixed dose)	Malaysia	Essential oil extract	2000 mg/kg	No any abnormal attributes	Dahham et al. (2016a)
12	*A. crassna*	Stem bark	Sub-chronic toxicity study	Malaysia	Essential oil extract	500–1000 mg/kg	No sign of toxicity	Dahham et al. (2016a)
13	*A. malaccensis*	Tea leaves	Sub-chronic oral toxicity study		Tea agarwood	130, 260, 390, 520 mg/kg	The dose is given up to 90 days and weakness and convulsion pattern observed at 390 and 520 mg/kg without any sign of death	Batubara et al. (2016)

16.6 Conclusion

The fragrant attribute of agarwood has chronically suppressed the medicinal importance of the plant in popular perception as well as scientific research. However, there is a significant divide among the fragrant and medicinal use of the plant along the Western and Eastern hemispheres. While in West Asia and Europe the fragrance of agarwood and its use in aromatherapy are valued, in East, particularly Southeast Asia and China, there is considerable traditional application of agarwood in medical conditions. The medicinal side of this fragrant plant is therefore as much interesting as formation of agarwood resin itself by complex environmental actions. This review presents the versatile nature of the plant with regard to its medicinal use. The favorable toxicity results also offer enough validation for the successful traditional use of the plant in treatment of diseases and symptoms. However, more comprehensive and cross-platform studies are required to establish the therapies based on agarwood. The aroma-medicinal synergy in agarwood can be an area of intense discussion and research for the future and can possibly generate new herbal therapies and drug formulations.

References

Adam AZ, Lee SY, Mohamed R. Pharmacological properties of agarwood tea derived from *Aquilaria* (Thymelaeaceae) leaves: An emerging contemporary herbal drink. J Herb Medicine. 2017;10:37–44.

Afiffudden SKN, Alwi H, Hamid KHK. Determination of 4′-hydroxyacetanilide in leaves extract of *Aquilaria malaccencis* by high pressure liquid chromatography. Procedia Soc Behav Sci. 2015;195:2726–33.

Akter S, Islam MT, Zulkefeli M, Khan SI. Agarwood production: a multidisciplinary field to be explored in Bangladesh. Int J Pharm Life Sci. 2013;2:22–32.

Alam J, Mujahid M, Rahman M, Akhtar J, Khalid M, Jahan Y, Basit A, Khan A, Shawwal M, Iqbal SS. An insight of pharmacognostic study and phytopharmacology of *Aquilaria agallocha*. J Appl Pharm Sci. 2015;5:173–81.

Alam J, Mujahid M, Jahan Y, Bagga P, Rahman MA. Hepatoprotective potential of ethanolic extract of *Aquilaria agallocha* leaves against paracetamol induced hepatotoxicity in SD rats. J Tradit Complement Med. 2017;7:9–13.

Alla T, Handral M, Nandakumar K, Venkatrao N, Shalam S, Shantakumar SM. Anxiolytic and anticonvulsant activity of alcoholic extract of heartwood of *Aquilaria agallocha* roxb, (Thymelaeceae) in mice. Pharmacology. 2007;2:218–25.

Alokail MS, Al-Daghri NM, Alarifi SA, Draz HM, Hussain T, Yakout SM. Long-term exposure to incense smoke alters metabolism in Wistar albino rats. Cell Biochem Funct. 2011;29:96–101.

Batubara R, Surjanto S, Sihombing TM, Ginting H. The safety of tea agarwood (*Aquilaria malaccensis*) from tree induction through test of toxicity subchronic oral 90 days. Biofarmasi. 2016;14(2):69–76.

Cabrera C, Artacho R, Gimenez R. Beneficial effects of green tea—a review. J Am Coll Nutr. 2006;25:79–99.

Chakrabarty K, Kumar A, Menon V. Trade in Agarwood. New Delhi: TRAFFIC India and WWF-India; 1994. p. 51.

Chen W, Ching-Hung C, Chieh-Ming JC, Bing-Chung L, Daina H. Supercritical carbon dioxide extraction of triglycerides from *Aquilaria crassna* seeds. Sep Purif Technol. 2010;73:135–41.

Chen D, Xu Z, Chai X, Zeng K, Jia Y, Bi D, Ma Z, Tu P. Nine 2-(2-Phenylethyl) chromone derivatives from the resinous wood of *Aquilaria sinensis* and their inhibition of LPS induced NO production in RAW 264.7 cells. Eur J Org Chem. 2012;27:5389–97.

Chitre T, Bhutada P, Nandakumar K, Somani R, Miniyar P, Mundhada Y, Gore S, Jain K. Analgesic and anti-inflammatory activity of heartwood of *Aquilaria agallocha* in laboratory animals. Pharmacology. 2007;1:288–98.

CITES, UNEP-WCMC Species Database: CITES-Listed Species; 2018. www.cites.org. Accessed 10 Sep 2018.

Dahham SS, Tabana YM, Iqbal MA, Ahamed MB, Ezzat MO, Majid AS, Majid AM. The anticancer, antioxidant and antimicrobial properties of the sesquiterpene β-caryophyllene from the essential oil of *Aquilaria crassna*. Mol. 2015;20:11808–29.

Dahham SS, Hassan LE, Ahamed MB, Majid AS, Majid AM, Zulkepli NN. *In vivo* toxicity and antitumor activity of essential oils extract from agarwood (*Aquilaria crassna*). BMC Complement Altern Med. 2016a;16:236.

Dahham SS, Tabana YM, Hassan LE, Ahamed MB, Majid AS, Majid AM. *In vitro* antimetastatic activity of Agar wood (*Aquilaria crassna*) essential oils against pancreatic cancer cells. Alex J Med. 2016b;52:141–50.

Dash M, Patra JK, Panda PP. Phytochemical and antimicrobial screening of extracts of *Aquilaria agallocha* Roxb. Afr J Biotechnol. 2008;7:3531–4.

Duan Z, Li W, Dou Z, Xie H, He A, Shi M. Extraction and antioxidant activity of flavonoids from *Aquilaria sinensis* (Lour.) Gilg leaves. J Food Sci. 2015;36:45–50.

Farber JL. Mechanisms of cell injury by activated oxygen species. Environ Health Perspect. 1994;102:17–24.

Feng J, Yang XW, Wang RF. Bio-assay guided isolation and identification of α-glucosidase inhibitors from the leaves of *Aquilaria sinensis*. Phytochemistry. 2011;72:242–7.

Fratkin J. Chinese herbal patent formulas: a practical guide. Colorado: Shya Publications; 1994.

Gao X, Xie M, Liu S, Guo X, Chen X, Zhong Z, Wang L, Zhang W. Chromatographic fingerprint analysis of metabolites in natural and artificial agarwood using gas chromatography-mass spectrometry combined with chemometric methods. J Chromatogr B. 2014;967:264–73.

Han W, Li X. Antioxidant activity of aloeswood tea *in vitro*. Spatula DD. 2012;2(1):43–50.

Haslett C, Chilvers ER, Boon NA, Colledge NR, Hunter JA. Side effects of NSAIDS. In: Davidson's Principles and Practice of Medicine. Edinburgh: Churchill Livingstone; 2002. p. 989–90.

Hendra H, Moeljopawiro S, Nuringtyas TR. Antioxidant and antibacterial activities of agarwood (*Aquilaria malaccensis* Lamk.) leaves. AIP Conf Proc. 2016;1755(1):140004.

Huang J, Chen H, Yu Z, Zhou Y, Ning G. Effects of different ratios of Aquilaria sinensis leaf meal on the growth performance, slaughter performance and nutrients digestibility of broiler. China Feed. 2016;11:36–42.

Huo HX, Gu YF, Sun H, Zhang YF, Liu WJ, Zhu ZX, Shi SP, Song YL, Jin HW, Zhao YF, Tu PF, Li J. Anti-inflammatory 2-(2-phenylethyl) chromone derivatives from Chinese agarwood. Fitoterapia. 2017;118:49–55.

Hussain T, Al-Attas OS, Al-Daghri NM, Mohammed AA, Rosas ED, Ibrahim S, Vinodson B, Ansari MG, El-Din KIA. Induction of CYP1A1, CYP1A2, CYP1B1, increased oxidative stress and inflammation in the lung and liver tissues of rats exposed to incense smoke. Mol Cell Biochem. 2014;391:127–36.

Ibrahim AH, Al-Rawi SS, Majid AA, Rahman NA, Abo-Salah KM, AbKadir MO. Separation and fractionation of *Aquilaria malaccensis* oil using supercritical fluid extraction and the cytotoxic properties of the extracted oil. Procedia Food Science. 2011;1(1):1953–9.

Ishihara M, Tsuneya T, Shiga M, Uneyama K. Three sesquiterpenes from agarwood. Phyrochem. 1991;30(2):563–6.

IUCN, IUCN Red List of Threatened Species; 2018. https://www.iucnredlist.org. Accessed 17 Nov 2018.

Jermsri P, Kumphune S. Ethyl acetate extract of *Aquilaria crassna* preserve actin cytoskeleton on simulated ischemia induced cardiac cell death. J Med Plants Res. 2012;6(23):4057–62.

Jermsri P, Jiraviriyakul A, Unajak S, Kumphune S. Effects of *Aquilaria crassna* crude extract on simulated ischemia induced cardiac cell death. Int J Pharm Bio Sci. 2012;3(3):604–13.

Jung D. The value of agarwood. Reflections upon its use and history in south Yemen. Extended Version of a talk given at the Workshop "The Use of Herbs in Yemeni Healing Practices," Halle, September 25–26, 2009. https://archiv.ub.uni-heidelberg.de/volltextserver/12039/.

Kakino M, Hara H. Pharmacological effects of *Aquilaria* spp. leaves and their chemical constituents. In: Mohamed R, editor. Agarwood-Science behind the fragrance. Singapore: Springer; 2016. p. 125–36.

Kakino M, Tazawa S, Maruyama H, Tsuruma K, Araki Y, Shimazawa M, Hara H. Laxative effects of agarwood on low-fiber diet-induced constipation in rats. BMC Complement Altern Med. 2010;10:1–8.

Kamonwannasit S, Nantapong N, Kumkrai P, Luecha P, Kupittayanant S, Chudapongse N. Antibacterial activity of *Aquilaria crassna* leaf extract against Staphylococcus epidermidis by disruption of cell wall. Ann Clin Microbiol Antimicrob. 2013;12:1–7.

Karimi I, Becker LA, Chalechale A, Ghashghaii A. Biochemical plasma profile of male rats exposed to smoke of agarwood (*Aquilaria* spp.). Comp Clin Pathol. 2012;21:1053–8.

Khalil AS, Rahim AA, Taha KK, Abdallah KB. Characterization of methanolic extracts of agarwood leaves. J Archaeol Sci. 2013;1:78–88.

Kim YC, Lee EH, Lee YM, Kim HK, Song BK, Lee EJ, Kim HM. Effect of the aqueous extract of *Aquilaria agallocha* stems on the immediate hypersensitivity reactions. J Ethnopharmacol. 1997;58:31–8.

Knecht DA, LaFleur RA, Kahsai AW, Argueta CE, Beshir AB, Fenteany G. Cucurbitacin I inhibits cell motility by indirectly interfering with actin dynamics. PLoS One. 2010;5:1–11.

Kumphune S, Prompunt E, Phaebuaw K, Sriudwong P, Pankla R, Thongyoo P. Anti-inflammatory effects of the ethyl acetate extract of *Aquilaria crassna* inhibits LPS-induced tumour necrosis factor-alpha production by attenuating P38 MAPK activation. Int J Green Pharm. 2011;5:43–8.

Li H, Jiang Z, Mei Q. Comparative study on the effect of *Aquilaria sinensis* leaf tea and agarwood on promoting small intestine propulsion. Asia-Pacific Tradit Med. 2013;9:24–5.

Liao G, Mei WL, Kong FD, Li W, Yuan JZ, Dai HF. 5,6,7,8-Tetrahydro-2-(2-phenylethyl) chromones from artificial agarwood of *Aquilaria sinensis* and their inhibitory activity against acetylcholinesterase. Phytochemistry. 2017;139:98–108.

Lin FH, Peng YH, Ke FF, Deng YL. Experimental study on the content, antioxidant activity *in vitro*, and delaying aging effect of tannins from the leaf of *Aquilaria sinensis* (Lour.) Gilg. J Guangdong Pharm Univer. 2012;3:011.

Liu MC, Bleecker ER, Lichtenstein LM, Kagey-Sobotka A, Niv Y, McLemore TL, Permutt S, Proud D, Hubbard WC. Evidence for elevated levels of histamine, prostaglandin D2, and other broncho constricting prostaglandins in the airways of subjects with mild asthma. Am Rev Respir Dis. 1990;142(1):126–32.

Maxwell SR, Prospects for the use of antioxidant therapies. Drugs. 1995;49(3):345–61

Miniyar PB, Chitre TS, Karve SS, Deuskar HJ, Jain KS. Anti-oxidant activity of ethyl acetate extract of *Aquilaria agallocha* on nitrite-induced methemoglobin formation. IJGP. 2008;2(1):43–5.

Naef R. The volatile and semi-volatile constituents of agarwood, the infected heartwood of *Aquilaria* species: A review. Flavour Fragr J. 2011;26:73–89.

Okugawa H, Ueda R, Matsumoto K, Kawanishi K, Kato A. Effects of agarwood extracts on the central nervous system in mice. Planta Med. 1993;59(01):32–6.

Oldfield S, Lusty C, MacKinven A. The word list of threatened trees. Cambridge: World Conservation Press; 1998. p. 650.

Pranakhon R, Pannangpetch P, Aromdee C. Antihyperglycemic activity of agarwood leaf extracts in STZ-induced diabetic rats and glucose uptake enhancement activity in rat adipocytes. Songklanakarin J Sci Technol. 2011;33(4):405–10.

Radosevic I. Uses and benefits for agarwood essential oil; 2018. http://www.balancemebeautiful.com/uses-and-benefits-for-agarwood-essential-oil. Accessed 15 Feb 2018.

Rahman H, Vakati K, Eswaraiah MC. *In-vivo* and *in-vitro* anti-inflammatory activity of *Aquilaria agallocha* oil. Int J Basic Med Sci Pharm. 2012;2:7–10.

Rahman H, Eswaraiah MC, Dutta AM. Anti-arthritic activity of leaves and oil of *Aquilaria agallocha*. Haya Saudi J Life Sci. 2016a;1:34–43.

Ritter JM. Anti-inflammatory and immunosuppressive drugs. In: Rang HP, Dale MM, editors. Pharmacology. Edinburgh: Churchill Livingston; 2000. p. 229–32.

Said F, Kamaluddin MT. Efficacy of the Aquilaria malaccensis leaves active fraction in glucose uptake in skeletal muscle on diabetic Wistar rats. IJHSR. 2016;6(7):162–7.

Saidana D, Mahjoub S, Boussaada O, Chriaa J, Mahjoub MA, Cheraif I, Daami M, Mighri Z, Helal AN. Antibacterial and antifungal activities of the essential oils of two saltcedar species from Tunisia. J Am Oil Chem Soc. 2008;85:817–26.

Sanchez-Moreno C, Larrauri JA, Saura-Calixto F. Free radical scavenging capacity an inhibition of lipid oxidation of wines, grape juices and related polyphenolic constituents. Food Res Int. 1999;32:407–512.

Sato M, Ramarathnam N, Suzuki Y, Ohkubo T, Takeuchi M, Ochi H. Varietal differences in the phenolic content and superoxide radical scavenging potential of wines from different sources. J Agri Food Chem. 1996;44:37–41.

Sattasai J, Bantadkit J, Aromdee C, Lattmann E, Airarat W. Antipyretic, analgesic and anti-oxidative activities of *Aquilaria crassna* leaves extract in rodents. J Ayurveda Integr Med. 2012;3(4):175–9.

Shao H, Mei WL, Kong FD, Dong WH, Gai CJ, Li W, Zhu GP, Dai HF. Fragrant sesquiterpenes of agarwood from *Gyrinops salicifolia*. Fitoterapia. 2016;113:182–7.

Singhal KG, Gupta GD. Hepatoprotective and antioxidant activity of methanolic extract of flowers of Nerium oleander against CCl4-induced liver injury in rats. Asian Pac J Trop Med. 2012;5(9):677–85.

Soehartono T, Newton AC. Reproductive ecology of *Aquilaria* spp. in Indonesia. Forest Ecol Manag. 2001;152(3):59–71.

Stajner D, Milic N, Mimica-dukic N, Lazic B, Igic R. Antioxidant abilities of cultivated and wild species of garlic. Phytother Res. 1998;12:513–4.

Strunin L. Metabolism of drugs by the liver. Ann R Coll Surg Engl. 1971;48:76–7.

Suhatri S, Putra DZ, Elisma E. Effect of aloe leaf extract (*Aquilaria malaccensis* Lamk.) on atherosclerosis in quail bull (Coturnix-coturnix japonica) (author's transl). J Farmasi Higea. 2017;6:174–82.

Sun J, Wang S, Xia F, Wang KY, Chen JM, Tu PF. Five new benzophenone glycosides from the leaves of *Aquilaria sinensis* (Lour.) Gilg. Chin Chem Lett. 2014;25:1573–6.

Sun J, Xia F, Wang S, Wang KY, Chen JM, Tu PF. Structural elucidation of two new megastigmane glycosides from the leaves of *Aquilaria sinensis*. Chin J Nat Med. 2015;13:0290–4.

Tajuddin SN, Muhamad NS, Yarmo MA, Yusoff MM. Characterization of the chemical constituents of agarwood oils from Malaysia by comprehensive two-dimensional gas chromatography–time-of-flight mass spectrometry. Mendeleev Commun. 2013;23:51–2.

Takemoto H, Ito M, Shiraki T, Yagura T, Honda G. Sedative effects of vapor inhalation of agarwood oil and spikenard extract and identification of their active components. J Nat Med. 2008;62(1):41–6.

Vakati K, Rahman H, Eswaraiah MC, Dutta AM. Evaluation of hepatoprotective activity of ethanolic extract of *Aquilaria agallocha* leaves (EEAA) against CCl4 induced hepatic damage in rat. Sch J App Med Sci. 2013;1:9–12.

Vogel GH, Vogel WH, Scholkens BA, Sandow J, Muller G, Vogel WF. Pharmacological assays. In: Drug discovery and evaluation. 2nd ed. Berlin; 2002. p. Springer-Verlag, 725–72.

Wang H. Determination of Genkwanin in the leaves of *Aquilaria sinensis* (Lour.) Gilg with HPLC. Guiding J Trad Chin Med Pharm. 2008;14:69–70.

Wang SC, Wang F, Yue CH. Chemical constituents from the petioles and leaves of *Aquilaria sinensis*. Biochem Syst Ecol. 2015;61:458–61.

Wang HN, Dong WH, Huang SZ, Li W, Kong FD, Wang H, Wang J, Mei WL, Dai HF. Three new sesquiterpenoids from agarwood of *Aquilaria crassna*. Fitoterapia. 2016;114:7–14.

White MV. The role of histamine in allergic diseases. J Allergy Clin Immunol. 1990;86(4):599–605.

Xiang P, Mei W, Chen H, Kong F, Wang H, Liao G, Zhou L, Dai H. Four new bi-phenylethylchromones from artificial agarwood. Fitoterapia. 2017;120:61–6.

Yagura T, Shibayama N, Ito M, Kiuchi F, Honda G. Three novel diepoxy tetrahydrochromones from agarwood artificially produced by intentional wounding. Tetrahedron Lett. 2005;46:4395–8.

Yang D, Wang J, Li W, Dong W, Mei W, Dai H. New guaiane and acorane sesquiterpenes in high quality agarwood "Qi-Nan" from *Aquilaria sinensis*. Phytochem Lett. 2016a;17:94–9.

Yang DL, Li W, Dong WH, Wang J, Mei WL, Dai HF. Five new 5, 11-epoxyguaiane sesquiterpenes in agarwood "Qi-Nan" from *Aquilaria sinensis*. Fitoterapia. 2016b;112:191–6.

Yang Y, Wen-Li M, Fan-Dong K, Hui-Qin C, Wei L, Zhi-Bao C, Hao-Fu D. Four new bi-2-(2-phenylethyl) chromone derivatives of agarwood from *Aquilaria crassna*. Fitoterapia. 2017;119:20–5.

Yang Y, Hui-Qin C, Fan-Dong K, Li-Man Z, Wei L, Wen-Hua D, Zhi-Bao C, Wen-Li M, Hao-Fu D. Dimeric sesquiterpenoid-4H-chromone derivatives from agarwood of *Aquilaria crassna* and their cytotoxicity. Phytochemistry. 2018;145:207–13.

Yoneda K, Yamaga-Ra E, Nakanishi T, Nagashima T, Kawasaki I, Yoshida T, Mori H, Miura I. Sesquiterpenoids in two different kinds of agarwood. Phytochemistry. 1984;23:2068–9.

Zhu Z, Zhao Y, Huo H, Gao X, Zheng J, Li J, Tu P. HHX-5, a derivative of sesquiterpene from Chinese agarwood, suppresses innate and adaptive immunity via inhibiting STAT signaling pathways. Eur J Pharmacol. 2016;791:412–23.

Zulkifle NL, Omar NAM, Tajuddin SN, Shaari MR. Anti-diabetic activities of Malaysian Agarwood (*Aquilaria* Spp.) Leaves extract conference on Industry–Academia joint initiatives in Biotechnology CIA. Biotech. 2013;13:5–7.

Processing and Potential Health Benefits of Betel Leaf (*Piper betle* L.)

17

Mitali Madhumita, Proshanta Guha, and Ahindra Nag

Contents

M. Madhumita · P. Guha
Department of Agricultural and Food Engineering, Indian Institute of Technology, Kharagpur, West Bengal, India

A. Nag (✉)
Department of Chemistry, Indian Institute of Technology, Kharagpur, West Bengal, India
e-mail: ahinnag@chem.iitkgp.ernet.in

S. Sen, R. Chakraborty (eds.), *Herbal Medicine in India*,
https://doi.org/10.1007/978-981-13-7248-3_17

17.1 Introduction

17.1.1 Betel Leaf: A Valuable Herbal Plant

Betel leaf (*Piper betle* L.) plant with heart-shaped deep green leaves is an important horticultural, medicinal and recreational cash crop of aesthetic and commercial values. It belongs to the family Piperaceae (black pepper family). It is known by different names across the country and abroad such as *Tamul* in Assamese, *Kavala* in Kannada, *Tambulam* in Sanskrit, *Bajjai* in Tulu and *Paan* in Hindi, Marathi, Punjabi and Urdu. It grows widely in the tropical humid climates of Southeast Asia (Ramji et al. 2002). It is commonly known as "*Paan*", a dioecious, perennial creeper, climbing by many short adventitious rootlets. It is widely cultivated in hotter and damper parts of India. As a herbal medicinal plant, it is used for the treatment of various disorders in various traditional systems (Khan et al. 2012). Mostly the leaves and roots are used for medicinal purposes. There are over 100 varieties of betel leaf across the world out of which 40 are present in India and 30 in West Bengal and Bangladesh (Guha 2006; Maiti and Shivashankara 1998). There are around 2000 species of *Piper betle* distributed worldwide out of which 10 species are available in Nepal. Betel vine is currently distributed in Africa, Western Asia, Himalaya, India, Southeast Asia, Malaysia, China, Nepal and Sri Lanka (Satyavati et al. 1987). Malaysia is the known place of origin of "*Paan*" (Chattapdayay and Maity 1967). Betel leaf contains some vitamins, minerals, protein, enzymes, essential oil and medicinal compounds for treatment of liver, brain and heart diseases. In regard to export, betel leaves have a good potential and India exports betel leaves to several countries, such as the UK, the USA, the UAE, Bahrain and Pakistan and many Western countries where it is consumed by the population descendent of Indian origin.

17.1.2 History and Cultivation of Betel Leaf

The betel plant originated from South and Southeast Asia but today the plants are also cultivated in India, Sri Lanka, Bangladesh, Philippine Islands, Burma, Malay Peninsula, East Africa and Nepal (Jayaweera 1982; Kumar et al. 2010). Currently, betel vine is cultivated broadly in India in almost all the states except Haryana, Punjab, Himachal Pradesh and J&K. In India, it is widely cultivated in West Bengal, Orissa, Tamil Nadu, Madhya Pradesh, Maharashtra and Uttar Pradesh. Different popular varieties of betel leaves cultivated in different states are listed in Table 17.1.

Betel vine is widely cultivated at altitudes of 02–1400 m in high land, moist, tropical as well as a subtropical region with a rainfall of about 2250–4750 mm, relative humidity 40–80% and temperature 15–40°C It requires tropical climate, high rainfall and a shady place for its vigorous growth. It is cultivated either under forest ecosystem with support for its weak stem or in artificially constructed shaded condition having high

Table 17.1 List of varieties of betel leaf popular in different states in India

State	Varieties of betel leaf available
Andhra Pradesh	Karapaku, Chennor, Tellaku, Bangla, Kalli Patti
Assam	Assam Patti, Awani Pan, Bangla, Khasi Pan
Bihar	Desi Pan, Calcutta, Paton, Maghai, Bangla
Karnataka	Kariyale, Mysoreale, Ambadiale
Kerala	Nadan, Kalkodi, Puthukodi
Madhya Pradesh	Desi Bangla, Calcutta, Deswari
Maharashtra	Kallipatti, Kapoori, Bangla
Odisha	Godi Bangla, Nova Cuttak, Sanchi, Birkoli
Tamil Nadu	Pachai Kodi, Vellaikodi
Uttar Pradesh	Deswari, Kapoori, Maghai, Bangla
West Bengal	Bangla, Sanchi, Mitha, Kali Bangla, Simurali Bangla

Source: Chaurasia and Johri 1990

humidity, rich soil moisture and nutrients. Betel vine requires light soil (loamy or sandy loam soil) with good organic matter and good drainage conditions. Red loamy soil, light with good soil depth and pH range of 5.6–8.2 are most suitable for the growth of betel vine whereas saline, alkali soils and waterlogged area are unsuitable and may be injurious (Balsubrahmanyam 1992). The cultivation of betel vine under controlled conditions is practised inside a covered structure, popularly known as *baraja* or *boroj* in Orissa and West Bengal. Planting seasons vary from state to state in India but the onset of monsoon and onset of winter (October) are the ideal time of planting under closed and open systems of cultivation, respectively. The peak harvesting season extends from July to December in West Bengal. In general, the life span of a betel vine ranges between 12 and 15 years. On average betel leaves can be plucked at least five times in a year from a vine. Based on the cultivation practices, betel vine can be classified into two groups, the plain land betel leaf "*Barajaj paan*" and tree betel leaf "*Gacha paan*" which naturally climbs on the adjacent trees. Also based on shape, size, brittleness and taste of leaf blade, betel vine is divided into pungent and non-pungent or sweet varieties. The annual turnover of betel vine is estimated at Rs. 9000 million (Guha and Jain 1997). It has good export potential and earns traders foreign exchange through exports. India exports betel leaves to many countries. Its cultivation is highly labour intensive and offers employments to millions of people for its cultivation, harvesting, packaging, preservation, transportation, marketing, etc.

17.1.3 Botanical Characteristics

Betel vine is a perennial dicotyledonous creeper, widely cultivated in tropical and subtropical countries particularly in South and Southeast Asia. It is an evergreen perennial plant with semi-woody stem that climbs with short adventitious roots. The leaves of the plant are dorsiventral with aromatic odour and pungent taste. And the leaves are also alternate, heart-shaped, smooth, shining and long-stalked, with pointed apex (acute or acuminate). Moreover, the leaves are petiolated with stout petioles of 2–2.5 cm or more long and 1.2–1.8 mm thick (Mabberley 1997). It has five to seven ribs arising from the base (Zakaria et al. 2010). The branches of the plant are strongly swollen at the nodes (Arambewela et al. 2005). Fruits are rarely produced, often sunk in the fleshy spike, forming nodule-like structures. Further, the female plants also rarely produce any flower or fruit in the Indian climate (Dassanayake and Fosberg 1987) except a few places like Bengaluru. Male spikes are cylindrical and dense and female spikes are 2.5–5.0 cm long and pendulous. There are many varieties of betel leaves recognized based on colour, size, taste and aroma. Some of the popular Indian varieties are Magadhi, Kauri, Venmony, Mysore, Salem, Bangla, Kapoori, Meetha, Sanchi, Ghanagete, Kasi, Banarasi, Desavari and Bagerhati (Zakaria et al. 2010).

17.1.4 Economic Status

The initial cost of cultivation of betel vine from boroj may be about Rs. 1–2 lakh/ha/year at the minimum during the first year which may come down to Rs. 0.5- 0.6 lakh/ha/year in the subsequent years due to several factors like location of the farm, variety, agro-climate, season and variation in wages of the workers. A minimum net profit of about Rs. 1.0 lakh/ha/year was reported to be very common which may go as high as Rs. 5.02 lakh/ha/year or more (Guha 2006). The marketing cost of betel leaves mostly depends on the packing and transportation expenses. From the economic status of 2011, after harvesting, betel leaves are bundled into ten leaves each and sold between Rs. 5.14 and 8.56 (Jan 2000). According to FAO, 2000 (Jan 2000), the betel leaf yield varies due to region, vine, variety and season and hence its profitability greatly fluctuates. The net income of the betel farms is expected to be Rs. 735 per 150 square feet (14 m^2) for every 6 months. Also from FAO study, it may be assumed that there are losses of perishable betel leaves in erratic weather, bad storage, high spoilage and costly transportation conditions. However, these losses are usually between 35 and 70% but at least 10%. In ideal conditions, some farms have net gross annual incomes after expenses of over Rs. 26,000 per 10 decimal farms. On the other hand, the demand for betel leaves has been dropping in India because of contagious acceptance of tobacco-based addictive "*Gutkha*" by consumers over betel leaf-based "*Paan*" preparations which ultimately reduces demand and profitability of betel leaf cultivation (Guha 2006).

17.2 Composition of Betel Leaf

17.2.1 Nutrients

Betel leaves mainly contain chlorophyll, water, protein, fat, fibre, carbohydrate, minerals and vitamins. The percentages of all nutritional constituents are mentioned in Table 17.2 (Guha 2006). Betel leaves contain several sugars including glucose, fructose, maltose and sucrose. The average content of free reducing sugars in different types of betel leaves generally varies from 0.38 to 1.46% (Tewari and Nayak 1991). The leaves contain good amounts of vitamins particularly nicotinic acid, ascorbic acid and carotenoids. These vitamins have an important role in the biochemical processes and a valuable impact on human body which exhibit anticancer effect, and antimicrobial and antioxidant properties. Carotenoids also increase the immune cell communication in human body. The leaves also contain significant amounts of all essential amino acids except lysine, histidine and arginine which help in breakdown of fats and reducing muscle generation. Large concentrations of asparagines with good amount of glycine and proline are present in betel leaves. It also contains the enzymes like diastase and catalase (Gopalan et al. 1984; CSIR 1969).

Table 17.2 Nutritional composition of fresh betel leaves

Constituents	Percentage
Water	85–90%
Protein	3–3.5%
Fat	0.4–1.0%
Minerals	2.3–3.3%
Fibre	2.3%
Chlorophyll	0.01–0.25%
Carbohydrate	0.5–6.10%
Nicotinic acid	0.63–0.89 mg/100 g
Vitamin C	0.005–0.01%
Vitamin A	1.9–2.9 mg/100 g
Thiamine	10–70 μg/100 g
Riboflavin	1.9–30 μg/100 g
Tannin	0.1–1.3%
Nitrogen	2.0–7.0%
Phosphorus	0.05–0.6%
Potassium	1.1–4.6%
Calcium	0.2–0.5%
Iron	0.005–0.007%
Iodine	3.4 μg/100 g
Essential oil	0.08–0.2%
Energy	44 kcal/100 gm

(Source: Guha 2006)

17.2.2 Extraction of Essential Oil

Essential oil (EO) is extracted from betel leaves by a "betel leaf oil extractor". Before placing the leaves with the required amount of water in round-bottom distillation flask, leaves are thoroughly washed and cut into small pieces. Heat is supplied by the heating mantle at 100 °C and the oil is extracted within 2–3 h. The steam and vaporized oil are condensed to liquid by a vertical condenser and collected in the receiver tube. Being immiscible and slightly lighter than water, the volatile oil is separated out as the upper layer in the receiver tube. The EO is then separated from water by a separating funnel, collected in a glass tube, dried over anhydrous sodium sulphate until the last trace of water is removed, labelled and stored in dark vials at 4 °C for further use.

Betel leaf oil, chief aromatic constituent of the betel leaves, gives it the characteristic flavour and is very much useful to health. The colour of the volatile oil is bright yellow to dark brown liquid and it possesses a clove-like flavour which consists of terpenes and phenols (Koff et al. 1971). The active ingredient of betel leaf oil is primarily a class of allyl benzene compounds, safrole, chavibetol, chavicol, allyl diacetoxy benzene, estragole, eugenol, methyl eugenol, hydroxycatechol, etc. Betel leaf oil is a very precious herbal commodity which is very effective for treating problems like dandruff, stress, memory loss, indigestion and moroseness. It is manufactured, exported, imported and supplied to the highly valued clients. The cost of 1 kg betel leaf oil currently ranges from Rs. 25,000 to Rs. 1,20,000 according to its quality. This oil provides quick relief from joint pain and headaches. It is also used for manufacturing medicines, perfumes, mouth fresheners, tonics, food additives, etc. (Guha 2006). Besides this, the oil also inhibits the growth of the deadly bacteria which cause typhoid, cholera, tuberculosis, etc. Betel leaf extract is also traditionally used in the eye and skin diseases (Amonkar et al. 1989).

17.2.3 Phenolic Compounds

Phenolics, secondary natural metabolites of plants, are aromatic benzene ring compounds with one or more hydroxyl groups and their derivatives produced by plants are used mainly for protection against stress. *Piper betle* leaf extract contains a large number of bioactive molecules like polyphenols, alkaloids, steroids, saponins, tannins, estragole, catechols, terpenes, limonene and cadinene (Prabu et al. 2012) which show diverse pharmacological activities. Both major phenolic compounds, i.e. hydroxychavicol (HC) and eugenol isolated from betel leaves, exhibit antimutagenic action against the mutagen dimethylbenzanthracene (DMBA) in the Ames test. HC reverses the mutagenic and carcinogenic activity of tobacco and also balances between the carcinogenic and anticarcinogenic activities of betel quid ingredients (Bhattacharya et al. 2005). Another major bioactive compound, i.e. allylpyrocatechol, is found in high concentration in betel leaf. It is a well-known antioxidant having a high degree of antioxidant power (Rastogi and Mehrotra 1993). Allylpyrocatechol, a phenolic compound, extracted from the leaves, showed a significant activity against obligate oral anaerobes which are responsible for bad breath (halitosis) (Dwivedi and Tripathi 2014). Also, some other chemical compounds of betel leaf were found to be polyphenols like eugenol, chavicol, carvacrol, chavibetol, catechol and vitamin C (Nouria et al. 2014). The benefits of these polyphenolic compounds present in plants are that they are helpful to regulate oxidation and stress-related chronic diseases, such as diabetes and cardiovascular diseases (Anonymous 2004; Chopra et al. 1982).

17.3 Medicinal Uses of the Herbal Plant

The leaf, the edible part of the plant, is the most valued medicinal, religious and ceremonial portion and consumed as a mouth freshener in its natural and raw condition. It has a strong pungent and peculiar taste and a strong aromatic clove-like flavour due to the presence of phenols and terpenes. In the past, to prevent halitosis, betel leaves were routinely used as a chewing agent by consumers and to obtain other health benefits. The leaves and leaf juice are also supposed to be useful in fever, indigestion, bronchitis, coughs, asthma, etc. and improve the vocalization, harden the gum, conserve the teeth and sweeten the breath. It is also used for the treatment of disorders of physiological function, endoparasites, skin diseases and even ENT (ear, nose and throat) diseases. Betel leaves possess analgesic as well as cooling properties and are used for several purposes and prophylactics. Betel leaves contain some components that are beneficial for the people with diabetes (Manigauha et al. 2004; Namburi et al. 2011) and different types of glycosuria. Betel leaf also possesses antimicrobial, anti-cariogenic, antiprotozoal, anti-allergic, anti-diabetic, anti-inflammatory, hepatoprotective, cardioprotective, antitumour and respiratory antidepressant effects (Chakraborthy and Shah 2011). Figure 17.1 gives a short description of health benefits of this herb.

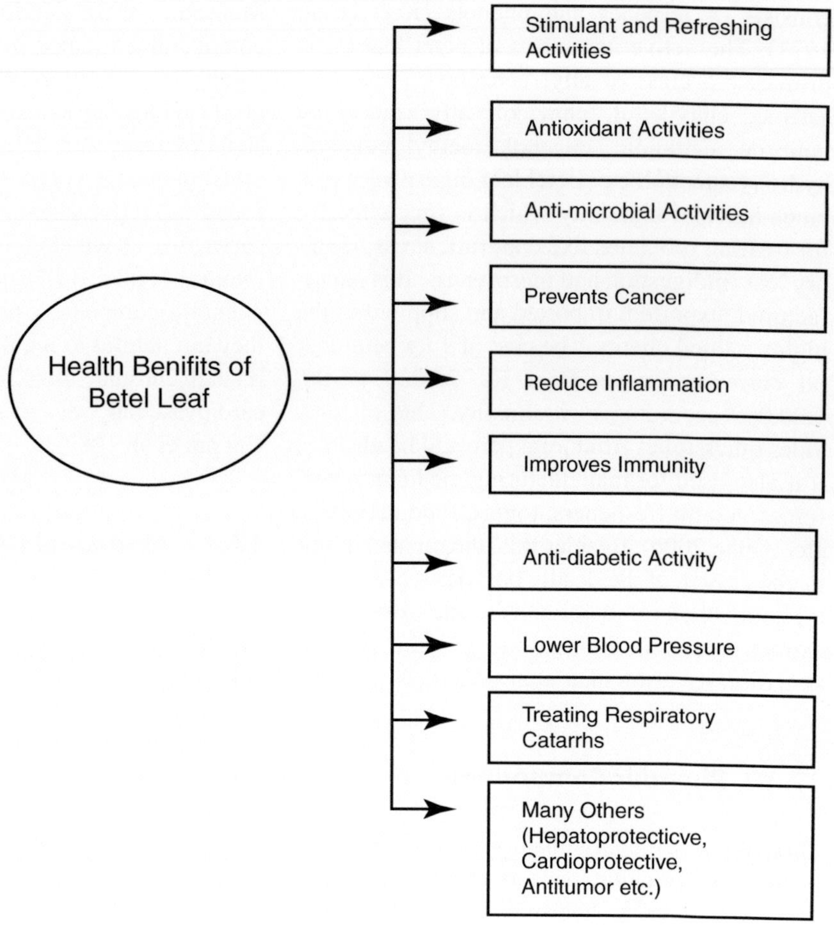

Fig. 17.1 Health benefits of betel leaf

17.4 Adverse and Toxic Effects

Betel leaf extract alone has not been shown to cause significant side effects. But there are some side effects associated with the use of betel quid which is the combination of betel leaf, areca nut, slaked lime and scented ingredients. Also, it contains tobacco in various forms that people use in excess which exerts extremely harmful effect due to the nicotinic compounds present in the tobacco preparations. Betel nuts, however, are known to cause mouth cancer and should not be chewed as it contains a harmful ingredient called arecaidine. It destroys the gums and leads to cancer. Half of the oral cancer cases in India and other Asian countries remain related to quid chewing. It accounts for the highest mortality rate in India from oral cancer in the age group of 30–69 years. There is no side effect of using betel leaves alone and it has the ability to prevent degeneration of cells and kill free radicals (Guha 2006; Roy and Vijayalaxmi 2013). It may even antidote tobacco-induced carcinogenesis (Guha 2006).

17.5 Pharmacological Activities

Several activities such as antimicrobial, anticaries, cardioprotective and gastroprotective have been done to validate traditional uses. However some others have been done on exploratory lines such as radioprotection, chemoprevention and immune modulation which have no traditional use for the performed pharmacological activity. Betel leaves possess activities like antimicrobial (Zakaria et al. 2010) antioxidative, anti-diabetic, antiulcer, cardiotonic, antitumour, detoxification, respiratory depressant, anthelmintic and wound healing properties (Chakraborthy and Shah 2011). Some of the above activities have been described in details in the following sections.

17.5.1 Antioxidant Activity

Antioxidants are compounds capable of inhibiting the oxidation of other compounds under the influence of atmospheric oxygen or reactive oxygen species. Several methods are available for analysis of antioxidant activity by using different assays including ORAC (oxygen radical absorption capacity) assay, HORAC (hydroxyl radical antioxidant capacity), CUPRAC (cupric reducing antioxidant power) assay, DPPH method (standard 2,2-diphenyl-1-picrylhydrazyl), FRAP (ferric reducing antioxidant power) assay and ABTS (2,2′-Azino-bis(3-ethylbenzothiazoline-6-sulfonic acid). EO serves as powerful antioxidants and prevents mutants and oxidants in cells. Due to their small molecular size, they have the capability of penetrating the membranes easily when oxygen deficiency is present. Betel leaves contain biologically active compounds whose concentration depends on the variety of the plant, season and climate. The various antioxidants and phytochemicals present in the betel plants are chavibetol, chavicol, hydroxychavicol, estragole, eugenol, methyl eugenol, hydroxycatechol, caryophyllene, eugenol, methyl ether, γ-lactone, allyl catechol, cepharadione, dotriacontanoic acid, tritriacontane, p-cymene, terpinene, eucalyptol, carvacrol, sesquiterpenes, cadinene, hentriacontane, pentatriacontane, stearic acid, n-triacontanol, triotnacontane, piperlonguminine, allylpyrocatechol diacetate, isoeugenol, 1, 8-cineol, α-pinene, β-pinene, sitosterol, β-sitosteryl palmitate, γ-sitosterol, stigmasterol, ursolic acid and ursolic acid 3β-acetate (Shah et al. 2016; Roy and Vijayalaxmi 2013; Zakaria et al. 2010).

17.5.2 Antimicrobial Activity

The EO of betel leaves has antibacterial properties, which can help fight infections that are caused by bacteria. Moreover, since it is filled with phenolic compounds and other phytochemicals, it can be very effective against the microbial activity. The fresh betel leaves possess antimicrobial compounds which act against ringworm and fungus, and have wound healing property. Thus, it acts as an antiseptic and anthelmintic. The extract of betel leaves increases salivation by which the amount of peroxidase and lysozyme increases and fights against bacterial growth in the oral cavity. The leaf has a significant antimicrobial activity against the microorganisms such as *Streptococcus pyrogen*, *Staphylococcus aureus*, *Proteus vulgaris*, *Escherichia coli* and *Pseudomonas aeruginosa* (Tewari and Nayak 1991). The betel leaves, roots and whole-leaf extract (mixture of volatile and non-volatile compounds) have also very strong antimicrobial activity.

In this research work, the antibacterial activity showed that the betel leaf EO has the potential antibacterial effect against *Staphylococcus aureus* and *Pseudomonas aeruginosa* at very low concentration. All the strains of *Staphylococcus aureus* and *Pseudomonas aeruginosa* were found to be sensitive to the betel leaf EO. From the result, it was clear that the betel leaf EO exerted its maximum bactericidal activity as evident by the significant reduction in microbial counts at 6- and 24-h exposure. There was a complete inhibition of cell viable counts at 24-h exposure. It has also been observed that the susceptibility of Gram-positive and Gram-negative bacteria to betel leaf EO has little influence on growth inhibition. The reason behind this work is that mycobacteria having the thickest hydrophobic cell wall hitherto protect themselves with an outer lipid bilayer. It blocks the penetration of hydrophobic oil and avoids the accumulation of essential oils in target cell membrane. The membrane, an effective permeability barrier, contains porins that serve functions analogous to those observed in Gram-negative bacteria. For the above reason, the *Mycobacterium smegmatis* bacteria were found to be more sensitive to the EO than Gram-negative bacteria.

17.5.3 Anticancer Activity

Although betel nuts can increase the risk of cancer, betel leaves have anticancer compounds in them. Betel leaves contain high amounts of phytochemicals, which can help fight cancer. Betel leaves also help fight oxidative stress and eliminate free radicals by which it can prevent cancer (Rai et al. 2011). Ascorbic acid, as an excellent antioxidant, is very useful to reduce the free radicals in the body and thus prevents cancer. Extracts of betel leaves have a gastroprotective activity which helps in preventing gastric ulcers (Namburi et al. 2011; Arawwawala et al. 2014). Also, to prevent dental caries, betel leaves have been traditionally used as a mouth freshener in India and other Southeast Asian countries.

17.5.4 Anti-diabetic Activity

Diabetes is defined as a heterogeneous and metabolic disorder of carbohydrate, lipid and protein metabolism characterized by high blood glucose levels due to an absolute deficiency of insulin. Due to this deficiency, body cells do not respond properly to insulin. Therefore, some antidiabetic drugs, as a medicine, are used to control the increased blood glucose level in the body. Some of the researchers reported that the oral administration of leaf suspension of betel leaf at 75 and 150 mg/kg of body weight for 30 consecutive days to streptozotocin-induced diabetic rats caused a significant decrease in blood glucose and glycosylated haemoglobin levels. Administering betel leaf to diabetic animals is also reported and in this report it was found that glucose-6-phosphatase and fructose-1,6-bisphosphatase levels decrease in the liver with an increase of hexokinase levels (Madan et al. 2014).

17.5.5 Anti-inflammatory Activity

Betel leaf has a great role in anti-inflammatory activity which has been used as a household remedy for the inflammation of the oral cavity (Dohi et al. 1989). Anti-inflammatory is the activity which helps in the treatment of inflammation or swelling. Inflammation is considered as a part of the complex biological response of vascular tissues to dangerous stimuli such as pathogens and damaged cells. It is also reported that the ethanolic extracts of betel leaf possess anti-inflammatory activities at non-toxic concentrations, in the complete Freund's adjuvant-induced model of arthritis in rats. Eugenol, a principal compound of betel leaf, also possesses anti-inflammatory effects in different animal models of studies with different inflammogens (Azuine et al. 1991). Besides eugenol, HC and α-tocopherol also enhance the levels of glutathione (GTH) in mouse skin and liver. These compounds act as important antioxidants in human body (Bhide et al. 1991). Due to the presence of high flavonoid content in betel leaves, the anti-ulcerogenic activity has also been attributed. Betel leaf extracts have the ability to cure gastric ulcers and peptic ulcers (Chaurasia and Johri 1990). The betel leaf is used as a household medicine for inflammation alone or with other medicinal plants, like turmeric and sandal wood paste.

17.6 Preservation Techniques

During storage and transportation, betel leaves can easily undergo quick spoilage due to its high perishable nature by several factors. These factors include microbial infections, pest attacks and discoloration. It may cause post-harvest loss ranging from 35 to 70% with a minimum of 10% every year (Jan 2000). In the rainy season, a large portion of the leaves remain unsold or are sold at a throwaway price. In view of the losses, different techniques are adopted to reduce the post-harvest losses of betel leaves such as drying including modern drying technologies, different chemical treatments, depetiolation, modifying surrounding atmosphere, advanced packaging technologies and extracting essential oil. Drying, such as solar drying, shade-drying, hot-air drying and thin-layer drying experiments (pilot plant cross-flow tunnel dryer and cabinet dryer), has been practised for removing moisture from betel leaves to a determined level. As a result, microbial spoilage, deterioration and chemical reactions are minimized due to these drying methods. Besides this, depetiolation method is also adopted to minimize the post-harvest losses which help in delaying senescence. It is the process in which petioles are removed from the leaves by which about 10–25% weight of leaves are reduced besides 10–40% reduction in length of leaves (Madan et al. 2014). The aim of MAP (modified atmospheric packaging) is to modify the atmosphere surrounding the leaves by changing the gaseous composition, mainly oxygen and carbon dioxide. Due to this MAP method, the quality of the leaves reduces and also the senescence process delays. Such wastage may also be reduced by bleaching of the leaves called curing.

The curing process for *Banarasi* variety of betel leaves was first invented at Varanasi, Uttar Pradesh, India. In a closed chamber, the fresh green betel leaves are treated with a required amount of smoke, high temperature and pressure. As a result, the green leaves are completely changed to white- or yellowish white-coloured leaves. Alternate heating at 50–60 °C for 6 h followed by cooling at room temperature for 12 h is applied on leaves. Aeration of the leaves is done two to three times by turning upside down and then stored under dark condition. After aeration, these leaves are incubated for 15–20 days for complete curing of the green betel leaves into white or yellowish form. By this curing process, the shelf life of cured betel leaves is increased to 30 days with respect to uncured leaves. This curing process improves the organoleptic properties and gives softness and sweet taste to betel leaves (Madan et al. 2014).

17.7 The Scope of Future Research

Post-harvest losses of betel leaves can be minimized by adopting above-mentioned proper preservation techniques which indicate a promising industrial future. To reduce these losses, more scientific research and technology inputs are required. The economy with a demand of employment opportunities will increase for the people if a well-co-ordinated effort has been achieved by the farmers, traders, scientists, technologists, administrators and policymakers. Waste and by-product utilization should be developed in the industries to get an economical solution. The government should take initiative steps in this area for funding various projects under skilled scientists and researchers which will be helpful for industry and people. The other critical undertaking for future research will be establishing a suitable quality control for betel leaves because on many occasions *Salmonella* contamination in the edible betel leaves created serious health problems like acute diarrhoea. This leads to cancellation of thousands of tons of foreign consignment causing huge losses to the traders who have to bear even the incineration charges of the contaminated leaves. To achieve a best possible synthesis of phytochemical, optimization of the growing conditions should be done and needs to be studied.

17.8 Conclusion

It is concluded from the above backgrounds that betel leaf contains phytochemicals, nutrients including water, fat, fibre, vitamins and minerals. which are helpful for various therapeutic and medicinal purposes. Betel leaf, as a herbal medicinal plant, can be used for the treatment of various disorders such as diabetes, microbial infection, fungal infection and inflammation. Further, studies should be aimed at understanding the ability and mechanism of action of the storage of the betel leaves and studying the biochemical changes during composition. Due to its low cost, availability and safety in consumption, more investigations and research activities should be done to get valuable applications for future use.

References

Amonkar AJ, Padma PR, Bhide SV. Protective effect of hydroxychavicol, a phenolic component of betel leaf, against the tobacco-specific carcinogens. Mutat Res. 1989;210:249–53.

Anonymous. The annual progress report of industrial technology institute, Colombo, Sri Lanka; 2004.

Arambewela LSR, Arawwawala LDAM, Ratnasooriya WD. Antidiabetic activities of aqueous and ethanolic extracts of *Piper betle* leaves in rats. J Ethnopharmacol. 2005;102:239–45.

Arawwawala LD, Arambewela LS, Ratnasooriya WD. Gastro protective effect of *Piper betle* Linn. Leaves grown in Sri Lanka. J Ayurveda Integr Med. 2014;5(1):38–42.

Azuine MA, Amonkar AJ, Bhide SV. Chemopreventive efficacy of betel leaf extract and its constituents on 7, 12-dimethylbenz(a)anthracene induced carcinogenesis and their effect on drug detoxification system in mouse skin. Indian J Exp Biol. 1991;29:346–51.

Balsubrahmanyam. Irrigating betel vine plantation the right way. Indian Horticulture. 1992;136(4)

Bhattacharya S, Subramanian M, Bauri A, Kamat JP. Radioprotecting property of the ethanolic extract of the *Piper betle* leaf. J Radiat Res. 2005;46:165–71.

Bhide SV, Zariwala MB, Amonkar AJ, Azuine MA. Chemopreventive efficacy of a betel leaf extract against benzo[a]pyrene-induced forestomach tumors in mice. J Ethnopharmacol. 1991;34:207–13.

Chakraborthy D, Shah B. Antimicrobial, antioxidative and anti-hemolytic activity of *Piper betle* leaf extracts. Int J Pharm Sci. 2011;3:192–9.

Chattapdayay SP, Maity S. Diseases of betel vine and species. New Delhi: ICAR; 1967.

Chaurasia RS, Johri JK. Production analysis of betel leaves. Agricultural Situation in India. 1990;44:23–5.

Chopra RN, Chopra IC, Handa KL, Kapur LD. Chopra's indigenous drugs of India. 2nd ed. New Delhi, Calcutta: AP; 1982.

CSIR (Council of Scientific and Industrial Research, New Delhi): The Wealth of India. 1969;8:84–94.

Dassanayake MD, Fosberg FR. A revised hand book to the flora of Ceylon. New Delhi: Amreind; 1987. p. 287–8.

Dohi T, Terada H, Anamura S, Okamoto H, Tsujimoto A. The anti-inflammatory effects of phenolic dental medicaments as determined by mouse ear edema assay. Jpn J Pharmacol. 1989;49:535–9.

Dwivedi V, Tripathi S. Review study on potential activity of *Piper betle*. J Pharmacogn Phytochem. 2014;3(4):93–8.

Gopalan C, Rama SBV, Balasubramanian SC. Nutritive value of Indian foods. New Delhi: National Institute of Nutrition, Hyderabad, Indian Council of Medical Research; 1984.

Guha P. Betel Leaf: The Neglected Green Gold of India. J Hum Ecol. 2006;19:87–93.

Guha P, Jain RK. Status Report on Production, Processing and Marketing of Betel Leaf (*Piper betle* L.). Kharagpur: Agricultural and Food Engineering Department, IIT; 1997.

Jan BO. Success Case Replication – A Manual for Increasing Farmer Household Income. 2000.

Jayaweera DMA. Medicinal Plants Used in Ceylon. National Science Council of Sri Lanka. Colombo. 1982;5:201.

Khan Z, Bashir O, Hussain JI, Kumar S, Ahmad R. Effects of ionic surfactants on the morphology of silver nanoparticles using *Paan* (*Piper betle*) leaf petiole extract. Colloids Surf B Biointerfaces. 2012;98:85–90.

Koff RS, Gordan G, Sabesin SM. D-Galactosamine hepatitis hepatocellular injury and fatty liver following a single dose. Proc Soc Exp Biol Med. 1971;137:696–701.

Kumar N, Misra P, Dube A. *Piper betle* Linn. A maligned Paan-Asiatic plant with an array of pharmacological activities and prospects for drug discovery. Curr Sc. 2010;99:922–32.

Mabberley DJ. The plant book, vol. 560. 2nd ed. Cambridge: Cambridge University Press; 1997.

Madan A, Balan N, Barma D. Reducing post-harvest losses of betel (*Piper betle* L.) leaves by various preservation techniques. J Agrisear. 2014;1(4):251–6.

Maiti S, Shivashankara KS. Betel vine research highlights. 1998.

Manigauha A, Patel S, Ali H, Chandy A, Maheshwari MU. Study the effect of phytochemical constituents of *Piper betle* leaves extracts on liver disorders by in vivo model. J Pharm Res. 2004;2:353–6.

Namburi SUR, Omprakash, Babu G. A review on management of warts in Ayu. 2011;32(1):100–2.

Nouria L, Nafchia AM, Karim AA. Phytochemical, antioxidant, antibacterial, and α-amylase inhibitory properties of different extracts from betel leaves. Ind Crop Prod. 2014;62:47–52.

Prabu SM, Muthumani M, Shagirtha K. Protective effect of *Piper betle* leaf extract against cadmium-induced oxidative stress and hepatic dysfunction in rats. Saudi J of Biological Sci. 2012;19:229–39.

Rai MP, Thilakchand KR, Palatty PL, Rao P, Rao S, Bhat HP, Baliga MS. *Piper betle* Linn. (Betel Vine), the Maligned Southeast Asian Medicinal Plant Possesses Cancer Preventive Effects: Time to Reconsider the Wronged Opinion. Asian Pac J Cancer Prev. 2011;12:2149–56.

Ramji N, Iyer R, Chandrasekaran S. Phenolic antibacterials from *Piper betle* in the prevention of halitosis. J Ethnopharmacol. 2002;83:149–52.

Rastogi RP, Mehrotra BN. Compendium of Indian Medicinal Plants. New Delhi: Publications and Information Directorate; 1993. p. 502–3.

Roy UB, Vijayalaxmi KK. Evaluation of Cytotoxic Activity of *Piper betle* Linn. using Murine and Human Cell Lines In Vitro. Int J Sci Eng Res. 2013;4(9):221–33.

Satyavati GV, Raina MK, Sharma. Medicinal Plants of India. New Delhi: Indian Council of Medical Research; 1987.

Shah SK, Garg G, Jhade D. *Piper betle*: Phytochemical, pharmacological and nutritional value in health management. Int J Pharm. 2016;38(2):181–9.

Tewari SN, Nayak M. Activity of four plant leaf extracts against three fungal pathogens of rice. Trop Agri Res. 1991;68:373–5.

Zakaria ZA, Patahuddin H, Mohamad AS, Israf D, Sulaiman MR. In vivo anti nociceptive and anti-inflammatory activities of the aqueous extract of the leaves of *Piper sarmentosum*. J Ethnopharmacol. 2010;128:42–8.

Part III

Phytochemicals & Drug Discovery

18 Spatio-Temporal Imaging and High-Resolution Mass Spectrometry Analysis: New Avenues in Herbal Drug Discovery and Plant Metabolomics

Yogini S. Jaiswal and Leonard L. Williams

Contents

18.1 Introduction

The advent and upsurge in the technological advancement of "omics" disciplines have led to great benefits to crops and therapeutically important medicinal plants. Identification of genes responsible for specific traits and secondary metabolites and their quantitative analysis have helped modification of several plants to confer them beneficial properties. Omics approaches have helped in modifying plants and making them resistant to diseases, tolerant to stressful environmental conditions, and enhancing their nutritive qualities (Khush 2001; Langridge and Fleury 2011). Compared to genomics and phenomics, metabolomics is still not extensively used for the study of plants and crops. Metabolomics is a versatile discipline with applications for analysis of microbial, animal, and plant metabolites, and the vast array of data output from small sample quantities makes it a valuable component in plant sciences (Sawada et al. 2009; Wuolikainen et al. 2016). Metabolite analysis of extracts of specific tissue or cell types helps identify the metabolic processes occurring

Y. S. Jaiswal · L. L. Williams (✉)
Center for Excellence in Post Harvest Technologies, The North Carolina Research Campus, North Carolina Agricultural and Technical State University, Kannapolis, NC, USA
e-mail: llw@ncat.edu; llw@ag.ncat.edu

S. Sen, R. Chakraborty (eds.), *Herbal Medicine in India*,
https://doi.org/10.1007/978-981-13-7248-3_18

in the target organs and cell types. Genetic modifications affecting metabolic processes can be depicted based on the metabolite profiles generated (Wen et al. 2016). Without the technological advancements, phenomics has been applied by agriculturalists to select best plant varieties with the traits based on morphological characteristics. With the recent advancements in imaging phenotypic variations, study of genomic traits has gained tremendous impetus.

Complimentary techniques of genomics, phenomics, transcriptomics, and metabolomics, when integrated together, provide a powerful tool to intersect molecular processes that occur within the plant system.

The methods employed in metabolomics often involve hyphenated chromatography and mass spectrometry techniques. Gas chromatography-mass Spectrometry (GC-MS), liquid chromatography-mass Spectrometry (LC-MS), matrix-assisted laser desorption ionization-time of flight mass spectrometry (MALDI-TOF/MS) are some of the most commonly used hyphenated mass spectrometry techniques. Metabolomics techniques enable one to analyze many known and unknown metabolites. However, annotation of unknown metabolites is still a challenge. Metabolomics and phenomics data analysis is complex, and often the visualization of the results obtained from tremendous amount of data requires application of statistics, bioinformatics, mathematics, and engineering. In this present chapter we describe mass spectrometry (MS) techniques, magnetic resonance imaging (MRI), and micro-computed tomography (μ-CT) used in metabolomics and phenomics analysis of plants (Issaq et al. 2009).

18.2 Hyphenated Mass Spectrometry Techniques and Their Applications

Mass spectrometry-based methods in metabolomics involve a complex sequence of steps in order to identify the detected compounds. Depending on the nature of the targeted analytes, respective solvents are selected for extraction of the analytes. Optimization of the concentration of the analytes to be detected is carried out to obtain good resolution and detection. After this step, the analytes are detected in the samples with a targeted approach or global profiling approach. Followed by detection, the generated data is cleaned up with specific thresholds and comparing the observed mass to charge ratios, relative intensities, and spectra to various compound and mass spectral databases (Dettmer et al. 2007; Go 2010; Kessler et al. 2014; Kind et al. 2009). A flowchart of typical steps involved in mass spectrometry analysis is depicted in Fig. 18.1.

18.2.1 LC-MS Analysis

Liquid chromatography-mass spectrometry (LC-MS) techniques are used widely for analysis of herbal supplements, forensic samples, and

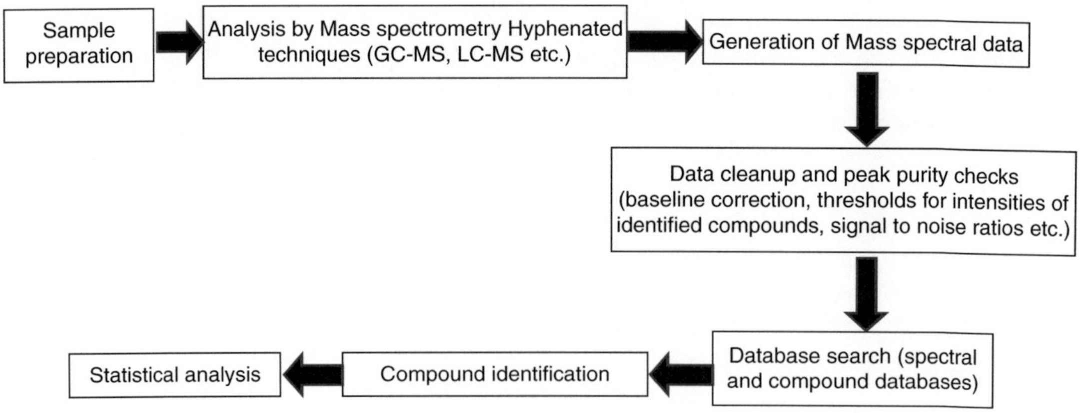

Fig. 18.1 Flowchart of steps involved in analysis and data interpretation in mass spectrometry analysis

pharmaceutical compounds due to the qualitative information obtained and their sensitivity in detection. For LC-MS analysis, despite the mass value information obtained, it is essential for the analytes to be well resolved and have baseline separation. Ultra-high-performance liquid chromatography systems (UHPLC) coupled with MS systems provide shorter run times, high peak capacity, sensitivity, and withstand high pressure up to 10,000 psi. UHPLC-MS systems are used widely in many applications because of these attributes (Chen et al. 2009; Nováková et al. 2006).

A wide range of mass analyzers from low to high resolution are available, depending on the sensitivity of the methods required. Some of these include triple quadrupole (QqQ), time-of-flight (TOF), quadrupole-time-of-flight (QqTOF), and ion trap (IT) mass spectrometers (Becue et al. 2011; Lau et al. 2003; Woo et al. 2013).

Mass spectrometry provides benefits of structural and mass identification to the separations obtained by LC methods. Mass spectrometry analyses can be performed in *single ion monitoring* (SIM), *multiple reaction monitoring* (MRM), or *tandem mass*(MS/MS) mode. In samples with high background noise of the matrix where the analyte and matrix mass to charge (*m/z*) ratios are closely related, *selected reaction monitoring* (SRM) mode is preferred. SRM mode helps to detect analytes at low detection values and thus requires less sample quantity and analysis time (Gross 2011). MRM analysis can be performed either by time-scheduled monitoring or product ion scanning. In product ion scanning the fragmentation spectra obtained after initial MRM screening is used. In reports published till date, it is recommended that for proper identification of analytes, it is important that the collision ion energy used in product ion scan should be used at low, medium, and high levels and the averaged spectra be used for analyte identification (Chen et al. 2009; Shou et al. 2005). Triple Q-TOF, TOF, and Fourier transform ion cyclotron resonance (FT-ICR) provide high accuracy and sensitivity in ultra-high-performance liquid chromatography techniques. When combined with electron spray ionization (ESI) and MALDI, these analyzers provide increased scanning rates and higher number of spectral identifications. ESI is the preferred technique when ionization of highly polar compounds is required. Atmospheric pressure chemical ionization (APCI) is used in the ionization of medium polarity compounds and MALDI for a wide range of compounds from polymers to proteins (Fenn 2003; Karas et al. 2000). A list of some compounds reported to be analyzed with these modern analyzers is provided in Table 18.1.

Table 18.1 List of some pharmaceutical drug compounds reported to be analyzed with hyphenated techniques

Compound class	MS system	Ionization mode	Reference
Nonsteroidal anti-inflammatory drug, flavonoids	Triple quadrupole	ESI+/SRM	Lau et al. (2003)
Anti-diabetics, analgesics, antidepressants, antibiotics	Triple quadrupole	ESI+ or ESI−/MRM	Bogusz et al. (2006)
Appetite suppressant	Quadrupole	ESI+/SIM	Huang et al. (2008)
Hypoglycemics	Quadrupole	ESI+/SIM	Wang et al. (2009)
Diuretic drugs	Triple quadrupole	ESI+ or ESI−/MRM	Woo et al. (2013)
Anti-hypertensives	Q-orbital IT	ESI+/full MS and MS/MS	Vaclavik et al. (2014)
Anti-lipidemic agents	triple quadrupole	ESI+ and ESI−/MRM	Kim et al. (2014)
Drugs for erectile dysfunction	Ion trap	ESI+/full MS and product ion scan	Park et al. (2012)
Drugs for erectile dysfunction	Triple Q-TOF	ESI+/full MS and MS/MS	Roh et al. (2011)
Steroidal compounds	Triple quadrupole	ESI−/full scan or ESI+	Becue et al. (2011)
Anti-hypertensive agents	Time of flight	ESI+/full MS	Kesting et al. (2010)
Central nervous system stimulants	Ion trap	APCI+/product ion scan	Deventer et al. (2007)
Anti-hypertensives	Quadrupole	ESI+ and ESI−/SIM	Lu et al. (2010)

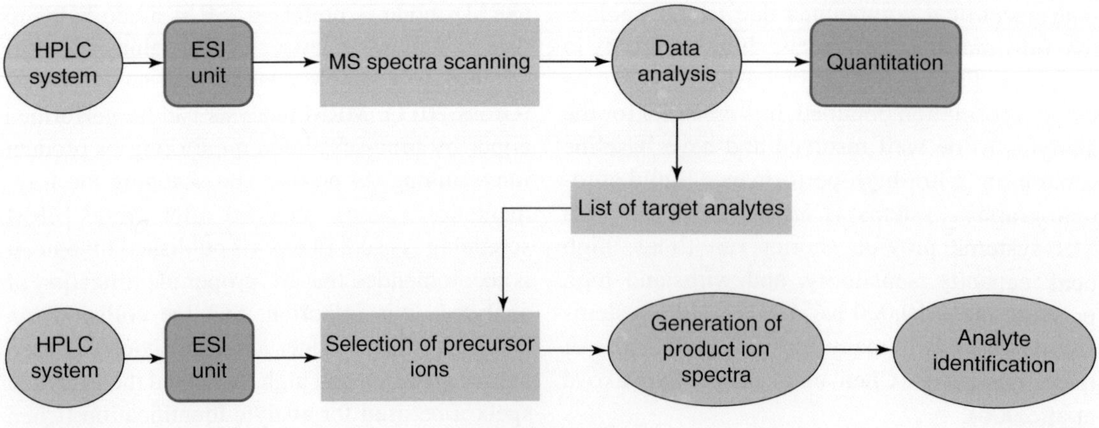

Fig. 18.2 Schematic representation of a typical LC-MS/MS system

A schematic representation of an LC-MS/MS system is shown in Fig.18.2.

Instruments of hyphenated mass spectrometry and liquid chromatography are equipped with powerful data analysis software, viz., Mass hunter, ChromaTOF, Met-Align, MET-XAlign, etc. (Lommen et al. 2012; de Souza et al. 2017). These software help in the initial screening of the data by peak alignment, deconvolution, base line correction, normalization, etc.

The screened list of compounds is then compared with libraries and databases to confirm the identity of the shortlisted compounds. Some of such databases include GOLM, NIST, METLIN, etc. Followed by confirmation from databases, the obtained list of compounds with their quantitative information is subjected to statistical analysis. In metabolomics the most commonly used statistical and visualization parameters include principal component analysis (PCA), heat map, cluster analysis, etc.

18.2.2 GC-MS Analysis

GC-MS analysis is applied to a wide range of analytes; however, the thermal stability and volatility of the analytes serve as the deciding factor for its selection as the method of analysis. Due to the well-established libraries, software, and low cost of analysis compared to an LC-MS method, GC-MS has become the method of choice in metabolomics (Geyer et al. 2008; Patel et al. 2014; Venhuis and de Kaste 2012). Helium is used as the carrier gas in GC-MS with methyl polysiloxane columns (either 100% or 95% with 5% phenyl) as the stationary phase (Patel et al. 2014). Columns generally used for higher resolution and greater number of analytes are 30 m in length, and for few analytes, columns up to 17 m length are used. Electron ionization (EI) and chemical ionization (CI) are two ionization techniques that are employed in GC-MS. EI is a "hard ionization" technique and thus for some molecules where molecular ions need to be ionized, CI is the preferred method of ionization (Hsu and Au 2001; Liu et al. 2001; Man et al. 2009).

For most GC-MS analysis, derivatization is performed to reduce the polarity of the analytes and improve their separation on columns with low polarity. There exists a wide range of derivatizing agents that can be used for influencing the polarity of target analytes. However, while selecting a derivatizing agent it is important to consider the additional molecular mass that will be added on the target analyte, as addition of high molecular mass (higher than the typical range m/z 650–1000) can pose an issue in its passage through the column. Trimethylsilylation or tert-butyldimethylsilylation are used frequently for derivatizing organic acid compounds. Prior to availability of trimethylsilyl (TMS) and tertbutyldimethylsilyl(TBDMS), diazomethane was the most commonly used derivatizing agent (Halket and Zaikin 2003; Jennings and Shibamoto 1980; Walton 1979).

Keto groups are derivatized by oximation to prevent the spectra from being complicated by multiple products formed by enolization reactions. TBDMS is the preferred derivatizing agent compared to TMS as it does not have the hydrolytic effects when exposure to moisture as is the case for TMS. However, TBDMS does increase the molecular mass significantly compared to TMS; thus the analyst has to choose the derivatizing agent based on the column properties and the nature of the target analyte (Birkemeyer et al. 2003).

For non-targeted analysis, analyte identification is carried out by applying an intensity threshold for all the peaks. The analyte peaks thus filtered are then identified based upon their mass spectral patterns and retention indices. A schematic representation of the analysis method selection based on various compound classes is provided in Fig. 18.3. In the analysis of biological samples, it is important to identify the matrix peaks and exclude the interferences that may be caused, thus demanding manual selection of analyte peaks. Commercially available software aid in this operation of data analysis. GC-MS spectral libraries with retention indices are of importance as it is crucial to correctly identify compounds with identical retention times but which may differ in their retention indices (Fiehn 2003). Chromatographic parameters such as stationary phase material, column length, and temperature affect the retention times for analytes; thus Kovats retention indices serve as a universal identification criterion in GC-MS.

The automated mass spectral deconvolution and identification system (AMDIS) has a comprehensive collection of retention indices of many compounds with a user-friendly interface which can be launched and used to clean up the data for database searching and further analyte identification. AMDIS was launched by the National Institute of Standards and Technology (NIST) (Stein 1999). There are several libraries and databases launched by the Max-Planck Institute for Plant Physiology, Agilent Technologies, HD Science, Bruker, Thermo Fisher, and other sources that are extensively used for mass spectral library searching. Despite the available software and algorithms for compound identification, GC-MS data requires an

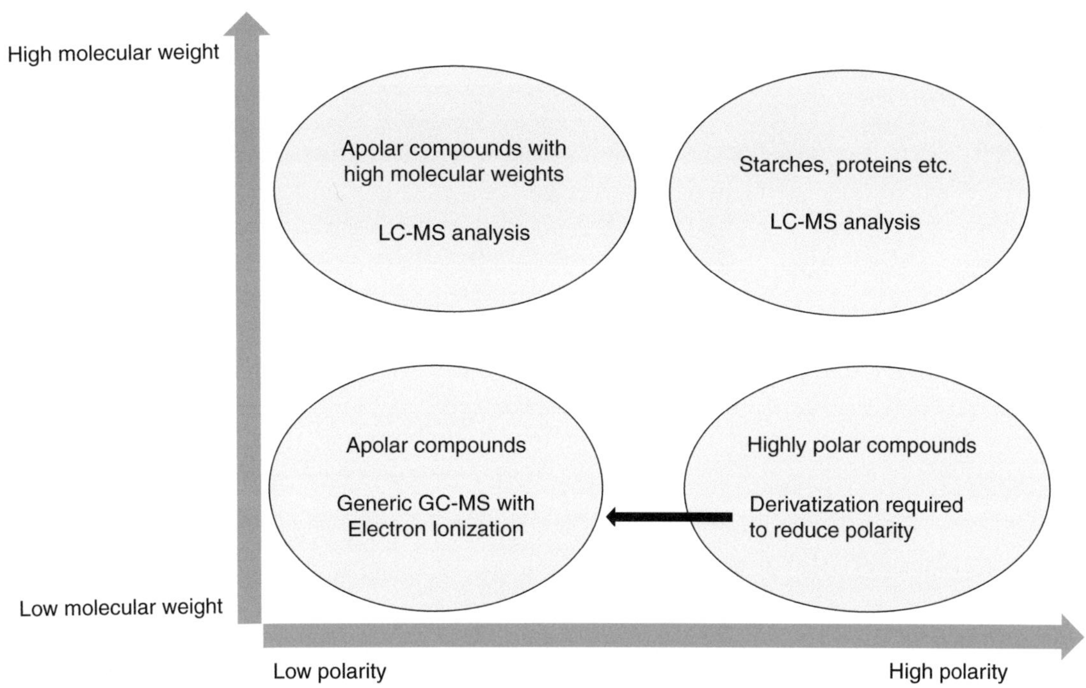

Fig. 18.3 Schematic representation of the analysis method selection based on various compound classes

extensive manual screening of the obtained data to correctly identify the compounds. For identification of unknown compounds, high resolution mass analyzers, study of MS/MS fragmentation patterns, and isotopes are required to support the identity of the compounds (Lee 1973; McLafferty et al. 1998).

18.3 Magnetic Resonance Imaging (MRI)

In the year 2003, Lauterbur and Mansfield were awarded a Nobel Prize in medicine for their invention of MRI. The popularity of MRI has grown due to its non-invasive nature in analysis. The human nuclear magnetic resonance (NMR) scanner is the basis of the development of MRI techniques for imaging of plants. The high instrumentation cost and long analysis time periods were the drawbacks due to which application of MRI for a multitude of sample types was limited. Since the past decade there have been advancements in MRI technology and application of other phenomics imaging techniques to study plants. Now MRI and NMR-MRI are extensively used in studying functions and structures of plant tissues. Popularity of MRI gained momentum due to its non-invasive nature as the prime benefit accompanied with the ability to study the static and dynamic features of samples. It enables researchers to study the morphological details of tissues in addition to their function and transport of nutrients (Van As 2007).

MRI can perform analysis on whole plant organs such as fruits, stems, and seeds and live imaging of intact live plants, unlike other conventional microscopy methods. Other imaging techniques such as matrix-assisted laser desorption/ionization (MALDI) and Raman spectroscopy require sectioning of the plant parts or sample pre-treatment with organic solvents (e.g., positron emission tomography, PET) to provide spatio-chemical distribution information (Holbrook 2001).

A typical MRI analysis system consists of three specific magnets to develop the magnetic field: (1) a static magnet, (2) a gradient coil to generate variable orthogonal magnetic field and, (3) a resonator to generate a variable magnetic field. The gradient coil and resonator are used to generate spatial and temporal magnetic fields, respectively. A diagrammatic representation of an MRI analysis unit is shown in Fig. 18.4. In

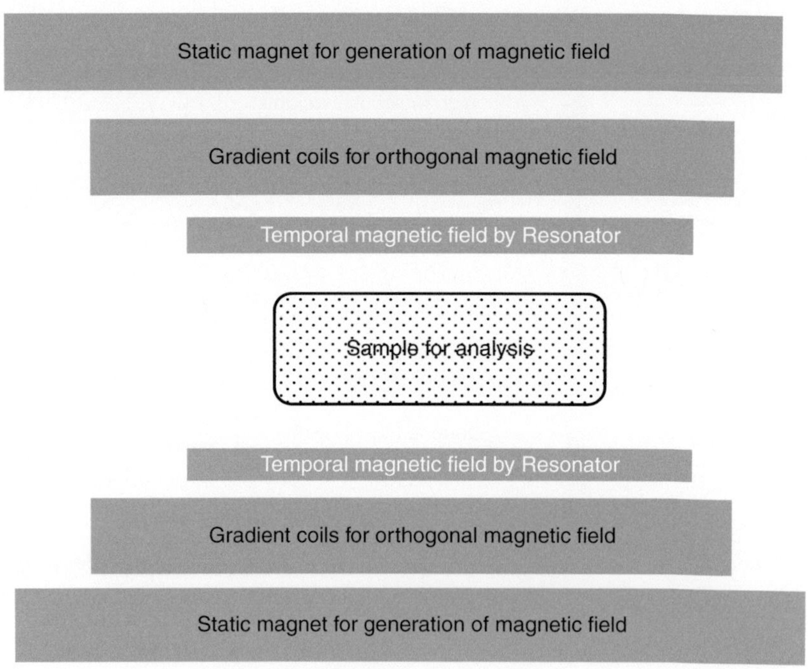

Fig. 18.4 Diagrammatic representation of an MRI analysis unit

MRI imaging, superconducting magnets with 21 Tesla (T) field strengths are used and spins with a non-zero value are detected (^1H, ^{23}Na, ^{13}C etc.). In plant tissue imaging, the protons in water molecules present in the tissues enable generation of spins.

The signals generated in MRI analysis do not provide any spatial data. The images acquired in Fourier space require reconstruction with Fourier transformation and encoding to obtain any spatial information from raw image files (Haase et al. 1986; Haishi et al. 2001).

It is a challenging task for biologists to develop protocols for analysis of plants by MRI, given their specific research focus on biological aspects. Thus, application of MRI imaging to plants requires integration of at least two disciplines: plant biology and physics. Optimization of resolution is critical in MRI imaging and is often achieved by a combination of high gradient and magnetic field strength (Ciobanu et al. 2002; Spragg 2017). Appropriate placement of RF resonators enhances resolutions and reduces imaging time. Given the interplay of several factors, it is a challenge to obtain high-quality images like optical microscopy through MRI analysis. Best resolution images are obtained when water is used as a target molecule, where the protons aid strong magnetization. Plants offer several advantages over human MRI imaging, and these include insensitivity to longer imaging times and variable/high excitation pulses. In live plants for experiments with longer durations, customized chambers are used to deliver water, light, and required nutrients (Van As 2007; Köckenberger 2001).

18.3.1 MRI Imaging in Plant Metabolomics

Metabolites have tissue specific distribution patterns in various tissues of plants. Being a non-invasive technique, MRI enables researchers to explore this compartmentalization of metabolites in plants. For biologists, the ability to study tissue specific distribution of metabolites helps in relating the histological and functional characteristics of specific plant parts. The most widely studied plant part to date is the seed which serves as a storage site with high concentrations of lipids (Tkáč et al. 1999; Vanhamme et al. 1997).

18.3.1.1 Imaging of Lipids and Other Metabolites

Imaging of lipid distribution in plant tissues is complex, and non-invasive techniques are preferred over the invasive techniques considering the physico-chemical characteristics of lipids. MRI utilizes the difference in frequencies of water and lipids for imaging. The small difference in between the frequencies of these two constituents provides good contrasts and imaging capabilities for this frequency-specific technique (Borisjuk et al. 2005; Neuberger et al. 2009). The ability to image tissue structure and lipid distribution enables researchers to relate structure to lipid metabolism functions. Seeds of oats, linseed, cotton, and several other plants have been studied by MRI imaging (Borisjuk et al. 2005; Hayden et al. 2011). Comparison of cultivar varieties based on their lipid distribution and correlating gene expression with metabolism of lipids have opened new avenues in plant research. MRI imaging is also being used to trace other single metabolites, of which sugars and amino acids have been reported to be successfully analyzed (Melkus et al. 2009; Rolletschek et al. 2011; Szimtenings et al. 2003).

For functional imaging in plants, combining MRI with NMR makes it more capable of experimental output. Flow-encoded NMR can measure movement of metabolites with velocities in mm h^{-1} range. As ^{12}C isotopes cannot be recorded in NMR, and ^{13}C is naturally low in its occurrence, additionally ^{13}C-labelled substrates are fed to the plant throughout the experimental duration. Application of this strategy has been found successful in tracking metabolite dynamics in plants (Bax et al. 1983; Fulmer et al. 2010).

MRI is now used as an effective tool in the study of systems biology. The information obtained from non-invasive analysis of the compartmentalization of metabolites between different tissues and organs of the plant is important in exploring the *in vivo* metabolic

Table 18.2 List of plants studied by application of imaging techniques

Plants	Study characteristics	Technique	Reference
Solanum lycopersicum (tomato) peduncle	Effect of heat girdling on xylem integrity	MRI	Van de Wal et al. (2017)
Vitis vinifera (grapevine)	Hydraulic integrity of stems	MRI	Hochberg et al. (2017)
Brassica napus seeds	Mapping of lipids	Matrix-assisted laser/desorption ionization-mass spectrometry imaging (MALDI-MSI)	Woodfield et al. (2017)
"Annurca Rossa del Sud" apple fruits	Metabolite analysis	NMR	D'Abrosca et al. (2017)
Cornus florida flower bud	Study effect of freezing on buds	MRI	Ishikawa et al. (2016)
Areca catechu seed	Alkaloid development patterns and their segregation	MRI	Srimany et al. (2016)
Hordeum vulgare	3D analysis of roots	MRI	van Dusschoten et al. (2016)
Zingiber officinale (ginger) cultivars	Water dynamics	NMR	Huang et al. (2016)
Vitis vinifera (grapevine) petioles	Hydraulic vulnerability in draught	MRI and microcomputed tomography	Hochberg et al. (2016)
Eucalyptus camaldulensis	Xylem embolism	Microcomputed tomography	Nolf et al. (2017)
Laurus nobilis stems	Xylem embolism	Microcomputed tomography	Nardini et al. (2017)
Physisporinus vitreus and *Xylaria longipes* wood	Degradation in wood	Synchrotron X-ray micro-tomography	Sedighi Gilani et al. (2014)
Coffea arabica Linn.	Microstructural properties of beans	Synchrotron X-ray micro-tomography	Pittia et al. (2011)
Piceaabies [L.] Karst.	Imaging of microstructure	Synchrotron X-ray micro-tomography	Trtik et al. (2007)

activities. A list of some plants studied by application of imaging techniques is provided in Table 18.2.

18.3.1.2 Other Applications of MRI Imaging

In addition to the study of lipids and plant metabolism, MRI can be applied for study of the below mentioned characteristics in plants:

1. *Development*: The growth features of fruits, roots, seeds, and bulbs have been studied by application of MRI imaging (Roh 2005; Roh et al. 1998; Yooyongwech et al. 2008, 2012).
2. *Water dynamics*: The flow of solutes and water in various transport tissues of plants is successfully studied through MRI imaging in combination with NMR (van der Weerd et al. 2002; Wojtyla et al. 2006).
3. *Stress response*: Exposure to stress (cold, drought) conditions leads to change in metabolism of the plants and the internal moisture status. MRI has been used as a diagnostic tool to identify acclimatized plants after exposure to stress, the hydration characteristics, and gene expression changes (Verslues et al. 2006; van der Weerd et al. 2001, 2002).
4. *Host-pathogen interaction*: Pathogen infections lead to blockage or disruption of tissues in plants. The infections may be lead to changes in parts of the plant above or below the ground. Changes in tissue structures lead to changes in the metabolic functions of the plants. Many studies in combination with NMR have been performed for MRI imaging of infected plants. This is a very important application of MRI as it helps support sustainability of plants and their conservation by imaging infected seeds, assessing their viability and moisture content,

and predicting their viability and regeneration characteristics (Enebak 2000; Lu et al. 2007; Salleo et al. 2004; Umebayashi et al. 2011).

18.4 Synchrotron Radiation Techniques

Several spectroscopic, spectrometry, and imaging techniques exist for study of plant structure and function. These techniques include electron microscopes, MALDI-MSI, X-rays, and optical IR. The application of synchrotron radiation (SR) techniques in plant research is attributed to its characteristics of unmatched nanosecond pulse properties, high brightness, polarization, and cohesiveness (Abo-Bakr et al. 2003; Duncan and Williams 1983; Miller and Dumas 2006). For imaging of plants with SR it is essential that the energy level selected for analysis can specifically interact with desired metabolites of the plants and the emerging radiation be detectable by the detectors without causing any physicochemical changes in the plant tissues. The SR can be effectively used to identify and localize elements in plant tissues and X-rays, and IR can be used to study the tissue-specific distribution of organic and inorganic metabolites. Beamlines with SR-X-ray have been developed to study cellular level changes in plant tissues (Goff et al. 2009; Lombi and Susini 2009; Schulze and Bertsch 1995). Computed microtomography (μ-CT) and phase contrast imaging with SR-X-ray are used to obtain spatial resolution up to 2 μm with sectioning time intervals in milliseconds.

In the instrumental setup, radiant energy is generated from the storage ring and is passed through two types of magnets, the bending magnets and the 'wiggler' or 'undulator' magnets (see Fig. 18.5). During this passage any energy lost from energy beam is compensated by other devices that maintain a constant flow of energy from the storage ring. To maintain constant beam intensities, fresh injections of electrons are done by the 'top up' technique. The passage of electrons near the bending magnet generates an electromagnetic radiation. This radiation can be used for extraction of IR, X-ray, and ultra-violet (UV) rays by use of monochromators, mirrors, and slits. Before focusing the selected beam on the target samples, the beam is collimated. The arrangement of the dipole magnet is critical in obtaining a discrete spectral with high brightness. The beamlines are designed to deliver the generated radiations to the end stations, where the target sample is illuminated. Recent advancements in beamline setups enable users to measure spectral data with a specific region of interest, desired surface area, and volume or monitor a chemical reaction (Graceffa et al. 2013; Kathuria et al. 2011; Sham and Rivers 2002).

In addition to synchrotron μ-computed tomography (SR-μCT), there are several other techniques that employed synchrotron radiations, viz., (1) synchrotron radiation-Fourier transform infrared (SR-FTIR), (2) X-Ray absorption spectroscopy,

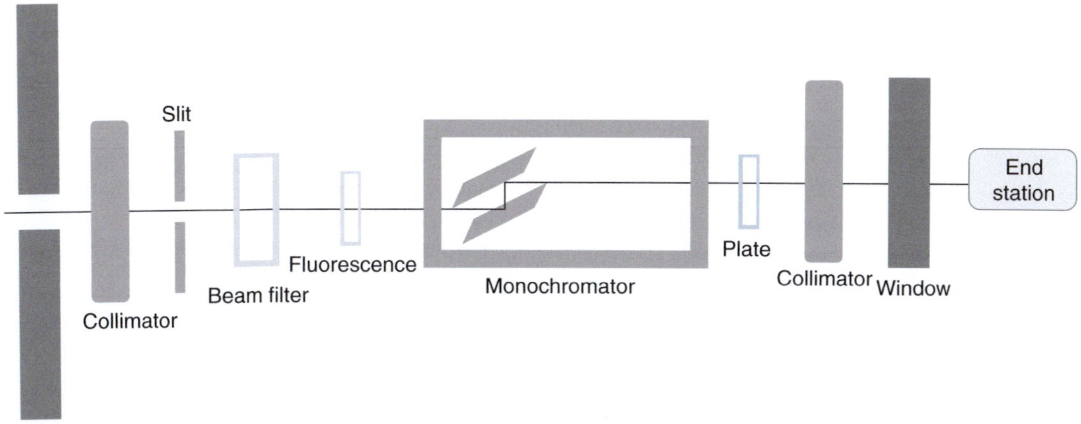

Fig. 18.5 Schematic representation of a typical synchrotron radiation instrument

and (3) X-Ray microfluorescence (m-XRF). SR-μCT is used in many applications in plant sciences. A comprehensive list of some applications is provided in Table 18.2.

18.4.1 Challenges in Application of SR Techniques in Plant Sciences

Although SR techniques provide an in-depth information of the *in-vivo* tissue structures of plants or any other materials there are several challenges to its application. Like any other technique, the analyst needs to optimize several factors to avoid the undesired effects of radiations on samples. Some issues which require careful consideration to explore the benefits of this technique with least sample damage are discussed here. The penetrating ability of X-rays can cause damage to the protein structure and dissociation of chemical bonds in certain metabolites if the sample is exposed at high temperatures and for a longer duration. Some researchers have reported use of cryogenic holders and fast scanning parameters to overcome this issue. Some samples may be prone to photoreduction and this issue can be managed by use of low radiation doses, faster scanning speeds, and freezing the samples by use of liquid helium (Hashizume et al. 1997; Rodriguez et al. 2015; Tanino et al. 2013). For samples where the scanning is to be performed repeatedly on the same sample with long exposure times, the loss of water content and cellular component delocalization should be critically considered. Damages can be reduced by reducing number of scans per sample, selecting optimum spatial resolutions, increasing the dwell time, and focusing the beam only on the region of interest of the sample.

18.5 Conclusions

The imaging techniques have only gained an upsurge in their application to plant sciences in the past decade. With significant advancements in their instrumentation, imaging and mass spectrometry techniques complement significant amount of research carried out in genomics, metabolomics, and proteomics. However, there is still a lot to be achieved as far as the resolution and sensitivity parameters are concerned. To explore the potential of these techniques, standardized protocols need to be developed. The versatile application of imaging techniques also requires financial support for researchers from various funding agencies as the techniques require long measurement periods and cost intensive instrumentation.

References

Abo-Bakr M, Feikes J, Holldack K, Kuske P, Peatman WB, Schade U, et al. Brilliant, Coherent Far-Infrared (THz) synchrotron radiation. Phys Rev Lett. 2003;90(9):4.

Bax A, Griffey RH, Hawkins BL. Correlation of proton and nitrogen-15 chemical shifts by multiple quantum NMR. J Magn Reson. 1983;55(2):301–15.

Becue I, Van Poucke C, Van Peteghem C. An LC-MS screening method with library identification for the detection of steroids in dietary supplements. J Mass Spectrom. 2011;46(3):327–35.

Birkemeyer C, Kolasa A, Kopka J. Comprehensive chemical derivatization for gas chromatography-mass spectrometry-based multi-targeted profiling of the major phytohormones. J Chromatogr A. 2003;993(1–2):89–102.

Bogusz MJ, Hassan H, Al-Enazi E, Ibrahim Z, Al-Tufail M. Application of LC-ESI-MS-MS for detection of synthetic adulterants in herbal remedies. J Pharm Biomed Anal. 2006;41(2):554–64.

Borisjuk L, Nguyen TH, Neuberger T, Rutten T, Tschiersch H, Claus B, et al. Gradients of lipid storage, photosynthesis and plastid differentiation in developing soybean seeds. New Phytol. 2005;167(3):761–76.

Chen Y, Zhao L, Lu F, Yu Y, Chai Y, Wu Y. Determination of synthetic drugs used to adulterate botanical dietary supplements using QTRAP LC-MS/MS. Food Addit Contam Part A Chem Anal Control Expo Risk Assess. 2009;26(5):595–603.

Ciobanu L, Seeber DA, Pennington CH. 3D MR microscopy with resolution 3.7 μm by 3.3 μm by 3.3 μm. J Magn Reson. 2002;158(1–2):178–82.

D'Abrosca B, Scognamiglio M, Corrado L, Chiocchio I, Zampella L, Mastrobuoni F, et al. Evaluation of different training systems on Annurca apple fruits revealed by agronomical, qualitative and NMR-based metabolomic approaches. Food Chem. 2017;222:18–27.

Dettmer K, Aronov PA, Hammock BD. Mass spectrometry-based metabolomics. Mass Spectrom Rev. 2007;26:51–78.

de Souza LP, Naake T, Tohge T, Fernie AR. From chromatogram to analyte to metabolite. How to pick horses for courses from the massive web resources for mass spectral plant metabolomics. Gigascience. 2017;6(7):1–20.

Deventer K, Van Thuyne W, Mikulčíková P, Van Eenoo P, Delbeke FT. Detection of selected stimulants as contaminants in solid nutritional supplements by liquid chromatography-mass spectrometry. Food Chem. 2007;103(4):1508–13.

Duncan WD, Williams GP. Infrared synchrotron radiation from electron storage rings. Appl Opt. 1983;22(18):2914–23.

Enebak SACWA. Evidence for induced systemic protection to fusiform rust in loblolly pine by plant growth-promoting rhizobacteria. Plant Dis. 2000;84(3):306–8.

Fenn JB. Electrospray wings for molecular elephants (Nobel lecture). Angew Chemie Int Ed Engl. 2003;42:3871–94.

Fiehn O. Metabolic networks of Cucurbita maxima phloem. Phytochemistry. 2003;62(6):875–86.

Fulmer GR, Miller AJM, Sherden NH, Gottlieb HE, Nudelman A, Stoltz BM, et al. NMR chemical shifts of trace impurities: Common laboratory solvents, organics, and gases in deuterated solvents relevant to the organometallic chemist. Organometallics. 2010;29(9):2176–9.

Geyer H, Parr MK, Koehler K, Mareck U, Schänzer W, Thevis M. Nutritional supplements cross-contaminated and faked with doping substances. J Mass Spectrom. 2008;43:892–902.

Go EP. Database resources in metabolomics: An overview. J Neuroimmune Pharmacol. 2010;5:18–30.

Goff KL, Quaroni L, Wilson KE. Measurement of metabolite formation in single living cells of Chlamydomonas reinhardtii using synchrotron Fourier-Transform Infrared spectromicroscopy. Analyst. 2009;134(11):2216.

Graceffa R, Nobrega RP, Barrea RA, Kathuria SV, Chakravarthy S, Bilsel O, et al. Sub-millisecond time-resolved SAXS using a continuous-flow mixer and X-ray microbeam. J Synchrotron Radiat. 2013;20(6):820–5.

Gross JH. Mass spectrometry: a textbook. 2nd ed. Heidelberg: Springer; 2011.

Haase A, Frahm J, Matthaei D, Hanicke W, Merboldt KD. FLASH imaging. Rapid NMR imaging using low flip-angle pulses. J Magn Reson. 1986;67(2):258–66.

Haishi T, Uematsu T, Matsuda Y, Kose K. Development of a 1.0 T MR microscope using a Nd-Fe-B permanent magnet. Magn Reson Imaging. 2001;19(6):875–80.

Halket J, Zaikin V. Review: derivatization in mass spectrometry—1. Silylation. Eur J Mass Spectrom. 2003;9(1):1.

Hashizume H, Shimomura S, Yamada H, Fujita T, Nakazawa H, Akutsu O. An X-ray diffraction system with controlled relative humidity and temperature. Rigaku J. 1997;14(1):1–4.

Hayden DM, Rolletschek H, Borisjuk L, Corwin J, Kliebenstein DJ, Grimberg A, et al. Cofactome analyses reveal enhanced flux of carbon into oil for potential biofuel production. Plant J. 2011;67(6):1018–28.

Hochberg U, Albuquerque C, Rachmilevitch S, Cochard H, David-Schwartz R, Brodersen CR, et al. Grapevine petioles are more sensitive to drought induced embolism than stems: evidence from in vivo MRI and microcomputed tomography observations of hydraulic vulnerability segmentation. Plant Cell Environ. 2016;39(9):1886–94.

Hochberg U, Windt CW, Ponomarenko A, Zhang Y-J, Gersony J, Rockwell FE, et al. Stomatal Closure, Basal Leaf Embolism, and Shedding Protect the Hydraulic Integrity of Grape Stems. Plant Physiol. 2017;174(2):764–75.

Holbrook NM. *In Vivo* observation of cavitation and embolism repair using magnetic resonance imaging. Plant Physiol. 2001;126(1):27–31.

Hsu R, Au AM. Gas chromatography-chemical ionization mass spectrometry for drug screen analyses. Bull Environ Contam Toxicol. 2001;66(2):178–83.

Huang Z, Xiao S, Luo D, Chen B, Yao S. Simultaneous determination of sibutramine and N-Di-desmethylsibutramine in dietary supplements for weight control by HPLC-ESI-MS. J Chromatogr Sci. 2008;46(8):707–11.

Huang C, Zhou Q, Gao S, Bao Q, Chen F, Liu C. Time-Domain nuclear magnetic resonance investigation of water dynamics in different ginger cultivars. J Agric Food Chem. 2016;64(2):470–7.

Ishikawa M, Ide H, Yamazaki H, Murakawa H, Kuchitsu K, Price WS, et al. Freezing behaviours in wintering Cornus florida flower bud tissues revisited using MRI. Plant Cell Environ. 2016;39(12):2663–75.

Issaq HJ, Van QN, Waybright TJ, Muschik GM, Veenstra TD. Analytical and statistical approaches to metabolomics research. J Sep Sci. 2009;31:2183–99.

Jennings W, Shibamoto T. Qualitative analysis of flavor and fragrance volatiles by glass capillary gas chromatography. New York: Academic Press; 1980.

Karas M, Glückmann M, Schäfer J. Ionization in matrix-assisted laser desorption/ionization: Singly charged molecular ions are the lucky survivors. J Mass Spectrom. 2000;35(1):1–12.

Kathuria SV, Guo L, Graceffa R, Barrea R, Nobrega RP, Matthews CR, et al. Minireview: Structural insights into early folding events using continuous-flow time-resolved small-angle X-ray scattering. Biopolymers. 2011;95:550–8.

Kessler N, Walter F, Persicke M, Albaum SP, Kalinowski J, Goesmann A, et al. Allocator: An interactive web platform for the analysis of metabolomic LC-ESI-MS datasets, enabling semi-automated, user-revised compound annotation and mass isotopomer ratio analysis. PLoS One. 2014;9(11):e113909.

Kesting JR, Huang JQ, Sørensen D. Identification of adulterants in a Chinese herbal medicine by LC-HRMS and LC-MS-SPE/NMR and comparative in vivo study with standards in a hypertensive rat model. J Pharm Biomed Anal. 2010;51(3):705–11.

Khush GS. Green revolution: the way forward. Nat Rev Genet. 2001;2(10):815–22.

Kim HJ, Lee JH, Park HJ, Cho S-H, Cho S, Kim WS. Monitoring of 29 weight-loss compounds in foods and dietary supplements by LC-MS/MS. Food Addit Contam Part A Chem Anal Control Expo Risk Assess. 2014;31(5):777–83.

Kind T, Wohlgemuth G, Lee DY, Lu Y, Palazoglu M, Shahbaz S, et al. FiehnLib: Mass spectral and retention index libraries for metabolomics based on quadrupole and time-of-flight gas chromatography/mass spectrometry. Anal Chem. 2009;81(24):10038–48.

Köckenberger W. Functional imaging of plants by magnetic resonance experiments. Trends Plant Sci. 2001;6(7):286–92.

Langridge P, Fleury D. Making the most of "omics" for crop breeding. Trends Biotechnol. 2011;29:33–40.

Lau A-J, Holmes MJ, Woo S-O, Koh H-L. Analysis of adulterants in a traditional herbal medicinal product using liquid chromatography-mass spectrometry-mass spectrometry. J Pharm Biomed Anal. 2003;31(2):401–6.

Lee JD. Interpretation of mass spectra. Talanta. 1973;20(10):1029–38.

Liu SY, Woo SO, Koh HL. HPLC and GC-MS screening of Chinese proprietary medicine for undeclared therapeutic substances. J Pharm Biomed Anal. 2001;24:983–92.

Lombi E, Susini J. Synchrotron-based techniques for plant and soil science: Opportunities, challenges and future perspectives. Plant Soil. 2009;320:1–35.

Lommen A, van der Kamp HJ, Kools HJ, van der Lee MK, van der Weg G, Mol HGJ. MetAlignID: A high-throughput software tool set for automated detection of trace level contaminants in comprehensive LECO two-dimensional gas chromatography time-of-flight mass spectrometry data. J Chromatogr A. 2012;1263:169–78.

Lu S, Sun YH, Amerson H, Chiang VL. MicroRNAs in loblolly pine (*Pinus taeda* L.) and their association with fusiform rust gall development. Plant J. 2007;51(6):1077–98.

Lu YL, Zhou NL, Liao SY, Su N, He DX, Tian QQ, et al. Detection of adulteration of anti-hypertension dietary supplements and traditional Chinese medicines with synthetic drugs using LC/MS. Food Addit Contam Part A Chem Anal Control Expo Risk Assess. 2010;27(7):893–902.

Man CN, Nor NM, Lajis R, Harn GL. Identification of sildenafil, tadalafil and vardenafil by gas chromatography-mass spectrometry on short capillary column. J Chromatogr A. 2009;1216(47):8426–30.

McLafferty FW, Zhang MY, Stauffer DB, Loh SY. Comparison of algorithms and databases for matching unknown mass spectra. J Am Soc Mass Spectrom. 1998;9(1):92–5.

Melkus G, Rolletschek H, Radchuk R, Fuchs J, Rutten T, Wobus U, et al. The metabolic role of the legume endosperm: a noninvasive imaging study. Plant Physiol. 2009;151(3):1139–54.

Miller LM, Dumas P. Chemical imaging of biological tissue with synchrotron infrared light. Biochim Biophys Acta Biomembr. 2006;1178:846–57.

Nardini A, Savi T, Losso A, Petit G, Pacilè S, Tromba G, et al. X-ray microtomography observations of xylem embolism in stems of Laurus nobilis are consistent with hydraulic measurements of percentage loss of conductance. New Phytol. 2017;213(3):1068–75.

Neuberger T, Rolletschek H, Webb A, Borisjuk L. Non-invasive mapping of lipids in plant tissue using magnetic resonance imaging. Methods Mol Biol. 2009;579:485–96.

Nolf M, Lopez R, Peters JMR, Flavel RJ, Koloadin LS, Young IM, et al. Visualization of xylem embolism by X-ray microtomography: a direct test against hydraulic measurements. New Phytol. 2017;214(2):890–8.

Nováková L, Matysová L, Solich P. Advantages of application of UPLC in pharmaceutical analysis. Talanta. 2006;68(3):908–18.

Park S, Lee JG, Roh SH, Kim G, Kwon CH, Park HR, et al. Determination of PDE-5 inhibitors and appetite suppressants in adulterated dietary supplements using LC/PDA and LC/MS. Food Addit Contam Part B Surveill. 2012;5(1):29–32.

Patel DN, Li L, Kee CL, Ge X, Low MY, Koh HL. Screening of synthetic PDE-5 inhibitors and their analogues as adulterants: Analytical techniques and challenges. J Pharm Biomed Anal. 2014;87:176–90.

Pittia P, Sacchetti G, Mancini L, Voltolini M, Sodini N, Tromba G, et al. Evaluation of microstructural properties of coffee beans by synchrotron X-ray microtomography: A methodological approach. J Food Sci. 2011;76(2):E222–31.

Rodriguez JA, Xu R, Chen CC, Huang Z, Jiang H, Chen AL, et al. Three-dimensional coherent X-ray diffractive imaging of whole frozen-hydrated cells. IUCrJ. 2015;2(Pt 5):575–83.

Roh MS. Flowering and inflorescence development of *Lachenalia aloides* "Pearsonii" as influenced by bulb storage and forcing temperature. Sci Hortic. 2005;104(3):305–23.

Roh MS, Grassotti A, Guglieri L. Storage and forcing temperatures affect inflorescence initiation, flowering and floret blast of *Lachenalia aloides* "Pearsonii". Acta Hortic. 1998;454:213–21.

Roh SH, Kang YP, Park S, Huh Y, Lee J, Park JH, et al. Determination of tadalafil and N-desmethylsibutramine in health and dietary supplements using ultra-performance liquid chromatography (UPLC) coupled with quadrupole-time-of-flight mass spectrometry (Q-TOF MS). Food Addit Contam Part A Chem Anal Control Expo Risk Assess. 2011;28(11):1475–82.

Rolletschek H, Melkus G, Grafahrend-Belau E, Fuchs J, Heinzel N, Schreiber F, et al. Combined noninvasive imaging and modeling approaches reveal metabolic compartmentation in the barley endosperm. Plant Cell. 2011;23(8):3041–54.

Salleo S, Lo Gullo MA, Trifilò P, Nardini A. New evidence for a role of vessel-associated cells and phloem in the rapid xylem refilling of cavitated stems of *Laurus nobilis* L. Plant Cell Environ. 2004;27(8):1065–76.

Sawada Y, Akiyama K, Sakata A, Kuwahara A, Otsuki H, Sakurai T, et al. Widely targeted metabolomics based on large-scale MS/MS data for elucidating metabolite accumulation patterns in plants. Plant Cell Physiol. 2009;50(1):37–47.

Schulze DG, Bertsch PM. Synchrotron X-Ray techniques in soil, plant, and environmental research. Adv Agron. 1995;55(C):1–66.

Sedighi Gilani M, Boone MN, Mader K, Schwarze FWMR. Synchrotron X-ray micro-tomography imaging and analysis of wood degraded by *Physisporinus vitreus* and Xylaria longipes. J Struct Biol. 2014;187(2):149–57.

Sham TK, Rivers ML. A brief overview of synchrotron radiation. Rev Mineral Geochemistry. 2002;49(1):117–47.

Shou WZ, Magis L, Li AC, Naidong W, Bryant MS. A novel approach to perform metabolite screening during the quantitative LC-MS/MS analyses of in vitro metabolic stability samples using a hybrid triple-quadrupole linear ion trap mass spectrometer. J Mass Spectrom. 2005;40(10):1347–56.

Spragg RA. Encyclopedia of Spectroscopy and Spectrometry. Encycl Spectrosc Spectrom 2017.

Srimany A, George C, Naik HR, Pinto DG, Chandrakumar N, Pradeep T. Developmental patterning and segregation of alkaloids in areca nut (seed of Areca catechu) revealed by magnetic resonance and mass spectrometry imaging. Phytochemistry. 2016;125:35–42.

Stein SE. An integrated method for spectrum extraction and compound identification from gas chromatography/mass spectrometry data. J Am Soc Mass Spectrom. 1999;10(8):770–81.

Szimtenings M, Olt S, Haase A. Flow encoded NMR spectroscopy for quantification of metabolite flow in intact plants. J Magn Reson. 2003;161(1):70–6.

Tanino KK, Kobayashi S, Hyett C, Hamilton K, Liu J, Li B, et al. *Allium fistulosum* as a novel system to investigate mechanisms of freezing resistance. Physiol Plant. 2013;147(1):101–11.

Tkáč I, Starčuk Z, Choi IY, Gruetter R. In vivo1H NMR spectroscopy of rat brain at 1 ms echo time. Magn Reson Med. 1999;41(4):649–56.

Trtik P, Dual J, Keunecke D, Mannes D, Niemz P, Stähli P, et al. 3D imaging of microstructure of spruce wood. J Struct Biol. 2007;159(1):46–55.

Umebayashi T, Fukuda K, Haishi T, Sotooka R, Zuhair S, Otsuki K. The Developmental Process of Xylem Embolisms in Pine Wilt Disease Monitored by Multipoint Imaging Using Compact Magnetic Resonance Imaging. Plant Physiol. 2011;156(2):943–51.

Vaclavik L, Krynitsky AJ, Rader JI. Targeted analysis of multiple pharmaceuticals, plant toxins and other secondary metabolites in herbal dietary supplements by ultra-high performance liquid chromatography-quadrupole-orbital ion trap mass spectrometry. Anal Chim Acta. 2014;810:45–60.

Van As H. Intact plant MRI for the study of cell water relations, membrane permeability, cell-to-cell and long distance water transport. J Exp Bot. 2007;58(4):743–56.

van Dusschoten D, Metzner R, Kochs J, Postma JA, Pflugfelder D, Buehler J, et al. Quantitative 3d analysis of plant roots growing in soil using magnetic resonance imaging. Plant Physiol. 2016;170:1176–88.

Van de Wal BAE, Windt CW, Leroux O, Steppe K. Heat girdling does not affect xylem integrity: an in vivo magnetic resonance imaging study in the tomato peduncle. New Phytol. 2017;215(2):558–68.

Vanhamme L, Van Den Boogaart A, Van Huffel S. Improved method for accurate and efficient quantification of MRS Data with use of prior knowledge. J Magn Reson. 1997;129(1):35–43.

Venhuis BJ, de Kaste D. Towards a decade of detecting new analogues of sildenafil, tadalafil and vardenafil in food supplements: A history, analytical aspects and health risks. J Pharm Biomed Anal. 2012;69:196–208.

Verslues PE, Agarwal M, Katiyar-Agarwal S, Zhu J, Zhu JK. Methods and concepts in quantifying resistance to drought, salt and freezing, abiotic stresses that affect plant water status. Plant J. 2006;45(4):523–39.

Walton DRM. Handbook of derivatives for chromatography. J Organomet Chem. 1979:C47.

Wang J, Yang D, Wang Z, Chen B, Yao S. Simultaneous of illegal additives in dietary supplements and traditional medicines by high performance liquid chromatography-electrospray ionization mass spectrometry. Food Chem. 2009;113(1):227–32.

van der Weerd L, Claessens MM, Ruttink T, Vergeldt FJ, Schaafsma TJ, Van As H. Quantitative NMR microscopy of osmotic stress responses in maize and pearl millet. J Exp Bot. 2001;52(365):2333–43.

van der Weerd L, Claessens M, Efde C, Vanas H. Nuclear magnetic resonance imaging of membrane permeability changes in plants during osmotic stress. Plant Cell Environ. 2002;25(11):1539–49.

Wen W, Liu H, Zhou Y, Jin M, Yang N, Li D, et al. Combining Quantitative Genetics Approaches with Regulatory Network Analysis to Dissect the Complex Metabolism of the Maize Kernel. Plant Physiol. 2016;170(1):136–46.

Wojtyla Ł, Garnczarska M, Zalewski T, Bednarski W, Ratajczak L, Jurga S. A comparative study of water distribution, free radical production and activation of antioxidative metabolism in germinating pea seeds. J Plant Physiol. 2006;163(12):1207–20.

Woo H, Kim JW, Han KM, Lee JH, Hwang IS, Lee JH, et al. Simultaneous analysis of 17 diuretics in dietary supplements by HPLC and LC-MS/MS. Food Addit Contam Part A Chem Anal Control Expo Risk Assess. 2013;30(2):209–17.

Woodfield HK, Sturtevant D, Borisjuk L, Munz E, Guschina IA, Chapman K, et al. Spatial and Temporal Mapping of Key Lipid Species in *Brassica napus* Seeds. Plant Physiol. 2017;173(4):1998–2009.

Wuolikainen A, Jonsson P, Ahnlund M, Antti H, Marklund SL, Moritz T, et al. Multi-platform mass spectrometry analysis of the CSF and plasma metabolomes of rigorously matched amyotrophic lateral sclerosis, Parkinson's disease and control subjects. Mol BioSyst. 2016;12(4):1287–98.

Yooyongwech S, Horigane AK, Yoshida M, Yamaguchi M, Sekozawa Y, Sugaya S, et al. Changes in aquaporin gene expression and magnetic resonance imaging of water status in peach tree flower buds during dormancy. Physiol Plant. 2008;134(3):522–33.

Yooyongwech S, Horigane AK, Yoshida M, Sekozawa Y, Sugaya S, Cha-Um S, et al. Hydrogen cyanamide enhances MRI-measured water status in flower buds of peach (*Prunus persica* L.) during winter. Plant Omics. 2012;5(4):400–4.

Drugs from Our Ancestors: Tradition to Innovation

19

Pulok K. Mukherjee, Subhadip Banerjee, Amit Kar, and Joydeb Chanda

Contents

19.1 Ancestors' Medicine

The history of medicine is ancient, the sum total of the knowledge, skills, and practices based on the theories, beliefs, and experiences indigenous to different cultures, used in the maintenance of health, as well as in the prevention, diagnosis, improvement, or treatment of physical and mental illnesses. The terms complementary/alternative/nonconventional drugs are used interchangeably with traditional medicine in some countries. The World Health Organization (WHO) acknowledges that ancient and practice of medicine are important parts of the healthcare system. The practices and public interest in natural therapies based on traditional practices have increased dramatically. This has raised the international trade of herbal medicine and attracted several pharmaceutical companies in commercializing herbal drugs (Heyman and Meyer 2012).

Ayurveda is an ancient healthcare system originated at the dawn of human civilization. It is based on experience over a long period of time, some of which has been proven experimentally. Several formulations and dosage forms

P. K. Mukherjee (✉) · S. Banerjee · A. Kar
J. Chanda
Department of Pharmaceutical Technology, School of Natural Product Studies, Jadavpur University, Kolkata, West Bengal, India
e-mail: pulok.mukherjee@jadavpuruniversity.in

S. Sen, R. Chakraborty (eds.), *Herbal Medicine in India*,
https://doi.org/10.1007/978-981-13-7248-3_19

play an important role in Ayurveda. Generally, Ayurvedic formulations are multicomponent mixtures, containing plant- and animal-derived products, minerals, and metals. The traditional Vedic text of Atharva-Veda was documented around 5000 years back that contains numerous references of Ayurvedic medicine and allied aspects of healthcare. The Sanskrit word "Ayurveda" consists of two words: "Ayus" suggesting life and "Veda" referring to knowledge or science. Thus "Ayurveda" in totality means "science of life." It integrates physical, psychological, spiritual, and social aspects of human life conferred in Ayurveda (Mukherjee et al. 2012).

Ancient texts starting from different "Samhita," "Nighantu," and other official compendia like Ayurvedic Pharmacopoeia and Ayurvedic Formulary showed a roadmap in natural product-based healthcare research (Mukherjee et al. 2017a, b). The Charak Samhita (900 B.C.) is considered as the first recorded treatise, devoted to the concepts and practice of Ayurveda which listed around 341 plants and plant products used in medicine. Most importantly, "Charak Samhita," an ancient text in Ayurveda classified the plant drugs into 50 groups based on their Sanskrit name. The next landmark in Ayurvedic literature was the Sushruta Samhita (600 B.C.), which has a special emphasis on surgery. It described 395 medicinal plants, 57 drugs of animal origin, and 64 minerals and metals as therapeutic agents. Sushruta, the father of surgery, lived and practiced surgery in Varanasi, India, approximately 2500 years ago. Another important authority in Ayurveda was Vagbhata, who practiced around 700 A.D. His work Ashtanga Hridaya is considered unrivaled for the principles and practice of medicine. The Madhava Nidana (800–900 AD) was the next important milestone; it is the most famous Ayurvedic work on the diagnosis of diseases. A celebrated writer on traditional Indian medicine, Bhava Mishra of Magadha, wrote Bhava Prakasha around 1550, which is held in high esteem by modern Ayurvedic practitioners for its descriptions of approximately 470 medicinal plants. Other than these monumental treatises, more than 70 "Nighantu Granthas" (pharmacy lexicons) were written, mostly between the seventh and sixteenth century AD. The ancient texts like "Raj Nighantu" by Narhari Pandit and "Madanpala Nighantu" by Madanpala are considered as masterpieces on medicinal plants. Thus, Ayurveda is believed to be a scientifically organized discipline from its origin. Most of the Ayurvedic texts are much respected in neighboring countries and were translated into Greek (300 B.C.), Tibetan, and Chinese (300 A.D.) and several other languages (Mukherjee et al. 2006).

19.1.1 Evidence Base of Ancient Knowledge

Since the Vedic era Indian scholars and sages have rigorously thought about health and wellness. Later, the texts like "Charak Samhita" and "Sushruta Samhita" were documented in about a thousand years B.C., where the uses of plants and poly-herbal formulations were highlighted in healthcare. In Charaka Samhita Sutrasthana, it has been mentioned that even if the most dangerous poison is used in a proper way, it will become a medicine. Similarly, the drugs, if used in an improper manner, will turn out to be poison. This presents the high ethical values of ancient health practices which advocated safety for patients (see Fig. 19.1).

The evolution of Ayurveda and plant-based remedies adopted in indigenous healthcare system is a part of cultural heritage in India. Indian *Materia Medica* includes about 2000 drugs of natural origin almost all of which are derived from different traditional systems and folklore practices (Mukherjee et al. 2017a, b). It provides a huge knowledge of traditionally inspired medicine based on folklore practices of India. Indian traditional medicine is based on AYUSH system, which has become an emerging interest of the world in adopting and studying traditional systems and healthcare perspectives. Nowadays, the Ministry of AYUSH, Government of India, has initiated several attempts to explore the possibil-

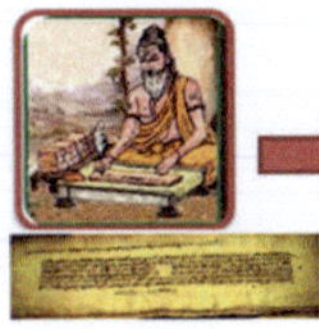

योगादपि विषं तीक्ष्णमुत्तमं भेषजं भवेत्।
भेषजं चापि दुर्युक्तं तीक्ष्णं सम्पद्यते विषम्॥

(च.सू– १/१२७)

तस्मान्न भिषजा युक्तं युक्तिबाह्येन भेषजम्।
धीमता किञ्चिदादेयं जीवितारोग्यकाङ्क्षिणा॥

(च.सू– १/१२८)
[Devanagari Script]

Yogadapi Visham tikshnamuttamam bheshajam bhabet |
Bheshajam chapi duryuktam tikshnam sampadyate visham | |
(Charaka Samhita Sutrasthana-1/127)
Tasmanna vishaja yuktam yuktivhayhena bheshajam |
Dhimita kinchidadyeyam jivitarogyakandikshana | |
(Charaka Samhita Sutrasthana-1/128)
[Diacritical Script]
"Even if the most dangerous poison is used in proper way will become a medicine. Similarly, the drugs if used in improper manner will turn out to be poison. So, if a person who wants health and Life should avoid receiving medicines from such physician who is ignorant about the proper use of drugs"

Fig. 19.1 Understanding of drug in Charaka Samhita

ity of evaluating TMs for their therapeutic potential as originally practiced, as well as to generate data to put them in national healthcare programs (Mukherjee et al. 2014).

In traditional systems of medicine, the medicinal plants play a major role and constitute their backbone. Indian *Materia Medica* includes about 2000 drugs of natural origin, almost all of which are derived from different traditional systems and folklore practices. The global market of trade associated with medicinal plants is estimated at around US$60 billion per year and is growing at the rate of 7% annually with varying shares of developed and developing countries. India has approximately 47,000 plant species and about 15,000 medicinal plants; among them 7000 plants are used in Ayurveda, 700 in Unani medicine, and 600 in Siddha medicine. Around 65% population of rural India uses Ayurvedic medicines. Traditionally, 2000 species in Ayurveda, Siddha, and Unani medicine (ASU) are used by classical traditions. Traditional village practitioners are practicing 4500–5000 species. A tribal and other traditional community uses 8000 plant species (Mukherjee et al. 2010).

Discovery of new drug is facing serious challenges due to rejection in several new drug approvals related with excessive cost. Combinatorial chemistry provided new expectation of higher achievement rates of new chemical entities (NCEs) but this scientific development has failed to improve the success rate in novel drug discovery. This scenario has prompted researchers to come out with a novel approach of integrated drug discovery from natural products. The starting point for plant-based new drug discovery should be identification of the right candidate plants by applying traditional documented use, tribal non-documented use, and exhaustive literature search. This integrated approach of bioassay-guided fractionation of medicinal plant leads to identification of novel active compounds as new drugs (Mukherjee et al. 2017a, b). The development of TM necessitates the merging of modern techniques and integrated approaches related to their evidence-based research in various fields of science through national and international collaboration (Mukherjee et al. 2015). The integrated strategies of drug development from TM have been enumerated in Fig. 19.2.

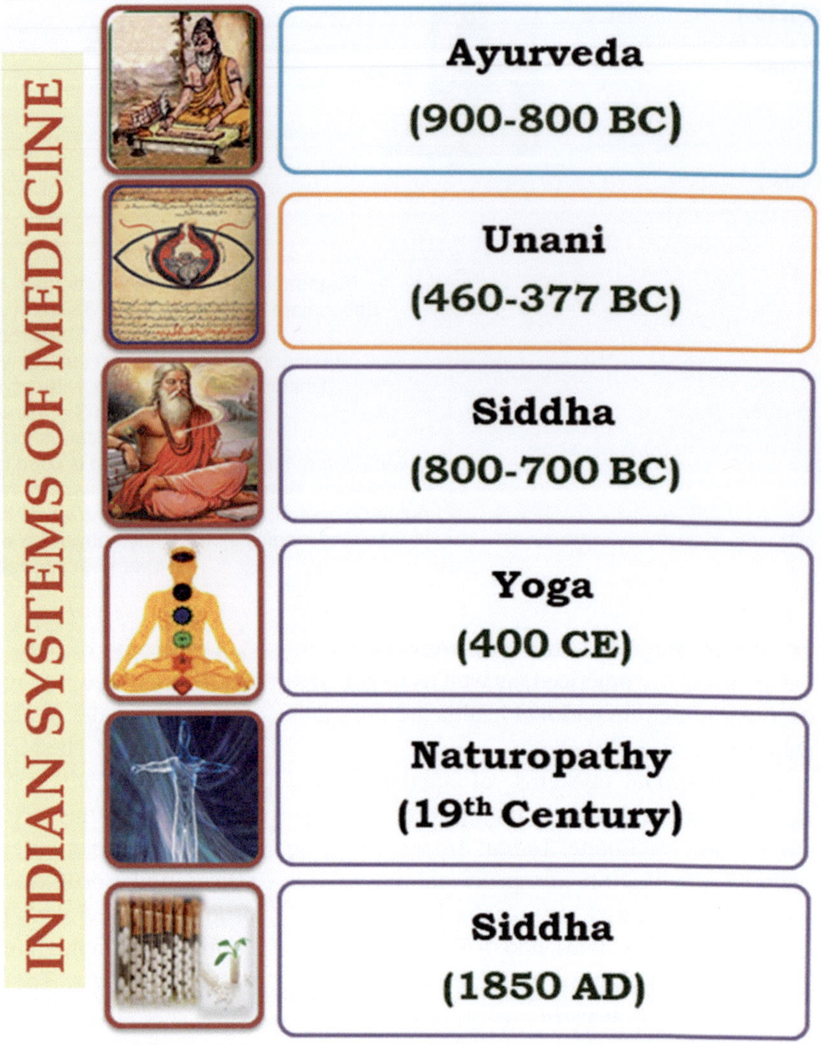

Fig. 19.2 Traditional medicine practiced in India

19.2 Ethnopharmacology in Health and Wellness

The term ethnopharmacology is an amalgamation of the bio-cultural perspective and the traditional indigenous knowledge of medicinal substances. The multiple disciplines that contribute to ethnopharmacological research are diverse, reflecting the discrete and overlapping investigational objectives of those disciplines. The importance of ethnopharmacology is growing to maintain well-being for improving quality of life. Ethnopharmacological information is often imparted to enhance the status of human health in the society. Ethnopharmacology focuses on the employment of traditional medicine in local communities, including its commercial applications. Today, it is employed for several types of research on medicinal, psychoactive, and toxic plants, and fungi or animals that are used by people worldwide. The ethnopharmacological approach is unique and it requires a contribution from the social and cultural sciences. It should be ensured that the medicine should work effectively and at the same time it is safe for human use. Ethically, it should not matter whether the medicine is an approved prescription product, over-the-counter medication, dietary supplement, phytopharmaceutical, or traditional medicine when human health is at stake. Thus, the scientific validation and quality control of TMs are critical and essential aspects confirm their therapeutic efficacy, safety, and rational uses in specific healthcare needs (Mukherjee et al. 2016). The ethnopharmacological approach toward the understanding and appraisal of ancient traditional medicines is characterized by the inclusions of the social as well as the natural sciences. Anthropological field study describing the local use of nature-derived medicines is the basis for ethnopharmacological inquiries. The multidisciplinary scientific validation of indigenous drugs is of great importance in modern societies to sustain local healthcare practices. Especially with respect to therapies related to aging and chronic and infectious diseases, TM offers favorable alternatives to synthetic drugs. Bioassay-guided investigation helps in the exploration of several therapeutically active molecules used to treat disease in variable depth and extent. The limitation of one-dimensional *in vitro* approach lies in the exploration of the complexity of human diseases and ignores the concept of polypharmacological synergies. The recent focus on synergy-driven system biology and reverse pharmacology approach in medicinal plant research helps in the understanding of complex multiparameter disease systems. Intensified economic process and economic liberalism presently accelerate the interchange between native and world pharmacopeias which depends on several medical practices based on the adopted historic-cultural perspective (Leonti 2013).

The demands of traditional medicines are rising increasingly due to its several therapeutic benefits in healthcare. It has been reported that the total global herbal market size is of 62.0 billion dollars, whereas India contributes only one billion dollars. As per the WHO reports, about three-quarters of the world's population presently use herbal medicine and other forms of traditional medicines. Even though the huge advancement occurred in allopathic system of medicines, there are many areas in which they have failed to prove its efficiency due to their adverse events. Nowadays, people have more faith toward traditional medicines than modern medicines due to occurrence of many side effects of modern medicines. The major reasons of popularity of traditional medicines are their accessibility, associability, and affordability in developing countries. As per WHO national policy on traditional medicine and guideline of herbal medications report, business of herbal medicines have increased from US$ 707 million in 1999 to US$ 1006 million in 2001 in nine countries (Republic of Islamic, Bhutan, the Czech Republic, Republic of Iran, Canada, Madagascar, Pakistan, Sweden, Sudan, and Malaysia). According to Global Industry Analysis, it was estimated that the global herbal market will reach $107 billion by the end of 2017. This shows that Ayurveda is one of the most noticeable expressions of substitute medication practiced throughout the world (Nirali and Shankar 2015).

19.3 Lead Development: Innovation in Traditional Medicine

Traditional medicines are considered as the sum of the ethnomedicinal knowledge, skills, and indigenous practices in different cultures. There is an urgent need of ensuring effective quality, safety, and efficacy of traditional medicine to direct natural product-inspired drug development research. A large number of people, suffering from cancer and rheumatic arthritis, use complementary and alternative medicine regularly.

For example, ispaghula, garlic, ginseng, ginger, gingko, St. John's wort, and saw palmetto are used by modern physicians. Nowadays, in most countries, allopathic and traditional systems of medicine are being practiced in a complementary way. So the efforts have been made to harmonize the process of the evaluation and quality control of the botanicals in drug discovery. In order to ensure the accurate identification and authentication of the herbs, the first crucial step is to avoid admixtures or adulterations in the botanicals. In regard to quality assurance, plant identification is vital for authentication which in terms ensures both safety and efficacy.

The identification is generally done by macroscopic and microscopic examination, chemical fingerprinting, DNA-based characterization, etc. The bioactive secondary metabolites used in medicinal preparation are of huge diversity, often present as a different chemical class of compound (Mukherjee and Houghton 2009). There are some important issues need to be considered for exact identification and authentication of traditional medicine plants (Mukherjee and Wahile 2006). In addition, there are several other integrated strategies being applied to the validation of traditional medicine and Ayurveda (Mukherjee et al. 2015). The global implementation of evidence-based validation of traditional medicine is required which can really transform the global healthcare system (Mukherjee et al. 2014). The development of traditional medicine requires the convergence of modern techniques based on "omics"-driven approaches in the various fields of natural product research. Botanical preparation is used to standardize based on the presence of known active ingredient or marker compounds. However this could facilitate in establishing the product's quality, depending on the characteristic chemical fingerprinting of it. Plants contain a large number of active substances in certain ratios which must be kept constant, within narrow limits, from one preparation to another. The unique processing methods followed for the manufacturing of traditional medicine products make the herbal ingredients into very complex mixtures. Owing to that, separation, identification, and estimation of chemical components become more challenging in some cases. Moreover, herbal medicine contains several phytoconstituents and in most of the cases the target compound responsible for the pharmacological activity is unexplored (Mukherjee et al. 2016).

India has an ancient system of Ayurvedic medicine which provides a wealth of information on the folklore practices and traditional aspects of therapeutically important natural products. One of the major challenges of Ayurvedic medicine is maintaining the quality, safety, and efficacy issues which should be given more priority during the ethnopharmacology-driven drug discovery program (Mukherjee et al. 2016). In this context, globalization of Ayurvedic medicine is necessary to establish the evidence-based healthcare claims. There has been a development in the dissemination of Ayurvedic knowledge which can now be interpretable in Western terminology and also a large variety of texts are now available online. The National Institute of Indian Medical Heritage (http://niimh.nic.in/) (CCRAS, Ministry of AYUSH) has published e-Samhitas of all the main classical works on Ayurveda, such as *Charaka Samhita, Sushruta Samhita, Ashtanga Sangraha, Astanga Hridaya,* and *Bhavaprakash Nighantu* which are available online. The Pharmacopoeial Laboratory of India (PLIM, http://www.plimism.nic.in/) has published monographs of 326 single drugs of plant origin and 83 compound formulations of Ayurveda which have been published in several volumes of Ayurvedic Pharmacopoeia of India (API). The Ayurvedic Formulary of India deals with drugs, their composition, and action in addition to the other aspects of the medical system. Essential Drug List of Ayurveda has also been published by the Ministry of AYUSH which contains 277 essential medicines of Ayurveda indicated in several diseases The *Materia Medica* of Ayurveda consists of an extremely rich armamentarium of natural drugs, derived from plants, minerals, animals, and marine sources. These drugs are used as monotherapies or in simple combinations, which are otherwise referred to as polypharmaceuticals. The forms in which these are used are varied, such as extracted juices, decoctions, infusions, distillates, powders, tablets, pills, confections, syrups, fermented liquids, medicated oil, bhasmas (resultant of incineration), and many more. The *Materia Medica* of Ayurveda is an exhaustive publication that describes simple, safe, and proven remedies for common ailments. The Indian Herbal Pharmacopeia (2002) contains 52 monographs on widely used medicinal plants in India with scientific evidences on therapeutic effects. In addition, the Pharmacopeia of India (1996) covers additional botanical monographs on clove, guggul, opium, mentha, senna, and ashwagandha (Mukherjee et al. 2017a, b). The AYUSH Research Portal (http://ayushportal.nic.in/) presents evidence-based research data of AYUSH systems at a global level. Some of the Ayurvedic books, known as *Nighantugranthas,* such as *Dhanvantarinighantu, Kaiyadevanighantu, Bhavaprakasanighantu,* and *Rajanighantu*, deal mainly with a single drug, representing their habitat, characteristics, and therapeutic action. The Ayurvedic drugs are derived from different vegetable, animal, and plant sources. Ayurvedic formulations, which are predominantly derived from plants, are known as "kasthausadhi, where the formulations are being made from extract or juice of plants" parts. These include several Ayurvedic formulations like "aristra," "avleha," "grafa," "churna," and "taila." Formulations which are predominantly derived from metal and minerals are known as "rasausadhi." The formulations are made mainly from minerals and in combinations of minerals and plants; these include "bhasma," "pishti," "lauha," "kapibadkva," "rasayana," and so on (Mukherjee et al. 2010). A detailed description of all these formulations has been provided elsewhere in this chapter. The Ministry of AYUSH has launched many authentic books on both groups of compound formulations. While Sarngadhara Samhita, Cakradatta, Bhaisajya Ratnavali, Sahasrayogam, and Bharat Bhaisajya Ratnakara deal with both the groups of formulations, others like Rasendra Sarasangraha, Rasarathna Samuccaya, Rasaprakasam Sudhakara, Ayurvedaprakasa, Rasatarangini, and Rasayogasagara only deal with the rasausadhi group of formulations. However, globally, there is a necessity to create molecular libraries for Ayurvedic phytoconstituents along with their probable mechanism of action and other databases regarding systems pharmacology, gene and target protein, and disease network (Mukherjee et al. 2012). Plant extract libraries are not available in the public domain which could serve as a reservoir of phytoconstituents to be used for high-throughput screening for relevant biological activities.

These traditional medicine-inspired drug development programs improve the quality of healthcare considerably. Virtually, the expedition of natural product discovery was started in 1785, with the English physician Withering. He proposed his observations on the use of the foxglove, *Digitalis purpurea*, for the treatment of heart disorders, and this eventually led to the isolation of the cardiotonic agent, digoxin, which inhibited sodium-potassium ATPase. Later, the isolation of morphine from *Papaver somniferum* by Serturner in 1806 opened a newer avenue for the use of pure chemicals as painkiller for cancer patients suffering from terminal pain. In 1875, salicylic acid was isolated from Willow bark and its acetyl salt known as aspirin was considered as an important milestone in drug discovery. The journey of drug discovery started with analgesic aspirin to anticancer drug taxol in the last century (Mukherjee et al. 2017b).

Malaria still continues to be one of the greatest health challenges in human civilization. In the history of the development of antimalarial drugs, the success stories have been attributed to natural products. After the serendipitous discovery of quinine (Fig 19.2a), it has been conserved as a vital antimalarial drug ever since its effectiveness was first documented. In 1820, it was first isolated from the bark of Cinchona species (e.g., *C. officinalis*) by two pharmacists from France. In the mid-twentieth century, its synthetic analog chloroquine and mefloquine showed higher potency and subsequently replaced quinine as a novel antimalarial agent. However as they are now becoming resistant against most of the pathogen, the evolution of *Artemisia annua* (qinghaosu) came up to prominence in antimalarial therapy. In 1971, a group of Chinese scientists developed artemisinin as a lead compound to treat malaria by utilizing ethnopharmacological data mining from ancient texts of traditional Chinese medicine (see Fig 19.2b) (Newman and Cragg 2007). The story of development of artemisinin was found very unconventional yet inspiring. They started working with more than 2000 Chinese herb preparations and identified 640 hits with possible antimalarial activities. After a long hit and trial, they identified qinghao (the Chinese name of *Artemisia annua* L.) to be effective against plasmodium parasites. In spite of getting non-reproducible results they still carry out searching of traditional Chinese literature and they found one reference stating that "A handful of qinghao immersed with 2 liters of water, wring out the juice and drink it all." This information gave them the key idea that perhaps there is some ambiguity in the extraction process in which heat is involved which should be avoided during extraction process. By doing this, they obtained a better result while extracting with lower temperature. Finally, after getting satisfactory preclinical results their team was volunteered for clinical study owing to unavailability of other clinical trial facilities. It was followed by large clinical trials conducted in Hainan province to examine its clinical efficacy in patients infected with both *Plasmodium vivax* and *P. falciparum*. After getting satisfactory results, the compound was first isolated in 1971 and the publication came out in the year of 1982. Due to their substantial therapeutic efficacy, World Health Organization (WHO) has recognized artemisinin-based combination therapies (ACTs) to combat malaria with significant effect. This significant natural product-based drug discovery led to acquire Noble Prize in 2015 in Physiology to fetch recognition to Professor Tu Youyou. Thus, the development of antimalarial drug generates a huge impact on global health and the paradigm shifts in ethnopharmacology-driven research (Mukherjee et al. 2017b) (Fig. 19.3).

Major thrust area for research in TM has been represented in Fig. 19.4. In the modern era, combinatorial chemistry and high-throughput screening are very useful methods to discover newer drug molecules from natural resources. Despite the huge diversity in synthetic and combinatorial chemistries over the past 50 years, the lead finding from natural products is extremely important in drug development. The natural products and related structures are likely to become more important due to a large variety of functionally relevant secondary metabolites obtained from microbial and plant species. The ultrafast DNA sequencing and related genomics and bioinformatics tools were found applicable to explore the genetic variety of medicinal plants. Heretofore, the identification and characterization of the active secondary metabolites have found inefficient and often tedious, but recent advances in "omics" technologies, viz. genomics, proteomics, and metabolomics, dramatically accelerate the pace of drug discovery and analysis. The sophisticated hyphenated modern chromatographic and spectrometric method can readily elucidate the metabolomes of cells, tissues, and even organisms. The multivariate statistical analysis and networking model assist in comprehensive identification and evaluation of natural product diversity and functionality. The integrative system pharmacology approach aids in profiling molecular changes attributed by mutation, pathogens, and some other environmental stressors, resulting in the prediction of targets and mode(s) of action and toxicities of natural products and derivatives (Mukherjee et al. 2013).

It was observed that the pharmaceutical companies are lacking enthusiasm for developing natural product nowadays due to several reasons.

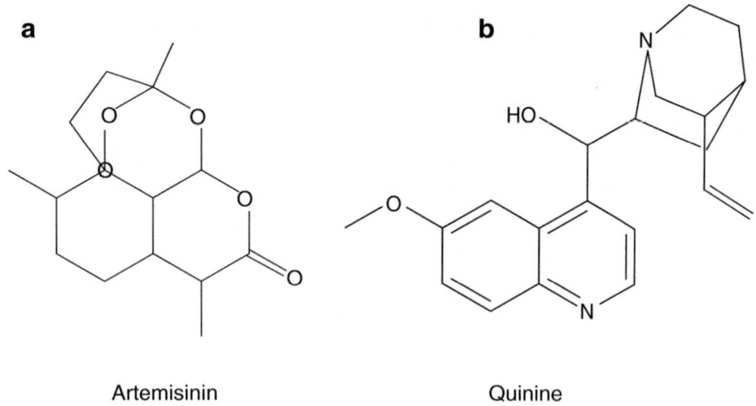

Fig. 19.3 Structures of artemisinin and quinine

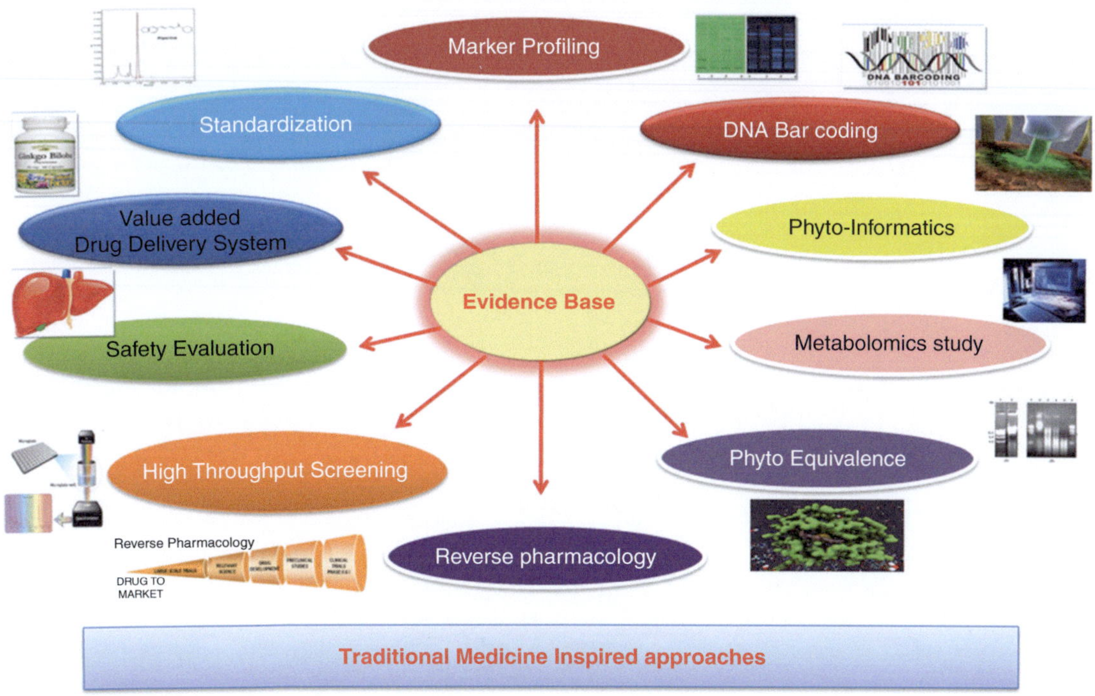

Fig. 19.4 Traditional medicine-inspired approaches for lead development

The United Nations Convention on Biological Diversity has mentioned some legitimate issues regarding the regulation of natural products and its international access. The natural product anthology offers an extensive range of pharmacophores with a high degree of stereochemistry. These assets can contribute to the ability to identify the difficult screening targets, such as protein–protein interactions (Mukherjee, 2017b). However, natural products may show several additional benefits over synthetic compounds owing to the fact that natural compounds show similar "metabolite-likeness" property (Hert et al. 2009). It implies that natural products can be explored as biologically active components and also likely to be substrates for one or more transporter systems which can deliver the compounds to their intracellular site of action. Several molecules have been derived from different traditional medicines as shown in Fig. 19.5 with the structures of the major active compounds (1 to 66). These advantages inspired a re-emerging interest in natural product research in drug discovery.

19.4 Synergy in Ethnomedicine

Nature presents various evolutionary evidences to molecular synergism. In nature, components perpetually interact with each other, creating a flow of energy between them. Synergy is when the sum of the whole system is greater than the sum of its parts. Synergism plays a significant role in therapeutic efficacy of herbs or herbal formulation. It is assumed that the effective concentration of combined ingredients is significantly increased with respect to that of each individual ingredient. In the last decade a rapid paradigm shift in chemotherapy was observed involving a gradual transition from monotherapy to multiple drug therapy. The major cause of the paradigm shift mainly lies in the ineffectiveness, resistance problems, and side effects which may appear from synthetic single-drug therapy, especially in the treatment of chronic diseases such as cancer, atherosclerosis, diabetes, and inflammation (Wagner and Ulrich-Merzenich 2009).

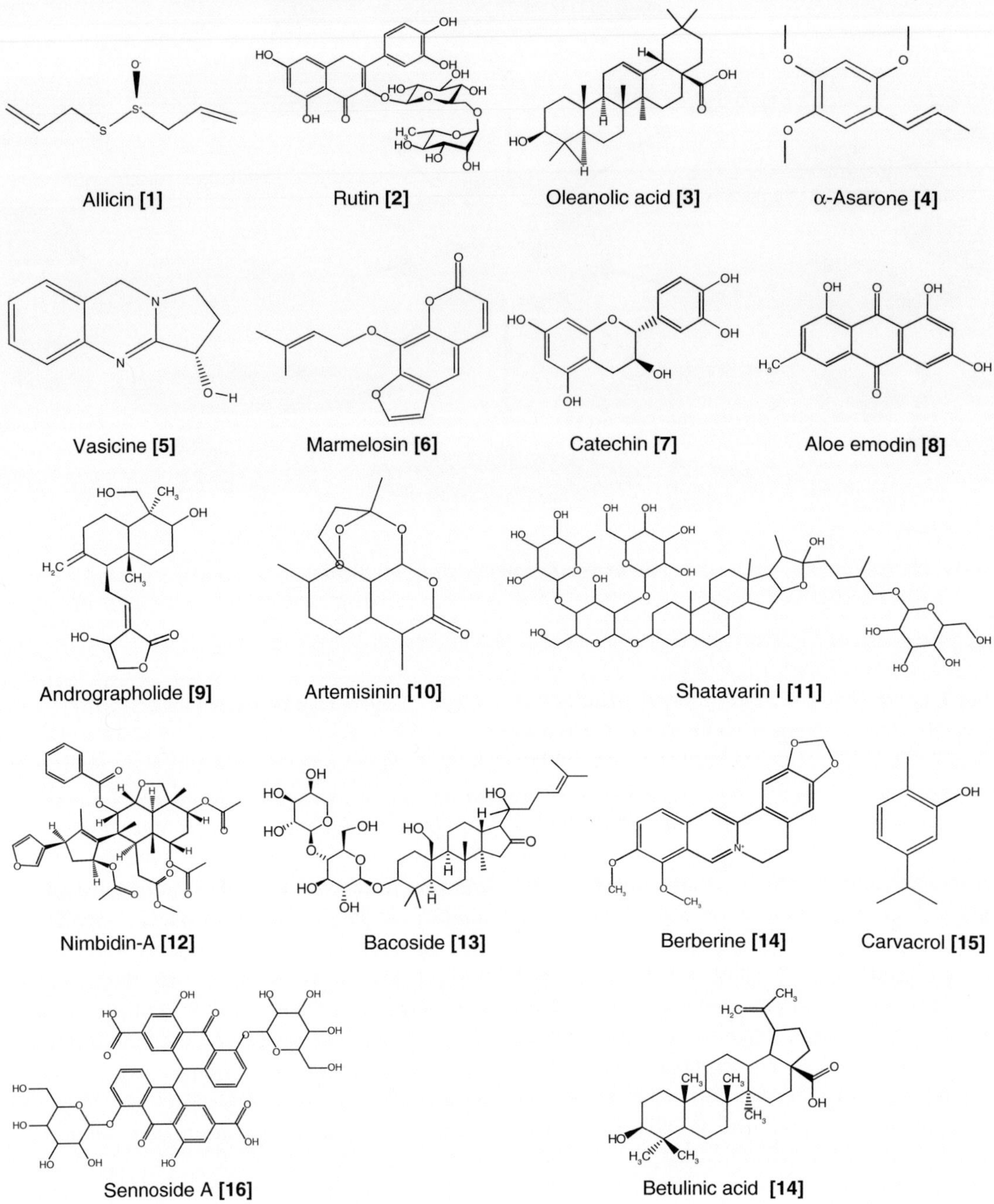

Fig. 19.5 Chemical constituents of traditional medicine

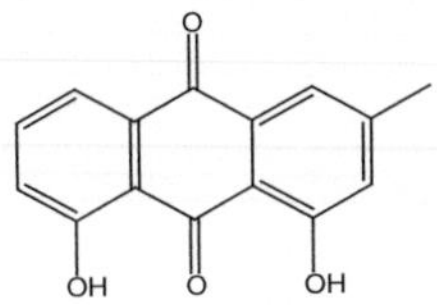

hrysophanol **[17]**

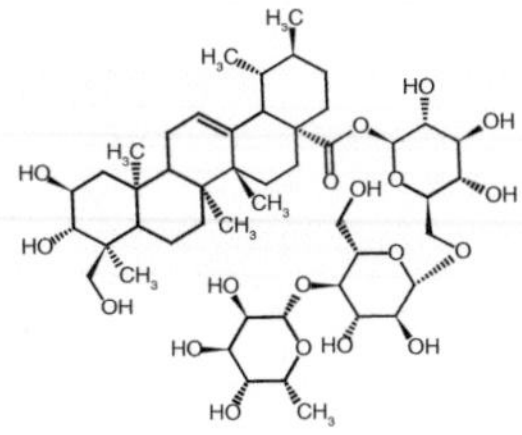

Asiaticoside **[18]**

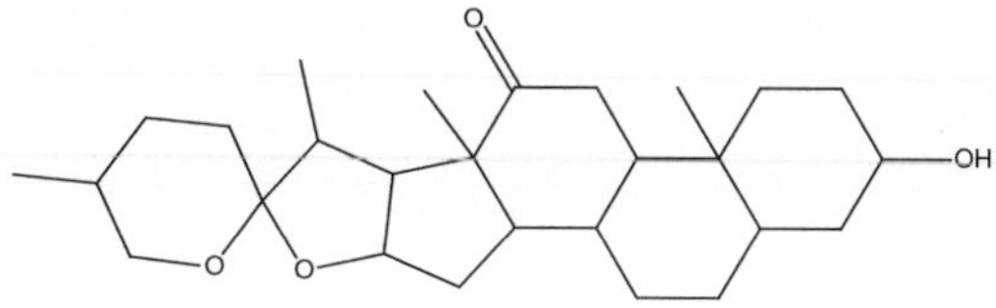

Hecogenin **[19]**

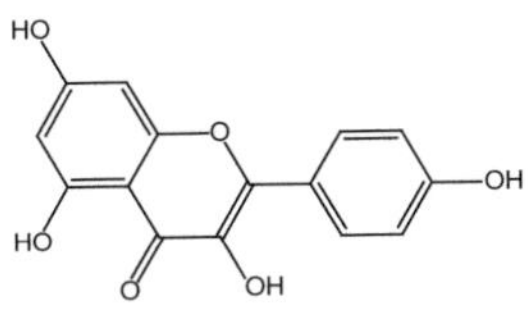

Kaempferol **[20]**

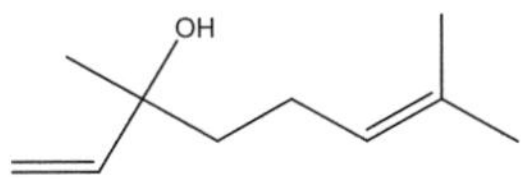

Linalool **[21]**

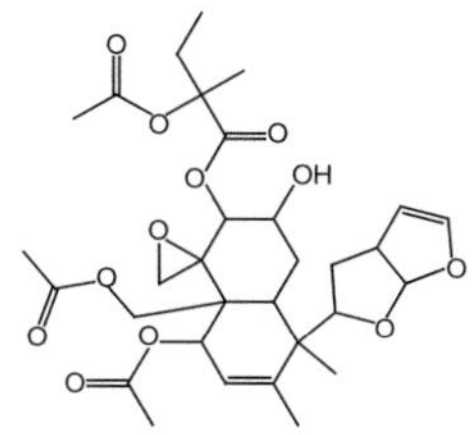

Clerodendrin A **[22]**

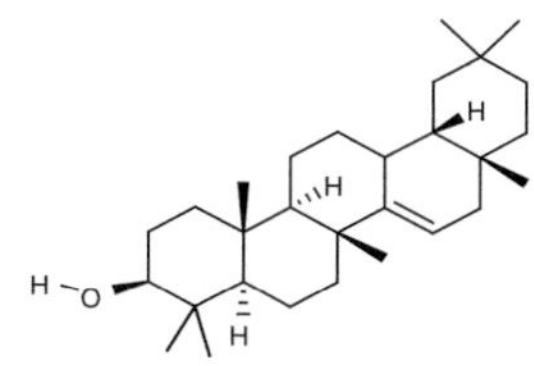

Taraxerol **[23]**

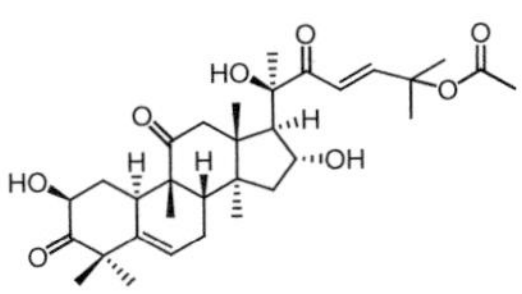

Cucurbitacin-B **[24]**

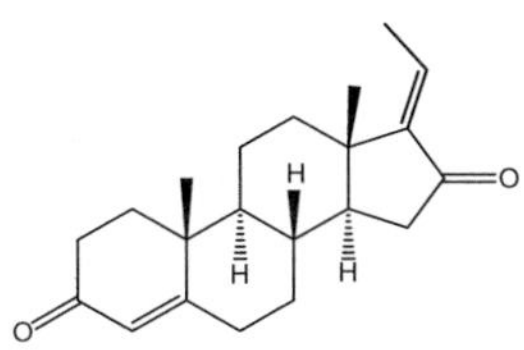

Guggulsterone- E **[25]**

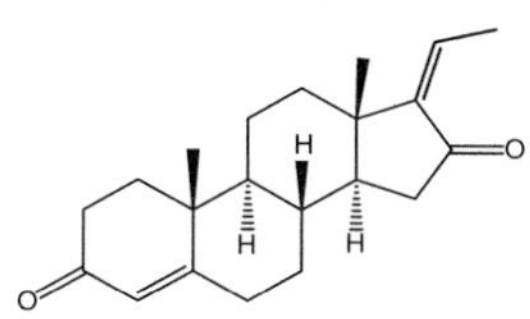

Guggulsterone-Z **[26]**

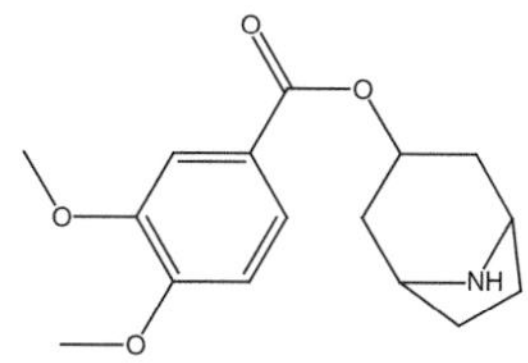

Convolvine **[27]**

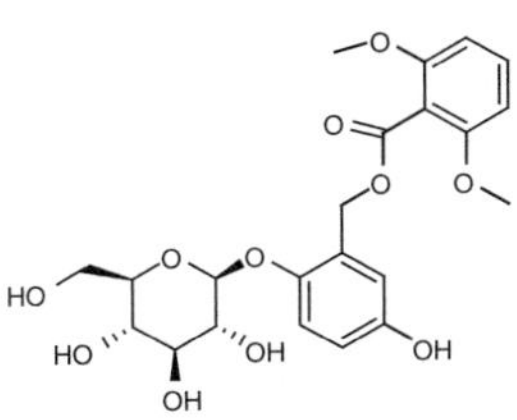

Curculigoside A **[28]**

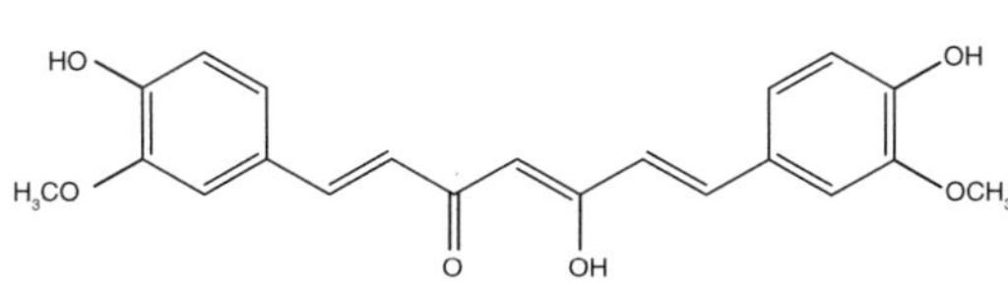

Curcumin **[29]**

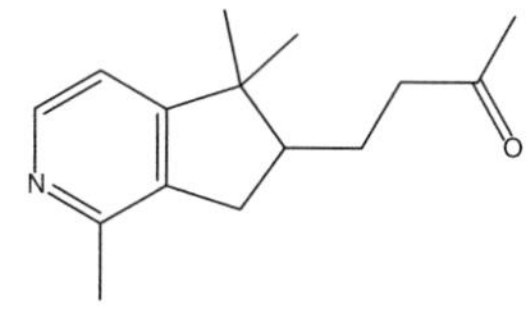

Rotundine A **[30]**

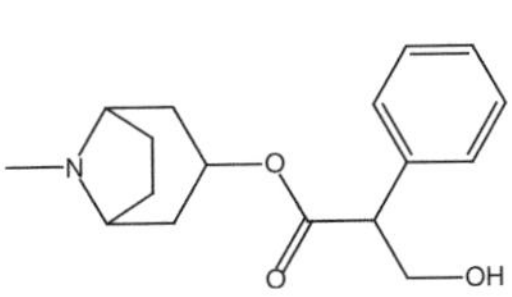

Hyoscyamine **[31]**

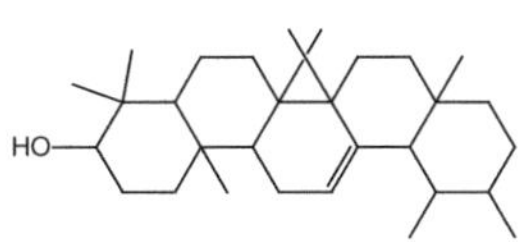

α-Amyrin **[32]**

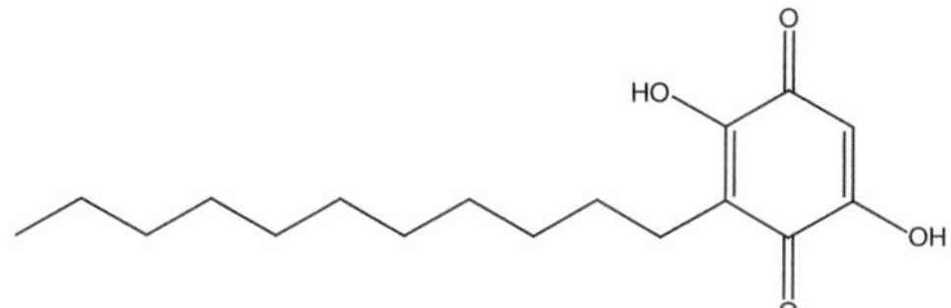

Embelin **[33]**

Fig. 19.5 (continued)

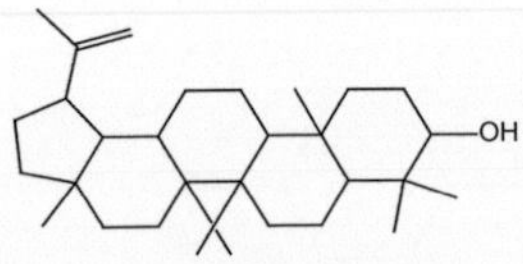
Lupeol **[34]**

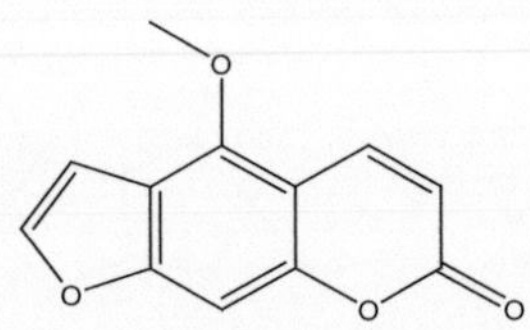
Bergapten **[35]**

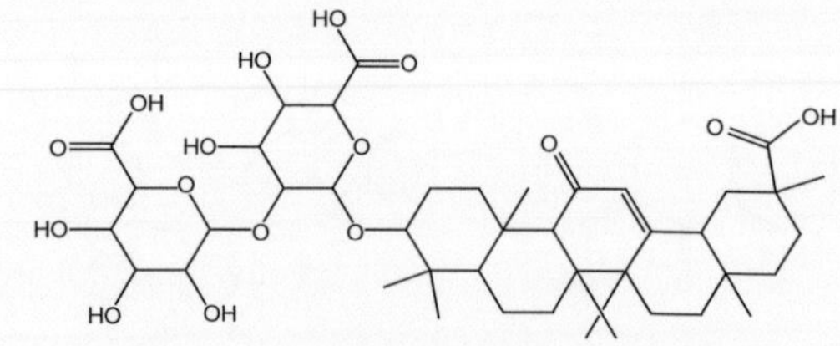
Glycyrrhizin **[36]**

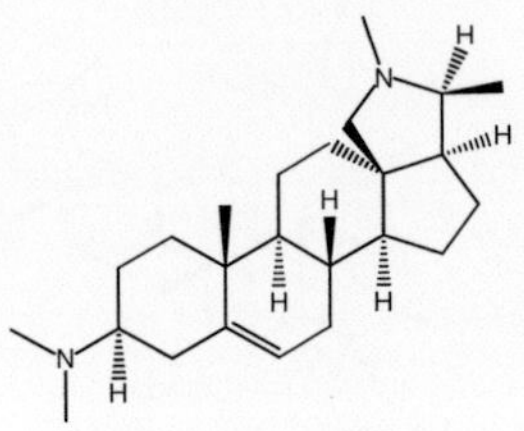
Conessine **[37]**

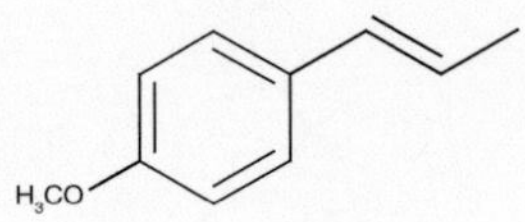
Anethole **[38]**

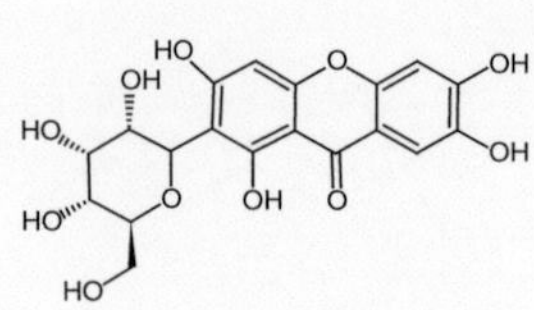
Mangiferin **[39]**

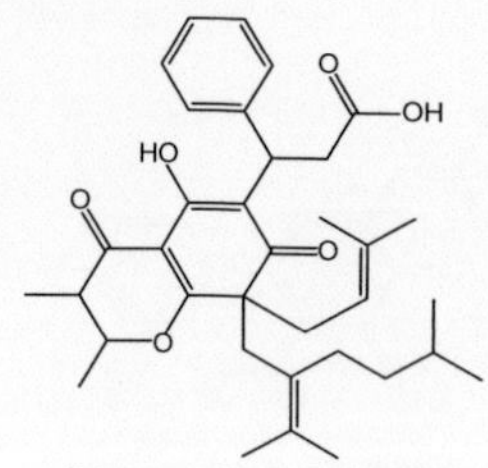
Mesuanic acid **[40]**

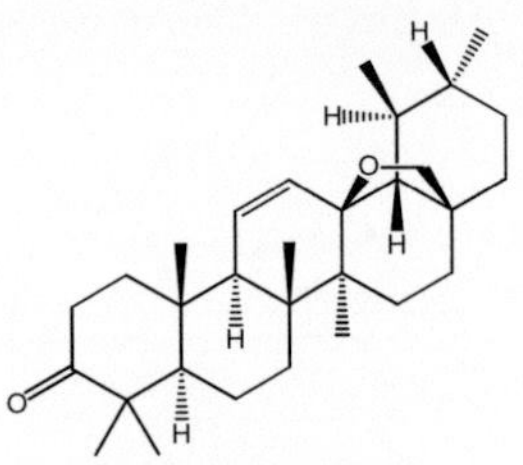
Momordicin **[41]**

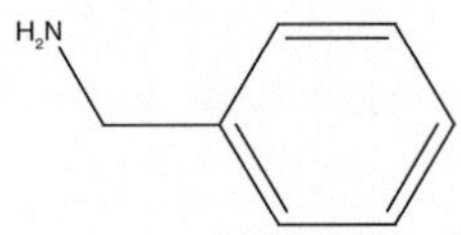
Moringine **[42]**

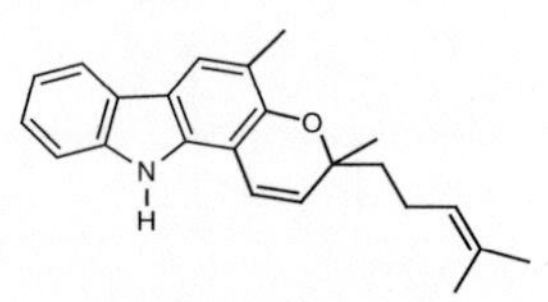
Mahanimbine **[43]**

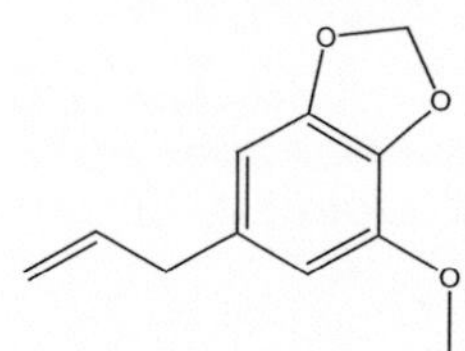
Myristicin **[44]**

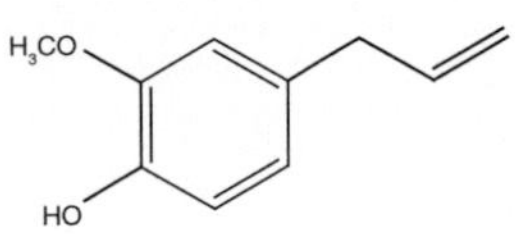
Eugenol **[45]**

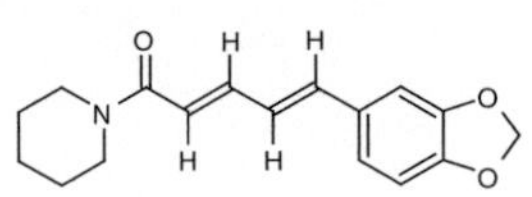
Piperine **[46]**

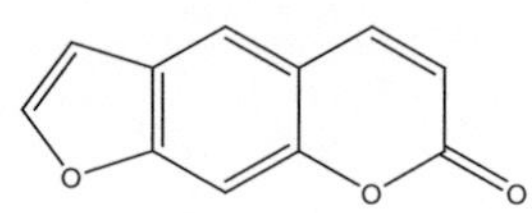
Psoralen **[47]**

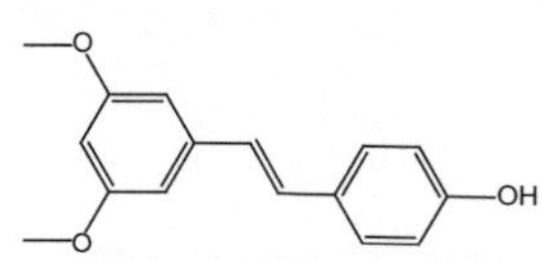
Pterostilbene **[48]**

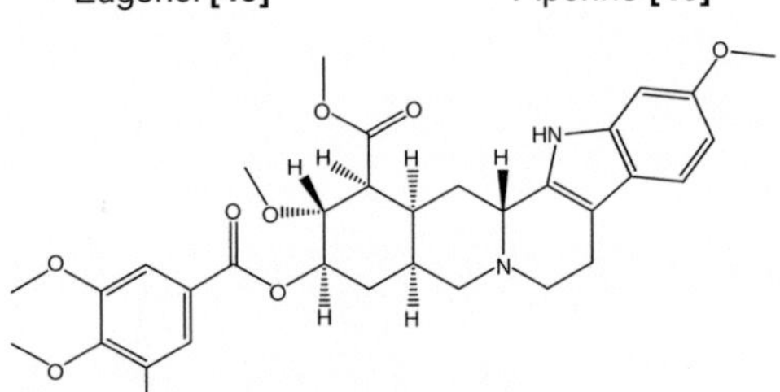
Reserpine **[49]**

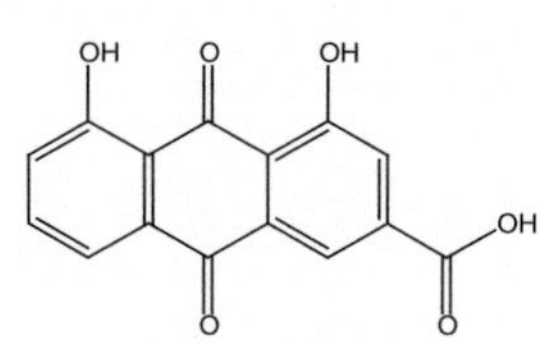
Rhein **[50]**

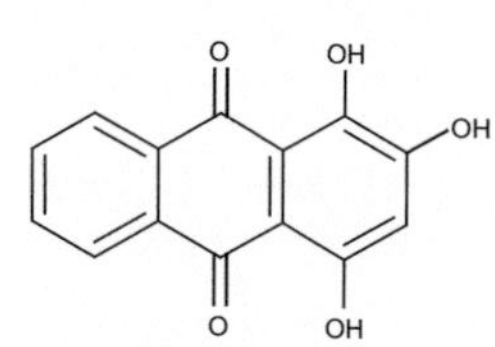
Purpurin **[51]**

Fig. 19.5 (continued)

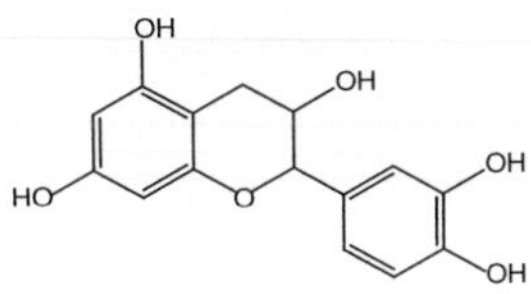
picatechin **[52]**

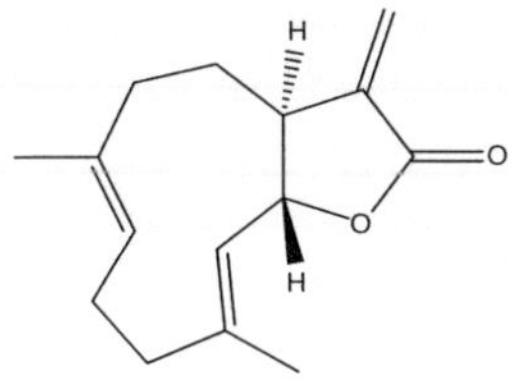
Costunolide **[53]**

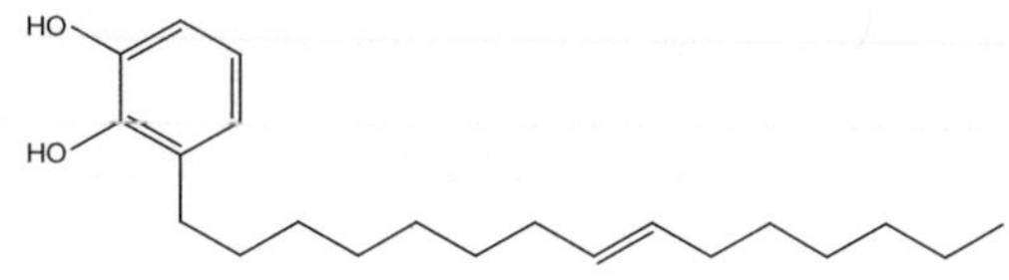
Bhilawanol A **[54]**

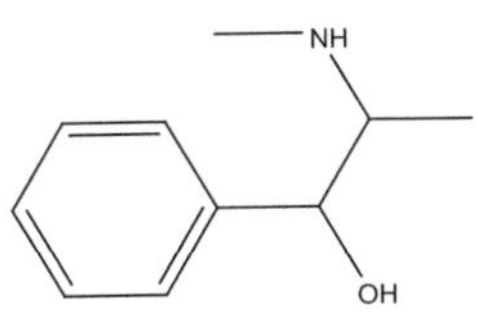
Ephedrine **[55]**

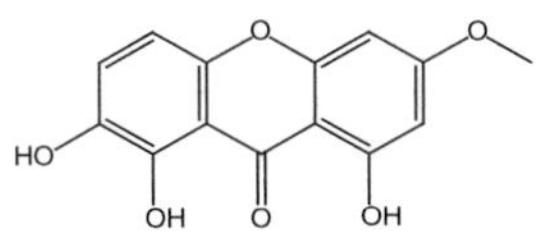
Swertianin **[56]**

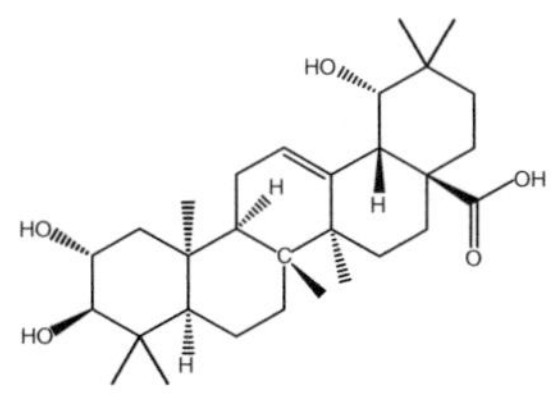
Arjunic acid **[57]**

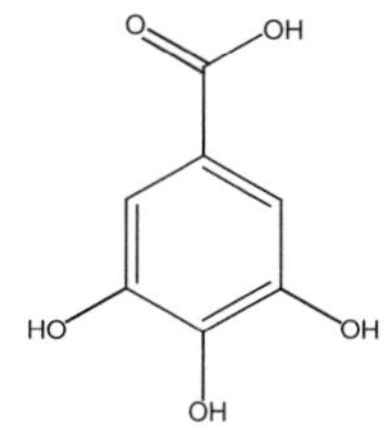
Gallic acid **[58]**

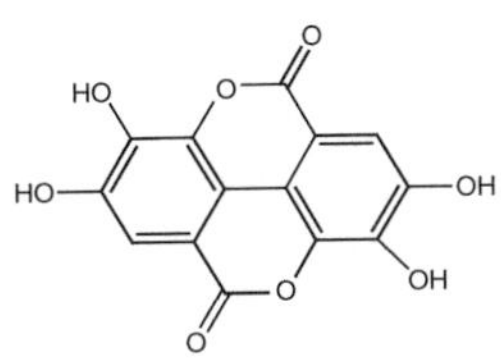
Ellagic acid **[59]**

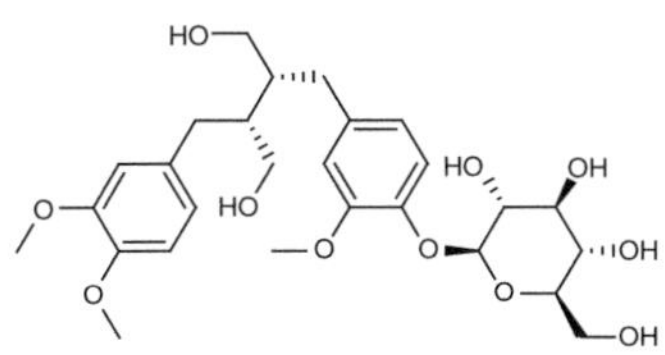
Tinosporoside A **[60]**

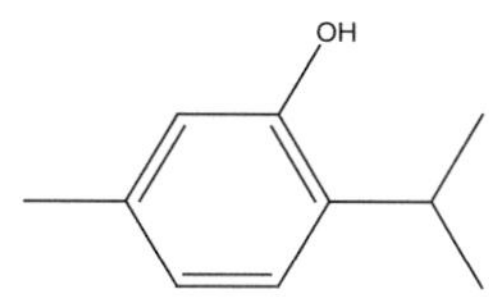
Thymol **[61]**

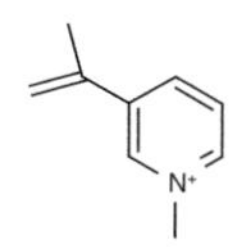
Trigonelline **[62]**

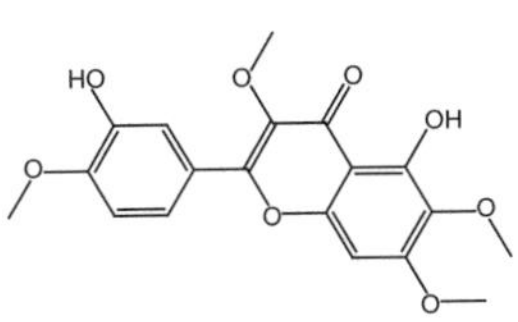
Casticin **[63]**

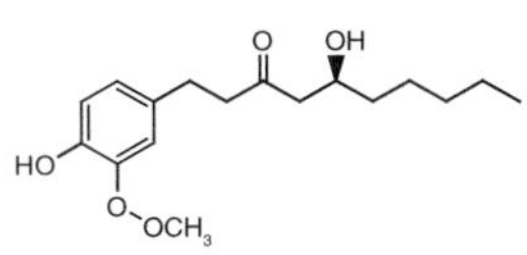
6-Gingerol **[64]**

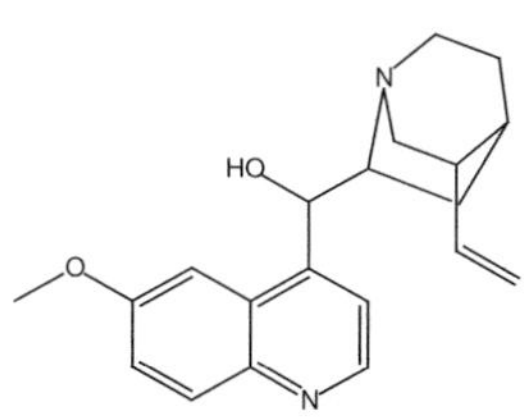
Quinine **[66]**

Fig. 19.5 (continued)

It has been observed that the cell surface receptor gets activated by extracellular signaling molecule and subsequently the signal transduction occurs with numerous actions of cellular messengers. Though the different compounds may affect various cellular messengers, the similar response may be observed in a cellular system. On the other hand, some of the chemical compounds may regulate the same target, and therefore act together in an agonistic, synergistic way (Yang et al. 2014).

Synergy research in phytomedicine was initiated during the past decade due to the development of analytical chemistry and molecular biology techniques. The other factor that escalated synergy research is the paradigm shift in chemotherapy from the mono-substance therapy toward a multidrug therapy (Mukherjee et al. 2011). Multidrug therapy is used in the treatment of AIDS and other infections, hypertension, cancer, and rheumatic diseases all over the world. The approach is to combat the diseases by a concerted action in a combinatorial approach (Wagner and Ulrich-Merzenich 2009). In phytotherapy, the paradigm shifting was very obvious as the therapy with drugs and the extract combinations has been favored for long past. The practice in traditional Chinese medicine and Ayurveda relies on the combination therapy based on the synergism among the bioactive phytoconstituents. Often there are some mono-extract preparations, which in most cases contain a majority of several bioactive constituents that exhibit synergistic effects. But the establishment of synergy in plant extract is sometimes difficult owing to the presence of minor concomitants, adulterants, and fibers, which can all be involved in the synergistic effects. Therefore, in order to prove synergy, the research strategy in phytomedicine should be different from that of classical medicine (Wagner and Ulrich-Merzenich 2009). Although the mechanism of action of many phytomedicines is still unknown, there are several instances of herbal extract showing a better efficacy than an equivalent dose of an isolated compound. The investigation of mechanism of action of isolated compounds and combination therapy, comprising newer molecular biology techniques, has been described by Wagner (1999). For example, pepper contains the alkaloid piperine, which is known to increase the bioavailability of a number of clinically used drugs. The unwanted interactions for tannin present in herbal drug may hinder the absorption of proteins and alkaloids, or the induction of enzymes such as cytochrome P450 which may accelerate the drug metabolism resulting in the increase of active metabolites in blood vessels. This could have more serious consequences, for example in the case of St John's wort, *Hypericum perforatum* extract, where the interactions with oral contraceptives have been reported.

In some traditional medicinal system, the mixtures of plants are used rather than one species and so the situation is even more complex, although the same concepts of synergy apply; that is, the mixture of the two (or more) species gives a better activity than either species on its own. The ancient formulation "Triphala," a well-known poly-herbal formulation (churna) in Indian system of medicine (ISM), contains several bioactive markers which are known to have potential therapeutic activity. The chemical fingerprinting of the Ayurvedic formulation has already been established. The churna (powdered preparation) is prepared in combination of dried fruits of *Emblica officinalis* Gaertn (family: Euphorbiaceae), *Terminalia belerica* Linn (family: Combretaceae), and *Terminalia chebula* Retz (family: Combretaceae), in equal proportions as described in Ayurvedic Formulary of India (AFI). Traditionally this formulation has been prescribed as a first-line treatment as a laxative (in chronic constipation), as a detoxifying agent of the colon, for digestive problems, as a rejuvenator of the body, etc. The mixture of the above three fruits acts as a poly-herbal formulation which has been considered as a classic example of the synergistic combination in Ayurveda. Another example in Ayurveda is *Ginkgo biloba*, in which both the ginkgolides A and B act as PAF antagonist and their synergistic interaction is proven for their anti-inflammatory activity. It was noticed that a dose of 120 mg of a standardized ginkgo extract containing only 6–7 mg of ginkgolides and when combined with bilobalide and flavonol glycosides produces an equivalent effect. The implications of these results are of course that an isolated ginkgolide would be less therapeutically effective than a mixture, despite the fact that ginkgolide B is known to be a specific PAF antagonist and has been the subject of many pharmacological experiments (Mukherjee et al. 2010). Kava is a well-known psychoactive herb used in the South Pacific as a ceremonial drink, sedative, and mild euphoriant. The synergism in anticonvulsant activity of the kava-lactones (such as yangonin and desmethoxyyangonin) was found more effective when combined with other kava constituents.

Liquorice affects absorption from the gut. It has been observed that bioavailability of glycyrrhizin was lower in case of extract compared to isolated compound. It has been reported that the crude extract of liquorice as well as isoliquiritin and related compounds inhibits angiogenesis, granuloma formation, and fluid exudation in a mouse model of inflammation, whereas glycyrrhizin and glycyrrhetinic acid tend to promote angiogenesis. In a poly-herbal formulation synergy exists between different herbs which is seen in formulation used against benign prostate hyperplasia where combination of nettle (*Urtica dioica*) and pygeum bark (*Pygeum africanum*) inhibits 5-reductase and aromatase more significantly than the sum of either alone. Several evidences of interaction between herbs were also observed in traditional Chinese medicine used to treat eczema. The evaluation of synergistic effects for most of the Chinese herbal formulations, consisting of up to seven or more herbs, was found very complicated by the fact that the concept of treatment in Chinese medicine differs in many respects from that of Western medicine. It is important to examine the synergistic effects by conducting clinical trials particularly in comparison with synthetic standard drugs, using the same indication and equivalent dosages. In the last 25 years, more than 200 comparative, double-blind, placebo-controlled trials have been performed using standardized mono- and multi-extract combinations against some well-known standard drugs. These standardized phyto-drugs showed therapeutic equivalence to the standard drugs, with the additional advantage of having fewer side effects relative to synthetic drugs (Mukherjee et al. 2010). There are some other examples of drug combinations with clinically proven synergistic effects as follows: Firstly, the phytopharmaceutical preparation Iberogast®, sold in Germany, consists of nine plant extracts and is used for the treatment of functional dyspepsia and motility-related disorders. The preparation showed therapeutic equivalence when compared with the synthetic drugs cisapride and metoclopramide, with fewer or no side effects. Secondly, the combinations of artemisinin (artesunate, artemether, arteether, and dihydroartemisinine) and mefloquine, lumefantrine, doxycycline, or tetracycline are usually prescribed in Thailand for the treatment of both uncomplicated and severe falciparum malaria (Wagner 2011).

Synergistic multi-target effects mean that the single constituents of a mono-extract or a multi-extract combination affect not only one single target, but also several targets, and therefore cooperate in an agonistic or a synergistic way (Ulrich-Merzenich et al. 2009). Imming et al. (2006) have listed possible important drug targets such as enzymes, substrates, metabolites and proteins, receptors, ion channels, transport proteins, DNA/RNA, ribosomes, and monoclonal antibodies. The multi-target principle will be especially effective and sometimes therapeutically auxiliary symptoms or "lateral damages" have been developed during a disease in negative concomitant. In this context, the polyvalent effect of numerous secondary constituents such as polyphenols and terpenoids should be considered. The phenolics and terpenoids can strongly bind to the different glycoproteins present in the cell membranes owing to their higher lipophilicity and thus it exhibits high potential to permeate through cell walls of the body or bacteria. Since many plant extracts are rich in these two groups of constituents, these compounds can strongly enhance the overall efficacy, if they possess a sufficiently high bioavailability (Wagner 2011). The latest scientific data presents mainly four mechanisms of synergy as follows:

- Combination of multi-target
- Pharmacokinetic or physicochemical effects
- Interaction agents
- Elimination or neutralization of adverse effects

19.5 Polypharmacology: A Paradigm Shift in Traditional Medicine Research

Due to the exponential growth of systems biology and allied molecular biology techniques, the efforts of drug discovery have been tremendously amplified. The philosophy of drug design has been transformed from "one drug one target" to "one drug multiple targets" which has been known as polypharmacology. Polypharmacology is an emerging field in the drug discovery process. Polypharmacological phenomenon includes: (a) single drug acting on multiple targets of a unique disease pathway, or (b) single drug acting on multiple targets pertaining to multiple disease pathways. In addition, polypharmacology for complex diseases is likely to employ multiple drugs acting on distinct targets, probably following a network model involved in various physiological responses.

The concept of polypharmacology has been practiced in traditional medicine systems, such as herbal medicine, for thousands of years (Verpoorte et al. 2009). It is characterized by the use of mixtures of several herbs into a single formula, in which the pharmacological activities of one single herb are either potentiated or prolonged, and/or its adverse effects reduced, by the addition of other herbs. A polypharmacological approach intends to explore the unknown off-targets for the existing drugs (also known as drug repurposing). The approach is based on the systematic integration of the data derived from different disciplines including computational modeling, synthetic chemistry, *in vitro/in vivo* pharmacological testing, and clinical studies (Reddy and Zhang 2013).

Traditional medicine generally employs herbs and herbal formulations which are mixture of numerous chemical ingredients, and it exhibits polypharmacological effects to act on multiple pharmacological targets, regulating different biological mechanisms related to several disease pathophysiologies. This complexity is impossible to deconvolute by the reductionist approach of extracting one active ingredient acting on one single biological target. One such example is aspirin which was derived from the willow meadowsweet and willow bark, often used as an analgesic to relieve minor pains or as an antipyretic to reduce fever; it also acts as an anti-inflammatory medication to treat rheumatoid arthritis, pericarditis, and Kawasaki diseases. Additionally, it has been used in the prevention of transient ischemic attacks, strokes, heart attacks, pregnancy loss, and even cancer. Another example is liquorice (*Glycyrrhiza glabra)* which has 73 bioactive components and 91 potential targets. These 91 targets are closely associated with a series of diseases of respiratory system, cardiovascular system, and gastrointestinal system (Liu et al. 2013).

However, the evolution of herbal medicine mostly relies on the accumulation of empirical evidence and subsequent deduction to form a series of complex theories, which can obviously prevent a herbal medicine system from being recognized by the modern scientific community. Thus, we need a promising systematic tool which could translate herbal evidence into scientific language settling the differences and misconceptions about traditional herbal medicine as an evidence-based science. Conventionally, the modern drug discovery process is based on separation, purification, and structure elucidation to identify and characterize discrete entities in herbal preparations and to find their corresponding biological activities. However, the complexity of herbal medicine offers unique experimental and theoretical challenges for this slow and troublesome process, even if sophisticated high-throughput screening technology was utilized. Firstly, most of the medicinal herbs contain dozens to thousands of constituents, but only a fraction of them are effective. Secondly, a certain ingredient might act on several biological targets but most of them are being unexplored. Thirdly, there is still a lack of clear understanding of how multiple ingredients act on multiple targets to produce synergistic effects. To understand the mechanism of herbal drugs or the active ingredients of herbal drug it is necessary to establish the link between the components with their molecular targets related to specific diseases. During the last decade, researchers have developed a set of systems biology strategies for systematically uncovering the molecular mechanisms related to the therapeutic efficacy of herbal medicines. The development of system pharmacology research has laid a foundation for a more comprehensive understanding of the pharmacological basis (Wang et al. 2012) and combinatorial effects of herbal medicine (Mukherjee et al. 2011). It also intends to understand several biological complexity by measuring different critical parameters as much as possible which could be helping to determine the effect of drug in extensive way. The major focus of systems biology is to inquire the dynamics of all genetic, regulatory, and metabolic processes in a cell and to uncover the complexity of cellular networks.

The interdisciplinary approaches of "omics" platform, viz. genomics, proteomics, and metabolomics, provide a powerful tool for the study on the essence of TM and its multifunctional benefits toward the human welfare (Mukherjee et al. 2010). Proteomics comprises the study of structural and functional aspects of proteins and metabolites. The term was coined to create an analogy with genomics. It was revealed by the Human Genome Project that there are fewer protein-coding genes in the human genome than there are proteins in the human proteome.

The genome initiatives can be complemented by proteomics-based approaches which examine the proteins of a tissue or cell type (Mukherjee et al. 2015). Proteins are the expressed form of genetic codes and hence more useful for quantitative determinations of biological endpoints. The "omics"-based disciplines like phytogenomics, proteomics, and metabolomics in medicinal plant research have started developing due to the application of the "omics" technologies where complex mixtures in medicine are used. In drug discovery and development of combination therapy concepts of polypharmacology are critical (Ulrich-Mezernich et al. 2009). The "omics" (proteomics, chemoinformatics, etc.) technologies are helping to understand the coverage of all targets which generates enormous molecular data. The polypharmacology research is now driven by the analysis of Big Data in systems biology in the post-genomic era. New off-targets are being frequently identified by these approaches. These enormous amounts of data are stored in public and private molecular databases which are growing in both size and number which integrate diverse information of molecular pathways, crystal structures, binding experiments, side effects, and drug targets. Small-molecule databases like ZINC, PubChem, Ligand Expo, and KEGG DRUG present enormous information about the disease relevance, chemical properties, and biological activities of the molecules which help in predicting the protein targets of a small molecule helping in designing of polypharmacological agents (Reddy and Zhang 2013). However the major challenges remain in understanding the pathways/mechanism of many diseases at the molecular levels. It is essentially impossible to derive the polypharmacological network without more accurate mining techniques and mapping methodologies for analyzing the complex data.

Acknowledgement The authors are thankful to the Department of Biotechnology, Government of India, New Delhi, for financial support through Tata Innovation fellowship to PKM.

Conflict of Interest: The authors declare that they have no conflict of interest.

References

Hert J, Irwin JJ, Laggner C, Keiser MJ, Shoichet BK. Quantifying biogenic Bias in screening libraries. Nat Chem Biol. 2009;5:479–83. https://doi.org/10.1038/nchembio.180.

Heyman HM, Meyer JJM. NMR-based metabolomics as a quality control tool for herbal products. S Afr J Bot. 2012;82:21–32.

Imming P, Sinning C, Meyer A. Drugs, their targets and the nature and number of drug targets. Drug Discov Today. 2006;5:821–34.

Leonti M. CasuL.Traditional medicines and globalization: current and future perspectives in ethnopharmacology. Front Pharmacol. 2013;4:1–13.

Liu H, Wang J, Zhou W, Wang Y, Yang L. Systems approaches and polypharmacology for drug discovery from herbal medicines: an example using licorice. J Ethnopharmacol. 2013;146:773–93.

Mukherjee PK, Houghton PJ. The worldwide phenomenon of increased use of herbal products: opportunity and threats. In: Evaluation of herbal medicinal products – perspectives on quality, safety and efficacy. 1st ed. London: Pharmaceutical Press; 2009. p. 3–12.

Mukherjee PK, Maiti K, Mukherjee K, Houghton PJ. Leads from Indian medicinal plants with hypoglycemic potentials. J Ethnopharmacol. 2006;106:1–28. https://doi.org/10.1016/j.jep.2006.03.021.

Mukherjee PK, Wahile A. Integrated approaches towards drug development from Ayurveda and other Indian system of medicines. J Ethnopharmacol. 2006;103:25–35.

Mukherjee PK, Venkatesh P, Ponnusankar S. Ethnopharmacology and integrative medicine – let the history tell the future. J Ayur Integr Med. 2010;1(2):100–9.

Mukherjee PK, Ponnusankar S, Venkatesh P. Synergy in herbal medicinal products: concept to realization. Indian J Pharma Res Edu. 2011;45(3):210–7.

Mukherjee PK, Nema NK, Venkatesh P, Debnath PK. Changing scenario for promotion and development of Ayurveda - way forward. J Ethnopharmacol. 2012;143:424–34.

Mukherjee PK, Bahadur S, Harwansh RK, Nema NK, Bhadra S. Development of traditional medicines: globalizing local knowledge or localizing global technologies. Pharma Times. 2013;45:39–42.

Mukherjee PK, Bahadur S, Harwansh RK, Chaudhary SK. Shifting paradigm for validation of medicinal plants in Indian traditional medicine. Indian Drugs. 2014;51:5–14.

Mukherjee PK, Chaudhary SK, Bahadur S, Debnath PK. Ethnopharmacology and integrative medicine: an Indian perspective. In: Heinrich M, Jäger AK, editors. Ethnopharmacology - a reader. Chichester: Wiley & Sons; 2015. p. 279–92.

Mukherjee PK, Harwansh R, Bahadur S, Banerjee S, Kar A. Evidence based validation of Indian traditional medicine – way forward. World J Trad Chin Med. 2016;2:48–61.

Mukherjee PK, Harwansh RK, Bahadur S, Banerjee S, Kar A, Chanda J, Biswas S, Ahmmed S, Katiyar CK. Development of Ayurveda – tradition to trend. J Ethnopharmacol. 2017a;197:10–24.

Mukherjee PK, Bahadur S, Harwansh RK, Biswas S, Banerjee S. Paradigm shift in natural product research: traditional medicine inspired approaches. Phytochem Rev. 2017b;1:24. https://doi.org/10.1007/s11101-016-9489-6.

Newman DJ, Cragg GM. Natural products as sources of new drugs over the last 25 years. J Nat Prod. 2007;70:461–77.

Nirali JB, Shankar MB. Global market analysis of herbal drug formulations. Int J Ayur Pharm Chem. 2015;4:59–65.

Reddy AS, Zhang S. Polypharmacology: drug discovery for the future. Expert Rev Clin Pharmacol. 2013;6 https://doi.org/10.1586/ecp.12.74.

Ulrich-Merzenich G, Panek D, Zeitler H, Wagner H, Vetter H. New perspectives for synergy research with the "omics" technologies. Phytomedicine. 2009;16:495–508.

Verpoorte R, Crommelin D, Danhof M, Gilissen L, Schuitmaker H, Vander Greef J, Witkamp R. A systems view on the future of medicine: inspiration from Chinese medicine? J Ethnopharmacol. 2009;121:479–81.

Wagner H. Synergy research: approaching a new generation of phytopharmaceuticals. Fitoterapia. 2011;82(1):34–7.

Wagner H, Ulrich-Merzenich G. Synergy research: approaching a new generation of phytopharmaceuticals. Phytomedicine. 2009;16:97–110.

Wang Y, Xiao J, Suzek TO, Zhang J, Wang J, Zhou Z, Han L, Karapetyan K, Dracheva S, Shoemaker BA, Bolton E, Gindulyte A, Bryant SH. PubChem's BioAssay database. Nucleic Acids Res. 2012;40(Database issue):D400–12.

Yang Y, Zhang Z, Li S, Ye X, Li X, He K. Synergy effects of herb extracts: pharmacokinetics and pharmacodynamic basis. Fitoterapia. 2014;92:133–47.

20 Phytochemical Analysis of Herbal Teas and Their Potential Health, and Food Safety Benefits: A Review

Patricia L. Mathivha, Titus A. M. Msagati, Vuyisile S. Thibane, and Fhatuwani N. Mudau

Contents

P. L. Mathivha · V. S. Thibane · F. N. Mudau (✉)
Department of Agriculture and Animal Health,
Florida Science Campus Florida Science Campus,
University of South Africa, Roodepoort, South Africa
e-mail: mudaufn@unisa.ac.za

T. A. M. Msagati
Nanotechnology and Water Sustainability Research
Unit, Florida Science Campus, University of South
Africa, Roodepoort, South Africa

S. Sen, R. Chakraborty (eds.), *Herbal Medicine in India*,
https://doi.org/10.1007/978-981-13-7248-3_20

20.1 Introduction

The consumption of herbal teas has increased significantly in recent years with most consumers cognizant of the health attributes of herbal teas (Hicks 2009; Al-Dalain et al. 2012). As the interest in natural plant remedies in reducing health problems around the world becomes greater, the consumption of herbal teas will continue to increase and the market for herbal teas will therefore grow larger. South Africa has proven to be a major player in the herbal tea industry, with local rooibos and honey bush tea, in particular, occupying a significant place in the global market. Studies on the introduction of other herbal teas that are not produced on a large scale and in respect of which the demand is exceeding the supply have already been started in South Africa. These include studies on bush tea, which is predominantly used to treat boils, sores, acne, infected wounds, cuts, headaches, colds, loss of voice and throat infections (Mudau and Mariga 2012). Special tea in South Africa is reported by Mamphiswana et al. (2011) to be used as a blood cleanser in combination with other herbs to cure sexually transmitted diseases and erectile disorders or to enhance male libido. In the light of the high demand for the plant species used for herbal teas, failure to ensure commercial propagation of these species could lead to their extinction, as has happened in the cases of the pepper-bark tree and wild ginger (Mander et al. 1999). This signals the need for research into commercial propagation, processing and value addition, especially in respect of herbal teas. The aim of this review is to look into the analysis, identification and quantification of phenolic compounds in herbal teas and their associated health and food safety benefits.

20.2 Free Radicals and Antioxidants in Biological Systems

The formation of free radicals such as the reactive oxygen species (ROS) and reactive nitrogen species (RNS) starts with the uptake of molecular oxygen. Reactive oxygen species such as the superoxide anion radical ($O_2^{\cdot -}$), singlet oxygen, hydroxyl radical ($HO^{\cdot}$), lipid peroxide and hydrogen peroxide (H_2O_2) are mainly formed as a result of monooxygenase activity of the oxygen molecule destined for normal metabolic process by energised electrons that escaped the electron transport chain. Reactive nitrogen species formed through the oxidation of L-arginine by nitric oxide synthase (NOS) further contribute to oxidative stress in biological systems. Nitric oxide ($^{\cdot}NO$) formed through these reactions contributes to the increase in lipoprotein oxidation and accumulation of oxidised lipids in vascular systems and atherosclerotic plaque formation due to the oxidation of proteins, lipids and carbohydrates (Bloodsworth et al. 2000). The excessive production of these radical species results in oxidative stress, resulting in oxidative damage. The presence of antioxidants counters the fatal action of this free radical by terminating the propagation of reactive chain reactions in biological systems. Therefore, antioxidants provide a protective function against proliferation of diseases associated with oxidative damage.

20.3 Analysis of Phenolic Composition and Antioxidant Activity of Herbal Tea

20.3.1 The Effect of Extraction Solvents on Phenolic Compounds

Different solvents of varying polarities such as water, ethanol, methanol, acetone and N,N-dimethylformamide (DMF) have been reported for extraction of phenolic compounds from different plant materials (Turkmen et al. 2006; Boulekbache-Makhlouf et al. 2013; Oh et al. 2013; Mokrani and Madani 2016). Studies have shown acetone effective at extracting high quantities of total phenols better than other solvents; however methanol was reported to extract effectively more of the anthocyanins compared to ethanol and acetone (Boulekbache-Makhlouf et al.

2013). Aqueous solutions of methanol, acetone and ethanol were reported by Martínez et al. (1997) for extraction of polyphenols in their study on phenolic distribution of flavonoids in *Aquifoliaceae*. Zhou and Yu (2004) reported the use of aqueous acetone for extraction of wheat bran phenolics and Wang and Helliwell (2001) reported aqueous ethanol to be more effective in extracting catechin from green and black teas. These aqueous solutions are found to be better solvents than their absolute counterparts as higher antioxidant activity was achieved with aqueous solution (50%) of acetone, methanol and ethanol (Metrouh-Amir et al. 2015). This effectively means that the polar nature of water allows for more leaching of antioxidants from the leaves. Furthermore, extraction solvents are not the only factors that affect the polyphenolic compounds extracted from teas. Sequential extraction method with multiple solvents of polar to acid nature was reported by Zou et al. (2002) as an effective method compared to single-extraction solvents which left residues. Mokrani and Madani (2016) demonstrated that increasing the extraction time and temperature further improved extraction of phenolic compounds. The least favourable method for extraction of phenolic compounds and subsequent antioxidant activity of teas is water as compared to other organic solvents. However, extraction of teas with hot or cold water is a convenient method due to the consumption nature of teas (Turkmen et al. 2006).

20.3.2 Quantification Methods for Phenolic Content of Herbal Teas

There are various analytical methods used for quantification studies of flavonoids and phenolic acids of teas. The most common method is by far liquid chromatography (LC). Other popular methods used include the column chromatography (CC), gas chromatography (GC), capillary electrophoresis (CE), thin-layer chromatography (TLC) and nuclear magnetic resonance (NMR) (Peterson et al. 2005; De Rijke et al. 2006).

20.3.2.1 Liquid chromatography

The quantification of phenolic compounds is usually performed using a reversed-phase mode using a C8- or C18-bonded silica column, with high-performance liquid chromatography (HPLC) being the preferred system. Recently, other phases such as silica, Sephadex and polyamide have been used (De Rijke et al. 2006). Water containing acetate or formate buffer and methanol or acetonitrile as an organic modifier is often what forms the binary solvent system for gradient elution. Because of the contamination of ion sources during mass spectrum (MS) detection, phosphate buffers have become less popular (Franke and Custer 1994). HPLC can be performed at temperatures ranging from room temperature to 40 °C. Higher temperatures are at times recommended to reduce running time and they also give good repeatability. For the isolation of mainly flavonoids, running times of between 30 min and 1 h are used. While running times of up to 2 h are used to isolate more complex compounds with these exhaustive runs, up to 30 compounds can be separated and identified together with many other conjugates such as glycosides, malonates and acetates (De Rijke et al. 2006). Various detectors can be used for HPLC. The first to consider may be the UV absorbance detector. Considering that all flavonoids contain at least one aromatic ring and efficiently absorb UV light, the UV absorbance detector is a commonly used detector (Mabry et al. 1970). This type of detection became popular several decades back and remains the preferred tool in most LC-based studies with multiple wavelength or diode-array UV detection as the norm. A limiting factor to diode-array UV detection is that most glycosides and acyl residues are poor chromophores and, therefore, no further discrimination can be achieved by this method of detection (De Rijke et al. 2006).

Another detection method is fluorescence detection. This method is commonly used because the numbers of flavonoids that possess native fluorescence are limited, thereby facilitating selective detection of complex mixtures (De Rijke et al. 2001). Flavonoids that have native fluorescence include isoflavones and flavonoids with an OH group in the 3-position such as catechins and methoxylated flavones. This makes the fluorescence detection method extremely selective, and it has been found to be tenfold more sensitive than UV detection. When used in combination with UV detection, a distinction can be made between fluorescent and non-fluorescent compounds (Rodríguez-Delgado et al. 2001). Lastly, another popular detection method is electrochemical detection, which is made possible by the electroactive nature of flavonoids due to the presence of phenolic groups. The levels of detection of this method can be quite low, possibly due to its low sensitivity (Zhong et al. 2003). Mass spectrometry is currently a state-of-the-art detection technique in LC, with single-stage MS being used in combination with UV detection to facilitate confirmation of the identified flavonoids in a sample with the help of standards and reference data (De Rijke et al. 2006).

20.3.2.2 Gas Chromatography

Gas chromatography was already used in the early 1960s for the analysis of flavonoids. Narasimhachari and von Rudloff (1962) managed to separate derivative flavonoids on a semi-preparative scale using a SE-30 silicone polymer column with thermal conductivity detection. With the introduction of LC, GC became less prominent but it has recently received renewed attention because of the developments in high-temperature GC, and improved derivatisation procedures (Morton et al. 1999; Fiamegos et al. 2004). The separation methods have not changed since the early 1960s, although recently fused silica capillary columns are used instead of packed glass columns. Most GC-based methods give a high resolution and low detection limits. However, they tend to be more labour intensive because derivatisation that occurs is unfavourable to the increase in volatility of these flavonoids and to their improved thermal stability (De Rijke et al. 2006). Flavonoids with more than one hydroxyl substituent methylation may occur, yielding several derivatives and making quantification more difficult.

A typical method of analysis of flavonoids by GC would have the flavonoids hydrolysed and converted into their trimethylsilyl (TMS) derivatives before they are injected onto a non-polar DB-5 or DB-1 column in the split or non-split mode and separated with a linear 30- to 90-min temperature programme of up to 300 °C. An improved derivatisation procedure for the GC-MS analysis of flavonoids and phenolic acids makes use of basic conditions so that the hydroxyl groups of the analytes are deprotonated (Fiamegos et al. 2004; Fiamegos et al. 2003). Interestingly, in conventional GC methods it is often difficult to analyse flavonoid glycosides, even after derivatisation. To overcome this challenge, Pereira et al. (2004) used high-temperature-high-resolution (HT-HR) GC-MS with columns that were not affected at temperatures of up to 400 °C for hesperidin. Unfortunately, the limit of detection was found to be as high as 50 mg/L; it took 72 h for derivatisation before analysis and this derivative showed severe peak tailing. This analysis was performed on both cold on-column and split-less injection at 370 °C.

20.3.2.3 Capillary Electrophoresis

The CE methods used are primarily capillary zone electrophoresis (CZE) and micellar electrokinetic chromatography (MEKC), typically with a phosphate or borate buffer, capillaries (50–100 μm I.D.), voltage (10–30 kV) and injection volumes of 10–50 mL. These analytical methods have mostly been used for natural products such as vegetables and herbs (Baumann et al. 2001). Detection is done using mostly UV, but fluorescence, ED and MS detectors are also used (Baumann et al. 2001; Chen et al. 2000).

20.3.3 Types of Antioxidants in True Tea

20.3.3.1 Phenolic and Polyphenolic Antioxidants

Different teas contain various types of antioxidants in different quantities and ratios. All these antioxidants have health benefits for consumers. The different major antioxidants in tea include phenolic and polyphenolic antioxidants, such as gallic acid (GA), gallocatechin (GC), catechin (CE), epigallocatechin

(EGC), epicatechin (EC), epicatechin gallate (ECG) and epigallocatechin gallate (EGCG). Epigallocatechin gallate (Fig. 20.1), ester of epigallocatechin and gallic acid, is the most abundant antioxidant in tea with other flavonols such as kaempferol, quercetin, theaflavins and myricetin (Fig. 20.2) and further present in significant amounts in green and black tea (Khan and Mukhtar 2013).

The structure-activity of flavonoids plays a critical role in their capacities to neutralise and reduce radical species. The chemistry of flavonoid antioxidants reveals that they have a general structure of a 15-carbon skeleton, consisting of two phenyl rings and a heterocyclic ring. Tea flavonoids are further grouped into isoflavonoids and neoflavonoids such as flavones and flavonols (Fig. 20.3).

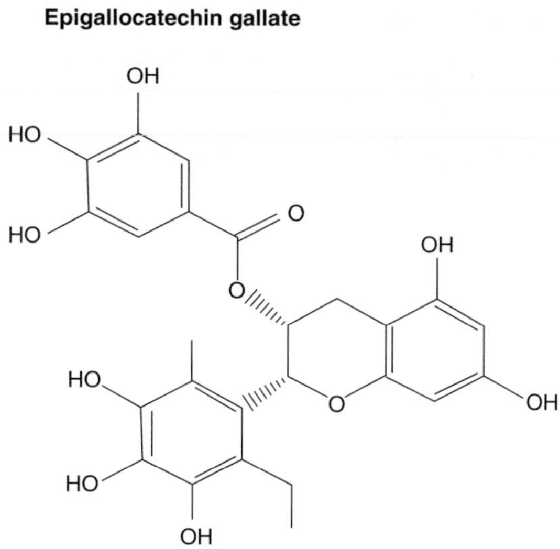

Fig. 20.1 The chemical structure of epigallocatechin gallate ([(2R,3R)-5,7-dihydroxy-2-(3,4,5-trihydroxyphenyl) chroman-3-yl] 3,4,5-trihydroxybenzoate)

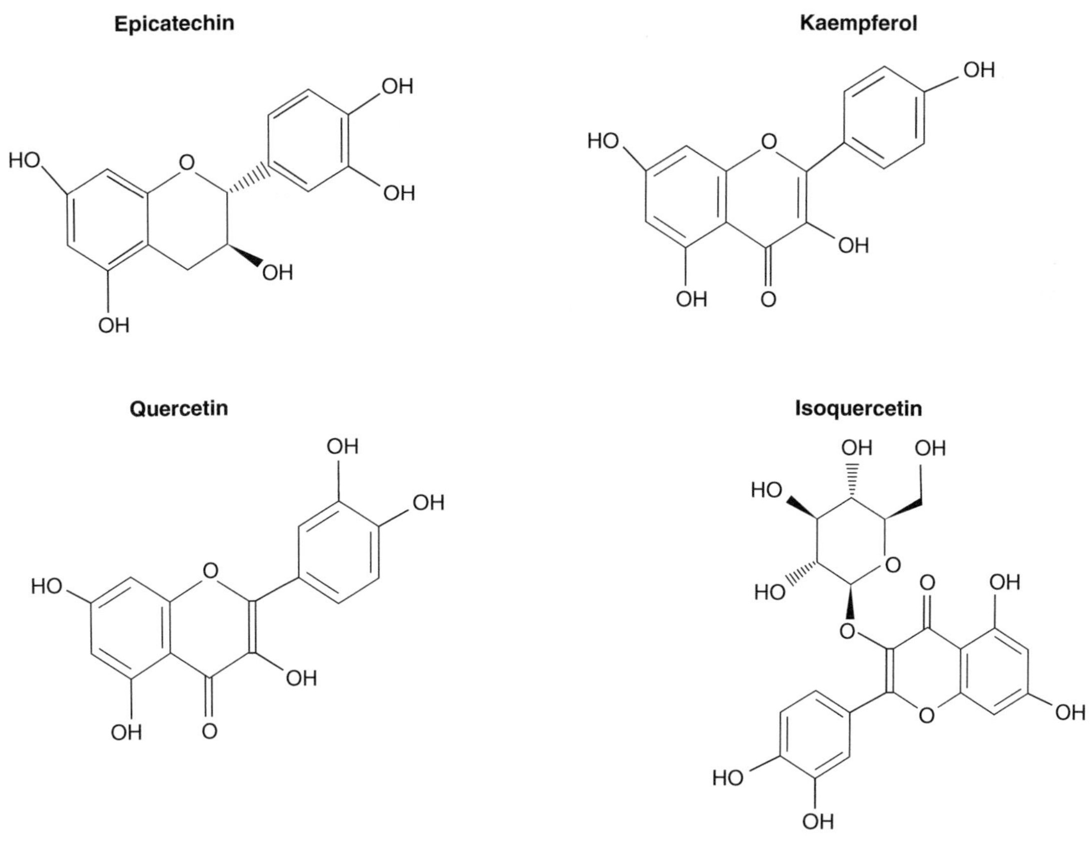

Fig. 20.2 The chemical structure of flavonols epicatechin ((2R,3S)-3,4-dihydro-2-(3,4-dihydroxyphenyl)-2H-chromene-3,57-triol), kaempferol (3,5,7-trihydroxy-2-(4-hydroxyphenyl)-4H-chromen-4-one), quercetin 2(-3,4-dihydroxyphenyl)-3,5,7-trihydroxy-4H-chromen-4-one) and isoquercetin (2-(3,4-dihydroxyphenyl)-5,7-dihydroxy-3-[(2S,3R,4S,5S,6R)-3,4,5-trihydroxy-6-(hydroxymethyl)oxan-2-yl)oxychromen-4-one) present in green and black tea at significant amounts

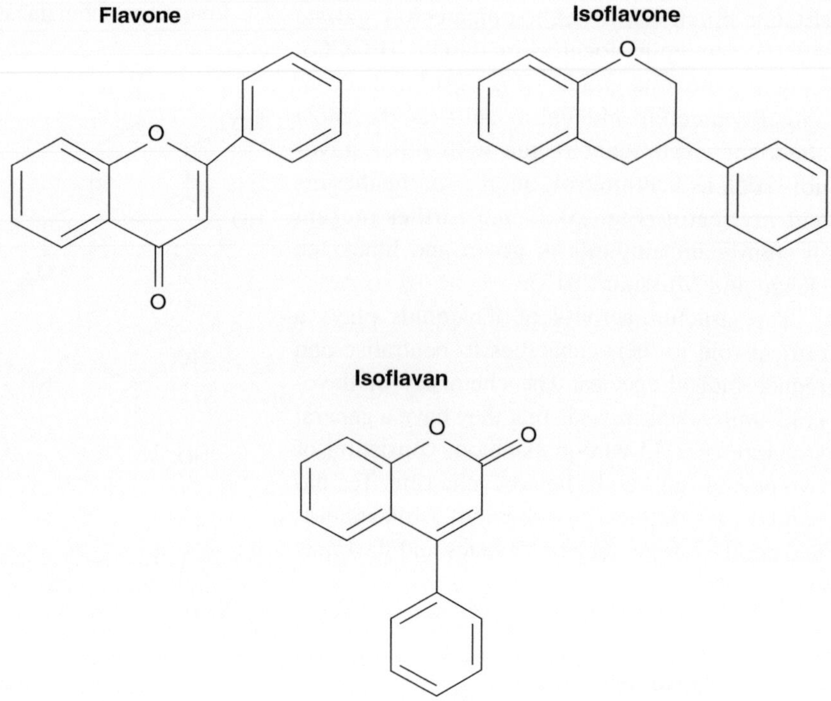

Fig. 20.3 Chemical structure of some of the known flavonoids in tea, flavone (2-phenyl-4H-chromen-4-one), isoflavone (3,4-dihydro-3-phenyl-2H-chromene) and isoflavan (4-phenyl-2H-chromen-2-one)

20.3.3.2 Epigallocatechin Gallate (EGCG) Mechanism of Action

The mechanism of action of EGCG involves the absorption of oxygen radicals, such that the radical anion gets transferred to the EGCG in a process that is catalysed by superoxide dismutase (SOD) (Fig. 20.4). Hydrogen peroxide, molecular oxygen and dimer radical are generated from this process. *The abundance of the hydroxyl (HO) group makes epigallocatechin gallate a powerful antioxidant*. Several genes are involved in coding for several processes that relate to the auto-oxidation process. The genes responsible for the various auto-oxidation mechanisms include those that code apoptotic proteins such as caspases 3, 7, 8, and 9; genes responsible for growth factors, TNF and IGF; genes responsible for protein kinases, PKA and PKC; genes that code for transcriptional factors, P53, AP-1 and AR; genes that are responsible for anti-apoptotic factors such as Bcl-2 and Bcl-XL; and genes that code for protein cell cycle, CDK-2,4,6, cyclins D1 and E.

20.3.4 Specific Antioxidants that Characterise Non-herbal Teas (from *Camellia sinensis*)

20.3.4.1 Catechin Antioxidants

Antioxidants that characterise non-herbal teas include epigallocatechin-3-gallate (EGCG), epicatechin (EC), epicatechin-3-gallate (ECg), epigallocatechin (EGC), catechin (CE) and gallocatechin (GC). The EGCG is regarded as the most important antioxidant with associated health benefits.

20.3.4.2 Theaflavin Antioxidants

There are several theaflavin compounds found in tea which are mainly theaflavin (TF-1), theaflavin-3-gallate (TF-2) and theaflavin-3,3′-digallate (TF-3) as represented in Fig. 20.5.

20.3.4.3 Tannin Antioxidants

Tannins are characterised by their astringent and bitter taste.

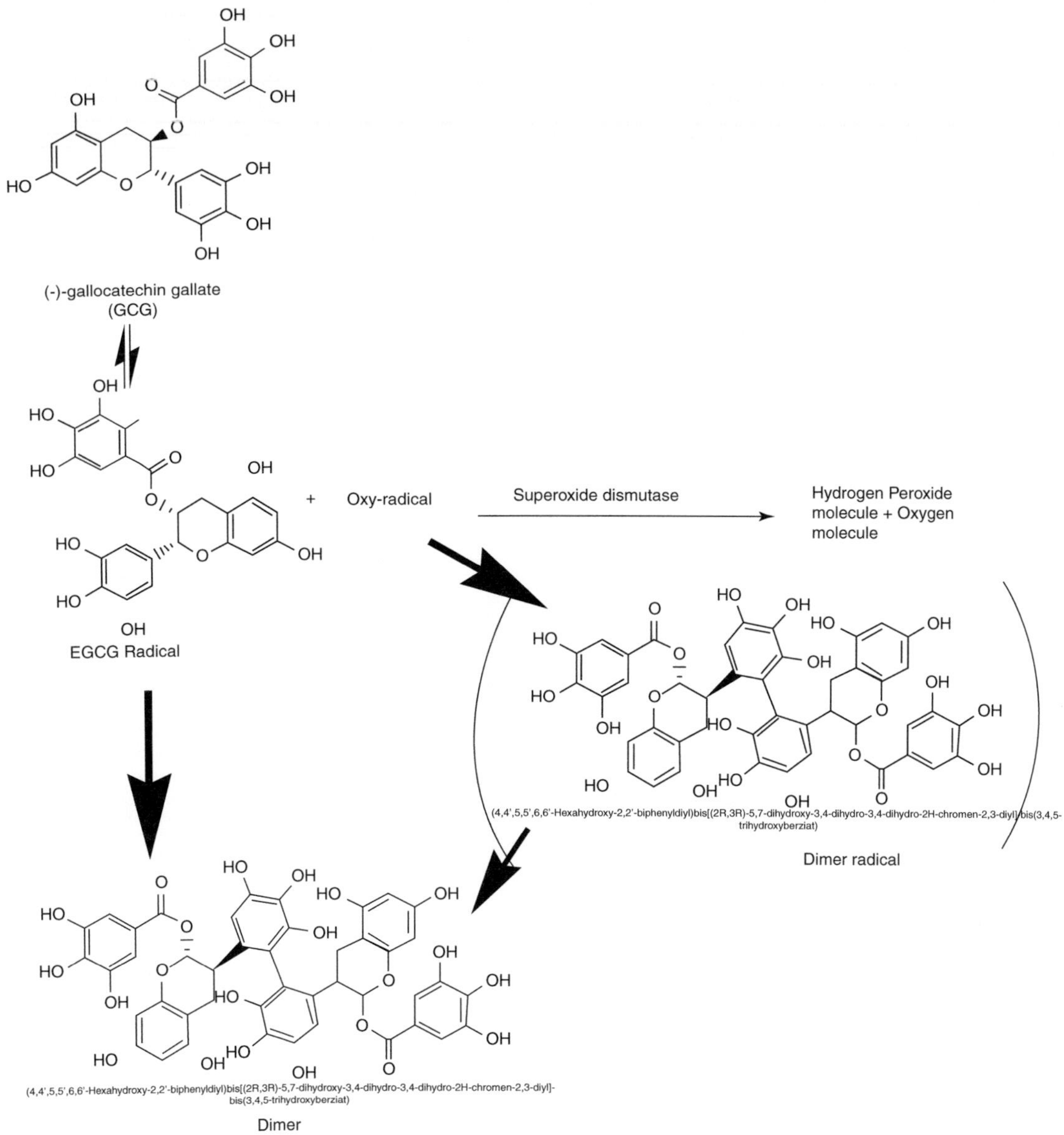

Fig 20.4 Schematic representation of the auto-oxidation mechanism of epigallocatechin gallate (EGCG)

20.3.4.4 Green Tea

Green tea is known to have epigallocatechin gallate in abundance, which is essential for protection against oxidative stress, as well as for inducing weight loss benefits; this is one of the reasons why many consumers prefer green tea to other teas.

20.3.4.5 White Tea

The composition of flavonoids in white tea is smaller compared to that of green tea and black tea, even though it has higher levels of EGCG than green tea. White tea is regarded to offer fewer health benefits compared to green tea and black tea because of its smaller content of flavonoids (Fig. 20.6).

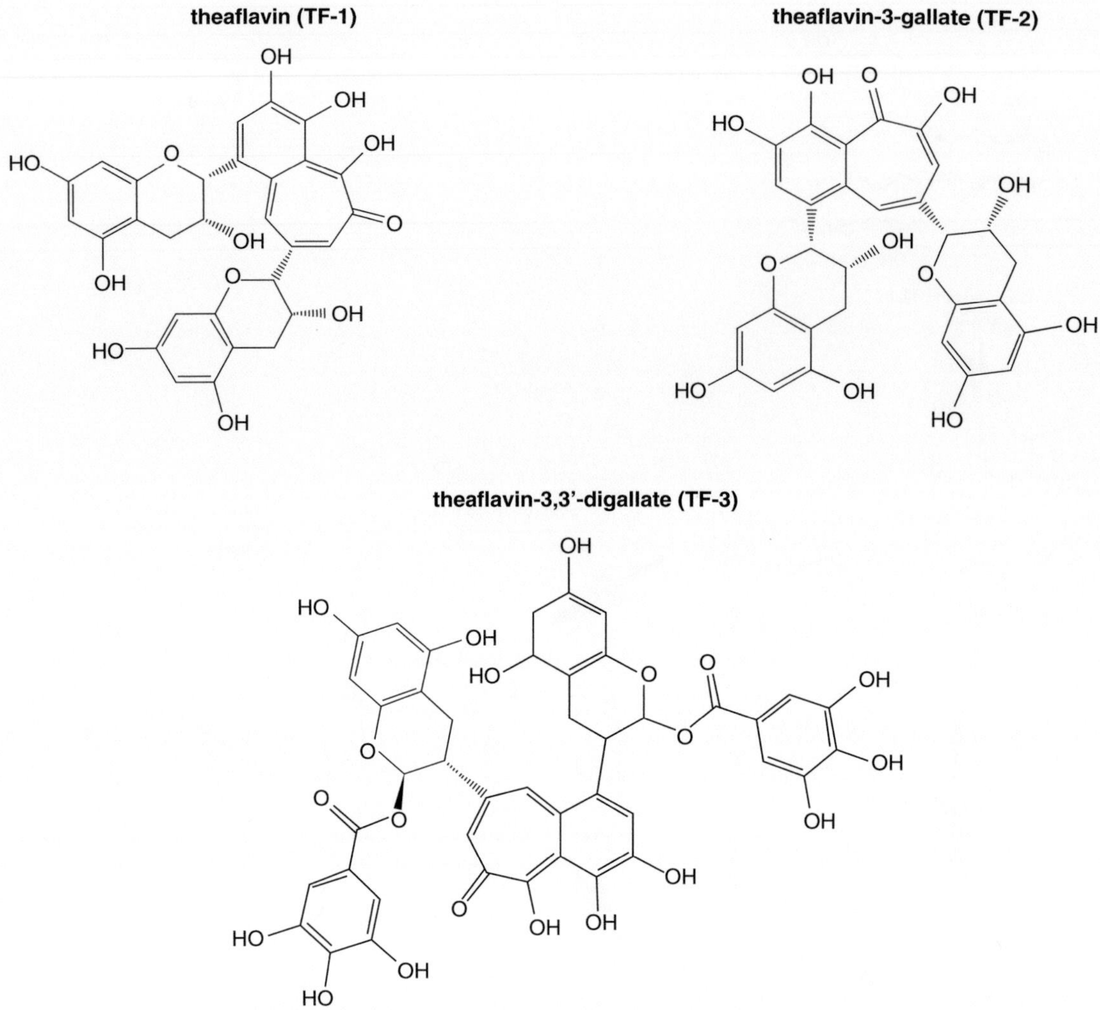

Fig. 20.5 Chemical structure of theaflavin compounds; (TF-1)-theaflavin ((4a*Z*,7*E*,9*Z*)-1-((2*R*,3*R*)-3,4-dihydro-3,5,7-trihydroxy-2*H*-chromen-2-yl)-3,4,5-trihydroxy-8-((2*R*,3*R*)-3,5,7-trihydroxychroman-2-yl)-6*H*-benzo[7] annulen-6-one); (TF-2)-theaflavin-3-gallate (3,4,6-trihydroxy-1,8-bis(3a,5,7-trihydroxy-2a-chromanyl)-5*H*-benzocyclohepten-5-one); (TF-3)-theaflavin-3,3′-digallate (3,4,5-trihydroxy-6-oxo-6*H*-benzo[7]annulene-1,8-diyl) bis[(2*R*,3*R*)-5,7-dihydroxy-3,4-dihydro-2*H*-chromene-2,3-diyl] bis(3,4,5-trihydroxybenzoate)

20.3.5 Specific Antioxidants that Characterise Herbal Teas

20.3.5.1 Rooibos Tea

There are a number of herbal teas, which include rooibos tea, rosemary tea, thyme tea and yerba tea. These herbal teas are known to be rich in different types of antioxidants. Rooibos tea, for example, is very rich in antioxidants known as nothofagin and aspalathin (Hillis and Inoue 1967; Bramati et al. 2002) (Fig. 20.7).

20.3.5.2 Antioxidants (Phenolic Diterpenes) in Rosemary (*Rosmarinus officinalis* L.)

Rosemary extracts are known to contain phenolic antioxidants (and flavonoids). The most active antioxidative ingredients of rosemary include phenolic diterpenes (carnosic acid, carnosol, rosmanol, rosmadial, 12-methoxycarnosic acid and epi- and isorosmanol) and phenolic acids (rosmarinic acid and caffeic acid) (Frankel 1991; Frankel et al. 1996; Richheimer et al. 1996; Nakatani 2003; Thorsen and Hildebrandt 2003;

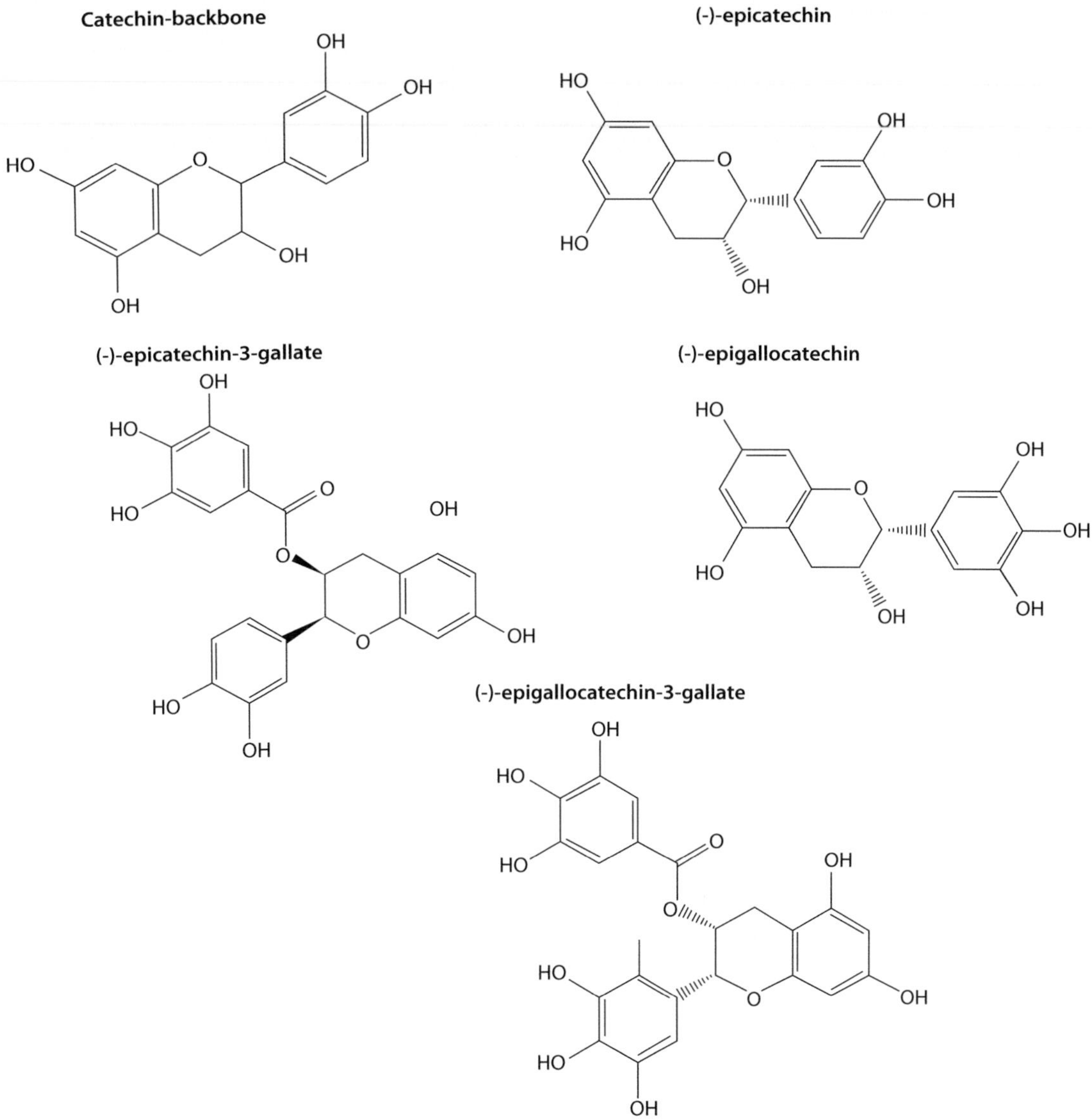

Fig. 20.6 The chemical structures of catechin compounds reported in green tea; (1) catechin backbone(2R,3S)-2-(3,4-dihydroxyphenyl)-3,4-dihydro-2H-chromene-3,5,7-trio; (2) (−)-epicatechin (2R,3R)-2-(3,4-dihydroxyphenyl)chroman-3,5,7-triol; (3) (−)-epicatechin-3-gallate ([(2S,3S)-2-(3,4-dihydroxyphenyl)-5,7-dihydroxy-3,4-dihydro-2H-chromen-3-yl] 3,4,5-trihydroxybenzoate; (4) (−)-epigallocatechin ((2R,3R)-2-(3,4,5-trihydroxyphenyl)-3,4-dihydro-2H-chromene-3,5,7-triol; (5) (−)-epigallocatechin-3-gallate[(2R,3R)-5,7-dihydroxy-2-(3,4,5-trihydroxyphenyl)-3,4-dihydro-2H-chromen-3-yl] 3,4,5-trihydroxybenzoate)

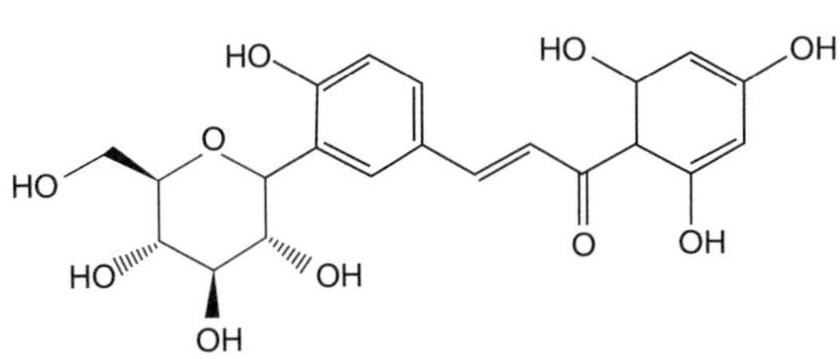

Fig. 20.7 The chemical structure of nothofagin

Carvalho et al. 2005). The chemical structures of these compounds are depicted in Fig. 20.8. Other names for eucalyptol are 1,8-cineol, 1,8-cineole, cajeputol, 1,8-epoxy-p-menthane, 1,8-oxido-p-menthane, eucalyptol, eucalyptole, 1,3,3-trimethyl-2-oxabicyclo[2,2,2]octane, cineol and cineole.

It should be noted that different herbal teas are composed of different ratios of chemical compounds as illustrated by Table 20.1 below.

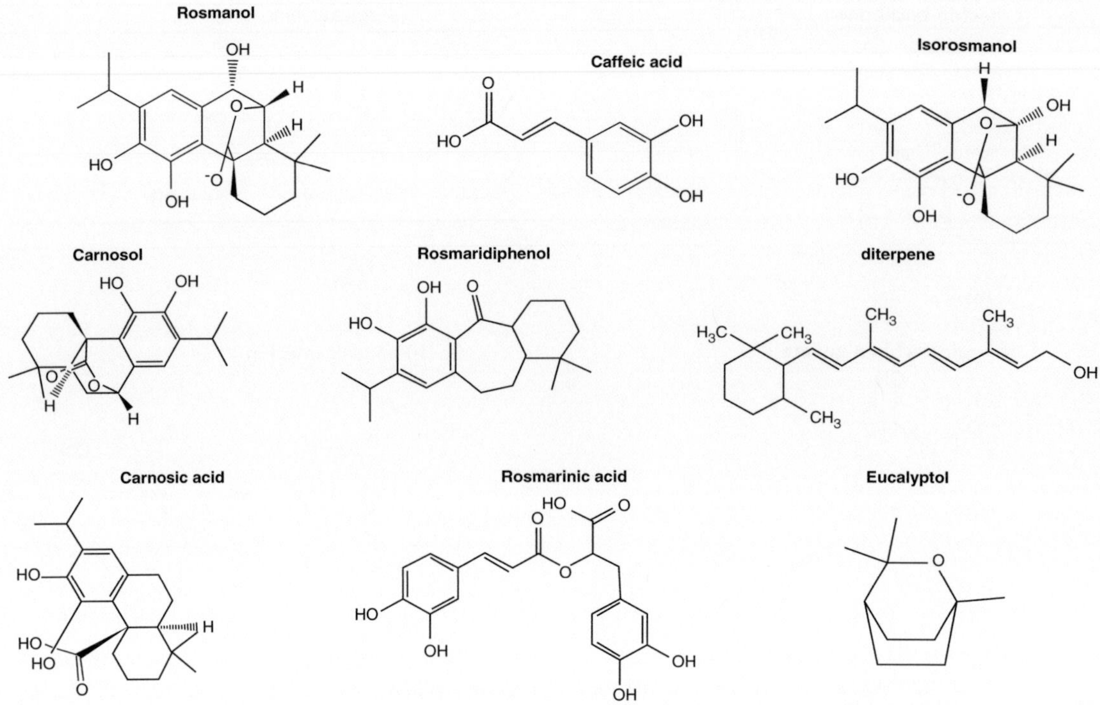

Fig. 20.8 The chemical structure of phenolic compounds found in rosemary extracts; (1) rosmanol ((4bR,8aS,9S,10S)-3,4,10-trihydroxy-2-isopropyl-8,8-dimethyl-6,7,8,8a,9,10-hexahydro-5H-9,4b-(epoxymethano)phenanthren-12-one); (2) Caffeic acid (3,4-dihydroxycinnamic acid; 331-39-5; 3-(3,4-dihydroxyphenyl)acrylic acid); (3) isorosmanol (6,11,12-trihydroxy-8,11,13-abietatrien-20,7-olide); (4) carnosol (1R,8S,10S)-3,4-dihydroxy-11,11-dimethyl-5-(propan-2-yl)-16-oxatetracyclo[6.6.2.0; {1,10}0.0; {2,7}] hexadeca-2,4,6-trien-1S-one); (5) rosmaridiphenol (14,15-dihydroxy-7,7-dimethyl-13-(propan-2-yl)tricyclo[9.4.0.0;{3,8}]pentadeca-1(11),12,14-trien-2-one); (6) diterpene (2E,4E,6E,8E)-3,7-dimethyl-9-(2,2,6-trimethylcyclohexyl) nona-2,4,6,8-tetraen-1-ol; (7) carnosic acid ((4aR,10aS)-5,6-dihydroxy-1,1-dimethyl-7-propan-2-yl-2,3,4,9,10,10a-hexahydrophenanthrene-4a-carboxylic acid); (8) rosmarinic acid (3-(3,4-dihydroxyphenyl)-2-{[(2E)-3-(3,4-dihydroxyphenyl)prop-2-enoyl]oxy}propanoicacid);(9)eucalyptol(1,3,3-trimethyl-2-oxabicyclo[2.2.2] octane

Table 20.1 Chemical composition of various herbal teas (excluding rooibos tea)

Oregano herbal tea	This tea contains phenolic antioxidants, mainly rosmarinic acid, phenolic carboxylic acids and glycosides.
Marjoram herbal tea	Marjoram contains phenolic antioxidants such as α-tocopherol, BHA, BHT, AA, epigallocatechin gallate, quercetin, or epicatechin, rosmarinic acid and carnosol, and essential oil, which can scavenge hydroxyl radicals (OH).
Sage herbal tea	Sage contains phenolic diterpene compounds, which are also found in rosemary, and they include carnosol, rosmanol and rosmadial. Moreover, sage contains methyl carnosate, rosmanol-9-ethyl ether, epirosmanol, isorosmanol and galdosol.
Thyme herbal tea	Thyme species such as *Thymus vulgaris*, *T. mastichina*, *T. caespititius* and *T. camphorate* are known to contain essential oil, α-tocopherol and BHT.
Basil herbal tea	In basil species such as the purple basil (*Ocimum basilicum*), the phenolic antioxidants form a high proportion of the compounds that are extractable. There is also a proportion of essential oils in basil species.

20.3.6 The Structure-Antioxidant Activity Relationship of Phenolic Compounds

A number of researches have been done into the contribution of flavonoids to the antioxidant activity of teas. This research has involved both *in vivo* and *in vitro* studies of black tea and green tea. Other studies have shown that the antioxidant activity of catechin and catechin gallate esters in green tea is more effective than that of vitamin C (Rice-Evans et al. 1997a). It therefore becomes important to understand what structural properties of these phenolic compounds make them more effective.

20.3.6.1 Flavonoids

Flavonoids are largely responsible for the distinctive taste, colour and aroma of tea, and are associated with the health benefits of tea. The most common flavonoids in tea are flavan-3-ols, namely, flavonols and flavans, which were reported to be present in very large amounts in tea when compared to other foods (A). These flavans are divided into subclasses according to the degree of polymerisation. These subclasses are the catechins, which are monomers and available as catechins, epicatechin, epicatechin gallate, epigallocatechin and epigallocatechin gallate. Again, there are the theaflavins, which are dimers and available as theaflavin, theaflavin-3-gallate, theaflavin-3′-gallate and theaflavin-3,3′-digallate. Oligomers are also present as arubigins, which are derived from tannins. The structures of these oligomers are unknown. Other flavonoids present in smaller amounts than flavan-3-ols are flavonols such as quercetin, kaempferol and myricetin, and flavones such as apigenin and luteolin (Peterson et al. 2005).

The Influence of the C-Ring on the Antioxidant Activity of Flavonoids

More studies have shown that the preferentially high antioxidant activities of flavonoids were due to their chemical structure. In comparing different -entahydroxy polyphenolic structures in a study by Rice-Evans et al. (1997b), it was clearly demonstrated that the unsaturated C-ring allowed for electron delocalisation across the molecule for stabilising the aryloxyl radical, resulting in higher antioxidant potential. Blocking this C-ring 3-hydroxyl group with a glycoside such as the structure of rutin, or completely removing it as in luteolin, significantly decreases the antioxidant activity.

The Influence of the B-Ring on the Antioxidant Activity of Flavonoids

Flavonoids such as naringenin and hesperetin, with only one hydroxyl group in the B-ring, have been suggested to possess little antioxidant activity, especially in lipid systems. The B-ring hydroxyl configuration was also described as the most significant determinant in antioxidant activity (Heim et al. 2002). The authors emphasise that the hydroxyl on the B-ring is the structure that donates hydrogen and an electron to the hydroxyl, peroxyl and peroxynitrite radicals. In this way it gives rise to a relatively stable flavonoid radical.

The Influence of Hydroxyl Groups on the Antioxidant Activity of Flavonoids

It is acknowledged that the spatial arrangement of substitutes is probably the greatest determinant of antioxidant activity in the flavan backbone alone (Heim et al. 2002). Free radical scavenging capacity is attributed to the reactive nature of the hydroxyl substitutes. This reaction can be illustrated as follows:

$$F-OH+R'\rightarrow F-O'+RH$$

Among structurally similar flavones and flavanones, peroxyl and hydroxyl scavenging activity increases in linear and curvilinear paths, respectively, according to the number of OH groups within the structure (Cao et al. 1997). Another example of the importance of the OH groups is noted in relation to luteolin and kaempferol. Luteolin exceeds kaempferol in antioxidant activity. Both these compounds have an identical structure, but kaempferol lacks the OH group on the B-ring (Heim et al. 2002).

The Role of O-Methylation on the Antioxidant Activity of Flavonoids

The antioxidant activity of quercetin is higher than that of its O-methylated and O-glycosylated derivatives due to the suppressed activity by O-methylation (Dugas Jr et al. 2000; Burda and Oleszek 2001; Arora et al. 1998). The differences in antioxidant activity between polyhydroxylated and polymethoxylated flavonoids are most likely due to the differences in hydrophobicity and molecular planarity (Arora et al. 1998). It should, however, be taken into consideration that the ratio of methoxy to hydroxyl substitutes does not in any way predict the scavenging ability of a flavonoid, although the B-ring is particularly sensitive to the position of this methoxy group. An example of this is demonstrated by Matthiesen et al. (1997), when the 6′-OH/4′-OMe configuration is alternated to 6′-OMe/4′-OH, resulting in the complete loss of the antioxidant activity against the DPPH radical. Similarly, the obstruction of the 3′4'-catechol structure by 4′-O-methylation greatly compromises the antioxidant activity (Dugas Jr et al. 2000). Multiple A-ring methoxy groups will also reverse any positive effects of the B-ring catechol. This is because the inhibition of the formation of the oxidation product malondialdehyde by the flavones with an A-ring ortho-dimethoxy or trimethoxy structure is not enhanced (Mora et al. 1990).

20.3.6.2 Phenolic Acids

Phenolic acids were known as secondary metabolites and are largely distributed throughout the plant kingdom. These compounds give plants their unique taste and flavour and additional health benefits (Dvorakova et al. 2008). The term "phenolic acids" designates phenols that possess one carboxylic acid functionality. These phenolic acids contain two distinctive carbon frameworks: the hydroxycinnamic and a hydroxybenzoic structures (Zhao et al. 2013) (Fig. 20.9).

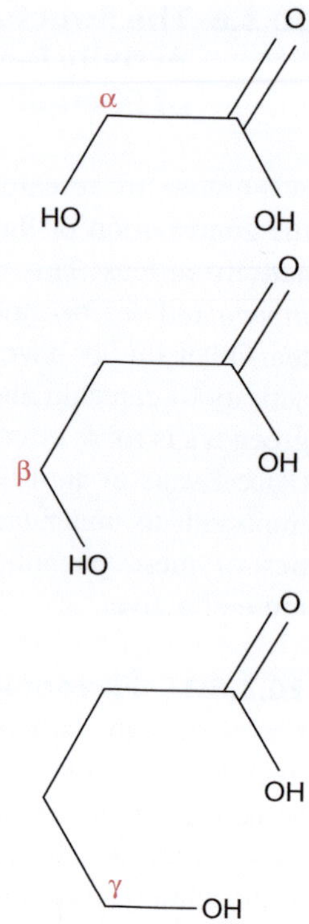

Fig. 20.9 The basic structures of hydroxy acids

The Influence of Hydroxybenzoic Acid on Antioxidant Activity

The monohydroxy benzoic acids show no antioxidant activity in the ortho and para positions in terms of hydrogen-donating capacity against radicals generated in the aqueous phase. This is consistent with the electron-withdrawing potential of the single carboxyl functional group on the phenol ring affecting the o- and p-positions (Heim et al. 2002). However, monohydroxybenzoates are more effective hydroxyl radical scavengers due to their propensity for hydroxylation and the highly reactive hydroxyl radical (Lien et al. 1999). The antioxidant activity of dihydroxybenzoic acid derivatives is dependent on the position of the hydroxyl group in the ring. In the ortho and meta positions, 2,3-dihydroxybenzoic acid gives a higher antioxidant activity compared to dihydroxylation in the meta and para positions, as in the case of protocatechuic acid (Heim et al. 2002). When hydroxyl substitution occurs in the ortho position to the carboxylate in the 2,5-dihydroxybenzoic acid, the antioxidant activity remains low. This concludes that the proximity of the -CO_2H to the orthodiphenolic substituents ultimately influences the availability of the hydrogen, with the m-position being the most effective position. This is supported by the fact that resorcylic acid possesses a much enhanced antioxidant activity compared to resorcinol, which has no CO_2H.

The Influence of Hydroxycinnamic Acid on Antioxidant Activity

The inclusion of an ethylenic group between a phenyl ring carrying the p-hydroxyl group and the carboxylate group is reported to greatly increase the reducing properties of the OH group (Rice-Evans et al. 1997b). This is supported by the electron-donating effects on the ring of the COOH–CH=CH– compared to COOH–CH_2– groups. The monohydroxyl groups in the cinnamic acids are more available as hydrogen donors than monohydroxyl groups in the phenylacetic acid. The glycosylation of the carboxylate group of the caffeic acid, similar to the structure of chlorogenic acid, has no effect on antioxidant activity. In contrast to this, substitution of the 3-hydroxyl group of a caffeic acid by a methoxy group, giving ferulic acid, significantly increases antioxidant activity. The presence of the –CH=CH–COOH groups within the cinnamic acid ensures a greater hydrogen-donating ability and radical stabilisation than the carboxylate group of the benzoic acids (Rice-Evans et al. 1997b). Caffeic acid, sinapic acid, ferulic acid and p-coumaric acid also display more activity than protocatechuic acid, syringic acid, vanillic acid and p-hydroxybenzoate (Cuvelier et al. 1992).

20.4 Herbal Tea Metabolites and Associated Health Benefits

Nutraceuticals are dietary supplements that have health benefits, such as prevention and treatment of disease. Nutraceuticals contain antioxidants and minerals as their major ingredients, providing the characterised nutritional and health benefits, which includes anti-inflammatory, anti-allergic, antiviral, anti-carcinogenic and antidiabetic activities and prevention of cardiovascular and Alzheimer's disease (Middleton Jr and Kandaswami 1992; Zieliński and Kozlowska 2000; Adom and Lui 2002; Willcox et al. 2004; Zhou et al. 2004; Moore et al. 2005; Udompataikul et al. 2009). Flavonoids are the major antioxidants present in teas and therefore contribute significantly to their nutraceutical potential. Of all the flavonoids, the flavones and catechins seem to be the most powerful in protecting the body against oxidative damage. The cells and tissues of the human body are under constant oxidative stress as a result of ROS produced during oxygen metabolism (Laughton et al. 1991; Hoult et al. 1994). These free radicals have been implicated in several studies as the cause of various human diseases (Siess et al. 1995; Cotelle et al. 1996). The modes of action with which antioxidants prevent and treat diseases are fully explained in sections to follow. Plant secondary metabolites are known for their antioxidative capacity through their preventive, radical scavenging and repair action. Antioxidants present at the site of radical attack break the chain of oxidation by being preferentially oxidised by the attacking radicals, thereby preventing oxidation of adjacent biomolecules (Willcox et al. 2004; Yu et al. 2002). Different groups of antioxidants during the formation and propagation of free radicals exhibit various modes of action in their effort of disease prevention. Proliferation of diabetics and cancer among young and old South Africans is burdening the country's healthcare system even though the country has a rich biodiversity of indigenous herbal teas that can aid combat diseases. These herbal teas have diverse compounds that have strong antioxidant properties with health benefits.

20.4.1 Phenolic Compounds on the Gastrointestinal and Cardiovascular Systems

Flavonoids have been reported for their anti-inflammatory and anti-ulceration activity, regulating metabolism of free arachidonic acid through the inhibition of cyclooxygenase and lipoxygenase activity (Glazer 1990; Sahu and Gray 1993). Flavonoids prevent endothelial dysfunction by promoting the vaso-relaxant process that leads to the reduction of arterial pressure. Endothelial dysfunction is the critical event in the development of cardiovascular disease and the major complication of atherosclerosis and arterial thrombus formation (Yoshida et al. 1994; Iwatsuki et al. 1995). Atherosclerosis is characterised by the accumulation of lipids and other fibrous elements within the large arteries. This is the single most important contributor to cardiovascular disease (Sato et al. 1992). During the onset of atherosclerosis, mononuclear cells adhere to the endothelium. This is triggered by a number of molecules such as P-selectin, E-selectin, vascular cell adhesion molecule-1 and intercellular adhesion molecule-1. These molecules are secreted by the human cells in the presence of stimuli such as oxidised LDL and oxidative free radicals (Hofnagel et al. 2007; Bonomini et al. 2008). This directly explains the role of antioxidants such as flavonoids in the prevention of atherosclerosis during its initial stages.

20.4.2 Phenolic Compounds as Anti-diabetic Agents

Diabetes mellitus is a complex metabolic disorder resulting from excess glucose in the biological system and exacerbated by the reduced secretion and action of insulin. There are two persistent types of diabetes: type 1, which occurs due to the absolute deficiency of insulin, and type 2,which occurs due to a combination of insulin resistance and inadequate insulin secretary response, with type 2 being the more prevalent of the two (Dewi and Maryani 2015). Therapeutic interventions of treating diabetes include the inhibition of α-amylase and α-glucosidase. The enzymes are responsible for the conversion of oligosaccharides and disaccharides into monosaccharides, such as glucose (Tarling et al. 2008; Dewi and Maryani 2015). Studies have shown that phenolic compounds of herbal plants such as *Camellia sinensis* (Wang et al. 2012), *Centella asiatica* (Dewi and Maryani, 2015), *Ligustrum robustum (*Yu et al. 2015), *Mallotus japonicus* (Indrianingsih et al. 2015) and *Quercus phillyraeoides* (Indrianingsih et al. 2015) have either α-glucosidase or α-amylase inhibitory properties, or both. Quercetin is the most reported flavonoid implicated in the successful management of diabetes through increased release of insulin (Halliwell and Gutteridge 1995). Quercetin stimulates insulin release and enhances Ca^{2+} uptake from pancreatic islet cells (Grisham 1992; Pieri et al. 1994).

20.4.3 Phenolic Compounds in Cancer Prevention and Treatment

Cai et al. (2004) carried out a study on 112 species of 50 plant families of Chinese medicinal plants that are associated with anticancer activity with extracts prepared from medicinally used plant parts. Flavonoids were found to be the largest class of phenols in the tested plant extracts. Furthermore, there was a positive relationship observed between the total phenolic content and the antioxidant activity of the tested herbs. In an older study by Cao et al. (1997) it was found that the flavonoids that contain multiple OH substitutions have very strong antioxidant activities against peroxyl radicals. For example, the ORACROOi activities of myricetin, quercetin, luteolin, fustin, eriodictyol and taxifolin were 4.32, 3.29, 3.57, 3.91, 3.41 and 3.59 Trolox equivalents, respectively, whereas α-tocopherol, ascorbic acid, β-carotene, GSH, uric acid and bilirubin were reported to have ORACROOi values of 1.0, 0.52–1.12, 0.64, 0.68, 0.92 and 0.84 Trolox equivalents, respectively. This further substantiates flavonoids as better anticancer agents than other common antioxidants, such as α-tocopherol and ascorbic acid since one of the possible modes of cancer prevention is the antioxidant stability of compounds. Due to radical species being generated through normal cellular metabolisms, the ability of flavonoids to remove these free radicals plays an important role in preventing chemical- and UV-induced carcinogenesis (Shiu-Ming 1997). Flavonoid antioxidants also possess the ability to chelate metal ions that possess redox potential. This activity enables flavonoids to play the role of preventing metal-induced membrane lipid damage.

Cancer is known as a hypoproliferative disorder that results in morphological cellular transformation, dysregulation of apoptosis, uncontrolled cell proliferation, invasion and metastasis (Hanahan and Weinberg 2000). Numerous clinical and epidemiological studies have shown a strong relationship between chronic infections, chronic inflammation, and cancer formation and progression (Coussens and Werb 2002; Dobrovolskaia and Kozlov 2005). This then strongly suggests that chronic inflammation is involved in tumour formation, promotion and progression. Several mechanisms have been suggested for flavonoids and their cancer-prevention ability such as anti-astrogenic and anti-proliferative activity, prevention of oxidation, regulation of the immune system, anti-inflammatory activity and induction of cell cycle arrest (Birt et al. 2001).

Other than their ability to directly inhibit the formation and development of cancer cells, flavonoids have also been found to inhibit the activity of enzymes that play a critical role in cancer development. One way in which they exhibit this ability is through their inhibition and/or modulation of several kinase pathways. Quercetin is vital in the general inhibiting activity of protein kinase C, mitogen-activated protein kinase (MAPK) and phosphorylase. This is largely significant because many molecular alterations associated with carcinogenesis occur in the cellular signalling pathways that include protein kinases, which are closely implicated in the inflammatory process. Abnormal activation of these kinases results in the uncontrolled cell growth that leads to malignant transformation (Fresco et al. 2006).

20.4.4 Phenolic Compounds on Skin Health and Ageing Process

The hallmarks of the skin ageing process are characterised by skin dryness, wrinkle formation, scarring, dark spot's formation and delays in wound healing. The consumption of teas can in many ways contribute to the reduction of the undesired ageing process the skin is programmed to undertake. This is mainly due to the photo-protective and oxidant-quenching activities enriched by antioxidants present in teas. Epigallocatechin-3-gallate, one of the most abundant catechins in tea, has been shown to have many beneficial health benefits. Oral administration and topical application of ECGC and other tea phenolic compounds have been reported to prevent the disruption of the skin's barrier function and ultimately strengthen the tolerance of the skin to UV-induced damage (Chiu et al. 2005; Janjua et al. 2009; Jeon et al. 2009). The protection of the skin against UV-induced damaged is one of the key strategies in ensuring the integrity of the skin's health and age. Furthermore, the characteristic enrichment of green tea and black tea with phenolic compounds such as catechin, kaempferol and quercetin during cultivation and processing plays a central role on the therapeutic capabilities of teas. Recently, Bloodsworth et al, 2000; Dewi and Maryani, 2015; Tanigawa et al. (2014) reported that catechins, which included ECGC, EGC, ECG and EC, accounted approximately 10% of the dry weight of green tea leaves. Therefore, the transdermal absorption of these phenolic compounds into the bloodstream is critical in realising their health benefits as it was reported by Miyazawa (2000).

Tea selection is one of the critical parameters to consider when exploiting the health benefits of phenolic compounds present in teas. Masaki (2010) reported that ROS can have a paradoxical action on the melanocyte cells due to their ability to enhance skin depigmentation and also increase pigmentation. The associated degeneration of melanocytes induced by the presence of H_2O_2 in the skin resulted in skin depigmentation while $NO^{\cdot}$ induced melanogenesis as a result of increased activity of tyrosinase-related protein 1, an enzyme responsible for melanin production. Therefore, achieving the desired skin complexion can be largely influenced by the activity of antioxidants present in tea towards H_2O_2 or $^{\cdot}NO$. Interestingly, even though EGCG has many reported beneficial effects due to its antioxidative potential, when present in biological systems it produces H_2O_2 (Kim et al. 2014) which has been reported to be responsible for depigmentation. Excessive levels of depigmentation will negatively affect the health of the skin, resulting in photodamage and skin-related diseases (i.e. vitiligo).

20.5 Herbal Tea Metabolites and Food Science

20.5.1 Phenolic Compounds as Food Additives

Synthetic antioxidants such as butylated hydroxyanisole (BHA), butylated hydroxytoluene (BHT) and tert-butylhydroquinone (TBHQ) have been used worldwide as antioxidants in food processing. However, due to safety concerns, there is a shift towards more natural antioxidants (Balasundram et al. 2006). The antioxidant activity of various phenolic compounds, especially flavonoids and hydrocinnamic acids, has been studied in various food model systems. Currently, green tea extracts have a generally recognised as safe (GRAS) status as food additives and have proven antioxidant properties in various food applications (Perumalla and Hettiarachchy 2011). The use of such extracts can also improve the marketing potential of various foods due to the associated health benefits (Lee et al. 2004). Tea catechins have demonstrated a significantly higher antioxidant activity compared to ginseng, rosemary, sage, vitamin C and BHA against lipid oxidation of cooked beef patties (O'Sullivan et al. 2004). This antioxidant activity is possible due to the ability of tea flavonoids, especially catechins, to bind the iron component of the myoglobin and to effectively help in delayed lipid oxidation by reacting with free radicals. Lipid oxidation inhibition in red meat, fish and poultry was found to be concentration dependent, with only catechin levels of 200–400 mg/kg having a significant inhibitory effect (Mitsumoto et al. 2005). At these levels, the catechins have no effect on the sensory attributes of the product such as flavour, tenderness, taste or overall acceptability (Tang et al. 2001), but actually delay the loss of redness in raw pork patties during storage (McCarthy et al. 2001).

The addition of certain plant extracts at 1 and 2% used to replace synthetic antioxidants in biscuits did not have any effect on the organoleptic acceptability of these products, while it had an excellent antioxidant effect as compared to the effect of BHA (Reddy et al. 2005). However, the use of these plant phenols as antioxidants has been met with challenges. Frankel et al. (1996) used plant extracts in corn, soybean, peanut and fish oils without any success. Instead, the plant polyphenol extracts acted as pro-antioxidants. Interestingly, in combination with BHT, they provided a more effective and synergistic protection in soybean oil. The pro-oxidant effect was attributed to the presence of chlorophyll by Wanasundara and Shahidi (1998) when they used green tea extracts in marine oils. This finding was furthermore emphasised by the use of dechlorophyllised green tea extracts, which had an antioxidant activity higher than that of the synthetic antioxidants.

20.5.2 Phenolic Compounds as Food Antimicrobials

The increasing demand for food with an extended shelf life, fewer chemical preservatives and an absence of food-borne risks has pushed food processors to explore naturally occurring preservatives (Sunilson et al. 2009). Herbal plants have been used since historic times as food preservatives (Dillon and Board 1994). Compounds that are naturally present in herbs and plants are generally hydrophobic and have membrane-rupturing characteristics (Brul and Coote 1999). This is possible since these plant extracts react with the protein of a microbial membrane and mitochondria, resulting in a disturbed structure and changes in their permeability (Mostafa et al. 2018). Some of the antimicrobial activities of plant extracts are based on the extracellular enzyme-inactivation ability of polyphenols (Brul and Coote 1999). Plant phenols also interact with microbial enzymes and protein on the surface of a microorganism, causing its disruption, and ultimately disperse a flux of protons towards the cell interior, which induces cell death or inhibition of enzymes for amino acid biosynthesis (Burt 2004).

Tea extracts have successfully demonstrated antimicrobial properties against various food-borne pathogens such as *E. coli, L. monocytogenes, Salmonella typhimurium, Staphylococcus aureus* and *Vibrio cholera* (An et al. 2004). A synergistic effect of tea extracts, bacteriocin and nisin, has been reported in respect of major food-borne pathogens (Sivarooban et al. 2008). Current studies have concluded that plant extracts can be used, and are potentially effective, as natural preservatives to control food poisoning and to assist in avoiding the application of chemical preservatives (Mostafa et al. 2018).

20.5.3 Phenolic Compounds in Food-Quality Applications

Green tea extracts have been found to successfully inhibit polyphenol oxidase (PPO) in white shrimp during storage. Polyphenol oxidase is responsible for the development of black spots in stored shrimp as phenols are oxidised to quinone. Although quinone in itself is colourless, it eventually undergoes non-enzymatic polymerisation, which gives rise to the black pigment. The pigment is not dangerous to human health but drastically reduces consumers' acceptability of the product, thereby resulting in poor quality and financial losses (Montero et al. 2006). Combining tea extracts with ascorbic acid not only lowers the formation of black spots on shrimp, but also retards microbial growth and lipid oxidation, thereby extending the shelf life of the shrimp without affecting the organoleptic properties of the product (Nirmal and Benjakul 2012).

Pectin-based edible coatings containing green tea extracts were also used to successfully improve the quality of pork patties. Sensory panellists preferred the appearance, odour and taste of raw patties with this pectin coat to the appearance, odour and taste of patties that were only vacuum packed and patties with a plain pectin-based coating (Kang et al. 2007). The use of green tea extracts in bread was found to decrease the brightness and sweetness of bread while increasing its hardness, stickiness and astringency properties. This is a significant finding since sweetness is an important desired sensory quality of bread and astringency is not (Lawless and Heymann 1999). Astringency is largely attributed to catechins, especially epigallocatechin gallate (Scharbert and Hofmann 2005). The increase in hardness is also a desirable attribute since hardness is used to determine bread quality (Spies 1990).

Green tea extracts have been successfully used and indicated as a feasible method of preservation for minimally processed lettuce when assessed against the nutrient markers ascorbic acid and carotenoid content of fresh-cut lettuce (Barry-Ryan et al. 2008). Unfortunately, at more concentrated forms, the extracts resulted in browning, which led to poor consumer acceptability.

Phenolic extracts from tea also help to improve the flavour attributes and fresh meat colour of fresh meat products (Namal Senanayake 2013). Green tea extracts also have no unfavourable flavour impact on beef burgers, because the extracts contribute to the "meaty" umami taste of meat (Namal Senanayake 2013). Studies have also shown that tea catechins in combination with nitrite and sodium ascorbate assist in remarkably maintaining the red colour of dry-cured sausages and standard ham, respectively (Moawad et al. 2012).

20.6 Conclusions

Phenolic compounds have been proven to be effective in the fight against chronic diseases. These medical benefits are due to the antioxidant capabilities of phenolic compounds. The structure and concentration of the individual phenolic compounds have a great influence on the effectiveness of the phenolic compounds to act as antioxidants. Flavonoids are the group of phenolic compounds known to have greater health benefits than the others. Flavonoids are found in abundance in herbal teas. Their antioxidant activity is influenced by the B-ring, the C-ring, hydroxyl groups, O-methylation groups and their positions on the flavan structure. Phenolic compounds also have benefits for the food industry and are gaining popularity as natural antimicrobials that enhance both the shelf life and the quality of products.

The main challenge currently is the lack of knowledge on the activities of individual phenolic compounds and the exact concentrations of these compounds that will give effect to their benefits. It therefore becomes critical to develop methods or to improve on the current analytical methods being used to identify, isolate and quantify these phenolic compounds.

References

Adom KK, Lui RH. Antioxidant activity of grains. J Agric Food Chem. 2002;50:6182–7.

Al-Dalain SYA, Abu-Darwish SM, Al-Fraihat AH, Al-Dabbas FM, Al-Dalin HK, Al-Hamaidah KD. Comparative studies of the trace elements content of some herbal tea consumed in Jordan. Pak J Nutr. 2012;11:916–8.

An BJ, Kwak JH, Son JH, Park JM, Lee JY, Jo C, Byun M-W. Biological and antimicrobial activity of irradiated green tea polyphenols. Food Chem. 2004;88:447–51.

Arora A, Nair MG, Strasburg GM. Structure–activity relationships for antioxidant activities of a series of flavonoids in a liposomal system. Free Radic Biol Med. 1998;24:1355–63.

Balasundram N, Sundram K, Samman S. Phenolic compounds in plants and agri-industrial by-products: antioxidant activity, occurrence, and potential uses. Food Chem Anal Nutri Clin Methods. 2006;99:191–203.

Barry-Ryan C, Martin-Diana A, Rico D. Green tea extract as a natural antioxidant to extend the shelf-life of fresh-cut lettuce. Innov Food Sci Emerg Technol. 2008;9:593–603.

Baumann D, Adler S, Hamburger MA. A simple isolation method for the major catechins in green tea using high-speed countercurrent chromatography. J Nat Prod. 2001;64:353–5.

Birt DF, Hendrich S, Wang W. Dietary agents in cancer prevention: flavonoids and isoflavonoids. Pharmacol Ther. 2001;90:157–77.

Bloodsworth A, O'Donnell VB, Freeman BA. Nitric oxide regulation of free radical-and enzyme-mediated lipid and lipoprotein oxidation. Arterioscler Thromb Vasc Biol. 2000;20:1707–15.

Bonomini F, Tengattini IS, Fabiano A, Bianchi R, Rezzani R. Atherosclerosis and oxidative stress. Histol Histopathol. 2008;23:381–90.

Boulekbache-Makhlouf L, Medouni L, Medouni-Adrar S, Arkoub L, Madini K. Effects of solvents extraction on phenolic content and antioxidant activity of the by product of eggplant. Ind Crop Prod. 2013;49:668–74.

Bramati L, Minoggio M, Gardana C, Simonetti P, Mauri P, Pietta P. Quantitative characterization of flavonoid compounds in rooibos tea *(Aspalathus linearis)* by LC-UV/DAD. J Agric Food Chem. 2002;50:5513–9.

Brul S, Coote P. Preservative agents in foods. Mode of action and microbial resistance mechanisms: a review. Int J Food Microbiol. 1999;50:1–17.

Burda S, Oleszek W. Antioxidant and antiradical activities of flavonoids. J Agric Food Chem. 2001;49:2774–9.

Burt S. Essential oils: their antibacterial properties and potential application in foods –a review. Int J Food Microbiol. 2004;94:223–339.

Cai Y, Luo Q, Sun M, Corke H. Antioxidant activity and phenolic compounds of 112 traditional Chinese medicinal plants associated with anticancer. Life Sci. 2004;74:2157–84.

Cao G, Sofic E, Prior RL. Antioxidant and pro-oxidant behavior of flavonoids: structure–activity relationships. Free Radic Biol Med. 1997;22:749–60.

Carvalho RN, Moura LS, Rosa PTV, Meireles MAA. Supercritical fluid extraction from rosemary (*Rosmarinus officinalis*): kinetic data, extract's global yield, composition, and antioxidant activity. J Supercrit Fluids. 2005;35:197–204.

Chen G, Zhang H, Ye J. Determination of rutin and quercetin in plants by capillary electrophoresis with electrochemical detection. Anal Chim Acta. 2000;423:69–76.

Chiu AE, Chan JL, Kern DG, Kohler S, Rehmus WE, Kimball AB. Double-blinded, placebo-controlled trial of green tea extractsin the clinical and histologic appearance of photoaging skin. Dermatol Surg. 2005;31:855–9.

Cotelle N, Bernier JL, Catteau JP, Pommery J, Wallet JC, Gaydou EM. Antioxidant properties of hydroxyflavones. Free Radic Biol Med. 1996;20:35–43.

Coussens LM, Werb Z. Inflammation and cancer. Nature. 2002;420:860–7.

Cuvelier M-E, Richard H, Berset C. Comparison of the antioxidative activity of some acid-phenols: structure–activity relationship. Biosci Biotechnol Biochem. 1992;56:324–5.

De Rijke E, Zafra-Gómez A, Ariese F, Brinkman UAT, Gooijer C. Determination of isoflavone glucoside malonates in *Trifolium pratense* L. (red clover) extracts: quantification and stability studies. J Chromatogr A. 2001;932:55–64.

De Rijke E, Out P, Niessen WMA, Ariese F, Gooijer C, Brinkman UAT. Analytical separation and detection methods for flavonoids. J Chromatogr A. 2006;1112:31–63.

Dewi RT, Maryani F. Antioxidant and α-glucosidase inhibitory compounds of *Centella asiatica*. Procedia Chem. 2015;17:147–52.

Dillon VM, Board RG, editors. Natural antimicrobial systems and food preservation. Wallingford: CAB International; 1994. p. 167–79.

Dobrovolskaia MA, Kozlov SV. Inflammation and cancer: when NF-kappaB amalgamates the perilous partnership. Curr Cancer Drug Targets. 2005;5:325–544.

Dugas AJ Jr, Castañeda-Acosta J, Bonin GC, Price KL, Fischer NH, Winston GW. Evaluation of the total peroxyl radical-scavenging capacity of flavonoids: structure–activity relationships. J Nat Prod. 2000;63:327–31.

Dvorakova M, Moreira MM, Dostalek P, Skulilova Z, Guido LF, Barros AA. Characterization of monomeric and oligomeric flavan-3-ols from barley and malt by liquid chromatography-ultraviolet detection-electrospray ionization mass spectrometry. J Chromatogr A. 2008;1189:398–405.

Fiamegos YC, Konidari CN, Stalikas CD. Cyanuric acid trace analysis by extractive methylation via phase-transfer catalysis and capillary gas chromatography coupled with flame thermoionic and mass-selective detection. Process parameter studies and kinetics. Anal Chem. 2003;75:4034–42.

Fiamegos YC, Nanos CG, Vervoort J, Stalikas CD. Analytical procedure for the in-vial derivatization–extraction of phenolic acids and flavonoids in methanolic and aqueous plant extracts followed by gas chromatography with mass-selective detection. J Chromatogr A. 2004;1041:11–8.

Franke AA, Custer LJ. High-performance liquid chromatography assay of isoflavonoids and coumestrol from human urine. J Chromatogr B. 1994;662:47–60.

Frankel EN. Recent advances in lipid oxidation. J Agric Food Chem. 1991;54:495–511.

Frankel EN, Huang S-W, Prior E, Aeschbach R. Evaluation of antioxidant activity of rosemary extracts, carnosol and carnosic acid in bulk vegetable oils and fish oil and their emulsions. J Sci Food Agric. 1996;72:201–8.

Fresco P, Borges F, Diniz C, Marques MPM. New insights on the anticancer properties of dietary polyphenols. Med Res Rev. 2006;26:747–66.

Glazer AN. Phycoerythrin fluorescence-based assay for reactive oxygen species. Methods Enzymol. 1990;186:161–8.

Grisham MB. Reactive metabolites of oxygen and nitrogen in biology and medicine. Austin, TX: R. G. Landes Company; 1992.

Halliwell B, Gutteridge JM. The definition and measurement of antioxidants in biological systems. Free Radic Biol Med. 1995;18:125–6.

Hanahan D, Weinberg RA. The hallmarks of cancer: the next generation. Cell. 2000;100:57–70.

Heim KE, Tagliaferro AR, Bobilya DJ. Flavonoid antioxidants: chemistry, metabolism and structure–activity relationships. J Nutr Biochem. 2002;13:572–84.

Hicks A. Current status and future development of global tea production and tea products. AU JT. 2009;12:251–64.

Hillis W, Inoue T. The polyphenols of *Nothofagus* species-II: the heartwood of *Nothofagus fusca*. Phytochemistry. 1967;6:59–67.

Hofnagel O, Luechtenborg B, Weissen-Plenz G, Robenek H. Statins and foam cell formation: impact on LDL oxidation and uptake of oxidized lipoproteins via scavenger receptors. Biochim Biophys Acta. 2007;1771:1117–24.

Hoult JRS, Moroney MA, Payá M. Action of flavonoids and coumarins on lipoxygenase and cyclooxygenase. Methods Enzymol. 1994;234:443–54.

Indrianingsih AW, Tachibana S, Itoh K. In vitro evaluation of antioxidant and α-glucosidase inhibitory assay of several tropical and subtropical plants. Procedia Environ Sci. 2015;25:639–48.

Iwatsuki M, Niki E, Stone D, Darley-Usmar VM. Alpha-tocopherol mediated peroxidation in the copper (II) and metmyoglobin induced oxidation of human low density lipoprotein: the influence of lipid hydroperoxides. FEBS Lett. 1995;360:271–6.

Janjua R, Munoz C, Gorell E, Rehmus W, Egbert B, Kern D, Chang ALS. A two-year, double-blind, randomized placebo-controlled trial of oral green tea polyphenols on the long-term clinical and histologic appearance of photoaging skin. Dermatol Surg. 2009;35:1057–65.

Jeon HY, Kim JK, Kim WG, Lee SJ. Effects of oral epigallocatechin gallate supplementation on the minimal erythema dose and UV-induced skin damage. Skin Pharmacol Physiol. 2009;22:137–41.

Kang HJ, Jo C, Kwon JH, Kim JH, Chung HJ, Byun MW. Effect of a pectin-based edible coating containing green tea powder on the quality of irradiated pork patty. Food Control. 2007;18:430–5.

Khan N, Mukhtar H. Tea and health: studies in humans. Curr Pharm Design. 2013;19:6141–7.

Kim H-S, Quon MJ, Kim J. New insights into the mechanisms of polyphenols beyond antioxidant properties; lessons from the green tea polyphenol, epigallocatechin 3-gallate. Redox Biol. 2014;2:187–95.

Laughton MJ, Evans PJ, Moroney MA, Hoult JRS, Halliwell B. Inhibition of mammalian 5-lipoxygenase and cyclo-oxygenase by flavonoids and phenolic dietary additives: relationship to antioxidant activity and to iron ion-reducing ability. Biochem Pharmacol. 1991;42:1673–81.

Lawless H, Heymann H. Sensory evaluation of food: principles and practices. Gaithersburg: Aspen Publishers; 1999.

Lee MJ, Lambert JD, Prabhu S, Meng XF, Lu H, Maliakal P, Ho CT, Yang CS. Delivery of tea polyphenols to the oral cavity by green tea levels and black tea extract. Cancer Epidemiol Biomark Prev. 2004;13:132–7.

Lien EJ, Ren S, Bui HH, Wang R. Quantitative structure–activity relationship analysis of phenolic antioxidants. Free Radic Biol Med. 1999;26:285–94.

Mabry TJ, Markham KR, Thomas MB, editors. The systematic identification of flavonoids. New York, NY: Springer-Verlag; 1970.

Mamphiswana ND, Mashela PW, Mdee LK. Accumulative capabilities of essential nutrient elements in organs of Monsonia burkeana. A J Biotechnol. 2011;10:16849–53.

Mander M, Steytler N, Lewis F, Rivers-Moore N. The economics of medicinal plant cultivation. Investigational report no. 206. Pietermaritzburg: Institute of Natural Resources; 1999.

Martínez MADP, Pelotto JP, Basualdo N. Distribution of flavonoid aglycones in Ilex species (Aquifoliaceae). Biochem Syst Ecol. 1997;25:619–22.

Masaki H. Role of antioxidants in the skin: anti-aging effects. J Dermatol Sci. 2010;58:58–90.

Matthiesen L, Malterud KE, Sund RB. Hydrogen bond formation as basis for radical scavenging activity: a structure–activity study of C-methylated dihydrochalcones from *Myrica gale* and structurally related acetophenones. Free Radic Biol Med. 1997;22:307–11.

McCarthy TL, Kerry JP, Kerry JF, Lynch PB, Buckley DJ. Evaluation of the antioxidant potential of natural food/plant extracts as compared with synthetic antioxidants and vitamin E in raw and cooked pork patties. Meat Sci. 2001;58:45–52.

Metrouh-Amir H, Duarte CMM, Maiza F. Solvent effect on total phenol contents, antioxidant, and antibacterial activities of *Matricaria pubescens*. Ind Crop Prod. 2015;67:249–56.

Middleton E Jr, Kandaswami C. Effects of flavonoids on immune and inflammatory cell functions. Biochem Pharmacol. 1992;43:1167–79.

Mitsumoto M, O'Grady MN, Kerry JP, Buckley DJ. Addition of tea catechins and vitamin C on sensory evaluation, colour and lipid stability during chilled storage in cooked or raw beef and chicken patties. Meat Sci. 2005;69:773–9.

Miyazawa T. Absorption, metabolism and antioxidative effects of tea catechin in humans. Bio Factors. 2000;13:55–9.

Moawad RK, Abozeid WM, Nadir AS. Effects of nitrite level and tea catechins on residual nitrite and quality indices of raw-cured sausages. J Applied Sci Res. 2012;8:815–22.

Mokrani A, Madani K. Effects of solvent, time and temperature on the extraction of phenolic compounds and antioxidant capacity of peach (Prunus persica L.) fruit. Sep Purfi Technol. 2016;162:68–76.

Montero P, Martínez-Álvarez O, Zamorano JP, Alique R, Gómez-Guillén MC. Melanosis inhibition and 4-hexylresorcinol residual levels in Deepwater pink shrimp (*Parapenaeus longirostris*) following various treatments. Eur Food Res Technol. 2006;223:1621.

Moore J, Hao Z, Zhou K, Luther M, Costa J, Yu LL. Carotenoid, tocopherol, phenolic acid, and antioxidant properties of Maryland-grown soft wheat. J Agric Food Chem. 2005;53:6649–57.

Mora A, Payá M, Ríos JL, Alcaraz MJ. Structure–activity relationships of polymethoxyflavones and other flavonoids as inhibitors of non-enzymic lipid peroxidation. Biochem Pharmacol. 1990;40:793–7.

Morton M, Arisaka O, Miyake A, Evans B. Analysis of phyto-oestrogens by gas chromatography-mass spectrometry. Environ Toxicol Pharmacol. 1999;7:221–5.

Mostafa AA, Al-Askar AA, Almaary KS, Dawoud TM, Sholkamy EN, Bakri MM. Antimicrobial activity of some plant extracts against bacterial strains causing food poisoning diseases. Suadi J Biol Sci. 2018;25:361–6.

Mudau F, Mariga IK. Bush tea as a herbal beverage and medicinal plant. In: Preedy VR, editor. Tea in health and disease prevention. 1st ed. Oxford, UK: Elsevier; 2012. p. 182–92.

Nakatani N. Biologically functional constituents of species and herbs. J Jpn Soc Nut Food Sci. 2003;56:389–95.

Namal Senanayake SPJ. Green tea extract: chemistry, antioxidant properties and food application–a review. J Funct Foods. 2013;5:1529–41.

Narasimhachari N, von Rudloff E. Gas–liquid chromatography of some flavonoid compounds and hydroxy diphenyls. Canadian J Chem. 1962;40:1123–9.

Nirmal NP, Benjakul S. Effect of green tea extract in combination with ascorbic acid on the retardation of melanosis and quality changes of Pacific white shrimp during iced storage. Food Bioprocess Tech. 2012;5:2941–51.

O'Sullivan CM, Lynch A, Lynch PB, Buckley DJ, Kerry JP. Assessment of the antioxidant potential of food ingredients in fresh, previously frozen and cooked chicken patties. Int J Poultry Sci. 2004;3:337–44.

Oh J, Jo H, Cho AR, Kim S-J, Han J. Antioxidant and antimicrobial activities of leafy herbal teas. Food Control. 2013;31:403–9.

Pereira ADS, Padilha MC, Neto FRDA. Two decades of high temperature gas chromatography (1983–2003): what's next? Microchem J. 2004;77:141–9.

Perumalla AS, Hettiarachchy NS. Green tea and grape seed extracts – potential applications in food safety and quality. Food Res Int. 2011;44:827–39.

Peterson J, Dwyer J, Bhagwat S, Haytowitz D, Holden J, Eldridge AL, Beecher G, Aladesanmi J. Major flavonoids in dry tea. J Food Comp Anal. 2005;18:487–501.

Pieri C, Marra M, Moroni F, Recchioni R, Marcheselli F. Melatonin: a peroxyl radical scavenger more effective than vitamin E. Life Sci. 1994;55:271–6.

Reddy V, Urooj A, Kumar A. Evaluation of antioxidant activity of some plant extracts and their application in biscuits. Food Chem Anal Nutri Clinical Methods. 2005;90:317–21.

Rice-Evans CA, Miller NJ, Paganga G. Antioxidant properties of phenolic compounds. Trends Plant Sci Rev. 1997a;2:152–9.

Rice-Evans CA, Miller NJ, Paganga G. Structure–antioxidant activity relationships of flavonoids and phenolic acids. Free Radic Biol Med. 1997b;20:933–56.

Richheimer SL, Bernart MW, King GA, Kent MC, Bailey DT. Antioxidant activity of lipid-soluble phenolic diterpenes from rosemary. J Am Oil Chem Soc. 1996;73:507–14.

Rodríguez-Delgado MA, Malovaná S, Pérez JP, Borges T, García Montelongo FJ. Separation of phenolic compounds by high-performance liquid chromatography with absorbance and fluorimetric detection. J Chromatogr A. 2001;912:249–57.

Sahu SC, Gray GC. Interactions of flavonoids, trace metals, and oxygen: nuclear DNA damage and lipid peroxidation induced by myricetin. Cancer Lett. 1993;70:73–9.

Sato K, Akaike T, Kohno M, Ando M, Maeda H. Hydroxyl radical production by H2O2 plus cu,Zn-superoxide dismutase reflects the activity of free copper released from the oxidatively damaged enzyme. J Biol Chem. 1992;267:25371–7.

Scharbert S, Hofmann T. Molecular definition of black tea taste by means of quantitative studies, taste reconstitution, and omission experiments. J Agric Food Chem. 2005;53:5337–84.

Shiu-Ming K. Dietary flavonoids and cancer prevention: evidence and potential mechanism. Crit Rev Oncog. 1997;8:47–69.

Siess MH, Leclerc J, Canivenc-Lavier MC, Rat P, Suschetet M. Heterogenous effects of natural flavonoids on monooxygenase activities in human and rat liver microsomes. Toxicol Appl Pharmacol. 1995;130:73–8.

Sivarooban Y, Hettiarachchy NS, Johnson MG. Transmission electron microscopy study of Listeria monocytogenes treated with nisin in combination with either grape seed or green tea extract. J Food Prot. 2008;71:2105–9.

Spies R. Application of rheology in the bread industry. In: Faridi H, Faubion JM, editors. Dough rheology and baked product texture. New York: Van Nostrand Reinhold; 1990. p. 343–61.

Sunilson JAJ, Suraj R, Rejitha G, Anandarajagopal K, Kumari AVAG, Promwichit P. In vitro antimicrobial evaluation of *Zingiber officinale, Curcuma longa and Alpinia galangal* extracts as natural food preservatives. Am J Food Technol. 2009;4:192–200.

Tanigawa T, Kanazawa S, Ichibori R, Fujiwara T, Magome T, Shingaki K, Miyata S, Hata Y, Tomita K, Matsuda K, Kubo T, Tohyama M, Yano K, Hosokawa K. (+)-Catechin protects dermal fibroblasts against oxidative stress-induced apoptosis. BMC Complement Altern Med. 2014;14:133–9.

Tang SZ, Kerry JP, Sheehan D, Buckley DJ, Morrisey PA. Antioxidative effect of added tea catechins on susceptibility of cooked red meat, poultry and fish patties to lipid oxidation. Food Res Int. 2001;34:651–7.

Tarling CA, Woods K, Zhang S, Brastianos HC, Brayer GD, Andersen RJ, et al. The search for novel human pancreatic α-amylase inhibitors: high-throughput screening of terrestrial and marine natural product extracts. Chembiochem. 2008;9:433–8.

Thorsen MA, Hildebrandt KS. Quantitative determination of phenolic diterpenes in rosemary extracts: aspects of accurate identification. J Chromatogr. 2003;9:119–25.

Turkmen N, Sari F, Velioglu S. Effects of extraction solvents on concentration and antioxidant activity of black and black mate tea polyphenols determined by ferrous tartrate and Folin–Ciocalteu methods. Food Chem. 2006;99:835–41.

Udompataikul M, Sripiroj P, Palungwachira P. An oral nutraceutical containing antioxidants, minerals and glycosaminoglycans improves skin roughness and fine wrinkles. Int J Cosmetic Sci. 2009;31:427–35.

Wanasundara UN, Shahidi F. Antioxidant and pro-oxidant activity of green tea extracts in marine oils. Food Chem. 1998;63:335–42.

Wang H, Helliwell K. Determination of flavonols in green and black tea leaves and green tea infusions by high-performance liquid chromatography. Food Res Int. 2001;34:223–7.

Wang YF, Huang SR, Shao SH. Studies on bioactivities of tea (Camellia sinensis L.) fruit peel extracts: antioxidant activity and inhibitory potential against α-glucosidase and α-amylase in vitro. Ind Crop Prod. 2012;37:520–6.

Willcox JK, Ash SL, Catignani GL. Antioxidants and prevention of chronic disease. Crit Rev Food Sci Nutr. 2004;44:275–95.

Yoshida Y, Tsuchiya J, Niki E. Interaction of alpha-tocopherol with copper and its effect on lipid peroxidation. Biochem Biophys Acta. 1994;1200:85–92.

Yu L, Haley S, Perret J, Harris M, Wilson J, Qian M. Free radical scavenging properties of wheat extracts. J Agric Food Chem. 2002;50:1619–24.

Yu Z-L, Gao H-X, Zhang Z, He Z, He Q, Jia L-R, Zeng W-C. Inhibitory effects of Ligustrum robustum (Rxob.) Blume extracts on α-amylase and α-glucosidase. J Funct Foods. 2015;19:204–13.

Zhao J, Deng JW, Chen YW, Li SP. Advanced phytochemical analysis of herbal tea in China. J Chromatogr A. 2013;1313:2–23.

Zhong DF, Yang DF, Chen XY, Li K, Xu JH. Determination of scutellarin in rat plasma by high-performance liquid chromatography with ultraviolet detection. J Chromatogr B Analyt Technol Biomed Life Sci. 2003;796:439–44.

Zhou K, Yu L. Effects of extraction solvent on wheat bran antioxidant activity estimation. LWT Food Sci Techn. 2004;37:717–21.

Zhou K, Su L, Yu L. Phytochemicals and antioxidant properties in wheat bran. J Agric Food Chem. 2004;52:6108–14.

Zieliński H, Kozlowska H. Antioxidant activity and total phenolics in selected cereal grains and their different morphological fractions. J Agric Food Chem. 2000;48:2008–16.

Zou Y, Chen H, Deng Y. Simultaneous determination of catechins, caffeine and gallic acids in green, oolong, black and pu-erh teas using HPLC with a photodiode array detector. Talanta. 2002;57:307–16.

Extraction, Isolation, and Quantitative Determination of Flavonoids by HPLC

21

Ashim K. Sen, Dhanya B. Sen, and Rajesh A. Maheshwari

Contents

21.1 Introduction

Throughout the world, herbal medicines (HMs) which form a major component of complementary and alternative medicine (CAM) are gaining popularity over conventional mainstream medicine in the treatment of diseases. Their use has been well documented in various ancient

A. K. Sen (✉) · D. B. Sen · R. A. Maheshwari
Department of Pharmacy, Sumandeep Vidyapeeth Deemed to be University, Vadodara, Gujarat, India

S. Sen, R. Chakraborty (eds.), *Herbal Medicine in India*, https://doi.org/10.1007/978-981-13-7248-3_21

texts and literature which have stood the test of time. The Western world is now embracing eastern philosophies and thereby adopting the practice of using herbal medicines which tend to have potent pharmacological action with minimalistic side effects and rare complications (Bansal et al. 2014).

The pressures of the modern world and the ailments that follow us with a busy working schedule make people susceptible to various ailments and burden them with huge health-care costs. This has made many to change their lifestyles and incorporate herbal medicine into their daily routine and the shift from symptomatic treatment to wellness has gained popularity. Looking at this rise in popularity for HMs, efforts are underway to standardize them and monitor their production. India as a country is not new to HMs or CAM. It's the land of ancient traditional practices like Ayurveda which is still practiced widely. Efforts are underway to popularize it further but the need of the hour is to standardize their production, implement stringent quality control practices, have extensive research and seize on the opportunity of increased interest among people regarding HMs over conventional treatments owing to the high cost and side effects of modern treatments (Pandey et al. 2013).

Plants have always formed the bedrock/backbone of treatment in various medicinal systems practiced across the globe. Of late many people across the globe are relying on plant-based medicine to maintain, manage and improve their health conditions in conjunction with conventional treatments. Various reports from the WHO state that a significant proportion of the world's population rely on HMs for the treatment of their ailments and which constitute various plant parts like leaves, bark, root etc. HMs also include various preparations like decoctions, teas, infusions etc. This rise in popularity of HMs across the globe is due to the fact that they do not cause much side effects or complications in comparison to conventional treatment options in the long run and also are seen as a ray of hope in the management of chronic ailments and as saviors in our fight against microbial resistance. We find that almost 75% of the therapeutic entities originated from plant sources which are used worldwide were mentioned in traditional/folk medicine. In India, about 70% of present-day drugs are derived from natural resources and synthetically engineered compounds from prototype substances extracted from plants. It was accounted that over 60% of antineoplastic drugs accessible to the mankind or in clinical trials are natural products. Presently, around 80% of antineoplastic, antimicrobial, cardiovascular and immunosuppressive medications are discovered from herbal sources. Natural products and its mimetics constitute nearly 70% drug candidates among 177 approved antineoplastic agents. It is further documented that between 2005 and 2007, there are 13 drugs of plant origin permitted in the United States and over 100 drugs based on natural product are undergoing clinical trials. Twenty-eight drugs out of 252 drugs published in Essential drug list by the WHO are exclusively of herbal origin. It was additionally assessed that 1200–1800 plants are used in Ayurveda, 500–900 plants are utilized in Siddha medicines, 400–700 medicinal plants are exploited in Unani and Amchi medicine which consumes 300 plants whereas 7500 medicinal plants are used by Indian folk healers. There is mention about 526, 573 and 902 number of plants in classical Ayurvedic texts such as Charaka Samhita, Sushruta Samhita and Astanga Hridaya, respectively (Pan et al. 2014; Sen and Chakraborty 2017; Wachtel-Galor and Benzie 2011; Pan et al. 2013; Debnath et al. 2015; Shankar and Majumdar 1997).

In spite of having such tremendous potential therapeutically, HMs have always faced issues relating to quality, safety and efficacy. Clinical and safety data concerning the dosage, side effects and toxicity have hindered HMs from being accepted into the mainstream treatment protocols. Looking at these issues, the World Health Organization (WHO) has given guidelines for the assessment of the quality of HMs. These guidelines help us maintain minimum standards for the manufacturing of quality herbal products (WHO 2000).

Assessment of quality and genuineness of HMs are of great concern in today's time, hence some substances called markers or pharmacologically active constituents in herbs or herbal mixtures are employed. Though this kind of determination does not reflect the true essence of HMs as they work in a holistic manner and the multiple constituents together help to give a synergistic effect which has to be embraced to realize their full potential (Juan and Tauler 2003; Liang et al. 2004).

Phytochemistry has developed into an independent discipline distinguishing itself from natural product organic chemistry, plant biotechnology and plant biochemistry in recent years. It has evolved from the parent discipline natural products chemistry and involves the study of plant constituents, their biosynthesis, metabolism, natural distribution and biological functions. The fact that just under 6% of around 6 lakh types of plants on earth has been explored demonstrates the opportunity offered and challenges tossed open to phytochemists. The assignment of phytochemist is built up in achieving the characterization of little amount of the mixes isolable from plants. Phytochemistry additionally appreciates the use of modern research for the scientific examination of familial observational learning. It has wide range of application in about all fields of life and development. Its direct contribution in the field of nourishment and sustenance, agribusiness, medication and cosmetics is notable for quite a long time (Miller 1973; Loewus and Ryan 1981; Reinhold et al. 1977; Harborne 1988; Dey 1989; Rahman 1989; Van Beek and Breteler 1993). Polyphenolics constitute a distinct group among the phytochemicals and they are characterized by the presence of an aromatic ring with one or more hydroxyl substituents or their ether or glycoside derivatives. Among the various secondary metabolites, they possess a great degree of structural diversity and widespread occurrence. They are also known to interact with primary metabolites such as polysaccharides and proteins. Flavonoids tend to be the most widespread naturally occurring phenolic compounds (Middleton and Kandaswami 1993).

Flavonoids comprise a vast collection of polyphenolic compounds which contain a benzo-ũFE;-pyrone structure and are universally found in plants. These compounds are synthesized through phenylpropanoid pathway. Accessible reports demonstrate that secondary metabolites of phenolic nature (for instance, flavonoids) are accountable for the wide range of pharmacological properties (Mahomoodally et al. 2005; Pandey 2007). Basically, flavonoids are hydroxylated phenolic compounds which are synthesized by plants in reaction to microbial infection (Dixon et al. 1983). The chemical nature of flavonoids relies upon their basic class, level of hydroxylation, different substitutions and conjugations and level of polymerization (Heim et al. 2002). As the antioxidant effect of flavonoid compounds provides with potential health benefits, recent interest in these compounds have been increased. The functional hydroxyl group in the flavonoids is responsible for their antioxidant activity by ROS scavenging and metal ion chelating ability (Kumar et al. 2013a, b; Kumar and Pandey 2013a, b). The metal chelation ability of flavonoids assumes a significant role in the prevention of free radical production which is responsible for the damage of target biomolecules (Leopoldini et al. 2006; Kumar et al. 2013a, b). Flavonoids are capable of inducing human defensive enzyme systems. Numerous studies have recommended defensive impacts of flavonoids against several irresistible (bacterial and viral illnesses) and degenerative infections, for example, cardiovascular maladies, malignancies and other age-related ailments (Pandey 2007; Kumar et al. 2013a, b; Cook and Samman 1996; Rice-Evans et al. 1995). Flavonoids additionally act as supplementary antioxidizing agents which protect the plant tissues go through various abiotic and biotic stresses. They are situated in the core of mesophyll cells and inside centers of ROS production. They additionally direct development factors in plants, for example, auxin (Agati et al. 2012). Biosynthetic qualities have been composed in a few microscopic organisms for increased formation of flavonoids (Du et al. 2011).

21.2 Chemistry of Flavonoids

Flavonoids are a group of plant-derived natural compounds having different phenolic structures. In early 1930, separation of oranges led to the discovery of a new substance which was labelled as vitamin P and it was thought to be a vitamin of a new class. This substance was proved to be flavonoids (rutin) later on and presently there are more than four thousand varieties of flavonoids identified so far. Chemical structure of flavonoids is founded upon a fifteen-carbon skeleton comprising two benzene rings (A and B as given in Fig. 21.1) connected through a heterocyclic pyran ring (C).

Flavonoids may be classified into various groups like flavones (e.g., apigenin, luteolin, chrysin), flavonols (e.g., kaempferol, quercetin, myricetin and isorhamnetin), flavanones (e.g., hesperetin, naringenin and eriodictyol), flavanols (catechins, gallocatechin and epicatechin) and others. General structures of flavonoids are shown in Table 21.1. The level of oxidation and substitution pattern of the C ring varies with different classes of flavonoids. However, single compounds in a class diverge in the pattern of substitution of the A and B rings (Middleton 1998). Flavonoids exist as aglycones, glycosides and methylated derivatives. Aglycone is the basic flavonoid structure (Fig. 21.1). Six-member ring condensed with the benzene ring is either a ũFC;-pyrone (flavonols and flavanones) or its dihydroderivative (flavonols and flavanones). The flavonoid class can be divided into flavonoids (2-position) and isoflavonoids (3-position) depending upon the position of the benzenoid substituent. Flavonols can be differentiated from flavanones by a hydroxyl group at the 3-position and a C2–C3 double bond (Narayana et al. 2001). Hydroxylation of flavonoids often occurs in positions 3, 5, 7, 2, 3′, 4′ and 5′. Methyl ethers and acetyl esters of the alcohol group are naturally existing. During the formation of glycosides, the glycosidic linkage is generally positioned at 3 or 7 and the carbohydrate might be L-rhamnose, D-glucose, glucorhamnose, galactose or arabinose (Middleton 1984).

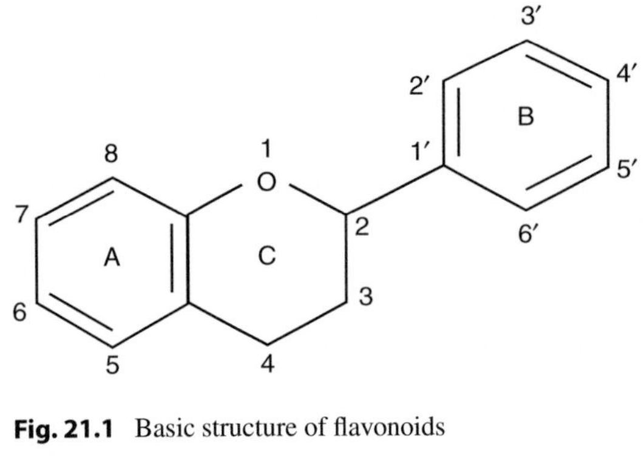

Fig. 21.1 Basic structure of flavonoids

21.3 Natural Sources of Flavonoids

Majority of plant parts contain flavonoids, predominantly the photosynthesizing plant cells and they are widely distributed group of plant phenolic compounds. Flavonoids are considered an essential component of human and animal diets (Harborne and Turner 1984; Clifford and Cuppett 2000). It is impossible to synthesize flavonoids by humans and animals as they are plant-derived phytochemicals. As the animals are incapable of biosynthesizing flavonoids in situ, plant-based animal feeds are the sole source of flavonoids found in animals. Around five thousand varieties of plant-derived flavonoids have been isolated from numerous plants (Cook and Samman 1996). The subgroups of flavonoids commonly found in the dietary sources are listed in Table 21.2 (Cook and Samman 1996; Bravo 1988; Aherne and Obrien 2002; Yao et al. 2004). The most plentiful flavonoids present in food are flavonols with the other three most common flavonoids being quercetin, kaempferol, and myricetin. Flavanones and flavones are primarily present in citrus fruits and in celery, respectively. Green and black teas together with red wine are rich sources of catechins, while anthocyanins are present in strawberries and other berries. Soy foods are an almost exclusive source of isoflavones. Flowering plants contain flavonoids as a major coloring component, which is present in all plant-based foods. Flavonoids present in food play a major role as they impart color and taste

Table 21.1 Chemical structure of some common flavonoids

Group of flavonoids	Structure backbone	Examples		
Flavones	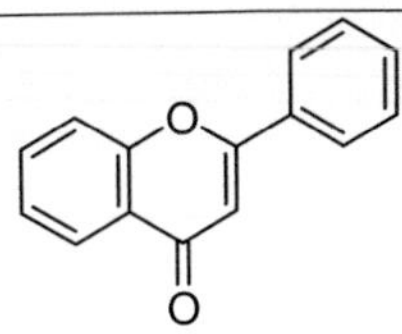	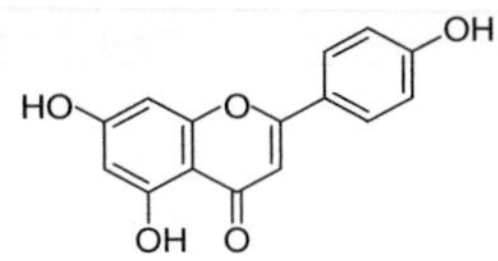 Apigenin	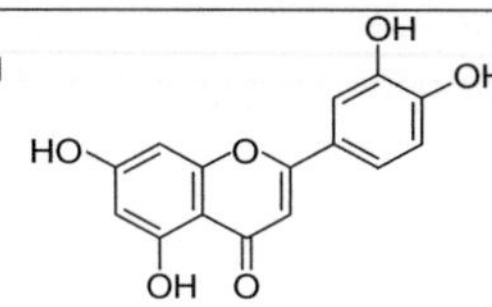 Luteolin	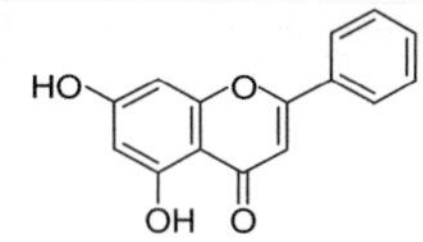 Chrysin
Flavonols	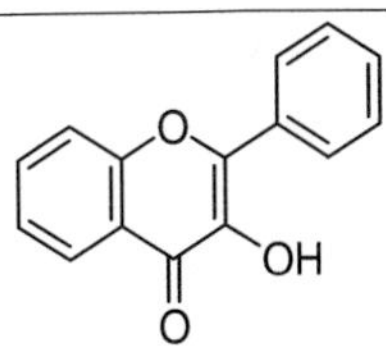	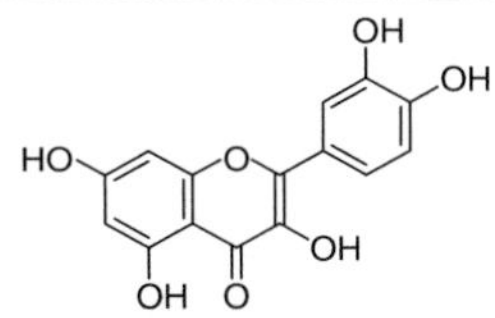 Quercetin	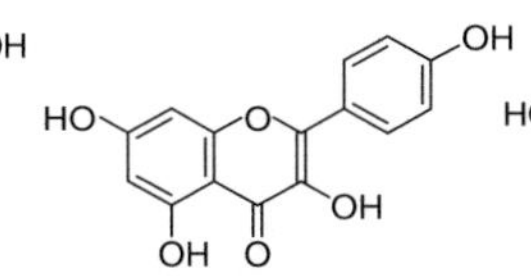 Kaempferol	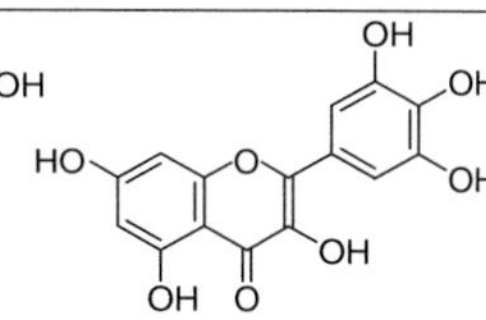 Myricetin
Flavanones	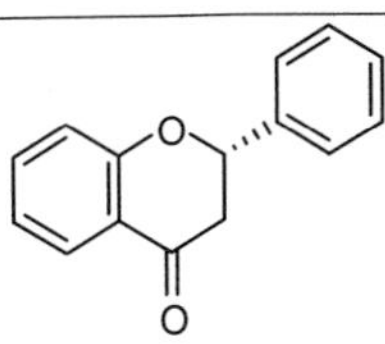	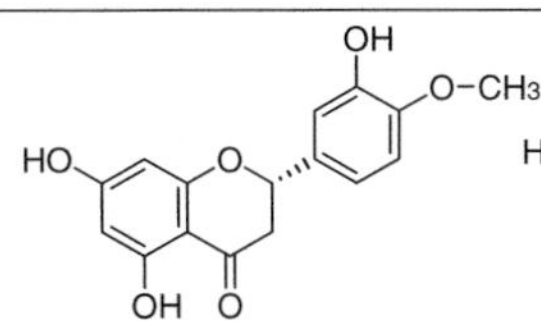 Hesperetin	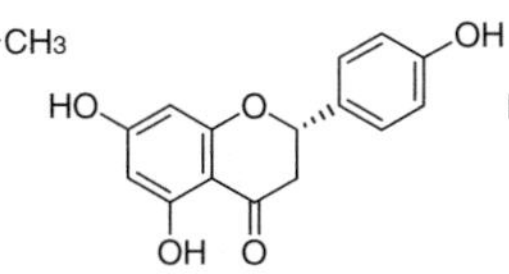 Naringenin	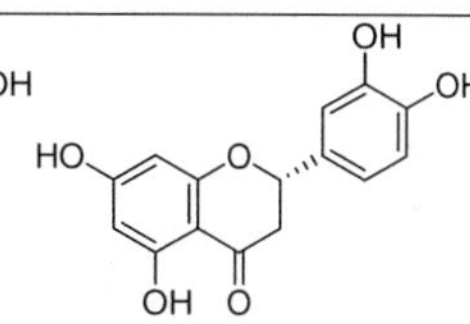 Eriodictyol
Flavanols	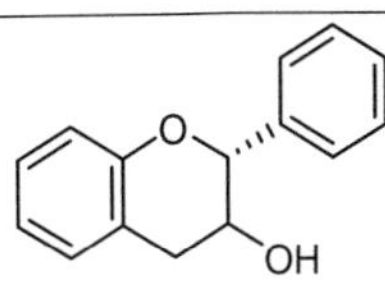	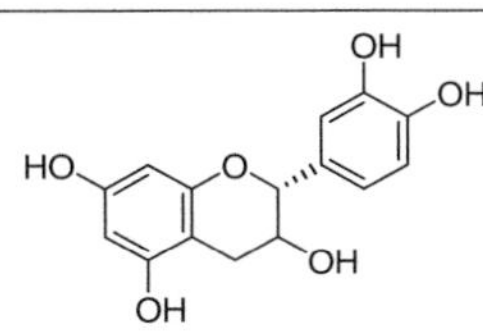 Catechin	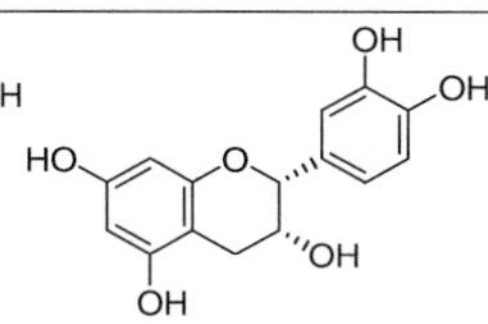 Epicatechin	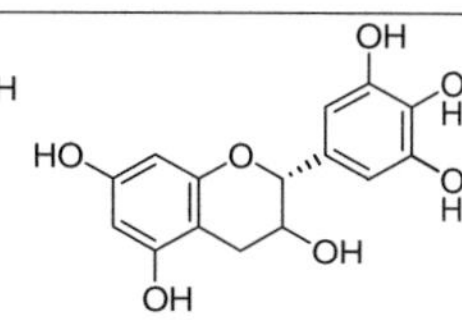 Gallocatechin
Isoflavones	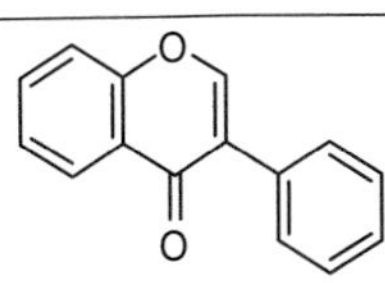	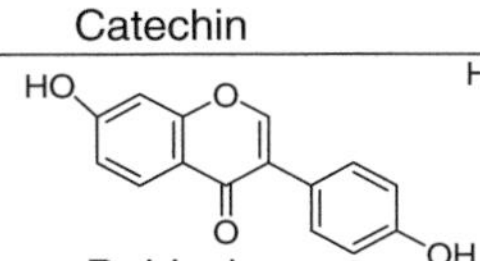 Daidzein	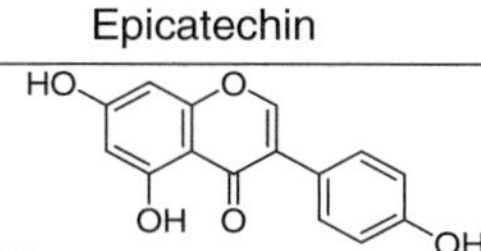 Genistein	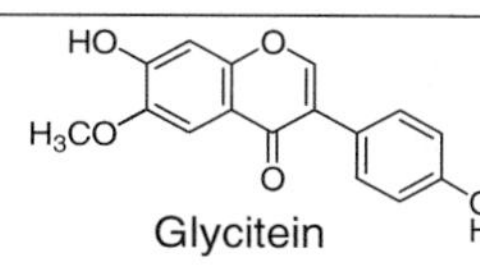 Glycitein
Anthocyanins	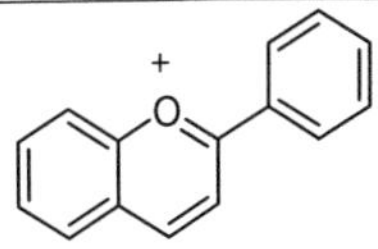	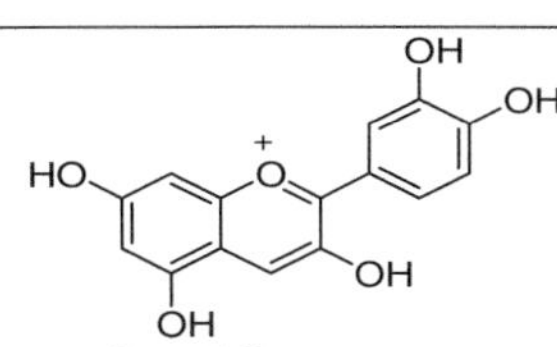 Cyanidin	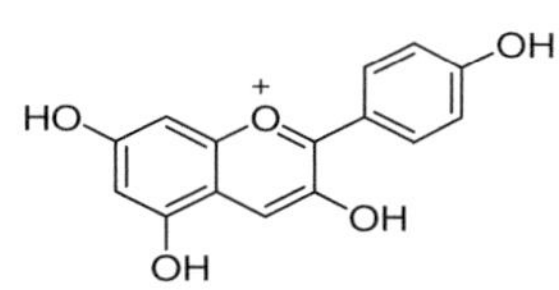 Pelargonidin	

to foods and also prevent oxidation of fat. Moreover, they protect vitamins and enzymes (Peterson and Dwyer 1998).

Numerous factors such as variation and the degree of light exposure affect the distribution of flavonoids in plants. Light accelerates the formation of oxidized flavonoids. Flavonoids functions as coloring agents. Therefore, foods with a natural flavor and coloring may contain flavonoids. Flavanones are the predominantly occurring coloring agents in citrus fruits, isoflavonoids in legumes and flavones primarily in herbs, whereas teas, fruits, and vegetables contain anthocyanins and catechins as coloring agents (Huang et al. 1994; Ho et al. 1994). Teas, fruits, and vegetables are excellent sources of natural

Table 21.2 Flavonoid subgroups, representative flavonoids and their sources

Class	Representative flavonoids	Food/dietary sources
Flavones	Apigenin, luteolin, chrysin, diosmetin, tangeretin	Herbs, fruits, vegetables, cereals, flowers parsley, thyme
Flavonols	Quercetin, kaempferol, myricetin, isorhamnetin, rutin, rhamnetin, isorhamnetin	Onions, tomatoes, cherries, tea, red wine apples, broccoli, kale, berries, tartary buckwheat
Flavanones	Hesperidin, naringenin, eriodictyol, neohesperidin	Citrus fruits, oranges, grapefruits, cumin, peppermint
Flavanols	Catechins, gallocatechin, epicatechin, epigallocatechin gallate, procyanidin, theaflavins	Apples, tea, beer, wine, fruit juice, black tea, hops
Isoflavones	Daidzein, genistein, glycitein, formononetin	Legumes (e.g. soybeans)
Anthocyanins	Cyanidin	Fruits and flowers

Table 21.3 Medicinal plants containing flavonoids

Plant	Family	Flavonoid
Aloe vera	Asphodelaceae	Luteolin
Acalypha indica	Euphorbiaceae	Kaempferol glycosides
Azadirachta indica	Meliaceae	Quercetin
Andrographis paniculata	Acanthaceae	5-hydroxy-7,8-dimethoxyflavone
Bacopa monnieri	Scrophulariaceae	Luteolin
Betula pendula	Betulaceae	Quercetin
Butea monospermea	Fabaceae	Genistein
Bauhinia monandra	Fabaceae	Quercetin-3-O-rutinoside
Byrsonima crassa	Malpighiaceae	(+)-Catechin
Calendula officinalis	Compositae	Isorhamnetin
Cannabis sativa	Compositae	Quercetin
Citrus medica	Rutaceae	Hesperidin
Clerodendrum phlomidis	Verbenaceae	Pectolinarigenin
Clitoria ternatea	Fabaceae	Kaempferol-3-neohesperidoside
Glycyrrhiza glabra	Leguminosae	Liquiritin
Mimosa pudica	Mimosoideae	Isoquercetin
Limnophila indica	Scrophulariaceae	3,4-Methlenedioxyflavone
Mentha longifolia	Lamiaceae	Luteolin-7-O-glycoside
Momordica charantia	Cucurbitaceae	Luteolin
Oroxylum indicum	Bignoniaceae	Chrysin
Passiflora incarnate	Passifloraceae	Vitexin
Pongamia pinnata	Fabaceae	Pongaflavonol
Tephrosia purpurea	Fabaceae	Purpurin
Tilia cordata	Tiliaceae	Hyperoside

phenolic compounds; however, red wine and coffee also contain some amounts of polyphenols (Ho et al. 1992). Flavanones, flavones, and flavonols are the major flavonoids found in citrus fruits (Benavente-Garcia et al. 1997), while citrus volatiles contain genistein (Saleh et al. 1998). French wines made from six grape varieties and three growing zones are found to have different types of anthocyanins and flavonoids (Etievant et al. 1988). Some of the medicinal plants (Kumar and Pandey 2013a, b) rich in flavonoids content are listed in Table 21.3.

21.4 Flavonoid-Rich Foods

21.4.1 Amount Present in Foods

Flavonoids present in large quantity in human diet comprise the flavones (luteolin and apigenin), soy isoflavones (biochanin A, genistein, daidzein) and flavonols (kaempferol, quercetin, myricetin) (Rosenberg et al. 2002). Genetic factors for example:- species, environmental surroundings like light, ripeness and post-harvest treatments like processing influence the level of individual and aggregate flavonoids in food (Bravo 1988; Duthie et al. 2000; Chu et al. 2000). Even though majority of fruits and some leguminous plants have catechins, the levels shift from 4.5 to 610 mg/kg for kiwifruit and dark chocolate, respectively (Arts et al. 2000a, b). Concentration of quercetin in the consumable portion of vegetables is normally under 10 mg/kg (Hertog et al. 1992, 1993a, b). The range of quercetin in black tea infusions varies from 10 to 25 mg/L, whereas myricetin and kaempferol range from 2 to 5 mg/L and 7 to 17 mg/L, respectively. Tea is the main beverage that has gallocatechin (GC), epicatechin gallate (ECG), epigallocatechin (EGC), and epigallocatechin gallate (EGCG), along with epicatechin (EC) and catechin (Arts et al. 2000a, b). Up to 35% of the dry matter of green tea constitutes of phenolic compounds which are highest among foods (Bravo 1988). It is believed that wine flavor is influenced by phenolic compounds and in total, wines have nearly 200 mg gallic acid equiv./L of phenolic content; on the other hand, young red table wines have nearly 750 mg/L anthocyanogenic tannins, 120 mg/L anthocyanins, 50 mg/L flavonols and 250 mg/L catechins (Singleton and Noble 1976). The differences in flavonoid content might be utilized to distinguish food types. Nevertheless, the method used for preparation and processing of food possibly will reduce concentration of flavonoid (Garcia-Viguera et al. 1997). For instance, in a latest research paper, orange juices contained 81–200 mg/L dissolvable flavanones, whereas the concentration in the cloud was 206–644 mg/L, proposing that the flavanones were concentrated and present in the cloud in the course of processing and storage (Gil-Izquierdo et al. 2001).

21.4.2 Dietary Intake

The plant pigments belonging to the flavonoid family consist of the most extensively scattered group of auxiliary plant foods consumed by humans. Due to the facts that flavonoids are available in wide varieties, are extensively distributed in numerous plants and also have varied consumptions by people, it is difficult to estimate the average dietary intake of flavonoids accurately (Tomas-Barberan and Clifford 2000). Therefore, the determination of flavonoid intake rests completely on the conditions of analysis, the technique utilized, and the reference substances chosen for investigation. Keeping this in consideration, the dietary admission of flavonoids has been varied from 100 to 1000 mg/day for assessment (Aherne and Obrien 2002). Despite the fact that the dietary information on dihydrochalcones and flavanones are not accessible until now, they may significantly contribute to the regular consumption of flavonoids. In spite of thermo-stable nature of flavonoids, they are easily destroyed during cooking process (Hertog et al. 1993a, b). By means of passive diffusion, flavonoids are absorbed after the glycosylated flavonoids are converted to respective aglycones. In this transformation, colon microflora plays a vital role. The bioavailability of flavonoids is only fractional, with the percentage of the consumed amount that is absorbed differing from 0.2 to 0.9 for tea catechins and 20% for quercetin and isoflavones (Hollman et al. 1995; Lee et al. 1995). Conjugation of flavonoids takes place in liver after absorption by phase II reactions and metabolized to smaller phenolic substances (Bravo 1988). Food source is also a major deciding factor for the bioavailability of certain flavonoids. For instance, when compared to apples or tea, quercetin found in onions shows a fourfold increase in absorption (Hollman et al. 1997).

21.5 Flavonoids and Their Biological Activities

21.5.1 Antioxidant Activity

Flavonoids have numerous biological and chemical properties, yet antioxidant property is found to be the most studied and acknowledged among all of them which rely on the arrangement of functional groups. Numerous mechanisms of antioxidant activity like free radical scavenging and metal ion chelation capacity depend on the arrangement, substitution and summative number of hydroxyl groups (Heim et al. 2002; Pandey et al. 2012). Suppression of reactive oxygen species (ROS) mediate majority of antioxidant action. This process can take place through inhibition of enzymes or by chelation of trace elements which are responsible for free radical production, scavenging ROS and upregulation of antioxidant defenses (Halliwell and Gutteridge 1998; Kumar and Pandey 2013a, b). Flavonoids restrain the proteins associated with ROS production, that is, microsomal monooxygenase, glutathione S-transferase, mitochondrial succinoxidase, NADH oxidase, etc. (Brown et al. 1998). Lipid peroxidation is a general outcome of oxidative pressure and flavonoid shield lipids from oxidative damage through different mechanisms (Kumar et al. 2013a, b; Kumar and Pandey 2012). Free metal ion reduces hydrogen peroxide by generating highly reactive hydroxyl radical thereby enhancing ROS formation.

On account of their ability to chelate metal particles (for instance, copper and iron), flavonoids prevent them from forming free radicals thus providing protection against oxidative stress (Mishra et al. 2013a, b). Previous studies demonstrated that flavonoids with unsaturated 2–3 bonds in conjugation with a 4-oxo functional groups are having more antioxidant effects than the flavonoids deficient in any of these features (Rice-Evans et al. 1996). Antioxidant activity of flavonoids is highly influenced by existence, location, structure and sugar moieties present in them (flavonoids glycosides). Thus, flavonoid contributes as antioxidant in prevention of many diseases caused due to oxidative stress (Ratty and Das 1988).

21.5.2 Hepatoprotective Activity

Numerous flavonoids which include quercetin, catechin, rutin, naringenin, venoruton and apigenin are pronounced for their hepatoprotective action (Tapas et al. 2008). Various chronic diseases like diabetes play a major role in developing alteration in liver function due to the changes in glutamate-cysteine ligase catalytic subunit (GCLC) expression, glutathione and ROS levels. Researcher depicted in previous studies that anthocyanin cyanidin-3-O-β-lucoside (C3G) enhances hepatic GCLC expression by increasing cAMP levels to stimulate protein kinase A (PKA), which in turn upsurges cAMP response element-binding protein (CREB) phosphorylation to encourage CREB-DNA binding and rise GCLC transcription. Upregulation of GCLC expression showed a significant reduction in ROS levels in liver and proapoptotic signaling. In addition, treatment of C3G reduces lipid peroxidation level in liver, along with inhibition of proinflammatory cytokines release, hence protecting against the progression of hepatic steatosis (Zhu et al. 2012). Silymarin is a flavonoid having three basic parts silibinin, silydianine and silychristine isolated from the seeds and fruits of milk thistle *Silybum marianum* (Compositae). It has been reported that silymarin stimulates enzymatic action of DNA-dependent RNA polymerase 1 thereby facilitating biosynthesis of RNA and protein. This results in DNA biosynthesis and cell multiplication eventually leading to liver regeneration only in liver damage (Sonnenbichler and Zetl 1986). Silymarin regulates the cell membrane penetrability and integrity, inhibits leukotriene, scavenging of ROS and suppresses NF-kB activity, protein kinases and collagen production. On account of the abovementioned mechanism, silymarin is useful in the management of cirrhosis, ischemic injury and toxic hepatitis induced by several toxins such as paracetamol and toxic mushroom (He et al. 2004; Saller et al. 2001). It was previously reported in several studies that flavonoids can be used safely and efficiently in GI complaints such as anorexia, nausea, abdominal pain and hepatobiliary diseases. *Equisetum arvense* flavonoids in addition to hirustrin and avicularin isolated from a few different sources is pronounced to offer protection from hepatotoxicity (chemically induced) in HepG2 cells (Spencer et al. 2009; Kim et al. 2011).

21.5.3 Antibacterial Activity

Flavonoids are substances which are produced by plants in reaction to microbial disease; along these lines, it ought not to be astonishing that they have been observed *in vitro* to be compelling antimicrobial agents which act on a wide exhibit of microorganisms. Plant extracts rich in flavonoids from various species have been accounted to have antibacterial action (Mishra et al. 2011, 2013a, b; Pandey et al. 2010). A few flavonoids like isoflavones, galangin, apigenin, flavone and flavonol glycosides, flavanones and chalcones have been appeared to have strong antibacterial action (Cushnie and Lamb 2005). Antibacterial flavonoids may have many cell targets, as opposed to one particular site of activity. In this manner, their method of antimicrobial activity might be identified with their capacity to deactivate enzymes, microbial adhesins, cell envelope transport proteins etc. Lipophilic flavonoids may likewise disturb microbial membrane (Cowan 1999; Mishra et al. 2009). Catechins have been accounted for their *in vitro* antibacterial action on *Shigella, Vibrio cholerae*, *Streptococcus mutans* and other bacteria (Borris 1996; Moerman 1996). Robinetin, myricetin, and (−)-epigallocatechin are responsible for inhibition of DNA synthesis in *Proteus vulgaris* (Mori et al. 1987). Quercetin, apigenin and 3,6,7,3′,4′-pentahydroxyflavone show inhibitory activity against *Escherichia coli* DNA gyrase (Ohemeng et al. 1993). Naringenin and sophoraflavanone G are found to have potent antibacterial action on methicillin-resistant *Staphylococcus aureus* (MRSA) and streptococci (Tsuchiya and Iinuma 2000). Haraguchi et al. reported licochalcones A and C flavonoids present in roots of *Glycyrrhiza inflata to* have antibacterial activity against *S. aureus* and *Micrococcus luteus* (Haraguchi et al. 1998).

21.5.4 Anti-inflammatory Activity

Tissue injury, infection caused by microbial pathogens and irritation due to chemicals may lead to inflammation which is a common biological and biochemical process. Immune cells migrate from blood vessels and release inflammatory mediators at injury site due to inflammation. This procedure is observed through inflammatory cells, release of ROS, reactive nitrogen species (RNS) and proinflammatory cytokines eradicating extraneous pathogens and restoring injured tissues. Normally, common inflammation is fast and self-restricted, yet aberrant evolution and continued infection cause several chronic ailments (Pan et al. 2010). The immune system may be altered by diet, environmental toxins, pharmacologic agents and naturally existing food chemical compounds. Some flavonoids play a major role in functioning of inflammatory cells and immune system (Middleton and Kandaswami 1992). A number of prominent flavonoids like quercetin, hesperidin, luteolin, and apigenin are known to have anti-inflammatory and pain-relieving properties. They may have an effect on function of enzyme systems unfavorably taking part in the progression of inflammatory procedures, mainly tyrosine and serine-threonine protein kinases (Nishizuka 1988; Hunter 1995). Flavonoids competitively bind with ATP at catalytic sites on the kinase enzymes thus inhibiting them. These enzymes are accountable for signal transduction and cell activation processes which involve cells of the immune system. Some studies also revealed that flavonoids are capable of inhibiting expression of isoforms of inducible nitric oxide synthase, cyclooxygenase and lipoxygenase which are accountable for the generation of an abundant quantity of nitric oxide, prostanoids, leukotrienes and additional intermediaries of the inflammatory process like cytokines, chemokines or adhesion molecules (Tunon et al. 2009).

21.5.5 Anticancer Activity

Dietary elements are having a vital role in preventing cancers. Flavonoids present in fruits and vegetables have shown anticancer activity (Mishra et al. 2013a, b; Ho et al. 1994). It is evident from the studies that consumption of apples and onions, which are major sources of the flavonol quercetin can prevent occurrence of cancer of the breast, prostate, stomach and lung. Moreover, epidemiological studies also suggest that moderate wine consumption also have a negative impact on development of the lung, stomach, esophagus, endometrium and colon cancer (Koen et al. 2005). The crucial relationship between consumption of fruits and vegetables and prevention of malignant growth has been widely reported and thus increasing consumption of foods containing flavonoids will unquestionably result in major public health benefits (Block et al. 1992). Mechanisms for the effect of flavonoids on the initial and advanced stages of the malignancy comprising impacts on developmental and hormonal actions have been put forth (Duthie et al. 2000). Flavonoids act by the following mechanisms of action.

(a) Downregulation of mutant p53 protein
(b) Cell cycle arrest
(c) Inhibition of tyrosine kinase
(d) Heat shock proteins inhibition
(e) Estrogen receptor binding capacity
(f) Inhibition of expression of Ras proteins

Commonly, genetic abnormalities are seen in human cancers due to the upregulation of mutant p53 protein. However, the downregulation of p53 protein expression may result in the arrest of the G2-M phase of the cancer cell cycle. Expression of mutant p53 protein can downregulate almost untraceable levels in breast cancer cell lines by the flavonoids (Davis and Matthew 2000). Tyrosine kinases are enzymes which take part in the transduction of growth factor signals to the nucleus. Researchers depicted in many studies that the expression of tyrosine kinase might be responsible for cancer cell growth and division. Tyrosine kinase inhibitors are effective in various malignancies without cytotoxic adverse effect seen with existing chemotherapy. The first tyrosine kinase inhibitor which undergone phase I clinical trial was quercetin (Ferry et al. 1996). Heat shock proteins are responsible for the progression of cancer cell. It was reported that flavonoids inhibit the production of heat shock proteins in numerous cancer cell lines such as breast cancer, leukemia and colon cancer. Quercetin is recognized to exert seizure of cell cycle in proliferating lymphoid cells (Davis and Matthew 2000). Quercetin may inhibit abnormal cell growth by interacting with nuclear type II estrogen binding sites (EBS) (Lamson and Brignall 2000; Markaverich et al. 1988).

21.5.6 Antiviral Activity

Plant-derived flavonoids are known to have antiviral activity since the 1940s and maximum research work done on antiviral agents was mainly restricted to inhibition of different enzymes related to the life cycle of viruses. Flavan-3-o1 was found to have better effect compared to flavones and flavonones in selective inhibition of HIV-1, HIV-2 and alike immunodeficiency virus infections (Gerdin and Srensso 1983). Baicalin is a flavonoid which was isolated from *Scutellaria baicalensis* (Lamiaceae) and is capable of inhibiting HIV-1 infection and its replication, whereas another study revealed that baicalein, robustaflavone and hinokiflavone have inhibitory effects on HIV-1 reverse transcriptase. Kaempferol and luteolin showed a significant synergic effect against herpes simplex virus (HSV). Concomitant administration of quercetin with 5-ethyl-2-dioxyuridine and acyclovir was shown superior effect against HSV and pseudorabies infection than monotherapy (Cushnie and Lamb 2005). Quercetin, hesperetin, naringin and daidzein have shown antidengue virus properties at various phases of dengue virus type-2 (DENV-2) infection and replication cycle. Other flavonoids like dihydroquercetin, dihydrofisetin, leucocyanidin, pelargonidin chloride and catechin show potential effect against HSV, respiratory syncytial virus, polio virus and sindbis virus (Gerdin and Srensso 1983). Some flavonoids and their activity (Kumar and Pandey 2013a, b) on viruses are given in Table 21.4.

Table 21.4 Flavonoids possessing antiviral activity

Flavonoid	Virus
Quercetin	Rabies virus, herpes virus, parainfluenza virus, polio virus, mengovirus and pseudorabies virus
Rutin	Parainfluenza virus, influenza virus and potato virus
Apigenin	Immunodeficiency virus infection, herpes simplex virus type and aujeszky virus
Naringin	Respiratory syncytial virus
Luteolin	Aujeszky virus
Morin	Potato virus
Galangin	Herpes simplex virus type

21.6 Extraction of Flavonoids

Irrespective of the physical nature (fresh or non-dried) of collected plant material, degradation of flavonoids (mainly glycosides) can occur by enzyme action. It is therefore desirable to use dry, lyophilized or frozen samples. The plant material is usually crushed into powder if it is in the dried form. The selection of solvent for extraction is based on the category of flavonoids required. Polarity of solvent plays an important role here. Solvents like ethyl acetate, dichloromethane, diethyl ether and chloroform are used for extraction of less polar flavonoids such as flavonols, isoflavones, flavanones and methylated flavones, whereas extraction of flavonoid glycosides and more polar aglycones is performed using alcohols or mixtures of alcohol and water. Since, the aqueous solubility of glycosides is high, aqueous alcoholic solutions can be used. Simple direct solvent extraction is preferred for extraction of flavonoid containing material.

Soxhlet apparatus can be utilized for the extraction of powdered plant material, initially with hexane to get rid of lipids and followed by ethyl acetate or ethanol to get phenolics. But thermolabile substances cannot be extracted using this method. Sequential solvent extraction method is the most appropriate and frequently employed. Firstly, dichloromethane will extract flavonoid aglycones along with less polar substance and subsequently flavonoid glycosides and polar constituents can be extracted using an alcohol.

Some flavanone and chalcone glycosides have less solubility in methanol, ethanol or alcohol-water mixtures and hence pH of water containing solutions will be the deciding factor for solubility of flavanone.

Flavonoids like catechins, proanthocyanidins, and condensed tannins (flavan-3-ols) are frequently extracted using water. The composition of the extract depends upon the solvents used, for instance, water, methanol, ethanol, acetone or ethyl acetate. However, methanol is proved to be the most appropriate solvent for the extraction of catechins and acetone (70%) for procyanidins (Hussein et al. 1990).

Extraction of anthocyanins is carried out using cold methanol acidified with around 7% acetic acid or 3% trifluoroacetic acid. However, the use of mineral acid is not recommended as it results in the removal of attached acyl groups.

Usually, extraction is achieved using magnetic stirring or shaking but so as to enhance the effectiveness and rate of the extraction procedure, technique like pressurized liquid extraction (PLE) has been introduced. By means of high temperature and high pressure employed in PLE, extraction can be faster due to the enhanced diffusivity of the solvent along with the option of working in an inert environment and safeguard from light. Research article claims that instruments carrying traction vessels with a capacity of 100 mL are available in the market that reduces solvent usage (Benthin et al. 1999). PLE showed improved extraction recovery of isoquercitrin and rutin from older (*Sambucus nigra*, Caprifoliaceae) flowers compared to maceration with the advantage of shorter duration of extraction and lesser quantity of solvent required (Dawidowicz et al. 2003). Catechin and epicatechin can be extracted from grape seeds and skins of wine making wastes with slight degradation with the help of PLE if temperature is kept under 130 °C (Pineiro et al. 2004).

Supercritical fluids are required to have solubilizing properties with lesser viscosities and increased diffusion rates in order to facilitate extraction of diffusion regulated matrices like plant tissues when supercritical fluid extraction (SFE) is used. The method has several benefits when compared to soxhlet extraction methods such as lower solvent utilization, manageable selectivity and low thermal or chemical degradation. For the extraction of flavonoids, numerous extraction procedures using supercritical carbon dioxide as extraction solvent have been suggested with polar solvents like methanol as modifiers. Therefore, selectivity is substantially reduced and this describes comparatively fewer applications to polyphenols in the texts. Yields of polyphenolic compound stays low even after incorporating pressure (up to 689 bar) and modifier (generally 20% methanol) as extraction liquid for marigold (*Calendula officinalis*, Asteraceae) and chamomile (*Matricaria recutita*, Asteraceae) (Bevan and Marshall 1994; Jarvis and Morgan 1997; Hamburger et al. 2004). Literature further suggests that fast techniques namely ultrasound-assisted extraction can be used for the extraction of Brazilian plant *Lychnophora ericoides* (Asteraceae) using an immiscible solvent system consisting of hexane with methanol-water (9:1). Sesquiterpene lactones and hydrocarbons with less polarity get extracted into the hexane layer, whereas flavonoids and more polar sesquiterpene lactones come into the alcohol water mixture (Sargenti and Vichnewski 2000).

Microwave-assisted extraction (MAE) is recognized to be a simple and rapid technique used for extracting numerous compounds from various matrices in which energy in the form of microwave radiation allowed to pass through a sample suspended in a solvent using a closed or open cell. However, more amount of samples can be extracted in open cell in which certain amount of heating is required (Ganzler et al. 1990; Kaufmann and Christen 2002).

21.7 Isolation or Separation of Flavonoids

It is always beneficial to do cleanup as soon as an appropriate polar plant extract is acquired. The established technique for isolating phenolics from extracted plant material is to precipitate by means of lead acetate or extract into carbonate or alkali and lastly acidification. The lead acetate method usually does not give good results because some phenolics do not precipitate and there may be co-precipitation of other compounds. Additionally, lead salts cannot be removed easily. Techniques such as solvent partition or countercurrent also can be applied. So as to get a portion of Erythrina species (Leguminosae) rich in flavonoid for purification, 90% methanol was used to dissolve organic solvent extract and first separated with hexane. Remaining part of methanol was adjusted to 30% by adding water and t-butyl methyl ether–hexane was added in the ratio of 9:1. This mixture was used as mobile phase (McKee et al. 1997).

Columns such as ion exchange resin, a short polyamide column or a Sephadex LH-20 column may be used. Crude extracts can also be absorbed onto Amberlite XAD-2 or Diaion HP-20 columns with subsequent elution using methanol-water as mobile phase for obtaining flavonoid-rich fractions.

21.7.1 Preparative Methods

Preparative separation of flavonoids creates difficulties due to the commonly used solvents in chromatography in which most of the flavonoids are sparingly soluble. Additionally, as the purification process speed up, solubility of flavonoids decreases. Decreased solubility of flavonoids in the mobile phase employed for separation can lead to the formation of precipitates at the top of the column and hence poor resolution, reduction in solvent flow and even blockage of the column may be observed.

It is necessary to avoid the use of acetonitrile and formic acid during the separation of anthocyanins or anthocyanin-rich fractions as acetonitrile does not evaporate easily and formic acid results in ester formation. Various isolation strategies and steps may require for the separation of flavonoids. Polarity of substance and sample quantity available play important roles during the selection of a method. Various preparative methods were reported by Hostettmann et al. (1998).

Simple techniques like conventional open-column chromatography are still used for initial separation of flavonoids. This technique can also be used in huge quantities of flavonoids obtained from crude plant extracts for preparative work. Materials such as silica gel, polyamide, cellulose, Sephadex LH-20 and Sephadex G-10, G-25 and G-50 are used for support. The recommended material for proanthocyanidin is Sephadex LH-20. Both partition and adsorption mechanisms work well with organic solvents for Sephadex and size exclusion. In spite of the fact that methanol and ethanol can be utilized as eluents for proanthocyanidins, acetone is a good option for polyphenols with high molecular weight with slow flow rates. There are chances that solute can be irreversibly adsorbed on the column due to some of the supports used such as silica gel and polyamide in open-column chromatography. Method can also be modified (vacuum liquid chromatography, VLC and dry-column chromatography, for instance) so that plant extracts can be fractionated rapidly. Flavonol glycosides have been separated with the help of VLC using a polyamide support (Carlton et al. 1990). Preparative TLC is an economical technique and the basic equipment. Quantities of sample in milligram are usually employed. However, gram quantities also can be employed if the sample mixture is simple. Even though techniques such as centrifugal TLC (Hostettmann et al. 1998) which is a modification of planar chromatography is used for the separation of flavonoids, preparative TLC combined with open-column chromatography remains a preferred simple method for isolation of natural products. Based on the separation criteria, obviously, different combinations also can be used. Complex separations can be performed using a combination of gel filtration with liquid chromatography (LC), liquid–liquid partition with liquid chromatography (LC) and chromatography on polymeric supports (Hostettmann et al. 1998). Depending on the pressure utilized for the separation, quite a few preparative pressure liquid chromatographic methods are available. Their classification is given below:

- High-pressure or high-performance LC (>20 bar/300 psi)
- Medium-pressure LC (5–20 bar/75–300 psi)
- Low-pressure LC (<5 bar/75 psi)
- Flash chromatography (ca. 2 bar/30 psi)

21.7.1.1 High-Performance Liquid Chromatography

HPLC is gaining momentum as the most widespread instrumental technique for the separation of flavonoids and preparative as well as analytical purpose. The technique is continuously improved by introducing changes in instrumentation, column technology and packing materials making it a more effective and attractive separation technique.

Analytical and preparative HPLC can be differentiated by the fact that analytical HPLC does not focus on sample recovery, while preparative chromatography emphasizes on isolation of pure material from a mixture as it is a purification method.

Columns with an internal diameter of 8–20 mm packed with 10 mm or smaller particle size particles can be used for samples of 1–100 mg in semipreparative HPLC separations while preparative installations are used for large samples.

Optimization can be achieved on analytical HPLC columns before reversal to semipreparative scale. In earlier days, preparative HPLC was not been utilized efficiently for isolation of flavonoids. But presently 80% of all flavonoid separations comprise a HPLC step. Octadecylsilyl phases with isocratic and gradient conditions are used in 95% of the reported HPLC methods.

21.7.1.2 Medium-Pressure Liquid Chromatography

MPLC consist of a closed column (usually glass) connected to a reciprocating pump or a compressed air source. It works as a substitute for flash chromatography or open-column chromatography with the advantage of high resolution and shorter separation time. Additionally, they have loading capacity of 1:25 sample-to-packing-material ratio making it suitable for flavonoid separation (Leutert and Von Arx 1984).

Particle sizes ranging from 25–200 mm are generally used (commonly used ranges are 15–25, 25–40 or 43–60 mm) in MPLC with slurry or dry packing and the column filling is usually done by the operator. A long column with small internal diameter provides more resolution in comparison with short column with large internal diameter using the same quantity of stationary phase (Zogg et al. 1989). Choosing of solvent systems may be achieved on analytical HPLC and TLC and can be reversed to MPLC directly (Schaufelberger and Hostettmann 1985).

21.7.1.3 Centrifugal Partition Chromatography

Countercurrent chromatography also found to be a successful technique applied for flavonoid separation in which sample is partitioned among two immiscible solvents and partition coefficients of components of solute is used to determine the amount of solute present in two phases. This method does not require a solid support as it is an all liquid technique, therefore when compared with other chromatographic methods, it has following advantages:

- Sample does not get adsorbed irreversibly.
- Complete recovery of the introduced sample.
- Significantly low risk of sample denaturation.
- Less utilization of solvents.
- Economically favorable.

Therefore, it is evident that such a procedure is perfect for flavonoids, which frequently suffer from difficulties in retention on solid supports, for example, silica gel and polyamide (Hostettmann et al. 1998).

21.8 Quantification of Flavonoids

Different traditional methods like UV/Visible absorption spectroscopy and separation techniques like thin-layer chromatography (TLC), paper electrophoresis and polyamide chromatography were commonly employed in earlier periods for flavonoid separation. Evidently, TLC is still a preferable method for flavonoid analysis, because of its simplicity, rapidity and versatility. On the other hand, significant portion of recently published work emphasizes on qualitative as well as quantitative determination of flavonoids by high-performance liquid chromatography (HPLC), liquid chromatography-nuclear magnetic resonance (LC-NMR), liquid chromatography-mass spectrometry (LC-MS) and capillary electrophoresis (CE). Flavonoids can be separated, identified and quantified in single operation by pairing HPLC with UV/Vis, MS or NMR detectors, especially if the study aims at determining individual flavonoids. Furthermore, HPLC enables the separation and quantification of the flavonoids simultaneously without initial derivatization. These factors have contributed to make HPLC analysis of flavonoids a commonly used technique. Liquid chromatography-based methods have been given special emphasis in this chapter because these are the most widely used and accepted techniques for flavonoid analysis (Fig. 21.2). Other techniques like thin-layer chromatography (TLC), gas chromatography (GC) and capillary electrophoresis (CE) will be elaborated later in this chapter.

21.8.1 Column Liquid Chromatography

Usually, flavonoid analysis is performed on bonded silica (C_8 or C_{18}) columns in reversed phase (RP) mode. Though, other phases like silica, polyamide and Sephadex are also used. Octadecylsilyl stationary phases coupled with hydrophilic end capping is preferred for the separation of very polar substances, which may not retain satisfactorily on regular reversed-phase columns. Moreover, they are found to be most suitable for the separation of flavonol and xanthone glycosides from mango (*Mangifera indica*, Anacardiaceae) peels (Careri et al. 1998). Occasionally unmodified silica gel (normal phase) is used to separate weakly polar flavonoid aglycones, polymethoxylated flavones, flavanones or isoflavones. The citrus fruits containing polymethoxylated flavones can be separated using silica gel columns, but the limitation is that

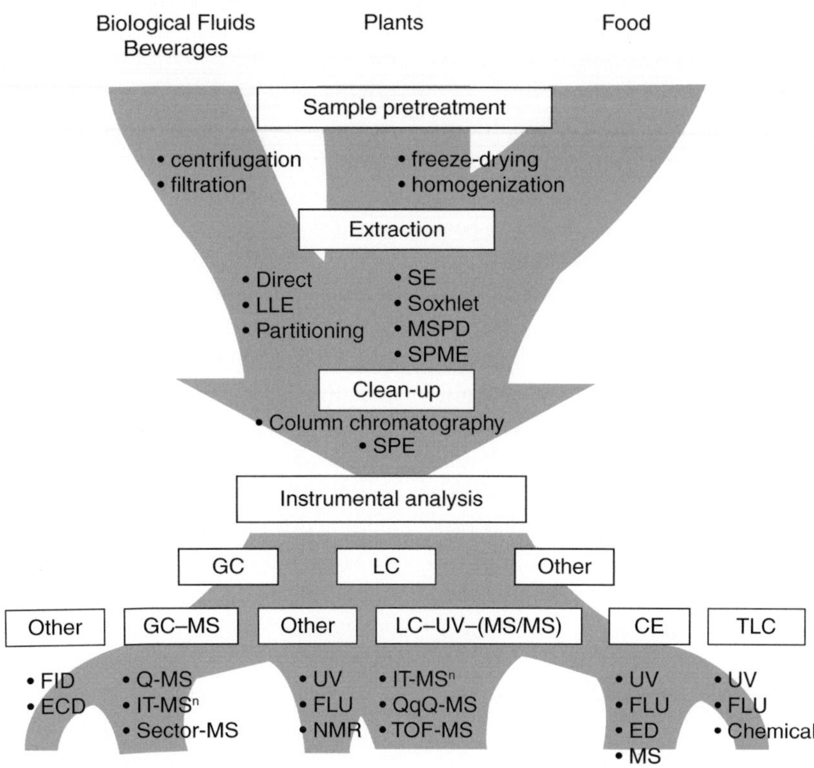

Fig. 21.2 Various approaches for the determination of flavonoids in biological fluids, beverages, plants, and food (Abbreviations: *LLE*, liquid–liquid extraction; *SE*, solvent extraction; *MSPD*, matrix solid-phase extraction; *SPME*, solid-phase micro-extraction; *SPE*, solid-phase extraction; *GC*, gas chromatography; *LC*, liquid chromatography; *MS*, mass spectrometry; *MS/MS*, tandem mass spectrometry; *CE*, capillary electrophoresis; *TLC*, thin-layer chromatography; *FID*, flame ionization detection; *ECD*, electron capture detection; *Q*, quadrupole; *QqQ*, triple-quadrupole; *IT*, ion trap, *FLU*, fluorescence; *NMR*, nuclear magnetic resonance; *TOF*, time-of-flight; and *ED*, electrochemical detection) (Reprinted from Journal of Chromatography A, 1112, De Rijke E, Out P, Niessen WM, Ariese F, Gooijer C, Brinkman UA, Analytical separation and detection methods for flavonoids, 31–63., Copyright (2006), with permission from Elsevier)

gradient solvent cannot be run with normal phases frequently. Gradient elution with binary solvent system containing acetate or formate buffer along with organic modifiers such as methanol or acetonitrile is preferred. Phosphate buffers are rarely used when MS is used for detection due to the higher possibility of contamination of ion sources. Solvents like isopropanol, tetrahydrofuran or n-propanol are also used occasionally. The ionization of phenolic hydroxyl groups can be suppressed by the addition of acid modifiers which results in sharper peaks with less tailing. Though, LC is operated at room temperature, thermostated columns (up to 40 °C) are preferred to bring down the run time. Depending on the number of flavonoids to be separated, run time may vary from 30 min to 2 h (Fabre et al. 2001; Franke and Custer 1994).

Retention time of flavone C-glycosides is usually short when compared to the corresponding O-glycosides. Therefore, vitexin (8-C-glucosylapigenin) shows lesser retention time compared to apigenin 7-O-glucoside. Moreover, 8-C-glycosylflavones are reported to elute faster as compared to corresponding 6-C-glycosylflavones. Isoflavones can also be successfully analyzed by HPLC using C_{18} columns (Zhong et al. 2003).

The anthocyanins exist in numerous structural arrangements in solutions which are pH and temperature dependent. Therefore, it is prerequisite to maintain the mobile phase pH and column temperature of HPLC with the help of thermostatically controlled columns in order to get precise results.

Further to attain sharp peaks with optimum resolution, anthocyanin equilibria have to be shifted towards their flavylium forms. This also helps to reduce peak tailing and improves peak sharpness. Then the detection of colored flavylium cations can be carried out at about 520 nm. It is remarkable that a previous study revealed that 90% of the separations from the methods explained the use of C_{18} columns. The significance of flavonoids in fruits, vegetables and grains prove that it is crucial to have appropriate analytical methods to determine their content (Mattila et al. 2000). Another review also provides an excellent summary of estimation of flavones, isoflavones, flavanones, flavonols and anthocyanidins by HPLC (Zhong et al. 2003).

21.8.1.1 Detectors Used in LC

UV Detection

As at least one aromatic ring is present in all flavonoid aglycones, they can absorb UV light efficiently. The first maximum is because of the A-ring which is observed in the range of 240–285 nm and the substitution pattern and conjugation of the C-ring is responsible for second maximum, which is in the range of 300–550 nm (Mabry et al. 1970). Usually minor shifting of absorption maxima is observed in the presence of substituent groups like methyl, methoxy and non-dissociated hydroxyl groups. Hence, for the detection and quantification of flavonoids, UV spectrophotometry was a commonly used technique decade ago. In recent times, UV detection is widely used in LC-based studies and even catechins and their respective glycosides in food are performed on RP-18 columns. Some of the reported methods have used C_8 packings for determination of aglycones and glycosides of isoflavone from soybean products (Watson et al. 2003) but these are uncommon.

LC coupled with diode array UV detection is highly preferred for screening and quantification of the main aglycones and their sub-group classification (Table 21.1). The above information is applicable for their conjugates too. In general, this enables the recognition of satellite sets, comprising of aglycones, glycosides, glycoside malonates and glycoside acetates. But it is very difficult to differentiate most of the glycosides and acyl residues using DD-UV detection because of their poor chromophoric characteristics. It should also be noted that chromophores having ionizable groups will exhibit pH dependency. LC–DAD UV is an appealing technique for distinguishing various flavonoid sub-classes and thus is an efficient complementary tool for structural characterization. Usually, detection of flavonoid is carried out at 250, 265, 290, 350, 370 and/or 400 nm (500–525 nm) range for anthocyanidins (Merken and Beecher 2000).

Most of the HPLC methods available have limitations such as requirement of pretreatment by hydrolysis which leads to loss of phenolic content because of decomposition and polymerization of polyphenols and inability to estimate aglycons without hydrolysis. At present, there is no existing HPLC method that can resolve all problems regarding flavonoid separation, though a method has been reported by Sakakibara et al. (2003) for identification and quantification of all polyphenol in both glycoside and aglycone forms present in fruits, vegetables and teas. The analysis was carried out using Hitachi HPLC (D-7000), Tokyo, Japan along with Hitachi chromatography data station software (D-7000), autosampler (D-7200), column oven (D-7300) and diode array detection system (D-7450) to monitor the entire wavelength range (200–600 nm). Capcell pak C_{18} UG120 (250 × 4.6 mm, S-5, 5 mm) main column combined with a guard column (10 × 4.0 mm i.d.) was kept at 35 °C. Solution A consisting of 50 mM sodium phosphate [pH 3.3] and 10% methanol and solution B containing 70% methanol were used for gradient elution which was proceeded as follows: beginning with 100% of solution A; for the following 15 min, 70% A; for 30 min, 65% A; for 20 min, 60% A; for 5 min, 50% A; and lastly 100% B for 25 min, employing 1 mL/min as flow rate run over 95 min. Injection volume of extract used was 10 μL. Dimethyl sulfoxide (DMSO) was used as diluent to solubilize commercially available pure polyphenols to get desired concentration (10 mM) and preserved in dark and low temperature (−20 °C) for a period of 3 months. Polyphenol solutions were further diluted in the range of 1.0–1000 μM using DMSO followed by construction of calibration curve. A characteristic HPLC profile for 28 reference polyphenols is depicted in Fig. 21.3. Thoroughly washed fresh vegetables and fruits were chopped and homogenized in liquid nitrogen by means of homogenizer, whereas teas, cacao and coffee beans were ground using a coffee mill. Lyophilization of homogenate and powdered material was carried out at 0.2 Pa for 48 h and preserved at low temperature (4 °C) in a desiccator prior to use. Stored powdered material (approximately 50 mg) were extracted with 2 mL solvent (90% methanol comprising 0.5% acetic acid) prior to the addition of flavone in DMSO as internal standard (50 nM). If the sample contains flavone, it can be replaced with flavonol or chalcone. Initially solutions were sonicated for 1 min and further centrifugation was done for 10 min at 3000 rpm and the supernatant was collected. Extraction was carried out three times and finally dried using centrifugal concentrator (VC-96 N, Taitec Co., Saitama, Japan). HPLC analysis was performed after dissolving the dried residue in DMSO (0.5 mL) followed by filtration (Millex-LG 0.2-μm membrane filter, Millipore Co., Bedford, MA). All polyphenol peaks of food extracts were compared with standard peaks in regard to retention time and spectra of aglycone stored in the library. In case the detected polyphenol did not match with a retention time of standards, food samples were hydrolyzed and analyzed once again with HPLC.

Diode array (DAD) and electrochemical (EC) detection yield different kinds of data which is

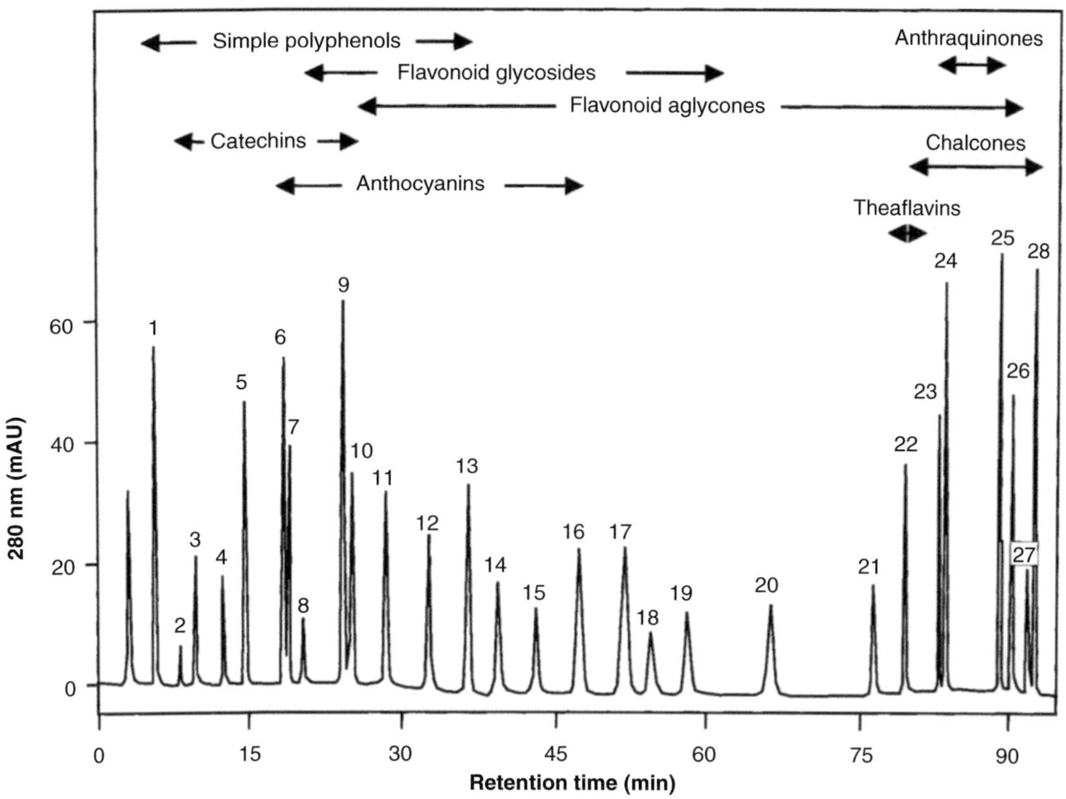

Fig. 21.3 HPLC separation of 28 different polyphenols using C_{18} column. Upper part of the chromatogram indicates class of compound (Reprinted with permission from Sakakibara H, Honda Y, Nakagawa S, Ashida H, Kanazawa K. Simultaneous Determination of All Polyphenols in Vegetables, Fruits, and Teas. J Agric Food Chem. 2003;51:571–581, Copyright (2003), American Chemical Society)

useful in recognizing the peaks of flavonoids present in plant materials. Estimation of catechin and other flavonoids have been reported by Mattila et al. (2000), using HPLC-DAD and HPLC-EC detection, respectively for qualitative and quantitative determination of 17 different flavonoids in plant-derived foods. Data obtained from spectral and voltammetric detection lead to specific, selective and precise flavonoid analysis. Flavonoid analysis was performed using HP HPLC system (1090 M Series II) coupled with DAD and an electrochemical coulometric array (eight-channel) detector (EC; ESA Inc., USA). Computer software program (HP 3D Chem Station) was used to monitor pumps, autosampler, column oven, DAD system and to assess analytical information. Catechins and other flavonoids were identified and quantified using DAD. (−)-Epigallocatechin, galangin and (−)-epigallocatechin gallate were detected at 270.4 nm; 280.4 nm was used for eriodictyol, naringenin, (+)-catechin, (−)-epicatechin, (−)-epicatechin gallate and hesperetin; 329.4 nm for luteolin, apigenin and tangeretin; 370.4 nm for myricetin, kaempferol, rhamnetin, quercetin and isorhamnetin, respectively. For flavonoids except catechins, gradient elution was accomplished with a mobile phase system comprising of 50 mM H_3PO_4, pH 2.5 (solution A) and acetonitrile (solution B) as follows: isocratic elution 95% A/5% B, 0–5 min; linear gradient from 95% A/5% B to 50% A/ 50% B, 5–55 min; isocratic elution 50% A/50% B, 55–65 min; linear gradient from 50% A/50% B to 95% A/5% B, 65–67 min; and post-time 6 min prior to next injection, whereas catechins were measured in isocratic mode (86% solution A and 14% solution B). For quantification of flavonoids, flow rate was kept at 0.7 mL/min and the injection volumes were fixed at 10 μL for standard and sample solutions. Quantification was carried out using peak area for DAD detection. All the standard stock solutions (5 mg/50 mL) were prepared using MeOH, except apigenin and luteolin (DMF/MeOH, 1:6, v/v) and isorhamnetin and rhamnetin (DMF/MeOH, 1:10, v/v). Necessary dilutions were made using methanol to get working standard solution (2–4 μg/mL) which was preserved in dark at −18 °C and remained in stable condition over 3 months. A characteristic HPLC profile for 17 flavonoids (Fig. 21.4) describes an HPLC-DAD method. Fresh samples of fruits and vegetables (excluding red wine and teas) were homogenized using blender and then freeze-dried and preserved at low temperature (−18 °C) prior to analysis, whereas tea samples were infused for 3 min in water at 90 °C and studied instantly. Dried samples (0.5 g) were extracted in a 100 mL Erlenmeyer flask using 40 mL of aqueous methanol (62.5% v/v) containing 2 g/L of 2,(3)-*tert*-butyl-4-hydroxyanisole (BHA). Then the mixture was ultrasonicated for about 5 min followed by addition of 10 mL HCl (6 M). Nitrogen gas was passed through the extract for 40–60 sec and flask was sealed tightly.

Hydrolysis was carried out in a shaking water bath at a temperature of 90 °C for 2 h. Thereafter the sample was cooled, filtered and methanol was added to make up the volume up to 100 mL and ultrasonicated for 5 min. Filtration of the sample was carried out using a membrane filter (0.2 μm) prior to quantification. For the sample preparation of red wine and tea, 25 mL of 62.5% methanol in water comprising BHA was added to a 15 mL sample and ultrasonicated for 5 min and 10 mL of HCl (6 M) was added. The remaining procedure was similar as that for the dried samples, but hydrolysis was carried out for 4 h at 90 °C. To 5 mL of black tea or red wine, 9 mL of ethyl acetate was added to extract catechins. The same procedure was repeated for 0.5 mL green tea sample. The samples were shaken for 1 min in a test tube fitted with a corkscrew cap for efficient extraction. The separated ethyl acetate layer was collected and evaporated till dry using nitrogen stream and then the residue was dissolved and made up the volume up to 20 mL with methanol. Finally extracted sample (approximately 2 mL) was filtered using membrane filter (0.2 μm) prior to HPLC study.

Flavonoids are present in Ginkgo extracts (leaves of *Ginkgo biloba* L.) used as phytomedicines which contain around 24% flavonoids and 6% terpene lactones and hence, the content of flavonoids and terpene lactones present in Ginkgo products is the basis of quality evaluation. Quality of Ginkgo preparation was assessed through fingerprint analysis which was described by Hasler

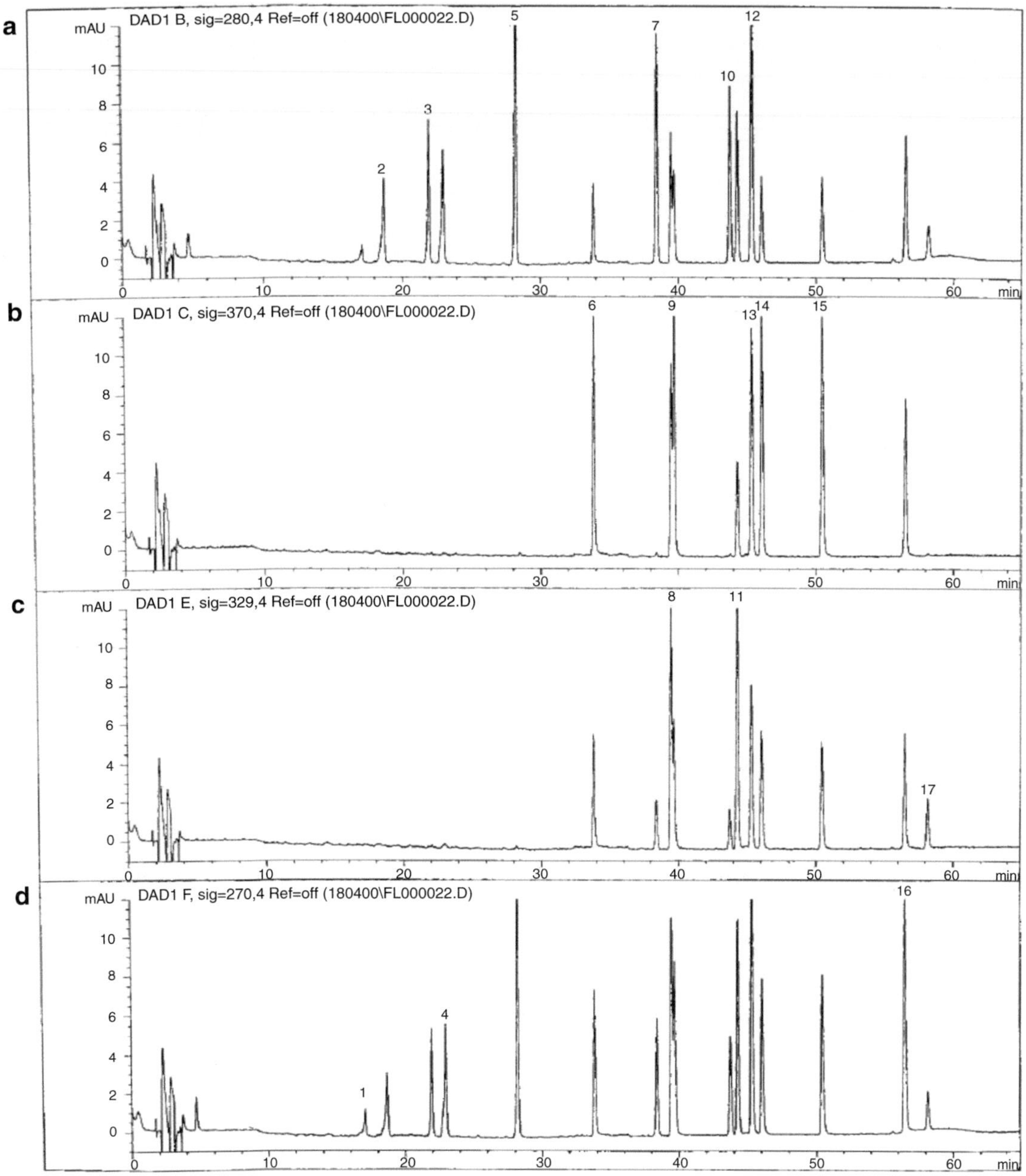

Fig. 21.4 Chromatograms of standard mixture containing 17 flavonoids using HPLC-DAD at 280.4 (**a**), 370.4 (**b**), 329.4 (**c**), and 270.4 (**d**) nm. (1) (−)-epigallocatechin; (2) (+)-catechin; (3) (−)-epicatechin; (4) (−)-epigallocatechin gallate; (5) (−)-epicatechin gallate; (6) myricetin; (7) eriodictyol; (8) luteolin; (9) quercetin; (10) naringenin; (11) apigenin; (12) hesperetin; (13) kaempferol; (14) isorhamnetin;(15) rhamnetin; (16) galangin; (17) tangeretin (Reprinted with permission from Mattila P, Astola J, Kumpulainen J. Determination of Flavonoids in Plant Material by HPLC with Diode Array and Electro-Array Detections. J Agric Food Chem. 2000;48:5834–5841, Copyright (2000), American Chemical Society)

et al. (1992). The study established the possibility of separating 6 flavonoid aglycones, 22 flavonoid glycosides and 5 biflavonoids in a single run (Fig. 21.5). This extraordinary task was accomplished on Hewlett-Packard system (Model 79994A Analytical Workstation, Model 1090 liquid chromatograph, Model 1040 diode-array detector). A Knauer (Berlin, Germany)

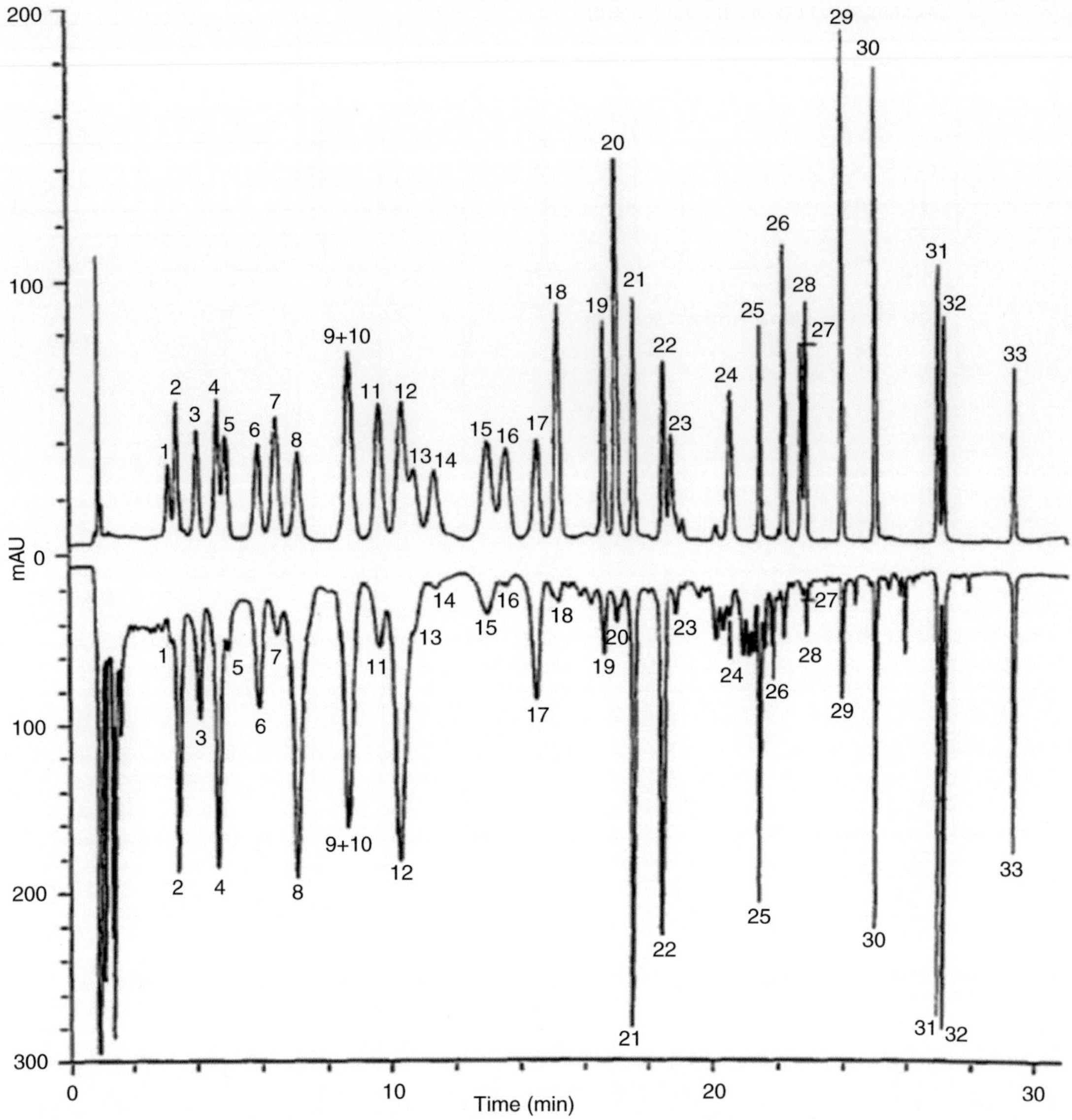

Fig. 21.5 HPLC chromatogram for fingerprint analysis of therapeutically used dry extract of *Ginkgo biloba* leaves. Chromatogram on the top shows pure reference flavonoids; chromatogram on the bottom shows leaf extract. Flavonoids are identified and numbered from 1 to 33 (Reprinted from Journal of Chromatography, 605, Hasler A, Sticher O, Meier B. Identification and determination of the flavonoids from *Ginkgo biloba* by high-performance liquid chromatography, 41–48, Copyright (1992), with permission from Elsevier)

prepacked column cartridge (100 × 4 mm I.D.) packed with Nucleosil 100-C_{18}, 3 μm (Macherey-Nagel, Duren, Germany) was used. All the compounds were eluted within 30 min with the help of a ternary mobile phase containing isopropanol-THF (25:65) (solvent A), acetonitrile (B) and 0.5% orthophosphoric acid (C). A solvent delivery arrangement containing three pumps was used to achieve a complex elution gradient (1 mL/min, detection at 350 nm) initially with 15.0% A, 1.5% B and 83.5% C and finally with 0% A, 78.0% B and 22% C.

A quantitative HPLC determination of two wild plant leaves, *Sonchus arvensis* and *Oenanthe linearis*, found in north eastern part of India was studied by Seal (2016) for ascorbic acid, flavonoids and phenolic acid content. The analysis was carried out on Dionex liquid chromatograph (Ultimate 3000), Germany, equipped with quaternary pump (LPG 3400 SD) and a diode array detector (DAD 3000) having 5 cm flow cell along with a loop injection valve (20 μL) and system manager (Chromelon 6.8) for data processing. A reverse phase Acclaim 120 C_{18} column (250 × 4.6 mm, 5 μm) was used for chromatographic separation and which was thermostatically controlled at 28° C. The stock solution (1 mg/mL) of ascorbic acid, phenolic acids and flavonoids were prepared using methanol and the mobile phase. Further dilutions were made to desired concentrations (5, 10, 20, 30,40, 60 μg/mL). The mobile phase constitutes acetic acid in water (1%) solution (solvent A) and acetonitrile (solvent B) for separation. A gradient elution was achieved at a flow rate of 0.7 mL/min by changing the proportion of solvent B to solvent A. The gradient elution was altered from 10 to 40% B in a linear fashion for 28 min, from 40 to 60% B in 39 min and from 60 to 90% B in 50 min. Initial mobile phase composition (solvent B/solvent A, 10:90) was brought back within 55 min and another sample was injected after running the mobile phase for 10 min. Total time taken for analysis of individual sample was 65 min. The chromatographic detection was carried out at 272, 280 and 310 nm using a photo diode array UV detector based on the absorption maxima of studied compounds. Identification of 17 compounds (Fig. 21.6) was done by comparing their retention time with standard by spiking under the similar settings. Peak area was measured for the quantification of the sample with the help of

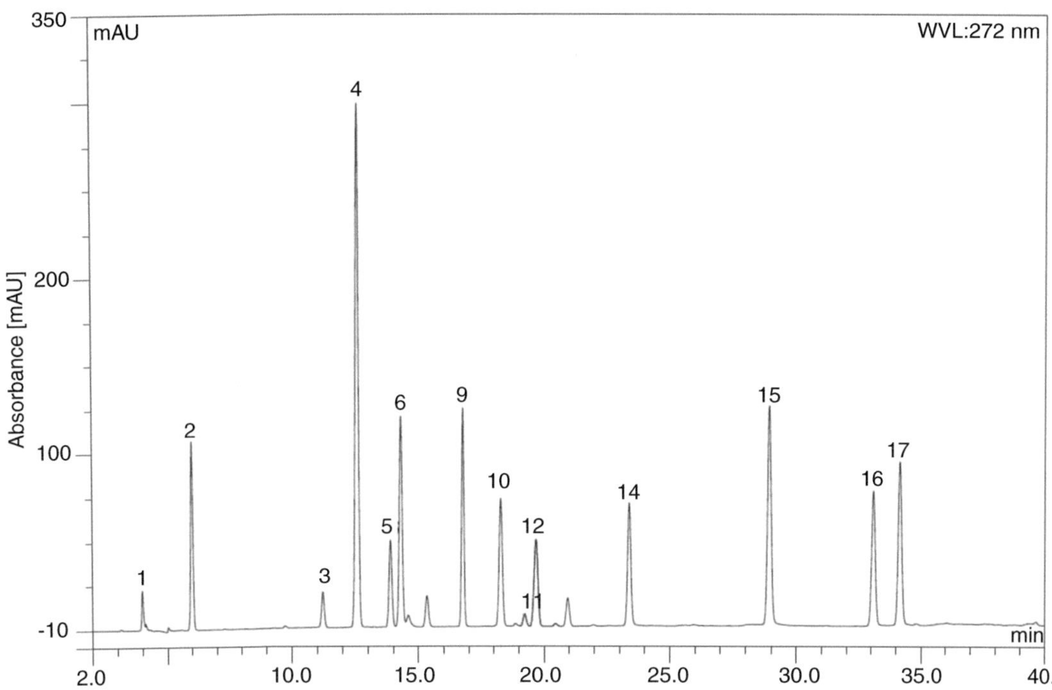

Fig. 21.6 HPLC chromatogram of standard ascorbic acid, phenolic acids, and flavonoids. (1) Ascorbic acid, (2) gallic acid, (3) catechin, (4) methyl gallate, (5) caffeic acid, (6) syringic acid, (9) rutin, (10) p-coumaric acid, (11) sinapic acid, (12) ferulic acid, (13) myricetin, (14) quercetin, (15) apigenin, (16) kaempferol (Reprinted with permission from Seal T. Quantitative HPLC analysis of phenolic acids, flavonoids and ascorbic acid in four different solvent extracts of two wild edible leaves, *Sonchus arvensis* and *Oenanthe linearis* of North-Eastern region in India. Journal of Applied Pharmaceutical Science. 2016;6(2):157–166, Copyright (2016), With permission from Open Science Publishers LLP)

standard calibration curve which was constructed by plotting peak area versus concentration. Plant samples were extracted using four solvents with different polarity. Firstly, extraction was carried out at ambient temperature using chloroform by stirring continuously for a day. The plant residue obtained after filtration of the extract was macerated using fresh solvent, stirred and filtered. The abovementioned procedure was performed three times. The combined extracts were lastly filtered using PVDF membrane and volume was brought to 10 mL. The same procedure was followed for sample extraction using methanol, aq. ethanol (80%) and aq. acetic acid (1%) solution.

Fluorescence Detection

Flavonoids which exhibit native fluorescence are less in number. Therefore, the scope of fluorescence detection in flavonoid analysis is very limited. Classes of flavonoids that exhibit inherent fluorescence comprise the isoflavones (De Rijke et al. 2002), flavonoids having an OH group in the 3-position [3-hydroxyflavone] (Sengupta and Kasha 1979), catechin [*trans*-3,3′,4′,5,7-pentahydroxyflavan] (Stoggl et al. 2004) and methoxylated flavones [3′,4′,5′-trimethoxyflavone] (Huck and Bonn 2001). Fluorescent as well as non-fluorescent compounds which co-elute simultaneously can be differentiated when fluorescence and UV detection techniques are combined (Rodriguez-Delgado et al. 2001; De Rijke et al. 2001). Generally, the type of the functional group present and pattern of their substitution is responsible for the fluorescence of flavonoids. For instance, among all the isoflavones, only those do not contain an OH group in 5-position exhibit strong natural fluorescence. In flavonols, OH group in the 3-position take part in excited state intramolecular proton transfer, which produces dual emission which is solvent dependent, resulting in strong native fluorescence (Sengupta and Kasha 1979; Wolfbeis et al. 1983; Bader et al. 2004). Non-fluorescent compounds can be converted into fluorescent ones by derivatization and were analyzed. Flavonoids like kaempferol, quercetin and morin, using their 3-OH, 4-keto substituents may produce highly fluorescent species due to the formation of complexes with metal cations (Hollman et al. 1996; Gutierrez and Gehlen 2002). Quercetin and kaempferol can make fluorescent complexes with Al (III) by post column derivatization which can lead to the increase in sensitivity of the method as LODs for kaempferol and quercetin were 0.05 and 0.15 ng/mL, respectively (Hollman et al. 1996). The method was helpful in studying the bioavailability of quercetin present in onions and apples consumed by humans. Quercetin levels in plasma were calculated for nine volunteers over a time period of 36 h. Peak plasma concentration was attained within 0.7 h after consumption of onions of concentration, 220 ng/mL, 2.5 h after intake of apples (90 ng/mL) and it took 9 h in the case of quercetin rutinoside (rutin) of concentration, 90 ng/mL (Hollman et al. 1997).

Electrochemical Detection

Majority of flavonoids are electro-active because they contain phenolic groups in them. This property of flavonoids can be used for their electrochemical detection. When compared to fluorescence detection, ED is not that much sensitive but it can provide LODs which are quite low: quantification of *trans*-resveratrol in rat blood gave LOD value of 2 μg/L with LC–multichannel ED (Zhong et al. 2003). A recent paper reveals determination of isoflavones in food containing soybean and human urine with the help of LC–coulometric array ED (Klejdus et al. 2004). Identification was done using LC–UV–MS. This detector is made up of a 6 μL flow-through analytical cell comprising an Ag/AgCl reference electrode, a counter-electrode made with platinum wire and eight working electrodes constructed with porous graphite (carbon paste). Standard solutions of daidzein and genistein showed highest signal at 450 mV, which is presumably matching with an oxidation signal. Genistein gave a linear calibration curve whereas calibration curve of daidzein was not linear probably because surface of electrode got saturated by the analyte. Daidzein and genistein showed LOD of 400 pg/mL with acetonitrile–acetate buffer as eluent when conditions were optimal. In quite a few soybean foods, daidzein and genistein were found in concentrations of 20–200 and

60–300 μg/g, respectively with 95–107% recovery. Another author explained the use of RPLC–ED for the assessment of the antioxidant action of phenolic compounds along with 11 different flavonoids, by determining the auto-oxidation of methyl linoleate in anhydrous dodecane, under accelerated and strongly oxidizing conditions (Peyrat-Maillard et al. 2000). A calibration graph was plotted using peak area vs. potential voltammograms. Out of two maxima, the first maximum represents oxidation of the phenolic substituents on ring B and the second one possibly arises from the other phenolic groups which are relatively less oxidizable. Due to different structural parameters, the antioxidant property of flavonoids found to be less linear with ED signal. For example, decrease in antioxidant or anti-radical activity was observed in flavonols due to the glycosylation of the 3-hydroxyl group, but their electrochemical behavior was unchanged. However, value of the first maximum which requires lowest energy to donate an electron is linked to the antioxidant efficiency for most of the analytes.

LC–MS

For assessment of flavonoids, MS is the contemporary detection technique used in LC. Table 21.5 sums up related evidence on selection of newer studies linked to LC–MS (De Rijke et al. 2006). In majority of cases, single-stage MS coupled with UV detector was used to identify several flavonoids present in a sample based on the standards and reference data available. However, for the identification of unknown compounds, tandem mass spectrometry (MS/MS or MS^n) is preferred. In recent times electrospray ionization (ESI) and atmospheric pressure ionization interfaces (APCI) are exclusively used in the LC–MS of flavonoids. Positive ionization and negative ionization are applied. ESI is preferred in flavonoid study; however, APCI too is gaining acceptance due to better results in that mode (De Rijke et al. 2003; Justesen et al. 1998; Boue et al. 2003). Most of the recent

Table 21.5 LC–MS methods used for flavonoids analysis

Sample	Flavonoids	Ionization mode	Concentration (mg/g)	LC eluents
Ginkgo biloba tablets	Kaempferol, quercetin, quercetin–glycoside, rutin, quercitrin, isorhamnetin	ESI (−)	0.005–0.330 gm/tablet	MeCN, FA
Genista tinctoria	16 flavone – and isoflavone – glycosides (−malonate) and aglycons	ESI (−)	0.003–15	MeCN, AcOH
Scutellaria baicalensis	Wogonin–5-*O*-glucoside, wogonoside, baicalin, wogonin, norwogonin, chrysin–6-*C*-arabinose-8-*C*-glucose, chrysin–6-*C*-glucose-8-*C*-arabinose	ESI (−)	–	MeCN, $AcONH_4$
Leguminosae (four species)	Isoflavone and flavonol-glucoside-(di)malonates and flavonol (di) glycosides	APCI (−)	0.03–65	MeOH, ammonium formate
Red clover	49 isoflavone–glucoside-malonates and –acetates, glycosides and aglycons	ESI (+)	–	MeCN, H_2O
Hypericum perforatum, *Rhodiola rosea*, red grape wine, orange juice, green tea	50 flavonols, flavanones, flavones, catechins and anthocyanins	ESI (+)	0.0002–0.01	MeOH, FA
Helichrysum stoechas	6 chalcones, flavanones and flavonols	APCI (±)	1.5–3	MeCN, ammonium formate

$AcONH_4$, ammonium acetate; *AcOH*, acetic acid; *MeOH*, methanol; and *FA*, formic acid

studies prove that NI mode delivers greatest sensitivity for APCI and ESI. Still, in the analysis associated with identification of unknown substance, PI mode plays major role in acquiring valuable complementary data. However, one should be aware that response of analyte may differ based on the mode of operation in one sub-class to another, and even within the same class (De Rijke et al. 2003; Rauha et al. 2001). Moreover, the significant impact in response can be observed depending on the gradient eluent composition, its pH and the type of buffer used (Rauha et al. 2001). Some frequently used additives for flavonoid analysis are acetic acid (Grayer et al. 2000), formic acid (Andlauer et al. 1999), ammonium acetate and ammonium formate (Hansen et al. 1999; De Rijke et al. 2003). Trifluoroacetic acid has also been used (Da Costa et al. 2000) even though it is responsible for suppression of ionization owing to ion pairing and surface tension effects. Resemblance in mass spectra was observed while analyzing flavonoids using ion trap and quadrupole instruments, but relative abundances of fragment ions and adducts showed variations (De Rijke et al. 2003). Therefore, spectral comparison is permitted for both the instruments directly. Ionization techniques like electron ionization (EI) (Harbone and Dey 1989), chemical ionization (CI) (Barbuch et al. 1989), fast atom bombardment (FAB) (Ma et al. 2000) and matrix-assisted laser desorption ionization (MALDI) (Wang and Sporns 1999; Wang and Sporns 2000a, b) are also used besides ESI and APCI. Recently, a potential technique namely off-line MALDI-TOF MS was also explored for the determination of flavonoids in soy products, red wine, fruit juices, green tea and onions (Wang and Sporns 1999; Wang and Sporns 2000a, b). Prior to MALDI-TOF MS analysis, pretreatment of sample was carried out through SPE and preparative LC followed by collection of various flavonoids and fractions containing anthocyanin. However, of the several MALDI matrices studied, 2,5-dihydroxybenzoic acid (DHB) was considered to be the preferred matrix for isoflavones from soy foods, anthocyanins from tea and onions and 2,4,6-trihydroxyacetophenone (THAP) for flavonol glycosides from fruit juices and red wine.

21.8.2 Other Methods

Separation techniques like CE, TLC and GC are not used regularly for analyzing flavonoids compared to LC. The consideration towards traditional techniques like TLC and GC can be termed rather surprising, but CE is a comparatively novel and versatile technique and has only been utilized in the past 10 years for flavonoid analysis. Use of supercritical fluid chromatography (SFC) and high-speed countercurrent chromatography (HSCCC) is restricted to flavonoid analysis (Tsao and Deng 2004).

21.8.2.1 Gas Chromatography

In early 1960, GC was used for the analysis of flavonoids (Narasimhachari and Rudloff 1962). Post-derivatization, flavonoids were isolated on a semi-preparative scale utilizing a SE-30 silicone polymer column followed by thermal conductivity detection; collected fractions were subjected to IR and UV/Vis spectroscopy. After LC analysis started gaining attention, flavonoid analysis by GC turned out to be less important, but of late it gained remarkable consideration (Morton et al. 1999; Deng and Zito 2003; Fiamegos et al. 2004), probably due to the advancements in high-temperature GC and the introduction of enhanced derivatization technique. However, in recent studies conventional derivatization methods and temperature programs are used. Even though GC-based methods offer high sensitivity and resolution, their derivatization procedures are laborious. But the derivatization process leads to the formation of trimethylsilyl ether (TMS) derivatives which may result in the enhancement of thermal stability and volatility. Quantification of flavonoids is difficult when multiple hydroxyl substituent methylations result in numerous derivatives. Nowadays, fused silica capillary columns are in use as alternative to packed glass columns which was popular in the early 1960s. Recent research articles on flavonoid analysis by GC are directed in the area of nutrition and biology and concentrated on metabolism, antioxidant activity and taxonomy. LC-based method development would have been a good option, but little attention has been paid in this regard.

Hydrolysis of flavonoids is carried out and subsequently they are transformed into TMS derivatives, injected onto a non-polar column (DB-5 or DB-1). The column was used in split or splitless mode and separation was performed with a linear temperature program (30–90 min) up to 300 °C. *N*-(*tert*-butyldimethylsilyl)-*N*-methyltrifluoroacetamide (TBDMS) and *N,O*-bis-(trimethylsilyl)-trifluoroacetamide (BSTFA) are the derivatizing agents which are most frequently used, along with detection in EI–MS mode with temperature of up to 250 °C employed. Detection was carried out with the molecular ion, $[M + H]^+$ and fragments produced by the loss of CH_3 and/or CO and retro-Diels–Alder (RDA) reactions. Genistein and daidzein present in fruits and nuts were determined by extraction of freeze-dried samples using methanol and subsequent hydrolysis with cellulase in acetate buffer. Extraction of aglycones with ethyl acetate and derivatization using TBDMS was performed followed by GC–MS analysis (Liggins et al. 2000). Out of 80 samples analyzed, only 37 found to have detectable quantities of isoflavones and 9 of them contained more than 100 μg/kg wet wt. Quantification limit was found to be 1 μg/kg. Several herbs have been analyzed by GC–MS for flavonoids and phenolic acids using an advanced derivatization procedure namely vial derivatization–extraction (Fiamegos et al. 2003, 2004). Alkaline conditions have to be maintained during derivatization to facilitate deprotonation of hydroxyl groups of the analytes. With the use of a phase transfer catalyst (PTC), transfer of anionic nucleophiles to organic phase was facilitated and then made to react with methyl iodide. One of the best PTC currently used is polymer-bound tri-*n*-butyl methyl phosphonium chloride. Flavonoids present in the extract showed LOD of 4–40 ng/mL in the SIM (Selected Ion Monitoring) mode. Determination of flavonoids in several food and food supplements like fruits and soy products and in serum using GC–MS has been reported recently, in which bioactivity and bioavailability of flavonoids and phyto-estrogens were studied (Morton et al. 1999; Liggins et al. 2000; Setchell et al. 2001; Rechner et al. 2004). An exciting part of the previous paper cited is that isotope dilution GC–MS was utilized in the study (Morton et al. 1999). Due to the high concentration of daidzein and genistein present in soy, their determination seems to be a non-challenging task. However, it is difficult to estimate the concentration of isoflavones accurately, since soy food consumption results in very low levels of isoflavones in the human body and some amount of them are also lost during sample treatment steps making the determination tougher. For an instance (Morton et al. 1999), phytoestrogens were determined in human serum by hydrolyzing samples using β-glucuronidase and then extracting aglycones using ethyl acetate followed by isolation of phyto-estrogen fraction on a Sephadex LH20 column and finally derivatization was done with BSTFA. Internal standards which are deuterated were utilized for the isotope dilution method, with detection in SIM mode. Daidzein and genistein levels in 42 human serum samples were found to be between 2 and 900 ng/mL (means, 80 and 160 ng/mL, respectively). It is difficult to go for further assessment due to lack of analytical performance data. Analysis of flavonoid glycosides using conventional GC have been found to be very tough even if derivatization is performed. Hence, Pereira et al. (2004) analyzed glucoside hesperidin using high-temperature–high-resolution (HT–HR) GC–MS, with columns that can bear temperatures up to 400 °C. However, standard solution of hesperidin showed very low sensitivity with a LOD of 50 mg/L with splitless and cold on-column injection at 370 °C. Additionally, the peaks showed severe tailing even after a lengthy derivatization procedure (72 h) of hesperidin using BSTFA. Interestingly, a research article described determination of mono-isoprenylated flavonoid aglycones (Branco et al. 2001) using HT–HRGC–MS with the help of cold on-column injection in an extract of *Vellozia graminifolia*. Positive fractions obtained from the fractionation using LC and TLC screening were then combined and studied by HT–HRGC–MS. Identification of six mono-isoprenylated flavonols was carried out based on their melting points, IR, MS, ^1H and ^{13}C NMR spectra. When comes to the determination of both flavonoid glycosides and aglycones, it is evident that GC will not easily substitute LC. Such studies require derivatization and there are chances that numerous derivatives are produced for one analyte. This is applicable even if HT-GC is used. The main advantages of SIM mode MS detection are effective in-vial derivatization and high sensitivity (low LODs). However, they cannot outweigh the speed of direct LC–MS(/MS) methods and the ease with which they screen samples for target analytes and unknowns.

21.8.2.2 Capillary Electrophoresis

CE is a known technique with efficient separation and short run time. Generally, when compared to HPLC, CE exhibits much lower sensitivity because of sample overloading and it provides quantitative data which is less precise (Weston and Brown 1997). It is well known that CE can be used for estimation of phytochemicals (Tomas-Barberan 1995; Issaq 1999). At higher pH values, flavonoids are negatively charged making it a suitable analytical technique for flavonoid separation (Tomas-Barberan 1995). A review by Suntornsuk (2002) clearly explained quantitative analysis and method validation of CE for flavonoids. CE can be a suitable alternative of HPLC when higher resolution and higher efficiency is a prerequisite. For instance, a study revealed CE is an appropriate method for analyses of passion flower when HPLC and TLC failed to give satisfactory separation of flavonoids (Marchart et al. 2003). Flavonoid glycosides of *Passiflora incarnata* (Passifloraceae) were separated using an uncoated fused-silica capillary having 50 mm internal diameter by using sodium borate buffer (25 mM) with 20% methanol (pH 9.5). The capillary was kept at 35 °C and a voltage of 30 kV was employed and a diode array detector was used for detection. Separation of twelve glycosides was carried out successfully within 13 min and glycosides were quantified using quercetin 3-*O*-arabinoside as internal standard. Then calibration curves were constructed for internal standardization. Ten commercial samples of *Passiflorae herba* were analyzed using this method. Flavonoid patterns exhibited by samples were similar but individual flavonoid glycosides varied quantitatively. The method showed good reproducibility, interday precision with a coefficient of variation (CV) of 2.83% and a mean CV of 1.26% for migration time (Marchart et al. 2003). Other examples of analysis also include quantitative estimation of flavonoids in *Hypericum perforatum* (Guttiferae) leaves and flowers with the help of online coupling of capillary isotachophoresis and CZE. In this method, flavonoid fractions were concentrated and pre-separated before introducing into the CZE capillary. Quercetin 3-Oglycosides showed detection limit of 100 ng/mL (Urbanek et al. 2002).

21.8.2.3 Thin-Layer Chromatography

TLC is a widely used analytical technique for flavonoid analysis since the 1960s. This technique is quite useful in preliminary screening of plant extracts before analyzing them using instrumental methods such as LC-UV as many samples can be estimated simultaneously. Silica is used extensively as stationary phase and a mixture of 2-(diphenylboryoxo) ethylamine and polyethylene glycol or $AlCl_3$ is used to develop the plates. Either UV light at 350–365 or 250–260 nm or densitometry using the same wavelengths can be used for detection. At present, TLC still is a preferred technique for flavonoid analysis which is evident from the list of papers summarized in Table 21.6 (De Rijke et al. 2006). One of the examples explains separation of rosmarinic acid from *Mentha piperita* (peppermint) and flavonoid glycosides using HPTLC plates (Fecka et al. 2004). Apart from different modified silica sorbents, numerous organic eluents like n-hexane to esters, ethers and methanol were tested. The combination of C_{18}-bonded silica with water-methanol (60:40, v/v) as eluent and aminopropyl-bonded silica column and acetone–acetic acid (85:15, v/v) as mobile phase results in better separation for all the six standard compounds. Peppermint extract was found to contain six standard substances which were isolated with the use of preparative LC and structural determination was carried out using different spectroscopic techniques. The chief flavonoid component found

Table 21.6 Representative studies on TLC of flavonoid

Method	Stationary phase	Eluents (v/v)	Detection	Sample	Flavonoids
HPTLC	Silica	EtAc-FA-H_2O (82:9:9)	Densitometry at 300 nm	*Passiflora* leaves	Orientin, isoorientin
HPTLC	Silica	EtAc-MeOH-FA (various v/v)	UV at 254 nm	Standard mixture	8 aglycons, 15 glycosides
HPTLC	Silica, aminopropyl, cyanopropyl-and C18-bonded silica	Various eluents were tested; Me_2O-AcOH 85:15 was the best	UV at 366 nm and (after isolation) IR	*Mentha piperita*	5 flavonoids
Double development	Silica	EtAc-FA-H_2O (85:15:0.5) and DCM-EtAc-FA (85:15:0.5)	Densitometry at 254 nm	Standard mixture	9 glycosides, 7 aglycones
TLC	Silica	EtAc-MeOH-FA (90:10:1)	Densitometry at 254	Standard mixture	6 flavonoid glycosides
TLC	Silica	Toluene-EtAc-FA-MeOH (3:3:0.8:0.2)	Densitometry at 355 nm	*Bacopa monnieri*, *Cuminum cyminum* fruit, *Achillea millefolium* flower	Luteolin
TLC	Silica	EtAc-FA-AcOH-H_2O (100:11:11:26) EtAc-FA-H_2O (8:1:1)	UV at 365 nm	5 *Hypericum* taxa plants	10 flavonoids
2D	Cyanopropyl-bonded silica	Several NP and RP systems	UV at 254 and 365 nm	Standard mixture	9 flavonoids
2D	Cyanopropyl-bonded silica	Me_2O-iPrOH (6:4) and 50% MeOH or THF or 1,4, dioxane	UV at 366 nm	*Sambucus nigra*	8 flavonoids
Numerical taxonomy	Silica	EtAc-MeOH-H_2O (75:15:0), EtAc-FA-H_2O (80:10:10), EtAc-FA-AcOH-H_2O (100:11:11:27)	Densitometry at 254 and 366 nm	Propolis	Flavonols, flavanones
Numerical taxonomy	Silica	Chloroform-MeOH-FA (various v/v) *n*-hexane-EtAc-AcOH (31:14:5)	UV at 366 nm	Propolis	Flavonoid and phenolic acid
Numerical taxonomy	Silica	EtAc-FA-H_2O (65:15:20)	UV at 366 nm	*Helleborus atrorubens*	Quercetin, kaempferol

EtAc, ethyl acetate; *Me_2O*, acetone; *FA*, formic acid; *AcOH*, acetic acid; *MeOH*, methanol; *DCM*, dichloromethane; *iPROH*, isopropanol

Reprinted from Journal of Chromatography A, 1112, Eva de Rijke, Pieter Out, Wilfried M.A. Niessen, FreekAriese, Cees Gooijer, Udo A.Th. Brinkman, Analytical separation and detection methods for flavonoids, 31–63., Copyright (2006), with permission from Elsevier

was eriocitrin; but quantification data was not provided. Further, Soczewinski et al. (2004) explained another method, which utilized double-development TLC for the separation of flavonoid mixture comprising seven aglycones and nine glucosides. Initially, using an eluent with high solvent strength, more polar glycosides were separated. Subsequently, the solvent was evaporated and separation of aglycones was done using a comparatively weak eluent. Many research articles (Medic-Saric et al. 2001; Males and Medic-Saric 2001; Jasprica et al. 2004; Rastija et al. 2004) used numerical taxonomy to compute the orthogonality of the retention factors of flavonoid mixtures. The optimum eluent composition for the determination of flavonoids in red wine

(Rastija et al. 2004) and in propolis (Jasprica et al. 2004) was studied. For this, 11 tertiary eluents were used.

The fact that, out of 19 standard compounds analyzed, for the optimum eluent combination, 10 were identified in 14 propolis samples of diverse origin demonstrates success of the method. Three flavonoids and numerous phenolic compounds were also identified in red wine (Rastija et al. 2004). Though TLC studies are not generally meant for quantification, densitometry has been utilized in several studies (Jamshidi et al. 2000; Janeczko et al. 2004). One of the research papers (Jamshidi et al. 2000) described estimation of kaempferol and quercetin in *Ginkgo biloba* leaf extract using HPTLC silica plates in the reflectance mode at 254 nm which gave a recovery of 94% using standard addition method. Kaempferol and quercetin concentrations in the extract were found to be 7 and 14 mg/L, respectively. Genistin and daidzin were also determined using a similar technique in soy cultivars (Janeczko et al. 2004). Genistin and daidzin concentrations were found to be 0.06–0.15% and 0.03–0.01%, respectively. Additionally, determination of phenolic acids, flavanones, flavonols and propolis was also carried out using two-dimensional (2D) TLC with densitometry at 254 and 366 nm (Medic-Saric et al. 2004). Again, good results were obtained with a concentration of 90–1440 mg/L. Wojciak-Kosior et al. (2004) studied hydrolysis of six flavonoid glycosides using TLC combined with densitometry. The flavonoids were analyzed in a time interval of every 15 min after heating under reflux using HCl. The pseudo-first-order hydrolysis of 3- and 7-glycosides proceeded at rate constants ranging between 1.7×10^{-2} and 1.1×10^{-2} min^{-1}; time taken for hydrolysis of 7-glycosides was 90–105 min. Rutin which is a diglycoside had a more complex hydrolysis mechanism which probably involves two steps. Another study (Hawryl et al. 2002) used cyanopropyl-bonded silica as stationary phase for the separation of three phenolic acids and eight flavonoids in *Flos sambuci* L. using two-dimensional TLC. From the abovementioned studies, it is evident that TLC is still in trend for flavonoid analysis. The stress should be given for analyzing the main flavonoids in real-life samples. For this, methods such as numerical taxonomy also can be useful.

References

Agati G, Azzarello E, Pollastri S, Tattini M. Flavonoids as antioxidants in plants: location and functional significance. Plant Sci. 2012;196:67–76.

Aherne SA, Obrien NM. Dietary flavonols: chemistry, food content and metabolism. Nutrition. 2002;18:75–81.

Andlauer W, Martena MJ, Furst P. Determination of selected phytochemicals by reversed-phase high performance liquid chromatography combined with ultraviolet and mass spectrometric detection. J Chromatogr A. 1999;849:341–8.

Arts IC, Van de Putte B, Hollman PC. Catechin contents of foods commonly consumed in the Netherlands. 1. Fruits, vegetables, staple foods, and processed foods. J Agric Food Chem. 2000a;48:1746–51.

Arts ICW, Van de Putte B, Hollman PC. Catechin contents of foods commonly consumed in the Netherlands. 2. Tea, wine, fruit juices, and chocolate milk. J Agric Food Chem. 2000b;48:1752–7.

Bader AN, Pivovarenko VG, Demchenko AP, Ariese F, Gooijer C. Excited state and ground state proton transfer rates of 3-hydroxyflavone and its derivatives studied by shpol'skii spectroscopy: the influence of redistribution of electron density. J Phys Chem B. 2004;108:10589–95.

Bansal A, Chhabra V, Rawal RK, Sharma S. Chemometrics: a new scenario in herbal drug standardization. J Pharm Anal. 2014;4:223–33.

Barbuch RJ, Coutant JE, Welsh MB, Setchell KDR. The use of thermospray liquid chromatography/tandem mass spectrometry for the class identification and structural verification of phytoestrogens in soy protein preparations. Biomed Environ Mass Spectrom. 1989;18:973–7.

Benavente-Garcia O, Castillo J, Marin FR, Ortuno A, Del-Rio JA. Uses and properties of citrus flavonoids. J Agric Food Chem. 1997;45:4505–15.

Benthin B, Danz H, Hamburger M. Pressurized liquid extraction of medicinal plants. J Chromatogr A. 1999;837:211–9.

Bevan CD, Marshall PS. The use of supercritical fluids in the isolation of natural products. Nat Prod Rep. 1994;11:451–66.

Block G, Patterson B, Subar A. Fruit, vegetables, and cancer prevention: a review of the epidemiological evidence. Nutr Cancer. 1992;18:1–29.

Borris RP. Natural products research: perspectives from a major pharmaceutical company. J Ethnopharmacol. 1996;51:29–38.

Boue SM, Carter-Wientjes CH, Shih BY, Cleveland TE. Identification of flavone aglycones and glycosides in soybean pods by liquid chromatography–tandem mass spectrometry. J Chromatogr A. 2003;991:61–8.

Branco A, Pereira AD, Cardoso JN, De Aquino Neto FR, Pinto AC, Braz R. Further lipophilic flavonols in Vellozia graminifolia (Velloziaceae) by high temperature gas chromatography: quick detection of new compounds. Phytochem Anal. 2001;12:266–70.

Bravo L. Polyphenols: chemistry, dietary sources, metabolism, and nutritional significance. Nutr Rev. 1988;56:317–33.

Brown JE, Khodr H, Hider RC, Rice-Evans CA. Structural dependence of flavonoid interactions with Cu2+ ions: implications for their antioxidant properties. Biochem J. 1998;330:1173–8.

Careri M, Mangia A, Musci M. Overview of the applications of liquid chromatography–mass spectrometry interfacing systems in food analysis: naturally occurring substances in food. J Chromatogr A. 1998;794:263–97.

Carlton RR, Gray AI, Lavaud C, Massiot G, Peter Waterman PG. Kaempferol-3-(2,3-diacetoxy-4-p-coumaroyl) rhamnoside from leaves of Myrica gale. Phytochemistry. 1990;29:2369–71.

Chu YH, Chang CL, Hsu HF. Flavonoid content of several vegetables and their antioxidant activity. J Sci Food Agric. 2000;80:561–6.

Clifford AH, Cuppett SL. Review: anthocyanins-nature, occurrence and dietary burden. J Sci Food Agric. 2000;80:1063–72.

Cook NC, Samman S. Review: flavonoids—chemistry, metabolism, cardioprotective effects, and dietary sources. J Nutr Biochem. 1996;7:66–76.

Cowan MM. Plant products as antimicrobial agents. Clin Microbiol Rev. 1999;12:564–82.

Cushnie TP, Lamb AJ. Antimicrobial activity of flavonoids. Int J Antimicrob Agents. 2005;26:343–56.

Da Costa CT, Dalluge JJ, Welch MJ, Coxon B, Margolis SA, Horton D. Characterization of prenylated xanthones and flavanones by liquid chromatography/atmospheric pressure chemical ionization mass spectrometry. J Mass Spectrom. 2000;35:540–9.

Dawidowicz AL, Wianowska D, Gawdzik J, Danuta H, Smolarz DH. Optimization of ASE conditions for the HPLC determination of rutin and isoquercitrin in *Sambucus nigra* L. J Liq Chromatogr Relat Technol. 2003;26:2381–97.

De Rijke E, Zafra-Gomez A, Ariese F, Brinkman UA, Gooije C. Determination of isoflavone glucoside malonates in Trifolium pratense L. (red clover) extracts: quantification and stability studies. J Chromatogr A. 2001;932:55–64.

De Rijke E, Joshi HC, Sanderse HR, Ariese F, Brinkman UA, Gooijer C. Natively fluorescent isoflavones exhibiting anomalous Stokes' shifts. Anal Chim Acta. 2002;468:3–11.

De Rijke E, Zappey H, Ariese F, Gooijer C, Brinkman UA. Liquid chromatography with atmospheric pressure chemical ionization and electrospray ionization mass spectrometry of flavonoids with triple-quadrupole and ion-trap instruments. J Chromatogr A. 2003;984:45–58.

De Rijke E, Out P, Niessen WM, Ariese F, Gooijer C, Brinkman UA. Analytical separation and detection methods for flavonoids. J Chromatogr A. 2006;1112:31–63.

Debnath PK, Banerjee S, Debnath P, Mitra A, Mukherjee PK. Ayurveda-opportunity for developing safe and effective treatment choice for the future. In: Mukherjee PK, editor. Evidence-based validation of herbal medicine. Amsterdam: Elsevier Science Publishing Co Inc; 2015. p. 427–54.

Deng F, Zito SW. Development and validation of a gas chromatographic-mass spectrometric method for simultaneous identification and quantification of marker compounds including bilobalide, ginkgolides and flavonoids in *Ginkgo biloba* L. extract and pharmaceutical preparations. J Chromatogr A. 2003;986:121–7.

Dey PM. Methods in plant biochemistry: plant phenolics. 1st ed. London: Academic Press Ltd; 1989.

Dixon RA, Dey PM, Lamb CJ. Phytoalexins: enzymology and molecular biology. Adv Enzymol Relat Areas Mol Biol. 1983;55:1–136.

Du F, Zhang F, Chen F, Wang A, Wang Q, Yin X, et al. Advances in microbial heterologous production of flavonoids. Afr J Microbiol Res. 2011;5:2566–74.

Duthie GG, Duthie SJ, Kyle JA. Plant polyphenols in cancer and heart disease: implications as nutritional antioxidants. Nutr Res Rev. 2000;13:79–106.

Etievant P, Schlich P, Bertrand A, Symonds P, Bouvier JC. Varietal and geographic classification of French red wines in terms of pigments and flavonoid compounds. J Sci Food Agric. 1988;42:39–54.

Fabre N, Rustan I, De Hoffman E, Quetin-Leclercq J. Determination of flavone, flavonol, and flavanone aglycones by negative ion liquid chromatography electrospray ion trap mass spectrometry. J Am Soc Mass Spectrom. 2001;12:707–15.

Fecka I, Kowalczyk A, Cisowski W. Optimization of the separation of flavonoid glycosides and rosmarinic acid from *Mentha piperita* on HPTLC plates. J Planar Chromatogr. 2004;17:22–5.

Ferry DR, Smith A, Malkhandi J, Fyfe DW, de Takats PG, Anderson D, et al. Phase I clinical trial of the flavonoid quercetin: pharmacokinetics and evidence for in vivo tyrosine kinase inhibition. Clin Cancer Res. 1996;2:659–68.

Fiamegos YC, Konidari CN, Stalikas CD. Cyanuric acid trace analysis by extractive methylation via phase transfer catalysis and capillary gas chromatography coupled with flame thermoionic and mass-selective detection. Process parameter studies and kinetics. Anal Chem. 2003;75:4034–42.

Fiamegos YC, Nanos CG, Vervoort J, Stalikas CD. Analytical procedure for the in-vial derivatization--extraction of phenolic acids and flavonoids in methanolic and aqueous plant extracts followed by gas chromatography with mass-selective detection. J Chromatogr A. 2004;1041:11–8.

Franke AA, Custer LJ. High performance liquid chromatographic assay of isoflavonoids and coumestrol from human urine. J Chromatogr B Biomed Sci Appl. 1994;662:47–60.

Ganzler K, Szinai I, Salgo A. Effective sample preparation method for extracting biologically active compounds from different matrices by a microwave technique. J Chromatogr. 1990;520:257–62.

Garcia-Viguera C, Bakker J, Bellworthy SJ, Reader HP, Watkins SJ, Bridle P. The effect of some processing variables on non-coloured phenolic compounds in port wines. Eur Food Res Technol. 1997;205:321–4.

Gerdin B, Srensso E. Inhibitory effect of the flavonoid O-(beta-hydroxyethyl)-rutoside on increased microvascular permeability induced by various agents in rat skin. Int J Microcirc Clin Exp. 1983;2:39–46.

Gil-Izquierdo A, Gil MI, Ferreres F, Tomas-Barberan FA. In vitro availability of flavonoids and other phenolics in orange juice. J Agric Food Chem. 2001;49:1035–41.

Grayer RJ, Kite GC, Abou-Zaid M, Archer LJ. The application of atmospheric pressure chemical ionization liquid chromatography–mass spectrometry in the chemotaxonomic study of flavonoids: characterization of flavonoids from *Ocimum gratissimum* var. *gratissimum*. Phytochem Anal. 2000;11:257–67.

Gutierrez AC, Gehlen MH. Time resolved fluorescence spectroscopy of quercetin and morin complexes with Al^{3+}. Spectrochim Acta A Mol Biomol Spectrosc. 2002;58:83–9.

Halliwell B, Gutteridge JMC. Free radicals in biology and medicine. 5th ed. Oxford: Oxford University Press; 1998.

Hamburger M, Baumann D, Adler S. Supercritical carbon dioxide extraction of selected medicinal plants--effects of high pressure and added ethanol on yield of extracted substances. Phytochem Anal. 2004;15:46–54.

Hansen SH, Jensen AG, Cornett C, Bjornsdottir I, Taylor S, Wright B, et al. High-performance liquid chromatography on-line coupled to high-field NMR and mass spectrometry for structure elucidation of constituents of *Hypericum perforatum* L. Anal Chem. 1999;71:5235–41.

Haraguchi H, Tanimoto K, Tamura Y, Mizutani K, Kinoshita T. Mode of antibacterial action of retrochalcones from Glycyrrhiza inflata. Phytochemistry. 1998;48:125–9.

Harborne JB. Phytochemical methods: a guide to modern techniques of plant analysis. 2nd ed. New York: Chapman and Hall; 1988.

Harborne JB, Turner BL. Plant chemosystematics. London: Academic Press; 1984.

Hasler A, Sticher O, Meier B. Identification and determination of the flavonoids from *Ginkgo biloba* by high-performance liquid chromatography. J Chromatogr A. 1992;605:41–8.

Hawryl M, Hawryl A, Soczewinski E. Application of normal- and reversed-phase 2D TLC on a cyanopropyl-bonded polar stationary phase for separation of phenolic compounds from the flowers of *Sambucus nigra* L. J Planar Chromatogr. 2002;15:4–10.

He Q, Kim J, Sharma RP. Silymarin protects against liver damage in BALB/c mice exposed to fumonisin B1 despite increasing accumulation of free sphingoid bases. Toxicol Sci. 2004;80:335–42.

Heim KE, Tagliaferro AR, Bobilya DJ. Flavonoid antioxidants: chemistry, metabolism and structure-activity relationships. J Nutr Biochem. 2002;13:572–84.

Hertog MGL, Hollman PCH, Katan MB. Content of potentially anticarcinogenic flavonoids of 28 vegetables and 9 fruits commonly consumed in the Netherlands. J Agric Food Chem. 1992;40:2379–83.

Hertog MG, Hollman PC, Katan MB. Intake of potentially anticarcinogenic flavonoids and their determinants in adults in the Netherlands. Nutr Cancer. 1993a;20:21–9.

Hertog MGL, Hollman PCH, Van de Putte B. Content of potentially anticarcinogenic flavonoids of tea infusions, wine sand fruit juices. J Agric Food Chem. 1993b;41:1242–6.

Ho CT, Lee CY, Huang MT. Phenolic compounds in food and their effects on health I: analysis. Occurrence & Chemistry: American Chemical Society; 1992.

Ho CT, Osawa T, Huang MT, Rosen RT. Food phytochemicals for cancer prevention II: teas, spices, and herbs. Oxford University Press: American Chemical Society; 1994.

Hollman PC, De Vries JH, Van Leeuwen SD, Mengelers MJ, Katan MB. Absorption of dietary quercetin in healthy ileostomy volunteers. Am J Clin Nutr. 1995;62:1276–82.

Hollman PCH, Van Trijp JMP, Buysman MNCP. Fluorescence detection of flavonols in HPLC by post column chelation with aluminium. Anal Chem. 1996;68:3511–5.

Hollman PC, Van Trijp JM, Buysman MN, Van Der Gaag MS, Mengelers MJ, De Vries JH, et al. Relative bioavailability of the antioxidant flavonoid quercetin from various foods in man. FEBS Lett. 1997;418:152–6.

Hostettmann K, Marston A, Hostettmann M. Preparative chromatography techniques: applications in natural product isolation. 2nd ed. Berlin: Springer-Verlag; 1998.

Huang MT, Osawa T, Ho CT, Rosen RT. Food phytochemicals for cancer prevention I: fruits and vegetables. 1st ed. Washington DC: Am Chem Society; 1994.

Huck CW, Bonn GK. Evaluation of detection methods for the reversed-phase HPLC determination of 3′,4′,5′-trimethoxyflavone in different phytopharmaceutical products and in human serum. Phytochem Anal. 2001;12:104–9.

Hunter T. Protein kinases and phosphatases: the yin and yang of protein phosphorylation and signalling. Cell. 1995;80:225–36.

Hussein L, Fattah MA, Salem E. Characterization of pure proanthocyanidins isolated from the hulls of faba beans. J Agric Food Chem. 1990;38:95–8.

Issaq HJ. Capillary electrophoresis of natural products-II. Electrophoresis. 1999;20:3190–202.

Jamshidi A, Adjvadi M, Husain SW. Determination of Kaempferol and Quercetin in the extract of Ginkgo biloba by high-performance thin layer chromatography (HPTLC). J Planar Chromatogr. 2000;13:57–9.

Janeczko Z, Krzek J, Pisulewska E, Sobolewska D, Dabrowska-Tylka M, Hubicka U, et al. Densitometric determination of genistin and daidzin in different cultivars of soy (Glycine max). J Planar Chromatogr. 2004;17:32–5.

Jarvis AP, Morgan ED. Isolation of plant products by supercritical fluid extraction. Phytochem Anal. 1997;8:217–22.

Jasprica I, Smolcic-Bubalo A, Mornar A, Medic-Saric M. Investigation of the flavonoids in Croatian propolis by thin-layer chromatography. J Planar Chromatogr. 2004;17:95–101.

Juan AD, Tauler R. Chemometrics applied to unravel multicomponent processes and mixtures: revisiting latest trends in multivariate resolution. Anal Chim Acta. 2003;500:195–210.

Justesen U, Knuthsen P, Leth T. Quantitative analysis of flavonols, flavones, and flavanones in fruits, vegetables and beverages by high-performance liquid chromatography with photo-diode array and mass spectrometric detection. J Chromatogr A. 1998;799:101–10.

Kaufmann B, Christen P. Recent extraction techniques for natural products: microwave assisted extraction and pressurized solvent extraction. Phytochem Anal. 2002;13:105–13.

Kim SM, Kang K, Jho EH, Jung YJ, Nho CW, Um BH, et al. Hepatoprotective effect of flavonoid glycosides from Lespedeza cuneata against oxidative stress induced by tert-butyl hyperoxide. Phytother Res. 2011;25:1011–7.

Klejdus B, Vacek J, Adam V, Zehnalek J, Kizek R, Trnkova L, et al. Determination of isoflavones in soybean food and human urine using liquid chromatography with electrochemical detection. J Chromatogr B Analyt Technol Biomed Life Sci. 2004;806:101–11.

Koen B, Ruth V, Guido V, Johannes VS. Induction of cancer cell apoptosis by flavonoids is associated with their ability to inhibit fatty acid synthase activity. J Biol Chem. 2005;280:5636–45.

Kumar S, Pandey AK. Antioxidant, lipo-protective and antibacterial activities of phytoconstituents present in *Solanum xanthocarpum root*. Int Review Biophys Chem. 2012;3:42–7.

Kumar S, Pandey AK. Chemistry and biological activities of flavonoids: an overview. Sci World J. 2013a;162750:16. https://doi.org/10.1155/2013/162750.

Kumar S, Pandey AK. Phenolic content, reducing power and membrane protective activities of Solanum xanthocarpum root extracts. Vegetos. 2013b;26:301–7.

Kumar S, Gupta A, Pandey AK. *Calotropis procera* root extract has the capability to combat free radical mediated damage. ISRN Pharmacol. 2013a;691372:8. https://doi.org/10.1155/2013/691372.

Kumar S, Mishra A, Pandey AK. Antioxidant mediated protective effect of *Parthenium hysterophorus* against oxidative damage using *in vitro* models. BMC Complement Altern Med. 2013b;13:120. https://doi.org/10.1186/1472-6882-13-120.

Lamson DW, Brignall MS. Antioxidants and cancer, part 3: quercetin. Altern Med Rev. 2000;5:196–208.

Lee MJ, Wang ZY, Li H, Chen L, Sun Y, Gobbo S, et al. Analysis of plasma and urinary tea polyphenols in human subjects. Cancer Epidemiol Biomark Prev. 1995;4:393–9.

Leopoldini M, Russo N, Chiodo S, Toscano M. Iron chelation by the powerful antioxidant flavonoid quercetin. J Agric Food Chem. 2006;54:6343–51.

Leutert T, Von Arx E. Praparative Mitteldruck-flussigkeitschromatographie (preparative medium-pressure liquid chromatography). J Chromatogr A. 1984;292:333–44.

Liang YZ, Xie P, Chan K. Quality control of herbal medicines. J Chromatogr B Analyt Technol Biomed Life Sci. 2004;812:53–70.

Liggins J, Bluck LJ, Runswick S, Atkinson C, Coward WA, Bingham SA. Daidzein and genistein content of fruits and nuts. J Nutr Biochem. 2000;11:326–31.

Loewus FA, Ryan CA. Recent advances in phytochemistry. 1st ed. New York: Springer US; 1981.

Ma YL, Vedernikova I, Heuvel HVD, Claeys M. Internal glucose residue loss in protonated O-diglycosyl flavonoids upon low-energy collision-induced dissociation. J Am Soc Mass Spectrom. 2000;11:136–44.

Mabry T, Markham KR, Thomas MB, editors. The systematic identification of flavonoids. 1st ed. New York: Springer-Verlag; 1970.

Mahomoodally MF, Gurib-Fakim A, Subratty AH. Antimicrobial activities and phytochemical profiles of endemic medicinal plants of Mauritius. Pharm Biol. 2005;43:237–42.

Males Z, Medic-Saric M. Optimization of TLC analysis of flavonoids and phenolic acids of Helleborus atrorubens Waldst. Et kit. J Pharm Biomed Anal. 2001;24:353–9.

Marchart E, Krenn L, Kopp B. Quantification of the flavonoid glycosides in *Passiflora incarnata* by capillary electrophoresis. Planta Med. 2003;69:452–6.

Markaverich BM, Roberts RR, Alejandro MA, Johnson GA, Middleditch BS, Clark JH. Bioflavonoid interaction with rat uterine type II binding sites and cell growth inhibition. J Steroid Biochem. 1988;30:71–8.

Mattila P, Astola J, Kumpulainen J. Determination of flavonoids in plant material by HPLC with diode-array and electro-array detections. J Agric Food Chem. 2000;48:5834–41.

McKee TC, Bokesch HR, McCormick JL, Rashid MA, Spielvogel D, Gustafson KR, et al. Isolation and characterization of new anti-HIV and cytotoxic leads from plants, marine, and microbial organisms. J Nat Prod. 1997;60:431–8.

Medic-Saric M, Stanic G, Bosnjak I. The use of information theory and numerical taxonomy methods for evaluating the quality of thin-layer chromatographic separations of flavonoid constituents of Matricariae flos. Pharmazie. 2001;56:156–9.

Medic-Saric M, Jasprica I, Mornar A, Smolcic-Bubalo A, Golja P. Quantitative analysis of flavonoids and phenolic acids in propolis by two-dimensional thin layer chromatography 2004.

Merken HM, Beecher GR. Measurement of food flavonoids by high-performance liquid chromatography: a review. J Agric Food Chem. 2000;48:577–99.

Middleton E. The flavonoids. Trends Pharmacol Sci. 1984;5:335–8.

Middleton EJ. Effect of plant flavonoids on immune and inflammatory cell function. Adv Exp Med Biol. 1998;439:175–82.

Middleton EJ, Kandaswami C. Effects of flavonoids on immune and inflammatory cell functions. Biochem Pharmacol. 1992;43:1167–79.

Middleton E, Kandaswami C. In: Harborne JB, editor. The flavonoids - advances in research since 1986. London: Chapman and Hall; 1993. p. 619.

Miller LP. Phytochemistry. California: Van Nostrand Reinhold; 1973.

Mishra AK, Mishra A, Kehri HK, Sharma B, Pandey AK. Inhibitory activity of Indian spice plant *Cinnamomum zeylanicum* extracts against *Alternaria solani* and *Curvularia lunata*, the pathogenic dematiaceous moulds. Ann Clin Microbiol Antimicrob. 2009;8:1–7. https://doi.org/10.1186/1476-0711-8-9.

Mishra A, Kumar S, Bhargava A, Sharma B, Pandey AK. Studies on in vitro antioxidant and antistaphylococcal activities of some important medicinal plants. Cell Mol Biol. 2011;57:16–25.

Mishra A, Kumar S, Pandey AK. Scientific validation of the medicinal efficacy of *Tinospora cordifolia*. Sci World J. 2013a;292934:8. https://doi.org/10.1155/2013/292934.

Mishra A, Sharma AK, Kumar S, Saxena AK, Pandey AK. *Bauhinia variegata* leaf extracts exhibit considerable antibacterial, antioxidant and anticancer activities. Biomed Res Int. 2013b;915436:10. https://doi.org/10.1155/2013/915436.

Moerman DE. An analysis of the food plants and drug plants of native North America. J Ethnopharmacol. 1996;52:1–22.

Mori A, Nishino C, Enoki N, Tawata S. Antibacterial activity and mode of action of plant flavonoids against *Proteus vulgaris* and *Staphylococcus aureus*. Phytochemistry. 1987;26:2231–4.

Morton M, Arisaka O, Miyake A, Evans B. Analysis of phyto-oestrogens by gas chromatography-mass spectrometry. Environ Toxicol Pharmacol. 1999;7:221–5.

Narasimhachari N, Rudloff EV. Gas–liquid chromatography of some flavonoid compounds and hydroxy diphenyls. Can J Chem. 1962;40:1123–9.

Narayana KR, Reddy MS, Chaluvadi MR, Krishna DR. Bioflavonoids classification, pharmacological, biochemical effects and therapeutic potential. Indian J Pharmacol. 2001;33:2–16.

Nishizuka Y. The molecular heterogeneity of protein kinase C and its implications for cellular regulation. Nature. 1988;334:661–5.

Ohemeng KA, Schwender CF, Fu KP, Barrett JF. DNA gyrase inhibitory and antibacterial activity of some flavones. Bioorg Med Chem Lett. 1993;3:225–30.

Pan MH, Lai CS, Ho CT. Anti-inflammatory activity of natural dietary flavonoids. Food Funct. 2010;1:15–31.

Pan S, Zhou S, Gao S, Yu Z, Zhang S, Tang M, et al. New perspectives on how to discover drugs from herbal medicines: CAM's outstanding contribution to modern therapeutics. Evid Based Complement Altern Med. 2013:25.

Pan S, Litscher G, Gao S, Zhou S, Yu Z, Chen H, et al. Historical perspective of traditional indigenous medical practices: the current renaissance and conservation of herbal resources. Evid Based Complement Alternat Med. 2014;525340:20. https://doi.org/10.1155/2014/525340.

Pandey AK. Anti-staphylococcal activity of a pantropical aggressive and obnoxious weed Parihenium histerophorus: an in vitro study. Natl Acad Sci Lett. 2007;30:383–6.

Pandey AK, Mishra AK, Mishra A, Kumar S, Chandra A. Therapeutic potential of C. zeylanicum extracts: an antifungal and antioxidant perspective. Int J Biol Med Res. 2010;1:228–33.

Pandey AK, Mishra AK, Mishra A. Antifungal and antioxidative potential of oil and extracts derived from leaves of Indian spice plant Cinnamomum tamala. Cell Mol Biol. 2012;58:142–7.

Pandey MM, Rastogi S, AKS R. Indian traditional ayurvedic system of medicine and nutritional supplementation. Evid Based Complement Alternat Med. 2013:12. https://doi.org/10.1155/2013/376327.

Pereira ADS, Padilha MC, Neto FRDA. Two decades of high temperature gas chromatography (1983-2003): what's next? Microchem J. 2004;77:141–9.

Peterson J, Dwyer J. Flavonoids: dietary occurrence and biochemical activity. Nutr Res. 1998;18:1995–2018.

Peyrat-Maillard MN, Bonnely S, Berset C. Determination of the antioxidant activity of phenolic compounds by coulometric detection. Talanta. 2000;51:709–16.

Pineiro Z, Palma M, Barroso CG. Determination of catechins by means of extraction with pressurized liquids. J Chromatogr A. 2004;1026:19–23.

Rahman A. Studies in natural products chemistry. 1st ed. Amsterdam: Elsevier Science Ltd; 1989.

Rastija V, Mornar A, Jasprica I, Srecnik G, Medic-Saric M. Analysis of phenolic components in Croatian red wines by thin-layer chromatography. J Planar Chromatogr. 2004;17:26–31.

Ratty AK, Das NP. Effects of flavonoids on nonenzymatic lipid peroxidation: structure-activity relationship. Biochem Med Metab Biol. 1988;39:69–79.

Rauha JP, Vuorela H, Kostiainen R. Effect of eluent on the ionization efficiency of flavonoids by ion spray, atmospheric pressure chemical ionization, and atmospheric pressure photoionization mass spectrometry. J Mass Spectrom. 2001;36:1269–80.

Rechner AR, Smith MA, Kuhnle G, Gibson GR, Debnam ES, Srai SK, et al. Colonic metabolism of dietary polyphenols: influence of structure on microbial fermentation products. Free Radic Biol Med. 2004;36:212–25.

Reinhold L, Harborne JB, Swain T. Progress in Phytochemlstry. 1st ed. Oxford: Pergamon Press; 1977.

Rice-Evans CA, Miller NJ, Bolwell PG, Broamley PM, Pridham JB. The relative antioxidant activities of plant-derived polyphenolic flavonoids. Free Radic Res. 1995;22:375–83.

Rice-Evans CA, Miller NJ, Paganga G. Structure-antioxidant activity relationships of flavonoids and phenolic acids. Free Radic Biol Med. 1996;20:933–56.

Rodriguez-Delgado MA, Malovana S, Perez JP, Borges T, Garcia Montelongo FJ. Separation of phenolic compounds by high-performance liquid chromatography with absorbance and fluorimetric detection. J Chromatogr A. 2001;912:249–57.

Rosenberg ZRS, Jenkins DJ, Diamandis EP. Flavonoids and steroid hormone-dependent cancers. J Chromatogr B Analyt Technol Biomed Life Sci. 2002;777:219–32.

Sakakibara H, Honda Y, Nakagawa S, Ashida H, Kanazawa K. Simultaneous determination of all polyphenols in vegetables, fruits, and teas. J Agric Food Chem. 2003;51:571–81.

Saleh MM, Hashem FAEM, Glombitza KW. Study of Citrus taitensis and radical scavenger activity of the flavonoids isolated. Food Chem. 1998;63:397–400.

Saller R, Meier R, Brignoli R. The use of silymarin in the treatment of liver diseases. Drugs. 2001;61:2035–63.

Sargenti SR, Vichnewski W. Sonication and liquid chromatography as a rapid technique for extraction and fractionation of plant material. Phytochem Anal. 2000;11:69–73.

Schaufelberger D, Hostettmann K. Analytical and preparative reversed-phase liquid chromatography of secoiridoid glycosides. J Chromatogr A. 1985;346:396–400.

Seal T. Quantitative HPLC analysis of phenolic acids, flavonoids and ascorbic acid in four different solvent extracts of two wild edible leaves, *Sonchus arvensis* and *Oenanthe linearis* of north-eastern region in India. J App Pharm Sci. 2016;6:157–66.

Sen S, Chakraborty R. Revival, modernization and integration of Indian traditional herbal medicine in clinical practice: importance, challenges and future. J Tradit Complement Med. 2017;7:234–44.

Sengupta PK, Kasha M. Excited state proton-transfer spectroscopy of 3-hydroxyflavone and quercetin. Chem Phys Lett. 1979;68:382–5.

Setchell KD, Brown NM, Desai P, Zimmer-Nechemias L, Wolfe BE, Brashear WT, et al. Bioavailability of pure isoflavones in healthy humans and analysis of commercial soy isoflavone supplements. J Nutr. 2001;131:1362S–75S.

Shankar D, Majumdar B. Beyond the biodiversity convention: the challenges facing the biocultural heritage of India's medicinal plants. In: Bodeker G, KKS B, Burley J, Vantomme P, editors. Medicinal plants for Forest conservation and health care. Rome: Food and Agriculture Organization (FAO); 1997. p. 87–99.

Singleton VL, Noble AC. Wine flavour and phenolic substances. In: Charalambous G, Katz I, editors. Phenolic, sulfur, and nitrogen compounds in food flavors. Chicago: American Chemical Society; 1976. p. 47–70.

Soczewinski E, Wojciak-Kosior M, Matysik G. Analysis of glycosides and aglycones of flavonoid compounds by double-development thin-layer chromatography. J Planar Chromatogr. 2004;17:261–3.

Sonnenbichler J, Zetl I. Biochemical effects of the flavonolignan silibinin on RNA, protein and DNA synthesis in rat livers. Prog Clin Biol Res. 1986;213:319–31.

Spencer JP, Vauzour D, Rendeiro C. Flavonoids and cognition: the molecular mechanisms underlying their behavioural effects. Arch Biochem Biophys. 2009;492:1–9.

Stoggl WM, Huck CW, Bonn GK. Structural elucidation of catechin and epicatechin in sorrel leaf extracts using liquid-chromatography coupled to diode array-, fluorescence-, and mass spectrometric detection. J Sep Sci. 2004;27:524–8.

Suntornsuk L. Capillary electrophoresis of phytochemical substances. J Pharm Biomed Anal. 2002;27:679–98.

Tapas AR, Sakarkar DM, Kakde RB. Flavonoids as nutraceuticals: a review. Trop J Pharm Res. 2008;7:1089–99.

Tomas-Barberan FA. Capillary electrophoresis: a new technique in the analysis of plant secondary metabolites. Phytochem Anal. 1995;6:177–92.

Tomas-Barberan FA, Clifford MN. Flavanones, chalcones and dihydrochalcones–nature, occurrence and dietary burden. J Sci Food Agric. 2000;80:1073–80.

Tsao R, Deng Z. Separation procedures for naturally occurring antioxidant phytochemicals. J Chromatogr B. 2004;812:85–99.

Tsuchiya H, Iinuma M. Reduction of membrane fluidity by antibacterial sophoraflavanone G isolated from Sophora exigua. Phytomedicine. 2000;7:161–5.

Tunon MJ, Garcia-Mediavilla MV, Sanchez-Campos S, Gonzalez-Gallego J. Potential of flavonoids as anti-inflammatory agents: modulation of pro-inflammatory gene expression and signal transduction pathways. Curr Drug Metab. 2009;10:256–71.

Urbanek M, Blechtova L, Pospisilova M, Polasek M. On-line coupling of capillary isotachophoresis and capillary zone electrophoresis for the determination of flavonoids in methanolic extracts of Hypericum perforatum leaves or flowers. J Chromatogr A. 2002;958:261–71.

Van Beek TA, Breteler H. Phytochemistry and agriculture (proceedings of phytochemical Society of Europe). Oxford: Clarendon Press; 1993.

Wachtel-Galor S, Benzie IFF. Herbal medicine: an introduction to its history, usage, regulation, current trends, and research needs. In: Benzie IFF, Wachtel-Galor S, editors. Herbal medicine: biomolecular and clinical aspects. 2nd ed. Boca Raton (FL): CRC Press/Taylor & Francis; 2011.

Wang J, Sporns P. Analysis of anthocyanins in red wine and fruit juice using MALDI-MS. J Agric Food Chem. 1999;47:2009–15.

Wang J, Sporns P. MALDI-TOF MS analysis of food flavonol glycosides. J Agric Food Chem. 2000a;48:1657–62.

Wang J, Sporns P. MALDI-TOF MS analysis of isoflavones in soy products. J Agric Food Chem. 2000b;48:5887–92.

Watson DG, Atsriku C, Oliveira EJ. Review role of liquid chromatography–mass spectrometry in the analysis of oxidation products and antioxidants in biological systems. Anal Chim Acta. 2003;492:17–47.

Weston A, Brown PR. HPLC and CE: principles and practice. Sun Diego: Academic Press; 1997.

WHO, General Guidelines for Methodologies on Research and Evaluation of Traditional Medicines, 2000, p. 1–74.

Wojciak-Kosior M, Matysik G, Skalska A. Densitometric determination of kinetics of hydrolysis of flavonoid glycosides. J Planar Chromatogr. 2004;17:286–9.

Wolfbeis OS, Knierzinger A, Schipfer R. pH-dependent fluorescence spectroscopy XVII: first excited singlet state dissociation constants, phototautomerism and dual fluorescence of flavonol. J Photochem. 1983;21:67–79.

Yao LH, Jiang YM, Shi J, Tomas-Barberan FA, Datta N, Singanusong R, et al. Flavonoids in food and their health benefits. Plant Foods Hum Nutr. 2004;59:113–22.

Zhong D, Yang B, Chen X, Li K, Xu J. Determination of scutellarin in rat plasma by high-performance liquid chromatography with ultraviolet detection. J Chromatogr B Analyt Technol Biomed Life Sci. 2003;796:439–44.

Zhu W, Jia Q, Wang Y, Zhang Y, Xia M. The anthocyanin cyanidin-3-O-β-glucoside, a flavonoid, increases hepatic glutathione synthesis and protects hepatocytes against reactive oxygen species during hyperglycemia: involvement of a cAMP-PKA-dependent signaling pathway. Free Radic Biol Med. 2012;52:314–27.

Zogg GC, Nyiredy S, Sticher O. Operating conditions in preparative medium pressure liquid chromatography (MPLC).II. Influence of solvent strength and flow rate of the mobile phase, capacity and dimensions of the column. J Liq Chromatogr. 1989;12:2049–65.

HPTLC Fingerprint in Herbal Drug Formulations

22

Tochhawng Lalhriatpuii

Contents

T. Lalhriatpuii (✉)
Department of Pharmacy, Regional Institute of Paramedical & Nursing Sciences (RIPANS), Aizawl, Mizoram, India

S. Sen, R. Chakraborty (eds.), *Herbal Medicine in India*,
https://doi.org/10.1007/978-981-13-7248-3_22

22.1 Introduction

The most widely used system of medicine in the world today and the earliest system of medicine is herbal medicine. It is medicine made exclusively from plant sources. It is widely used in all community and is common to all cultures and traditions. Herbal drugs are medicines made from plant sources. The term can refer to any of hundreds of herbal remedies sold as dietary supplements and for therapeutic purposes. According to WHO assessment, there are three different types of herbal medicines: raw plant material, processed plant material and medicinal herbal products (Choudhary and Sekhon 2011). Herbal medicines are complex phytochemical mixtures obtained from plant sources which are widely used in the management of healthcare system in both developed and developing countries (Amit et al. 2007). It is no wonder that the world's one-fourth population is using traditional medicines for the treatment of various ailments (Jena et al. 2011). However, one of the impediments to the acceptance of the Ayurvedic or herbal medicines is the lack of standard quality control profiles (Bagul and Rajani 2005). Due to the complex nature and inherent variability of the chemical constituents of the plant-based drugs, it is difficult to establish a quality control parameter (Jeganathan and Kannan 2008). Quality assurance of herbal medicine is an important factor and basic requirement for the herbal drug industry and other drug development organisations (Saraswathy et al. 2009). There are several problems which influence the quality of herbal drugs.

- Variable sources of the raw material.
- The phytochemical constituents of herbs and herbal products may vary depending on the stage and duration of collection, parts of the plant collected, harvest seasons, plant origins (regional status), drying processes and other factors (Ahirwal et al. 2006).
- Plant extracts are mixtures of many phytochemical constituents.
- The active principle(s) is (are) in most cases unknown.
- Selective analytical methods or reference compounds may not be easily available commercially (Wani et al. 2007; Ekka et al. 2008; Bele and Khale 2011).

Analysis of pharmaceutical and natural compounds and newer drugs is commonly used in all the stages of drug discovery and development process. High-performance thin-layer chromatography is one of the sophisticated instrumental techniques based on the full capabilities of thin-layer chromatography. The advantages of automation, scanning, full optimisation, selective detection principle, minimum sample preparation, hyphenation and so on enable it to be one of the most powerful analytical techniques for chromatographic information of complex mixtures of pharmaceuticals, natural products, herbal formulation, clinical samples, food stuffs and so on (Attimarad et al. 2011).

HPTLC remains one of the most flexible, reliable, accurate, sensitive and cost-efficient separation technique ideally suited for the analysis of botanicals and herbal drugs. Used with standardised procedures, it guarantees reproducible results, a vital element in the routine identification and authentication of complex fingerprint profiles of plant extracts and pharmaceutical products and formulations. It has established itself as the method of choice for handling complex analytical tasks involving herbal drugs and botanicals. The unique combination of state-of-the-art instrumentation, standardised procedures and solid theoretical foundations enables it to deliver reliable, cGMP-compliant results time after time (Arup et al. 1993).

Unlike other analytical methods, HPTLC produces visible chromatograms' complex information about the entire sample. Multiple samples can be analysed simultaneously, so that reference and test samples can be compared for proper identification since similarities and differences are immediately apparent and with the help of the image comparison. Several chromatograms can be compared directly, even from different plates. In addition to the visible chromatograms, analogue peak data are also available from the chromatogram. They can be evaluated either by the image-based software Video scan or by scanning densitometry with TLC Scanner, measuring the absorption and/or fluorescence of the substances on the plate. TLC is an offline technique: the subsequent steps are relatively independent, allowing parallel treatment of multiple samples during chromatography (Andola and Purohit 2010).

Standardised manufacturing procedures and suitable analytical tools are required to establish the necessary framework for quality control in herbals. Among those tools, high-performance liquid chromatography (HPLC), high-performance thin-layer chromatography (HPTLC) and capillary electrophoresis are the most widely used to establish reference fingerprints of herbs, against which raw materials can be evaluated and finished products can be assayed. High-performance thin-layer chromatography, also known as planar chromatography, is a modern technique with high separation power and reproducibility superior to classical TLC. Main difference of HPTLC and TLC is in particle and pore size of sorbents. Salient features of HPTLC are given as follows:

- Simultaneous processing of sample and standard—better and reliable analytical precision and accuracy and less need for internal standard
- Several analysts can work simultaneously
- Lower analysis time and less cost per analysis
- Low maintenance cost
- Simple sample preparation—one can handle samples of divergent nature
- No prior treatment for solvents like filtration and degassing
- Low mobile-phase consumption per sample
- No interference from previous analysis—fresh stationary and mobile phases for each analysis, no contamination involved
- Visual detection possible—open system
- Non-UV-absorbing compounds can be detected by post-chromatographic derivatisation (Shinde et al. 2011)

22.2 Common Methodology for HPTLC Analysis

Method development in thin-layer (planar) chromatography is one of the most significant steps for a qualitative and quantitative analysis of drugs and gerbil medicines. During establishing a new analytical procedure, always start with wide literature survey (Nyiredy 2002), i.e. primary information about the physic-chemical characteristics of sample and nature of the sample (structure, polarity, volatility, stability and solubility, viscosity). It involves considerable trial-and-error procedures (Koll et al. 2003). General steps involved in HPTLC method developments are as follows (Patel et al. 2012).

Basic steps:

- Selection of the stationary phase
- Activation of pre-coated plates
- Mobile-phase selection and optimisation
- Sample preparation and application
- Preconditioning chamber saturation
- Chromatogram development (separation)
- Derivatisation
- Detection
- Quantification

22.2.1 Basic Steps

22.2.1.1 Selection of the Stationary Phase

Stationary-phase selection should be based on the type of compounds to be separated at the time of method development (Scott 1973). HPTLC uses smaller plates (10 × 10 or 10 × 20 cm) with significantly decreased development distance (typically 6 cm) and analysis time (7–20 min). HPTLC plates provide improved resolution, higher detection sensitivity and improved in situ quantification and are used for industrial pharmaceutical densitometric quantitative and qualitative analysis (Sethi 1996; Sherma 2007). The pre-coated plates with different supporting materials (glass, aluminium, plastic, etc.) and with different sorbent layers are available in different formats and thicknesses. Usually, plates with a solvent thickness of 100–250 mm are used for quantitative and qualitative analysis. Commonly available pre-coated plates are listed below:

Silica gel 60F: More than 80% of analysis is done on these plates.

Aluminium oxide: Basic substances, alkaloids, steroids.

Microcrystalline cellulose: Amino acids, sugars, antibiotics.

RP-2, RP-8 and RP-18: These are the chemically modified silica gel plates.

Commonly used for analysis of fatty acids, carotenoids, steroids and cholesterol and its esters (Shinde et al. 2011).

22.2.1.2 Activation of Pre-coated Plates

Freshly open box of plates does not require activation. Plates which are exposed to high humidity or kept on hand for a longer time require activation. Activation of the plates can be done by placing the pre-coated plates in an oven at 110–120 °C for 30 min prior to spotting. Aluminium sheets should be placed in between two glass plates and kept in an oven at 110–120 °C for 15 min (Shinde et al. 2011).

22.2.1.3 Mobile-Phase Selection and Optimisation

The selection of mobile phase is based on adsorbent material used as stationary phase and physical and chemical properties of analyte (Wagner 1996). Table 22.1 shows the detail of mobile phase generally used in detection of some chemical compounds. Poor grade of solvent used in preparing mobile phases has been found to decrease resolution, spot definition and Rf value reproducibility. Mobile phase commonly called solvent system is traditionally selected by controlled process of trial and error and also based on one's own experience and literature. Mobile phase should be chosen taking into consideration chemical properties of the analytes and sorbent layer. Use of mobile phase containing more than three or four components should normally be avoided as it is often difficult to get the reproducible ratios of different components. If normal stationary phase is polar and mobile phase selected is nonpolar, then nonpolar compounds are eluted first because of lower affinity with stationary phase and polar compounds retained because of higher affinity with the stationary phase and vice versa (Shinde et al. 2011).

Table 22.1 Generally used mobile phase in detection of some chemical compounds

Sl. no.	Chemical compounds	Mobile phase
1	Polar compounds like anthraglycosides, arbutin, alkaloids, cardiac glycosides, bitter principles, flavonoids, saponin	Ethyl acetate:methanol:water [100:13.5:10]
2	Lipophilic compounds like essential oils, terpenes, coumarin, naphthoquinons, valepotriate	Toluene:ethyl acetate [93:7]
3	Alkaloids	Toluene:ethyl acetate:diethyl amine [70:20:10]
4	Flavonoids	Ethyl acetate:formic acid:glacial acetic acid:water [100:11:11:26]
5	Saponin	Chloroform:glacial acetic acid:methanol:water [64:32:12:8]
6	Coumarin	Diethyl ether:toluene [1:1] saturated with 10% acetic acid
7	Bitter drug	Ethyl acetate:methanol:water [77:15:8]
8	Cardiac glycosides	Ethyl acetate:methanol:water [100:13.5:10] OR [81:11:8]
9	Essential oil	Toluene:ethyl acetate [93:7]
10	Lignans	Chloroform:methanol:water [70:30:4], chloroform:methanol [90:10], toluene:ethyl acetate [70:30]
11	Pigments	Ethyl acetate:formic acid:glacial acetic acid:water [100:11:11:26]
12	Pungent testing	Toluene:ethyl acetate [70:30]
13	Terpenes	Chloroform:methanol:water [65:25:4]
14	Triterpenes	Ethyl acetate:toluene:formic acid [50:50:15], toluene:chloroform:ethanol [40:40:10]

22.2.1.4 Sample Preparation and Application

Perfect solvent system used in HPTLC will be the one that moves all components of the mixture off the baseline but does not put anything on the solvent front. The peaks of interest should be resolved within Rf 0.15 and Rf 0.85. The elution power of the mobile phase depends on a property called eluent strength which is related to the polarity of the mobile-phase components (Patel et al. 2012). The more nonpolar the compound, the faster it will elute (or the less time it will remain on the stationary phase) and the more polar the compound the slower it will elute (or more time on the stationary phase). The following table is useful in predicting the order of elution for solute in solvent system (Shewiyo et al. 2012; Srivastava 2011).

Any sample to be analysed which is having sufficiently high concentration of analyte is simply dissolved in a suitable solvent that will completely solubilise the analyte and leave excipients undissolved to yield a test solution that can be directly applied on HPTLC plate (Koll et al. 2003; Sherma 2007). It is a fact that application of the sample is the most critical step to obtain good resolution for quantification in HPTLC. Sample application technique depends on factors such as the type of sample matrix, workload and time constraints (Jaenchen and Reich 2000; Patel et al. 2012). Usual concentration range is 0.1–1 mg/mL; ranges above this lead to poor separation. Sample and standard can be applied by using an automatic sample applicator with nitrogen gas sprays on TLC plates as bands or spots. Band-wise application has an advantage of better separation, high resolution, better accuracy and high response to densitometer (Shinde et al. 2011).

22.2.1.5 Preconditioning Chamber Saturation

Chamber saturation has a pronounced influence on the separation profile. Unsaturated chamber causes high Rf values. Saturated chamber by lining with filter paper for 30 min prior to development leads to uniform distribution of solvent vapours and requires less solvent for the sample to travel (Shinde et al. 2011).

Table 22.2 Common mobile phases listed by increasing polarity

Sl. no.	Solvent	Eluent strength
1	N-pentane	0.00
2	Hexane	0.01
3	Cyclohexane	0.04
4	Carbon tetrachloride	0.18
5	Toluene	0.29
6	Chloroform	0.40
7	Methylene chloride	0.42
8	Tetrahydrofuran	0.45
9	Acetone	0.56
10	Ethyl acetate	0.58
11	Aniline	0.62
12	Acetonitrile	0.65
13	Ethanol	0.88
14	Methanol	0.95
15	Acetic acid	Large

22.2.1.6 Chromatogram Development (Separation)

Chromatogram development is the most difficult and crucial step in the HTLC procedure since important parameters are generally overlooked (Srivastava 2011). HPTLC plates are developed in twin-trough chambers or horizontal-development chambers. In general, saturated twin-trough chambers fitted with filter paper offer the best reproducibility and sample resolution. Twin-trough chamber avoids solvent vapour preloading and humidity (Renger 1993, 1998; Wall 2005) (Table 22.2).

22.2.1.7 Derivatisation

Derivatisation can be defined as a procedural technique that primarily modifies an analyte's functionality in order to enable chromatographic separations. Derivatisation can be performed either by immersing the plates or by spraying the plates with a suitable spraying reagent (Table 22.3) (Srivastava 2011; Wagner 1996; Knapp 1979; Jork and Funk 1990). For better reproducibility, immersion method is the preferred derivatisation technique.

22.2.1.8 Detection

Detection of separated compounds on the sorbent layers is enhanced by quenching of fluorescence due to UV light (ranged normally at 200–400 nm). This process is commonly called fluorescence quenching.

Table 22.3 List of common derivatisation reagents

Sl. no.	Colour reagent	Chemical compounds	Colour
1	Dragendorff reagent: It forms complex reaction with some nitrogen-containing compounds	Alkaloids	Red-brown zone (vis)
2	Natural products: polyethylene glycol reagent, i.e. diphenylboric acid-2-aminoethyl ester forms complexes with 3-hydroxyflavones via condensation reaction	Flavonoids	Intense yellow, orange and green fluorescent zones in UV 366 nm
3	Vanillin sulphuric acid OR anisaldehyde sulphuric acid	Bitter principle	Red-brown, yellow-brown, dark green zone (vis)
		Essential oil	Blue, brown or red zones (vis)
4	10% Ethanolic KOH	Anthraquinones (emodin, rhein)	Red zones (vis), red fluorescence (UV 366 nm)
		Anthrones (aloin, cascarosides)	Yellow zones (vis), yellow fluorescence (UV 366 nm)
		Coumarins, scopoletin, umbelliferone	Bright blue fluorescent zone (UV 366 nm)
5	Ninhydrin reagent	Amino acids, peptides, amines and amino sugars	Yellow, brown to pink and violet (vis)
6	Iodine: It produces iodine reaction possibly resulting in an oxidative product	Indole, quinoline derivative, thiols and all organic compounds	Dark zone (UV 254)

(a) **Visualisation at UV 254 nm**: F254 should be described as phosphorescence quenching. In this instance, the fluorescence remains for a short period after the source of excitation is removed. It is very short-lived, but longer than 10 s (Wall 2005). F254 fluorescent indicator is excited with UV wavelength at 254 nm and emits green fluorescence (Sherma 1991). Compounds that absorb radiation at 254 nm reduce this emission on the layer, and a dark violet spot on a green background is observed where the compound zones are located (Patel et al. 2012; Brainthwaite et al. 1999). This quenching is caused by all compounds with conjugated double bonds. Anthraglycosides, coumarins, flavonoids, propylphenols in essential oils, and some alkaloid types such as indole, and isoquinoline and quinoline alkaloids, should be detected under 254 nm (Wagner 1996).

(b) **Visualisation at UV 366 nm**: F366 should be described as fluorescence quenching. In this instance the fluorescence does not remain after the source of excitation is removed (Wall 2005). This quenching is shown by all anthraglycosides, coumarins, flavonoids, phenol carboxylic acids and some alkaloid types like Rauwolfia and Ipecacuanha alkaloids (Wagner 1996).

(c) **Visualisation at white light**: Zone containing separated compounds can be detected by viewing their natural colour in daylight, i.e. white light (Sherma 2007).

22.2.1.9 Quantification

Generally, densitometer or scanner with a fixed sample light beam in the form of a rectangular slit can be used for quantitative evaluation by measuring the zones of samples and standards. The chromatogram can be scanned in reflectance or in transmittance mode by absorbance or by fluorescent mode; scanning speed is used up to 100 mm/s (Patel et al. 2012; Srivastava 2011). Due to scanning spectra calibration of single and multiple levels of linearity, linear and nonlinear regression equations are possible. Scanning has been done by two methods, i.e. slit scanning and video scanning (Shewiyo et al. 2012).

(a) **Slit scanning and documentation**: Slit-scanning densitometry is now relatively mature although limited to absorption and fluorescence detection in the UV–visible range. It consists of a fibre-optic bundle for illumination of sample zones and collection of reflected light (or fluorescence). Photodiode-array detector is used for simultaneous length detection and spectral recording (Srivastava 2011).
(b) **Video scanning and documentation**: Video densitometry is a fast and simultaneous data acquisition from the whole plate, in which optical scanning takes place electronically, using a computer with video digitiser, light source, monochromators and appropriate optics to illuminate the plate and focus the image onto a charge-coupled device (CCD) video camera. It is also useful in two-dimensional separations for thin-layer chromatography with image analysis (Srivastava 2011).

22.2.2 HPTLC Method Validation for Pharmaceutical/Herbal Product Analysis

Specificity: Specificity is the ability to assess unequivocally the analyte in the presence of components which may be expected to be present. Typically these might include impurities, degradants, matrix, etc. It includes identification, purity tests and assay (International Conference on Harmonisation 1996). The specificity of the method was ascertained by analysing standard drug and sample. The peak purity of chemical compound was assessed by comparing the spectra at three different levels, i.e. peak start (S), peak apex (M), and peak end (E) positions of the spot (Srivastava 2011).

Linearity: The linearity of an analytical procedure is its ability (within a given range) to obtain test results which are directly proportional to the concentration (amount) of analyte in the sample (International Conference on Harmonisation 1996). The linearity is usually documented as the ordinary least squares (OLS) curve or simply as linear regression curve of the measured responses (peak area or height) as a function of increasing analyte concentrations (Ermer 2005).

Range: The range of an analytical procedure is the interval between the upper and lower concentration (amounts) of analyte in the sample (including these concentrations) for which it has been demonstrated that the analytical procedure has a suitable level of precision, accuracy and linearity (International Conference on Harmonisation 1996). In most of the pharmaceutical industry, usually a range from 80 to 120% of the target concentrations was tested (Patra et al. 2010).

Accuracy: The accuracy of an analytical procedure expresses the closeness of agreement between the value which is accepted either as a conventional true value or an accepted reference value and the value found (International Conference on Harmonisation 1996). For bioanalytical method, accuracy should be performed for at least three quality control (QC) samples (low, medium and high) in triplicate, and the accuracy was expressed as % recovery (Shah et al. 2000).

Precision: Precision of the analytical method can be divided into three categories, i.e. repeatability, intermediate precision and reproducibility. Repeatability or intra-assay within-day precision is determined when the analysis is done in one laboratory by one analyst with same conditions (equipment, TLC plate, reagents) and performed within 1-day work. Intermediate precision is obtained when the analysis was performed within a laboratory by different analysts, equipment, reagents and plates over a number of days or weeks. Reproducibility represents the precision obtained from some laboratories with the aim to verify whether the method can yield the same results in different laboratories (International Conference on Harmonisation 1996). For bioanalytical method, it is recommended to test the precision using a minimum of five determinations per concentration. A minimum of three levels of concentrations in the expected range is recommended; RSD is not permitted more than 15%, and at the maximum limit lower concentration RSD of 20% is acceptable (Garofolo 2004; International Organization for Standardization, Accuracy 1994).

Detection limit and quantitation limit: The detection limit of an individual analytical procedure is the lowest amount of analyte in a sample which can be detected but not necessarily quantitated as an exact value. The quantitation limit (QL) of an individual analytical procedure is the lowest amount of analyte in a sample which can be quantitatively determined with suitable precision and accuracy (International Conference on Harmonisation 1996). Generally, QL can be estimated at 2–3 times of detection limit (DL). DL and QL for instrumental (chromatographic) analytical methods can be defined in terms of the signal-to-noise ratio (2:1–3:1 for DL and 10:1 for QL) or in terms of the ratio of the standard deviation of the blank response, the residual standard deviation of the calibration line or the standard deviation of intercept (s) and slope (S) (Yuwono and Indrayanto 2005; Lee 2004).

Robustness: The robustness of an analytical procedure is a measure of its capacity to remain unaffected by small, but deliberate, variations in method parameters and provides an indication of its reliability during normal usage. Some important parameters for testing of the robustness evaluation for HPTLC methods are mobile-phase composition, pH of the mobile phase, temperature, humidity, development distance, spot shape, spot size, batch of the plates, volume of samples, drying condition (temperature, time) and condition of spot visualisation like spraying reagents, dipping reagents and UV detection (Van der Hyden et al. 2001).

22.3 HPTLC Fingerprinting Applications in Herbal Drug Formulations

HPTLC plays a major role in the characterisation of the phytoconstituents from herbal medicines for the development of the standardisation parameters of different plant extracts. To strengthen this comment some examples have been cited in the following section with some potent plant species from the reference.

22.3.1 Determination and Quantification of Gymnemagenin and *β*-Sitosterol in Marketed Herbal Formulation by Validated Normal-Phase HPTLC Method

Gymnemic acid is isolated from the leaf extract of the plant named *Gymnema sylvestre* which is responsible for its antidiabetic action. Gymnemagenin is an aglycone of gymnemic acids, produced after acidic and basic hydrolysis. *β*-Sitosterol is a waxy, white phytosterol with antidiabetic and antioxidant property as well as activity. Though individual analytical methods are available for gymnemagenin and *β*-sitosterol, no HPTLC method is available for their concurrent analysis. In this prospective, the research study was undertaken to develop and validate new, rapid, accurate, precise, robust and sensitive procedure for estimation of gymnemagenin and *β*-sitosterol quantitatively in a polyherbal formulation with densitometric detection. A Camag (Camag, Muttenz, Switzerland) HPTLC system made up of a Linomat V sample applicator, a twin-trough plate development chamber, a model III TLC scanner and winCATS software (Version 1.4.4) integration software were used. Chromatographic separation was made on Merck aluminium HPTLC plates pre-coated with silica gel 60 F254. The selected and optimised solvent system consisted of toluene:ethyl acetate:methanol (6.5:2.5:1.4, v/v/v) after so many trial-and-error search for the most suitable solvent system. Developed plates were derivatised with 5% sulphuric acid reagent followed by heating at 110 °C for 4 min in a preheated oven and scanned at 423 nm in reflectance-absorbance mode. The retention factor for gymnemagenin and *β*-sitosterol was found to be 0.27 ± 0.02 and 0.78 ± 0.02, respectively. The proposed densitometric method was validated according to ICH Q2 (R1) guidelines. Results were found

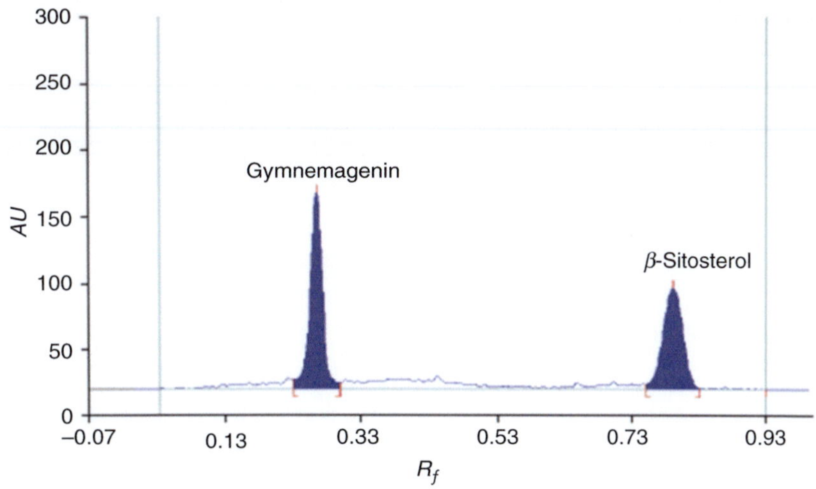

Fig. 22.1 Densitogram obtained from mixed standard solution of gymnemagenin and *β*-sitosterol scanned at 423 nm

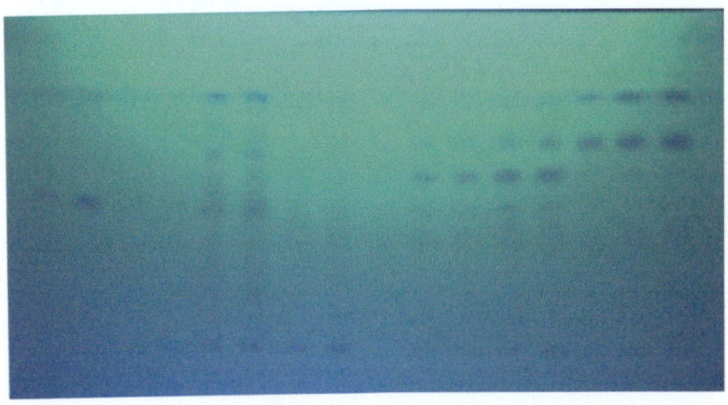

Fig. 22.2 TLC chromatogram of glycyrrhetic acid at 254 nm

to be linear over a range of 100–1200 ng band−1 and 200–1200 ng band−1 for gymnemagenin and *β*-sitosterol, respectively. The percent content of gymnemagenin and *β*-sitosterol in the marketed polyherbal formulation was found to be 0.0405% and 0.1377%, respectively. This developed method can be used for estimation and quantification of gymnemagenin and *β*-sitosterol in marketed polyherbal formulations as well as in other pharmaceutical dosage forms (Potawale et al. 2014) (Figs. 22.1 and 22.2).

22.3.2 Estimation of Hesperidin by HPTLC in Different Varieties of Citrus Peels Quantitatively

Hesperidin is a flavanone glycoside, a bioflavonoid and an abundant and inexpensive by-product of citrus cultivation. A deficiency of this substance in the diet has been linked with abnormal capillary leakiness as well as pain in the extremities causing aches, weakness and night leg cramps. It is found in citrus fruits and possesses anti-allergy, anti-inflammatory, analgesic, anticancer and antioxidant activities. High-performance thin-layer chromatography (HPTLC) method was developed which can be used for routine analysis of hesperidin in crude drug as well as in herbal and pharmaceutical dosage form containing citrus fruits as an ingredient. The method was carried out in aluminium-backed silica gel 60 F254 plates with ethyl acetate:methanol:water 15:3:2 (%, v/v) as mobile phase. The developed HPTLC method was simple, reliable, sensitive and accurate which can be used to quantify hesperidin in different varieties of citrus fruits (Fig. 22.3).

A compact band was obtained for hesperidin at Rf value of (0.40 ± 0.04). The calibration plot was linear in the range of 100–800 ng/spot of hesperidin and the correlation coefficient of 0.9986 was indicative of good linear dependence of peak area on concentration. Limit of detection (8.87 ng/spot), limit of quantification (23.21 ng/spot), accuracy (less than 2%) and recovery (ranging from 98.55 to 99.38) were found satisfactory (Alam et al. 2014) (Fig. 22.4).

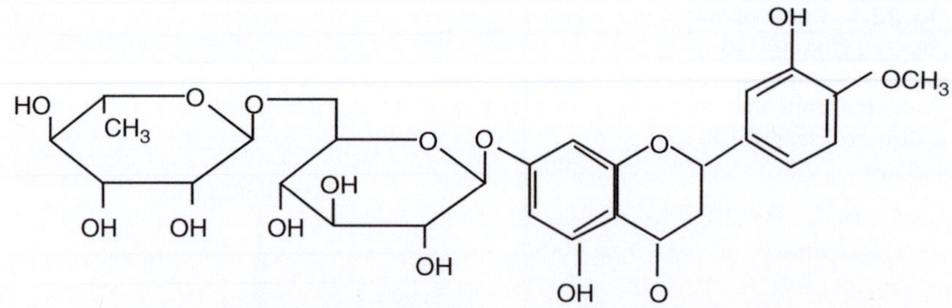

Fig. 22.3 Structure of hesperidin

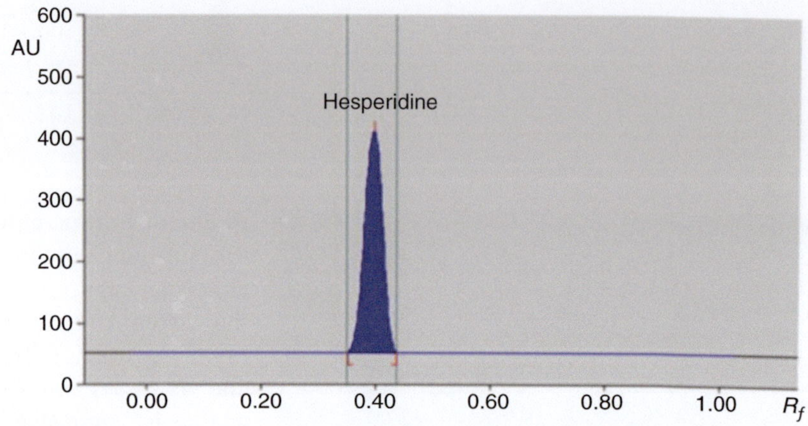

Fig. 22.4 HPTLC chromatogram of standard hesperidine

22.3.3 Quantitative Analysis of 8-Gingerol in *Zingiber officinale* Extract and Ginger-Containing Dietary Supplements, Teas and Commercial Creams Using HPTLC Densitometric Method (Fig. 22.5)

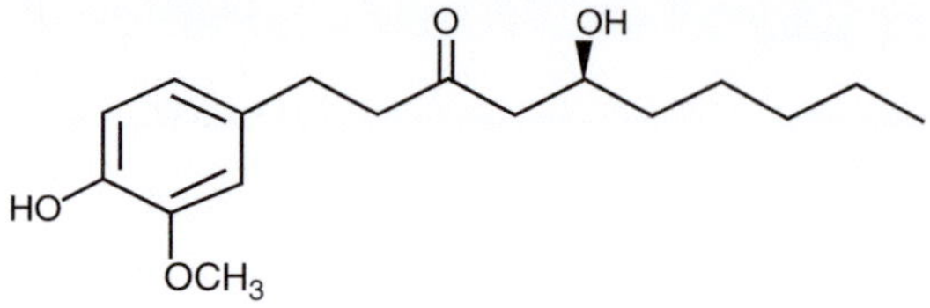

Fig. 22.5 Structure of 8-gingerol

Ginger [*Zingiber officinale* Roscoe (*Z. officinale*)] is widely used as a dietary supplement as well as a spice and flavouring agent in foods and beverages around the world. For decades, it has been an important ingredient in Chinese, Ayurvedic and Tibb-Unani and Indian systems of medicine and widely used in the treatment of unrelated ailments like arthritis, rheumatism, sprains, muscular aches, pains, sore throats, cramps, fever, infectious diseases and helminthiasis. Ginger has a very long history of use in various forms of traditional/alternative medicine. It has been used to help digestion, reduce nausea and help fight the flu and common cold. It can be used fresh, dried or powdered, or as an oil or juice, and is sometimes added to processed foods and cosmetics. The unique fragrance and flavour of ginger come from its natural oils, the most important of which is gingerol, the main bioactive compound in ginger, responsible for much of its medicinal properties since it has powerful anti-inflammatory and antioxidant effects.

The different pungent and biologically active compounds found in ginger include 6-gingerol, 8-gingerol, zingerone and paradol. 8-Gingerol, the structure shown above, is one of the most principal pungent components of ginger. Many researchers proved that 8-gingerol possesses various pharmacological functions, such as anti-platelet aggregation activities, spasmolytic activity, modulation of macrophage functions, inhibition of LPS-induced PGE 2 production and LPS-induced COX-2 expression, 5-HT3 receptor blocking activity and immunosuppressive activity. Because of the widespread use of ginger as a spice, dietary supplements, tea, cream, household remedy as well as an ingredient of various herbal formulations, it is essential to standardise ginger formulations in various forms. Many analytical methods like HPLC have been reported for the analysis of 8-gingerol in its extract, commercial formulations and biological fluids. The developed method was simple, economical, selective, precise and sensitive HPTLC technique for analysis of 8-gingerol in its methanolic extract, dietary supplements, teas and commercial creams and was validated using International Conference on Harmonisation Guidelines (ICH Guideline 1996). The analysis was performed on 10 × 20 cm aluminium-backed plates coated with 0.2 mm layers of silica gel 60 F254 (E-Merck, Germany) with n-hexane:ethyl acetate 60:40 (v/v) as mobile phase. Camag TLC Scanner III was used for the UV densitometric scanning at 569. This system was found to give a compact spot of 8-gingerol at retention factor (Rf) value of (0.39 ± 0.04) and linearity was found in the ranges 50–500 ng/spot (r2 = 0.9987). Limit of detection (12.76 ng/spot), limit of quantification (26.32 ng/spot), accuracy (less than 2%) and recovery (ranging from 98.22 to 99.20) were found satisfactory (Alam 2013) (Figs. 22.6, 22.7, 22.8, 22.9, 22.10, 22.11 and 22.12).

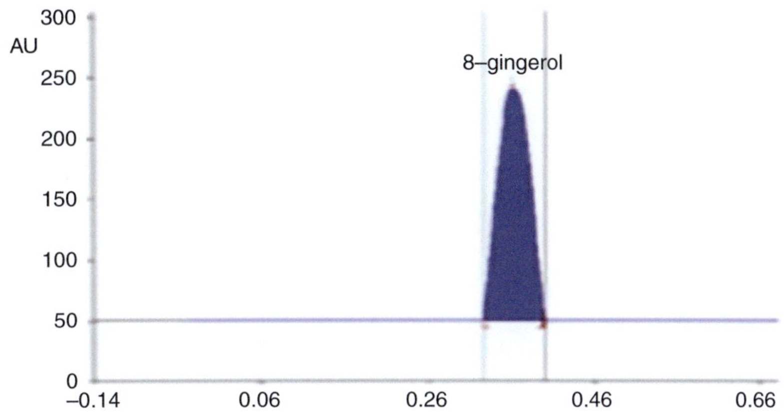

Fig. 22.6 HPTLC densitogram of methanolic extract of *Z. officinale*

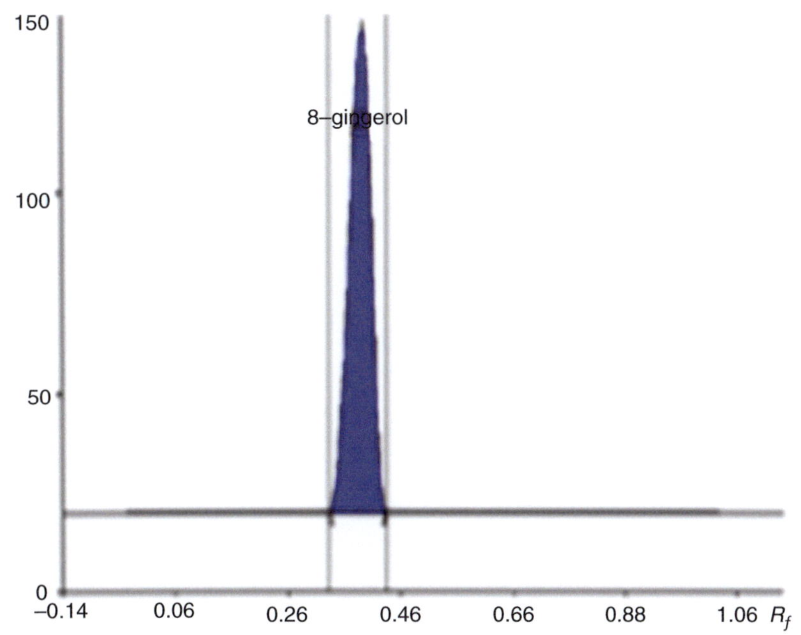

Fig. 22.7 HPTLC densitogram of standard 8-gingerol

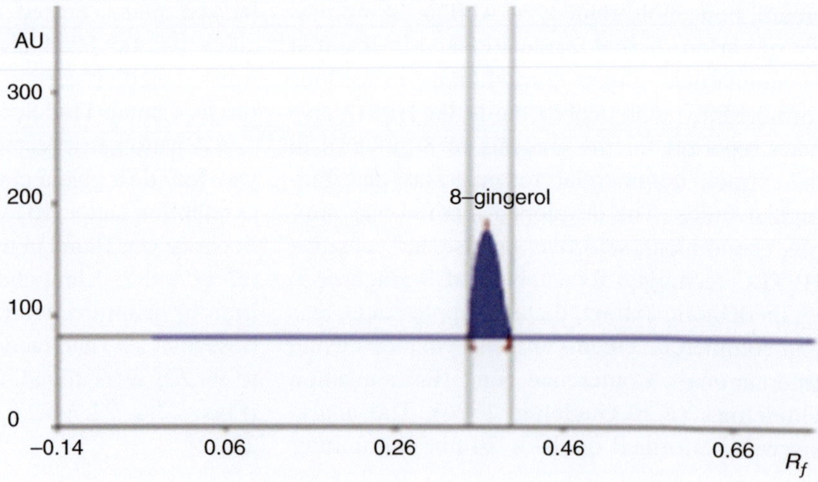

Fig. 22.8 HPTLC densitogram of cream A

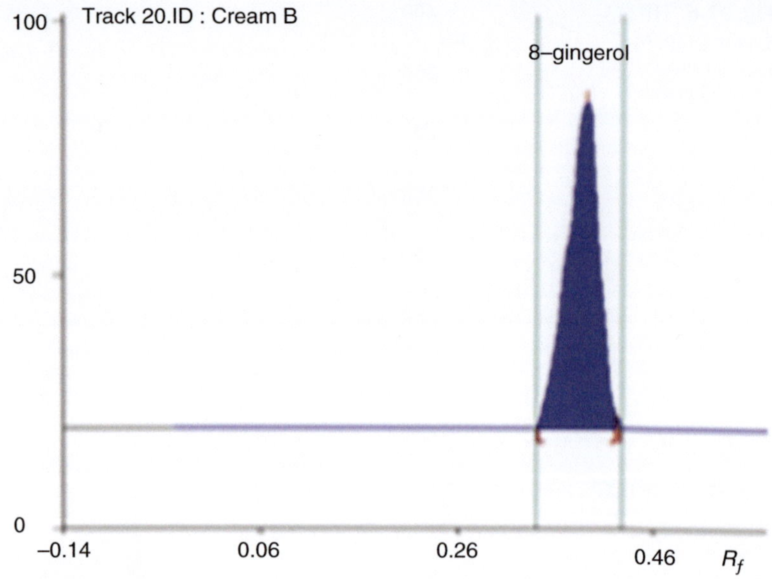

Fig. 22.9 HPTLC densitogram of cream B

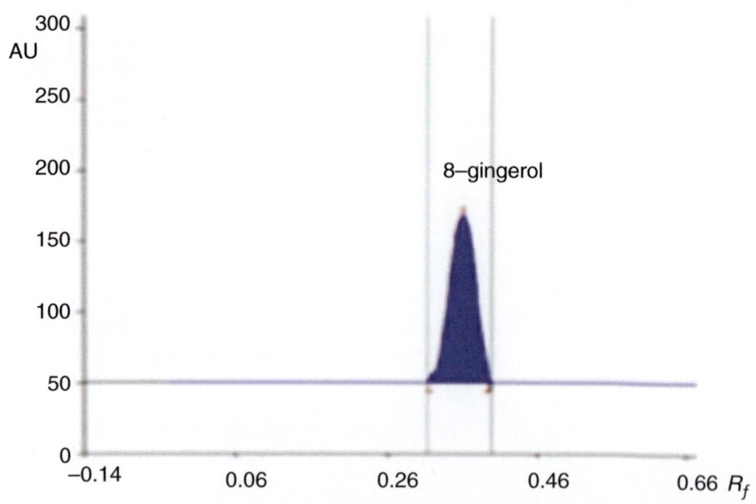

Fig. 22.10 HPTLC densitogram of tea (TG 1)

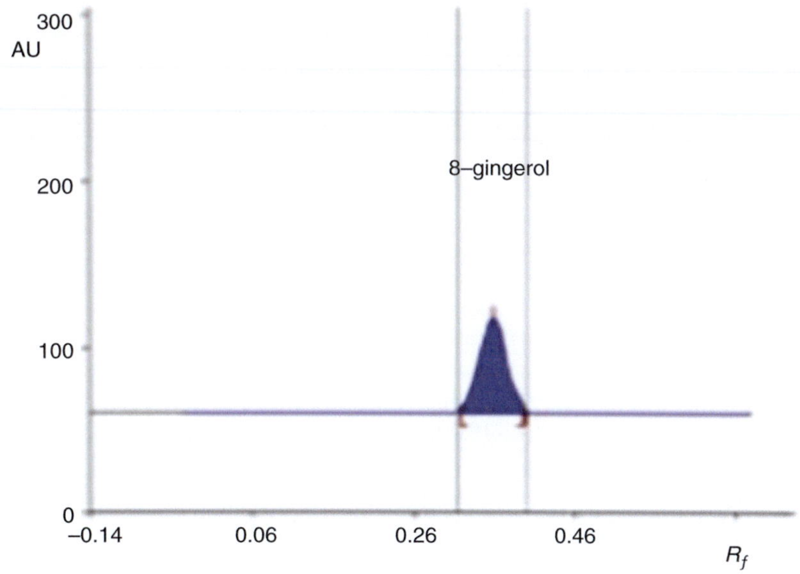

Fig. 22.11 HPTLC densitogram of tea (TG 2)

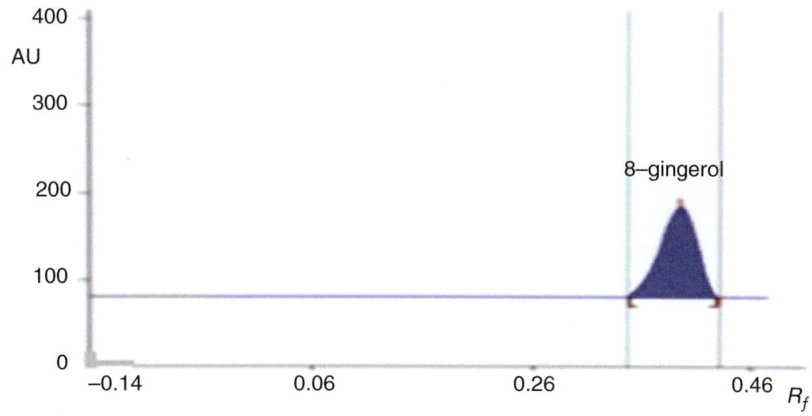

Fig. 22.12 HPTLC densitogram of dietary supplement

22.3.4 Simultaneous Densitometric Analysis of Glycyrrhetic Acid and Solasodine in Herbal Drug Formulation Using HPTLC Techniques (Fig. 22.13)

Glycyrrhetic acid is an aglycone of glycyrrhizin, a triterpenoid compound isolated from *Glycyrrhiza glabra*. It possesses various activities like anti-inflammatory, analgesic and anti-asthmatic. Solasodine is a steroidal glycoalkaloid, isolated from *Solanum xanthocarpum* which possesses anti-asthmatic and mucolytic activities; hence they form one of the most important constituents of almost each and every polyherbal formulation used for the management of asthmatic conditions. Few HPTLC and HPLC methods are available for estimation of glycyrrhetic acid individually and in combination with other marker compounds in the same plant. Even though both of these compounds are most commonly used together, there were no reports found for simultaneous estimation of glycyrrhetic acid and solasodine. Hence the objective of the work was to develop and validate a sensitive, reliable, simple, accurate and reproducible method for the simultaneous HPTLC analysis of glycyrrhetic acid and solasodine in polyherbal formulations. The method was developed using HPTLC silica gel GF_{254} pre-coated aluminium plate as the stationary phase and chloroform:methanol

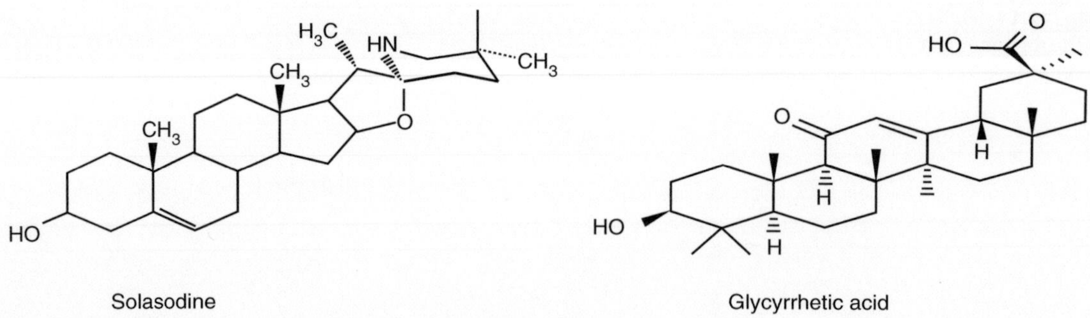

Fig. 22.13 Structure of solasodine and glycyrrhetic acid

(9:1 v/v) as the mobile phase. Quantification of glycyrrhetic acid was achieved by determining the area under the curve at 267 nm using CAMAG TLC Scanner and CATS 3 software. Since the structure of solasodine lacks conjugated double bond, it does not give any fluorescence either in the absorbance mode or reflectance mode; hence solasodine was derivatised using 0.5% anisaldehyde sulphuric acids which gave a bluish spot as seen on TLC plate. These spots were scanned at 546 nm wavelength using CAMAG TLC Scanner and CATS 3 software. The retention factors for glycyrrhetic acid and solasodine were found to be 0.52 ± 0.01 and 0.40 ± 0.01% w/w, respectively. The developed HPTLC method was validated using parameters described in International Conference on Harmonisation (ICH) guideline. The developed method shows good linearity in the range of 400–2000 ng spot-1 for glycyrrhetic acid as well as for solasodine. The contents of glycyrrhetic acid and solasodine in marketed polyherbal formulation were found to be 0.67% ± 0.8 and 0.10 ± 0.35%w/w, respectively (Patel and Bhatt 2017).

22.3.5 Quantification of Markers of Dhatrinisha Churna Using HPTLC Method Development and Validation

Traditionally Dhatrinisha churna has been used in the Ayurveda, Siddha and Unani systems of medicine in India to treat hyperlipidaemia. A sensitive, reliable, selective, precise and accurate densitometric high-performance thin-layer chromatography (HPTLC) fingerprinting method has been developed for the simultaneous estimation and quantification of curcumin and ellagic acid in Dhatrinisha churna. Validation of method was performed in order to demonstrate its sensitivity, selectivity, accuracy, precision, repeatability and recovery study. All calibration curves showed good linear correlation coefficient ($r^2 > 0.997$) within the tested ranges. The chromatogram of Dhatrinisha churna was quantified with respect to curcumin (1.072% w/w) and ellagic acid (0.867%w/w). Intra- and inter-day RSDs of retention time and peak area were less than 1.92%. The recoveries were between 96.60 and 101.40%. The developed HPTLC method was found to be reliable, sensitive, simple, precise and accurate and can be used for the quality control of the raw materials as well as formulations (Patel and Patel 2012) (Figs. 22.14 and 22.15).

22.3.6 Determination of Caffeine in Stimulant Herbal Products and Power Drinks Using HPTLC Validation Method

Caffeine, 1,3,7-trimethylxanthine, is the major alkaloid ingredient in about 60 herbs, including *Thea sinensis* (tea leaves), *Coffea arabica* (coffee beans), *Theobroma cacao, Paullinia cupana* (guarana seeds) and *Cola nitida* (kola nuts), in which their CNS stimulant is attributed. The pharmacological effect of caffeine can be achieved when it is consumed in the form of herbal extract or pure ingredient added to various food products. Hot tea and coffee drinks are among the most popular sources for obtain-

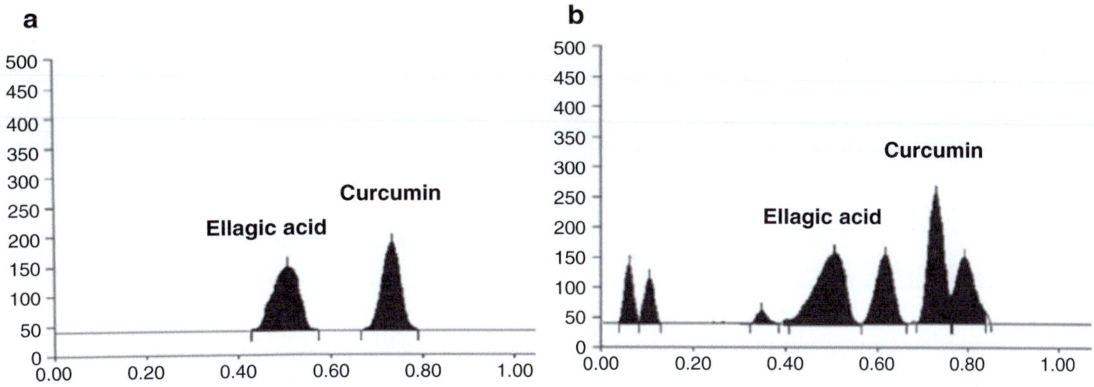

Fig. 22.14 (**a**) HPTLC chromatogram of curcumin and ellagic acid, (**b**) HPTLC chromatogram of Dhatrinisha churna

Fig. 22.15 Structure of ellagic acid and curcumin

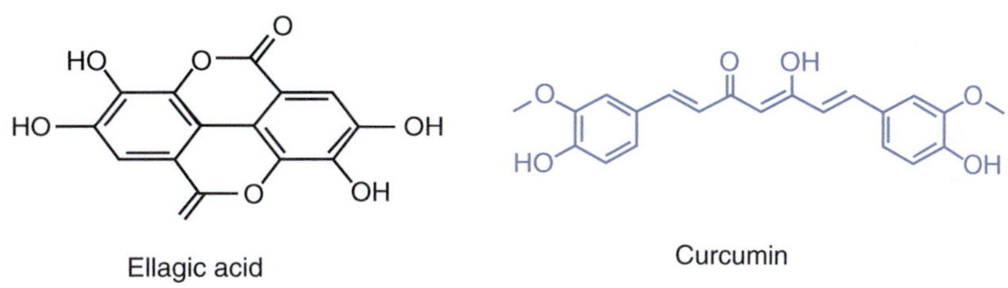

ing the desired effect of caffeine, providing ca 50 and 100 mg caffeine per cup, respectively. Caffeine is also a vey common ingredient in many pain killers and antimigraine drug formulations. With the recent re-emergence of medicinal herbs as a major player in the global dietary supplement product, such new products containing caffeine have been introduced. Of these, dry extracts of caffeine-containing herbs and carbonated beverages, known as power or energy drinks, enriched with pure caffeine extracts are becoming popular around the world. The levels of caffeine in different forms (biological, pharmaceutical and herbal) are determined by numerous techniques, including spectroscopic and chromatographic method. Planar chromatography and its high performance (HPTLC) coupled with densitometric detection are among the various methods reported for the quality control of pharmaceutical products containing caffeine. It has the advantage of simplicity, speed, reproducibility and cost-effectiveness and can thus provide an affordable and reliable alternative to other analytical techniques such as HPLC or GC. As such, HPTLC may be utilised as an effective analytical tool for the quality control of caffeine-containing dietary supplements. In this study, the caffeine content of selected herbal products and energy drinks available in the Saudi market was determined by HPTLC-UV densitometric analysis. Pre-coated HPTLC silica gel plates (20 cm × 10 cm) were used for the analysis. The solvent system consisted of ethyl acetate:methanol (85:15 v/v), and caffeine was detected at 275 nm. The developed method was validated for specificity, repeatability (CV < 5%), recovery (98.90 ± 3.46) and accuracy (99.84 ± 2.87). The levels of caffeine were 4.76–13.29% (w/w) and 0.011–0.032% (w/v) for the herbal products and the energy drinks, respectively (Fig. 22.16).

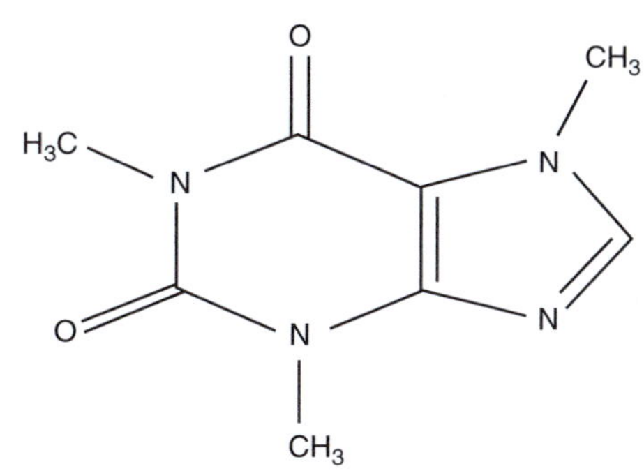

Fig. 22.16 Structure of caffeine

The developed HPTLC method was validated for specificity, linearity of calibration, recovery, accuracy and precision (repeatability) and was used to determine the levels of caffeine in stimulant herbal products and power drinks (Abourashed and Mossa 2004).

22.3.7 Estimation of Curcumin Content in Turmeric Powder Using HPTLC Validation Method

Curcuma longa Linn. (turmeric) belongs to the family Zingiberaceae. Extensive literature reveals its anti-inflammatory, cholagogue, hepatoprotective, blood purifier, antioxidant, detoxifier and regenerator of liver tissue, anti-asthmatic, antitumour, antiprotozoal, stomachic and carminative properties. It reduces high level of cholesterol in plasma. Its antiplatelet activity offers protection to heart and vessels. It also prevents DNA damage in lymphocytes. Several constituents present in this plant include curcumin (a flavonoid), demethoxycurcumin, bisdemethoxy, volatile oils like turmerone, atlantone, zingiberene, sesquiphellandrene, terpinolene, phellandrene, p-cymene, cineol, caryophyllene, nerolidol, curlone, dehydrozingerone, zerumbone, germacrene, sesquiterpenes, etc. Curcumin has a molecular formula ($C_{21}H_{30}O_6$), molecular weight 368.91 and melting point 183 °C. It is the main active constituent of *Curcuma longa* having broad spectrum of activities including antioxidant, anti-inflammatory, anticarcinogenic, hypocholesterolaemic, antibacterial, wound healing, antispasmodic, anticoagulant, antitumour and hepatoprotective. It is also a potent free radical scavenger, having superoxide anions, singlet oxygen, hydroxyl radical scavenging and lipid peroxidation inhibitory activities. High-performance thin-layer chromatography (HPTLC) method has been developed for determination of curcumin in several marketed spice sample of turmeric powder and has been compared with an in-house turmeric powder. The HPTLC separation was performed on pre-coated aluminium-backed HPTLC plates of 0.2 mm layer thickness with silica gel 60 F with dichloromethane and methanol (99:1) combination as mobile phase. The plate was developed up to 80 mm at temperature of 20 ± 4 °C with 10 min of chamber saturation. Under this condition the retardation factor (R_f) of curcumin is 0.43 and the compound was quantified at its absorbance maxima (λ_{max}) at 427 nm. The limit of detection and limit of quantification were found to be 49 ng and 148 ng per spot, respectively. The response of curcumin was linear over the range of 0.8 μg to 1.3 μg per spot with correlation coefficient 0.995395 indicating good relationship between peak area and concentration. Recovery values from 99.60 to 99.73 showed that the reliability and reproducibility of the developed method were excellent (Gantait et al. 2011) (Fig. 22.17).

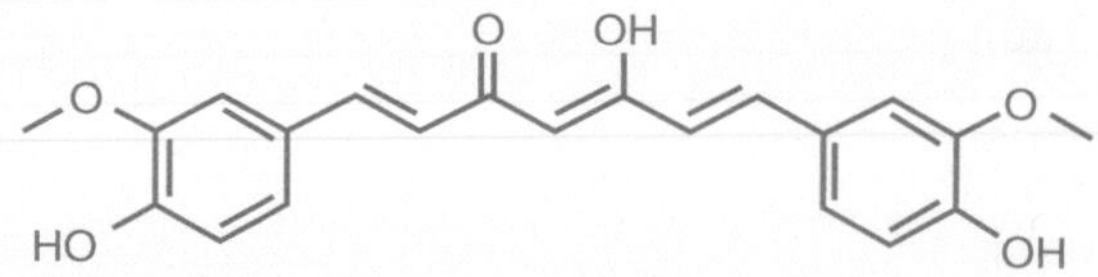

Fig. 22.17 Structure of curcumin

22.3.8 Standardisation of Sulaharan Yoga: An Ayurvedic Tablet Formulation Using HPTLC Fingerprinting Method

Sulaharan yoga consists of (1) *Terminalia chebula* (Combretaceae, dried fruit), (2) *Zingiber officinale* (Zingiberaceae, dried rhizome), (3) *Piper nigrum* (Piperaceae, dried fruit), (4) *Piper longum* (Piperaceae, dried fruit), (5) *Strychnos nux-vomica* (Fabaceae, dried seed), (6) *Ferula foetida* (oleo-gum-resin), (7) sulphur and (8) rock salt (Saindhava lavana). In-house formulation of sulaharan yoga was prepared as per Ayurvedic Formulary of India. The ingredients number 1–4 were washed, dried and powdered and passed through 80# sieve. The ingredients number 5, 6, 7 and 8 were cleaned and powdered individually and passed through 80# sieve. All the ingredients were mixed thoroughly in specified ratio (1 parts each) to obtain a homogeneous blend. The blended mass was fed through tablet punch machine fitted with suitable die. The rolled vatis (tablets) were dried in a tray-dryer at a temperature not exceeding 60 °C. One marketed sample of sulaharan yoga (Sarmayu) was chosen for the present study. Sarmayu and the in-house preparation were standardised based on their fingerprint profiles using HPTLC method (Fig. 22.18).

The methanolic extracts of the individual ingredients, in-house formulation and marketed formulation were compared with the different marker compounds like gingerol, brucin, gallic acid, umbelliferone and piperine corresponding to the active ingredients to ensure the presence of active ingredients in the Ayurvedic tablet formulations for this developed HPTLC method. For HPTLC fingerprint profile, 2 g of each sample was extracted with 25 mL of methanol on boiling water bath for 25 min successively three times using fresh portion of 25 mL methanol filtered and concentrated. The chromatograph was performed by spotting standards and extracted samples on pre-coated silica gel aluminium plate 60F-254 (10 cm × 10 cm with 250 μm thickness) using Camag Linomat IV sample applicator and 100 μL Hamilton syringe. The samples, in the form of bands of length 5 mm, were spotted 15 mm from the bottom, 10 mm apart, at a constant application rate of 15 nl/s using nitrogen aspirator. Subsequent to the development, TLC plates were dried in a current of air with the help of a hairdryer. Densitometric scanning was performed on Camag TLC scanner III in the absorbance/reflectance mode (Fig. 22.19).

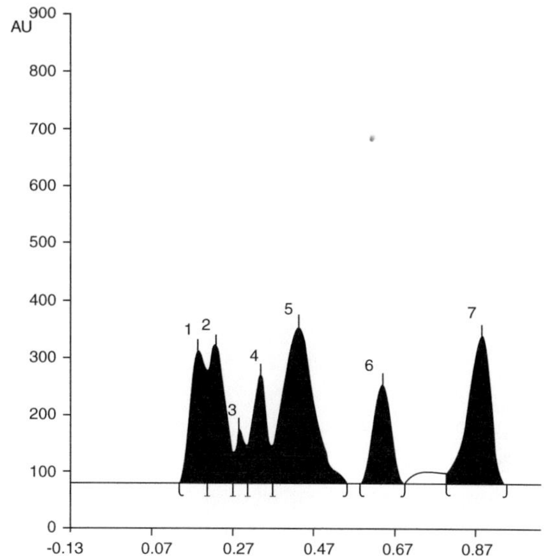

Fig. 22.19 HPTLC fingerprinting of sulaharan yoga

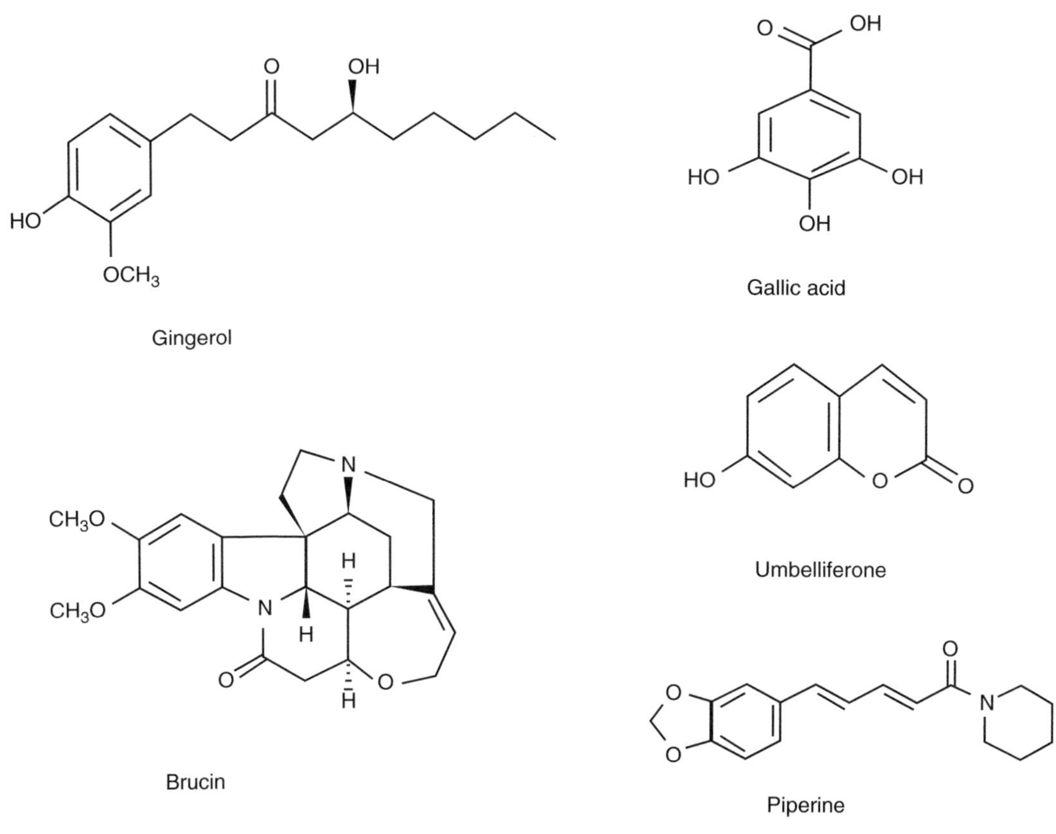

Fig. 22.18 Structure of gingerol, brucin, gallic acid, umbelliferone, piperine

From superimposition study, a band (R_f 0.44) corresponding to gallic acid is visible in both *Terminalia chebula* and *sulaharana yoga* formulations, indicating the presence of *Terminalia chebula* in the formulations. Band (R_f 0.35) corresponding to gingerols is visible in both the ingredient and formulations, indicating the presence of *Zingiber officinale*. Similarly, bands with R_f values 0.50 corresponding to piperine indicate the presence of both *Piper nigrum* and *Piper longum* in the formulations. Bands (R_f 0.15 and 0.33) corresponding to brucine and strychnine are visible in both the ingredient and formulations indicating the presence of *Strychnos nux-vomica*. A band (R_f 0.40) corresponding to umbelliferone is visible in both the ingredient and formulations, indicating the presence of *Ferula foetida* in the formulations. The TLC profiles of both the formulations are superimposable indicating the presence of all the constituents in the marketed and in-house formulation (Pattanaya et al. 2010).

22.3.9 Selected HPTLC Fingerprinting Profile of *Melothria heterophylla* (Lour.) and *Vitex peduncularis* Wall.

22.3.9.1 HPTLC Fingerprinting Profile of *Melothria heterophylla* (Lour.)

The results from HPTLC fingerprint scanned at wavelength 254 nm for the ethanol leaf extracts showed the presence of eight polyvalent phytoconstituents and corresponding ascending order of Rf values starting from 0.15 to 1.07 in which the highest concentration of the phytoconstituents was found to be 35.12% and its corresponding Rf value was found to be 0.15 and is recorded in Table 22.4 (Figs. 22.20, 22.21 and 22.22).

22.3.9.2 HPTLC Fingerprinting Profile of *Vitex peduncularis* Wall.

The results from HPTLC fingerprint scanned at wavelength 254 nm for the methanol leaf extracts of *Vitex peduncularis* Wall. showed the presence of four polyvalent phytoconstituents and corresponding ascending order of Rf values starting from 0.11 to 0.87 in which the highest concentration of the phytoconstituents was found to be 83.95% and its corresponding Rf value was found to be 0.11 and is recorded in Table 22.5 (Figs. 22.23, 22.24 and 22.25).

22.3.9.3 HPTLC Fingerprinting Profile of *Ilex khasiana*

HPTLC fingerprint scan at wavelength 366 nm for methanol extract of *Ilex khasiana* was performed at the concentration of 5 μL using toluene:ethyl acetate:acetic acid (6:1:2) as a mobile phase. The results revealed the presence of six unknown bioactive compounds with the corresponding Rf values of 0.27, 0.37, 0.46, 0.62, 0.71 and 0.75, respectively. The highest concentration of the phytoconstituent was found to be 45.57% and its corresponding Rf value was found to be 0.51 (Figs. 22.26 and 22.27).

From the present HPTLC fingerprinting profile study, we can conclude that certain significant phytochemical constituents were present in those selected extracts that might be responsible for their ethnomedicinal use. The present study is to report the HPTLC fingerprint of ethanol/methanol leaf extracts (viz. *Melothria heterophylla* (Lour.), *Vitex peduncularis* Wall.) and *Ilex Khasiana*). From the HPTLC studies, it has been found that the above extracts contain a mixture of compounds. This densitometric HPTLC fingerprint profile may be used as a marker for quality evaluation and standardisation of the drug. Thus, HPTLC fingerprint profile along with their Rf values was recorded, which would serve as a reference standard for the scientist engaged in research on various medicinal properties of the selected plants. HPTLC fingerprint analysis not only gives the idea for the authentication of the plant extracts and its constituents but also provides the parameters for quality of herbal formulations (Table 22.6).

In HPTLC technique, as the sample is applied as a rectangular band it provides more resolution and better separation of spots as compared to the TLC technique because of the shape of the area in which the compounds are present on the plate. The chromatographic fingerprint is suit-

Table 22.4 Rf values of chloroform extract of *Melothria heterophylla* (Lour.)

Peak	Start Rf	Start Height	Max Rf	Max Height	Max %	End Rf	End Height	Area	Area %	Assigned substance
1	−0.03	6.2	0.02	717.3	34.29	0.15	77.8	22694.7	35.12	Unknown[a]
2	0.19	76.7	0.23	110.2	5.27	0.28	50.1	4742.8	7.34	Unknown[a]
3	0.34	46.3	0.44	569.3	27.21	0.49	57.0	19837.7	30.70	Unknown[a]
4	0.49	57.2	0.53	259.5	12.41	0.55	96.0	5954.0	9.21	Unknown[a]
5	0.56	98.4	0.58	212.8	10.17	0.64	39.7	5955.7	9.22	Unknown[a]
6	0.64	40.6	0.67	185.6	8.87	0.72	8.4	4502.4	6.97	Unknown[a]
7	0.80	11.7	0.82	23.0	1.10	0.85	12.2	555.9	0.86	Unknown[a]
8	0.99	0.6	1.03	14.2	0.68	1.07	2.6	376.6	0.58	Unknown[a]

[a] Denotes the detected unassigned unknown peak in the chromatograph

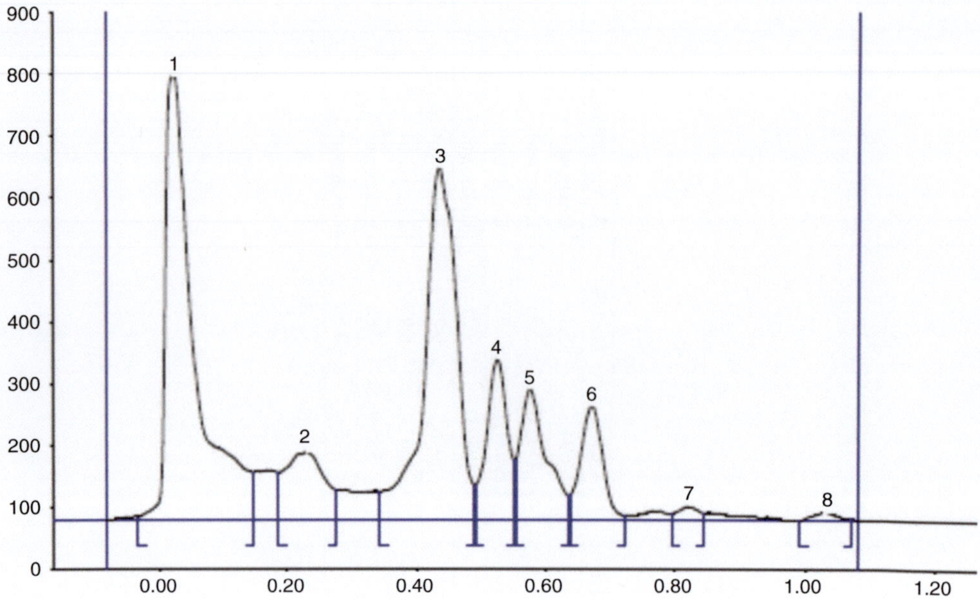

Fig. 22.20 Peak densitogram display of ethanol extract of *Melothria heterophylla* (Lour.)

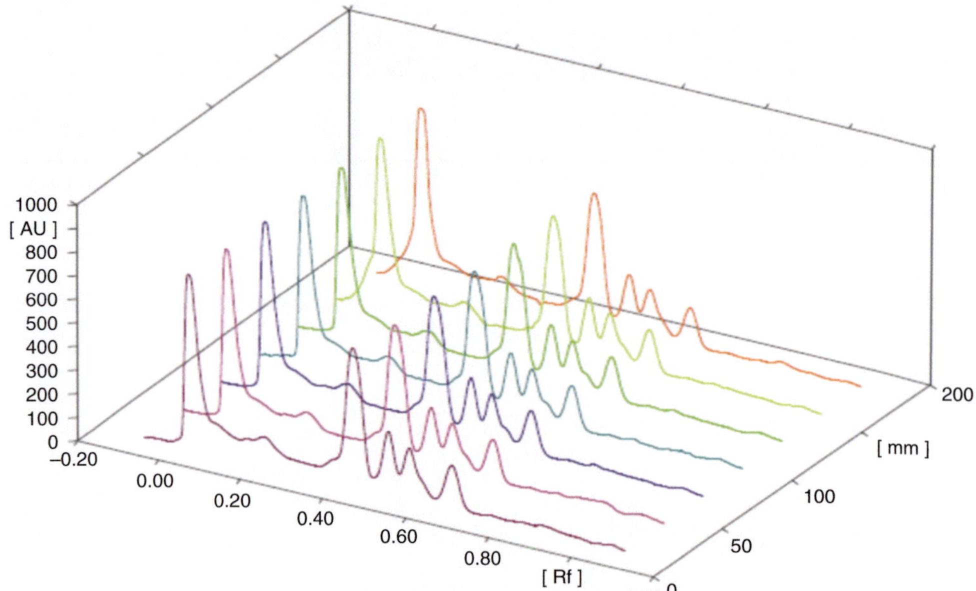

Fig. 22.21 Three-dimensional (3D) representation of HPTLC chromatogram of methanol extracts of *Melothria heterophylla* (Lour.)

Fig. 22.22 HPTLC plate seen at 254 nm for ethanol extract of *Melothria heterophylla* (Lour.)

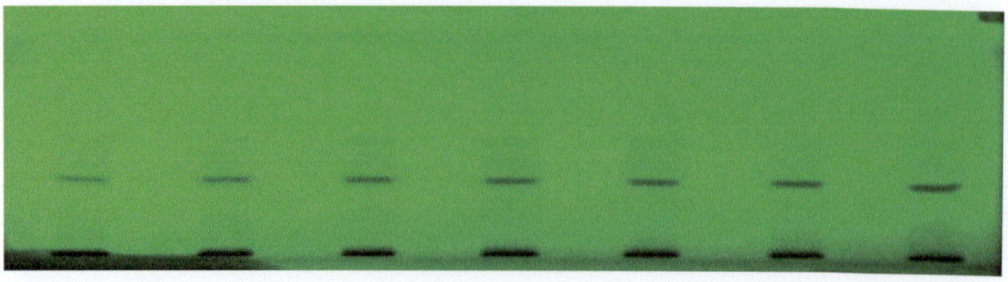

Table 22.5 Rf values of methanol extract of *Vitex peduncularis* Wall

Peak	Start Rf	Start Height	Max Rf	Max Height	Max %	End Rf	End Height	Area	Area %	Assigned substance
1	−0.05	4.8	0.00	448.6	83.74	0.11	20.7	12514.3	83.95	Unknown[a]
2	0.28	8.7	0.33	19.4	3.61	0.35	14.2	586.4	3.93	Unknown[a]
3	0.40	17.0	0.43	48.6	9.07	0.48	6.9	1323.5	8.88	Unknown[a]
4	079	0.1	0.83	19.1	3.57	0.87	3.3	483.0	3.24	Unknown[a]

[a] Denotes the detected unassigned unknown peak in the chromatograph

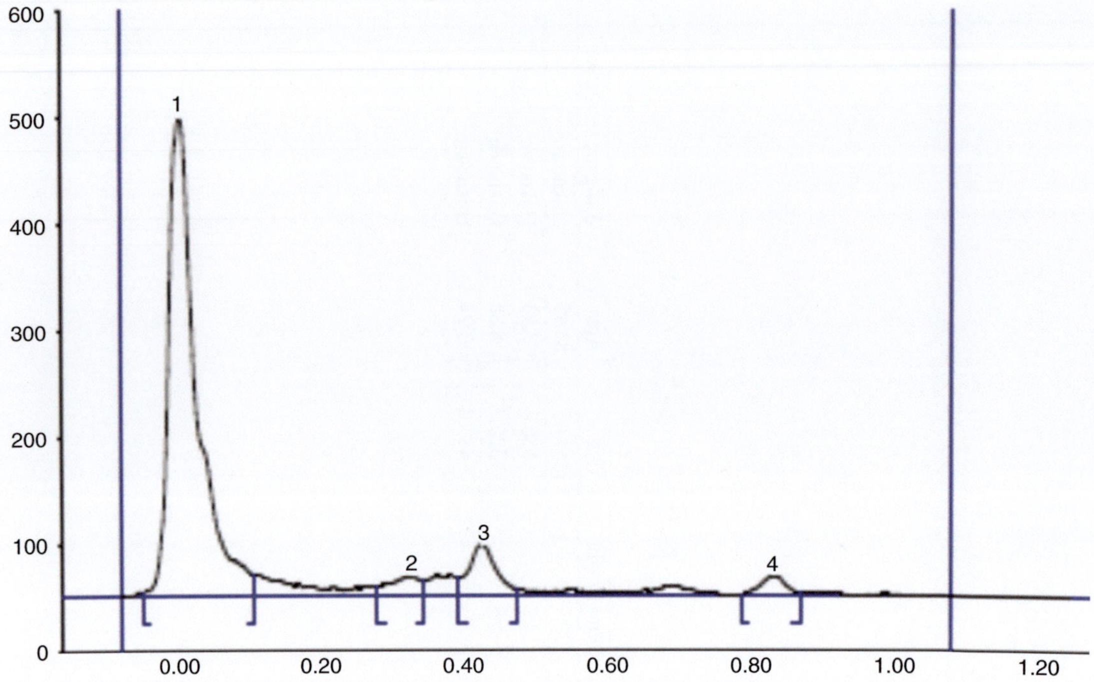

Fig. 22.23 Peak densitogram display of methanol extract of *Vitex peduncularis* Wall

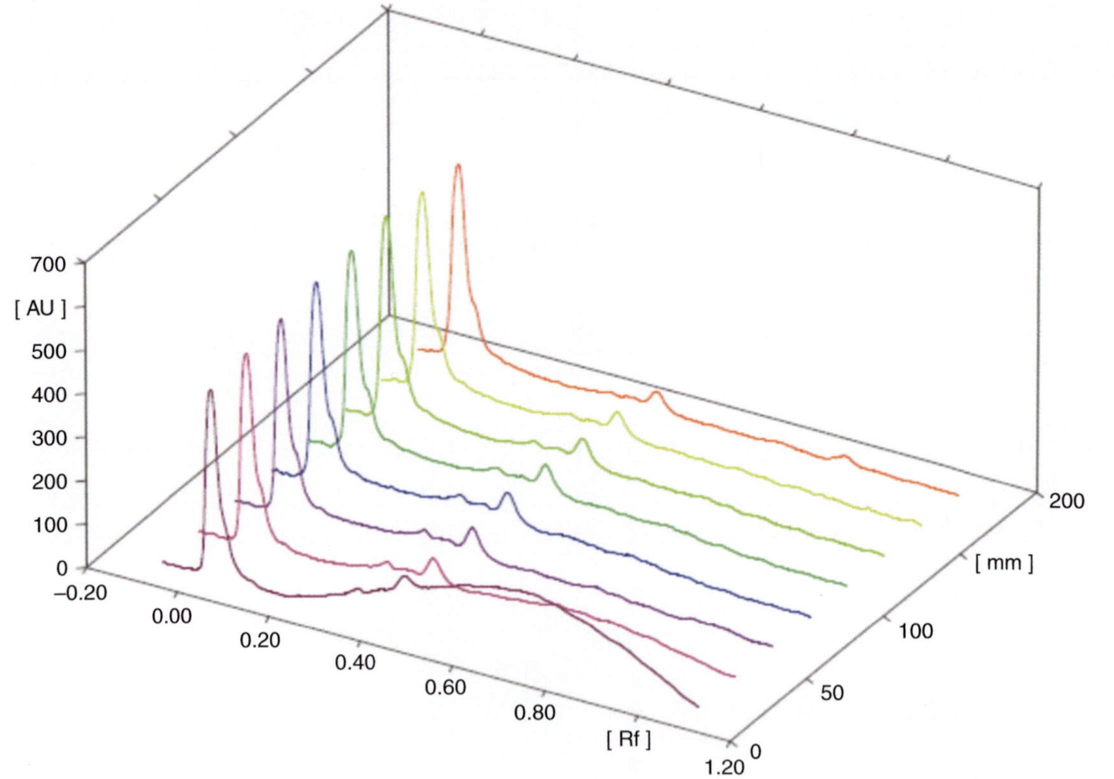

Fig. 22.24 Three-dimensional (3D) representation of HPTLC chromatogram of methanol extracts of *Vitex peduncularis* Wall

Fig. 22.25 HPTLC plate seen at 254 nm for methanol extract of *Vitex peduncularis* Wall

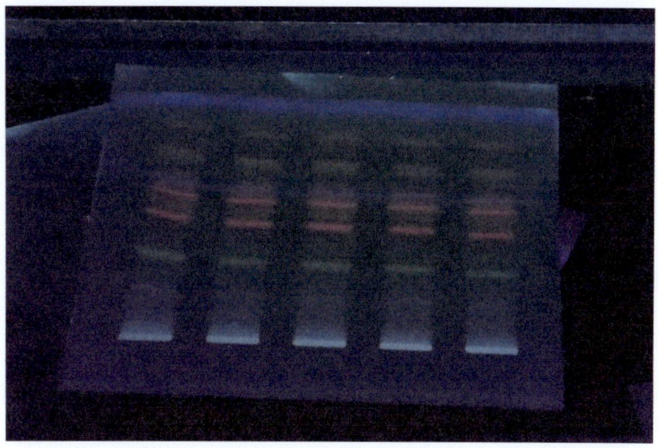

Fig. 22.26 HPTLC plate seen at 366 nm for methanol extract of *Ilex khasiana*

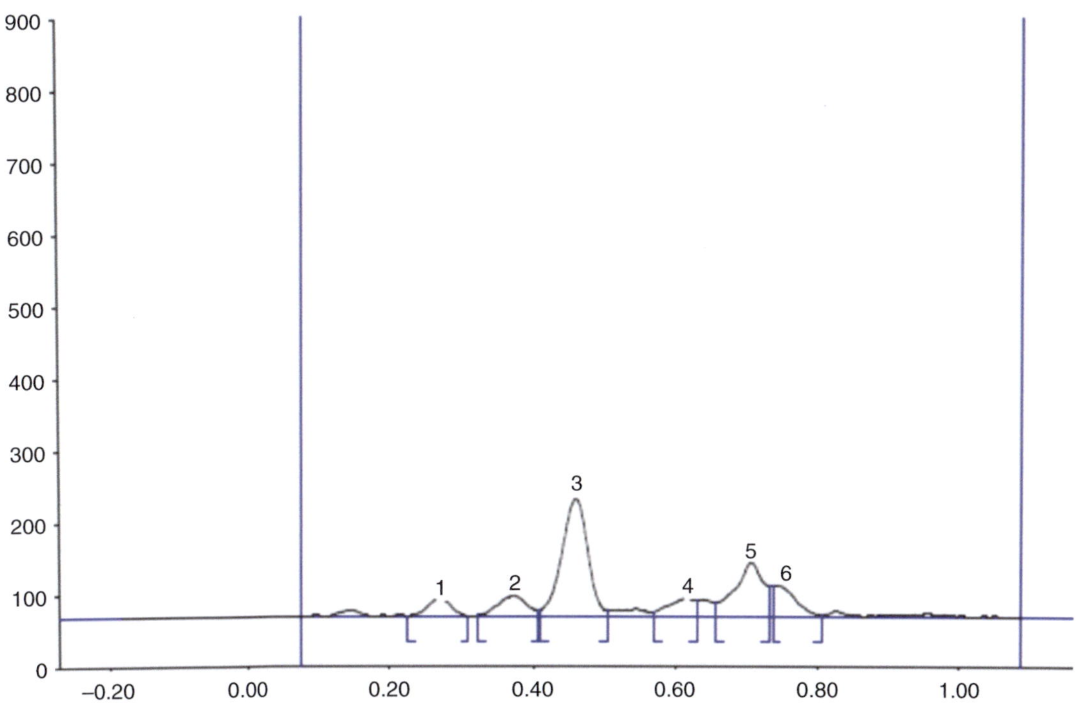

Fig. 22.27 Peak densitogram display of methanol extract of *Ilex khasiana* showing six unknown bioactive compounds

Table 22.6 Rf values of methanolic extract of *Ilex khasiana*

Peak	Start Rf	Start Height	Max Rf	Max Height	Max %	End Rf	End Height	Area	Area %	Assigned substance
1	0.23	0.5	0.27	22.8	6.35	0.31	0.5	490.8	5.80	Unknown[a]
2	0.32	1.0	0.37	28.5	7.97	0.41	8.6	729.0	8.62	Unknown[a]
3	0.41	8.8	0.46	163.0	45.53	0.51	8.5	3847.8	45.47	Unknown[a]
4	0.57	6.3	0.62	24.9	6.95	0.63	22.2	601.0	7.10	Unknown[a]
5	0.66	18.6	0.71	75.2	20.99	0.73	42.5	1920.0	22.69	Unknown[a]
6	0.74	42.6	0.75	43.7	12.20	0.81	2.4	873.2	10.32	Unknown[a]

[a] Denotes the detected unassigned unknown peak in the chromatograph

able for monitoring the identity and purity profile of a plant extract. In addition to qualitative detection, HPTLC technique also provides semi-quantitative information about the major active phytoconstituents present in a plant extract, thus enabling an assessment of plant extract quality. HPTLC fingerprint analysis can be used as a diagnostic tool for the correct identification of the plant. Further work to characterise the other chemical constituents and perform quantitative estimation with marker compounds is yet necessary; these present data can also be considered along with the other values for fixing standards to this plant. For conclusion, the results obtained from qualitative evaluation of HPTLC fingerprint images will be helpful in the identification and quality control of the drug and ensure therapeutic efficacy.

It can be concluded that HPTLC fingerprint analysis of the selected leaf extracts can be used as a diagnostic tool for the correct identification of the plant and it is useful as a phytochemical marker and also a good estimator of genetic variability in plant population. HPTLC fingerprint enables a particular plant to be identified and distinguished from closely related species.

References

Abourashed AA, Mossa JS. HPTLC determination of caffeine in stimulant herbal products and power drinks. J Pharm Biomed Anal. 2004;36:617–20.

Ahirwal B, Ahirwal D, Ram A. Evaluation of standards and quality control parameters of herbal drugs, Souvenir, recent trends in herbal therapy 2006: 25–29.

Alam P. Densitometric HPTLC analysis of 8-gingerol in Zingiber Officinale extract and ginger- containing dietary supplements, teas, and commercial creams. Asian Pac J Trop Biomed. 2013;3(8):634–8.

Alam P, Alam A, Anwer MK, Alqasoumi SI. Quantitative estimation of hesperidin by HPTLC in different varieties of citrus peels. Asian Pac J Trop Biomed. 2014;4(4):262–6.

Amit J, Sunil C, Vimal K, Anupam P. Phytosomes: a revolution in herbal drugs. Pharma Rev. 2007:11–3.

Andola HC, Purohit VK. High performance thin layer chromatography (HPTLC): a modern analytical tool for biological analysis. Nat Sci. 2010;8(10):58–61.

Arup U, Ekman S, Lindblom L, Mattsson JE. High performance thin layer chromatography (HPTLC), an improved technique for screening lichen substances. Lichenologist. 1993;25:61–71.

Attimarad M, MA KK, Aldhubaib BE, Harsha S. High-performance thin layer chromatography: a powerful analytical technique in pharmaceutical drug discovery. Pharma Methods. 2011;2(2):71–4.

Bagul MS, Rajani M. Phytochemical evaluation of classical formulation: a case study. Indian Drugs. 2005;42:15–9.

Bele AA, Khale A. Standardisation of herbal drugs: an overview. Int Res J Pharm. 2011;2(12):56–60.

Brainthwaite A, Smith FJ, Stock R, Rice CBF. Chromatographic methods. 5th ed. London: Kluwer Academic Publishers; 1999.

Choudhary N, Sekhon BS. An overview of advances in the standardization of herbal drugs. J Pharm Educ Res. 2011;2(2):55–70.

Ekka NR, Namdeo KP, Samal PK. Standardization strategies for herbal drugs: an overview. Res J Pharm Tech. 2008;1(4):310–2.

Ermer J. Linearity. In: Ermer J, Miller JHMB, editors. Method validation in pharmaceutical analysis. Weinheim: Wiley-VCH; 2005.

Gantait A, Barman T, Mukherjee PK. Validated method for estimation of curcumin in turmeric powder. Int J Trad Knowled. 2011;10(2):247–50.

Garofolo F. Bioanalytical method validation. In: Chan CC, Lam H, Lee YC, Zhang X-U, editors. Analytical method validation and instrument performance verification. Hoboken, NJ: Wiley-Interscience; 2004. p. 105–38.

International Conference on Harmonisation (ICH) of Technical Requirements for the Registration of Pharmaceuticals for Human Use. Validation of analytical procedures: methodology. Geneva: ICH-Q2B; 1996.

International Organization for Standardization. Accuracy (trueness and precision) of measurement methods and results. Geneva: ISO:DIS 5725–1 to 5725–3; 1994.

Jaenchen DE, Reich E. Planar chromatography: instrumentation. In: Encyclopedia of separation science. New York: Academic Press; 2000. p. 839–47.

Jeganathan NS, Kannan K. HPTLC method for estimation of ellagic acid and gallic acid in Triphala churnam formulations. Res J Phytochem. 2008;2(1):1–9.

Jena A, Saha D, Biswal B, Jana SB, Koley A, Sur D, Battacharya A. Pharmacognostic studies of leaves of *Pterospermum suberifolium*. Int J Res Pharma Biomed Sci. 2011;2(1):2229–3701.

Jork H, Funk W. TLC reagents & detection methods – physical & chemical detection methods: fundamentals. Hoboken: Wiley; 1990. p. 15–40.

Knapp DR. Handbook of analytical derivatization reactions. Hoboken: Wiley-Interscience; 1979. p. 2–24.. 449-453, 482

Koll K, Reich E, Blatter A, Veit M. Validation of standardized high-performance thin-layer chromatographic methods for quality control and stability testing of herbals. J AOAC Int. 2003;86:909–15.

Lee YC. Method validation for HPLC analysis of related substances in pharmaceutical products. In: Chan CC, Lam H, Lee YC, Zhang X-U, editors. Analytical method validation and instrument performance verification. Hoboken, NJ: Wiley-Interscience; 2004. p. 27–9.

Nyiredy S. Planar chromatographic method development using the PRISMA optimization system and flow charts. J Chromatogr Sci. 2002;40:553–63.

Patel K, Bhatt C. Development and validation of a HPTLC method for simultaneous densitometric analysis of Glycyrrhetic acid and Solasodine in herbal drug formulation. Int J Curr Pharm Res. 2017;9(4):29–32.

Patel VR, Patel RK. HPTLC method development and validation for quantification of markers of Dhatrinisha churna. Pharmacog J. 2012;4(29):26–9.

Patel R, Patel M, Dubey N, Dubey N. Patel B. HPTLC method development and validation: strategy to minimize methodological failures. J Food Drug Anal. 2012;20(4):794–804.

Patra KC, Pareta SK, Harwansh RK, Kumar JK. Traditional approaches towards standardization of herbal medicines -a review. J Pharm SciTechnol. 2010;2(11):372–9.

Pattanaya P, Jena RK, Panda SKHPTLC. Fingerprinting in the standardisation of sulaharan yoga: an Ayurvedic tablet formulation. Int J Pharma Sci Review Res. 2010;3(2):33–6.

Potawale SE, Gabhe SY, Mahadik KR. Quantification of gymnemagenin and β-sitosterol in marketed herbal formulation by validated normal phase HPTLC method. Chromatogr Res Int. 2014:1–6.

Renger B. Quantitative planar chromatography as a tool in pharmaceutical analysis. J AOAC Int. 1993;76:7–13.

Renger B. Contemporary thin layer chromatography in pharmaceutical quality control. J AOAC Int. 1998;81:333–9.

Saraswathy A, Rukmani S, Ariyanathan S. Analysis of Hinguvachadi Churna. Indian J Tradit Knowl. 2009;8(3):319–25.

Scott RM. The stationary phase in thin layer chromatography. J Chromatogr Sci. 1973;2:129–35.

Sethi PD. Quantitative analysis of pharmaceutical formulations, high performance thin layer chromatography. New Delhi: CBS Publishers and Distributors; 1996. p. 1–30.

Shah VP, Midha KK, Findlay JWA, Hill AM, Hulse JD, Mc-Gilveray IJ, McKay G. Bioanalytical method validation – a revisit with a decade progress. Pharma Res. 2000;17(12):1551–8.

Sherma J. Basic techniques, materials and apparatus in handbook of thin-layer chromatography. New York: Marcel Dekker; 1991. p. 3–41.

Sherma J. Chromatographic methods of analysis: thin layer chromatography. In: Swarbrick J, editor. Encyclopedia of pharmaceutical technology. 3rd ed. Swarbrick: Informa Healthcare; 2007. p. 538–50.

Shewiyo DH, Kaaleb E, Rishab PG, Dejaegherc B, Verbekec JS, Heydenc YV. HPTLC methods to assay active ingredients in pharmaceutical formulations: a review of the method development and validation steps. J Pharm Biomedical Anal. 2012;66:11–23.

Shinde DB, Chavan MJ, Wakte PS. HPTLC in herbal drug quantification. In: Srivastava MM, editor. High-performance thin-layer chromatography (HPTLC). Berlin: Springer; 2011. p. 117–21.

Srivastava MM. High-performance thin-layer chromatography (HPTLC). Berlin: Springer; 2011. p. 32–60.

Van der Hyden Y, Nijhuis A, Smayers-Verbeke J, Vandeginste BMG, Massart DL. Guidance for robustness/ruggedness test in method validation. J Pharm Biomed Anal. 2001;24:723–53.

Wagner H. Plant drug analysis: a thin layer chromatography atlas. 2nd ed. Berlin: Springer; 1996.

Wall PE. Thin-layer chromatography: a modern practical approach. Chromatography: a modern practical journal of scientific and innovative research 1096 approach. Cambridge: Royal Society of Chemistry; 2005. p. 100–50.

Wani MS, Parakh SR, Dehghan MHG, Polshettiwar SA, Chopade VV, Chepurwar S. Herbal medicine and its standardization. Pharma Info. 2007;5(6):1–6.

Yuwono M, Indrayanto G. Validation of chromatographic methods of analysis. In: Brittain G, editor. Profiles of drugs substances, excipients and related methodology, vol. 32. San Diego: Academic Press Elsevier Inc; 2005. p. 243–58.

Drug Discovery and Herbal Drug Development: A Special Focus on the Anti-diarrheal Plants of Bangladesh

23

Rownak Jahan, Khoshnur Jannat, Jannatul Ferdoes Shoma, Md. Arif Khan, Hossain Uddin Shekhar, and Mohammed Rahmatullah

Contents

23.1 Introduction

Human beings have probably suffered from diseases since their advent. Evidence of small pox and poliomyelitis has been found from 3000-year-old Egyptian mummies and papyrus paintings (Brachman 2003). It has been postulated that diseases in humans increased with the advent of agriculture and domestication of animals. The two factors in combination led to settlements of more densely populated human population, thus facilitating the transfer of pathogens. At the same time, domesticated animals became sources of transmission of diseases to humans, a process that is still ongoing; for instance measles may have come from rinderpest and small pox from cow pox (Pearce-Duvet 2006).

Medicinal plants have always formed a therapeutic source for treatment of human diseases since time immemorial. Evidence indicates that plants may have been cultivated as drugs approximately 60,000 years ago (Solecki and Shanidar 1975). Even with the advent of allopathic medicine, the dependency on plants for new and effective drugs have not decreased. Each plant contains phytochemicals or secondary

R. Jahan · K. Jannat · J. F. Shoma · M. A. Khan
Department of Biotechnology & Genetic Engineering, University of Development Alternative, Dhaka, Bangladesh

H. U. Shekhar
Department of Biochemistry & Molecular Biology, University of Dhaka, Dhaka, Bangladesh

M. Rahmatullah (✉)
Department of Pharmacy, University of Development Alternative, Dhaka, Bangladesh
email: rahmatm@uoda.edu.bd

S. Sen, R. Chakraborty (eds.), *Herbal Medicine in India*,
https://doi.org/10.1007/978-981-13-7248-3_23

metabolites with widely diverse pharmacological activities. And while some of these activities may be detrimental to human health, other activities can be beneficial and be of therapeutic value. What allopathic medicine does is basing on the principle of 'one drug one therapy', it isolates and identifies the relevant bio-active component from the plant, and following further tests and clinical trials on toxicity, efficacy, and any short- or long-term adverse effects approves the drug for therapeutic uses. This has paid rich dividends in the isolation of a number of important allopathic drugs from plants. Examples of important allopathic drugs obtained from plants include digoxin, quinine, artemisinin, vincristine, vinblastine, atropine, morphine, codeine, and reserpine (only a few examples are cited) (Rates 2001).

Herbal medicine, on the other hand, can be crude extract of a plant (monoherbal formulation) or multiple plants (polyherbal formulation) or enriched fractions like tinctures, powders, or pills. Herbal medicine is also often called traditional medicine, because all traditional medicinal systems are essentially plant based. The Traditional Medicine Division of the World Health Organization (WHO) recognizes that if a plant has been used traditionally as a medicine for centuries, the plant can be taken as a credible proof for its therapeutic efficacy for the disease that it has been used for and is still in use (Gilbert et al. 1997). Controversies, however, abound in the literature regarding the use and efficacy of herbal medicines versus allopathic medicines. A substantial section of modern scientists question the efficacy of using herbal medicines because even a monoherbal formulation may contain dozens of ingredients with diverse pharmacological activities. Moreover, it is technically difficult if not impossible to standardize a herbal formulation because the phytochemicals present in a certain plant may change depending on the region of where it is grown, whether the plant is cultivated or collected from the wild, the maturity (age) of the plant when it is collected, any stresses faced by the plant (drought, insect pests) while growing, and the mode of preservation from field to factory.

On the other hand, recent attention has been focusing more and more on herbal medicines. It has been estimated that in the USA, plant drugs may constitute up to 25% of total drugs. In countries like India and China, it may go as high as 80% (Qazi and Molvi 2016). This has happened due to a number of factors. Allopathic medicines, because they comprise of a single active ingredient, can quickly develop drug resistance. Antibiotic (allopathic products) resistance of microorganisms is rapidly becoming a severe menace to human civilization (Chandra et al. 2017). Allopathic drugs are perceived to have more adverse effects; in fact even common over-the-counter pain alleviating allopathic drugs like aspirin or paracetamol can give rise to serious adverse effects like gastric ulceration or hepatotoxicity (More 2016). Emerging infectious diseases (EIDs) like a host of viral diseases (Nipah, MERS, Hanta, Ebola, bird flu) to which allopathy has no answer are forcing scientists to look for new drugs, the plant kingdom being considered an excellent possible source for such drugs (Shakya 2016). Finally, diseases like atherosclerosis, diabetes, and Alzheimer's and a host of other neurodegenerative disorders are yet to find cures, and once again plants may hold the key to their cures.

Herbal drug development can prove its efficacy not only in finding new plants and formulations, which can lead to more effective treatment of diseases, but also through more effective means of standardization of formulations, maintaining good manufacturing practices, collection and storage of medicinal plants, toxicity studies, and establishing a control center for reporting adverse effects, help in bringing back herbal drugs within mainstream treatment, and restore confidence among allopathic doctors and their patients about the safety of using them. At the same time, the establishment of the efficacy of a plant formulation will definitely encourage scientists to look for the active ingredient(s), which in turn can become the new generation of allopathic drugs. From this viewpoint, herbal drug development and drug discovery goes hand in hand with each section complementing the other.

Ethnopharmacology is the key to successful drug discovery from medicinal plants. First, one has to collect relevant data from the traditional medicinal practitioners about phytotherapeutic uses and ascertain from patients that the treatment methods are successful. Information on any therapeutic uses of a given medicinal plant then needs to be checked against similar uses both within the country and outside the country. Corroborative evidence would give credence to the idea that the plant may prove to be a potential source for lead compounds and new drugs. Bioactivity-guided fractionation can lead to isolation and identification of the active component(s). Pharmacological activity and other clinical studies can then follow leading to final approval of the active component(s) (if new) as a new drug.

Bangladesh is a country with a scarcity of data on the traditional uses of plants. Apart from the three established traditional systems of medicine, namely, Ayurveda, Unani, and homeopathy, documentation of medicinal plants used by folk and tribal medicinal practitioners, folk herbalists, and home remedies is largely absent. Recent years have seen a growth of interest in the collection of ethnic information on phytotherapeutic uses, but still neither the Government nor the general people appear to be much interested in the creation of a herbal pharmacopoeia. Continuation of this process will lead to loss of both plants and knowledge. Plants are becoming endangered or extinct as a result of increase of human habitat. And paradoxically, when the more educated or knowledgeable section of the population are becoming re-interested in herbal medicine, the majority of the population (who are poor and illiterate) including the tribal people are switching over to allopathic medicine, believing allopathic medicine is the panacea to all sicknesses.

Towards a complete documentation of the medicinal plants of Bangladesh, we had been collecting information on the medicinal uses of plants from folk medicinal practitioners (FMPs), tribal medicinal practitioners (TMPs), folk herbalists (FHs), and persons with knowledge on home remedies for over a decade. This has resulted in primary data collection from over 400 FMPs (spread throughout all 64 districts of the country) and interviews along with data collection from TMPs of more than 30 tribes, besides dozens of FHs and people dispensing home remedies. Although this is only the tip of the iceberg (for instance, Bangladesh has 86,000 villages with at least one FMP in practically every village), our medicinal plant database already contains considerable medicinal use information on more than 1500 medicinal plants of the country. This is in contrast to the popular belief even 5 years ago that the total medicinal plant species of the country does not exceed 600. The other interesting feature that has come out from our studies is that traditional medicinal use of most plants can be to some extent scientifically validated based on existing scientific reports on their phytochemical constituents and pharmacological activities. Thus the potential for discovery of new drugs from the medicinal plants of Bangladesh is quite high. A highly selective list of our various publications on ethnic uses of plants of Bangladesh is given (Rahmatullah et al. 2009, 2010a, b, 2011a, b, 2012a, b, c, d, 2013a, b, 2014a, b; Seraj et al. 2011, 2012; Malek et al. 2012; Rahmatullah and Biswas 2012; Das et al. 2013a, b; Mukti and Rahmatullah, 2013; Hossan et al. (2014); Kabir et al. 2014; Khan et al. 2015).

To explore the potential for drug discovery from the medicinal plants of Bangladesh, we have selected diarrhea, which we deem to be important, and have listed the medicinal plants used in folk and tribal medicine to treat this disease. The medicinal plants given are from our database only. Although this may have limited the number of medicinal plants used by some extent, it is our belief that the extent of limitation will be very small and probably less than 2%. Our belief is based on perusals of the literature available in Google Scholar, SCOPUS, and PubMed, which clearly indicates that the number of papers published by us far outnumbers the publications by the other authors combined. On the other hand, information on plants from our database means that sources of information, location of source, and the information collected and produced in this work can be given in details.

Diarrhea is generally defined as having three or more liquid or loose bowel movements in a 24-hour period. Diarrhea can be caused by a variety of organisms including bacteria, viruses, parasitic worms, and protozoa. Diarrhea prevails, particularly in rural Bangladesh and urban slums of cities like Dhaka and Chittagong, due to a combination of lack of quality water for drinking and cooking, poor sanitary facilities, and unhygienic conditions of living. Although a number of organisms can cause dysentery and diarrhea, the major pathogens responsible for these two conditions in Bangladesh are reportedly *Vibrio cholerae*, rota virus, enterotoxigenic *Escherichia coli*, and *Shigella* (Ferdous et al. 2015). Not only in Bangladesh, but diarrhea is prevalent in many countries of the world with a rural population that is predominantly poor and living in unhygienic conditions. According to the World Health Organization (WHO), every year diarrhea kills around 525,000 children below 5 years of age, children being more vulnerable to diarrhea than adults. Again according to the WHO, globally there are 1.7 billion cases of childhood diarrheal disease every year. As such it is expected that the list of anti-diarrheal plants as given in Table 23.1 will spur scientific interest and lead to discovery of readily available and affordable drugs.

Over-the-counter (OTC) anti-diarrheal medicines include loperamide (Imodium) and

Table 23.1 List of medicinal plants used in Bangladesh folk medicine for treatment of diarrhea

Botanical name	Family	Local name	Parts use	Disease and dosage
Abutilon indicum (L.) sweet syn. *Abutilon indicum* (L.) sweet var. *guineense* (Schumach.) Feng, *Sida indica* L. **English:** Indian abutilon, Indian mallow, monkey bush	Malvaceae	Flur-bang (Marma[a])	Root	Diarrhea and gastrointestinal disorders in humans and cattle
Acacia arabica (Lam.) Willd. var. *indica* Benth., syn. *Acacia nilotica* (L.) Delile var. *indica* (Benth.) A.F. Hill, *Acacia nilotica* (L.) Willd. ex Del. subsp. *Indica* (Benth) Brenan **English:** Indian gum Arabic tree	Leguminosae-Mimosoideae alt. Fabaceae	Babla	Leaf, root, bark, flower, seed	Diarrhea. The five parts are taken together and boiled in eight volumes of water till the volume is reduced to ¼ of the original. The decoction is then strained and heated over a low flame till the decoction turns the texture of pitch. To every kilogram of the decoction, 8–10 g of shohaga (borax) or 3–5 g of sodium benzoate is added. It is then applied to eyes during eye inflammation or to scalp to strengthen and blacken hair and prevent hair loss. The decoction can be orally taken to improve stomach functions and to stop diarrhea

Table 23.1 (continued)

Botanical name	Family	Local name	Parts use	Disease and dosage
Acacia catechu (L. f.) Willd., syn. *Acacia catechu* (L. f.) Willd. var. *catechuoides* (Roxb.) Prain, *Acacia catechuoides* (Roxb.) Benth., *Acacia sundra* (Roxb.) Bedd., *Acacia wallichiana* DC., *Mimosa catechu* L. f., *Mimosa catechuoides* Roxb. **English:** Black catechu, black cutch, catechu, catechu tree, cutch tree, khair tree (India), wadalee gum tree	Fabaceae	Khoyer	Flower	Diarrhea, cholera. Leaves of *Catharanthus roseus*; stems of *Eleusine coracana* and *Vitex negundo*; leaves of *Clerodendrum viscosum*, *Justicia adhatoda*, and *Myristica fragrans*; flowers of *Acacia catechu*; and fruits of *Morus alba* are macerated together and made into pills. The pills are taken daily till cure (Garo[a])
Acalypha australis L., syn. *Acalypha chinensis* L., *Acalypha pauciflora* Hornem.,*Acalypha virgata* Thunb. non L. **English:** Australian acalypha	Euphorbiaceae	Muktaborshi	Whole plant	Diarrhea
Acalypha indica L., syn. *Acalypha ciliate* Wall., *Acalypha canescens* Wall., *Acalypha spicata* Forsk. **English:** Indian acalypha, Indian nettle	Euphorbiaceae	Denari shak	Leaf, root	Diarrhea in children
Acorus calamus L., syn. *Acorus americanus* Raf. **English:** Sweet flag, myrtle flag, calamus, flagroot, sweet sedge, sweet myrtle	Acoraceae alt. Araceae	Boch (Khasia[a])	Rhizome of young plants	Diarrhea
Adenanthera pavonina L., syn. *Adenanthera gersenii* Scheffer. **English:** Bead tree, coral bean tree, coralwood, false wiliwili, peacock flower-fence, Polynesian peanut, red bead tree, red sandalwood tree	Fabaceae	Rokto-chondon gach	Gota (nodule)	Diarrhea. Gota is taken
Aegle marmelos (L.) Corr., syn. *Belou marmelos* (L.) A. Lyons, *Crataeva marmelos* L., *Crateva marmelos* L., *Cydonia indica*Spach., *Feronia pellucida* Roth **English:** Bengal quince, golden apple, stone apple	Rutaceae	Bel	Fruit, flower	Diarrhea, dysentery. Powdered fruit is taken for diarrhea and dysentery. Flowers are orally taken to relieve excessive thirst, vomiting, and diarrhea
Ageratum conyzoides L., syn. *Ageratum latifolium* Cavanilles, *Ageratum cordifolium* Roxb., *Ageratum hirtum* Lam., *Ageratum humile* Salisbury, *Ageratum odoratum* Vilmorin, *Carelia conyzoides* (L.) Kuntze, *Eupatorium conyzoides* (L.) E.H.L. Krause **English:** Billy goat weed, tropical white weed	Asteraceae	Waila (Murong[a])	Leaf, root	Diarrhea. Decoction of leaves and roots are taken orally

(continued)

Table 23.1 (continued)

Botanical name	Family	Local name	Parts use	Disease and dosage
Alocasia macrorrhizos (L.) G. Don., syn. *Alocasia alba* Schott, *Alocasia crassifolia* Engl., *Alocasia indica* (Lour.) Spach, *Alocasia plumbea* Van Houtte, *Alocasia macrorrhiza* (L.) Schott, *Colocasia indica* (Lour.) Kunth **English:** Giant taro	Araceae	Maan kochu	Whole plant	Diarrhea
Alstonia scholaris (L.) R.Br., syn. *Echites scholaris* (L.) English: Blackboard tree, Indian devil tree, Dita bark	Apocynaceae	Khaka-singh (Murong[a])	Bark	Diarrhea. Bark decoction is orally taken
Amaranthus spinosus L., syn. *Amaranthus caracasanus* H.B. and K., *Amaranthus diacanthus* Raf., *Galliaria spinosa* Nieuwl. **English:** Prickly amaranth, spiny amaranth, thorny amaranth, thorny pigweed	Amaranthaceae	Kanta-khudurey	Whole plant	Diarrhea. Juice obtained from crushed whole plant is orally taken
Amomum aromaticum Roxb., syn. *Amomum subulatum* Roxb. **English:** Bengal cardamom, Nepal cardamon	Zingiberaceae	Elach	Fruit	Diarrhea. Fruits are eaten with seeds
Amorphophallus campanulatus Blume ex Decne syn. *Amorphophallus paeoniifolius* (Dennst.) Nicolson., *Dracontium paeoniifolium* Dennst. **English:** Elephant-yam, leopard palm, Stanley's washtub, telinga potato, white-spotted giant arum	Araceae	Ol	Tuber, tuber root	Diarrhea. Tubers and tuber roots are eaten in the cooked form
Annona squamosa L., syn. *Annona asiatica* L., *Anona cinerea* Dunal, *Anona forskahlii* DC., *Annona glabra* Forssk., *Guanabanus squamosus* M. Gómez, *Xylopia frutescens* Sieb. ex Presl. **English**: Custard apple, sugar apple, sweetsop	Annonaceae	Ata-phol	Fruit	Diarrhea. Fruits are eaten without seeds
Anthocephalus chinensis (Lam.) A. Rich. ex Walp., syn. *Neolamarckia cadamba* (Roxb.) Bosser, *Anthocephalus chinensis* A. Rich, *Anthocephalus indicus* A. Rich, *Nauclea cadamba* Roxb., *Sarcocephalus cadamba* (Roxb.) Kurz., *Anthocephalus cadamba* (Roxb.) Miq., *Samama cadamba* (Roxb.) Kuntze, *Anthocephalus morindifolius* Korth., *Nauclea megaphylla* S. Moore, *Neonauclea megaphylla* (S. Moore) S. Moore **English:** Bur-flower tree	Rubiaceae	Kodom gach	Leaf, flower	Cow's/goat's diarrhea

Table 23.1 (continued)

Botanical name	Family	Local name	Parts use	Disease and dosage
Areca catechu L., syn. *Areca catechu* L. **English:** Betel palm	Arecaceae	Supari	Leaf	Diarrhea in cattle. Leaves of *Areca catechu* and *Tamarindus indica* are boiled in water and then fed to cattle with rhizomes of *Zingiber officinale* and seeds of *Piper nigrum* 2–3 times daily
Argyreia speciosa (L.f.) sweet syn. *Argyreia nervosa* (Burm. F.) Bojer **English:** Hawaiian baby woodrose	Convolvulaceae	Ruphtola (Chakma-1[a])	Whole plant	Diarrhea
Artemisia indica Willd., syn. *Artemisia asiatica* (Pamp.) Nakai ex Kitamura, *Artemisia vulgaris* auct., non L., *Artemisia vulgaris* auct. var. indica (Willd.) Maxim. **English:** Asian mugwort	Asteraceae	Nagdana	Leaf	Diarrhea, stomach pain. Leaves are macerated with water. ½ poa of the mix is taken thrice daily on an empty stomach or till cure
Artemisia nilagirica (Clarke) Pamp., syn. *Artemisia vulgaris* auct. non. Linn. **English**: Indian wormwood	Asteraceae	Nag duma	Leaf	Diarrhea. Juice obtained from macerated leaves is mixed with water and bottled. 1 teaspoonful of the mixture is taken twice daily for 1 day
Artocarpus heterophyllus Lam. syn. *Artocarpus integer* auct., *Artocarpus integrifolia* auct., *Artocarpus jaca* Lam. **English:** Jackfruit, jackfruit tree	Moraceae	Gathra (Santal[a]) Thimbrongh (Garo-3[a])	Whole plant Leaf, root, fruit, seed	Cow's/goat's dysentery or diarrhea Diarrhea
Asparagus racemosus Willd., syn. *Asparagus rigidulus* Nakai, *Asparagus schoberioides* Kunth, *Asparagus volubilis* Buch.-Ham., *Protasparagus racemosus* (Willd.) Oberm. **English:** Indian asparagus, shatavari white, shatavari yellow, wild asparagus	Liliaceae	Shotomul	Whole plant	Gulmo-otishar (diarrhea)
Averrhoa carambola L., syn. *Averrhoa pentandra* Blanco **English:** Carambola, Coromandel gooseberry, five-corner fruit, star apple, starfruit, star fruit	Oxalidaceae	Kamarangha (Garo[a])	Fruit	Diarrhea
Azadirachta indica A. Juss., syn. *Antelaea azadirachta* (L.) Adelb., *Antelaea javanica* Gaertn., *Melia azadirachta* L., *Melia indica* (A. Juss.) Brandis **English:** Neem, bead tree, Burmese neem tree, chinaberry, Indian cedar	Meliaceae	Neem	Leaf	Diarrhea. Stems of *Leucas aspera* are mixed with leaves of *Azadirachta indica* and leaves and fruits of *Coccinia cordifolia* and taken
Barleria prionitis L., syn. **English:** Porcupine flower	Acanthaceae	Shonjiboni	Leaf	Diarrhea. Juice from macerated leaves is taken twice for diarrhea

(continued)

Table 23.1 (continued)

Botanical name	Family	Local name	Parts use	Disease and dosage
Barringtonia acutangula (L.) Gaertn. syn. *Eugenia acutangula* L. **English:** Cut nut, wild almond, kandu almond	Lecythidaceae	Hijol	Leaf	Diarrhea
Barringtonia racemosa (L.) Roxb. syn. *Eugenia racemosa* L., *Barringtonia racemosa* (L.) Blume ex DC. *Barringtonia racemes* (L.) Spreng. **English:** Fish-killer tree, fish-poison tree, fish-poison wood, freshwater mangrove, small-leaved barringtonia	Lecythidaceae	Moha shomudro (Bede[a])	Root	Sutika (symptoms: diarrhea, indigestion, wasting of body). Roots of *Barringtonia racemosa* (L.) Roxb. (Lecythidaceae) are mixed with fruits of *Myristica fragrans* Houtt. (Myristicaceae), *Phyllanthus emblica*, *Terminalia belerica*, and *Terminalia chebula*, macerated and mixed with ½ kg water and a little more than a handful of molasses prepared from date palm [*Phoenix sylvestris* L. (Arecaceae)] sap, and boiled for 30 minutes. The decoction is taken twice daily for 7 days
Bauhinia variegata L. syn. *Bauhinia candida* Ait., *Bauhinia purpurea* auct. **English:** Butterfly tree, mountain ebony, orchid tree, Poor man's orchid	Fabaceae	Rokto-kanchon	Leaf, bark, root, flower	Diarrhea
Bischofia javanica Blume syn. *Bischofia cummingiana* Decne, *Bischofia oblongifolia* Decne, *Bischofia roperiana* Decne, *Bischofia toui* Decne, *Bischofia trifoliata* (Roxb.) Hook, *Microelus roeperianus* Wight and Arn., *Stylodiscus trifoliastus* Benn. **English:** Bishop wood, Java cedar	Euphorbiaceae	Kanchol-Bhadhi	Leaf, stem, root	Diarrhea
Blumea lacera DC., syn. *Blumea axillaris* (Lam.) DC, *Conyza lacera* Burm. f. **English:** Malay Blumea	Asteraceae	Sheal moti	Root	Crushed roots are taken for diarrhea
Bombax ceiba L., syn. *Bombax malabaricum* Candolle, *Bombax malabaricum* DC. *Gossampinus malabarica* (Candolle) Merrill, *Salmalia malabarica* (Candolle) Schott and Endlicher. *Salmalia malabarica* (DC.) Schott and Endl. **English:** Indian cottonwood, Indian kapok, Kapok tree, red cottontree, red-flowered silk-cotton tree, red silk-cotton, red silk-cotton tree, shaving brush, silk cottontree, simal tree	Bombacaceae	Shimul	Seed	Bhuri basanta (diarrhea with smelly feces, may sometimes contain blood) in cattle. Seeds of *Bombax ceiba* and *Piper nigrum* are mixed with hirapor and water and fed 2–3 times daily

Table 23.1 (continued)

Botanical name	Family	Local name	Parts use	Disease and dosage
Caesalpinia digyna Rottler **English:** Teri pod	Leguminosae	Mukhoi-chechai (Tripura[a])	Root	Frequent diarrhea
Cajanus cajan (L.) Millsp. syn. *Cytisus cajan*L., *Cajanus cajan*(L.) Druce., *Cajanus cajan* (L.) Huth, *Cajanus cajan* (L.) Merr., *Cajanus indicus* Sprengl. **English:** Pigeon pea; Congo pea; Congo bean; Angola pea	Fabaceae	Orhor-kolai	Leaf juice	Diarrhea
Callicarpa macrophylla Vahl., syn. *Callicarpa incana* Roxb., *Callicarpa tomentosa* J. Koenig ex Vahl, nom. Inval. **English:** Beauty berry	Lamiaceae alt. Verbenaceae	Jama-thoi (Tripura[a])	Root	Diarrhea
Calotropis gigantea (L.) Ait.f., syn. *Calotropis procera* (Ait.) R. Brown, *Asclepias gigantea* L. **English:** Giant milkweed	Asclepiadaceae	Akondo	Leaf, flower	Diarrhea
Cassia alata L., syn. *Senna alata* (L.) Roxb., *Herpetica alata* (L.) Raf., *Cassia bracteata* L.f., *Cassia herpetica* Jacq. **English:** Guajava, candlebush, candlestick senna, Christmas candle, ringworm bush, ringworm senna, ringworm shrub, seven golden candlesticks	Fabaceae	Sada-kodom (Chakma[a])	Leaf, stem	Diarrhea
Cassia sophera L., syn. *Senna sophera* (L.) Roxb. *Cassia canca* Cav., *Cassia esculenta* Roxb., *Cassia frutescens* Miller, *Cassia geminiflora* Schrank, *Cassia linearis* Michaux, *Cassia linneata* Michaux, *Cassia occidentalis* L. var. *glabra* DC., *Cassia occidentalis* L. var. *sophera* (L.) Kuntze, *Cassia patula* Aiton, *Cassia proboscidea* Pollard, *Cassia sophera* L. var. *ligustrinoides* Benth., *Cassia torosa* Cav., *Chamaefistula sophera* G. Don, *Ditremexa sophera* (L.) Britton and Wilson **English:** Senna, Senna sophera, African senna	Fabaceae	Kal-kashundae	Leaf	Diarrhea. 15–20 ml of juice obtained from macerated leaves of *Cassia sophera* is mixed with 1 glass of coconut water (water within the fruits of *Cocos nucifera*) and taken 3–4 times daily till cure
Cassia tora L., syn. *Senna tora* (L.) Roxb., *Cassia obtusifolia* L. **English:** Ringworm plant, foetid cassia, Sickle senna, wild senna	Fabaceae	Chetki	Leaf	Diarrhea

(continued)

Table 23.1 (continued)

Botanical name	Family	Local name	Parts use	Disease and dosage
Casuarina equisetifolia L., syn. *Casuarina litorea* L. ex Fosberg and Sachet **English:** Australian pine, beach sheoak, common ironwood	Casuarinaceae	Zhau	Whole plant	Diarrhea
Catharanthus roseus (L.) G. Don syn. *Vinca rosea* L., *Ammocallis rosea* (L.) Small, *Lochnera rosea* (L.) Reichenb. ex Spach **English:** Vinca, Madagascar periwinkle	Apocynaceae	Noyon tara (Garo[a])	Leaf	Diarrhea, cholera. Leaves of *Catharanthus roseus*; stems of *Eleusine coracana* and *Vitex negundo*; leaves of *Clerodendrum viscosum*, *Justicia adhatoda*, and *Myristica fragrans*; flowers of *Acacia catechu*; and fruits of *Morus alba* are macerated together and made into pills. The pills are taken daily till cure
Cayratia trifolia (L.) Domin., syn. *Cissus trifolia* (L.) K. Schum., *Vitis trifolia* L., *Cissus carnopa* Lam., *Vitis carnosa* (Roxb.) Wall. **English:** Three-leaf cayratia	Vitaceae	Mundi	Leaf	Diarrhea
Centella asiatica (L.) Urb., syn. *Hydrocotyle asiatica* L., *Hydrocotyle erecta* L. f. **English:** Asian pennywort, Asiatic coinwort, Asiatic pennywort, Indian pennywort, Indian water navelwort, marsh penny, marsh pennywort, pennyweed, sheep-rot, spadeleaf, thick-leaved pennywort, water pennywort, white rot	Umbelliferae alt. Apiaceae	Chasta (Tripura[a]) Teka thankuni, Thankuni pata (Bede[a])	Leaf Leaf	Diarrhea Diarrhea and flatulency in children. Leaves of *Centella asiatica* are macerated with rice. Pithas (a Bangladesh dish) made from the mixture is taken twice daily in the morning and evening for 7 days
Chenopodium ambrosioides L., syn. *Ambrina ambrosioides* (L.) Spach, *Atriplex ambrosioides* Crantz, *Blitum ambrosioides* (L.) Beck, *Chenopodium suffruticosum* Willd., *Dysphania ambrosioides* (L.) Mosyakin and Clemants, *Teloxys ambrosioides* (L.) W. A. Weber **English:** American wormseed, bluebush, Indian goosefoot, Jerusalem tea, Jesuit's tea, Mexican tea, Spanish tea, wormseed	Chenopodiaceae	Nag dana	Leaf, stem	Diarrhea
Cinnamomum iners Reinw. ex Blume syn. *Cinnamomum malabathrum* sensu Gamble, *Cinnamomum malabathrum* auct. **English:** Wild cinnamon	Lauraceae	Tej-bohul	Leaf, fruit	Diarrhea

Table 23.1 (continued)

Botanical name	Family	Local name	Parts use	Disease and dosage
Cinnamomum tamala (Buch.-Ham.) Nees and Eberm., syn. *Cinnamomum tejpata* hort., *Laurus tamala* Buch.-Ham. **English:** Indian bay-leaf, Indian cassia, Indian cassia bark, Tamala cassia, tejpat (India)	Lauraceae	Tejpata (Garo[a])	Leaf	Diarrhea
Citrus aurantiifolia (Christm.) Swingle syn. *Citrus acida* Roxb., *Citrus aurantium* L. subsp. *aurantiifolia* Guillaumin, *Citrus excelsa* Wester, *Citrus hystrix* DC. subsp. *Acida* (Roxb.) Engl., *Citrus javanica* Blume, *Citrus lima* Lunan, *Citrus limetta* auct., non Risso, *Citrus limetta* Risso var. *aromatica* Wester, *Citrus limonellus* Hassk., *Citrus medica* L. subsp. *Acida* (Roxb.) Engl., *Citrus medica* L. var. *acida* Hook. f., *Citrus notissima* Blanco, *Citrus spinosissima* Meyer, *Limonia acidissima* Houtt., *Limonia aurantiifolia* Christm **English:** Acid lime, Egyptian lime, Indian lime, kagzi lime, lime, Mexican lime, West Indian lime, sour lime, large lime, key lime	Rutaceae	Lebu	Leaf, fruit	Fruit juice is taken like a sherbet for diarrhea, and dysentery and to keep stomach cool
Citrus aurantium L. syn. *Citrus amara* Link, *Citrus aurantium* L. subsp. *Amara* (L.) Engl., *Citrus aurantium* L. subsp. *Aurantium*, *Citrus aurantium* L. var. *amara* Engl., *Citrus bigarradia* Loisel., *Citrus florida* Salisb., *Citrus vulgaris* Risso, *Citrus sinensis* (L.) Osbeck **English:** Bigarade, bitter orange, Oranger à fruit amer, Seville orange, sour orange	Rutaceae	Komla	Skin of fruit	Diarrhea in young children. Crushed skin of fruit is taken
Clerodendrum viscosum Vent., syn. *Clerodendrum infortunatum* auct., *Volkameria infortunata* Roxb. **English:** Glorybower	Verbenaceae alt. Lamiaceae	Ghatho (Santal[a]) Baik (Garo[a])	Leaf, root Leaf	Cow's/goat's diarrhea. Diarrhea, cholera. Leaves of *Catharanthus roseus*; stems of *Eleusine coracana* and *Vitex negundo*; leaves of *Clerodendrum viscosum*, *Justicia adhatoda*, and *Myristica fragrans*; flowers of *Acacia catechu*; and fruits of *Morus alba* are macerated together and made into pills. The pills are taken daily till cure

(continued)

Table 23.1 (continued)

Botanical name	Family	Local name	Parts use	Disease and dosage
Coccinia grandis (L.) J. Voigt syn. *Bryonia alceifolia* Willd, *Bryonia grandis* L., *Coccinia cordifolia* sensu auct. non (L.) Cogn., *Cephalandra indica* Naud., *Coccinia cordifolia* (L.) Cogn. var. *alceifolia* (Willd.) Cogn., *Coccinia cordifolia* (L.) Cogn. var. *wightiana* (M.Roem.) Cogn., *Coccinia grandis* (L.) Voigt var. *wightiana* (M.Roem.) Greb., *Coccinia indica* Wight and Arn., *Coccinia loureiriana* M. Roem., *Coccinia wightiana* M.Roem., *Cucumis pavel* Kostel., *Momordica bicolor* Blume, *Momordica covel* Dennst., *Momordica monadelpha* Roxb. **English**: Ivy gourd, scarlet gourd, scarlet-fruited gourd, kowai fruit	Cucurbitaceae	Telakochu	Leaf	Diarrhea, dysentery. Juice obtained from macerated leaves of *Coccinia grandis* (L.) J. Voigt (Cucurbitaceae) is mixed with salt. 2 teaspoonful of the mixture is taken once daily for 5–7 days
Cocos nucifera L. syn. *Palma cocos* Miller **English**: Bahia coconut palm (Brazil), coconut, coconut palm, copra (product)	Arecaceae	Narikhol (Garo-4[a])	Fruit	Diarrhea (fruit juice)
Coffea arabica L. syn. **English:** Arabian coffee, Arabica coffee, coffee	Rubiaceae	Coffee	Leaf	Otishar (diarrhea)
Coix lacryma-jobi L. syn. *Coix agrestis* Lour., *Coix arundinacea* Lamk, *Coix lacryma* L., *Coix exaltata* Jacq. **English:** Job's tears, Adlay, Adley, Adlay millet, Coix millet, Gromwell reed	Poaceae	Rikesire (Garo[a])	Root, seed	Diarrhea
Colocasia esculenta (L.) Schott syn. *Arum esculentum* L., *Caladium esculentum* (L.) Vent., *Colocasia antiquorum* Schott, *Colocasia antiquorum* Schott var. *esculenta* (L.) Schott **English:** Cocoyam, dasheen, eddo, elephant's ear, taro, taro potato	Araceae	Kochu-mannhe (Santal[a])	Whole plant	Diarrhea
Commelina benghalensis L. syn. English: Benghal dayflower, tropical spiderwort	Commelinaceae	Kandha lota	Whole plant	Diarrhea
Corchorus capsularis L., syn. *Corchorus cordifolius* Salisb., *Corchorus marua* Buch.-Ham., nom. Nudum **English:** Bangla white jute (India), jute, white jute	Tiliaceae	Pata (Santal[a])	Whole plant	Cow's/goat's dysentery or diarrhea
Crataeva nurvala Buch-Ham., syn. *Crateva religiosa* f. var. Forster *nurvala* f. Hook. and Thomson, *Crateva lophosperma* Kurz, *Crataeva magna* (Lour.) DC **English:** Three-leaf caper	Capparaceae	Burum	Fruit	Diarrhea

Table 23.1 (continued)

Botanical name	Family	Local name	Parts use	Disease and dosage
Crinum asiaticum L. syn. *Crinum amabile* Donn ex Ker Gawl **English:** Poison bulb, Asiatic poison bulb	Liliaceae	Gurunda	Leaf, root	Diarrhea in cattle
Curcuma longa L., syn. *Curcuma domestica* Valeton **English:** Turmeric	Zingiberaceae	Holud	Rhizome	Diarrhea
Curcuma zedoaria (Christm.) Roscoe syn. *Amomum zedoaria* Christm. **English:** Red-leaf spice ginger	Zingiberaceae	Kalo holud (Khasia)	Rhizome	Diarrhea
Cuscuta reflexa Roxb. syn. *Cuscuta verrucosa* sweet **English:** Giant dodder	Cuscutaceae	Ore-rui (Murong) Shorno lota (Khasia)	Vine, fruit Shoot	Diarrhea Diarrhea, shoots are crushed with a little amount of water and taken orally
Cynodon dactylon (L.) Pers., syn. *Capriola dactylon* (L.) O. Kuntze, *Panicum dactylon* L., *Digitaria dactylon* Scopoli, *Dactylon officinale* Villars, *Paspalum umbellatum* Lamarck **English:** Bermuda grass, Bahama grass	Poaceae	Durba (Chakma)	Whole plant	Diarrhea
Cyperus rotundus L., syn. *Pycreus rotundus* (L.) Hayek, *Cyperus tuberosus* Roxn., *Cyperus olivaris* Targioni-Tozzetti **English:** Nut grass, purple nutsedge	Cyperaceae	Mutha, Bada	Tuber	Diarrhea
Dalbergia sissoo Roxb. ex DC. syn. *Amerimnom sissoo* (Roxb. ex DC.) Kuntze, *Dalbergia pseudo-sissoo* Miq. **English:** Indian rosewood	Fabaceae	Shishu (Santal)	Young stem	Diarrhea
Datura stramonium L., syn. *Datura tatula* L., *Datura laevis* L.f., *Datura stramonium* L. Var. *Inermis* (Jacq.) Lundstr. **English:** Devil's trumpet, jimsonweed	Solanaceae	Konok dhutra	Leaf, fruit, seed	Diarrhea
Desmodium gangeticum (L.) DC., syn. *Desmodium gangeticum* (L.) DC. Var. *Maculatum* (L.) Baker, *Hedysarum gangeticum* L., *Hedysarum maculatum* L., *Desmodium natalitum* Sond., *Desmodium polygonoides* Baker	Fabaceae	Shalpani	Whole plant	Diarrhea
Dillenia indica L., syn. *Dillenia speciosa* Thunb. **English:** Chulta, Hondapara tree, elephant apple	Dilleniaceae	Chalta	Leaf	Diarrhea, dysentery. Macerated young leaves are taken with a little honey to restore appetite. Juice obtained from fruits is taken to prevent stomach upsets and for treatment of diarrhea and dysentery

(continued)

Table 23.1 (continued)

Botanical name	Family	Local name	Parts use	Disease and dosage
Dioscorea bulbifera L., syn. *Dioscorea sativa* Thumb auct. Non LD **English:** Air potato, air yam, bitter yam	Dioscoreaceae	Kukur bicha	Fruit	Diarrhea, indigestion. Boiled fruits are mixed with salt and boiled rice and pills are made from the mixture the size of marbles. 1 pill is taken thrice daily
Diospyros peregrina (Gaertn.) Gürke., syn. *Diospyros malabarica* (Desr.) Kostel., *Diospyros embryopteris* Pers. **English:** Indian persimmon	Ebenaceae	Gaab	Bark	Diarrhea in cattle. Barks of *Psidium guajava*, *Mangifera indica*, *Lannea coromandelica*, *Syzygium cumini*, *Diospyros peregrina*, and *Ficus religiosa* are mixed together and boiled in 10 kg water till the amount has been reduced to around 2 kg. ½ chatak (local measure, approximates 30 g) is fed to large-sized cattle (cow/buffalo) thrice daily. A little less than ½ chatak is fed to medium-sized cattle thrice daily. 2–3 spoonfuls of the decoction are fed to small-sized cows and buffaloes or goats or calves thrice daily
Diplazium esculentum (Retz.) Sw. syn. *Anisogonium esculentum* Retz., *Athyrium esculentum* (Retz.) Copeland **English:** Vegetable fern	Woodsiaceae	Dheki shak	Root	Diarrhea in cattle. 250 g juice obtained from macerated root is fed to cattle three times for cattle dysentery. 50 g juice obtained from macerated root is fed three times for human dysentery. Juice obtained from macerated leaves is given to cattle for cattle diarrhea
Drynaria quercifolia (L.) J. Smith syn. *Polypodium quercifolium* L. **English:** Oak leaf basket fern	Polypodiaceae	Ponkhi Raj	Rhizome	Diarrhea. Juice obtained from crushed rhizomes is taken 2–3 times daily till cure
Eclipta alba (L.) Hassk., syn. *Eclipta prostrata* L. **English:** False daisy	Asteraceae / Compositae	Khot-kushte	Leaf juice	Diarrhea
Eleusine coracana (L.) Gaertn., syn. *Cynosurus coracanus* L., *Eleusine quatic* (Kenn.-O'Byrne) Hilu and de Wet., *Eleusine tocussa* Fresen **English**: Finger millet, African millet	Poaceae	Dutle (Garo[a])	Stem	Diarrhea, cholera. Leaves of *Catharanthus roseus*; stems of *Eleusine coracana* and *Vitex negundo*; leaves of *Clerodendrum viscosum*, *Justicia adhatoda*, and *Myristica fragrans*; flowers of *Acacia catechu*; and fruits of *Morus alba* are macerated together and made into pills. The pills are taken daily till cure

Table 23.1 (continued)

Botanical name	Family	Local name	Parts use	Disease and dosage
*Eleutherine plicata*Herb. Alho do Mato., syn. **English:** Small-flowered Marica	Iridaceae alt. Liliaceae	Sulusu (Chak[a]) Chinisam (lal) (Garo[a])	Leaf, onion like tubers Leaf	Diarrhea Diarrhea
Eryngium foetidum L., syn. **English:** Long cilantro, Javanese cilantro, Mexican cilantro, long coriander	Apiaceae	Dhonia pata	Whole plant	Diarrhea
Erythrina variegata L. syn. *Erythrina indica* Lam., *Erythrina orientalis* (L.) Merr. **English:** Tiger's claw	Fabaceae	Krong-singh (Murong[a]) Madar gach	Leaf, bark Leaf, bark	Diarrhea Diarrhea. Cuts and wounds to stop bleeding. ½ kg bark of *Erythrina variegata* is combined with ½ kg bark of *Diospyros ebenum* and is boiled in 2 kg water till the volume is reduced to 1 kg. 3–4 teaspoonful of the decoction is taken thrice daily for 15–20 days for lower abdominal pain or diarrhea. To stop bleeding from cuts and wounds, macerated leaves of the plant are applied
Eupatorium odoratum L. syn. *Chromolaena odorata* (L.) R. M. King and H. Rob., syn. *Osmia odorata* (L.) Schultz **English:** Baby bush	Asteraceae alt. Compositae	Fuler-chorie	Leaf, flower	Diarrhea
Euphorbia hirta L., syn. *Euphorbia pilulifera* (L.), *Chamaesyce hirta* (L.) Millsp. **English:** Cats hair, asthma weed	Euphorbiaceae	Khatre-phang (Garo[a])	Whole plant	Diarrhea
Euphorbia milii "Lutea" Hort syn. *Euphorbia splendens* Bojer ex Hook English: Crown of thorns, Christ thorn, Christ plant	Euphorbiaceae	Dodhi-kata	Whole plant	Diarrhea
Euphorbia prostrata Aiton syn. *Chamaesyce prostrata* (Aiton) Small **English:** Prostrate spurge, spurge	Euphorbiaceae	Choto-kheworoi	Whole plant	Diarrhea
Euryale ferox Salisb., syn. **English:** Euryale	Nymphaeaceae	Makhna	Whole plant	Diarrhea
Feronia elephantum Corrêa., syn. *Feronia limonia* (L.) Swingle, *Limonia acidissima* L., *Schinus limonia* L. **English:** Elephant apple, wood apple, monkey fruit	Rutaceae	Kothbel	Leaf, bark, fruit	Diarrhea

(continued)

Table 23.1 (continued)

Botanical name	Family	Local name	Parts use	Disease and dosage
Ficus benghalensis L., syn. *Ficus indica* L., *Ficus benghalensis* Bailey and Bailey "Krishnae," *Ficus krishnae* C.DC. English: Banyan fig, Banyan tree, East Indian fig tree, Indian banyan, weeping Chinese banyan	Moraceae	Bot (Bede[a]) Botia (Garo[a])	Aerial root, leaf stalk Leaf bud	Diarrhea (any type). Whitish sap obtained from leaf stalks and aerial roots of *Ficus benghalensis* is taken with a little batasha (a Bangladesh sweet product made from flour and sugar) twice daily on a full stomach for 7 days. Note that the amount of sap in both cases cannot be more than 3 drops; otherwise it will heat up the body. Diarrhea. Juice obtained from squeezed leaf buds is orally taken
Ficus hispida L.f., syn. *Ficus compressa* S. S. Chang, *Ficus heterostyla* Merr. **English:** Rough-leaved fig	Moraceae	Khoksa	Leaf, root, fruit	Diarrhea
Ficus racemosa L., syn. *Covellia glomerata* (Roxb.) Miq., *Ficus glomerata* Roxb., *Ficus goolereea* Roxb. **English:** Cluster fig, cluster tree, country fig, gular fig, redwood fig	Moraceae	Dumur	Leaf	Diarrhea. Juice obtained from combination of macerated leaves and roots is taken for diarrhea
Ficus religiosa L., syn. **English:** Bo tree, Bodhi tree, peepul tree (Nepal), pipal tree (India), pippala (India), po tree (Thailand), sacred fig, sacred fig tree	Moraceae	Pakur	Bark	Diarrhea in cattle. Barks of *Psidium guajava*, *Mangifera indica*, *Lannea coromandelica*, *Syzygium cumini*, *Diospyros peregrina*, and *Ficus religiosa* are mixed together and boiled in 10 kg water till the amount has been reduced to around 2 kg. ½ chatak (local measure, approximates 30 g) is fed to large-sized cattle (cow/buffalo) thrice daily. A little less than ½ chatak is fed to medium-sized cattle thrice daily. 2–3 spoonfuls of the decoction are fed to small-sized cows and buffaloes or goats or calves thrice daily
Garcinia cowa Roxb. syn.	Clusiaceae	Kau-pata	Leaf	Diarrhea

Table 23.1 (continued)

Botanical name	Family	Local name	Parts use	Disease and dosage
Glycyrrhiza glabra L., syn. *Glycyrrhiza echinata* Lepech., *Glycyrrhiza yaline*L., *Glycyrrhiza officinalis* Lepech., *Glycyrrhiza yalin* Boiss. and Noe, *Glycyrrhiza violacea* Boiss. and Noe., *Liquiritia officinarum* Medik., *Liquiritia officinalis* Moench **English:** Common liquorice, cultivated licorice, licorice, liquorice, Russian liquorice, Spanish liquorice, sweet licorice, sweet wood, true licorice	Fabaceae	Josthi-modhu (Khasia[a])	Root	Diarrhea
Grewia microcos L. syn. *Microcos paniculata* L. **English:** Panicled Indian linden	Tiliaceae	Pichondi gach (Khasia[a])	Bark	Diarrhea. Juice obtained from crushed bark is mixed with ½ cup water and taken orally thrice daily
Grewia paniculata Roxb. ex DC., syn. English: False brandy bush	Tiliaceae	Gota pata	Leaf, root, fruit	Diarrhea
Grewia subinaequalis DC., syn. *Grewia asiatica* L., *Grewia vestita* Wall **English:** Phalsa	Tiliaceae	Folsha	Seed, fruit	Diarrhea
Hedyotis corymbosa (L.) Lam. syn. *Oldenlandia corymbosa* L. **English:** Old world diamond flower	Rubiaceae	Khet-papra	Leaf	Diarrhea
Hemidesmus indicus R. Br., syn. *Periploca indica* Willd, *Periploca yalin* Retz., *Asclepias pseudosarsa* Roxb. English: Indian sarsaparilla	Apocynaceae	Boisthofa (Mandai[a])	Root	Diarrhea. Paste or pill prepared from a mixture of gum of *Streblus asper* Lour. (Moraceae) and root of *Hemidesmus indicus* R. Br. (Apocynaceae) is taken for 2–3 days
Heritiera fomes Wall., syn. *Amygdalus minor* Kuntze, *Balanopteris minor* Gaertn., *Fometica punctata* Rafin. **English:** Sundri tree	Sterculiaceae	Sundari	Leaf, bark	Diarrhea
Hibiscus rosa sinensis L., syn. **English:** China rose, Chinese hibiscus	Malvaceae	Rokto-joba (Khasia[a]) Rokto joba (Chakma[a]) Rokto joba (Patro[a])	Flower	Diarrhea Diarrhea. Juice obtained from macerated flower petals is taken with water for diarrhea. Crushed flower petals are topically applied to palm infections For diarrhea, juice obtained from three macerated flowers (a little less than half cup) is mixed with tal mishri (crystalline sugar prepared from sap of *Borassus flabellifer*) and taken for 3 days in the morning on an empty stomach

(continued)

Table 23.1 (continued)

Botanical name	Family	Local name	Parts use	Disease and dosage
Holarrhena pubescens Wall. Ex G. Don syn. *Chonemorpha antidysenterica* (Roxb. ex Fleming) G. Don, *Echites antidysenterica* Roxb. ex Flem., *Echites antidysentericus* Roth, nom. Illeg., *Echites pubescens* Buch.-Ham., *Holarrhena antidysenterica* (L.) Wall. Ex A. DC., *Holarrhena antidysenterica* (Roxb. ex Fleming) Wall. Ex A. DC., *Holarrhena febrifuga* Klotzsch, *Nerium antidysentericum* L., *Wrightia antidysenterica* R. Br., *Wrightia zeylanica* R. Br. **English:** Cavessi bark, common holarrhena, Conessi bark, easter tree, ivory tree, tellicherry bark, white angel	Apocynaceae	Kutishwer	Bark, seed	Diarrhea. Juice obtained from macerated bark and seeds is taken twice daily with honey until cure
Ipomoea aquatica Forssk., syn. *Ipomoea reptans* (L.) Poiret, nom. Invalid **English:** Chinese water spinach, water convolvulus, water spinach, swamp cabbage, swamp morning glory, tropical spinach	Convolvulaceae	Kolmi shak	Root	Macerated roots are taken with honey for jaundice and diarrhea till cure
Ipomoea batatas (L.) Lam. Var. *Batatas* syn. *Convolvulus batatas* L., *Convolvulus edulis* Thunb., *Batatas edulis* (Thunb.) Choisy, *Ipomoea batatas* (L.) Lam. Var. *edulis* (Thunb.) Kuntze **English:** Sweet potato, sweetpotato (USA), yam (USA), kumara (NZ)	Convolvulaceae	Shakha-alu	Leaf, tuber root	Diarrhea
Ipomoea lacunosa L. **English:** Whitestar, small white morning glory	Convolvulaceae	Kamli rong (Patro[a])	Leaf, stem	Diarrhea. Juice obtained from macerated leaves is taken. Dosage is 4 spoonfuls of juice taken on an empty stomach
Ixora athroantha Bremek.	Rubiaceae	Ludi choulla (Chakma[a])	Bark	Diarrhea. Macerated bark is dried in the sun and then taken with cold water
Ixora coccinea L., syn. *Ixora yaline* (Blume) DC., *Ixora grandiflora* Bot., *Ixora bandhuca Roxb.* **English:** Flame of the world, jungle flame, jungle geranium, flame of the woods	Rubiaceae	Fema (Chakma[a])	Leaf, stem, flower	Diarrhea

Table 23.1 (continued)

Botanical name	Family	Local name	Parts use	Disease and dosage
Justicia adhatoda L., syn. *Adhatoda* (L.) Huth, *Adhatoda pubescens* Moench., *Adhatoda vasica* Nees, *Adhatoda zeylanica* Medik., *Dianthera latifolia* Salisb., *Gendarussa adhatoda* Steud., *Justicia adhathoda* L. **English:** Malabar nut tree	Acanthaceae	Hong-shu-bang (Marma[a]) Bashok (Garo[a])	Leaf Leaf	Diarrhea Diarrhea, cholera. Leaves of *Catharanthus roseus*; stems of *Eleusine coracana* and *Vitex negundo*; leaves of *Clerodendrum viscosum*, *Justicia adhatoda*, and *Myristica fragrans*; flowers of *Acacia catechu*; and fruits of *Morus alba* are macerated together and made into pills. The pills are taken daily till cure
Kalanchoe pinnata (Lam.) Pers., syn. *Bryophyllum pinnatum* (Lam.) Oken, *Cotyledon pinnata* Lam., *Bryophyllum calycinum* Salisb., *Bryophyllum germinans* Blanco, *Cotyledon calycina* Salisb. Roth, *Cotyledon calyculata*Solander ex De Candolle, *Cotyledon rhizophilla* Roxb., *Crassuvia floripendia* Commers. Ex Hiern, *Crassula pinnata* L.f., *Sedum madagascariense* (H.Perrier) H. Obla, *Verea pinnata* (Lam.) Spreng. **English:**Air plant, cathedral bells, life plant	Crassulaceae	Pathorkuchi	Leaf	Diarrhea (symptoms: frequent and watery bowel movements), irregular urination, dysuria, or urinary tract infection (symptoms: sudden abdominal pain, burning sensations in urinary tract). Juice obtained from macerated leaves is taken orally with salt in the morning on an empty stomach thrice daily for 21 days
Lagerstroemia speciosa (L.) Pers., syn. *Lagerstroemia reginae* Roxb. **English:** Queen's flower, Queen's cape myrtle, pride of India	Lythraceae	Jarul	Bark, seed	Diabetes
Lallemantia royleana (Benth.) Benth. Syn. *Dracocephalum royleanum* Benth. (basionym) **English:** Black psyllium	Lamiaceae	Tokhma	Seed	Diarrhea. Seeds are orally taken for the aforementioned gastrointestinal disorders

(continued)

Table 23.1 (continued)

Botanical name	Family	Local name	Parts use	Disease and dosage
Lannea grandis (Dennst.) Engl., syn. *Lannea coromandelica* (Houtt.) Merr. **English:** Indian ash tree	Anacardiaceae	Jiga	Bark	Diarrhea in cattle. Barks of *Psidium guajava*, *Mangifera indica*, *Lannea coromandelica*, *Syzygium cumini*, *Diospyros peregrina*, and *Ficus religiosa* are mixed together and boiled in 10 kg water till the amount has been reduced to around 2 kg. ½ chatak (local measure, approximates 30 g) is fed to large-sized cattle (cow/buffalo) thrice daily. A little less than ½ chatak is fed to medium-sized cattle thrice daily. 2–3 spoonfuls of the decoction are fed to small-sized cows and buffaloes or goats or calves thrice daily
Leea macrophylla Roxb. ex Hornem syn. *Leea diffusa* M.A. Lawson, *Leea robusta* Roxb. **English:** Elephant ear	Leeaceae	Pituri	Leaf, stem	Diarrhea
Leonurus sibiricus L. syn. *Leonurus artemisia* auct. Non Lour. **English:** Honeyweed	Lamiaceae	Dondo-kolosh	Leaf, flower	Diarrhea
Lepisanthes tetraphylla (Vahl) Radlk. Syn. *Cupania canescens* **English**: Torchwood, four-leaved soapnut	Sapindaceae	Sapindaceae (Mro)	Root	Diarrhea. The barks of *Mangifera indica* L. (Anacardiaceae) and *Ziziphus mauritiana* Lam. (Rhamnaceae), which are yet to bear fruits, are collected and combined with roots of *Lepisanthes tetraphylla* (Vahl) Radlk. (Sapindaceae) and gall bladder of *Varanus indicus* (monitor lizard) and thoroughly mixed by rubbing with a stone. A portion of the mixture is taken thrice daily till cure
Leucas aspera (Willd.) Link, syn. *Leucas plukenetii* (Roth) Spreng., *Phlomis aspera* Willd. (basionym), *Phlomis plukenetii* Roth. **English:**Common leucus	Lamiaceae alt. Labiatae	Dondo kolosh	Stem	Diarrhea, blood purifier, loss of appetite, indigestion. Stems of *Leucas aspera* are mixed with leaves of *Azadirachta indica* and leaves and fruits of *Coccinia cordifolia* and taken

Table 23.1 (continued)

Botanical name	Family	Local name	Parts use	Disease and dosage
Lippia javanica (Burm.f.) Spreng **English:** Fever tea	Verbenaceae	Jongli chitki (Bede)	Leaf	Diarrhea and flatulency in children. Macerated leaves of *Lippia javanica* are applied to middle of head twice daily for 2 hours each time for 7 days. After 2 hours of application, the head is thoroughly washed
Litchi chinensis Sonn., syn. *Nephelium litchi* Cambess. **English:** Lychee	Sapindaceae	Lichu	Fruit, seed	Diarrhea
Litsea chinensis Lam. syn. *Litsea geminata* Blume, *Litsea glabraria* A.L. Juss., *Litsea glutinosa* (Lour.) C.D.Robins., *Litsea littoralis* (L.) Vill.,*Litsea tetranthera* (Willd.) Pers. **English:** Common tallow laurifolia	Lauraceae	Khara jora (Kuch)	Bark, leaf	Diarrhea (stomach pain, frequent urge for defecation). Leaves are soaked in water for 60–90 minutes followed by crushing of the leaves in water. The water is taken orally
Litsea sebifera Pers., syn. *Tetranthera laurifolia* Roxb. **English:** Soft bollygum	Lauraceae	Chapat pata	Leaf	Diarrhea
Ludwigia adscendens (L.) H. Hara syn. *Jussiaea adscendens* L., *Jussiaea fluviatilis* Bl., *Jussiaea repens* (non Forst.) L. **English:** Creeping water primrose	Onagraceae	Kejer pata	Whole plant	Diarrhea
Ludwigia hyssopifolia (G. Don) Exell apud A.R. Fernandessyn. *Jussiaea hyssopifolia* G. Don (basionym) **English:** Seedbox, primrose willow	Onagraceae	Rakhal-fota	Leaf, root, flower	Diarrhea
Luffa cylindrica M. Roem syn. *Luffaaegyptiaca* Mill. **English:** Sponged luffa	Cucurbitaceae	Dhundol	Leaf, bark, seed	Diarrhea
Lygodium flexuosum (L.) Sw., syn. *Ophioglossum flexuosum* L. (basionym) **English:** Maidenhair creeper	Lygodiaceae alt. Schizaeaceae	Bhaluk jan (Mandai).	Root	Diarrhea. One teaspoonful of paste prepared from macerated roots of *Lygodium flexuosum* (L.) Sw. (Lygodiaceae) and a little water is taken once daily

(continued)

Table 23.1 (continued)

Botanical name	Family	Local name	Parts use	Disease and dosage
Mangifera indica L., syn. *Mangifera domestica* Gaertn., *Mangifera sativa* Roem. and Schult. **English:** Mango	Anacardiaceae	Aam	Bark	Diarrhea in cattle. Barks of *Psidium guajava*, *Mangifera indica*, *Lannea coromandelica*, *Syzygium cumini*, *Diospyros peregrina*, and *Ficus religiosa* are mixed together and boiled in 10 kg water till the amount has been reduced to around 2 kg. ½ chatak (local measure, approximates 30 g) is fed to large-sized cattle (cow/ buffalo) thrice daily. A little less than ½ chatak is fed to medium-sized cattle thrice daily. 2–3 spoonfuls of the decoction are fed to small-sized cows and buffaloes or goats or calves thrice daily
Marsilea quadrifolia L. syn. *Marsilea quadrifoliata* **English:** Four-leaf clover	Oxalidaceae	Amrul	Whole plant	Diarrhea
Melastoma malabathricum L., syn. **English:** Indian rhododendron, Malabar melastome	Melastomataceae	Ustalog (Chak[a]) Tai-tong (Tripura[a])	Leaf, root Root	Diarrhea Diarrhea
Mentha piperita **English:** Peppermint	Labiatae/ Lamiaceae	Pudina (Khasia)	Oil from whole plant	Diarrhea
Mimosa pudica L., syn. *Mimosa hispidula* Kunth **English:** Shame plant	Fabaceae	Laal lojjaboti (Bongshi[a]).	Root	Diarrhea in children. Roots are tied to the hand or leg on a Tuesday or Saturday
Mimusops elengi L., syn. *Mimusops parviflora* R. Br. **English:** Spanish cherry, bullet wood	Sapotaceae	Bokul	Leaf, flower, seed	Diarrhea
Mirabilis jalapa L., syn. *Mirabilis jalapa* ssp. *Lindheimeri* Standl., *Mirabilis lindheimeri* (Standl.) Shinners **English:** Common four-o-clock, marvel of Peru	Nyctaginaceae	Shondha-maloti	Leaf, root, flower	Diarrhea
Momordica charantia L., syn. *Momordica indica* L., *Momordica muricata* Willd., *Momordica ceylanicum* Mill. **English:** Balsam pear, bitter cucumber, bitter gourd, bitter melon, carilla plant	Cucurbitaceae	Korola	Fruit	Two teaspoonfuls of juice obtained from macerated leaves is taken orally for 7 days

Table 23.1 (continued)

Botanical name	Family	Local name	Parts use	Disease and dosage
Morinda citrifolia L. syn. *Morinda angustifolia* Roth, *Morinda aspera* Wight and Arn., *Morinda bracteata* Roxb., *Morinda chachuca* Buch.-Ham., *Morinda chrysorhiza* (Thon.) DC., *Morinda citrifolia* var. *bracteata* (Roxb.) Hook.f., *Morinda citrifolia* var. *bracteata* (Roxb.) Kurz, *Morinda citrifolia* var. *elliptica* Hook.f., *Morinda citrifolia* forma *potteri* (O.Deg.) H.St.John, *Morinda citrifolia* var. *Potteri* O.Deg., *Morinda coreia* var. *Stenophylla* (Spreng.) Chandrab., *Morinda elliptica* (Hook.f.) Ridl., *Morinda ligulata* Blanco, *Morinda littoralis* Blanco, *Morinda macrophylla* Desf., *Morinda mudia* Buch.-Ham., *Morinda multiflora* Roxb., *Morinda nodosa* Buch.-Ham., *Morinda quadrangularis* G.Don, *Morinda stenophylla* Spreng., *Morinda teysmanniana* Miq., *Morinda tinctoria* Noronha, *Morinda tinctoria* var. *Aspera* (Wight and Arn.) Hook.f., *Morinda tinctoria* var. *Multiflora* (Roxb.) Hook.f., *Morinda tomentosa* B.Heyne ex Roth, *Morinda zollingeriana* Miq., *Platanocephalus orientalis* Crantz, *Psychotria chrysorhiza* Thonn., *Samama citrifolia* (L.) Kuntze, *Sarcocephalus leichhardtii* F.Muell. **English:** Awl tree, beach mulberry, canary wood (Australia), cheese fruit, great morinda, Indian mulberry, Indian-mulberry, large-leaved morinda, noni, noni (Hawaii), noni fruit, noni plant, Nonu (Samoa), pain killer tree (Caribbean), rotten cheesefruit, rotten cheesefruit (Aust)	Rubiaceae	Boro-chad	Leaf, fruit	Diarrhea

(continued)

Table 23.1 (continued)

Botanical name	Family	Local name	Parts use	Disease and dosage
Moringa oleifera Lam., syn. *Guilandina moringa* L., *Hyperanthera arborea* J.F. Gmel., *Hyperanthera decandra* Willd., *Hyperanthera moringa* (L.) Vahl, *Moringa erecta* Salisb., *Moringa* (L.) small, *Moringa octogona* stokes, *Moringa parvifolia* Noronha, *Moringa polygona* DC., *Moringa pterygosperma* Gaertn., nom. Illeg., *Moringa zeylanica* Pers. **English:** Horseradish tree	Moringaceae	Sajna	Leaf, fruit	Diarrhea
Morus alba L., syn. *Morus atropurpurea* Roxb., *Morus indica* L., *Morus macrophylla* Moretti, *Morus morettiana* Jacq. Ex Burr., *Morus multicaulis* Perr., *Morus nervosa* Deless. Ex Spach. **English:** Black-fruited mulberry, mulberry tree, mulberry bush, mulberry, Russian mulberry, silkworm mulberry, silkworm tree, Chinese white mulberry, white-fruited mulberry, white mulberry	Moraceae	Tuth (Garo[a])	Fruit	Diarrhea. Leaves of *Catharanthus roseus*; stems of *Eleusine coracana* and *Vitex negundo*; leaves of *Clerodendrum viscosum*, *Justicia adhatoda*, and *Myristica fragrans*; flowers of *Acacia catechu*; and fruits of *Morus alba* are macerated together and made into pills. The pills are taken daily till cure
Murraya exotica L., syn. *Murraya paniculata* (L.) Jack, *Chalcas exotica* (L.) Millsp., *Chalcas paniculata* auct. Non L. **English:** Chinese box	Rutaceae	Bashuri (Bede[a])	Leaf	Diarrhea (presence of slight mucus but no blood in stool). Crushed leaves of *Murraya paniculata*are taken twice daily in the morning and evening for 7–14 days depending on the severity of diarrhea
Murraya koenigii (L.) Spreng syn. *Bergera koenigii* L., *Chalcas koenigii* (L.) Kurz **English:** Curry leaf tree	Rutaceae	Keri pata	Leaf, stem	Diarrhea
Musa sapientum L., syn. **English:** Banana	Musaceae	Acchi-mio-bong (Rakhain[a])	Fruit (ripe)	Diarrhea, stomach disorders (ripe fruit)

Table 23.1 (continued)

Botanical name	Family	Local name	Parts use	Disease and dosage
Myristica fragrans Houtt., syn. *Myristica officinalis* L. f. **English:** Nutmeg	Myristicaceae	Jaifol, Joyotri (Bede[a]). Dai fol, Jai fol (kernel of fruit known in English as nutmeg), Jayatri (a thin leathery tissue between the stone and the pulp known in English as mace) (Garo[a])	Seed kernel, aril (seed coat) Leaf, seed kernel	Sutika (symptoms: diarrhea, indigestion, wasting of body). Roots of *Barringtonia racemosa* (L.) Roxb. (Lecythidaceae) are mixed with seeds (seed kernel) of *Myristica fragrans* Houtt. (Myristicaceae), *Phyllanthus emblica*, *Terminalia belerica*, and *Terminalia chebula*, macerated and mixed with ½ kg water and a little more than a handful of molasses prepared from date palm [*Phoenix sylvestris* L. (Arecaceae)] sap and boiled for 30 minutes. The decoction is taken twice daily for 7 days Diarrhea, cholera. Leaves of *Catharanthus roseus*; stems of *Eleusine coracana* and *Vitex negundo*; leaves of *Clerodendrum viscosum*, *Justicia adhatoda*, and *Myristica fragrans*; flowers of *Acacia catechu*; and fruits of *Morus alba* are macerated together and made into pills. The pills are taken daily till cure

(continued)

Table 23.1 (continued)

Botanical name	Family	Local name	Parts use	Disease and dosage
Nymphaea nouchali Burm.f., syn. *Castalia acutiloba* (DC.) Hand.-Mazz., *Castalia stellaris* Salisb., *Castalia stellata* (Willd.) Blume, *Leuconymphaea stellata* (Willd.) Kuntze, *Nymphaea acutiloba* DC., *Nymphaea cahlara* Donn, nom. Inval., *Nymphaea cyanea* Roxb., *Nymphaea edgeworthii* Lehm., *Nymphaea henkeliana* Rehnelt, *Nymphaea hookeriana* Lehm., *Nymphaea malabarica* Poir., *Nymphaea membranacea* Wall. Ex Casp., nom. Inval., *Nymphaea minima* F. M. Bailey, *Nymphaea punctata* Edgew., *Nymphaea rhodantha* Lehm., *Nymphaea stellata* Willd., *Nymphaea stellata* var. *albiflora* F. Henkel et al., *Nymphaea stellata* var. *cyanea* (Roxb.) Hook. f. and Thomson, *Nymphaea stellata* var. *parviflora* Hook. f. and Thomson, *Nymphaea stellata* var. *versicolor* (Sims) Hook. f. and Thomson, *Nymphaea tetragona* var. *acutiloba* (DC.) F. Henkel et al., *Nymphaea versicolor* Sims, *Nymphaea voalefoka* Lat.-Marl. Ex W. Watson, nom. Nud **English:** Blue lotus	Nymphaeaceae	Aphlak (Garo[a])	Whole plant	Diarrhea
Ocimum basilicum L., syn. *Ocimum americanum* Jacq., *Ocimum barrelieri* Roth, *Ocimum basilicum* L. var.*glabratum* Benth., *Ocimum basilicum* L. var. *majus* Benth., *Ocimum bullatum* Lam., *Ocimum thyrsiflorum* L., *Plectranthus barrelieri* (Roth) Spreng. **English:** Basil, common basil, garden basil, Roman basil, sweet basil	Labiatae/ Lamiaceae	Babui tulshi	Seed	Diarrhea
Ocimum gratissimum L., syn. *Geniosporumdiscolor* Baker, *Ocimum dalabaense* A. Chev., *Ocimum gratissimum* L. subsp. *Iringense* A.J. Paton, *Ocimum superbum* Busc. and Muschl., *Ocimum trichodon* Baker ex Gürke **English:** African basil, Caribbean basil, clove basil, East Indian basil, pale-yellow-flowered basil, Russian basil, shrubby basil, Southeast Asian tree basil, tree basil	Lamiaceae/ Labiatae	Boro tulshi	Leaf	Diarrhea

Table 23.1 (continued)

Botanical name	Family	Local name	Parts use	Disease and dosage
Ocimum sanctum L. **English:** Basil	Lamiaceae/ Labiatae	.Krishno-tulshi Shada-tulshi	Leaf Whole plant	Diarrhea Diarrhea
Ocimum tenuiflorum L., syn. *Geniosporum tenuiflorum* (L.) Merr. *Ocimum album* Blanco, *Ocimum brachiatum* Hassk, non Blume, *Ocimum flexuosum* Blanco, *Ocimum frutescens* sensu Burm. F., non L., *Ocimum gratissimum* sensu Lour., non L., *Ocimum hirsutum* Benth., *Ocimum inodorum* Burm. F., *Ocimum monachorum* L., *Ocimum sanctum* L., *Ocimum sanctum* L. var. *aculat* (Benth.) Hook. f., *Ocimum tomentosum* Lam., *Ocimum villosum* Roxb., *Ocimum virgatum* Blanco, non Thunb., *Plectranthus monachorum* (L.) Spreng., *Plectranthus striatus* sensu Muschler and Hosseus, non Benth. **English:** Holy basil, monks' basil, red basil, rough basil, sacred basil, sacred Thai basil, Siamese basil, Thai basil	Lamiaceae/ Labiatae	Krishna-tulshi (Chakma[a])	Whole plant	Diarrhea
Opuntia dillenii (Ker-Gawl.) Haw., syn. *Opuntia stricta* var. *dillenii* (Ker-Gawl.) L. Benson, *Cactus dillenii* Ker-Gawl., *Opuntia atrocapensis* Small, *Opuntia nitens* Small, *Opuntia tunoidea* Gibbes, *Opuntia zebrina* Small **English:** Erect prickly pear	Cactaceae	Phoni-raaz	Whole plant	Diarrhea
Oroxylum indicum (L.) Vent., syn. *Bignonia indica* L., *Calosanthes indica* Blume **English:** Indian trumpet, tree of Damocles	Bignoniaceae	Aklong-singh, Hanghoal	Leaf, bark, fruit	Diarrhea
Oxalis lobata Sims syn. **English:** South American Oxalis	Oxalidaceae	Amrul	Whole plant	Diarrhea
Paederia foetida L., syn. *Paederia scandans* (Lour.) Merr. **English:** Skunk vine, stink vine	Rubiaceae	Gondho badail (Bede[a]).	Leaf	Diarrhea and flatulency in children. Leaves of *Paederia foetida* are crushed with rice and pills or pithas (Bangladesh dish made from flour and oil) made from the mixture and are taken twice daily in the morning and evening for 7 days

(continued)

Table 23.1 (continued)

Botanical name	Family	Local name	Parts use	Disease and dosage
Passiflora coccinea Aubl. Syn. *Passiflora miniata* Vanderplank **English:** Red passion flower, red granadilla, scarlet passion flower	Passifloraceae	Jhumko lota	Whole plant	Diarrhea
Pedilanthus tithymaloides (L.) Poit., syn. *Euphorbia tithymaloides* L. **English:** Devil's backbone, redbird flower	Euphorbiaceae	Roilabang (Rakhain[a])	Leaf	Diarrhea
Peperomia pellucida (L.) Kunth., syn. *Piper pellucidum* L.. *Peperomia exigua* (Blume) Miquel, *Peperomia translucens* Trelease **English:** Man to man, shiny bush, pepper elder	Piperaceae	Shamol-phang (Garo)	Whole plant	Diarrhea
Pergularia extensa (Jacq.) N.E. Br., syn. Pergularia *daemia* (Forssk.) Chiov., *Cynanchum cordifolium* Retz., *Ascelpias daemia* Forssk., *Cynanchum echinatum* Thunb., *Cynanchum extensum* Jacq., *Daemia cordifolia* (Retz.) Schum., *Daemia extensa* (Jacq.) R. Br., *Gomphrocarpus volubilis* Moon **English:** Trellis vine	Asclepiadaceae	Azoshringi	Leaf	Diarrhea
Persicaria laphatifolia (L.) Gray syn. *Polygonum lapathifolium*L. **English:** Pale persicaria, willow weed, pale smartweed, green smartweed	Polygonaceae	Aagrha	Whole plant	Diarrhea
Phoenix sylvestris L. syn. *Elate sylvestris* L. **English:** Silver date palm	Arecaceae	Khejur (Bede[a]).	Molasses made from juice	Sutika (symptoms: diarrhea, indigestion, wasting of body). Roots of *Barringtonia racemosa* (L.) Roxb. (Lecythidaceae) are mixed with fruits of *Myristica fragrans* Houtt. (Myristicaceae), *Phyllanthus emblica*, *Terminalia belerica*, and *Terminalia chebula*, macerated and mixed with ½ kg water and a little more than a handful of molasses prepared from date palm [*Phoenix sylvestris* L. (Arecaceae)] sap and boiled for 30 minutes. The decoction is taken twice daily for 7 days

Table 23.1 (continued)

Botanical name	Family	Local name	Parts use	Disease and dosage
Phyla nodiflora (L.) Greene syn. *Lippia canescens* Kunth, *Lippia acula* (Small) Tidestrom, *Lippia reptans* Kunth, *Phyla acula* Small, *Lippia nodiflora* (L.) Michx. English: Turkey tangle fogfruit, creeping lip plant	Verbenaceae	Bokon	Leaf	Cattle diarrhea. Leaves are fed to cattle
Phyllanthus amarus Schumach. and Thonn. **English:** Stone breaker plant	Euphorbiaceae	Voiyom gach	Leaf	Boiled leaves are taken for loss of diarrhea
Phyllanthus niruri L., syn. *Diasperus niruri* (L.) Kuntze, *Phyllanthus fraternus*Webster, *Phyllanthus filiformis* Pavon ex Baillon **English:** Small gooseberry	Euphorbiaceae	Bhui-amloki	Whole plant, root	Diarrhea, dysentery (whole plant)
Phyllanthus reticulatus Poir., syn. *Kirganelia reticulata* (Poiret) Baillon, *Phyllanthus multiflorus* Willd. **English:** Roast potato plant	Euphorbiaceae	Chitki pata	Whole plant	Diarrhea
Piper betle L., syn. *Chavica betle* Miq. *Chavica auriculata* Miq. **English:** Betel, betel pepper, betelvine, betel vine	Piperaceae	Paan (Patro[a])	Leaf	Diarrhea. Leaves of pira rong (unidentified) are held upwards so that the leaf stalk is slightly broken. The sap that oozes out is taken with betel leaves (leaf of *Piper betle* L., local name: paan, Piperaceae)
Piper cubeba L.f. syn. *Cubeba officinalis* Raf. **English:** Cubeb pepper, Java pepper, Javanese peppercorn, West African black pepper	Piperaceae	Moha-potting (Chakma[a])	Whole plant	Diarrhea
Piper longum L., syn. *Chavica roxburghii*Miq.,*Piper jaborandii* Vell. **English:** Indian long pepper, jaborandi pepper, long pepper	Piperaceae	Pipul	Whole plant	Diarrhea, 8 chatak plants are crushed thoroughly, mixed with salt or gondhok lobon (sulfur containing salt), and fed in the mornings and evenings
Piper nigrum L., syn. *Piper aromaticum* Lam. **English:** Pepper, black pepper, white pepper	Piperaceae	Gul morich	Seed	Diarrhea in cattle. Leaves of *Areca catechu* and *Tamarindus indica* are boiled in water and then fed to cattle with rhizomes of *Zingiber officinale* and seeds of *Piper nigrum* 2–3 times daily
Piper sarmentosum Roxb. **English**: Lolo pepper	Piperaceae	Buno paan	Leaf	Diarrhea. One tablespoonful of juice obtained from macerated leaves is taken in the morning before meal

(continued)

Table 23.1 (continued)

Botanical name	Family	Local name	Parts use	Disease and dosage
Plumeria acutifolia Poir.,syn. *Plumeria rubra* L., *Plumeria tricolor* Ruiz and Pav. **English:** Frangipani, temple tree	Apocynaceae	Kath-gulap, Lal guloncho	Leaf, root, bark, flower	Diarrhea
Psidium guajava L., syn. *Guajava pyrifera* (L.) Kuntze, *Guajava pyriformis* Gaertn., *Psidium aromaticum* L., *Psidium guayava* Raddi, *Psidium pomiferum* L., *Psidium pyriferum* L., *Psidium sapidissimum* Jacq. English: Guava	Myrtaceae	Taam-rash (Santal[a]) Piyara gach	Leaf, fruit Leaf	Diarrhea Diarrhea. Juice from crushed leaf is taken for menstrual problems or diarrhea. Leaves of the plant are burnt with *Syzygium cumini* leaves and mixed with salt and teeth brushed with the mixture (45)
Pteridium aquilinum (L.) Kuhn syn. *Pteris aqulina* L. **English:** Western bracken fern, brake, bracken, Northern bracken fern, brackenfern	Polypodiaceae	Dheki shak	Root	Diarrhea
Punica granatum L., syn. *Granatum punicum* St.-Lag., *Punica florida* Salisb., *Punica multiflora*hort. Ex Siebold and Voss, *Punica nana* L., *Punica spinosa* Lam. **English:** Pomegranate	Lythraceae	Dalim-phang (Garo[a])	Root, fruit	Diarrhea
Quisqualis indica L., syn. *Combretum indicum* (L.) DeFilipps **English:** Rangoon creeper	Combretaceae	Madhobi lota	Leaf, root, flower	Diarrhea
Rauwolfia serpentina (L.) Benth.ex Kurz syn. *Ophioxylon serpentinum* L., *Rauvolfia serpentine* (Gaertn.) Baill. **English:** Ajmalicine (drug), Ajmaline (drug), Java devil pepper, rauwolfia, serpentine wood, snakeroot, snakewood	Apocynaceae	Shorpogondha	Root, fruit	Diarrhea
Ricinus communis L., syn. *Ricinus africanus* Willd., *Ricinus communis* L. var. *viridis* (Willd.) Müll. Arg., *Ricinus inermis* Jacq., *Ricinus lividus* Jacq., *Ricinus macrocarpus* G. Popova, *Ricinus microcarpus* G. Popova, *Ricinus persicus* G. Popova, *Ricinus speciosus* Burm., *Ricinus viridis* Willd., *Ricinus vulgaris* Mill., *Ricinus zanzibaricus* G. Popova	Euphorbiaceae	Valla	Seed	Diarrhea

Table 23.1 (continued)

Botanical name	Family	Local name	Parts use	Disease and dosage
Scoparia dulcis L., syn. *Scoparia grandiflora* Nash., *Scoparia aculat* Forssk., *Capraria dulcis* Kuntze, *Gratiola micrantha* Nutt. **English:** Licorice weed, sweetbroom	Scrophulariaceae	Bon-dhonnyo (Tripura[a]) Bakhor gach, Chini pata (Khasia[a]) Saam-kuchuk (Garo[a]) Oshto modh (Bongshi[a]).	Whole plant, root Whole plant, leaf Whole plant Whole plant	Diarrhea Diarrhea Diarrhea in children Diarrhea
Semecarpus anacardium L.f., syn. *Anacardium latifolium* Lam., *Anacardium officinarum* Gaertn., *Anacardium orientale* auct. Ex Steud., *Semecarpus latifolia* Pers. **English:** Indian marking nut tree, marany nut, marking nut tree, marsh nut, oriental cashew nut, phobi nut tree, varnish tree	Anacardiaceae	Bhela	Leaf, root	Diarrhea (cattle)
Solanum melongena L., syn. *Solanum cumingii* Dunal, *Solanum pressum* Dunal, *Solanum undatum* Poiret sensu Ochse **English**: Aubergine (UK), Eggplant (USA), brinjal (India), large-fruit eggplant, melange (Caribbean Trinidad)	Solanaceae	Misinachol (Garo[a])	Leaf, root, fruit	Diarrhea
Solanum nigrum L., syn. *Solanum nigrum* L. Var. *Vulgare*L. **English:** Black nightshade, garden nightshade, small-fruited black nightshade, petty morel, hound's berry, wonderberry	Solanaceae	Kack-machie, Tit baegun	Fruit	Diarrhea
Solanum torvum Swartz syn. *Solanum ferrugineum* Jacq., *Solanum largiflorum* C. White, *Solanum ficifolium* Ortega **English:** Green-fruited pea eggplant, pea aubergine, Thai pea eggplant, Thai cultivated nightshade, Devil's fig, water nightshade, gully bean (Jamaica), susumber (Jamaica), turkeyberry (USA), plate brush	Solanaceae	Jhuri-tabra, Guti-baegun	Whole plant	Diarrhea
Sonneratia apetala Buch.-Ham., syn. *Blatti apetala* O.K., *Kambala apetala* Rafin. **English:** Mangrove apple	Euphorbiaceae	Keowra	Leaf, bark juice, fruit	Diarrhea
Stephania japonica (Thunb.) Miers syn. **English:** Snake vine	Menispermaceae	Muich-chali lota (Tripura[a])	Leaf	Diarrhea in children

(continued)

Table 23.1 (continued)

Botanical name	Family	Local name	Parts use	Disease and dosage
Streblus asper Lour., syn. **English:** Siamese rough bush, khoi, toothbrush tree	Moraceae	Uli-phang (Chak[a]) Sarwa (Tripura[a]) Shora gach (Mandai[a]).	Leaf, stem Bark Gum	Diarrhea Diarrhea Diarrhea. Paste or pill prepared from a mixture of gum of *Streblus asper* Lour. (Moraceae) and root of *Hemidesmus indicus* R. Br. (Apocynaceae) is taken for 2–3 days
Synedrella nodiflora (L.) Gaertn. Syn. *Ucacou nodiplorum* (L.) Hitchcock, *Verbesina dichotoma* Sieber ex Steud **English:** Cinderella weed, pig's grass	Asteraceae	Megh pata (Patro[a]).	Leaf	Diarrhea in children. ½ spoonful of juice obtained from macerated leaf is taken twice daily in the morning and evening for 2 days
Syzygium cumini (L.) Skeels syn. *Consolida major* Gilib., *Eugenia cumini* (L.) Druce, *Eugenia jambolana* Lam., *Eugenia jouat* Perr., *Myrtus cumini* L., *Calyptranthes jambolana* Willd., *Syzygium jambolanum* DC., *Syzygium jambolana* DC. **English:** Black plum, damson plum, duhat plum, jambolan, jambolan plum, Java plum, Malabar plum, Portuguese plum	Myrtaceae	Cha-briishi (Rakhain[a]) Jaam (Bede[a])	Leaf, seed Bark, leaf, seed	Diarrhea Diarrhea in children accompanied with loss of appetite and lack of movement. Juice obtained from macerated leaves of *Syzygium cumini* is taken once daily for 7 days
Syzygium jambos (L.) Alston syn. *Eugenia jambos* L., *Jambosa jambos* Millsp., *Jambosa vulgaris* DC., *Caryophyllus jambos* Stokes **English:** Malabar plum, plum rose, rose apple, water apple	Myrtaceae	Pang-mishing (Murong[a])	Leaf, bark, fruit	Diarrhea
Syzygium malaccense (L.) Merr. and L. M. Perry syn. *Caryophyllus malaccensis* (L.) Stokes *Eugenia malaccensis* L. English: Malacca apple, Malay apple, Malay rose apple, mountain apple, otaheite cashew, otaheite apple, rose apple, water apple	Myrtaceae	Jamrul	Fruit	Diarrhea
Tamarindus indica L., syn. *Tamarindus occidentalis* Gaertn., *Tamarindus officinalis* Hook., *Tamarindus umbrosa* Salisb. **English:** Indian date, sweet tamarind, tamarind	Fabaceae	Tiintile-phang (Garo-3[a]) Tetul gach	Stem, fruit, seed Leaf	Pig/cow diarrhea Diarrhea. Three leaves are mixed with three mustard seeds and fed in the morning for 3 days. Alternately, leaves are boiled in water and the water fed to cattle

Table 23.1 (continued)

Botanical name	Family	Local name	Parts use	Disease and dosage
Tectaria heterosora (Baker) Ching	Dryopteridaceae	Baidya nath86 (Chakma[a])	Root	Diarrhea in infant. One spoonful of water is fed in which roots have been boiled
Terminalia arjuna (Roxb. ex DC.) Wight and Arn., syn. *Pentaptera angustifolia* Roxb., *Pentaptera arjuna* Roxb. ex DC., *Pentaptera glabra* Roxb., *Terminalia berryi* Wight and Arn., *Terminalia glabra* Wight and Arn., *Terminalia ovalifolia* Rottl. Ex C.B. Clarke **English:** Arjuna, white marudah, white murdh	Combretaceae	Arjun-phang (Garo[a])	Bark	Diarrhea
Terminalia belerica (Gaertn.) Roxb., syn. *Myrobalanus bellirica* Gaertn., *Myrobalanus laurinioides* Kuntze, *Terminalia angustifolia* Blanco, non Jacq., *Terminalia aculate* Edgew., *Terminalia edulis* Blanco, *Terminalia moluccana* Roxb., *Terminalia punctata* Roth **English**: Bastard myrobalan, behere, belleric myrobalan	Combretaceae	Bohera (Bede[a])	Fruit	Sutika (symptoms: diarrhea, indigestion, wasting of body). Roots of *Barringtonia racemosa* (L.) Roxb. (Lecythidaceae) are mixed with fruits of *Myristica fragrans* Houtt. (Myristicaceae), *Phyllanthus emblica*, *Terminalia belerica*, and *Terminalia chebula*, macerated and mixed with ½ kg water and a little more than a handful of molasses prepared from date palm [*Phoenix sylvestris* L. (Arecaceae)] sap, and boiled for 30 minutes. The decoction is taken twice daily for 7 days Diarrhea in cattle. Dried fruits of *Phyllanthus emblica*, *Terminalia belerica*, and *Terminalia chebula* are mixed, boiled in water with molasses, and fed to cattle

(continued)

Table 23.1 (continued)

Botanical name	Family	Local name	Parts use	Disease and dosage
Terminalia chebula Retz. syn. *Myrobalanus chebula* Gaertn., *Myrobalanus gangetica* Kostel., *Terminalia acuta* Walp., *Terminaliagangetica* Roxb., *Terminalia parviflora* Thwaites, *Terminalia reticulata* Roth, *Terminalia zeylanica* Heurck and Muell. Arg. **English:** Black myrobalan, chebulic myrobalan, gali nut, Indian gall nut, ink nut, yellow myrobalan	Combretaceae	Horitoki (Bede[a])	Fruit	Sutika (symptoms: diarrhea, indigestion, wasting of body). Roots of *Barringtonia racemosa* are mixed with fruits of *Myristica fragrans*, *Phyllanthus emblica*, *Terminalia belerica*, and *Terminalia chebula*, macerated and mixed with ½ kg water and a little more than a handful of molasses prepared from date palm [*Phoenix sylvestris* L. (Arecaceae)] sap, and boiled for 30 minutes. The decoction is taken twice daily for 7 days
Tinospora crispa (L.) Hook.f. and Thoms., syn. *Menispermum crispum* L. (basionym), *Tinospora rumphii* Boerl. **English:** Chinese Tinospora	Menispermaceae	Aam guruz	Leaf, stem	Diarrhea in cattle. For cows, 250 g leaf and stem is fed with 1 liter water; for goats, 70 g leaf and stem is fed with 250 ml water. This is continued every day till the diarrhea is healed
Trema orientalis (L.) Blume syn. *Celtis orientalis* L., Sponia orientalis (L.) Decne, *Trema hoseiate* (Hochst.) Blume, *Trema guineensis* (Schum. Et Thonn.) Ficalho, *Trema guineensis* (Schum. Et Thonn.) Ficalho var. *hochstetteri* (Planchon) Engl. **English:** Charcoal tree, Indian charcoal tree, Indian nettle tree, pigeon wood	Ulmaceae	Gulan pata	Leaf, stem, root	Diarrhea. Boiled leaves are orally administered for diarrhea
Urena lobata L., syn. *Urena trilobata* Vell., *Urena sinuata* L. **English:** Aramina, Caesar weed, burr mallow	Malvaceae	Shanta, Lilonchi (Tripura[a]) Fou-fi-bang (Rakhain[a])	Root Root	Diarrhea Diarrhea
Vernonia cinerea (L.) Less., syn. *Blumea chinensis* (L.) DC., *Conyza chinensis* L., *Conyza cinerea* L., *Cyanthillium cinereum* (L.) H. Rob., *Serratula cinerea* (L.) Roxb. *Vernonia arguta* Baker, *Vernonia betonicaefolia* Baker, *Vernonia exilis* Miq., *Vernonia vialis* DC. **English:** Ash-colored fleabane, ash-colored ironweed, little ironweed, purple fleabane, purple-flowered fleabane	Asteraceae alt. Compositae	Shial mutra, Lal mutra	Leaf, whole plant	Juice obtained from squeezed leaves is taken orally after meal thrice daily for diarrhea

Table 23.1 (continued)

Botanical name	Family	Local name	Parts use	Disease and dosage
Vitex negundo L. syn. *Vitex arborea* Desf., *Vitex bicolor* Willd., *Vitex paniculata* Lam. **English:** Chinese chastetree, five-leaf chastetree	Verbenaceae alt. Lamiaceae	Nimondha Nishinda (Garo[a]).	Leaf Stem	Diarrhea Diarrhea, cholera. Leaves of *Catharanthus roseus*; stems of *Eleusine coracana* and *Vitex negundo*; leaves of *Clerodendrum viscosum*, *Justicia adhatoda*, and *Myristica fragrans*; flowers of *Acacia catechu*; and fruits of *Moruș alba* are macerated together and made into pills. The pills are taken daily till cure
Xanthium indicum J. Koenig ex Roxb., syn. *Xanthium strumarium* L., *Xanthium occidentale* Bertol., *Xanthium pungens* Wallr., *Xanthium vulgare* Hill **English:** Cocklebur, large cocklebur	Asteraceae	Hagra	Root	Diarrhea. Macerated roots are taken with water twice daily for 7 days
Zingiber officinale Roscoe syn. *Amomum zingiber* L., *Zingiber* (L.) Karst. **English:** Garden ginger	Zingiberaceae	Ada (Khasia[a])	Rhizome	Diarrhea
Zizyphusjujube Mill. var. spinosa (Bunge) Hu ex F. H. Chen, syn. *Ziziphus spinosa* (Bunge) Hu ex F. H. Chen, nom. Illeg., *Ziziphus vulgaris* Lam., nom. Illeg. Var. spinosa Bunge **English:** Spiny jujube, sour-fruited jujube	Rhamnaceae	Khankare (Garo[a])	Leaf, root, bark, fruit, seed	Diarrhea, pig/cow diarrhea
Ziziphus mauritiana Lam., syn. *Rhamnus jujube* L., *Ziziphus jujube* (L.) Gaertn.,nom. Illeg. **English:** Chinese date	Rhamnaceae	Kul (Chakma[a]).	Leaf, bark	Diarrhea. Macerated leaves or barks are mixed with a small amount of water and applied to head during fever. Juice obtained from macerated leaves is taken twice daily for flatulence or diarrhea
Ziziphus oenoplia (L.) Mill., syn. *Rhamnusoenoplia* L. **English:** Jackal jujube, small-fruited jujube, wild jujube	Rhamnaceae	Deshi boroi (Kole[a])	Root	Diarrhea. Juice obtained from macerated roots of *Ziziphus oenoplia* (L.) Mill. (Rhamnaceae) is administered twice daily

Note: Names of tribes are indicated

[a]A tribal name indicates that a given plant was used by that particular tribe

bismuth subsalicylate (Kaopectate or Pepto-Bismol). However, these medications are not indicated for diarrhea caused by microorganisms. Moreover, loperamide may cause abdominal pain, constipation, nausea, dizziness, or vomiting. Bismuth subsalicylate can cause constipation, blackened stools or tongue, and tinnitus. For a country like Bangladesh, lacking qualified doctors among the rural population, who are mostly illiterate, even choosing an OTC drug can be a problem. Moreover, the question remains as to whether for a diarrheal patient, OTC drugs or antibiotics are the proper remedy. From that viewpoint, even a crude herbal remedy may prove useful provided scientific experiments have validated the use.

23.2 Drug Discovery Potential

Table 23.1 presents a list of plants used in Bangladesh for the treatment of diarrhea. The list is not inclusive of all plants. It is very certain that more surveys among the folk and tribal medicinal practitioners of Bangladesh will lead to expansion of the list through inclusion of newer plant species. A number of the plants have been shown in scientific studies to possess anti-diarrheal properties. Space limitations will preclude a full discussion; however some of the plants will be discussed.

Antibacterial effects of aqueous and organic extracts of bark of *Terminalia arjuna* have been found against a number of diarrhea-causing bacteria like *Shigella*, *Salmonella*, *Escherichia coli*, *Bacillus*, and *Staphylococcus* species (Panda et al. 2011). *Acorus calamus* contains α- and β-asarone, which among other properties also have anti-diarrheal activities (Mukherjee et al. 2007). Thus these two compounds can be potential anti-diarrheal drugs of the future. Both leaf extract and fruits of *Aegle marmelos* have been found to be useful for stopping diarrhea (Rao and Lakshmi 2012; Sukumaran et al. 2009). Anti-diarrheal activity of aqueous extract of leaves of *Ageratum conyzoides* has been shown in Wistar rats (Emudainohwo et al. 2015)

The above few examples suggest that the anti-diarrheal plants of Bangladesh may prove to be useful not only as herbal remedies but also towards discovery of new drugs against diarrhea. To give just one example, one of the most used anti-diarrheal plants of Bangladesh, namely, *Holarrhena antidysenterica*, is known to contain the compounds conessine, holarrhenine, and kurchessine (Sinha et al. 2013). Molecular docking studies of these three compounds with capsid protein VP6 of Group A rotavirus gave docking energies (kcal/mol) of −10.3, −10.2, and −10.5, respectively. These values suggest that the compounds can bind tightly to the rotavirus capsid protein and so prevent further viral replication and thus may be effective compounds against rotavirus-induced diarrhea. The binding of holarrhenine to capsid protein VP6 of Group A rotavirus is shown in Fig. 23.1.

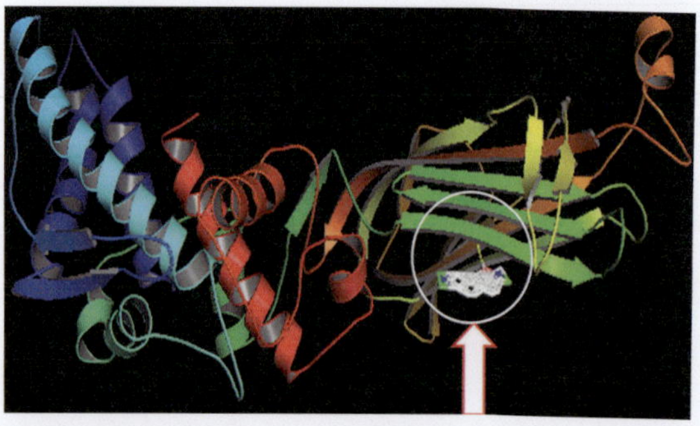

Fig. 23.1 Graphical Representation of Molecular Docking Study between Capsid Protein VP6 of Group A Rotavirus and Holarrhenine. White circle and arrow indicates Holarrhenine

23.3 Conclusion

In conclusion, there is an excellent possibility of discovering new anti-diarrheal drugs from medicinal plants of Bangladesh. Additionally, these plants or plant parts can serve as herbal remedies or crude drugs. Since the plants have been used for untold number of years (which can be thousands of years), the chances of any adverse effects from the plants are possibly minimal. As such, the plants can be a readily available and affordable means for phytotherapy, which can not only be lifesaving for the people but also save on medical costs. Herbal drugs are slowly entering the mainstream therapy with allopathic drugs under various terms like integrative medicine, functional foods, and nutraceuticals. Because of the multi-component nature of the herbal drugs, they have the potential to mitigate a number of factors, which may be associated with the main disease, and so can prove better than allopathy.

References

Brachman PS. Infectious diseases – past, present, and future. Int J Epidemiol. 2003;32:684–6.

Chandra H, Bishnoi P, Yadav A, Patni B, Mishra AP, Nautiyal AR. Antimicrobial resistance and the alternative resources with special emphasis on plant-based antimicrobials – A review. Plan Theory. 2017;6:16. https://doi.org/10.3390/plants6020016.

Das PR, Islam MT, Jahan R, Rahmatullah M. Ethnomedicinal plants used by the Nag clan of the Rai Ghatual tribe of Moulvibazar district, Bangladesh. Anc Sci Life. 2013a;32:217–21.

Das PR, Islam MT, Mostafa MN, Rahmatullah M. Ethnomedicinal plants of the Bauri tribal community of Moulvibazar District, Bangladesh. Anc Sci Life. 2013b;32:144–9.

Emudainohwo JOT, Erhirhie EO, Moke EG. Antidiarrheal activity of the aqueous leaf extract of *Ageratum conyzoides* in Wistar rats. J Appl Sci Environ Manag. 2015;19:169–75.

Ferdous F, Ahmed S, Farzana FD, Das J, Malek MA, Das SK, Salam MA, Faruque AS. Aetiologies of diarrhoea in adults from urban and rural treatment facilities in Bangladesh. Epidemiol Infect. 2015;143:1377–87.

Gilbert B, Ferreira JLP, Almeida MBS, Carvalho ES, Cascon V, Rocha LM. The official use of medicinal plants in public health. Ciência e Cultura. J Brazil Assoc. Adv Sci. 1997;49:339–44.

Hossan S, Hanif A, Jahan R, Rahmatullah M. Ethnomedicinal plants of the Bawm tribal community of Rowangchhari in Bandarban district of Bangladesh. J Altern Complement Med. 2014;20:581–9.

Kabir MH, Hasan N, Rahman MM, Rahman MA, Khan JA, Hoque NT, Bhuiyan MR, Mou SM, Jahan R, Rahmatullah M. A survey of medicinal plants used by the Deb barma clan of the Tripura tribe of Moulvibazar district, Bangladesh. J Ethnobiol Ethnomed. 2014;10:19. https://doi.org/10.1186/1746-4269-10-19.

Khan MA, Islam MK, Siraj MA, Saha S, Barman AK, Awang K, Rahman MM, Shilpi JA, Jahan R, Islam E, Rahmatullah M. Ethnomedicinal survey of various communities residing in Garo Hills of Durgapur, Bangladesh. J Ethnobiol Ethnomed. 2015;11:44. https://doi.org/10.1186/s13002-015-0033-3.

Malek I, Islam T, Hasan E, Akter S, Rana M, Das PR, Samarrai W, Rahmatullah M. Medicinal plants used by the Mandais--a little known tribe of Bangladesh. Afr J Tradit Complement Altern Med. 2012;9:536–41.

More B. Overview of medicine – Its importance and impact. DJ Int J Med Res. 2016;1:1–8.

Mukherjee PK, Kumar V, Mal M, Houghton PJ. *Acorus calamus*: Scientific validation of Ayurvedic tradition from natural resources. Pharm Biol. 2007;45:651–66.

Mukti M, Rahmatullah M. Treatment with aquatic plants by a Bagdi tribal healer of Rajbari District, Bangladesh. Anc Sci Life. 2013;33:22–6.

Panda SK, Dutta SK, Bastia AK. Antidiarrheal activity of *Terminalia arjuna* Roxb. from India. J Biol Active Prod. Nature. 2011;1:236–47.

Pearce-Duvet JMC. The origin of human pathogens – evaluating the role of agriculture and domestic animals in the evolution of human disease. Biol Rev. 2006;81:369–82.

Qazi MA, Molvi KI. Herbal medicine: A comprehensive review. Int J Pharm Res. 2016;8:1–5.

Rahmatullah M, Biswas KR. Traditional medicinal practices of a Sardar healer of the Sardar (Dhangor) community of Bangladesh. J Altern Complement Med. 2012;18:10–9.

Rahmatullah M, Ferdausi D, Mollik AH, Jahan R, Chowdhury MH. Haque WM. A survey of medicinal plants used by Kavirajes of Chalna area, Khulna district, Bangladesh. Afr J Tradit Complement Altern Med. 2009;7:91–7.

Rahmatullah M, Mollik AH, Rahman S, Hasan N, Agarwala B, Jahan R. A medicinal plant study of the Santal tribe in Rangpur district, Bangladesh. J Altern Complement Med. 2010a;16:419–25.

Rahmatullah M, Rahman MA, Hossan MS, Taufiq-Ur-Rahman M, Jahan R, Mollik MA. A pharmacological and phytochemical evaluation of medicinal plants used by the Harbang clan of the Tripura tribal community of Mirsharai area, Chittagong district, Bangladesh. J Altern Complement Med. 2010b;16:769–85.

Rahmatullah M, Jahan R, Azam FM, Hossan S, Mollik MA, Rahman T. Folk medicinal uses of Verbenaceae family plants in Bangladesh. Afr J Tradit Complement Altern Med. 2011a;8:53–65.

Rahmatullah M, Haque ME, Mondol MR, Mandal A, Azad MA, Seraj S, Jahan R. Medicinal plants of the Hodis: a disappearing tribe of Bangladesh. J Altern Complement Med. 2011b;17:1103–8.

Rahmatullah M, Hasan A, Parvin W, Moniruzzaman M, Khatun A, Khatun Z, Jahan FI, Jahan R. Medicinal plants and formulations used by the Soren clan of the Santal tribe in Rajshahi district, Bangladesh for treatment of various ailments. Afr J Tradit Complement Altern Med. 2012a;9:350–9.

Rahmatullah M, Khatun Z, Hasan A, Parvin W, Moniruzzaman M, Khatun A, Mahal MJ, Bhuiyan MS, Mou SM, Jahan R. Survey and scientific evaluation of medicinal plants used by the Pahan and Teli tribal communities of Natore district, Bangladesh. Afr J Tradit Complement Altern Med. 2012b;9:366–73.

Rahmatullah M, Azam MN, Khatun Z, Seraj S, Islam F, Rahman MA, Jahan S, Aziz MS. Medicinal plants used for treatment of diabetes by the Marakh sect of the Garo tribe living in Mymensingh district, Bangladesh. Afr J Tradit Complement Altern Med. 2012c;9:380–5.

Rahmatullah M, Ayman U, Akter F, Sarker M, Sifa R, Sarker B, Chyti HN, Jahan FI, Chowdhury MH, Chowdhury SA. Medicinal formulations of a Kanda tribal healer--a tribe on the verge of disappearance in Bangladesh. Afr J Tradit Complement Altern Med. 2012d;10:213–22.

Rahmatullah M, Khatun Z, Barua D, Alam MU, Jahan S, Jahan R. Medicinal plants used by traditional practitioners of the Kole and Rai tribes of Bangladesh. J Altern Complement Med. 2013a;19:483–91.

Rahmatullah M, Pk SR, Al-Imran M, Jahan R. The Khasia tribe of Sylhet District, Bangladesh, and their fast-disappearing knowledge of medicinal plants. J Altern Complement Med. 2013b;19:599–606.

Rahmatullah M, Khatun Z, Saha S, Tuly MA, Hossain A, Roy A, Jahan R. Medicinal plants and formulations of Tribal healers of the Chekla clan of the Patro tribe of Bangladesh. J Altern Complement Med. 2014a;20:3–11.

Rahmatullah M, Haque ME, Mondol MR, Hasan M, Aziz T, Jahan R, Seraj S. Medicinal formulations of the Kuch tribe of Bangladesh. J Altern Complement Med. 2014b;20:428–40.

Rao HJ, Lakshmi P. Evaluation of antidiarrheal activity of extract from leaves of *Aegle marmelos*. J Appl Pharm Sci. 2012;2(2):75–8.

Rates SMK. Plants as source of drugs. Toxicon. 2001;39:603–13.

Seraj S, Rahmatullah M, Monjur-E-Khudha M, Aporna SA, Khan MS, Jahan R. Amulets and other uncommon treatments prescribed by traditional medicinal practitioners of the Bede community residing in Porabari village of Dhaka district, Bangladesh. J Altern Complement Med. 2011;17:987–93.

Seraj S, Jahan FI, Chowdhury AR, Monjur-Ekhuda M, Khan MS, Aporna SA, Jahan R, Samarrai W, Islam F, Khatun Z, Rahmatullah M. Tribal formulations for treatment of pain: a study of the Bede community traditional medicinal practitioners of Porabari Village in Dhaka District, Bangladesh. Afr J Tradit Complement Altern Med. 2012;10:26–34.

Shakya AK. Medicinal plants: future source of new drugs. Int J Herbal Med. 2016;4:59–64.

Sinha S, Sharma A, Reddy PH, Rathi B, Prasad NVSRK, Vashishtha A. Evaluation of phytochemical and pharmacological aspects of *Holarrhena antidysenterica* (Wall.): A comprehensive review. J Pharm Res. 2013;6:488–92.

Solecki R, Shanidar IV. A Neanderthal flower burial in northern Iraq. Science. 1975;190:880–1.

Sukumaran B, Daswani P, Tetali P, Antia N, Birdi T. Studies on the antidiarrhoeal activity of *Aegle marmelos* unripe fruit. BMC Complement Alternat Med. 2009;9:47. https://doi.org/10.1186/1472-6882-9-47.

Diversity of Antimutagenic Phytocompounds from Indian Medicinal Plants

24

Mohammad Shavez Khan and Iqbal Ahmad

Contents

24.1 Introduction

Mutations are the cause of inborn errors of metabolism and also due to effect of certain environmental agents, resulting in morbidity and mortality in a living organism. Including genetic metabolic disorders, a spectrum of human diseases along with cancer is caused by mutations (Shon et al. 2004). A mutagen can be described as an agent, having the capacity to destroy or interfere with genomic integrity and hereditary mechanism of a cell or an organism. External factors including physical and chemical agents are considered as a major contributor to mutations. On the other hand, due to error in DNA replication, repair, and recombination events, mutations can occur spontaneously. Mutations in germline cells can be forwarded to future generation, while somatic mutations may be associated with pathogenesis of various disease conditions including cancer (Weakley et al. 2010). Antimutagenic agents are able to counter the effect of mutagens. These antimutagenic compounds are able to decrease or completely annul the effect of harmful chemicals and have ability to diminish the rate of induced or spontaneous mutation frequency. This group includes both natural and synthetic compounds. Antimutagens can be further classified into desmutagens and bioantimutagens. Desmutagens are

M. S. Khan · I. Ahmad (✉)
Faculty of Agricultural Sciences, Department of Agricultural Microbiology, Aligarh Muslim University, Aligarh, India

S. Sen, R. Chakraborty (eds.), *Herbal Medicine in India*,
https://doi.org/10.1007/978-981-13-7248-3_24

antimutagenic agents that function extracellularly and are able to eliminate or inactivate mutagenic agents before they reach DNA, while bioantimutagens are those antimutagens which act inside the cell and preferably reverse the action of mutagens. On the basis of their mechanism of action, several classes of antimutagens can be distinguished such as compounds with antioxidant activity, compounds inhibiting the activation of mutagens, blocking agents, and compounds with multiple modes of action (Bhattacharya 2011; Słoczyńska et al. 2014).

The plant kingdom comprises large number of species, producing a vast diversity of bioactive compounds with unique or chemically distinct structural scaffolds (Rodrigues et al. 2016). However, according to earlier observations, only about 6% of existing plant biodiversity has been systematically investigated for their pharmacological properties including antimutagenic properties and around 15% of the total plant diversity has been characterized chemically (Harvey et al. 2015). Wide range of pharmacologically active moieties with high degree of stereochemistry is an important characteristic feature of natural products. Additionally, natural products have the advantage over synthetic compounds by virtue of their being natural metabolites. Medicinal plants in its virtue as whole or bioactive compounds obtained from them are not only biologically active but also likely to be a substrate for one or more transporter systems that can deliver them to their intracellular site of action. Medicinal plants have continued to enter modern scientific investigation in search of lead compounds that might developed particularly as antimutagens and anticancer (Harvey et al. 2015; Khan et al. 2018).

Antimutagenic and DNA-protective chemicals from medicinal and edible plants are of particular importance as they may be used effectively as anticancer agents and have no undesirable xenobiotic effects on the living organism (Bacanli et al. 2017). There is increasing evidence that cancer and other mutation-related disorders can be prevented by intake of DNA-protective agents. The identification of antimutagenic agents in plants is considered as an effective strategy to inhibit pathogenic process resulting from exposure to mutagenic/genotoxic substances present in the environment (Gautam et al. 2016). Encouraging reports on the antimutagenic potential of plants have led to increased interests in search of phytoantimutagens from different parts of the world including India. Majority of the Indian medicinal plants used in traditional system of medicine are considered as safe to treat a number of ailments. However, scientific evaluation on the mechanism of actions of bioactive compounds in herbal formulations and their therapeutic contribution is largely less understood (Chakraborty 2018). Considering the global recognition of herbal medicines in treatment of various ailments, traditionally used medicinal plants have been exploited for search of novel antimutagenic compounds as well as to understand the mechanism of pharmacological action. Therefore, in this chapter, an attempt have been made to reveiw the antimutagenic activity of different chemical compounds originating from Indian medicinal plants, with special focus on their mechanisms of action.

24.2 Mutagens

Mutagen refers to physical or chemical agent that can induce changes in the hereditary material of an organism, consequently complementing background mutation frequency and increasing the overall mutation frequency. Mutagens act through different mechanisms, based on their action; several major classes of them such as base analogs, intercalating agents, alkylating agents, can be classified.

N-methyl-N′-nitrosoguanidine (MNNG), ethyl methanesulphonate (EMS) and methyl methanesulphonate are able to interact and transfer an alkyl group to DNA which results in the formation of monoadducts. Monoadduct formation leads to DNA strand breaks, causing specific mispairing (Ralhan and Kaur 2007). Guanine base in the nucleic acid is the most frequent location of adduct formation leading to O6-alkylguanine (Sanderson and Shield 1996). Base analogs have similar structure to normal DNA bases. Due to this structural similarity, base analogs can substitute normal bases in genetic material leading to transition or tautomerization. For instance, 2-amino-purine is an analog of adenine, while 5-bromouracil is an analog of thymine. Taking into account, these base analogs or antimetabolites are also used as therapeutic agents against different types of cancers and as immunosuppressant agents as well (Galmarini et al. 2002). Another group of largely recognized mutagens are intercalators such as acridine (acridine mutagen ICR-91) that are able to intercalate or insert between DNA bases. The intercalation by such agents at the core of DNA double helix results in insertions or deletion of single nucleotide pair (Martinez and Chacon-Garcia 2005).

Direct-acting mutagens are those mutagenizing agents which affect genetic material directly. For example, sodium azide interaction with DNA leads to structural damage directly, while, on the other hand, certain chemical compounds such benzo(a)pyrene act on DNA rather indirectly which are known as indirect mutagens. During the process of indirect mutagenesis, promutagen or parent compound transformed into active mutagen by the action of different cellular enzymes.

24.3 Antimutagens and Their Mechanisms

Antimutagens are a group of specific natural and synthetic chemical compounds which are able to lower or even completely annul the mutagenic effect of potentially harmful mutagens. According to Novick and Szilard (1952), the term "antimutagen" is applied to those chemical agents having the ability to reduce the rate of externally induced or naturally occurring spontaneous mutations. Antimutagens can be broadly classified into two different categories, i.e., desmutagens and bioantimutagens. Antimutagenic agents that function outside of the cells and are able to interact with mutagen which results in the inactivation of mutagens before they can enter the cell or interact with DNA are termed as desmutagens, whereas those antimutagenic agents which are able to act within the cell after DNA damage preferably via participating in genome repair and replication are known as bioantimutagens (Sangwan et al. 1998).

Antimutagens may also be distinguished in several classes based on their mode of actions. Antioxidant activity of the compounds is largely associated with their antimutagenic potential. As various mutagenic chemicals affect the genetic material through the production of reactive oxygen species, scavenging the free radicals represents one of the important mechanisms in the process of antimutagenesis (Simic 1988). Previously various plant-derived phytocompounds have been reported for their antimutagenic property which have been associated with their antioxidant potential such as curcumin (Parvathy et al. 2010), Lisosan G polyphenols (Frassinetti et al. 2012), bichalophenes (El-Sayed et al. 2013), lipoic acid (Rochette et al. 2013), etc. Thus, it can be concluded on the basis of the current knowledge that antioxidant activity is an anticipated property as it can be directly linked with the antimutagenic effects of compounds.

Natural antimutagens are also able to inhibit the metabolic activation of promutagens, thus ceasing the process of mutagenesis. The metabolic activation of promutagens is mediated by phase I metabolic enzymes such as the cytochrome P450 family of enzymes. Antimutagenic phytocompounds or plant extracts such as isothiocyanates (Hamilton and Teel 1996), certain phytoconstituents of *Terminalia arjuna* (Kaur et al. 2010), and lichen extracts (Nardemir et al. 2015) are able to inhibit the metabolic activation of mutagens, via influencing the activity of cytochrome P450.

Certain phytocompounds and plant extracts were characterized with another important protective mode of action against chemical-induced mutagenesis which is their ability to directly interact with mutagenic agents. These structural/chemical modifications of the harmful mutagens by antimutagenic agents protect the genetic material from mutagenic damage. For example, compounds containing sulphahydryl groups such as cysteine was used to inactivate 3-chloro-4-(dichloro)-5-hydroxy-2(5H)-furanone, a DNA damage-inducing agent (Watanabe et al. 1994). Similarly, antimutagenic action of bichalcohenes was attributed to its ability to prevent mutagenic chemicals from reaching target sites as well due to its possible interaction with mutagens, leading to the reduction in their damaging response (Watanabe et al. 1994; Marnewick et al. 2000). Other blocking agents such as gallic acid and extract of *Acanthopanax divaricatus* were also studied for a similar mechanistic response against chemical-induced mutagenesis (Hour et al. 1999; Hong et al. 2011).

Moreover, various plant-derived multifunctional antimutagens act through more than one mechanism simultaneously to provide protection against a variety of mutagens. These compounds simultaneously affect mutagens in several different ways which significantly increase the antimutagenic potency. Plant-derived phenolic compounds have the ability to act via both intracellular and extracellular mechanism against different direct- and indirect-acting mutagens in addition to their well-established antioxidant potential (Masuoka et al. 2012). Moreover, antimutagenic action of these polyphenols is also related to their DNA-protecting ability or providing a protective shield to DNA against the electrophilic or nucleophilic attack of mutagens (Marnewick et al. 2000; Mladenović et al. 2013). Similarly various polyphenols such as luteolin and rutin (Orhan et al. 2013; Khan et al. 2018), xanthones and flavones derived from *Syngonanthus* (De Oliveira et al. 2013), and caffeine and other methyl xanthines (Ulanowska and Węgrzyn 2006; Ulanowska et al. 2007) are reported with dual mechanisms in preventing mutagenic action of different harmful chemical mutagens.

24.4 Antimutagenicity Screening Assays

Appropriate mutagenicity/genotoxicity assays are required for the evaluation of antimutagenic property of the selected phytocompounds. Antimutagenic assays differ from mutagenicity testing as the tested models (cells) are treated with both the candidate compound and standard mutagens simultaneously. During initial development of antimutagenicity testing of different chemicals including those derived from plants, short-term bacterial assays are used. These short-term bacterial assays are intensively used for primary antimutagenic testing as they are relatively fast, simple, sensitive, and flexible (De Flora et al. 1992). In this section listed below is a brief description of those antimutagenic assays that are frequently used to screen synthetic chemicals, plant-derived compounds, and plant extracts for their antimutagenic potential.

The Ames/*Salmonella* histidine reversion assay (Ames test) also known as Ames/Salmonella microsome assay was developed by Maron and Ames for testing diverse chemicals for their mutagenic/antimutagenic activity (Maron and Ames 1983). Ames test is one of the widely used short-term assays based on different mutant strains of *Salmonella typhimurium*. In this assay, different mutant strains of *S. typhimurium* detect the mutagenicity of tested substance via induction of the histidine (His) operon (Maron and Ames 1983; Mortelmans and Zeiger 2000). Different mutation mechanisms such as base pair substitution and frameshift mutations of a mutagen could be detected by this assay. Furthermore, by employing tester strains of different genotypes, the antimutagenic action of tested phytocompounds against different mutagenic agents can be assessed (Mortelmans and Zeiger 2000). To date, numerous Indian medicinal plant extracts and various phytocompounds have been evaluated for their antimutagenic potential using Ames test as a primary screening assay. The major advantages of this bacterial-based antimutagenic assay are that vast diversity of mutagens can be employed, it is easy to perform, and no special apparatus are needed; however, this assay could not detect the mutagens specific to eukaryotic targets.

A similar test assay based on the genetically modified strain of *Escherichia coli* WP2 is also used primarily for the detection of A/T base pair damage. The tester strain *E. coli* WP2 utilized tryptophan instead of histidine as in the case of Ames test (Mortelmans and Riccio 2000). This assay is rather simpler as only one tester strain is required; however, like that of Ames test, this test also could not utilize for eukaryotic specific mutagen testing.

In the last two decades, numerous mutagenicity/antimutagenicity assays based on bacteria have been introduced and optimized. One such assay is based on the marine bacterium *Vibrio harveyi* which was optimized by different workers (Podgórska et al. 2005; Ulanowska and Węgrzyn 2006; Słoczyńska et al. 2010; Kamiński et al. 2013). In the *V. harveyi* test, a series of different mutant strains of *V. harveyi* is utilized. The ability of mutagens to influence the resistance profile of the bacterium against neomycin via interfering the genetic makeup forms the basis of this test. The number of mutants in a population increases in the presence of mutagens in a concentration-dependent fashion. The major advantage of the test is its high sensitivity, and it may detect significantly smaller doses of chemical mutagens with that of Ames test.

Another important tool for testing antimutagenic potential and an alternative to the Ames test is SOS chromotest (Quillardet and Hofnung 1985). This assay allows the calorimetric assessment of DNA alterations produced by different mutagens by measuring the expression of a reporter gene, β-galactosidase, via employing *Escherichia coli* PQ37 mutant strain (Quillardet et al. 1985). The SOS chromotest is rather simpler, utilizes only one tester strain, is versatile, and can detect a large number of differentially acting antimutagenic compounds.

Besides bacteria-based assays, another popular antimutagenic assessment assay based on yeast *Saccharomyces cerevisiae* is frequently used for the search of new antimutagenic compounds. The distinctive feature of the yeast assay is the fact that as eukaryotes, *S. cerevisiae* are characterized with chromosomal structure and different repair enzymes structurally similar to higher organisms including mammals. Additionally, *Saccharomyces cerevisiae* D7 tester strains also harbor endogenous cytochrome P450, and hence no prior activation is required for indirect promutagens (Zimmermann et al. 1975).

24.5 Antimutagenic Phytocompounds

Plant represents vast reservoirs of antimutagenic and protective chemical entities. India represents a vast diversity of plants which are used for the medicinal purpose since ancient times. Diverse medicinal properties of Indian medicinal plants attract scientist for the exploration of principal components and their evaluation using various *in vitro* and *in vivo* strategies. A large number of Indian medicinal plants have been also screened for their antimutagenic properties (Zahin et al. 2010, 2017, 2018; Satish et al. 2013; Devi et al. 2015; Nag et al. 2015; Kaur et al. 2015; Sharma et al. 2016; Pandey et al. 2017). Listed below are certain phytocompounds with antimutagenic activity identified from Indian medicinal plants.

24.5.1 Curcumin

Curcumin (1,7-bis(4-hydroxy-3methoxyphenyl)-1,6-heptadien-3,5-dione) is a yellow-colored polyphenol, an active constituent of the rhizome of *Curcuma longa* L. Apart from the rhizome of *Curcuma longa*, curcumin is also purified and characterized from other members of the genus *Curcuma* (Rauf et al. 2018). *Curcuma longa* has been extensively used in Indian traditional medicine, and it is used as an anti-inflammatory, blood purifier, hepatoprotective, detoxifier, and stomachic (Khare 2008). Modern scientific investigations revealed numerous bioactivities of its constituent curcumin including anticancer (Aggarwal et al. 2003), antibacterial (Gunes et al. 2016), antioxidant (Menon and Sudheer 2007), antimutagenic (Puliyappadamba et al. 2015), and anti-inflammatory activities (Kant et al. 2014) utilizing more test systems/models (Fig. 24.1).

Antimutagenic activity of curcumin has been extensively investigated and found to possess multiple modes of action against diverse chemical mutagens. Moreover, curcumin was also found to be active against chemical-induced mutagenesis in higher mammalian models. Nagabhushan et al. (1987) investigated

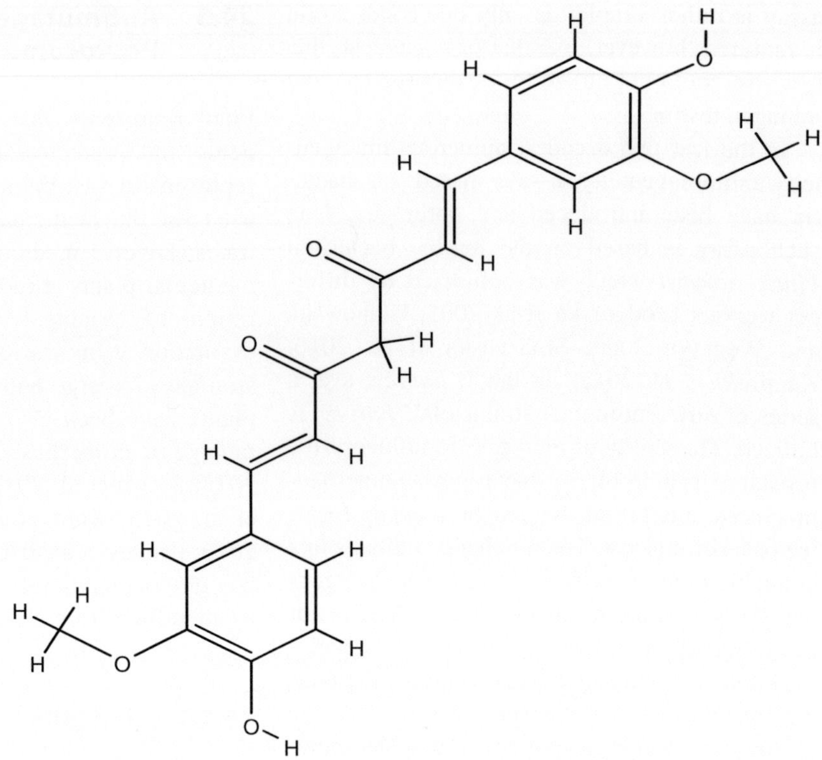

Fig. 24.1 Chemical structure of curcumin

the effect of curcumin on the mutagenicity of different environmental mutagenic chemicals in the Salmonella/microsome assay with or without S-9 mix activation. Curcumin was found to be active against cigarette smoke condensates, tobacco extracts, benzo[α]pyrene, and dimethyl benzo[α]anthracene in a concentration-dependent manner. However, in the study, no influence of curcumin was observed against direct-acting mutagens such as sodium azide and monoacetylhydrazine. Authors thus speculate the possible alteration of metabolic activation and detoxification of mutagens as an underlying mechanism for the observed activity. Curcumin was also evaluated for antimutagenic activity via *in vivo* chromosomal aberration assay in Wistar rats against cyclophosphamide-induced chromosomal damage. It was observed that in curcumin-supplemented animals, no significant chromosomal aberrations or change in mitotic index was evident (Shukla et al. 2002). Chromosomal aberrations induced by sodium azide in root tips of *Allium cepa* was also found to be significantly lowered when co-treated with up to 5 μg/mL of curcumin (Ragunathan and Panneerselvam 2007).

Antimutagenic activity of curcumin against promutagens benzo[α]pyrene induced carcinogenesis in lungs of Swiss albino mice was evaluated (Puliyappadamba et al. 2015). The treatment of curcumin significantly lower various cancer-related parameters such as downregulation of tumor necrosis factor kappa NF-kB, MAPK signalling, and Cox-2 transcription as well as number of tumor nodules in lung tissues of mice. Thus it can be concluded that curcumin is effective against variety of mutagenic chemicals in a different test systems including plant and animal models.

Structural activity relationship of curcumin reveals the presence of a) unsaturation of the side chain, b) substitution of methoxy group on the benzene ring, and c) central backbone β-diketone moiety in the curcumin molecule are the important requirement for the antimutagenic potential of curcumin against different chemical mutagens (cooked food heterocyclic amines) (Kaur 2008). Additionally, studies also showed that with modification in the chemical structure of curcumin, either with glycosylation or addition of amino acid group at specific positions, the antimutagenic activity was found to be enhanced against direct-acting mutagens (Parvathy et al. 2009, 2010). Moreover, these modifications also enhance the water solubility of otherwise insoluble curcumin pigments.

24.5.2 Punicalagin and Ellagic Acid

Punica granatum L. (pomegranate) is one of the important edible plants, cultivated throughout India, and is known for various ethnopharmacological uses. Punicalagin and ellagic acid are considered as major bioactive polyphenols of *Punica granatum* (Singh et al. 2018). Punicalagin (2,3-(S)-hexahydroxydiphenoyl-4,6-(S,S)-gallagyl-D-glucose), a most abundant pomegranate ellagitannin with the highest molecular weight among other polyphenols of pomegranate. Ellagic acid (2,3,7,8-tetrahydroxy-chromeno[5,4,3-cde] chromene-5,10-dione) a dilactone of hexahydroxydiphenic acid represents another polyphenolic active constituent of *Punica granatum* and also isolated from other edible plants. Punicalagin and ellagic acid have been shown to have numerous biological activities including anti-radical (Seeram et al. 2005), anti-inflammatory (BenSaad et al. 2017), anticancer, and antimutagenic activity (Zahin et al. 2014).

Antimutagenic properties punicalagin was investigated against benzo[α]pyrene-induced DNA adducts formation *in vitro* and *in vivo* (Aqil et al. 2012). Punicalagin inhibits DNA adduct formation in a dose-dependent protective activity when co-treated with benzo[α]pyrene along with appropriate activation factors (liver microsome). However, no inhibition was observed when the non-microsomal system was employed suggesting that the inhibition of DNA adduct formation was mediated through inactivation of cytochrome P450 enzymes by punicalagin. Moreover, when tested under *in vivo* conditions, it was observed that punicalagin significantly inhibits the DNA adduct formation; however, increase in the concentration of ellagic acid in serum of female rat indicated conversion of punicalagin into ellagic acid which produces an overall effect (Aqil et al. 2012) (Fig. 24.2).

Zahin et al. (2014) reported similar inhibitory activity of punicalagin and ellagic acid against DNA adduct formation by benzo[α]pyrene *in vitro*. Additionally, authors also evaluated both pomegranate tannins against panel of mutagens (direct and indirect) in Ames test and found significant (90%) antimutagenic activity. Varshney et al. (2015) evaluated antimutagenic potential of ellagic acid using *in vitro* (Ames test) and *in vivo* (mouse bone marrow micronucleus) assays. It was found that ellagic acid co-treatment results in decrease in revertant frequency of *S. typhimurium* tester strain TA100 against benzo[α]pyrene-induced mutation as well as a reduction in mean number of polychromatic erythrocytes in micronucleus test. Moreover, Western blotting results indicate downregulation of cytochrome P450 (1A1) isoform which prevented activation of benzo[α]pyrene.

24.5.3 Quercetin and Rutin

Other important phytoantimutagens reported from numerous Indian medicinal plants are quercetin and rutin. Quercetin and rutin are structurally similar flavonoids found ubiquitously in vegetables, fruit, herbs, leaves, seed, and several medicinal plants (Harborne 1986) (Fig. 24.3).

The basic structure consists of benzopryan ring (C_6-C_3-C_6) with different substitution patterns; rutin is glycoside-substituted quercetin (Chen et al. 2018). These flavonoids are reported to have numerous bioactive effects including anti-oxidant (Rice-Evans et al. 1996), anti-cancer (Raffa et al. 2017), antimicrobial (Cushnie and Lamb 2005), anti-inflammatory (González-Gallego et al. 2014), anti-diabetic (Vinayagam and Xu 2015), as well as antimutagenic activity (Snijman et al. 2007).

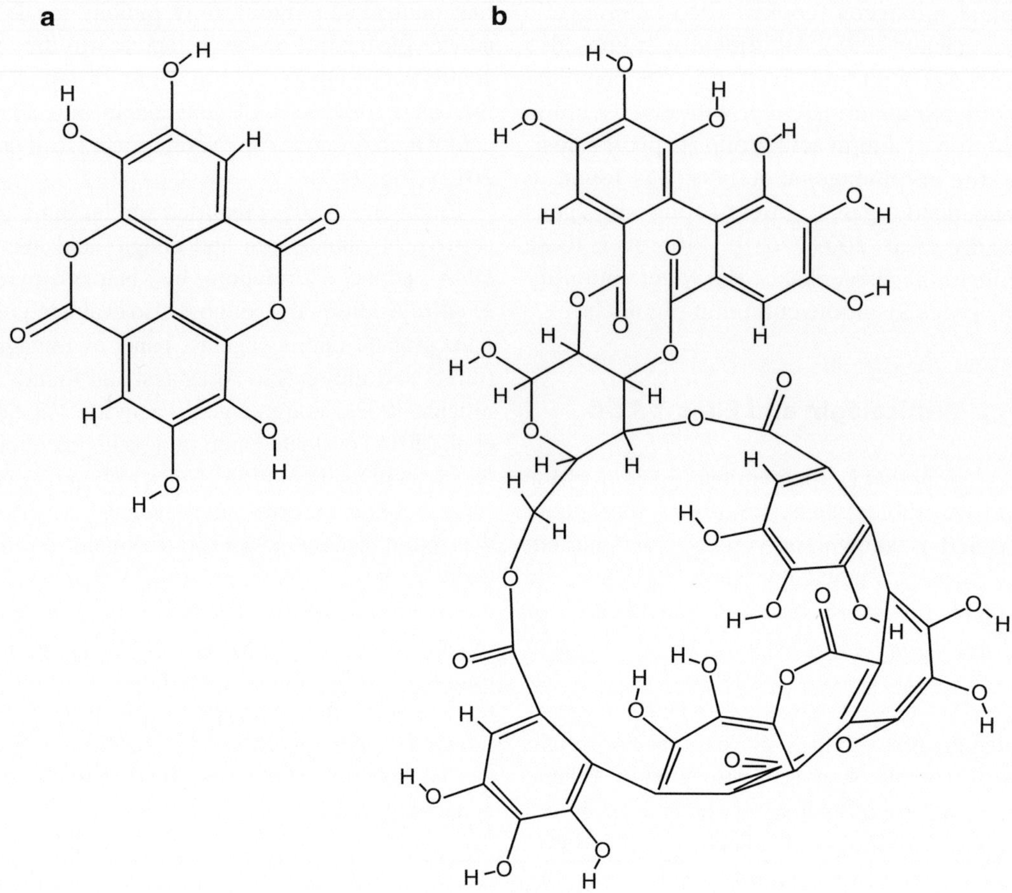

Fig. 24.2 Chemical structure of (**a**) ellagic acid and (**b**) punicalagin

Antimutagenic active flavonoids have been detected and characterized from numerous Indian medicinal plants such as *Bauhinia variegata*, *Bacopa monnieri*, *Centella asiatica*, *Ginkgo biloba*, *Lonicera japonica*, *Rosa bourbonia*, *Rosa brunii*, *Rosa damascena*, *Psidium guajava*, *Aegle marmelos*, and *Rhododendron* species (Bhandari et al. 2007; Sharma et al. 2010; Nair et al. 2017). The antimutagenic activity of flavonoids is closely related to their strong antioxidant properties (Korkina and Afanas' Ev 1996). Geetha et al. (2005) observed a strong correlation between the antimutagenic activity of quercetin and its antioxidant potency. However, the authors concluded that the overall antimutagenic activity of quercetin observed against oxidative mutagen (t-butyl hydroperoxide) was not solely dependent upon the anti-radical activity of the flavonoids; rather, other distinctive mechanisms were involved. Another study evaluated antimutagenic and antioxidant activity of quercetin against diethylnitrosamine (hepatocarcinogen) in rat liver (Gupta et al. 2010). Quercetin displayed remarkable protective activity when co-administered with the mutagen. Furthermore, quercetin administration also improved in various *in vivo* antioxidant parameters such as plasma aspartate transaminase (AST), plasma alanine transaminase (ALT), as well as glutathione levels in liver cells as evident from single-cell gel electrophoresis assay. Along with antioxidant efficacy, polyphenols are also known for their DNA-protecting activity chiefly attributed to their ability to act as a protective barrier between DNA and harmful mutagens (Mladenović et al. 2013). Khan et al. (2018) detected and quantified rutin form

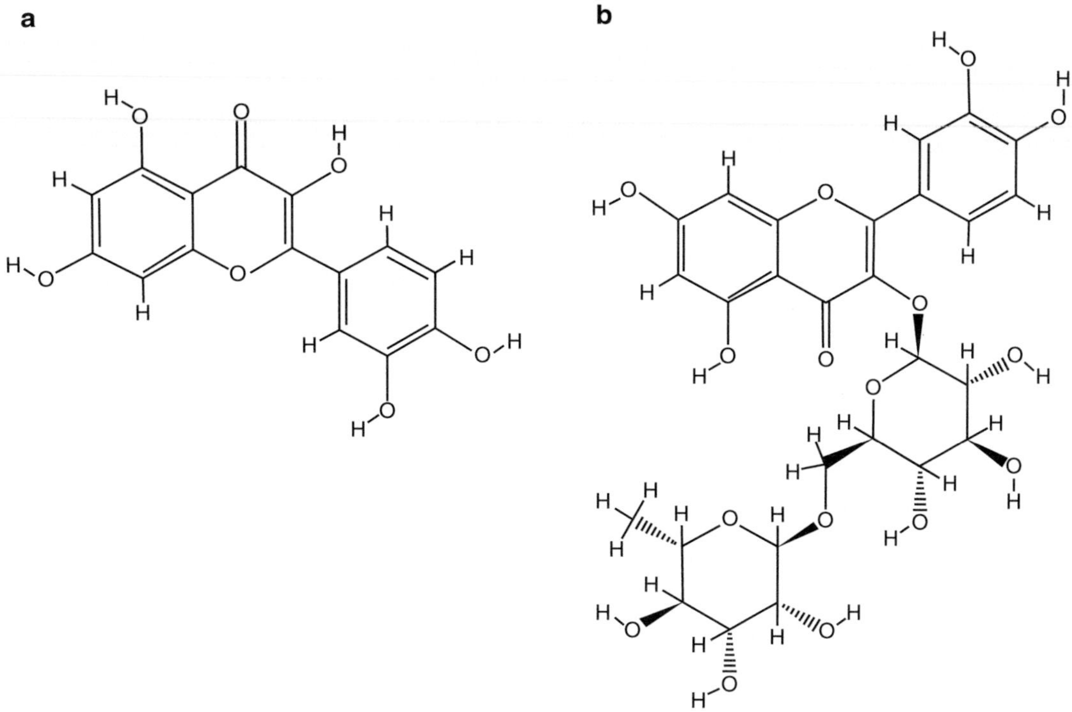

Fig. 24.3 Chemical structure of (**a**) quercetin and (**b**) rutin

extract of *Syzygium cumini*, an Indian medicinal plant of great importance, showing significant antioxidant and antimutagenic activity. Further, rutin as a pure compound was evaluated for antimutagenic and DNA-protective efficacy and showed significant activity in different *in vitro* systems. Through different biophysical techniques and molecular modelling tools, authors further confirm the DNA-protective role of rutin against mutagenic chemicals.

24.6 Conclusion

Mutations play important role in the onset and progression of various degenerative diseases including various types of cancer. Numerous harmful chemicals are capable of inducing mutations thus leading to alteration of the genetic makeup of an organism. On the other hand, antimutagenic compounds may partially or completely remove the harmful effect of mutagens, acting through diverse mechanistic pathways. Owing to rich biodiversity and well-recorded history of ethnomedicinal uses, searching antimutagenic principles from Indian medicinal plants will remain in focus of future scientific research, although there is an urgent need to focus antimutagenicity research on understanding the mechanism of action of active phytocompounds. Furthermore, antimutagenic effects of most active phytoantimutagens need to be evaluated in appropriate *in vivo* models to develop effective therapeutics.

References

Aggarwal BB, Kumar A, Bharti AC. Anticancer potential of curcumin: preclinical and clinical studies. Anticancer Res. 2003;23(1/A):363–98.

Aqil F, Vadhanam MV, Gupta RC. Enhanced activity of punicalagin delivered via polymeric implants against benzo [a] pyrene-induced DNA adducts. Mutat Res. 2012;743(1):59–66.

Bacanli M, Aydin S, Başaran AA, Başaran N. Are all phytochemicals useful in the preventing of DNA damage? Food Chem Toxicol. 2017;109(Pt 1):210–7.

BenSaad LA, Kim KH, Quah CC, Kim WR, Shahimi M. Anti-inflammatory potential of ellagic acid, gallic acid and punicalagin A&B isolated from *Punica granatum*. BMC Complement Altern Med. 2017;17(1):47.

Bhandari P, Kumar N, Gupta AP, Singh B, Kaul VK. A rapid RP-HPTLC densitometry method for simultaneous determination of major flavonoids in important medicinal plants. J Sep Sci. 2007;30(13):2092–6.

Bhattacharya S. Natural antimutagens: a review. Res J Med Plant. 2011;5(2):116–26.

Chakraborty P. Herbal genomics as tools for dissecting new metabolic pathways of unexplored medicinal plants and drug discovery. Biochimie Open. 2018;6:9–16.

Chen L, Teng H, Xie Z, Cao H, Cheang WS, Skalicka-Woniak K, Georgiev MI, Xiao J. Modifications of dietary flavonoids towards improved bioactivity: an update on structure–activity relationship. Crit Rev Food Sci Nutr. 2018;58(4):513–27.

Cushnie TT, Lamb AJ. Antimicrobial activity of flavonoids. Int J Antimicrob Agents. 2005;26(5):343–56.

De Flora S, Bronzetti G, Sobels FH. Assessment of antimutagenicity and anticarcinogenicity. Mutat Res. 1992;267:153–5.

De Oliveira AP, De Sousa JF, Da Silva MA, Hilário F, Resende FA, De Camargo MS, Vilegas W, dos Santos LC, Varanda EA. Estrogenic and chemopreventive activities of xanthones and flavones of Syngonanthus (Eriocaulaceae). Steroids. 2013;78(11):1053–63.

Devi HP, Mazumder PB, Devi LP. Antioxidant and antimutagenic activity of *Curcuma caesia* Roxb. rhizome extracts. Toxicol Rep. 2015;2:423–8.

El-Sayed WM, Hussin WA, Al-Faiyz YS, Ismail MA. The position of imidazopyridine and metabolic activation are pivotal factors in the antimutagenic activity of novel imidazo [1, 2-a] pyridine derivatives. Eur J Pharmacol. 2013;715(1–3):212–8.

Frassinetti S, Della Croce CM, Caltavuturo L, Longo V. Antimutagenic and antioxidant activity of Lisosan G in *Saccharomyces cerevisiae*. Food Chem. 2012;135(3):2029–34.

Galmarini CM, Mackey JR, Dumontet C. Nucleoside analogues and nucleobases in cancer treatment. Lancet Oncol. 2002;3(7):415–24.

Gautam S, Saxena S, Kumar S. Fruits and vegetables as dietary sources of antimutagens. J Food Chem Nanotechnol. 2016;2(3):97–114.

Geetha T, Malhotra V, Chopra K, Kaur IP. Antimutagenic and antioxidant/prooxidant activity of quercetin. Indian J Exp Biol. 2005;43(1):61–67.

González-Gallego J, García-Mediavilla MV, Sánchez-Campos S, Tuñón MJ. Anti-inflammatory and immunomodulatory properties of dietary flavonoids. In: Polyphenols in human health and disease; 2014. p. 435–52.

Gunes H, Gulen D, Mutlu R, Gumus A, Tas T, Topkaya AE. Antibacterial effects of curcumin: an *in vitro* minimum inhibitory concentration study. Toxicol Ind Health. 2016;32(2):246–50.

Gupta C, Vikram A, Tripathi DN, Ramarao P, Jena GB. Antioxidant and antimutagenic effect of quercetin against DEN induced hepatotoxicity in rat. Phytother Res. 2010;24(1):119–28.

Hamilton SM, Teel RW. Effects of isothiocyanates on cytochrome P-450 1A1 and 1A2 activity and on the mutagenicity of heterocyclic amines. Anticancer Res. 1996;16(6B):3597–602.

Harborne JB. Nature, distribution and function of plant flavonoids. Prog Clin Biol Res. 1986;213:15–24.

Harvey AL, Edrada-Ebel R, Quinn RJ. The re-emergence of natural products for drug discovery in the genomics era. Nat Rev Drug Dis. 2015;14(2):111.

Hong CE, Cho MC, Jang HA, Lyu SY. Mutagenicity and anti-mutagenicity of *Acanthopanax divaricatus* var. *albeofructus*. J Toxicol Sci. 2011;36(5):661–8.

Hour TC, Liang YC, Chu IS, Lin JK. Inhibition of eleven mutagens by various tea extracts (−) epigallocatechin-3-gallate, gallic acid and caffeine. Food Chem Toxicol. 1999;37(6):569–79.

Kamiński K, Obniska J, Chlebek I, Liana P, Pękala E. Synthesis and biological properties of new N-Mannich bases derived from 3-methyl-3-phenyl-and 3, 3-dimethyl-succinimides. Eur J Med Chem. 2013;66:12–21.

Kant V, Gopal A, Pathak NN, Kumar P, Tandan SK, Kumar D. Antioxidant and anti-inflammatory potential of curcumin accelerated the cutaneous wound healing in streptozotocin-induced diabetic rats. Int Immunopharmacol. 2014;20(2):322–30.

Kaur IP. Antimutagenicity of curcumin and related compounds against genotoxic heterocyclic amines from cooked food: the structural requirement. Food Chem. 2008;111(3):573–9.

Kaur S, Kumar S, Kaur P, Chandel M. Study of antimutagenic potential of phytoconstituents isolated from *Terminalia arjuna* in the Salmonella/Microsome Assay. Am J Biomed Sci. 2010;2(2):164–77.

Kaur A, Kaur D, Arora S. Evaluation of antioxidant and antimutagenic potential of *Justicia adhatoda* leaves extract. African J Biotech. 2015;14(21):1807–19.

Khan MS, Qais FA, Ahmad I, Hussain A, Alajmi MF. Genotoxicity inhibition by *Syzygium cumini* (L.) seed fraction and rutin: understanding the underlying mechanism of DNA protection. Toxicol Res. 2018;7(2):156–71.

Khare CP. Indian medicinal plants: an illustrated dictionary. Berlin: Springer; 2008.

Korkina LG, Afanas' Ev IB. Antioxidant and chelating properties of flavonoids. In: Advances in pharmacology, vol. 38. Cambridge: Academic Press; 1996. p. 151–63.

Luc Rochette, Stéliana Ghibu, Carole Richard, Marianne Zeller, Yves Cottin, Catherine Vergely. Direct and indirect antioxidant properties of α-lipoic acid and therapeutic potential. Mol Nutr Food Res. 2013;57(1):114–25.

Marnewick JL, Gelderblom WC, Joubert E. An investigation on the antimutagenic properties of South African herbal teas. Mutat Res. 2000;471(1):157–66.

Maron DM, Ames BN. Revised methods for the Salmonella mutagenicity test. Mutat Res. 1983;113(3–4):173–215.

Martinez R, Chacon-Garcia L. The search of DNA-intercalators as antitumoral drugs: what it worked and what did not work. Curr Med Chem. 2005;12(2):127–51.

Masuoka N, Matsuda M, Kubo I. Characterisation of the antioxidant activity of flavonoids. Food Chem. 2012;131(2):541–5.

Menon VP, Sudheer AR. Antioxidant and anti-inflammatory properties of curcumin. In: The molecular targets and therapeutic uses of curcumin in health and disease. Boston, MA: Springer; 2007. p. 105–25.

Mladenović M, Matić S, Stanić S, Solujić S, Mihailović V, Stanković N, Katanić J. Combining molecular docking and 3-D pharmacophore generation to enclose the in vivo antigenotoxic activity of naturally occurring aromatic compounds: Myricetin, quercetin, rutin, and rosmarinic acid. Biochem Pharmacol. 2013;86(9):1376–96.

Mortelmans K, Riccio ES. The bacterial tryptophan reverse mutation assay with *Escherichia coli* WP2. Mutat Res. 2000;455(1):61–9.

Mortelmans K, Zeiger E. The Ames Salmonella/microsome mutagenicity assay. Mutat Res. 2000;455(1):29–60.

Nag D, Ghosh M, Mukherjee A. Antimutagenic and genoprotective effects of *Saraca asoca* bark extract. Toxicol Ind Health. 2015;31(8):696–703.

Nagabhushan M, Amonkar AJ, Bhide SV. *In vitro* antimutagenicity of curcumin against environmental mutagens. Food Chem Toxicol. 1987;25(7):545–7.

Nair CJ, Ahamad S, Khan W, Anjum V, Mathur R. Development and validation of high-performance thin-layer chromatography method for simultaneous determination of polyphenolic compounds in medicinal plants. Pharm Res. 2017;9(Suppl 1):S67.

Nardemir G, Yanmis D, Alpsoy L, Gulluce M, Agar G, Aslan A. Genotoxic, antigenotoxic and antioxidant properties of methanol extracts obtained from *Peltigera horizontalis* and *Peltigera praetextata*. Toxicol Ind Health. 2015;31(7):602–13.

Novick A, Szilard L. Anti-mutagens. Nature. 1952;170:926–7.

Orhan F, Gulluce M, Ozkan H, Alpsoy L. Determination of the antigenotoxic potencies of some luteolin derivatives by using a eukaryotic cell system, *Saccharomyces cerevisiae*. Food Chem. 2013;141(1):366–72.

Pandey A, Sekar KC, Tamta S, Rawal RS. Assessment of phytochemicals, antioxidant and antimutagenic activity in micropropagated plants of *Quercus serrata*, a high value tree species of Himalaya. Plant Biosystems. 2017;15:1–8.

Parvathy KS, Negi PS, Srinivas P. Antioxidant, antimutagenic and antibacterial activities of curcumin-β-diglucoside. Food Chem. 2009;115(1):265–71.

Parvathy KS, Negi PS, Srinivas P. Curcumin–amino acid conjugates: synthesis, antioxidant and antimutagenic attributes. Food Chem. 2010;120(2):523–30.

Podgórska B, Chec E, Ulanowska K, Węgrzyn G. Optimisation of the microbiological mutagenicity assay based on genetically modified *Vibrio harveyi* strains. J Appl Genet. 2005;46(2):241–6.

Puliyappadamba VT, Thulasidasan AK, Vijayakurup V, Antony J, Bava SV, Anwar S, Sundaram S, Anto RJ. Curcumin inhibits B [a] PDE-induced procarcinogenic signals in lung cancer cells, and curbs B [a] P-induced mutagenesis and lung carcinogenesis. Biofactors. 2015;41(6):431–42.

Quillardet P, Hofnung M. The SOS Chromotest, a colorimetric bacterial assay for genotoxins: procedures. Mutat Res. 1985;147(3):65–78.

Quillardet P, de Bellecombe C, Hofnung M. The SOS Chromotest, a colorimetric bacterial assay for genotoxins: validation study with 83 compounds. Mutat Res. 1985;147(3):79–95.

Raffa D, Maggio B, Raimondi MV, Plescia F, Daidone G. Recent discoveries of anticancer flavonoids. Eur J Med Chem. 2017;142:213–28.

Ragunathan I, Panneerselvam N. Antimutagenic potential of curcumin on chromosomal aberrations in *Allium cepa*. J Zhejiang Univ Sci B. 2007;8(7):470–5.

Ralhan R, Kaur J. Alkylating agents and cancer therapy. Exp Opin Ther Pat. 2007;17(9):1061–75.

Rauf A, Imran M, Orhan IE, Bawazeer S. Health perspectives of a bioactive compound curcumin: a review. Trends Food Sci Technol. 2018:7.

Rice-Evans CA, Miller NJ, Paganga G. Structure-antioxidant activity relationships of flavonoids and phenolic acids. Free Radic Biol Med. 1996;20(7):933–56.

Rodrigues T, Reker D, Schneider P, Schneider G. Counting on natural products for drug design. Nat Chem. 2016;8(6):531.

Sanderson BJ, Shield AJ. Mutagenic damage to mammalian cells by therapeutic alkylating agents. Mutat Res. 1996;355(1):41–57.

Sangwan NS, Shanker S, Sangwan RS, Kumar S. Plant-derived products as antimutagens. Phytother Res. 1998;12(6):389–99.

Satish A, Kumar RP, Rakshith D, Satish S, Ahmed F. Antimutagenic and antioxidant activity of *Ficus benghalensis* stem bark and *Moringa oleifera* root extract. Int J Chem Analyt Sci. 2013;4(2):45–8.

Seeram NP, Adams LS, Henning SM, Niu Y, Zhang Y, Nair MG, Heber D. *In vitro* antiproliferative, apoptotic and antioxidant activities of punicalagin, ellagic acid and a total pomegranate tannin extract are enhanced in combination with other polyphenols as found in pomegranate juice. J Nutr Biochem. 2005;16(6):360–7.

Sharma N, Sharma UK, Gupta AP, Sinha AK. Simultaneous determination of epicatechin, syringic acid, quercetin-3-O-galactoside and quercitrin in the leaves of Rhododendron species by using a validated HPTLC method. J food Com Ana. 2010;23(3):214–9.

Sharma S, Sharma S, Vig AP. Evaluation of antimutagenic and protective effects of *Parkinsonia aculeata* L. leaves against H_2O_2 induced damage in pBR322 DNA. Physiol Mol Biol Plants. 2016;22(1):17–31.

Shon MY, Choi SD, Kahng GG, Nam SH, Sung NJ. Antimutagenic, antioxidant and free radical scavenging activity of ethyl acetate extracts from white, yellow and red onions. Food Chem Toxicol. 2004;42(4):659–66.

Shukla Y, Arora A, Taneja P. Antimutagenic potential of curcumin on chromosomal aberrations in Wistar rats. Mutat Res. 2002;515(1):197–202.

Simic MG. Mechanisms of inhibition of free-radical processes in mutagenesis and carcinogenesis. Mutat Res. 1988;202(2):377–86.

Singh B, Singh JP, Kaur A, Singh N. Phenolic compounds as beneficial phytochemicals in pomegranate (*Punica granatum* L.) peel: a review. Food Chem. 2018;261:75–86.

Słoczyńska K, Pękala E, Wajda A, Węgrzyn G, Marona H. Evaluation of mutagenic and antimutagenic properties of some bioactive xanthone derivatives using *Vibrio harveyi* test. Lett Appl Microbiol. 2010;50(3):252–7.

Słoczyńska K, Powroźnik B, Pękala E, Waszkielewicz AM. Antimutagenic compounds and their possible mechanisms of action. J App Genet. 2014;55(2):273–85.

Snijman PW, Swanevelder S, Joubert E, Green IR, Gelderblom WC. The antimutagenic activity of the major flavonoids of rooibos (*Aspalathus linearis*): Some dose–response effects on mutagen activation–flavonoid interactions. Mutat Res. 2007;631(2):111–23.

Ulanowska K, WZgrzyn G. Mutagenic activity of 1-methyl-4-phenyl-1, 2, 3, 6-tetrahydropyridine. J Appl Genet. 2006;47(1):85–7.

Ulanowska K, Piosik J, Gwizdek-Wiśniewska A, Węgrzyn G. Impaired mutagenic activities of MPDP+ (1-methyl-4-phenyl-2, 3-dihydropyridinium) and MPP+ (1-methyl-4-phenylpyridinium) due to their interactions with methylxanthines. J Geriatr Psychiatry Neurol. 2007;15(15):5150–7.

Varshney M, Vijayan V, Meshram GP. Chemopreventive effects of ellagic acid against genotoxicity induced by benzo (a) pyrene. Toxicol Environ Chem. 2015;97(6):786–98.

Vinayagam R, Xu B. Antidiabetic properties of dietary flavonoids: a cellular mechanism review. Nutr Metab (Lond). 2015;12(1):60.

Watanabe M, Kobayashi H, Ohta T. Rapid inactivation of 3-chloro-4-(dichloromethyl)-5-hydroxy-2 (5H)-furanone (MX), a potent mutagen in chlorinated drinking water, by sulfhydryl compounds. Mutat Res. 1994;312(2):131–8.

Weakley SM, Jiang J, Kougias P, Lin PH, Yao Q, Brunicardi FC, Gibbs RA, Chen C. Role of somatic mutations in vascular disease formation. Exp Rev Mol Diag. 2010;10(2):173–85.

Zahin M, Aqil F, Ahmad I. Broad spectrum antimutagenic activity of antioxidant active fraction of *Punica granatum* L. peel extracts. Mutat Res. 2010;703(2):99–107.

Zahin M, Ahmad I, Gupta RC, Aqil F. Punicalagin and ellagic acid demonstrate antimutagenic activity and inhibition of benzo [a] pyrene induced DNA adducts. Biomed Res Int. 2014;2014:467465.

Zahin M, Ahmad I, Aqil F. Antioxidant and antimutagenic potential of *Psidium guajava* leaf extracts. Drug Chem Toxicol. 2017;40(2):146–53.

Zahin M, Khan MS, AbulQais F, Abulreesh HH, Ahmad I. Antioxidant properties and anti-mutagenic potential of Piper Cubeba fruit extract and molecular docking of certain bioactive compounds. Drug ChemToxicol. 2018;41(3):358–67.

Zimmermann FK, Kern R, Rasenberger H. A yeast strain for simultaneous detection of induced mitotic crossing over, mitotic gene conversion and reverse mutation. Mutat Res. 1975;28(3):381–8.

Health Benefits of Octacosanol and Other Long-Chain Aliphatic Fatty Alcohols from Plants

25

Yearul Kabir

Contents

25.1 Introduction

Octacosanol, a long-chain aliphatic alcohol, is the predominant part of a natural wax product having physiological activity found in wheat germ oil, rice bran oil, fruits, leaves, surface of plants, and whole seeds (de Oliveira et al. 2012). Most studies that evaluated the efficacy of octacosanol used either a wheat germ oil extract or a natural combination of primary aliphatic alcohols (policosanol) isolated from sugar cane wax (*Saccharum officinarum* L.), of which octacosanol is the major component. Octacosanol occupies 60–70% of total aliphatic alcohols present in policosanol (Marinangeli et al. 2007). Because only a little amount can be obtained from diets, octacosanol has to be supplied extra in order to gain health benefits.

Octacosanol has been recognized to show a variety of important biological and pharmacological functions in humans and animals, including antioxidant activities (Ohashi et al. 2011; Sengupta et al. 2018), cholesterol-lowering effects, and lipid peroxidation (Keller et al. 2008; Ohashi et al. 2011). In addition, studies also demonstrated beneficial effects of octacosanol such as improving neurological function (Norris et al.

Y. Kabir (✉)
Department of Biochemistry and Molecular Biology, University of Dhaka, Dhaka, Bangladesh

S. Sen, R. Chakraborty (eds.), *Herbal Medicine in India*,
https://doi.org/10.1007/978-981-13-7248-3_25

1986), antiparkinsonism (Wang et al. 2010, 2012), antiangiogenic and antitumour activity (Thippeswamy et al. 2008), and prevention of pain and inflammation (Fernandez-Arche et al. 2009; de Oliveira et al. 2012). Further, antifatigue function (Kim et al. 2003), ergogenic properties (Shimura et al. 1987), and improving athletic and running performance in exercise-trained rats (Kabir and Kimura 1991; Kim et al. 2003; Saint-John and McNaughton 1986) have also been reported for octacosanol. Because of these beneficial biological activities and its high stability as a compound, octacosanol has been widely used in health food, medicine, and cosmetics.

Policosanol, the purified natural product, was initially described by Cuban researchers and consists of a mixture of eight very-long-chain aliphatic alcohols obtained from the wax of sugar cane (Hernandez et al. 1992). The main component of policosanol is octacosanol (C28) (60–70%), followed by hexacosanol (C26) (3.0–10.0%), triacontanol (C30) (10.0–15.0%), and dotriacontanol (C32) (5.0–10.0%). Other alcohols, like tetracosanol (C24), heptacosanol (C27), nonacosanol (C29), and tetratriacontanol (C34) are minor components (Laguna et al. 1997).

Policosanol shows primarily cholesterol-lowering and antiplatelet effects in experimental models (Lee et al. 2016; Molina et al. 2011; Wong et al. 2016), healthy volunteers (Abdul et al. 2010; Illnait et al. 2013; Lopez et al. 2010), and patients with type II hypercholesterolaemia (Castano et al. 2000; Tedeschi-Reiner et al. 2005). Besides, experimental and clinical studies have shown that oral treatment with policosanol inhibit cholesterol biosynthesis (Banerjee et al. 2011; Lee et al. 2016) and produce antioxidant effects *in vivo* (Sengupta et al. 2018; Kitts et al. 2012) as well as *in vitro* (Menendez et al. 2000a, b; Rodríguez et al. 2010). The related studies dealing with lowering of cholesterol and serum lipids, antiplatelet and antioxidant properties of policosanol, and policosanol as nutraceuticals have been extensively reviewed (Berthold and Berthold 2002; Viola et al. 2008). Besides cholesterol-lowering and antiplatelet effects, policosanol has been reported to exhibit a variety of important biological activities in humans and rodents, including anti-cardiovascular (Herrera et al. 1994; Noa et al. 1994), hepatoprotective (Noa et al. 2003; Ohta et al. 2008), and neurological activities (Molina et al. 2017; Sanchez et al. 2012, 2013) and anti-inflammation properties (Perez et al. 2015b) and reduction of markers of oxidative stress (Molina et al. 2013; Sanchez et al. 2013).

Several studies (Pons et al. 1994; Rodriguez and Garcia 1998) have indicated that policosanol is safe and well tolerated amongst the population. Long-term clinical studies also have demonstrated that policosanol is well suited and safe (Canetti et al. 1997). Toxicological studies in rats have shown that doses as high as 500 mg/kg body weight per day, which is 1724 times the recommended therapeutic dose, resulted in no reports of toxicity (Aleman et al. 1994a). Studies on carcinogenicity (Aleman et al. 1994b, 1995), reproduction, and teratogenicity (Rodriguez et al. 1997; Rodriguez and Garcia 1994) did not show any side effects.

25.2 Health Benefits and Functional Properties

25.2.1 Lipid-Lowering Effect

Policosanol is a well-studied nutraceutical for the management of blood cholesterol levels. Numerous studies have performed to elaborate its lipid-lowering effect especially reducing total cholesterol (TC), triglycerides (TG), and low-density lipoprotein cholesterol (LDL-C) as well as increasing serum high-density lipoprotein cholesterol (HDL-C) in human and animal cases (Castano et al. 2002a; Hernandez et al. 1992; Liu et al. 2012; Lopez et al. 2010; Keller et al. 2008; Xu et al. 2007).

In a randomized, double-blind, placebo-controlled crossover study, policosanol supplement (10 mg/day) for 8 weeks significantly reduced plasma TC and increased apoprotein AI but did not alter plasma triglycerides, HDL, oxidized LDL, Lp (a), and apoprotein S in patients with moderate hypercholesterolaemia (Tedeschi-Reiner et al. 2005). Illnait et al. (2013) reported that policosanol (5 and 10 mg/day) administered for 12 weeks in adults lowered serum LDL-C and TC and raised HDL-C. In another study, policosanol therapy (5 mg /day) for 12 weeks significantly decreased LDL-C, TC, and TC/HDL-C and LDL-C/HDL-C ratios and increased HDL-C without affecting TG (Castano et al. 2002b). Cuban policosanol was effective in lowering TC and LDL-C along with HDL-C elevation by inhibiting cholesterol synthesis (Lee et al. 2016). A summary of recent human studies on lipid-lowering effects of policosanol is presented in Table 25.1.

Martino et al. (2013) investigated the effects of glucomannan (GM) combination of low-dose chromium-polynicotinate (CP) or policosanol (PC) in hypercholesterolaemic children in a double-blind study and reported that GM combined treatment with low-dose CP or PC reduced total cholesterol and LDL-C without changing HDL-C, TG, and FBG. Concurrent therapy with policosanol 5 mg/kg and omega-3 FA 250 mg/kg lowered LDL-C, TC, and TG and increased HDL-C in male rabbits (Gamez 2005). Haim et al. (2012) reported that esterification of policosanol with oleic acid improves policosanol bioavailability and serum lipid profile in normocholesterolaemic rats by inactivating HMG-CoA.

Short-term dietary supplement of red yeast rice extract and policosanols combination in a group of children with known history of heterozygous familial hypercholesterolaemia and familial combined hyperlipidaemia significantly reduced TC, LDL-C, and apolipoprotein B levels without effecting HDL-C and apolipoprotein AeI levels compared to placebo (Guardamagna et al. 2011). In another, randomized, prospective, parallel group, single-blind study, combined pill containing berberine, red yeast rice, and policosanol significantly reduces cholesterolaemia and achieved acceptable plasma LDL-C levels in elderly hypercholesterolaemic patients previously intolerant to statins (Marazzi et al. 2011).

Hypertension is another fatal risk factor for the development of cardiovascular disease (CVD), which is often linked to other risk factors such as dyslipidaemia (Kim et al. 2017). In a randomized, double-blinded, and placebo-controlled study, policosanol was supplemented (10 mg, 20 mg, or placebo) for 24 weeks, wherein policosanol 20 mg group significantly reduced the aortic systolic blood pressure (SBP) and diastolic blood pressure (DBP) up to 9% as well as significantly reduced the TC and increased the serum HDL-C compared with first week (Kim et al. 2018). Thus, policosanol supplementation is effective in patients with hypertension and hypercholesterolaemia history (Kim et al. 2018), although, until now, there has been no *in vivo* or human study on the HDL-C/TC ratio and HDL functionality in relation to the central BP-lowering effect of policosanol.

Exact mechanism of hypocholesterolaemic effect of policosanol has not been established yet. Several studies describe the possible mechanism of lowering cholesterol effect like suppression of HMG-CoA reductase activity (Singh et al. 2006), CETP inhibition (Kim et al. 2017, 2018), and renin–angiotensin–aldosterone system that might help in reducing lipid and blood pressure level (Rozza et al. 2009). In a hypercholesterolaemic (1.25% cholesterol in diet) rat model, policosanol supplementation (8.0 mg/kg body weight) for 6 weeks significantly decreased the TC, TG, LDL-C, and HMG-CoA reductase activity in the liver compared to the control group (Lee et al. 2016). Singh et al. (2006) reported that treatment of hepatoma cell line with policosanol generated a 55% HMG-CoA reductase activity as well as threefold increase of AMP kinase phosphorylation. Oliaro-Bosso et al. (2009) have compared the effect of octacosadienol (octacosa-10,19-dien-1-ol) and policosanol on the regulation of HMG-CoA reductase in HUVEC and HepG2 human hepatoma cells, wherein both were found effective in inhibiting the upregulation of HMG-CoA reductase as well as inducing the AMPK phosphorylation, as AMP kinase, which is well known to inactivate acetyl-CoA carboxylase, is also the major regulator of HMG-CoA reductase phosphorylation (Carling et al. 1987).

Besides, policosanol inhibits cholesterol biosynthesis by indirect enhancement of receptor-dependent LDL processing (Menendez et al. 2001). Thus, there are multiple pathways by which policosanol might generate elevated hepatic acyl-CoA and AMP levels to activate

Table 25.1 Recent studies on human determining the effects of policosanol on total, LDL, and HDL cholesterol levels

Reference	Study subjects	Study design	Dosage (mg/d) duration	Physiological effects	P value*
Kim et al. (2018)	61 healthy Korean Placebo ($n = 18$) Policosanol 10 mg ($n = 18$) Policosanol 20 mg ($n = 25$)	Parallel, randomized, double-blind, placebo-controlled	10; 24 weeks 20; 24 weeks	–TC: 8%; –LDL-C: 14% +HDL-C: 16% –TC: 10% –LDL-C: 20% +HDL-C: 12%	$p < 0.05$ NS $p < 0.01$ $p < 0.001$ $p < 0.05$ $p < 0.05$
Kim et al. (2017)	25 healthy male volunteers YN: young non-smoker ($n = 7$, 24.0 ± 2.4 years) YS: young smoker ($n = 7$, 26.3 ± 1.5 years) MN: middle-aged subjects ($n = 11$, 52.5 ± 9.8 years)		10; 8 weeks	MN group –TC: 6% +HDL-C YN: 36% YS: 35% MN: 8%	NS NS $p < 0.05$
Sanchez et al. (2016)	60 recent ischemic stroke patients Policosanol ($n = 30$) Placebo ($n = 30$)	Parallel, randomized, double-blind, placebo-controlled	20; 12 weeks	–TC: 9.7% –LDL-C:17.8% +HDL-C: 12.6%	$p < 0.01$ $p < 0.01$ $p < 0.05$
Lopez et al. (2015)	83 hypercholesterolaemic patients with serum TC ≥5.2	Parallel, randomized, double-blind, comparative study.	5; 3 months increased to 20; 12 months	–TC: 19.5% –LDL-C: 39.0% +HDL: 7.4%	$p < 0.0001$ $P < 0.0001$ $P < 0.01$
Guo et al. (2014)	15 healthy volunteers Policosanol ($n = 7$) Placebo ($n = 8$)	Randomized, controlled, open-label, prospective study	20; 12 weeks	TC: n/c LDL-C: n/c HDL-C: n/c	NS NS NS
Illnait et al. (2013)	90 subjects with serum TC ≤5.9 mmol/L. Policosanol 5 mg ($n = 30$) Policosanol 10 mg ($n = 30$) Placebo ($n = 30$)	Parallel, randomized, double-blind, placebo-controlled	5; 12 weeks 10; 12 weeks	–TC: 13.1% –LDL-C: 17.6% +HDL-C: 11.3% –TC: 17.4% –LDL-C: 19.7% +HDL-C: 14.8%	$P < 0.00001$ $P < 0.00001$ $P < 0.00001$ $P < 0.00001$ $p < 0.00001$ $P < 0.00001$
Liu et al. (2012)	72 hyperlipidaemia patients Policosanol ($n = 36$) Placebo ($n = 36$).	Randomized, open study	20; 16 weeks	–TC: 19.4% –LDL-C: 22.5% +HDL-C: n/c	$P < 0.01$ $P < 0.01$ NS
Swanson et al. (2011)	54 clinically stable HIV-infected people (91% black) with at least one lipid abnormality. Policosanol ($n = 28$) Placebo ($n = 26$)	Crossover, randomized, double-blind, placebo-controlled	20; 12 weeks	TC: n/c LDL-C: n/c HDL-C: n/c	NS NS NS
Lopez et al. (2010)	55 subjects with serum TC ≤5.9 mmol/L. Policosanol ($n = 27$) Placebo ($n = 28$)	Parallel, randomized, double-blind, placebo-controlled	10; 12 weeks	–TC: 11.7% –LDL-C: 22.1% +HDL-C: 9.6%	$p < 0.00001$ $p < 0.00001$ $p < 0.05$

Physiological effects: the difference in percentage changes between experimental groups; – net effect was a decrease; + net effect was an increase. *TC* total cholesterol, *LDL-C* low-density lipoprotein cholesterol, *HDL-C* high-density lipoprotein cholesterol, *NS* non-significant, *n/c* no change, * percentage difference from baseline to end value

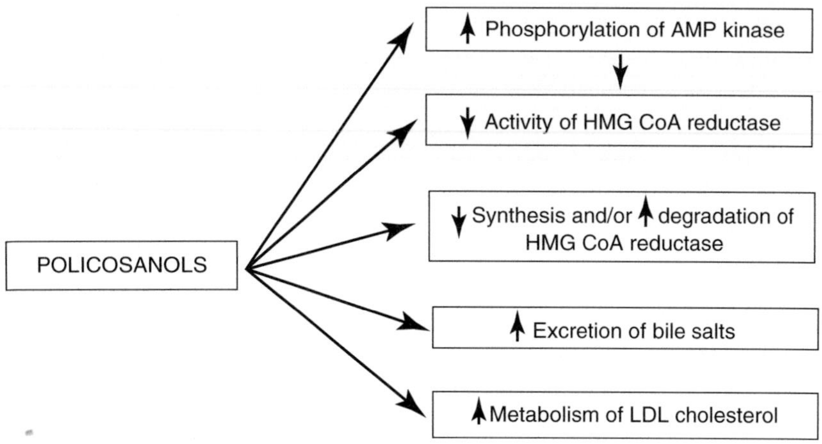

Fig. 25.1 Proposed mechanisms for the cholesterol lowering effect of policosanols

AMP-kinase and suppress cholesterol synthesis. Policosanol and/or policosanol metabolites may inhibit cholesterol absorption across intestinal cells by partially oxidizing cholesterol ester fatty acids (Li et al. 2011) or policosanol-increased bile acid excretion as shown by Chi et al. (2005). This will reduce the blood cholesterol level by making the liver utilize cholesterol to synthesize more bile. A summary of the proposed mechanisms for cholesterol-lowering effect of policosanol is outlined in Fig. 25.1.

Although several studies described the controversial result of policosanol efficacy in hypercholesterolaemic subjects especially sugar cane policosanol (SCP) supplementation. Kassis and Jones (2008) studied SCP supplementation (10 mg/day) in healthy hypercholesterolaemic subjects for 28 days in a randomized double-blind crossover study and found no significant change in LDL cholesterol and cholesterol synthesis compared to control, which failed to support prior research regarding policosanols efficacy and mode of action.

Reiner et al. (2005) reported that rice policosanol has much fewer effects on TC and no significant effect on LDL-C, HDL-C, TG, Ox-LDL, HDL2-C, HDL3-C, apoprotein B, homocysteine, and C-reactive protein. Further, it is found that policosanol does not reduce cholesterol level in Caucasian patients (Berthold et al. 2006). Also policosanol derived from rice, sunflower, and sugar cane wax had no significant effect on plasma lipid levels in hamsters (Wang et al. 2003) or rabbits (Murphy et al. 2008). In a randomized, placebo-controlled, double-blind study, Greyling et al. (2006) reported that 20 mg/d policosanol for 12 weeks consumption had no significant effect on serum lipid improvements in hypercholesterolaemic and heterozygous familial hypercholesterolaemic patients when compared with placebo intake.

25.2.2 Other Possible Benefits

25.2.2.1 Reduction of Platelet Aggregation

Molina et al. (2011) investigated the effects of policosanol and grape seed extract (GSE) on platelet aggregation induced ex vivo by ADP and collagen in plasma rich in platelets of rats and found that both substances significantly inhibited ADP- and collagen-induced platelet aggregation compared with the control group. In rat model, 5–20 mg/kg of policosanol causes an antiaggregatory effect by inhibiting arachidonic acid metabolism (Arruzazabala et al. 1993). Another, randomized, double-blind, placebo-controlled study using healthy volunteers investigated the effects of policosanol and aspirin on platelet aggregation (Arruzazabala et al. 1996). Castano et al. (2006) reported that policosanol (10 mg/d) administered concomitantly with omega-3FA to adults with type II hypercholesterolaemia that significantly enhanced the inhibition of platelet aggregation to arachidonic acid and collagen without enhancing the effect of omega-3FA on bleeding time. Gamez et al. (2005) investigated the effect of combined therapy of policosanol with omega-3 FA on platelet aggregation in rabbits and reported that treatment with policosanol + omega-3 FA inhibited platelet aggregation much better compared to policosanol or omega-3 FA alone.

Wong et al. (2016) showed that crude rice bran policosanol extract (RBE) could inhibit *in vitro* platelet adhesion, aggregation, and secretion upon activation using agonists. RBE reduced ex vivo ADP-induced platelet aggregation without any adverse effects. Antiplatelet effect of RBE was evident after 30 days of oral administration of RBE. The exact aggregation inhibitory mechanisms are yet to be known, although policosanol was shown to inhibit cyclooxygenase enzyme activity (Perez et al. 2013) and was reported to lower the production of serum thromboxane (Arruzazabala et al. 1993; Carbajal et al. 1998).

25.2.2.2 Analgesic and Anti-inflammatory Activity

de Oliveira et al. (2012) reported that octacosanol isolated from *Sabicea grisea* var. *grisea* leaves possesses the anti-inflammatory activities through mediating the alpha 2-adrenergic receptors, which could be of relevance for the pharmacological control of pain and inflammatory processes. Furthermore, this compound significantly reduced the total leukocyte count and neutrophils influx, as well as TNF-α level in the carrageenan-induced pleurisy. Based on these findings, de Oliveira et al. (2012) concluded that octacosanol may be useful in developing new strategies for preventing pain and inflammation. Other study also reported a reduction of TNF-α production by fatty alcohols in both *in vitro* and *in vivo* (Fernandez-Arche et al. 2009; Saito et al. 2006).

25.2.2.3 Anticardiovascular and Antiangiogenic Activity

Noa et al. (1994) reported that prior intake of policosanol in isoprenaline-induced myocardial infarction reduced the cardiac cell damage in the rat by decreasing the number of polymorphonuclear neutrophils (PMN) and mast cells in the damaged areas. Several other studies also described the beneficial effect of policosanol in isoprenaline-induced myocardial necrosis (Herrera et al. 1994; Noa et al. 1994). Thippeswamy et al. (2008) found that octacosanol purified from the medicinal plant *Tinospora cordifolia* inhibited tumour-induced angiogenesis *in vivo* by inhibiting vascular endothelial growth factor (VEGF) gene expression by Nf-Kb-dependent pathway.

25.2.2.4 Hepatoprotective Activity

Policosanol has a good safety profile and is well tolerated and is shown to have hepatoprotective effect. Policosanol (25 mg/kg and 100 mg/kg) protected against the CCl4-induced acute hepatic injury in rat model via increasing liver enzymes (Noa et al. 2003). In another study, Ohta et al. (1997) reported that orally administered octacosanol also prevents CCl4-induced acute liver injury in rats through improvement of hepatic TG accumulation. Ohta et al. (2008) also reported octacosanol attenuates hepatic oxidative stress associated with acute liver injury progression in rats intoxicated once with CCl4 through its indirect antioxidant action by increasing tissue GSH level rather than its direct antioxidant action.

25.2.2.5 Neurological Activity

Molina et al. (2017) reported that the repeated oral doses of policosanol (100 and 200 mg/kg) and omega-3 fish oil (1.25 and 2.5 g/kg) for 7 days significantly reduced the global cerebral ischemia in Mongolian gerbils with greater policosanol efficacy. These anti-ischemic effects of policosanol have been associated with its ability to reduce the oxidative stress markers (Molina et al. 2013; Sanchez et al. 2013) and inflammation (Perez et al. 2015a). Further, oral policosanol pretreatment (50–400 mg/kg) protected against blood-brain barrier (BBB) damage induced by cerebral ischemia-reperfusion (I/R) in rats and attenuated the increase of myeloperoxidase (MPO), a marker of inflammation, in the brain tissue (Perez et al. 2015b).

Long-term (5 years) policosanol and aspirin intake therapy was associated to a very good neurological recovery in patients, who suffered an ischemic stroke and had the previous history of transient ischemic attacks (TIA) (Sanchez et al. 2010). Likewise, two double-blind, placebo-controlled studies demonstrated that the administration of policosanol + aspirin (AS) therapy improved the neurological recovery and favourably modified plasma oxidative markers as compared to placebo + As in patients with recent (≤30 days) ischemic stroke (Sanchez et al. 2012, 2013).

In another study, orally administered single doses of policosanol (200 mg/kg) and atorvastatin (10 and 20 mg/kg) was found effective against hyperlocomotion and neurological damage of hippocampal CA1 neurons in gerbils with ischemia-reperfusion-induced global cerebral ischemia on experimental brain ischemia (IR-induced GCI) in gerbils (Molina et al. 2013). Sanchez et al. (2016) compared the efficacy of policosanol (20 mg/day) in combination with atorvastatin (20 mg/day) for 12 weeks, wherein this combination improved the functional outcome of the patients with recent ischemic stroke treated with aspirin compared to placebo and atorvastatin combination.

25.2.2.6 Protective Effects on Parkinsonism

Octacosanol has anti-parkinson effect. Wang et al. (2010) showed that oral administration of octacosanol (35–70 mg/kg) significantly ameliorated 6-hydroxydopamine (6-OHDA)-induced motor and behavioural impairments in rats by decreasing oxidative stress markers, for example MDA, SOD, CAT, and GSHPx. Octacosanol inhibited the 6-OHDA- and proNGF-p75NTR/sortilin-mediated cell death as well as activated the nerve growth factor (NGF)-TrkA-mediated cell survival. Octacosanol treatment also effectively improved the morphological appearances of tyrosine hydroxylase (TH)-positive neuronal cells in nigrostriatal systems.

In another study, Wang et al. (2012) reported that protective effects of octacosanol against Parkinson might be mediated by blocking the phosphorylation of p38 mitogen-activated protein kinase (p38 MAPK) and c-jun N-terminal kinase (JNK) on the signal transduction *in vivo* in 1-methyl-4-phenyl-1,2,3,6-tetrahydropyridine (MPTP)-treated C57BL/6 N mice. Although they could not elucidate the exact mechanism underlying how octacosanol might interfere with MAPKs signalling, they thought that it was not directly related to the chemical structure of octacosanol.

25.2.2.7 Antidiabetic Activity

Ohashi et al. (2011) have reported that dietary administration of octacosanol (10 or 50 mg/kg BW for 5 weeks) can ameliorate hypertriglyceridemia, hypercholesterolaemia, and oxidative stress in type 2 diabetic KKAy (Spontaneous Mouse Model for Type 2 Diabetic Nephropathy) mice without affecting obesity, hyperglycaemia, and hyperinsulinemia condition. However, dietary supplementation of octacosanol (50 mg/kg BW) reduced the elevated hepatic cholesterol concentration but not serum total-cholesterol level in diabetic KKAy mice by inhibiting cholesterol synthesis in HMG-CoA reductase-independent manner. Saito et al. (2006) investigated the effects of N-hexacosanol on streptozotocin-induced rat diabetic nephropathy and reported that diabetic rats treated with N-hexacosanol (2 mg/kg and 8 mg/kg i.p. every day) for 8 weeks prevent the increase of malonaldehyde and transform growth factor beta-1 (TGF-beta1) concentrations as well as the protein kinase C (PKC) activities in the diabetic kidney and ameliorate diabetic-induced nephropathy.

25.2.2.8 Antibacterial and Antioxidant Activity

Recently, Sengupta et al. (2018) reported antibacterial activities of octacosanol against *Escherichia coli*, *Pseudomonas aeruginosa*, and *Bacillus subtilis* as observed by disc assay against concentrations of 1 mg/mL and 2 mg/mL.

Togashi et al. (2007) investigated the antibacterial activity of long-chain fatty alcohols against *Staphylococcus aureus* and found that 1-dodecanol and 1-tridecanol had the highest antibacterial activity amongst the long-chain fatty alcohols tested, although the antibacterial activity varied with the length of the aliphatic carbon chain. Antibacterial activity of long-chain alcohol against *Streptococcus mutans* (Kubo et al. 1993) and upper-airway respiratory tract bacteria (Tanaka et al. 2002) was also reported. Kitts et al. (2012) examined the effect of feeding a mixture of high-molecular-weight alcohols derived from sugar cane (SCA), both alone and in combination with phytosterols (PS), on changes in plasma lipids, organ cholesterol accumulation, and antioxidant status of Wistar rats, and reported that plasma oxygen radical scavenging capacity values significantly decreased when rats were fed the atherogenic diets that contained the combination of PS and SCA.

25.2.3 Anti-stress Activity

Kaushik et al. (2017) reported that octacosanol improved sleep by increasing number of sleep episodes and decreasing wake episode duration. Octacosanol (200 mg/kg) administration significantly lowered plasma corticosterone levels, which would decrease the mental stress. Administration of octacosanol mitigates stress in mice by inducing changes in sleep-wake parameters that was reflected in terms of restored non-rapid eye movement (NREM) sleep. Although octacosanol does not alter normal sleep, it clearly lessens stress and restores stress-affected sleep (Kaushik et al. 2017). Oliaro-Bosso et al. (2009) reported that anti-stress ability of octacosanol in an animal may be due to the activation of AMP-activated protein kinase (*AMPK*), which rapidly increases the supply of ATP *in vivo* and thus maintains the balance of energy metabolism and relieve stress.

25.2.4 Ergogenic Properties

Octacosanol supplementation (0.75% in diet) for 28 days significantly increased the running performance in exercise-trained rats by elevating creatine phosphokinase activity in plasma as well as citrate synthase activity in the muscles (Kim et al. 2003). Thus, the ergogenic properties of octacosanol include the sparing of muscle glycogen stores and upregulate the oxidative capacity in the muscle of exercise-trained rats (Kim et al. 2003). Kabir and Kimura (1991) also reported an increase in voluntary exercise in rats supplemented with dietary octacosanol for 28 days. Further, Shimura et al. (1987) found that dietary supplementation of octacosanol (about 40% purity) in mice not only enhances the motor endurance like swimming endurance but also affects the concentrations of hepatic and serum lipids (Shimura et al.1987).

25.2.5 Body Weight

Long et al. (2016) revealed that octacosanol (24 mg/kg diet) improved the growth performance of broiler chicks. Long et al. (2015) also reported that dietary octacosanol supplementation increased the average daily growth by 6.45% and significantly improved feed conversion ratio by 6.35% compared to control diet in weaning piglets. On the other hand, Long et al. (2016) also reported that the abdominal fat percentage decreased in response to the increase in the dietary addition of octacosanol in broiler chicks. Lee et al. (2016) investigated the effects of policosanol supplementation in Wistar male rats for 42 days and reported significantly decreased body weight in the policosanol-treated group compared to control groups after 42 days (Lee et al. 2016). Besides, Ohashi et al. (2011) reported that octacosanol administered at a dose of 10 or 50 mg/kg BW for 5 weeks to KKAy mice had no effect on the increase in body weight.

25.3 Toxicity Studies

To date, no study has described any toxic or carcinogenic effects secondary to octacosanol or policosanol supplementation. The toxicity of policosanol supplement has been evaluated in different animal models including mice (Aleman et al. 1995), rats (Aleman et al. 1994a, b; Rodriguez et al. 1997; Rodriguez and Garcia 1998), rabbits (Rodriguez et al. 1994), dogs (Mesa et al. 1994), and monkeys (Rodriguez-Echenique et al. 1994), using doses ranging from 0.25 to 500 mg/kg. Toxicological studies on animals show policosanol is safe up to 500 mg/kg/day for 18 months, a dose that is 1500 times the normal human dose of 20 mg/day (Aleman et al. 1995). Besides, policosanol supplementation did not accelerate tumour growth (Aleman et al. 1995). Up to 180 mg/kg/day given to beagle dogs for 1 year showed no adverse effects (Mesa et al. 1994), and in monkey, 25 mg/kg/day for 54 months had no signs of adverse effects (Rodríguez-Echenique et al. 1994). Policosanol supplementation (500 mg/kg/day) shows no adverse effects on fertility, reproduction, teratogenesis, or development, providing to rat model from the 15th day of pregnancy to 21 days post-parturition (Rodriguez and Garcia 1998). Besides, policosanol supplementation (500 mg/kg/day) in rat model before 2 weeks of mating, pregnancy, or even 21 days into lactation showed no adverse effects observed on postnatal growth and behaviour (Rodriguez and Garcia 1994). Male rats given policosanol 500 mg/kg/day for 60 days prior to mating or even examined for three successive generations showed no adverse effects on fertility, reproduction, or development (Rodriguez and Garcia 1994; Rodriguez et al. 1997).

25.4 Metabolism of Octacosanol

There is little information regarding octacosanol and other fatty alcohols metabolism. Kabir and Kimura, who elaborately examined systemic distribution and metabolism of radiolabeled octacosanol in rat model after oral dosing (Kabir and Kimura 1993, 1994, 1995a). They investigated the *in vivo* conversion of octacosanol to its corresponding acid by administering ^{14}C-octacosanol to rats and examining the recoveries of radioactivity in different liver fractions (Kabir and Kimura 1993, 1994, 1995b). Thus, octacosanol is firstly converted to fatty acids (FA) in the liver and then incorporated into TGs, sterols, and phospholipids (Kabir and Kimura 1995b). However, an abundant level of radioactivity was found in the muscle which proved that either octacosanol itself or metabolic products notably FA were utilized for energy production via β-oxidation in the muscle (Kabir and Kimura 1995a).

Octacosanoic acid was postulated as the active metabolite of octacosanol, which was found the elevated amount in the liver and plasma after oral administration of octacosanol to rats (Menendez et al. 2005). Ohta et al. (2008) described a possible mechanism of octacosanoic acid production from octacosanol oxidation in the liver of rats after CCl_4 intoxication. Menendez et al. (2005) also demonstrate the octacosanoic acid production after human fibroblasts cultured in the presence of ^{3}H-octacosanol and after oral dosing with policosanol to rats. Although these results indicate a conversion of octacosanol to octacosanoic acid in rat fibroblast, to date, this metabolism has not been confirmed in humans. Besides, shortened saturated (myristic, palmitic, and stearic) and unsaturated (oleic, palmitoleic) fatty acids are also formed after oral dosing with policosanol to monkeys (Menendez et al. 2005). Thus, octacosanol metabolism is linked to FA metabolism via β-oxidation.

On the contrary, Menendez et al. (1996) found the faecal excretion of fatty alcohols after [^{3}H]-octacosanol loading in healthy volunteers. Keller et al. (2008) reported significant increase in faecal octacosanol after supplementation, although a baseline excretion of octacosanol was found in all study participants which may be due to the bacterial synthesis of fatty alcohols in the colon or even a dietary intake. In the study of Keller et al. (2008), they could not confirm the octacosanol metabolites in the faecal and serum samples, although a serum concentration of octacosanoic acid below the limit of detection cannot be excluded.

25.5 Conclusion

Octacosanol and other long-chain aliphatic alcohols have the potential to treat various health conditions without major side effects and thus would be beneficial to many patients and normal healthy individuals. In spite of the limited information available on the health benefits of octacosanol and other long-chain aliphatic alcohols, the chapter has tried to present a comprehensive picture of the available information. Although a number of functional properties and benefits have been documented in this chapter, more long-term studies and a great deal of further research are needed, including clinical trials, before substantially establishing their purported health benefits. Further studies with high throughput techniques as well as well-designed human controlled trials focused on the mechanism of action, rate and amount of absorption, and different compositions of policosanol sources are required to scientifically substantiate claims for health benefits of octacosanol. Finally, due to excellent safety and tolerability, the search for lipid-lowering compounds based on octacosanol and policosanol is of great importance and interest, especially in children, elderly persons, and other special populations.

References

Abdul MIM, Jiang X, Williams KM, Day RO, Roufogalis BD, Liauw WS, Xu H, Matthias A, Lehmann RP, McLachlan AJ. Pharmacokinetic and pharmacodynamic interactions of echinacea and policosanol with warfarin in healthy subjects. Br J Clin Pharmacol. 2010;69(5):508–15.

Aleman CL, Mas R, Hernandez C, Rodeiro I, Cerejido E, Noa M, Capote A, Menendez R, Amor A, Fraga V, Sotolongo V, Jimenez S. A 12-month study of policosanol oral toxicity in Sprague Dawley rats. Toxicol Lett. 1994a;70(1):77–87.

Aleman CL, Mas R, Puig MN, Guerra IR, Ortega CH, Capote A. Carcinogenicity of policosanol in Sprague Dawley rats: a 24 month study. Teratog Carcinog Mutagen. 1994b;14(5):239–49.

Aleman CL, Puig MN, Elias EC, Ortega CH, Guerra IR, Ferreiro RM, Brinis F. Carcinogenicity of policosanol in mice: an 18-month study. Food Chem Toxicol. 1995;33:573–8.

Arruzazabala ML, Carbajal D, Molina V, Valdes S, Mas R. Effect of policosanol on cerebral ischemia in Mongolian gerbils: role of prostacyclin and thromboxane A2. Prostaglandins Leukot Essent Fatty Acids. 1993;49(3):695–7.

Arruzazabala ML, Valdes S, Mas R, Fernandez L, Carbajal D. Effects of policosanol successive dose increases in platelet aggregation in healthy volunteers. Pharmacol Res. 1996;34:181–5.

Banerjee S, Ghoshal S, Porter TD. Activation of AMP-kinase by policosanol requires peroxisomal metabolism. Lipids. 2011;46:311–21.

Berthold IG, Berthold HK. Policosanol: clinical pharmacology and therapeutic significance of a new lipid-lowering agent. Am Heart J. 2002;143:356–65.

Berthold HK, Unverdorben S, Degenhardt R, Bulitta M, Gouni-Berthold I. Effect of policosanol on lipid levels among patients with hypercholesterolemia or combined hyperlipidemia – a randomized controlled trial. J Am Med Assoc. 2006;295(19):2262–69.

Canetti MM, Moreira M, Mas R, Illnait J, Fernandez L, Fernandez JC. Effects of policosanol on primary hypercholesterolemia: a 3-year open-extension follow-up. Curr Ther Res. 1997;58:868–75.

Carbajal D, Arruzazabala ML, Valdes S, Mas R. Effect of policosanol on platelet aggregation and serum levels of arachidonic acid metabolites in healthy volunteers. Prostagl Leukotr Essent Fatty Acids. 1998;58(1):61–4.

Carling D, Zammit VA, Hardie DG. A common bicyclic protein kinase cascade inactivates the regulatory enzymes of fatty acid and cholesterol biosynthesis. FEBS Lett. 1987;223:217–22.

Castano G, Mas R, Feranadez L, Fernandez JC, Illnait J, Lopez LE, Alvarez E. Effects of policosanol on postmenopausal women with type II hypercholesterolemia. Gynecol Endocrinol. 2000;14(3):187–95.

Castano G, Mas R, Fernandez JC, Fernandez L, Illnait J, Lopez E. Effects of policosanol on older patients with hypertension and type II hyperlipoproteinaemia. Drugs R D. 2002a;3:159–72.

Castano G, Mas R, Fernandez L, Illnait J, Hernández E, Fernandez JC, Gamez R, Gutierrez C, Alvarez E. A randomized, double-blind, placebo-controlled study of the efficacy and tolerability of policosanol in adolescents with type II hypercholesterolemia. Curr Ther Res. 2002b;63(4):286–303.

Castano G, Arruzazabala ML, Fernandez L, Mas R, Carbajal D, Molina V, Illnait J, Mendoza S, Gamez R, Mesa M, Fernandez J. Effects of combination treatment with policosanol and omega-3 fatty acids on platelet aggregation: A randomized, double-blind clinical study. Curr Ther Res. 2006;67:174–92.

Chi HN, Ka YL, Yu H, Zhen YC. Policosanol has no antioxidant activity in human low-density lipoprotein but increase excretion of bile acids in hamsters. J Agr Food Chem. 2005;53:6289–93.

de Oliveira AM, Conserva LM, de Souza Ferro JN, de Almeida Brito F, Lyra Lemos RP, Barreto E. Antinociceptive and anti-inflammatory effects of octacosanol from the leaves of *Sabicea grisea* var. *grisea* in mice. Int J Mol Sci. 2012;13:1598–611.

Fernandez-Arche A, Marquez-Martin A, de la Puerta Vazquez R, Perona JS, Terencio C, Perez-Camino C, Ruiz-Gutierrez V. Long-chain fatty alcohols from pomace olive oil modulate the release of proinflammatory mediators. J Nutr Biochem. 2009;20:155–62.

Gamez R, Maz R, Arruzazabala ML, Mendoza S, Castano G. Effects of concurrent therapy with policosanol and omega-3 fatty acids on lipid profile and platelet aggregation in rabbits. Drugs RD. 2005;6(1):11–9.

Greyling A, De Witt C, Oosthuizen W, Jerling JC. Effects of a policosanol supplement on serum lipid concentrations in hypercholesterolaemic and heterozygous familial hypercholesterolaemic subjects. Br J Nutr. 2006;95(5):968–75.

Guardamagna O, Abello F, Baracco V, Stasiowska B, Martino F. The treatment of hypercholesterolemic children: efficacy and safety of a combination of red yeast rice extract and policosanols. Nutr Metab Cardiovasc Diseases. 2011;21:424–9.

Guo YL, Xu RX, Zhu CG, Wu NQ, Cui ZP, Li JJ: Policosanol attenuates statin-induced increases in serum proprotein convertase subtilisin/kexin type 9 when combined with atorvastatin. Evid Based Complement Alternat Med 2014. http://dx.doi.org/10.1155/2014/926087.

Haim D, Valenzuela A, Branes MC, Fuenzalida M, Videla LA. The oleic acid esterification of policosanol increases its bioavailability and hypocholesterolemic action in rats. Grasas Aceites. 2012;63(4):345–54.

Hernandez F, Illnait J, Mas R, Castano G, Fernandez L, Gonzalez M, Cordovi N, Fernandez J. Effect of policosanol on serum lipids and lipoproteins in healthy volunteers. Curr Ther Res. 1992;51:568–75.

Herrera MN, Magraner J, Mas R. Effect of policosanol on isoprenaline-induced myocardial necrosis in rats. J Pharm Pharmacol. 1994;46:282–5.

Illnait J, Lopez E, Fernandez L, Mas R, Gamez R, Mesa M, Mendoza S, Fernandez JC. Effects of policosanol (5 and 10 mg/day) in adults with serum cholesterol levels ≤ 5.9 mmol/L. Int J Pharm Sci Rev Res. 2013;22(2):303–9.

Kabir Y, Kimura S. Biochemical effect of octacosanol on voluntary exercise in rats. Dhaka Univ Studies (Part E). 1991;6:77–85.

Kabir Y, Kimura S. Biodistribution and metabolism of orally administered octacosanol to rats. Ann Nutr Metab. 1993;37:33–8.

Kabir Y, Kimura S. Distribution of radioactive octacosanol in response to exercise in rats. Nahrung. 1994;4:373–7.

Kabir Y, Kimura S. Tissue distribution of (8-14C)-octacosanol in liver and muscle of rats after serial administration. Ann Nutr Metab. 1995a;39:279–84.

Kabir Y, Kimura S. Metabolism of octacosanol in liver and muscle of rat. Acta Aliment. 1995b;24:39–46.

Kassis AN, Jones PJH. Changes in cholesterol kinetics following sugar cane policosanol supplementation: a randomized control trial. Lipids Health Dis. 2008;7:17.

Kaushik MK, Aritake K, Takeuchi A, Yanagisawa M, Urade Y. Octacosanol restores stress affected sleep in mice by alleviating stress. Sci Rep. 2017;7:8892.

Keller S, Gimmler F, Jahreis G. Octacosanol administration to humans decreases neutral sterol and bile acid concentration in feces. Lipids. 2008;43:109–15.

Kim H, Park S, Han DS, Park T. Octacosanol supplementation increases running endurance time and improves biochemical parameters after exhaustion in trained rats. J Med Food. 2003;6:345–51.

Kim JY, Kim SM, Kim SJ, Lee EY, Kim JR, Cho KH. Consumption of policosanol enhances HDL functionality via CETP inhibition and reduces blood pressure and visceral fat in young and middle-aged subjects. Int J Mol Med. 2017;39:889–99.

Kim S-J, Yadav D, Park H-J, Kim J-R, Cho K-H. Long-term consumption of Cuban policosanol lowers central and brachial blood pressure and improves lipid profile with enhancement of lipoprotein properties in healthy Korean participants. Front Physiol. 2018;9:412.

Kitts DD, Kopec A, Zawistowski J, Popovich DG. Effects of high molecular weight alcohols from sugar cane fed alone or in combination with plant sterols on lipid profile and antioxidant status of Wistar rats. Appl Physiol Nutr Metab. 2012;37(5):938–46.

Kubo I, Muroi H, Kubo A. Antibacterial activity of long-chain alcohol against *Streptococcus mutans*. J Agric Food Chem. 1993;41:2447–50.

Laguna A, Magraner J, Carbajal D, Arruzazabala ML, Mas R, Garcıa M. A mixture of higher primary aliphatic alcohols, its obtention from sugar cane wax and its pharmacological uses. U.S. Patent 5663156, 1997.

Lee J-Y, Choi H-Y, Kang Y-R, Chang H-B, Chun H-S, Lee M-S, Kwon Y-I. Effects of long-term supplementation of policosanol on blood cholesterol/glucose levels and 3-hydroxy-3-methylglutaryl coenzyme a reductase activity in a rat model fed high cholesterol diets. Food Sci Biotechnol. 2016;25(3):899–904.

Li Q, Thomson AB, Clandinin MT. Cholesterol ester and free fatty acids are modulated by policosanol in CaCo-2 intestinal cell. J Am Coll Nutr. 2011;30:201–9.

Liu S, Tan MY, Zhao SP, Rong H. Effects of policosanol on serum lipids and heme oxygenase-1 in patients with hyperlipidemia. Zhonghua Xin Xue Guan Bing Za Zhi. 2012;40:840–3.

Long L, Gao MZ, Peng K, Sun J, Wang SX. Effects of octacosanol extracted from rice bran on production performance and blood parameters in weanling piglets. J Chin Cereals Oils Assoc. 2015;30:94–100. [in Chinese]

Long L, Wu SG, Yuan F, Wang J, Zhang HJ, Qi GH. Effects of dietary octacosanol on growth performance, carcass characteristics and meat quality of broiler chicks. Asian Australas J Anim Sci. 2016;29:1470–6.

Lopez E, Illnait J, Fernandez JC, Fernandez L, Gamez R, Mesa M, Mendoza S, Mas R, Ruiz D, Jardines Y. Effects of sugarcane wax alcohols in subjects with normal or borderline serum cholesterol levels. Rev CENIC Cien Biol. 2010;41:31–7.

Lopez E, Fernandez L, Mas R, Illnait J, Mendoza S, Ramirez Y, Fernández JC, Ruiz ID. A comparison of the long-term (1 year) lipid modifying effects of D-003 (sugarcane wax acids) and policosanol: A randomized, double-blind study. Int J Pharm Sci Rev Res. 2015;33(1):171–8.

Marazzi G, Cacciotti L, Pelliccia F, Iaia L, Volterrani M, Caminiti G, Sposato B, Massaro R, Grieco F, Rosano G. Long-term effects of nutraceuticals (berberine, red yeast rice, policosanol) in elderly hypercholesterolemic patients. Adv Ther. 2011;28(12):1105–13.

Marinangeli CP, Kasis AN, Jain D, Ebine N, Gunnane SC, Jones PJ. Comparison of composition and absorption of sugarcane policosanols. Br J Nutr. 2007;97(2):381–8.

Martino F, Puddu PE, Pannarale G, Colantoni C, Martino E, Niglio T, Zanoni C, Barillà F. Low dose chromium-polynicotinate or policosanol is effective in hypercholesterolemic children only in combination with glucomannan. Atherosclerosis. 2013;228:198–202.

Menendez R, Sotolongo V, Fraga V, Amor AM, Gonzalez R, Del Rio A, Jimenez S, Perez N, Mas R. Plasma levels and total radioactivity excretion in healthy volunteers after oral 3H-octacosanol administration. Rev CENIC Cien Biol. 1996;27:32–5.

Menendez R, Más R, Amor AM, Fernandez JC, Gonzalez RM. Effects of policosanol on the susceptibility of low-density lipoprotein isolated from hypercholesterolemic patients at high coronary risk to *in vitro* copper-mediated lipid peroxidation: a randomized, double-blind pilot study. Curr Ther Res. 2000a;61(9):609–20.

Menendez R, Mas R, Amor AM, Gonzalez RM, Fernandez JC, Rodeiro I, Zayas M, Jimenez S. Effects of policosanol treatment on the susceptibility of low density lipoprotein (LDL) isolated from healthy volunteers to oxidative modification *in vitro*. Br J Clin Pharmacol. 2000b;50(3):255–62.

Menendez R, Amor A, Rodeiro I, Gonzalez RM, Gonzalez PC, Alfonso JL, Mas R. Policosanol modulates HMG-CoA reductase activity in cultured fibroblasts. Arch Med Res. 2001;32(1):8–12.

Menendez R, Marrero D, Mas R, Fernandez I, Gonzalez L, Gonzalez RM. In vitro and in vivo study of octacosanol metabolism. Arch Med Res. 2005;36(2):113–9.

Mesa AR, Mas R, Noa M, Hernandez C, Rodeiro I, Gamez R, Garcia M, Capote A, Aleman CL. Toxicity of policosanol in beagle dogs: one-year study. Toxicol Lett. 1994;73(2):81–90.

Molina V, Carbajal D, Arruzazabala ML, Ravelo Y, Mas R. Comparative study of policosanol and grape seed extract on platelet aggregation in rats. Rev CENIC Cienc Biol. 2011;42(1):3–6.

Molina V, Ravelo Y, Noa M, Mas R, Perez Y, Oyarzabal A, Mendoza N, Valle M, Jimenez S, Sánchez J. Therapeutic effects of policosanol and atorvastatin against global brain ischaemia-reperfusion injury in Gerbils. Indian J Pharm Sci. 2013;75(6):635–41.

Molina V, Ravelo Y, Mena L, Noa M, Perez Y, Oyarzaba A, Valle M, Jimenez S. Therapeutic effects of policosanol and omega-3 fish oil against global brain ischemia reperfusion in *Mongolian gerbils*. Int J Pharm Sci Rev Res. 2017;42(2):179–85.

Murphy KJ, Saint DA, Howe PR. Lack of effect of sugarcane and sunflower seed policosanols on plasma cholesterol in rabbits. J Am Coll Nutr. 2008;27:476–84.

Noa M, Herrera M, Magraner J, Mas R. Effect of policosanol on isoprenaline-induced myocardial necrosis in rats. J Pharm Pharmacol. 1994;46:282–5.

Noa M, Mendoza S, Más R, Mendoza N. Effect of policosanol on carbon tetrachloride-induced acute liver damage in Sprague-Dawley rats. Drugs Res Develop. 2003;4:29–35.

Norris FH, Denys EH, Fallat RJ. Trial of octacosanol on amyotrophic lateral sclerosis. Neurology. 1986;36(9):1263–4.

Ohashi K, Ishikawa H, Ohta Y. Octacosanol ameliorates hyperlipidemia and oxidative stress in KKAy mice with type 2 diabetes. J Anal Bio Science. 2011;34(3):223–33.

Ohta Y, Sasaki E, Ishiguro I. Effect of oral octacosanol administration on hepatic triglyceride accumulation in rats with carbon tetrachloride-induced acute liver injury. Med Biol. 1997;134:185–9.

Ohta Y, Ohashi K, Matsura T, Tokunaga K, Kitagawa A, Yamada K. Octacosanol attenuates disrupted hepatic reactive oxygen species metabolism associated with acute liver injury progression in rats intoxicated with carbon tetrachloride. J Clin Biochem Nutr. 2008;42:118–25.

Oliaro-Bosso S, Calcio E, Mantegna S, Giraudo E, Meda C, Viola F, Cravotto G. Regulation of HMG-CoA reductase activity by policosanol and octacosadienol, a new synthetic analogue of octacosanol. Lipids. 2009;44(10):907–16.

Perez Y, Mas R, Oyarzabal A, Jimenez S, Molina V. Effects of policosanol (sugar cane wax alcohols) and D-003 (sugarcane wax acids) on cyclooxygenase (COX) enzyme activity *in vitro*. Int J Pharm Sci Rev Res. 2013;19(2):18–23.

Perez Y, Mas R, Oyarzábal A, Jimenez S, Molina V. Effects of octacosanol and triacontanol alcohols on cyclooxygenase and 5-lipoxygenase enzyme activities in vitro. Rev Cubana Farm. 2015a;49(1):117–31.

Perez Y, Molina V, Mas R, Oyarzabal A, Jiménez S. Effects of policosanol pre-treatment on blood-brain barrier damage induced by ischemia-reperfusion in rats. Int J Pharm Sci Rev Res. 2015b;32(1):1–6.

Pons P, Rodriguez M, Mas R, Illnait J, Fernandez L, Robaina C, Fernandez JC. One-year efficacy and safety of policosanol in patients with type II hypercholesterolaemia. Curr Ther Res. 1994;55(9):1084–92.

Reiner Z, Tedeschi-Reiner E, Romic Z. Effects of rice policosanol on serum lipoproteins, homocysteine, fibrinogen and C-reactive protein in hypercholesterolaemic patients. Clin Drug Invest. 2005;25(11):701–7.

Rodriguez MD, Garcia H. Teratogenic and reproductive studies of policosanol in the rat and rabbit. Teratog Carcinog Mutagen. 1994;14(3):107–13.

Rodriguez MD, Garcia H. Evaluation of peri- and post-natal toxicity of policosanol in rats. Teratog Carcinog Mutagen. 1998;18(1):1–7.

Rodriguez I, Illnait J, Molina V, Oyarzábal A, Fernándezl MM, Mas R, Mendoza S, Gamez R, Jiménez S, Ruiz D. Comparison of the antioxidant effects of D-002 (beeswax alcohols) and grape seed extract (GSE) on plasma oxidative variables in healthy subjects. Lat Am J Pharm. 2010;29:255–62.

Rodriguez MD, Sanchez M, Garcia H. Multigeneration reproduction study of policosanol in rats. Toxicol Lett. 1997;90:97–106.

Rodríguez-Echenique C, Mesa R, Mas R, Noa M, Menendez R, Gonzalez RM, Amor AM, Fraga V, Sotolongo V, Laguna A. Effect of policosanol chronically administered in male monkeys (Macacaarctoides). Food Chem Toxicol. 1994;32(6):565–75.

Rozza F, de Simone G, Izzo R, De Luca N, Trimarco B. Nutraceuticals for treatment of high blood pressure values in patients with metabolic syndrome. High Blood Press Cardiovasc Prev. 2009;16(4):177–82.

Saint-John M, McNaughton L. Octacosanol ingestion and its effects on metabolic responses to submaximal cycle ergometry, reaction time and chest and grip strength. Int Clin Nutr Rev. 1986;6:81–7.

Saito M, Kinoshita Y, Satoh I, Shinbori C, Kono T, Hanada T, Uemasu J, Suzuki H, Yamada M, Satoh K. n-hexacosanol ameliorates streptozotocin-induced diabetic rat nephropathy. Eur J Pharmacol. 2006;544:132–7.

Sanchez J, Mas R, Mendoza S, Fernandez J, Ruiz D. Effects of policosanol on patients with ischemic stroke with previous transient ischemic attack: a long-term follow-up. Rev CENIC Cien Biol. 2010;41:23–9.

Sanchez J, Fernandez L, Illnait J, Arruzazabala ML, Molina V, Mas R. Effects of policosanol on the recovery of ischemic stroke: a randomized controlled study. IOSR J Pharm. 2012;2(6):14–24.

Sanchez J, Illnait J, Mas R, Perez Y, Mendoza S, Cabrera L, Fernandez L, Mesa M, Fernandez J, Oyarzabal A, Molina V, Jimenez S, Reyes P. Effects of policosanol plus aspirin therapy on the neurological recovery and plasma oxidative markers of patients with ischemic stroke. IOSR J Pharm. 2013;3(4):31–40.

Sanchez J, Illnait J, Mas R, Mendoza S, Vega H, Fernandez L, Mesa BM, Fernandez J, Reyes P, Ruiz D. Policosanol versus atorvastatin on the functional recovery of patients with ischemic stroke. Int J Pharm Sci Rev Res. 2016;37(1):7–14.

Sengupta S, Nandi I, Bhattacharyya DK, Ghosh M. Anti-oxidant and anti-bacterial properties of 1-octacosanol isolated from rice bran wax. J Plant Biochem Physiol. 2018;6:1. https://doi.org/10.4172/2329-9029.1000206.

Shimura S, Hasegawa T, Takano S, Suzuki T. Studies on the effect of octacosanol on motor endurance in mice. Nutr Rep Int. 1987;36:1029–38.

Singh DK, Li L, Porter TD. Policosanol inhibits cholesterol synthesis in hepatoma cells by activation of AMP-kinase. J Pharmacol Exp Ther. 2006;318(3):1020–6.

Swanson B, Keithley JK, Sha BE, Fogg L, Nerad J, Novak RM, Adeyemi O, Spear GT. Policosanol for managing human immunodeficiency virus–related dyslipidemia in a medically underserved population: a randomized, controlled clinical trial. Altern Ther Health Med. 2011;17(2):30–35.

Tanaka Y, Fukuda S, Kikuzaki H, Nakatani N. Antibacterial activity of aliphatic long-chain compounds against upper-airway respiratory tract pathogens. ITE Lett Batter New Technol Med. 2002;1:777–80.

Tedeschi-Reiner E, Reiner Z, Romic Z, Ivankovic D. A randomized, double blind, placebo-controlled study of the antilipemic efficacy and tolerability of food supplement policosanol in patients with moderate hypercholesterolemia. Lijec Vjesn. 2005;127:273–9.

Thippeswamy G, Sheela MI, Salimath BP. Octacosanol isolated from *Tinospora cordifolia* downregulates VEGF gene expression by inhibiting nuclear translocation of NF-kappaNB and its DNA binding activity. Eur J Pharmacol. 2008;588:141–50.

Togashi N, Shiraishi A, Nishizaka M, Matsuoka K, Endo K, Hamashima H, Inoue Y. Antibacterial activity of long-chain fatty alcohols against *Staphylococcus aureus*. Molecules. 2007;12(2):139–48.

Viola F, Oliaro S, Binello A, Cravotto G. Policosanol: updating and perspectives. Mediterr J Nutr Metab. 2008;1:77–83.

Wang YW, Jones PJH, Pischel I, Fairow C. Effects of policosanols and phytosterols on lipid levels and cholesterol biosynthesis in hamsters. Lipids. 2003;38(2):165–70.

Wang T, Liu YY, Wang X, Yang N, Zhu HB, Zuo PP. Protective effects of octacosanol on 6-hydroxydopamine-induced Parkinsonism in rats via regulation of ProNGF and NGF signaling. Acta Pharmacol Sin. 2010;31:765–74.

Wang T, Liu Y, Yang N, Ji C, Chan P, Zuo P. Anti-parkinsonian effects of octacosanol in 1-methyl-4-phenyl-1,2,3,6 tetrahydropyridine-treated mice. Neural Regen Res. 2012;7(14):1080–7.

Wong W-T, Ismail M, Tohit ERM, Abdullah R, Zhang Y-D. Attenuation of thrombosis by crude rice (*Oryza sativa*) bran policosanol extract: *Ex vivo* platelet aggregation and serum levels of arachidonic acid metabolites. Evidence Based Compl Altern Med. 2016;2016:8. Article ID 7343942

Xu ZY, Fitz E, Riediger N, Moghadasian MH. Dietary octacosanol reduces plasma triacylglycerol levels but not atherogenesis in apolipoprotein E-knockout mice. Nutr Res. 2007;27:212–7.

Folk Medicine of North East India and Drug Discovery: Way to Look Forward

26

Raja Chakraborty

Contents

26.1 North East India and Its Biodiversity

Assam, Meghalaya, Tripura, Manipur, Mizoram, Arunachal Pradesh, and Sikkim are considered as North East Indian states. The area comprises only 8% of the total geographical area of India with 262,179 sq. km. Arunachal Pradesh is the largest and Sikkim is the smallest state of North East India with a geographical area of 83,743 sq. km and 7098 sq. km, respectively. Nearly 450 tribes residing in India and out of 225 tribes are from North East India. The area is also considered one of the biodiversity hotspots with a richest reservoir of plant diversity comprising about 50% of the total Indian biodiversity. The eastern range of North East India is covered with foothills of the Himalayas and is surrounded by Bangladesh, Nepal, Myanmar, China, and Bhutan (Lokho 2012; Chakraborty et al. 2012). Geographically the region can be divided into Meghalaya plateau, Brahmaputra valley, and north-eastern hills and basin. The region experience diverse climatic conditions in respect of variation in temperature (minimum 0 °C to maximum 38 °C) and rainfall (minimum 1650 mm to maximum 6320 mm).

R. Chakraborty (✉)
NEF College of Pharmacy Lokhra, Guwahati, Assam, India

S. Sen, R. Chakraborty (eds.), *Herbal Medicine in India*,
https://doi.org/10.1007/978-981-13-7248-3_26

The area can be divided into two climatic zones i.e. Alpine or Montane zone and Humid subtropical. The Alpine or Montane zone is especially for Arunachal Pradesh and Sikkim as they are situated near the Himalayas and have a montane climate with cold, mild summers and snowy winters, while the other states experience tropical climate with high humidity, low to moderate temperature. The region consists of plain plateaus, mountains, and valleys with immense climatic, altitudinal, and edaphic variety making it different with a diverse ecological habitat with richest biological values compared to other parts of India (Chatterjee et al. 2006; Mao et al. 2009; Bhutani 2008). There are different types of forests found in this region which include subtropical forests, tropical wet evergreen forests, tropical moist deciduous forests, temperate forests, alpine forests, and subtropical forests The area is rich with flora and fauna as a total of nine vegetation are found in India, six important vegetation found in North East region, and out of fifteen thousand flowering plant eight thousand found in this region which include 500 species of pteridophytes, 40 species of gymnosperms, 825 species of orchids, 80 species of rhododendrons, 60 species of bamboo, and 25 species of canes, 50 molluscs, 3624 species of insects, 236 fishes, 137 reptiles, 64 amphibians, 160 mammalian, and 850 birds species that have been reported so far. A lot of species are yet to be described (Dutta and Dutta 2006; Chatterjee et al. 2006; Eyzaguirre 1995; Forest Survey of India 2009).

26.2 North East Indian Traditional Knowledge

The region is comprised of a number of tribes from different group ethnic peoples with full of traditional knowledge. These peoples always create, harvest refines, and pass on the traditional information from one generation to another. This information is based on their instinct, need trial, and observation and experience. The information is sometimes important for their cultural identity. In this modern era still, the traditional knowledge plays an important role in their daily life health management, food, shelter, and rituals. The practice made them highly efficient to select plant parts, mode of application, dose, etc. depending on the severity and category of disease (Mao et al. 2009). It was observed that more than 250 tribes are residing in North East India that speaks more than 200 tongues. During the last 40–50 years, the researchers and government policies are finding keen interest to study about the tribes and their traditional knowledge (Mao and Roy 2016). A number of review and systemic surveys reveal that maximum medicinal plants used by the tribal peoples are locally available. Nearly 90% of the medicinal plants are from forest habitats, and few are from grasslands, agricultural pastures, and wasteland and in and around freshwater bodies, etc. The tribal peoples are having a great experience to identify and use of these medicinal plants. In spite of vast importance, the traditional knowledge is suffering a setback due to modern civilization, industrialization, and lost investment especially in urban areas. The modern world is gaining interest towards the herbal medicines, cosmetics, and supplements due to better compatibility, less side effect, cost-effectiveness, and safer treatment compared to synthetic competitors. Study and documentation of tribal traditional medicines can add new dimensions in the disease management with herbal medicine (Chakraborty et al. 2012).

26.3 Traditional Medicinal Knowledge, Medicinal Plants of India, and Drug Discovery

26.3.1 Herbal Medicine

Since the inception of modern technology and science, traditional knowledge is guiding the mankind in the discovery of new medicines. Nature bestowed its kindness on us by providing food, shelter, and other resources including medicine. It was observed that advancement of science and technology has helped us in the discovery of new medicine, but nature has provided us with the resources and traditional knowledge guiding us in this process (Chakraborty and Sen 2017). Some of the key points related to herbal medicine are as follows:

- Only 5–15% among the total 250,000 species of higher plants were investigated systematically (Sen et al. 2011).
- Still a large proportionate of Indian population are seeking the help of traditional medicine mainly in remote and rural areas (Sen et al. 2011).
- Peoples living in the cities/urban areas where the full-flagged facility of modern medicine are available also use traditional medicine particularly herbal medicine with the hope of better activity due to its lesser side effect and cost-effectiveness (Sen et al. 2011).
- In India, more than 8000 species of plants are used by around 4500 ethnic communities for medicinal purpose. In rural, peoples are using nearly 25,000 effective medicinal formulations (majorly plant based) (Sen and Chakraborty 2017).
- Development of around 80% of antimicrobial, cardiovascular, anticancer, and immunosuppressive drugs is linked with plant sources (Sen and Chakraborty 2017).
- More than 70% entities among approved 177 anticancer are connected with herbal sources (Sen and Chakraborty 2017).
- In the USA, 13 drugs were approved during 2005–2007 that are from natural origin, and clinical trials of more than 100 entities (natural source) are going on (Sen and Chakraborty 2017).

26.3.2 Medicinal Plants of India and Drug Discovery

India is known for its rich heritage of traditional medicinal knowledge and practice. Ayurveda is one of the oldest systems of medicine in medicinal literature (5000 BC–1000 BC) and considered as "Science of Life". Siddha system of medicine was developed and nurtured mainly in southern parts of India by 18 Siddhas (traditional and ancient Siddha practitioners).

In the pre-Vedic period (approx. 3000 BC–2000 BC), the Siddha system of medicine originated in the southern part of India. "Siddhas" (ancient practitioners of Siddha medicine) are believed to have developed this system which is written (Sen and Chakraborty 2015, 2017). Unani medicine originated in Greece by the great philosopher and physician Hippocrates (460–377 BC); in subsequent time, Galen (130–201 AD) and other contributors enriched this system of medicine. In 1350 AD, Arabs were instrumental in bringing Unani medicine in India (Ravishankar and Shukla 2007). Amchi and folk medicine were also practiced widely in India since the ancient time. The basic foundation of all systems is linked with nature particularly plant sources. Indian medicinal plants and medicinal knowledge always guided the mankind in the discovery of medicine. For example, use of chaulmoogra oil in leprosy is known in India since the ancient time. It is believed that the Asian Indians spared medicinal importance of chaulmoogra oil during their migration to America via Russia across the Bering Strait to Alaska (Ravina 2011). Few classic instances that involved drug discovery from Indian medicinal plants or using Indian traditional knowledge are (Mukherjee et al. 2007; Sen et al. 2011; Sen and Chakraborty 2015, 2017):

- Antihypertensive effect of Rauwolfia and isolation of alkaloid with hypotensive and CNS depressant activity
- Isolation and development of a cardiac glycoside (Peruvoside) from *Thevetia peruviana*
- Isolation of taxol (an anticancer drug) from *Taxus brevifolia.*
- *Acorus calamus, Asparagus recemosus, Azadirachata indica, Bacopa monnieri, Catharanthus roseus, Centella asiatica, Aegle marmelos, Aloe barbadensis, Boerhavia diffusa, Boswellia serrata, Cinnamomum zeylanicum, Holarrhena antidysenterica, Piper longum, Curcuma longa, Evolvulus alsionoids, Emblica officinalis, Nardostachys jatamansi, Ocimum sanctum, Rauvolfia serpentine, Zingiber officinale* and many more are well known among traditional/folk medicinal

practitioners since the ancient time, and subsequently plants were investigated and numerous new phytochemicals are isolated and used as leads to the discovery of new medicine.

- Isolation of *Bacosoides* (*Bacopa monnieri*), tylophorine (*Tylophora indica*), camptothecin (*Camptotheca acuminate*), conessine (*Holarrhena antidysenterica*), morphine and codeine (*Papaver somniferum*), sarsasapogenin and asparanin (*Asparagus adscendens*), glycyrrhizin (*Glycyrrhiza glabra*), shatavari (*Asparagus racemosus*), atropine (*Atropa belladonna*), trigonelline (*Trigonella foenum graecum*), withanolides (*Withania somnifera*), aegelin and marmelosin (*Aegle marmelos*), boeravinones (*Boerrhavia diffusa*), jatamansone (*Nardostachys jatamansi*), gingerols (*Zingiber officinale*), nimbidin (*Azadirachta indica*), diosgenin (plants of *Dioscorea* species and *T. foenumgraecum*), and vasicine and vasicinone (*Adhatoda vasica*).
- Flavopiridol and P-276-00 (semisynthetic derivatives of rohitukine) undergoing clinical trial as anticancer drug (rohitukine isolated from *Amoora rohituka* and *D. binectariferum*).

26.4 Approach Towards the New Drug Discovery in North East India

Apart from codified traditional medicinal text like Ayurveda, Siddha, and Unani, folk medicinal knowledge can play a big role in drug discovery. North East India is the habitat of a large number of ethnic groups, and a majority of populations of this area are still living in rural and comparatively rural areas away from the modern medical facility. Since the ancient time, they are utilizing their natural resources for healthcare need. Ethnic and rural communities are the hub of folk medicinal knowledge which is still largely not known to the outer world. Of course since the last few decades, researchers are focusing in this area, and documentation of folk medicinal knowledge and research based on such knowledge are going on. But such efforts constitute very small part compared to the hidden treasure of medicinal knowledge and plants available in this part, and such informations are mostly segregated not compiled together. Therefore, a systemic approach (Fig. 26.1) can make a difference in drug discovery and development in North East India which in turn also boosts the socio-economic condition of the people and state.

26.4.1 Collection of Folk Medicinal Information and Database Preparation

Collection of folk medicinal information in a systemic way is essential in current days. Ethnobotanical survey is a foremost approach to collect the data from folk medicinal practitioners or old age people. During such approach proper documentation is essential considering the following points:

- Method of folk formulation and ingredients
- Details medicinal use (single plant and combination)
- Proper authentication of plant species
- Mode of applications
- Part used
- Whether any specific season or time for collecting pant part is required
- Adjuvant approaches (like food or any other precautions during treatment)

During the survey, listing our endangered species could also be helpful for conservation purpose. Of course, a multidisciplinary approach could help in this regard. After collection of data, it should be documented systemically, and it could help to address any IPR-related issue if arises in the future. Published books, folk medicinal text written in vernacular languages, and published ethnobotanical information can also be the source of such folk knowledge of North East India and can be the source to identify important medicinal plants for further investigation/conservation. A database preparation is truly required which will include all the information of medicinal plants and folk medicinal knowledge of North East India, and subsequent research, documentation of new knowledge, and further and the new ethnobotanical survey will

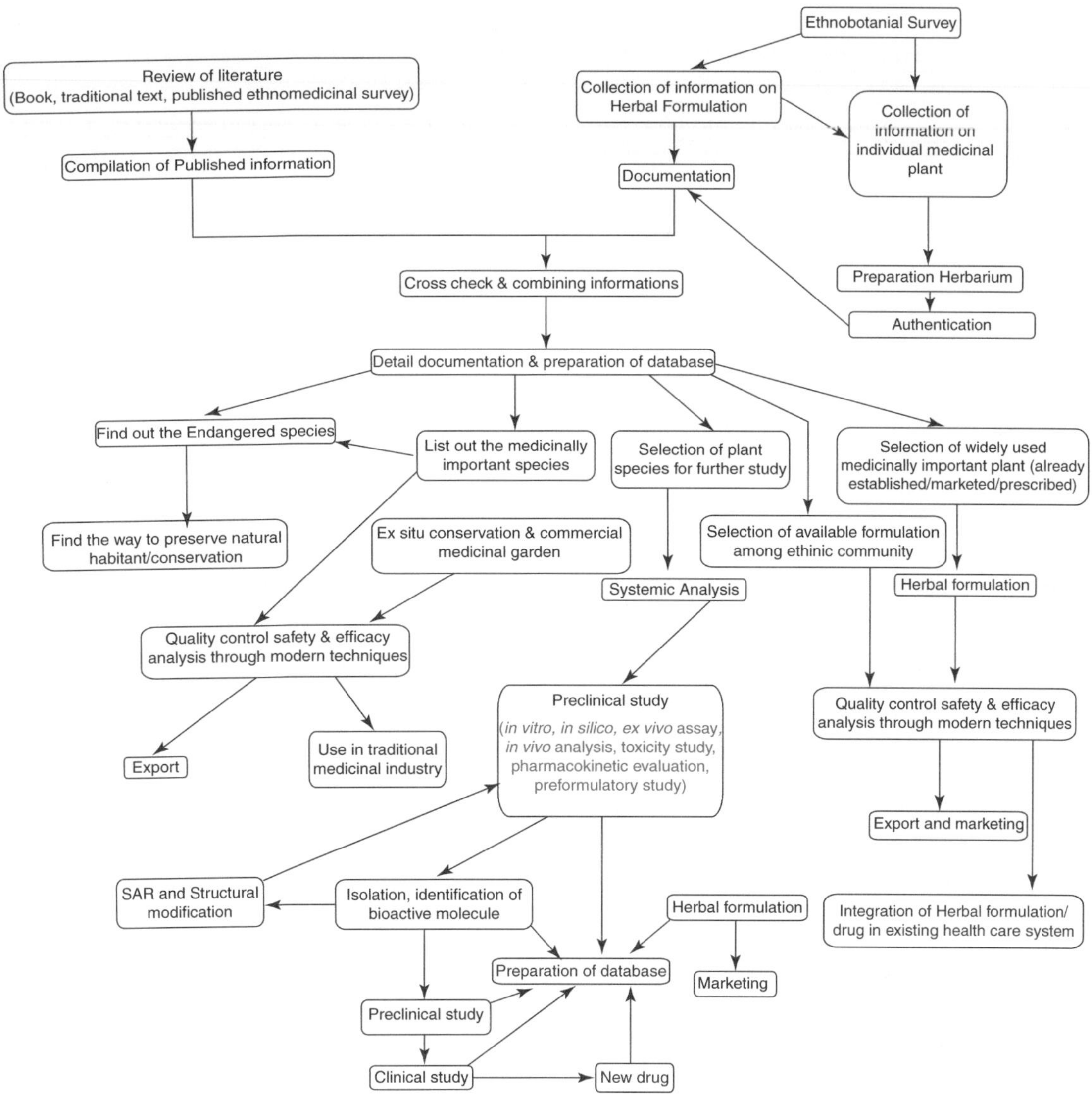

Fig. 26.1 Systemic approach towards the documentation and research on traditional medicinal plants

enrich this database. Traditional Knowledge Digital Library is a unique approach from Government of India (Sen and Chakraborty 2014), and that can guide us in preparation of such a database.

26.4.2 The Journey of Medicine from Forest to Market: A Systemic Approach

The journey of a medicine to market is an adventurous process which required time, money, knowledge, and labour. But traditional information along with reverse pharmacology and new technologies like computer-aided drug design, smart screening methods, high-throughput screening, robotic separation with structural investigation, metabolic engineering Sen and Chakraborty 2017; Li and Vederas 2009), and use of computer-based software could be helpful to save time, money, and labour.

Preclinical studies of extract, fraction, isolated biomolecules, or formulations are required before clinical trial. *In vitro*, in situ, ex vivo, and *in vivo* assays are essential along with toxicity study, pharmacokinetic and pharmacodynamic evaluation, and preformulatory study as a part of preclinical evaluation. Successful analysis of drug through clinical trial (Phase I, II, and II) is required for marketing. Of course, for traditional herbal preparation, such approaches can be minimized based on the traditional evidence. But exporting the drug and commercialization of herbal formulation in global level required strict quality control, evidence from a study on human, and research using modern techniques (Fig. 26.1). A preparation of database including the plant name, habitat, traditional knowledge, pharmacological activity, and isolated biomolecules along with therapeutic potency could help the scientists involved in such research, and this could also be useful to save time, money, and repetition of work. Recently, Mohanraj et al. (2018) came with a comprehensive, manually curated, online database named as IMPPAT which includes information of 1742 Indian medicinal plants, 9596 phytochemicals, and 1124 medicinal uses. Such an approach is truly essential in current time.

26.4.3 Future Approach and Goal to Achieve

North East India is a gold mine of traditional knowledge and medicinal plants. So, systemic documentation and research could make a lot of difference. In the current age, in spite of the discovery of new synthetic medicine and technology, we are facing a lot of problems like drug resistance, side effect and adverse effect exerted by drugs, etc. Therefore, exploration of the medicinal hidden treasure of North East India could help to find new drug molecule which is better, safer, and cost effective. Herbal formulations also can be useful for their curative and preventive purpose when people are seeking the help from traditional medicine. Integration of such traditional formulation/medicine in existing healthcare system particularly in rural areas can make a difference when all of us try to achieve the goal "Health for All". Including some herbal formulation in the National Reproductive & Child Health Programme, appointing AYUSH doctor in primary health centre under the National Rural Health Mission, and adoption of National AYUSH Mission are some essential steps in promoting herbal medicine. Identifying endangered and medicinally important species will be helpful in the conservation process. In situ and ex situ conservation and medicinal plant garden for commercial production will also help local people for socioeconomic development.

26.5 Conclusion

An interdisciplinary and multidisciplinary approach is essential to discover medicine or medicinal formulation. Treasure of medicinal plants in North East India needs special attention and a systemic collaboration and approach are needed for this purpose. IPR issue can be solved and the right of ethnic people can be preserved through documentation and preparation of the database. Besides new drug discovery protecting medicinal plants, this ensures their sustainable use and uninterrupted supply, and economic development is some key benefit of such process. We are living in a world where we can find continuous scientific advancement. Incorporation of knowledge obtained from scientific research and utilizing modern techniques will speed up the process. In conclusion, systemic and collaborative research on medicinal knowledge and medicinal plants of North East India can help to achieve a new dimension in the healthcare system.

References

Bhutani KK. Herbal Wealth of North-East India database and appraisal. Panjab: National Institute of Pharmaceutical Science and Research; 2008.

Chakraborty R, Sen S. Drug discovery – traditional medicine enthused approach. In: Das N, editor. Natural products' chemistry. New Delhi: Write & Print Publications; 2017. p. 190–205.

Chakraborty R, De B, Devanna N, Sen S. North-East India an ethnic storehouse of unexplored medicinal plants. J Nat Prod Plant Resour. 2012;2(1):143–52.

Chatterjee S, Saikia A, Dutta P, Ghosh D, Pangging G, Goswami AK. Biodiversity significance of North East

India. Forest conservation programme. New Delhi: WW-India; 2006. http://mdoner.gov.in/writereaddata/sublink3images/13Biodiversity9583338441.pdf

Dutta BK, Dutta PK. Potential of ethnobotanical studies in North East India: an overview. Indian J Tradit Knowl. 2006;4:7–14.

Eyzaguirre P. Ethnobotanical information in plant genetic resources collecting and documentation. International Plant Genetic Resources Institute (IPGRI). Unpubl; 1995.

Forest Survey of India. India State Forest Report, Govt. of India; 2009.

Li JW, Vederas JC. Drug discovery and natural products: end of an era or an endless frontier? Science. 2009;325:16. https://doi.org/10.1126/science.1168243.

Lokho A. The folk medicinal plants of the Mao Naga in Manipur, North East India. Int J Sci Res Pub. 2012;2(6):1–8.

Mao AA, Roy DK. Ethnobotanical studies in North East India: a review. In: Jain AK, editor. Indian ethnobotany: emerging trends. New Delhi: Scientific; 2016. p. 99–112.

Mao AA, Hynniewta TM, Sanjappa M. Plant wealth of Northeast India with reference to ethnobotany. Indian J Tradit Knowl. 2009;8:96–103.

Mohanraj K, Karthikeyan BS, Vivek-Ananth RP, et al. IMPPAT: a curated database of Indian medicinal plants, phytochemistry and therapeutics. Sci Rep. 2018;8:4329.

Mukherjee PK, Rai S, Kumar V, Mukherjee K, Hylands PJ, Hider RC. Plants of Indian origin in drug discovery. Expert Opin Drug Discov. 2007;2(5):633–57.

Ravina E. The evolution of drug discovery: from traditional medicines to modern drugs. Weinheim: WILEY-VCH Verlag GmbH & Co. KGaA; 2011.

Ravishankar B, Shukla VJ. Indian systems of medicine: a brief profile. Afr J Trad CAM. 2007;4(3):319–37.

Sen S, Chakraborty R. Traditional Knowledge Digital Library (TKDL): a distinctive approach to protect and promote Indian indigenous medicinal treasure. Curr Sci. 2014;106(10):1340–3.

Sen S, Chakraborty R. Towards the integration and advancement of herbal medicine: a focus on traditional Indian medicine. Bot Targ Ther. 2015;5:33–44.

Sen S, Chakraborty R. Revival, modernization and integration of Indian traditional herbal medicine in clinical practice: importance, challenges and future. J Trad Complemen Med. 2017;7:234–44.

Sen S, Chakraborty R, De B. Challenges and opportunities in the advancement of herbal medicine: India's position and role in global context. J Herb Med. 2011;1(3–4):67–75.

Part IV

Herbal Nutraceuticals and Today's Life

Wild Edible Fruits of Northeast India: Medicinal Values and Traditional Practices

27

Lalduhsanga Pachuau and Rajat Subhra Dutta

Contents

L. Pachuau (✉)
Department of Pharmaceutical Sciences, Assam University, Silchar, Assam, India

R. S. Dutta
Department of Pharmacy, Regional Institute of Paramedical and Nursing Sciences, Aizawl, Mizoram, India

S. Sen, R. Chakraborty (eds.), *Herbal Medicine in India*,
https://doi.org/10.1007/978-981-13-7248-3_27

27.1 Introduction

Wild edible fruits and vegetables are rich sources of dietary fibers, macronutrients, vitamins and, minerals, having a potential to provide healthy and balanced diet (Agrahar-Murugkar and Subbulakshmi 2005). Among the indigenous communities, wild edible fruits have always occupied a significant place, and play an important role in supplementing the diet of rural people (Sharma et al. 2015). According to the Food and Agriculture Organisation (FAO), at least one billion people around the globe are utilizing wild plants as vital part of their daily diet routine (Burlingame 2000). Studies have shown that several wild fruits contain bioactive compounds including anthocyanins and flavonoids, and elicit various activities such as free radical scavenging, antioxidant, anti-inflammatory, antimicrobial, and anticancer (Li et al. 2016). Nutritional qualities of foods from wild plants are also reported to be comparable to or even superior to their counterparts amongst the domestic cultivars (Aberoumand and Deokule 2009). As a result, these under-utilized, highly nutritious wild fruits have received renewed interest, over the past few decades, as sources of healthy balanced diet (Fig. 27.1). Significant progress has also been made in understanding their chemistry, nutritional status, and biological activities.

Northeast India comprised of eight different states – Arunachal Pradesh (AP), Assam (AS), Manipur (MN), Meghalaya (ML), Mizoram (MZ), Nagaland (NL), Sikkim (SK) and Tripura (TR). It represents about 8% of India's geographical area (Fig. 27.2). Being part of both Himalaya and Indo-Myanmar biodiversity hotspots, Northeast India has a wealth of natural resources and supports about 50% of India's plant diversity (Asati and Yadav 2004; Mao et al. 2009). The region is inhabited by extremely diverse ethnic tribal groups, and each of them has their own methods and practices in making use of the wealth of plant resources as food articles. The wild edible plants and fruits occupy a significant place in the life and traditional practices of the indigenous people living in Northeast India. Their food requirement, especially during famines and other hardship situations, have been mainly met and supplemented through produce obtained from various wild plants. Recently, more than 60 wild fruits belonging to 35 plant families from Mizoram were reported to be utilized in traditional medicine for curing various ailments including gastrointestinal disorders, dermatological and respiratory problems, cardiovascular compliance, bone diseases, allergy and malaria (Hazarika et al. 2012). Wild berries and fruits consumed by Khasi tribes of Meghalaya states were also reported to contain highly nutritious components including vitamins, minerals and healthy fibers (Agrahar-Murugkar and Subbulakshmi 2005). The antioxidant activities, the flavonoid contents and other physicochemical properties of wild edible fruits from Manipur have also been described in recent times (Sharma et al. 2015). Nutraceutical and dietary qualities of wild fruits have also been reported from Assam and Sikkim (Sarmah et al. 2018; Sundriyal and Sundriyal 2001).

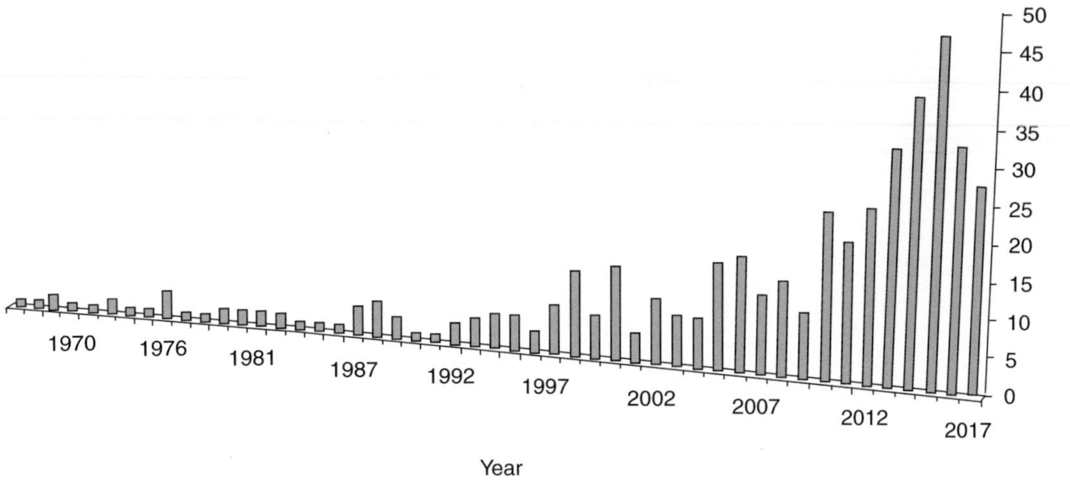

Fig. 27.1 Number of publications on 'Wild Fruits' from Pubmed search

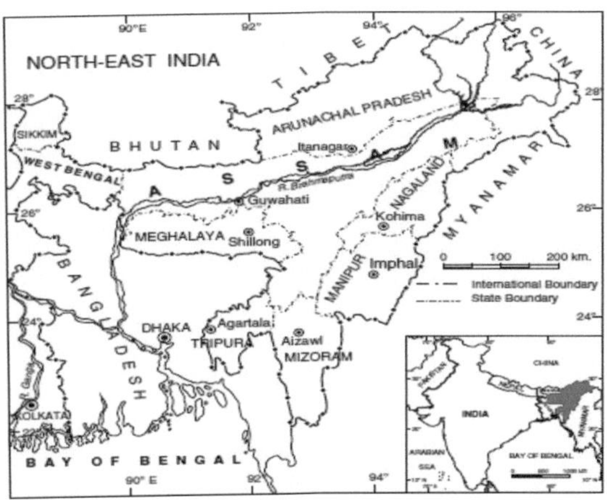

Fig. 27.2 Map of Northeast India with constituent states and capitals (Reproduced with permission from Springer Nature, Singapore ©2014)

Northeast Indian (NEI) states have been impressive in various health performance indicators. Compared to the rest of India, Northeast Indian states show much better life expectancy at birth and lower Infant Mortality Rates (IMRs) (Ghatak and Lalitha 2018). Better nutritional status in general, a lower rate of stunting, wasting and underweight among children of NEI states as compared to the rest of India has been attributed to the diversity of diet and traditional knowledge of the different tribal communities of NEI (Longvah 2013). The diet system has also been considered to be the main reason for the lower prevalence of mortality from cardiovascular diseases and the lower percentage of obesity among men and women population as shown in Table 27.1 (Longvah 2013; Ghatak and Lalitha 2018).

This chapter will discuss various traditional practices on the utilization of wild fruits from Northeast India. The prospects of these underutilized wild species of nutritious and functional dietary foods in promoting the health and economy of the region will be addressed.

27.2 Indigenous Knowledge and Practices on Wild Fruits of Northeast India

Northeast India is a land of diversity. Situated at the meeting point of the Indian, Indomalayan and Indo-Chinese biogeographical realms, it harbors unique habitats befitting biodata with illustrious endemism (Chatterjee et al. 2006). Boasting of the Himalayan and Indo-Burma Biodiversity Hotspots, the region is home to numerous plants and animals, and a paradise to ethnobotanists and anthropologists (Mao and Roy 2016). The wealth of the region towards wild relatives of crop plants has been well recognized by the National Bureau of Plant Genetic Resources (NBPGR), India and its Regional Centre in Shillong has already

Table 27.1 Body mass index (BMI) and percent obese among NEI states by gender (Ghatak and Lalitha 2018)

States	Women with BMI below normal (%)	Men with BMI below normal (%)	Women overweight or obese (%)	Men overweight or obese (%)
Arunachal Pradesh	16.4	15.2	8.8	7.1
Assam	36.5	35.6	7.8	5
Manipur	14.8	16.3	13.3	9.2
Meghalaya	14.6	14.1	5.3	5.9
Mizoram	14.4	9.2	10.6	11.4
Nagaland	17.4	14.2	6.4	5.7
Tripura	11.2	12.2	15.4	11.9
Sikkim	36.9	41.7	7.1	4.8
All India	**35.6**	**34.2**	**12.6**	**9.3**

collected over 10,000 accessions of wild relative crop plants. Out of these, about 132 are economically important crop plants such as citrus, banana, rice, and sugarcane (Mao et al. 2009). The region is, thus, a proud home to the famous citrus fruits.

Consumption of a diet rich in diversity, with emphasis on plant food, is the most universally accepted dietary recommendation for maintenance of human health (Gold and McBurney 2010). Traditional diets of the indigenous people are always rich in diversity. Due to their direct interaction with the forest over generations, the indigenous people of Northeast India, which comprised of more than 200 tribes and ethnic groups, have developed plenty of knowledge and practices for sustainable consumption of wild foods from forest resources. Out of the 300 edible plant species found in the region, large numbers of them are rich in vitamins, minerals and other bioactive components (Deka et al. 2012). These highly nutritious plant foods are an integral part of the indigenous diets.

Among the wild plants, indigenous fruits are highly important for rural communities in the developing world. They play essential roles in food security, maintenance of health and nutrition, and also their economic welfare (Cheikhyoussef and Embashu 2013). In fact, foods collected from the wild plants have an important place even in the developed world (Burlingame 2000). Gathering wild fruits and mushroom from the forest is so popular in countries such as Italy that a daily limit has to be imposed on their collection. In as much as the more exotic and domesticated fruits are, the lesser known and underutilized wild fruits are also rich in minerals like Ca, Fe, P, Mn, organic acids, vitamins and other nutrients like carbohydrates, proteins, and fats (Patel et al. 2010). The indigenous fruits of Northeast India range from tropical and sub-tropical to temperate fruits and the tribals of the region have their systems of consuming these fruits (Deka et al. 2012). Minor fruits are mostly eaten raw or prepared them into beverages, pickled or cooked with some other dishes (Patel et al. 2010). Apart from providing the much-needed nutrition, the wild fruits also serve as an additional source of income to the community (Fig. 27.3).

27.3 Wild Fruits and Their Medicinal Use in Northeast India

The multiple nutritional properties of exotic fruits such as dragon fruit, durian, apple, mango, grapes, kiwifruit and others are well known and documented (Dembitsky et al. 2011). The polyphenols, flavonoids, ascorbic acid, minerals and anthocyanin along with other bioactive components are responsible for various antioxidant radical scavenging and other medicinal properties. Strong evidence was also observed on the protective effect of fruits and vegetables on various types of cancers, especially on the pancreas and stomach cancers (Block et al. 1992). However, the major drawback with these exotic fruits is that they are highly expensive and out of reach to the common people living in the cancer-prevalent Northeast Indian regions. In this regards, wild fruits serve a potential candidate for cost-effective functional food supplements to the more costly

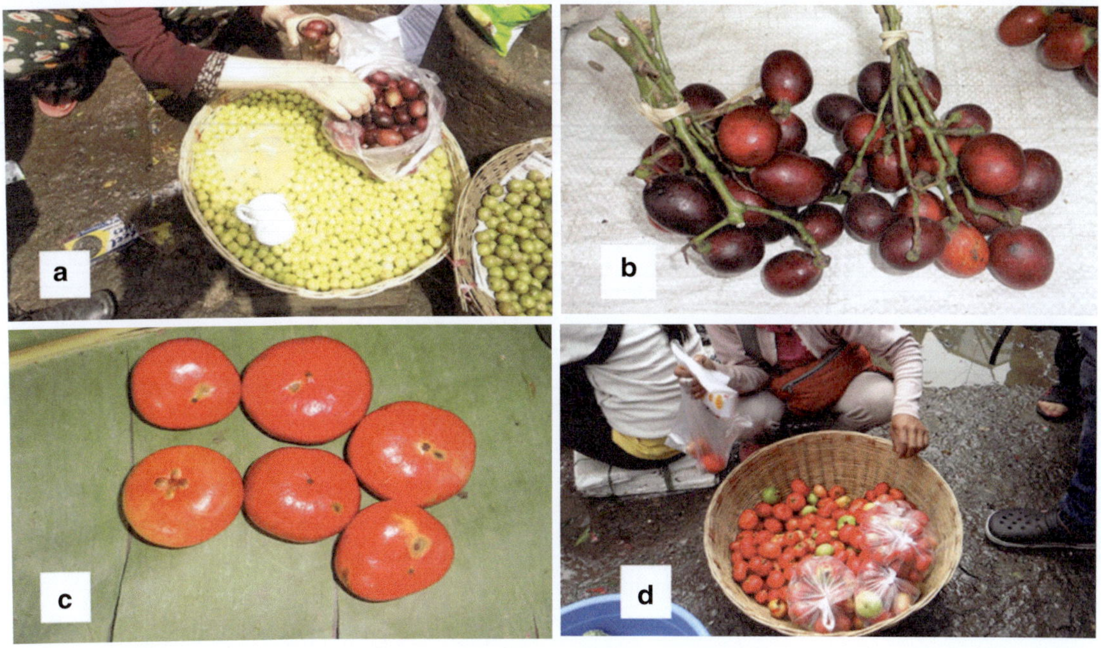

Fig. 27.3 A Mizo women selling wild fruits at a market in Zemabawk, Aizawl (Pictures were taken on 12th May, 2018. Picture (**a**) Fruits of *Phyllanthus acidus*, *P. emblica* & *Haematocarpus validus*; (**b**) Fruits of *Haematocarpus validus*; (**c**, **d**) *Garcinia lanceifolia*)

exotic fruits and vegetables. More emphasis is, therefore, needed towards the scientific exploration of the wild edible fruits of Northeast India and formulates a systematic strategy for their popularization and conservation.

There are more than 60 different wild fruits that have been used by the indigenous people of Northeast India to treat various kinds of diseases and conditions. These plant species distributed across a wide range of genera and families. Those wild fruits, the medicinal uses of which are documented in at least four different Northeastern states are only included in the current chapter.

27.3.1 *Aegle marmelos Correa*

Family: Rutaceae
Common name: Wood apple
Local/Vernacular names: Bilva (AR), Bel (AS), Heiri-khagok (MN), Soh-bel (ML), Bel-thei (MZ), Bael (SK, TR)
Description: It is a small deciduous tree. Flowering and fruiting time is between September and February.

Ethnomedicinal uses: Across the northeast region, the fruits of *E. marmelos* have been used in the treatment of various gastric problems. Both the ripe and unripe fruits are used to cure diarrhoea, stomach ulcer, dyspepsia and dysentery. In Assam, Manipur and Meghalaya, the fruit pulp is also used as a laxative. In Assam, 'Bel tea' is also prepared from the dried fruit which is used for the treatment of heart weakness (Hazarika and Singh 2018; Lalfakzuala et al. 2007; Majumdar and Datta 2009; Patiri and Borah 2007; Shankar and Rawat 2008).

27.3.2 *Annona squamosa* L.

Family: Annonaceae
Common name: Custard Apple
Local/Vernacular names: Miklang (AP), Atlas, Ata-Kathal (AS), Ata bol (ML), Thei-arbawm (MZ), Seeta phala, Swarupa, Ata (TR)
Description: It is a small tree, often cultivated, but more or less running wild. Flowering and fruiting season ranges from March to October.

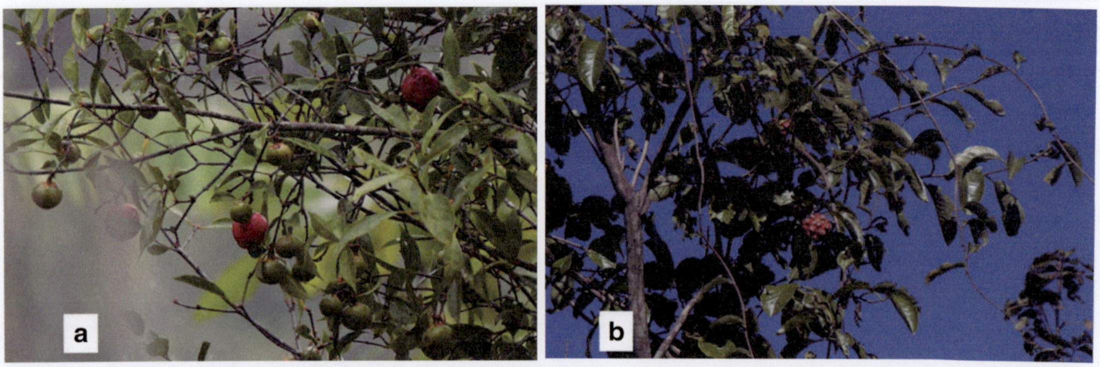

Fig. 27.4 Fruits bearing trees of (**a**) *G. lanceifolia*; (**b**) *Annona squamosa* L.

Ethnomedicinal uses: Diverse medicinal use of the fruit has been reported from different states. In ML, the fruit juice is used against indigestion. The sweet and aromatic ripe fruit is considered invigorating, sedative to heart, antiemetic and expectorant in Assam. The fruit juice is used as muscle tonic, removal of burning sensation and antiemetic in Mizoram. The fruits are also useful in diarrhoea and dysentery. In Arunachal Pradesh, the powdered seeds are taken along with fresh leaves of *Polygonum perfoltatum* in warm water to treat diabetic conditions (Hazarika et al. 2012; Majumdar and Datta 2009; Patiri and Borah 2007; Sharma et al. 2001; Tag et al. 2012; Sankaran et al. 2006; Shankar and Rawat 2008) (Fig. 27.4).

27.3.3 *Artocarpus lakoocha* Roxb.

Family: Moraceae
Common name: Monkey Jack, Lakooch
Local/Vernacular names: Belang (AR), Dewa Chali, Bohot (AS), Heiri kokthong, Keitat (MN), Armu (ML), Thei-tat (MZ), Sungyen-kung, Badar (SK), Borta, Deua (TR).
Description: Deciduous tree with a spreading crown, often cultivated but more or less running wild. Flowering and fruiting season ranges from March to October.
Ethnomedicinal uses: The ripe fruit is eaten raw and also used for the preparation of pickle. The fruit pulp is used during constipation and fever, and also as an anthelmintic. The seed is used as purgative. The powdered stem bark and the bark infusion are also applied externally for wounds, pimples and crack skins (Hazarika and Singh 2018; Lalfakzuala et al. 2007; Patiri and Borah 2007; Sharma et al. 2001)

27.3.4 *Averrhoa carambola* L.

Family: Averrhoaceae
Common name: Star fruit
Local/Vernacular names: Tanyak, Kordoi, Kurangi (AR), Kardoi (AS), Heinoujom (MN), Soh-pyrsong (ML), Thei-her-awt (MZ), Charkona (NL), Kamranga (TR).
Description: A small tree. Flowering/fruiting time is August to January.
Ethnomedicinal uses: Both the ripe and unripe fruits are eaten raw and also used for preparing jelly, pickles and squash. The fruit is used treating jaundice, kidney stone and bleeding piles. In Arunachal Pradesh, the fruit is used for treatment of diabetes (Das and Deb 2011; Hazarika and Singh 2018; Lalfakzuala et al. 2007; Patiri and Borah 2007; Sharma et al. 2001; Sharma et al. 2015; Tag et al. 2012).

27.3.5 *Baccaurea ramiflora* Lour.

Synonym: *Baccaurea sapida* (Roxb.)
Family: Euphorbiaceae
Common name: Burmese grape
Local/Vernacular names: Lateku, Khiju (AR, AS), Moktokhei (MN), Soh-ram-dieng (ML), Pangkai (MZ), Tangshi (NL), Latkan, Bhubi (TR)

Description: Middle-sized evergreen tree. Flowering/fruiting time is April to July.
Ethnomedicinal uses: The ripe fruit is eaten raw and is delicious. The fruit is used as digestive and the bark for various skin diseases. The fruit is also used for the treatment of arthritis in Nagaland. The bark and the leaves are also used for constipation and toothache, respectively (Devi et al. 2012; Hazarika and Pongener 2018; Patiri and Borah 2007; Sawian et al. 2007; Sawmliana 2013; Singh and Asha 2017).

27.3.6 *Citrus indica* Yu. Tanaka

Family: Rutaceae
Common name: Indian wild orange
Local/Vernacular names: Tsalum (AR), Narak Komla, Biurengthai (MN), Soh-kumphlair, Memang narang (ML), Ram-ser, Zawng-ser (MZ), Mejem naring (NL), Chaksi (SK).
Description: It is a shrub armed with spines.
Ethnomedicinal uses: The fruit of *C. indica* is highly valued especially in ML, due to its culinary and medicinal properties. It is used as an antidote for any kind of food poisoning, for curing hypertension, jaundice, and smallpox. The fruit juice helps in gaining appetite and possesses anthelmintic activities (Birjit et al. 2016; Hazarika and Pongener 2018; Upadhaya et al. 2016; Sawmliana 2013).

27.3.7 *Citrus grandis* L.

Synonym: *Citrus maxima* (Burm.) Merr.
Family: Rutaceae
Local/Vernacular names: Madhu Arkati (AR), Nobab (MN), Ser-tawk (MZ), Chempen (NL), Jambura, Batabi (TR).
Description: A small, evergreen tree. Flower/fruiting is year round.
Ethnomedicinal uses: The ripe fruit is fleshy, nutritive with flavor and serve as a good refrigerant. The fruit juice is used for constipation, digestive problems, cough, high blood pressure, jaundice and cardiotonic. The Mizo people use the seeds of this fruit to reduce blood sugar level in diabetes (Hazarika and Pongener 2018; Hazarika and Singh 2018; Majumdar and Datta 2009; Sankaran et al. 2006; Sawmliana 2013).

27.3.8 *Citrus macroptera* Montrouz.

Family: Rutaceae
Local/Vernacular names: Satkora (AS, TR), Heiribop (MN), Hatkora (MZ), Soh Kwit, Chambal (ML).
Description: A small evergreen tree. Flowering occurs in the months of March to May.
Ethnomedicinal uses: The fruit pulp, peels and juices are highly cherished in ML for their culinary properties. The fruit juice is used to get immediate relief from stomach disorders and fever. It is also applied as an antiseptic to cuts and wounds (Hazarika and Singh 2018; Malik et al. 2013; Upadhaya et al. 2016).

27.3.9 *Citrus medica* L.

Family: *Rutaceae*
Common name: Citron, Bara Nimbu
Local/Vernacular names: Tanyum, Narang (AR), Jara Tenga (AS), Heijaang (MN), Ser-pui (MZ), Nasu, Ongshe (NL), Bimbira (SK), Jamir, Pat lebu (TR).
Description: A small tree. Flowering/fruiting takes place from June to September.
Ethnomedicinal use: Ripe fruit is consumed raw or made into pickle. In Assam, Manipur, Mizoram and Nagaland, the fruit is considered medicinal and used against various gastric problems. The fruit and the seeds are anti-inflammatory, carminative and cardiac stimulant, and also used in blood problems and skin diseases (Angami et al. 2006; Deka et al. 2012; Hazarika and Pongener 2018; Hazarika and Singh 2018; Majumdar and Datta 2009; Patel et al. 2010; Sawmliana 2013).

27.3.10 *Dillenia indica* L.

Family: *Dilleniaceae*
Common name: Dillenia, Chalta

Local/Vernacular names: Yayo (AR), Outenge (AS), Heigri (MN), Kawrthingdeng (MZ), Ramphal, Chalta (SK), Chalta (TR).
Description: A moderate size, evergreen tree. Flowering occurs in May–June and fruiting during December–March.
Ethnomedicinal use: The mature fruit is eaten raw and also cooked as vegetable. The fruit is laxative, carminative and the mucilage obtained from the fruit is used as shampoo and drug delivery excipient. The fruit juice is used in cough, cancer and diabetes mellitus (Khatoon et al. 2012; Majumdar and Datta 2009; Patiri and Borah 2007; Sharma et al. 2001; Tag et al. 2012).

27.3.11 *Eleagnus* spp. (*E. caudate* *Schlidt Syn. E. latifolia* L., *E. pyriformis, E. umbellata* Thunb., *E. parviflora*)

Family: Eleagnaceae
Local/Vernacular names: Ganyamrap, Makhachi (AR), Selegni (AS), Heiyai (MN), Soh-shang (ML), Sar-zuk (MZ), Kotarangjang (NL).
Description: These are large, evergreen shrub. It flowers in November–January and fruiting takes place in February–May.
Ethnomedicinal use: The ripe fruits are eaten raw and used as a refreshing drink. The fruit is digestive. In Manipur, the seed is used for curing cough. In Mizoram, the root juice of *E. caudata* is given orally in rheumatic pain and also to remove retained placenta (Hazarika and Singh 2018; Kayang 2007; Sawmliana 2013; Seal 2011; Sharma et al. 2001).

27.3.12 *Euphoria longan* (Lour) (*Syn.: Dimocarpus longan* Lour, *Nephelium longana* Camb.)

Family: Sapindaceae
Common name: Litchi
Local/Vernacular names: Naga lichu, Tokra, Mirgoch (AS), Nonganhei (MN), Theifeimung (MZ), Pakojang (NL).
Description: A middle size, evergreen tree. Flowers in March–April, fruiting in July–September.
Ethnomedicinal use: The fresh fruit juice is taken against stomach problems. It is also consumed for insomnia and mental disorders in Nagaland (Hazarika and Pongener 2018; Patiri and Borah 2007; Singh et al. 2014).

27.3.13 *Ficus glomerata* Roxb. (*Syn. F. racemosa*)

Family: Moraceae
Common name: Cluster fig tree
Description: A large deciduous tree. Fruiting takes place in May–July.
Local/Vernacular names: Indung, Jagyadimoru (AP), Adumbra (AS), Charongyan (MN), Thei-chek (MZ), Mama, Yiurthi (NL), Jagga damur (TR).
Ethnomedicinal use: The fruits are eaten raw. The fruit pulp is taken for lung disease, excessive appetite, diabetes, leucoderma and menorrhagia (Angami et al. 2006; Devi et al. 2012; Hazarika and Pongener 2018; Kar et al. 2008; Singh et al. 2014; Takatemjen et al. 2009).

27.3.14 *Ficus hispida* L.

Family: Moraceae
Common name: Devil fig
Local/Vernacular names: Kukto belo, Taku, Mukongpong (AR), Dimoru (AS), Asiheibong (MN), Thamusa (ML), Thei-thawt (MZ), Nithutong, Poksok (NL), Damur (TR).
Description: A small tree; fruiting takes place throughout the year.
Ethnomedicinal use: The ripe fruits are eaten raw. The green fruits may also be cooked as vegetable. The fruits, bark and leaves are used in dysentery, diabetes and skin diseases (Kayang 2007; Mozhui et al. 2011; Sharma et al. 2001; Singh et al. 2014; Tag et al. 2012).

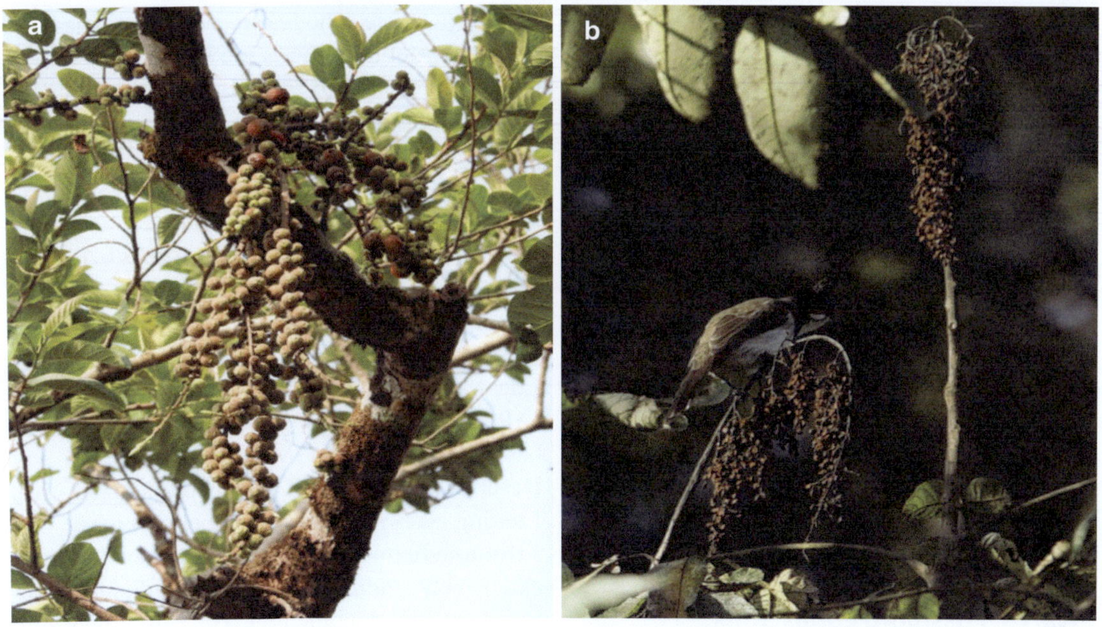

Fig. 27.5 Fruits bearing trees of (**a**) *Ficus semicordata*; (**b**) *Rhus chinensis*

27.3.15 *Ficus semicordata* (Syn. *F. cunia*)

Family: Moraceae
Common name: Drooping fig
Description: A small or middle-sized tree. Fruiting time is throughout the year.
Local/Vernacular names: Sorbek gulo, Takop (AR), Taikhro (AS), Thei-pui (MZ), Khyingothi, Koro nem (NL), Khasrey khaneu (SK).
Ethnomedicinal use: The ripe fruit is eaten raw. The fruit, latex, leaf and bark are medicinal. The latex and bark are applied on boils to check infection. The bark and the leaves are also used in jaundice, hepatitis and diabetes (Hazarika and Pongener 2018; Patiri and Borah 2007; Sawmliana 2013; Singh and Asha 2017) (Fig. 27.5).

27.3.16 *Garcinia cowa* Roxb.

Family: Clusiaceae
Common name: Cowa
Local/Vernacular names: Kau thekera (AS), Rengran (ML), Dang-kha (MZ), Aghatsa (NL), Kok (TR).
Description: A small/medium-sized tree. Fruiting occurs in November–January.
Ethnomedicinal use: Ripe fruits are sweet in taste and consumed raw or made into pickles. The fruit and leaves are used for treating dysentery and other stomach ailments (Hazarika et al. 2012; Majumdar and Datta 2009; Mozhui et al. 2011; Patiri and Borah 2007).

27.3.17 *Garcinia pedunculata* Roxb.

Family: Clusiaceae
Common name: Indian Rhubarb
Local/Vernacular names: Tabing (AR), Bor thekera (AS), Heibung (MN), Soh-danae, Thizou (ML), Vawm-vapui (MZ), Mijen, Sangselasu (NL), Baikal (TR).
Description: A large, evergreen tree. Fruiting takes place during May–June.
Ethnomedicinal use: The ripened fruits are consumed raw. The fruits are also taken orally for cardiovascular problems, dysentery, diarrhoea, dyspepsia and jaundice (Hazarika and Pongener 2018; Kagyung et al. 2010; Singh et al. 2014; Takatemjen et al. 2009).

27.3.18 *Myrica esculenta*

Family: Myricaceae
Common names: Bay berry
Local/Vernacular names: Noga tenga (AS), Dieng-soh-phie (ML), Keifang (MZ), Metiong (NL), Katusi (SK).
Description: Middle-sized evergreen tree. Fruiting occurs from April to June.
Ethnomedicinal use: The ripe fruits are eaten raw or made into pickle. It is also used to make a refreshing drink in hot weather. The fruit is consumed for indigestion. The bark juice is also used for various purposes such as antiseptic, asthma, cough, diarrhoea and dysentery (Kala 2005; Patiri and Borah 2007; Sawmliana 2013; Seal 2011).

27.3.19 *Passiflora edulis* Sims; *P. foetida* L.

Family: Passifloraceae
Common name: Passion fruit
Local/Vernacular names: Bel (AR), Soh-brap (ML), Sap-thei, Ram-sap-thei (MZ), Entsulashi (NL), Farendal, Ganlum pat (SK).
Description: A wide spreading, perennial climber. Fruiting takes place in May.
Ethnomedicinal use: The fruit is delicious, taken raw and medicinal. The fruit juice is used to make a refreshing squash drink. In Mizoram, the inner part of the fruit is taken orally in jaundice. In Arunachal, the fruit of *P. foetida* is taken for respiratory disorders. The leaves are also medicinal (Kala 2005; Sharma et al. 2001).

27.3.20 *Phyllanthus acidus* L. Roxb.

Family: Euphorbiaceae
Common name: Gooseberry
Local/Vernacular names: Pora amlokhi, Pom lokhi (AS), Kihori (MN), Kawl-sunhlu (MZ), Tsumar-lozu (NL), Hara bari, Param lakhi (TR).
Description: Small deciduous tree. Fruiting in April–June.
Ethnomedicinal use: Ripe fruits are eaten raw or used for making pickle. The fruit is consumed raw for jaundice. The leaves are used in measles, while the root decoctions are used in snake bites (Hazarika et al. 2012; Hazarika and Pongener 2018; Sankaran et al. 2006).

27.3.21 *Phyllanthus emblica* L. (Syn. *Emblica officinalis* L.)

Family: Euphorbiaceae
Common name: Amla
Local/Vernacular names: Am lokhi (AS), Amla (AR, SK, TR), Heikru (MN), Soh-mylleng, Bon bakeri (ML), Sun-hlu (MZ), Lozu (NL).
Description: A small to medium-sized tree. Fruiting takes place in November–February.
Ethnomedicinal use: Amla is one of the most extensively studied fruit and its medicinal properties are well documented. The fruit grows wild and also domesticated in most of the Northeast Indian states. The fruit is used for a variety of diseases and problems including dysentery, nose and gum bleedings, diarrhoea, liver cirrhosis, respiratory problems, indigestion, diabetes, jaundice, cough, etc. (Bhardwaj and Gakhar 2005).

27.3.22 *Prunus domestica* L. (Syn. *P. communis*)

Family: Rosaceae
Common name: Plum
Local/Vernacular names: Ahom bogori (AS), Heikha (MN), Thei-te (MZ).
Description: A small tree. Fruiting in May–July.
Ethnomedicinal use: The ripe fruit is eaten raw and is considered medicinal. The fruit is used against constipation and to enhance appetite. The crushed fruit is also used for treating asthma (Hazarika et al. 2012; Singh et al. 2014).

27.3.23 *Prunus persica* L.

Family: Rosaceae
Common name: Peach

Local/Vernacular names: Takung (AR), Nara bogori (AS), Chumbrei (MN), Thei-te-hmul (MZ), Mokori (NL).
Description: A small tree. Fruiting in May–July.
Ethnomedicinal use: The fruit is taken raw with delicacy and helps to increase appetite. Other parts of the plant such as the leaves are consumed in mild constipation and also used as anthelmintic (Hazarika and Singh 2018).

27.3.24 *Rhus semialata* Murray (*Syn. R. chinensis* Miller)

Family: Anacardiaceae
Common name: Chinese sumac
Local/Vernacular names: Amashi, Tamo (AR), Naga tenga (AS), Heimang (MN), Dieng-soh-ma (ML), Khawm-hma (MZ), Aomah, Tangmo (NL)
Description: A small, middle-sized deciduous tree. Fruiting takes place in December–January.
Ethnomedicinal use: The fruit infusion is taken as cool drink in the summer. The sour fruit is also taken raw. The fruit is used as medicine for gastro-intestinal problems, diarrhea, colic, dysentery, kidney problems, etc. (Kala 2005; Pradheep et al. 2016; Sawmliana 2013).

27.3.25 *Rubus ellipticus* Smith

Family: *Rosaceae*
Common name: Yellow Himalayan Raspberry
Local/Vernacular names: Aingku shi, Komrupsiang (AR), Borjetulipoka (AS), Heijampet (MN), Soh-pero (ML), Hmu-tau (MZ), Masujemben (NL), Aeiselu (SK).
Description: A straggling, thorny shrub. Fruiting in April–May.
Ethnomedicinal use: The fruit is eaten raw and possess excellent flavor. The fruit is highly nutritious and mildly astringent. Other parts of the plant such as leaves, shoots and roots are also used for medicinal purposes (Patiri and Borah 2007).

27.3.26 *Solanum indicum*

Family: Solanaceae
Common name: Poison berry, Bush tomato
Local/Vernacular names: Bake, Fisuk (AR), Bhot bengena, Bhekuri (AS), Soh-ngan (ML), Sam-tawk-te (MZ)
Description: Errect, perennial herb or branched shrub. Fruiting in October–January.
Ethnomedicinal use: The green fruit is cooked as a vegetable and also used as medicine to treat various conditions. The fruit juice is applied externally in herpes and also applied over painful sores. The fruit is also used against worm infection and skin diseases (Namsa et al. 2011; Sharma et al. 2001).

27.3.27 *Solanum nigrum* L.

Family: Solanaceae
Common name: Black nightshade berry
Local/Vernacular names: Bhul potting (AR), Kochi (AS), An-hling (MZ), Kalobehi (SK)
Description: An annual branching herb fruiting in the summer.
Ethnomedicinal use: The fruit, roots and leaves of this plant are used in dysentery, vomiting, asthma, bronchitis, fever, liver tonic, urinary discharge, etc. The juice of the green berry is also applied to boils, ringworms, etc. (Kala 2005; Sawmliana 2013).

27.3.28 *Spondias pinnata* (*Syn. S. mangifera* Willd.)

Family: Anacardiaceae
Common name: Hog-plum, Amra
Local/Vernacular names: Amora (AR, AS, TR), Heining (MN), Dieng-soh-pier (ML), Tawi-taw (MZ), Pako (NL).
Description: Middle-sized, deciduous tree. Fruiting in November–February.
Ethnomedicinal use: The ripe fruit is eaten raw or made into pickles. The fruit and other parts of the

plant are used for diabetes, gastrointestinal disorders, gonorrhea, liver tonic, etc. (Tag et al. 2012).

27.3.29 *Syzygium cumini* L. Skeels (Syn. *Eugenia jambolana* Lam.)

Family: Myrtaceae
Common name: Black plum, Black berry
Local/Vernacular names: Aamun (AR), Kolajamu (AS, TR), Len-hmui (MZ), Longchen (NL), Bor jam (TR).
Description: A middle-sized or large evergreen tree. Fruiting during June–July.
Ethnomedicinal use: The fruit is used for stomach problems, gums diseases, etc. The fermented liquor of the fruit is used as laxative. Seeds, leaves and barks are used for various diseases including diabetes (Sawmliana 2013).

27.3.30 *Tamarindus indica* L.

Family: Caesalpiniaceae
Common name: Tamarind, Imli
Local/Vernacular names: Teteli (AS, AR), Mange (MN), Dieng-soh-kyntoi (ML), Teng-te-re (MZ), Imli, Tentul, Amlaka (TR).
Description: A middle-sized evergreen tree. Fruiting during February–April.
Ethnomedicinal use: The sour fruit is eaten fresh or prepared as jelly pickles. In Arunachal Pradesh, the paste of the ripen pods and seeds are used in diabetes. The fruit is also taken for various gastrointestinal problems (Tag et al. 2012).

27.3.31 *Terminalia chebula* Retz.

Family: Combretaceae
Common name: Myrobalan
Local/Vernacular names: Logyo, Hilikha (AR, AS), Manakhi (MN), Re-raw (MZ), Lingka chang (NL), Haritoki (TR).
Description: Middle-sized deciduous tree. Fruiting during February–March.
Ethnomedicinal use: Both the ripe and unripe fruits are eaten raw or used as medicine. In Assam, the fruit is boiled, sliced and dried which was chewed after meal as digestive. In Arunachal Pradesh, the pulp of the fruit is chewed after meal for at least 10 days to treat diabetes. It is also used in malaria, chest pain, asthma, tooth-ache and bleeding gums (Das and Tag 2006; Tag et al. 2012; Tangjang et al. 2011).

27.3.32 *Ziziphus mairitiana* Lam. (*Syn. Z. jujube* Mill.)

Family: Rhamnaceae
Common name: Indian plum
Local/Vernacular names: Bogori, Thakri (AS), Soh-broi (ML), Borai, Kawr-sun-hlu (MZ), Pokori (NL), Kul (TR).
Description: Middle-sized, branched, deciduous tree. Fruiting during December–February.
Ethnomedicinal use: The fruit is eaten raw, dried and preserved. It is used in the preparation of curries and pickles. The fruit is used for gastrointestinal problems such as dysentery and constipation.

27.4 Conclusion

The present study showed ethnomedicinal properties of various wild fruits from Northeast India. Only fruits that are documented to have been used in at least four different states are selected. Indigenous people living in the Northeast India depend on these wild fruits as their source of nutritional supplement and a cure in times of illness. Most of the wild fruits are utilized for gastro-intestinal problems such as diarrhoea, dysentery and constipation. The mineral and fiber contents of these fruits may be attributed to their medicinal and nutritional properties. Many of the fruits, in combination with other plant parts, have also been used in the treatment of diabetes and other chronic diseases. Moreover, these wild fruits are not only medicinal and nutritious, many are rare and highly delicious. A proper chemical and pharmacological evaluation will help in getting recognition of their veritable values and help in their popularization. Systematic conservation policy will also make sure that these invaluable fruits see the future and survive the human onslaught on our environment.

Acknowledgement We are grateful to Ms. Lalnunpuii Khawlhring, Aizawl and ASEP, Mizoram, for providing us with their photographs of different wild fruits.

References

Aberoumand A, Deokule SS. Determination of elements profile of some wild edible plants. Food Anal Methods. 2009;2:116–9.

Agrahar-Murugkar D, Subbulakshmi G. Nutritive values of wild edible fruits, berries, nuts, roots and spices consumed by the Khasi tribes of India. Ecol Food Nutr. 2005;44:207–23.

Angami A, Gajurel PR, Rethy P, et al. Status and potential of wild edible plants of Arunachal Pradesh. Ind J Tradit Know. 2006;5:541–50.

Asati BS, Yadav DS. Diversity of horticultural crops in North Eastern Region. ENVIS Bull Himalayan Ecol. 2004;12:4–14.

Bhardwaj S, Gakhar SK. Ethnomedicinal plants used by the tribals of Mizoram to cure cut and wounds. Ind J Trad Know. 2005;4:75–80.

Birjit RK, Khonachand S, Sony N et al. Report of the rapid biodiversity assessment field survey at Longku forest, Dailong village, Tamenglong District, Manipur. Government of Manipur: Manipur Biodiversity Board; 2016

Block G, Patterson B, Subar A. Fruit, vegetables, and cancer prevention: a review of the epidemiological evidence. Nutr Cancer. 1992;18:1–29.

Burlingame B. Wild nutrition. J Food Compos Anal. 2000;13:99–100.

Chatterjee S, Saikia A, Dutta P, et al. Biodiversity significance of Northeast India. Forests Conservation Programme. New Delhi: WWF-India; 2006.

Cheikhyoussef A, Embashu W. Ethnobotanical knowledge on indigenous fruits in Ohangwena and Oshikoto regions in Northern Namibia. J Ethnobiol Ethnomed. 2013;9:34.

Das AK, Tag H. Ethnomedicinal studies of the Khamti tribes of Arunachal Pradesh. Ind J Tradit Know. 2006;5:317–22.

Das SC, Deb AK. Studies of bio-diversity of medicinal plants and their prospects and problems in Tripura. Ann Pharm Pharm Sci. 2011;2:62–71.

Deka BC, Thirugnanavel A, Patel RK, et al. Horticultural diversity in North-East India and its improvement for value addition. Indian J Genet. 2012;72:157–67.

Dembitsky VM, Poorvarodom S, Leontowicz H, et al. The multiple nutrition properties of some exotic fruits: biological activity and active metabolites. Food Res Int. 2011;44:1671–701.

Devi N, Sarma GC, Baishya SK. Wild edible fruits of Pakke Tiger Reserve in Arunachal Pradesh, India. Pleione. 2012;6:348–52.

Ghatak A, Lalitha N. Health in north-eastern states of India: an analysis of economic vulnerabilities. In: De UK, Pal M, Bharati P, editors. Issues on health and healthcare in India—focus on the north eastern region. Singapore: Springer Nature; 2018. p. 127–62.

Gold K, McBurney RPH. Conservation of plant biodiversity for sustainable diets. In: Burlingame B, Dernini S, editors. Sustainable diets and Biodiversity. Rome: FAO; 2010. p. 108–14.

Hazarika TK, Lalramchuana, Nautiyal BK. Studies on wild edible fruits of Mizoram, India used as ethnomedicine. Genet Resour Crop Evol. 2012;59:1767–76.

Hazarika TK, Pongener M. Potential wild edible fruits of Nagaland, North-east India and its significance in the livelihood and nutritional security of rural, indigenous people. Genet Resour Crop Evol. 2018;65:199–215.

Hazarika TK, Singh TS. Wild edible fruits of Manipur, India: associated traditional knowledge and implications to sustainable livelihood. Genet Resour Crop Evol. 2018;65:319–32.

Kagyung R, Gajurel PR, Rethy P, et al. Ethnomedicinal plants used for gastro-intestinal diseases by *Adi* tribe of Dehang-Debang biosphere reserve in Arunachal Pradesh. Indian J Tradit Know. 2010;9:496–501.

Kala CP. Ethnomedicinal botany of the Apatani in the Eastern Himalayan region of India. J Ethnobiol Ethnomed. 2005;1:11.

Kar A, Borkataki S, Borthakur SK. Wild edible fruits of the Karbi's of Karbi Anglong district of Assam, India. Pleione. 2008;2:175–81.

Kayang H. Wild edible fruits of Manipur, India: associated traditional knowledge and implications to sustainable livelihood. Indian J Tradit Know. 2007;6:177–81.

Khatoon R, Singh PK, Das AK, et al. Indigenous wild edible fruits for Kom tribe in Manipur, India. Pleione. 2012;6:268–72.

Lalfakzuala R, Lalramnghinglova H, Kayang H. Ethnobotanical usages of plants in western Mizoram. Ind J Tradit Know. 2007;6:486–93.

Li Y, Zhang JJ, Xu DP, et al. Bioactivities and health benefits of wild fruits. Int J Mol Sci. 2016;17:1258.

Longvah T. Biodiversity, food systems and nutritional status of the indigenous people of Northeast India. Ann Nutr Metab. 2013;63.(Suppl. 1:125.

Majumdar K, Datta BK. Traditional wild edible fruits for the forest dwellers of Tripura, India. Pleione. 2009;3:167–78.

Malik SK, Uchoi A, Kumar S, et al. Molecular characterization of *Citrus macroptera* Montr.(Satkara): an endangered wild species from northeast India. Plant Biosyst. 2013;147:857–63.

Mao AA, Hynniewta TM, Sanjappa M. Plant wealth of Northeast India with reference to ethnobotany. Indian J Tradit Know. 2009;8:96–103.

Mao AA, Roy DK. Ethnobotanical studies in North East India: a review. In: Jain AK, editor. Indian ethnobotany: emerging trends. Jodhpur: Scientific Publishers; 2016. p. 99–112.

Mozhui R, Rongsensashi L, et al. Wild edible fruits used by the tribals of Dimapur district of Nagaland, India. Pleione. 2011;5:56–64.

Namsa ND, Mandal M, Tangjang S, et al. Ethnobotany of the Monpa ethnic group at Arunachal Pradesh, India. J Ethnobiol Ethnomed. 2011;7:31.

Patel RK, De LC, Singh A, et al. Lesser known edible fruits of North Eastern India. In: Peter KV, editor. Underutilized and underexploited horticultural crops, vol 5. New Delhi: New India Publishing Agency; 2010. p. 163–73.

Patiri B, Borah A. Wild edible plants of Assam. Assam: Director Forest Communication, Forest Department; 2007.

Pradheep K, Soyimchiten PA, et al. Wild edible plants used by Konyak tribe in Mon district of Nagaland: survey and inventorisation. Indian J Nat Prod Resour. 2016;7:74–81.

Sankaran M, Prakash J, Singh NP, et al. Wild edible fruits of Tripura. Nat Prod Rad. 2006;5:302–5.

Sarmah P, Dutta S, Sarma A. Phyto-chemical properties of *Momordica cochinchinensis* Spreng: an underutilised wild edible fruit from Cachar Hills, Assam. Agrofor Syst. 2018;92:85–9.

Sawian JT, Jeeva S, Lyndem FG, et al. Wild edible plants of Meghalaya, Northeast India. Nat Prod Rad. 2007;6:410–26.

Sawmliana M. The book of Mizoram plants. Aizawl: P. Zakhuma; 2013.

Seal P. Antioxidant activity of some wild edible fruits of Meghalaya state in India. Adv Biol Res. 2011;5:155–60.

Shankar R, Rawat MS. Medicinal plants used in traditional medicine in Lohit and Dibang valley districts of Arunachal Pradesh. Ind J Tradit Know. 2008;7:288–95.

Sharma HK, Chhangte L, Dolui AK. Traditional medicinal plants in Mizoram, India. Fitoterapia. 2001;72:146–61.

Sharma PB, Handique PJ, Devi HS. Antioxidant properties, physico-chemical characteristics and proximate composition of five wild fruits of Manipur, India. J Food Sci Technol. 2015;52:894–902.

Singh AV, Asha H. Wild edible fruits of Arunachal Pradesh. Int J Innov Res Sci Eng Technol. 2017;6:12203–9.

Singh SR, Phurailatpam AK, Wangchu L, et al. Traditional medicinal knowledge of underutilized minor fruits as medicine in Manipur. Int J Agri Sci. 2014;4:241–7.

Sundriyal M, Sundriyal RC. Wild edible plants of the Sikkim Himalaya: nutritive values of selected species. Econ Bot. 2001;55:377–90.

Tag H, Kalita P, Dwivedi P, et al. Herbal medicines used in the treatment of diabetes mellitus in Arunachal Himalaya, northeast, India. J Ethnopharmacol. 2012;141:786–95.

Takatemjen, Jamir NS, Deb MS. Wild edible fruits of Wokha District of Nagaland, India. Pleione. 2009;3:59–62.

Tangjang S, Namsa ND, Aran C, et al. An ethnobotanical survey of medicinal plants in the Eastern Himalayan zone of Arunachal Pradesh, India. J Ethnopharmacol. 2011;134:18–25.

Upadhaya A, Chaturvedi SS, Tiwari BK. Utilization of wild *Citrus* by *Khasi* and *Garo* tribes of Meghalaya. Ind J Tradit Know. 2016;15:121–7.

Fruits of Indian Subcontinent and Their Health Benefits

28

Jiwan S. Sidhu and Tasleem A. Zafar

Contents

J. S. Sidhu (✉)
Masters' Program in Food and Environmental Toxicology, Department of Food Science and Nutrition, College of Life Sciences, Kuwait University, Safat, Kuwait

T. A. Zafar
Masters' Program in Food Science & Nutrition, Department of Food Science & Nutrition, College of Life Sciences, Kuwait University, Safat, Kuwait

S. Sen, R. Chakraborty (eds.), *Herbal Medicine in India*,
https://doi.org/10.1007/978-981-13-7248-3_28

28.1 Indian Gooseberry (*Phyllanthus emblica*)

Amla or Indian Gooseberry (*Emblica officinalis* Gaertn or *Phyllanthus emblica* L.) is a deciduous tree that commonly grows in several Asian countries such as in the tropical and subtropical parts of India, China, Indonesia, and Malaysia. Amla tree can grow well even on soils of low fertility level and with little rainfall. Amla fruit is one of the richest sources of vitamin C (Raghu et al. 2007), and it can be processed into various products such as pickles, jam, preserve (*murabba*) in thick sugar syrup, candy, powder, and as juice or beverages (Chinprahast et al. 2013). Health-promoting nutraceuticals such as polyphenols, tannins, and pectin have been reported from many of the edible fruits grown in the Indian Himalayan region (Tsai et al. 2014; Bhatt et al. 2017; Kumar et al. 2017). The antioxidants from amla have been used as a film coating on roasted cashew nuts to enhance their shelf life (Suppakul et al. 2016). An exhaustive review is available on the chemistry and technology of amla fruit in one of the earlier publications (Sidhu and Zafar 2012) (Fig. 28.1).

28.1.1 Medicinal Uses

Amla fruit, being rich in many health-promoting nutraceuticals, has been used for treating many medical conditions such as improving cardiorespiratory status among people with smoking history (Biswas et al. 2014), providing gastroprotective effects in patients with gastrointestinal disorders (Iqbal et al. 2017b), and providing protective effects on retinal degeneration in a well-characterized animal model of Alzheimer disease (Jang et al. 2017). Cardiovascular dis-

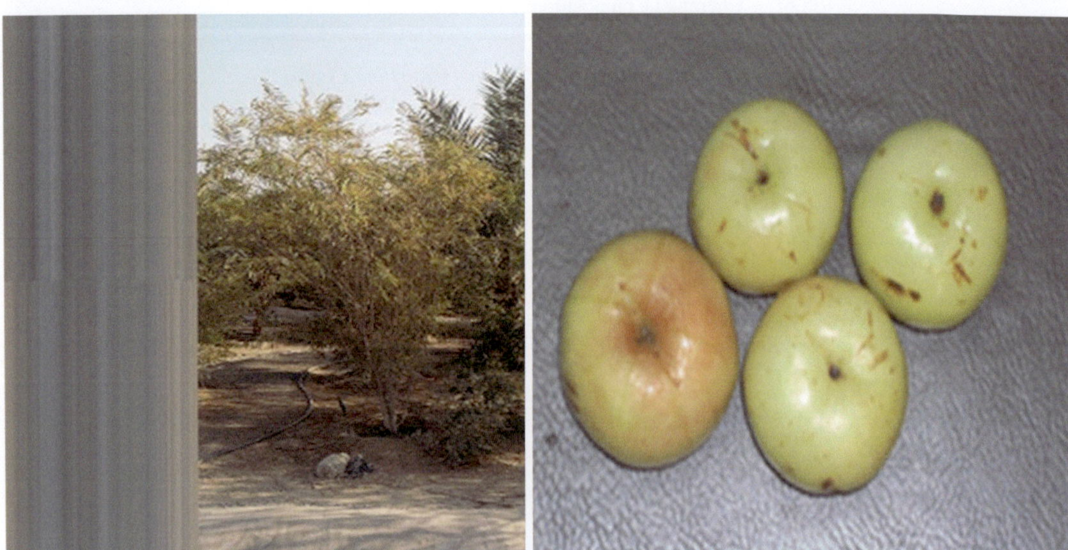

Fig. 28.1 Amla tree and fruits (Photo source: Prof. Jiwan S. Sidhu)

eases in patients with diabetes are a leading cause of morbidity and mortality, all due to multiple risk factors. Fatima et al. (2014) have used amla extracts in combination with clopidogrel and ecosprin in patients with type-II diabetes to inhibit platelet aggregation. In a recent study, Srinivasan et al. (2018) have investigated the antidiabetic activity of quercetin extracted from amla fruit, especially, with various diabetes-related protein targets, such as glycogen phosphorylase and peroxisome proliferator-activated receptor gamma. According to their findings, quercetin is a potential drug with antidiabetic and antihyperglycemic actions mediated by changes in the level of glucose, cholesterol, and triglycerides in diabetic animals.

The incidences of various types of cancers, such as breast, uterus, ovarian, and colon, have been on the rise the world over. These diseases have been associated with various risk factors such as hormones, high fat intake, and reactive oxygen species. Amla fruit is one of the best natural sources of vitamin C, and contains many health-promoting phytochemicals, which can provide protection against these diseases. Vaithiyanathan and Mirunalini (2013) have confirmed by histopathology and immunohistochemistry analysis that the active constituents in amla fruit could suppress mammary tumors, and this fruit can be used as a pharmaceutical tool in cancer subjects. Lately, Vadde et al. (2016) have evaluated the antiproliferative and pro-apoptotic mechanism of amla fruit extract on human colon cancer stem cells (HCCSC) and indicated that this may be due to its effect on Wnt/β-catenin signaling. Their results showed that amla fruit extract suppresses HCCSC proliferation and induces apoptosis independent of p53 status through potentially targeting the Wnt/β-catenin signaling pathway, thus proving amla to be a useful functional food for consumers to obtain protection against colon cancer.

Some of the cancer treatment drugs (used in chemotherapy) have been shown to have side effects. Nephrotoxicity is the major limitation of one of the important drugs, cisplatin. Purena et al. (2018) have studied the use of hydroethanolic amla leaf extract in preventing cisplatin-induced nephrotoxicity in rats. According to their results, the leaf extract of amla significantly attenuated the renal damage by decreasing serum creatinine and blood urea nitrogen, enhanced the activities of catalase, superoxide dismutase, glutathione peroxidase, glutathione reductase, and decreased renal MDA levels compared with the chemo drug cisplatin. The extract of amla fruit in combination with *Alpinia galanga* rhizomes have been used to reduce the hydrogen peroxide-induced oxidative stress and lipid peroxidation in human epithelial cell lines (Chansriniyom et al. 2018).

Another common condition of injury to the liver with histopathological abnormalities including steatosis with inflammation and fibrosis is known as nonalcoholic steatohepatitis (NASH). Methionine and a choline-deficient diet, oxidative stress, lipid peroxidation, and pro-inflammatory cytokines are implicated in the progression of NASH to fibrosis, but the administration of amla fruit extract has been suggested to ameliorate the rapid progression of NASH (Lu et al. 2016; Tung et al. 2018). In an interesting study, Khan et al. (2018a, b) have recently compared the efficacy of amla fruit extract with procaine penicillin in the treatment of subclinical mastitis in dairy buffaloes. Their results showed that amla fruit extract is an inexpensive source in the treatment of subclinical mastitis in dairy animals and can be used as an alternative to procaine penicillin therapy.

28.2 Pomegranate (*Punica granatum* L.)

Pomegranate (*Punica granatum* L.) is a unique fruit belonging to the family of Punicaceae. Pomegranate grows well in semi-arid, mild-temperate to subtropical climates and is naturally adapted to regions with cool winters and hot summers. The tree size ranges from a large shrub to a small tree and grows 5–8 m tall. Although pomegranate is native to Persia and Himalayan regions, it is widely cultivated since ancient times throughout the Mediterranean regions of Asia, Africa and Europe. The most important growing countries include Iran, Afghanistan, Azerbaijan, Pakistan, India,

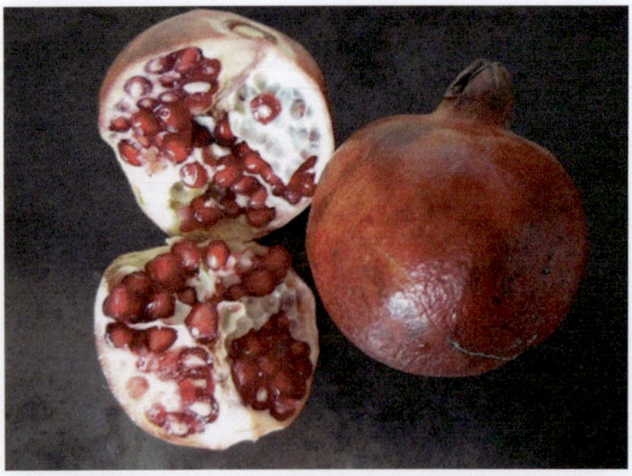

Fig. 28.2 Pomegranate fruit with arils (Photo source: Prof. Jiwan S. Sidhu)

Table 28.1 Phytochemicals in various parts of pomegranate fruit

Pomegranate part	Active phytochemical	Reference
Seed, bark, and leaves	Lignins, sterols, and terpenoids	Lansky and Newman (2007)
Seed oil	Fatty acids and triglycerides	Lansky and Newman (2007)
Juice	Organic acids	Ender et al. (2002)
Rind	Flavonols	Kim et al. (2002)
Fruit	Flavonols	Mirdehghan and Rahemi (2007)
Juice, seeds, and peel extracts	Estrogens	Kho et al. (2010)

Bangladesh, Egypt, Iraq, China, Burma, Malaysia, Turkey, Yemen, and Saudi Arabia. The Spanish settlers introduced this tree to the United States in 1769, and these are grown mainly in California and Arizona for juice production (Anon 2018; Mustafa and Dogan 2018).

The fruit is nearly round but crowned at the tip ranging from 2½ to 5 in. in diameter with tough leathery skin, with rind having yellowish to red color (Fig. 28.2). The interior of the fruit is separated by whitish spongy membranous walls into compartments that are packed with juicy arils. Pomegranate arils are pinkish to red in color. The tartness or sweetness varies depending upon the cultivars and region from where the fruit comes. Depending on the cultivar, each aril may contain a soft to hard white or red angular seed, which accounts for about 52% of the weight of the whole fruit (Morton 1987a).

28.2.1 Antioxidants in Pomegranate

Pomegranate fruit is known to have very high antioxidant activity as it is rich in total phenolics, flavonoids, and flavonols (Table 28.1). The peel is richer in these phenolic compounds than even the seeds and juice (Derakhshan et al. 2018). The ultrasound-assisted extraction of polyphenolic compounds from pomegranate peel has been employed to obtain higher amounts of biologically active phenolics than seeds or juice (Zivkovic et al. 2018). Ambigaipalan et al. (2017) have identified several bioactive phenolic antioxidants from pomegranate juice and seeds using HPLC-DAD-ESI-MS technique. These phenolics inhibited the DNA damage due to hydroxy and peroxyl radicals, copper-induced LDL-cholesterol peroxidation, and α-glucosidase and lipase activities. As the pomegranate peel contains 10-fold higher content of phenolics than the pulp, green extraction of polyphenols from whole fruit with cyclodextrins has been employed by Diamanti et al. (2017) and obtained 20% higher yield. Extraction techniques have been reported to have a significant effect on the antioxidant capacities and phytochemical composition of polyphenol-rich extracts from pomegranate fruits (Castro-Lopez et al. 2017; Xi et al. 2017). Determination of the quality of pomegranate fruit using surface microstructure, surface roughness, and glossiness by noninvasive luster sensor technology has been suggested by Czieczor et al. (2018) which can be used in the postharvest technology of this fruit. Using 25% maltodextrin level and at 124 °C temperature, a nutritionally rich, spray-dried pomegranate juice powder with high water solubility index of 95%, high density of 0.889 g cm^{-3}, and anthocyanin content of 8 mg L^{-1} has been produced, which can find uses in the development of functional foods (Jafari et al. 2017).

Derakhshan et al. (2018) carried out an evaluation of antioxidant activity using different pomegranate cultivars.

- Total flavonols, total flavonoids, total phenolics, and antioxidant activity of Natanz peel is 25 ± 5.43 mg rutin/g, 36 ± 3.56 mg rutin/g, 276 ± 12.69 mg GAE/g, and 45 ± 9.9%, respectively.
- Total flavonols, total flavonoids, total phenolics, and antioxidant activity of Natanz seed is 8.02 ± 1.58 mg rutin/g, 30.5 ± 6.38 mg rutin/g, 72.4 ± 10.02 mg GAE/g, and 34 ± 4.06%, respectively.
- Total flavonols, total flavonoids, total phenolics, and antioxidant activity of Natanz seed is 1.5 ± 1.0 mg rutin/g, 1.8 ± 1.03 mg rutin/g, 23.8 ± 6.74 mg GAE/g, and 10 ± 3.24%, respectively.
- Total flavonols, total flavonoids, total phenolics, and antioxidant activity of Shahreza peel is 37 ± 8.51 mg rutin/g, 45 ± 6.25 mg rutin/g, 361 ± 12.87 mg GAE/g, and 50 ± 10.86%, respectively.
- Total flavonols, total flavonoids, total phenolics, and antioxidant activity of Shahreza seed is 3.4 ± 1.24 mg rutin/g, 7.55 ± 2.12 mg rutin/g, 73 ± 13.35 mg GAE/g, and 26 ± 6.14%, respectively.
- Total flavonols, total flavonoids, total phenolics, and antioxidant activity of Shahreza seed is 1.5 ± 0.9 mg rutin/g, 2.14 ± 0.92 mg rutin/g, 215.8 ± 5.81 mg GAE/g, and 9 ± 2.84%, respectively.

Research carried out by Derakhshan et al. (2018) showed that of peel extract, seed extract and juice of different pomegranate cultivar possess significant total flavonols, total flavonoids, total phenolics and showed potent antioxidant activity.

28.2.2 Medicinal Applications

Antioxidant capacity, immune-boosting, and anticarcinogenic properties are the major reasons for pomegranate to have risen to such fame for its medical applications. Recently, nanotechnology applications of pomegranate for biosynthesizing different nanoparticles and developing newer drug delivery systems, such as nanoemulsion, nanoparticles, nanoliposomes, phytosomes, nanovesicles, and niosomes; along with pomegranate's chemical compositions; antibacterial properties and their mechanisms; anticancer properties; and its medicinal applications have been reviewed by Karimi et al. (2017). A food-grade self-nano-emulsifying delivery system for enhancing the oral bioavailability of ellagic acid from pomegranate has been developed by Wang et al. (2017).

Elzayat et al. (2018) have studied the wound-healing activity of henna, pomegranate, and myrrh herbal ointment blend, which showed antimicrobial activity against *Candida*, *Staphylococcus aureus*, *E. coli*, and mucous membrane infections. Pomegranate fruit extract has been shown to inhibit pro-inflammatory cytokines (TNF-α and IL-6) and anti-angiogenic factors (sFlt-1 and sEng) due to plasma stimulus of patients suffering from severe preeclampsia (Ambarwati et al. 2017; Nasifah et al. 2017). A chitin-binding lectin found in pomegranate juice has been reported to possess antifungal activity against *Candida albicans* and *Candida krusei* (da Silva et al. 2018). The action mechanism involved in this activity is oxidative stress, energetic collapse, and damage to the cell wall, leading to the rupture of yeast cells. Pomegranate peel extract when used at higher concentrations killed cariogenic bacteria, *Streptococcus mutans*; however, at sub-bactericidal concentrations, it did reduce the biofilm formation and acid and extracellular polysaccharide production (Gulube and Patel 2016). Wafa et al. (2017) have investigated the use of pomegranate peel, seeds, juice, and flowers against *Salmonella enterica* in chicken meat. They reported that the peel extract had the highest antimicrobial activity against this pathogen than the other parts.

The pomegranate peel extract has recently been studied for its anticoccidial activity for controlling the incidence of coccidiosis in poultry birds (Ahad et al. 2018). They found that the ethanol extract of pomegranate peel has an active ingredient which offers a significant potential to control coccidian parasites in chicken. An active ingredient, quercetin, has been identified through HPLC and GC-MS analysis in pomegranate peel which can be effectively used to control *Microcerotermes beesoni* (a termite). Pomegranate peel being a waste material from the processing industry and easily available can, thus, be utilized as a natural termite-managing agent by farmers around the world (Mishra et al. 2017). Pomegranate peel extracts have been shown to exhibit anthelmintic activity against *Ascaridia galli* (Aziz et al. 2018).

The inhibitory effect of an antitumor polysaccharide (a galactomannan) from pomegranate peel on metastasis has also been reported by Varghese et al. (2017). The extract from pomegranate peel has also been shown to induce apoptosis and impairs metastasis of prostate cancer cells (Deng et al. 2017). In another study, pomegranate wine polyphenols have been shown to affect Nef2 activation and antioxidant enzyme expression in human neuroblastoma cells (SH-SY5Y) by increasing heme oxygenase (HO-1) expression and SOD activity (Li et al. 2017a). Thus, pomegranate polyphenolics may have a protective effect on neurons by increasing Nrf2 and inhibiting NF-κβ signaling. The mesocarp extract from pomegranate has been shown to suppress the advanced glycation end products (AGEs) and H_2O_2-induced oxidative stress and pro-inflammatory biomarkers, such as NF-κβ, iNOS, and IL-6, and reduced adipose tissue inflammation with the propensity to mitigate obesity-related insulin resistance and type II diabetes (Les et al. 2017; Ramlagan et al. 2017). Pomegranate peel as a food industry waste material can be used as a low-cost natural source of biologically active phytochemicals for their antioxidant, antidiabetic, and antineurodegenerative properties (Savikin et al. 2018). Pomegranate peel extract has been shown to suppress colon cancer by downregulating Wnt/β-catenin in rat model (Ahmed et al. 2017). Pomegranate seeds have been reported to possess the highest antioxidant activity when compared with tomato and grape seeds (Dureante et al. 2017). Pomegranate pulp silage when fed to dairy cows up to 150 g/kg DM did not affect the milk yield and chemical composition but improved the milk fatty acid profile and blood plasma antioxidant status (Kotsampasi et al. 2017). Punicalagin, a polyphenolic compound from pomegranate fruit, is shown to induce growth inhibition and apoptosis in human PC-3 and LNCaP prostate cancer cells (Adaramoye et al. 2017).

Most urinary calculi (stones) are usually made of calcium oxalate, occurring mainly in two crystalline forms: calcium oxalate monohydrate and calcium oxalate dihydrate. Pomegranate juice was found to be highly effective in the prevention of urinary calculi (Kachkoul et al. 2018). Punicalagin extracted from pomegranate peel has shown inhibitory effects against type II collagenase-induced osteoarthritis (Lee et al. 2018). They suggested the use of punicalagin from pomegranate peel as an active ingredient for developing functional foods for knee-related diseases. A systematic review and meta-analysis of randomized controlled trials on the effects of pomegranate juice on blood pressure have recently been published (Sahebhar et al. 2017). This meta-analysis suggested the consistent benefits of pomegranate juice consumption on blood pressure, and the review suggested the inclusion of pomegranate juice in the heart-healthy diet as a prudent approach.

Pomegranate has also been investigated to improve the quality of a few processed products. The impact of adding lyophilized pomegranate peel nanoparticles (LPP-NPs) as an antioxidant and antimicrobial agent in meatballs during storage at chilling temperatures for 5 days has recently been investigated by Morsy et al. (2018). According to their results, the LPP-NPs were found to be more effective in retarding lipid oxidation and improving the microbial quality and cooking characteristics of meatballs. Jam prepared from pomegranate peel was found to be less firm than the commercial pectin but had more reddish color and better sweetness score (Abid et al. 2018). Lan et al. (2017) have investigated the antioxidant properties and flavor profile of pomegranate wine using E-nose and E-tongue to monitor odor and taste changes during the brewing process. They have suggested the use of this technology for improving the functional features and quality control of pomegranate wine manufacture.

28.3 Jamun (*Syzygium cumini*), the Indian Blackberry

Syzygium is a large genus from the Myrtaceae family, having many species of evergreen flowering plants, and is native to the Indian subcontinent but now widespread in the tropical and subtropical regions of Southeast Asia, Africa, and Australia. The tree has a long duration up to 100 years and can grow up to a height of 30 m. In India, it bears fruits during the month of July–August. Even the leaves have good nutritional value and are used as cattle feed. The mature fruit has dark purple color, sweet, slightly sour and astringent flavor, but when eaten makes the tongue turn purple (Fig. 28.3).

28.3.1 Antioxidants in Jamun

The jamun fruit is rich in carotenoids, vitamin C, terpenoids, and phenolic compounds as reported by Faria et al. (2011) when analyzed for antioxidant capacity using HPLC-DAD-MS/MS. The anthocyanin composition was characterized by the presence of 3,5-diglucosides. The major carotenoids were found to be all-trans-lutein and all-trans-β-carotene. The trolox equivalent antioxidant capacity (TEAC) values indicated that the hemiacetals/chalcones and quinonoidal bases species possessed higher free-radical scavenging capacity as compared to flavylium cations. New triterpenoid compounds, 2-O-cis-p-coumaroyl maslinic acid along with other thirteen known terpenoids, have been reported by Li et al. (2017b). According to their results, the triterpenoid may play an important role in the antidiabetic properties of the jamun fruit. Nutritional profile and molecular fingerprinting of locally grown black jamun from western parts of India have been reported by Gajera et al. (2018). Large fruits had higher amount of moisture, total fat, sugar, protein, starch and free amino acids, whereas small fruits contained higher amounts of ascorbic acid, anthocyanins, crude fiber, and total phenolics in their fruit pulp and seed part. One of the methanolic extract fraction from jamun fruit was found to be rich in rutin and ellagic acid and exhibited highly significant antioxidant activity as well as antibacterial activity against *Escherichia coli*, *Salmonella typhi*, and *Staphylococcus aureus* at 100 mg/ml concentrations (Sathyanarayanan et al. 2018). The stability of anthocyanins and anthocyanidins from jamun fruit pulp has been investigated by Sharma et al.

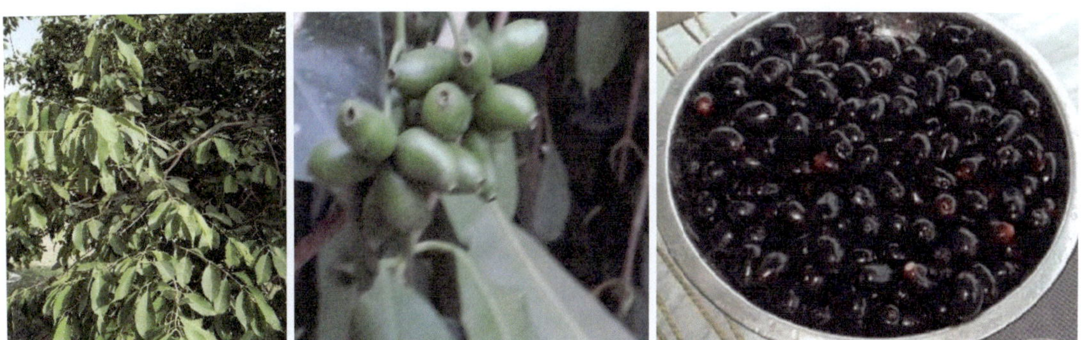

Fig. 28.3 Jamun tree and fruit at green stage of maturity (Photo source: Prof. Kuldip S. Minhas)

(2016) who reported lesser degradation at 5 °C and low pH, but higher degradation at high H_2O_2 concentration.

The jamun fruit and seeds are known to be rich in phenolic compounds. Balyan and Sarkar (2016) have successfully developed an integrated membrane process for the purification and concentration of aqueous jamun seed extract with enhanced purity and antioxidant activity. The safety of jamun seed extract has been evaluated by Sankhari et al. (2010) using acute and subchronic toxicity assays in Swiss albino mice and concluded that orally administered jamun fruit extract is safe up to a 10-fold higher dose than its reported therapeutic dose. The antibacterial potential of jamun seeds against multidrug resistant human bacterial pathogens has been investigated by Bag et al. (2012). They found that the phenolics were the major active phytoconstituents having maximum antibacterial effect against all the test isolates. Apart from antihyperlipidemic and anti-allergic properties, and good performance as an antimicrobial agent against bacteria, fungi and protozoa, the jamun essential oils, mainly the –pinene, exhibited significant anti-Leishmania activity modulated by macrophage activation with acceptable levels of cytotoxicity (Rodriguez et al. 2015). Fruit and leaf extracts from *Syzygium australe* and *Syzygium luehmannii* exhibited potent growth inhibition against all *Shewanella* spp., reported using disc and liquid diffusion assays (Murhekar et al. 2017). The potent antibacterial properties and lack of toxicity from *S. australe* fruit extracts indicated their potential for use as natural fish and seafood preservatives. Prabhu et al. (2018) have studied the use of jamun leaf powder on the growth and nonspecific immunity of *Litopenaeus vannamei* against a virulent strain of *Vibrio parahaemolyticus* pathogen. The jamun leaf powder added to the diet protected the shrimp effectively against virulent strains of *V. parhaemolyticus* through both the continuous- and day-feeding regimes. Singh et al. (2016) have reported that jamun fruit polyphenol extract exhibited a broad spectrum antimicrobial activity against *Staphylococcus aureus*, methicillin-resistant *S. aureus* (MRSA), *Escherichia coli*, *Klebsiella pneumonia*, and *Candida albicans*.

28.3.2 Medicinal Value

During last few years, numerous studies have appeared in the literature bringing out the novel benefits of jamun fruit pulp and seeds as a medicinal plant. Baliga et al. (2011b) have exhaustively reviewed the phytochemistry, traditional uses, and pharmacology of jamun fruit. Ayyanar et al. (2013) have reviewed antidiabetic effects of different parts of jamun tree and the active constituents present in therein. Jana et al. (2015) have compared the antidiabetic effect of the ethyl acetate fraction of jamun seed extract with glibenclamide, a standard antidiabetic drug in streptozotocin-induced diabetic albino rats. Their results provided information about the antihyperglycemic effect of this fraction through the *hepatic hexokinase*-1 gene regulation. The aqueous extracts of jamun seed possess liver protective effects by significantly lowering the contents of live enzymes (SGOT, SGPT, bilirubin) as well as serum glucose levels in alloxan-induced diabetic mice (Sharma et al. 2013). Raza et al. (2017) evaluated the potential of both jamun seed and fruit extracts in hyperglycemic rats and found that both have a potent prophylactic role against hyperglycemia. In another study, Nahid et al. (2017) have evaluated the cardio- and hepatoprotective potential of methanolic extract of jamun seeds in rats. An oral dosage of 200 mg/kg of methanolic extracts of jamun seeds reversed the cardiac and liver damage caused by alloxan. Jamun fruit has been identified to have antidiabetic, anti-inflammatory, antipyretic, and antioxidant activities. Yadav et al. (2011a) have tested the methanolic fraction of alcoholic extract from jamun seed for its anticancer properties. They reported that this fraction showed significantly positive anticancer potential effects on various types of human cancer cell lines.

28.3.3 Processing of Jamun Fruit

Pasteurization techniques have successfully been applied to jamun fruit pulp by Branco et al. (2016). The total soluble solids, phenolic compounds, and flavonoids were increased in levels to the tune of 6.7, 7.2, and 16.4%, respectively after pasteurization. Anthocyanins content was largely preserved to the extent of 91%. The jamun fruit pulp after pasteurization showed cytostatic activity in kidney (786–0) and ovary (OVCAR-3) lineages of human tumor cell lines. Thus, the thermal treatment (70 °C) can beneficially be applied to the jamun fruit pulp for preserving the product with a longer shelf life. Carvalho et al. (2017) have produced a powder from jamun fruit juice using foam mat drying. Elevation of dehydration temperature negatively affected the anthocyanin content of the products, and they recommended a processing temperature of 70 °C as the most suitable to produce high-quality dried product from jamun juice. Peixoto and Freitas (2012) have successfully prepared a jamun seed extract powder by spray-drying technique, which showed antihyperglycemic action in alloxan-induced experimental diabetes. In another study, Santhalakshmy et al. (2015) investigated the effect of inlet air temperature (from 140 to 160 °C) on the physicochemical properties of spray-dried jamun fruit juice powder. Lower inlet temperature produced jamun juice powder with desirable bright purple color and smoother particle surfaces than the higher temperature. Bezerra et al. (2015) have developed frozen yoghurt with fresh and spray-dried jamun fruit pulp supplemented with a probiotic strain, *Bifidobacterium animalis*. About 97% of the probiotic bacteria survived during 90 days of frozen yoghurt storage. The frozen yoghurt made with jamun fruit pulp proved to be an efficient carrier for *B. animalis subsp. Lactis* BI-07 still having desirable bioactive and technological qualities.

28.4 Bilva, Sriphal, or Bel (*Aegle marmelos*)

Aegle marmelos, commonly known as bel, sriphal, or bilva is indigenous to India but also grows in Pakistan, Burma, Vietnam, Sri Lanka, and Bangladesh.

28.4.1 Chemical Composition

The fruit pulp of bel is reported to contain many bioactive compounds, such as pectin, alkaloids, phenolics, tannins, flavonoids, coumarins, carotenoids, and terpenoids. The total, soluble, and insoluble dietary fiber in Thai bel fruit were 19.84, 11.22, and 8.62% on dry basis, respectively. Among volatile flavor compounds, monoterpenes and sesquiterpenes were the major ones. The characteristic bel flavor was attributed to the major component, limonene. The other major phytochemicals present in *Aegle marmelos* are limonene, citronella, citral, bphellandrene, linalool, p-cymene, 3,5-octadiene, trans-p-mentha-2,8-dienol, α-cubebene, cineole, citronellal, cuminaldehyde, hexadecane, β-cubebene, α-humulene, β-caryophyllene, pulegone, carvylacetate, carvone, verbenone, (E)-6,10-dimethyl-5,9-undecadien-2-one, dihydro-β-ionone, β-ionone, humulene oxide, hexadecenoic acid, and caryophyllene oxide (Charoensiddhi and Anprung 2008). Using bel leaves as an eco-friendly and cost-effective method, green synthesis of NiO nanoparticles have been synthesized by Ezhilarasi et al. (2018). These nanoparticles were confirmed as pure face-centered cubic phase and single crystalline in nature by X-ray diffraction. They evaluated these nanoparticles for cytotoxicity towards A549 cell cultures, antibacterial activity, and photocatalytic degradation of 4-chlorophenol, an endocrine-disrupting chemical. Their results showed not only better antibacterial activity towards Gram-positive strains but an efficient and better photocatalyst stability towards the degradation of 4-chlorophenol (Fig. 28.4).

A water-soluble antioxidative arabinogalactan protein gum from bel fruit has been prepared by Bera et al. (2017), who also investigated its structural details. It contained β-1,3-linked galactopyranosyl main chain substituted at the O-6 position with side chains consisting of arabinose and galactose residues. This arabinogalactan gum showed antioxidant potential quite like standard antioxidants. It is expected to serve as an important raw material for food industry as an antioxidative gum with the ability to produce stable water-soluble complex with β-lactoglobulin. Sandeep et al. (2017) have extracted and characterized a fiber obtained from bel bark. When this fiber was treated with 10% NaOH solution, the tensile strength and chemical composition of bel bark fibers were comparable to those of other natural fibers. They suggested the use of bel bark fiber as a reinforcement in composites.

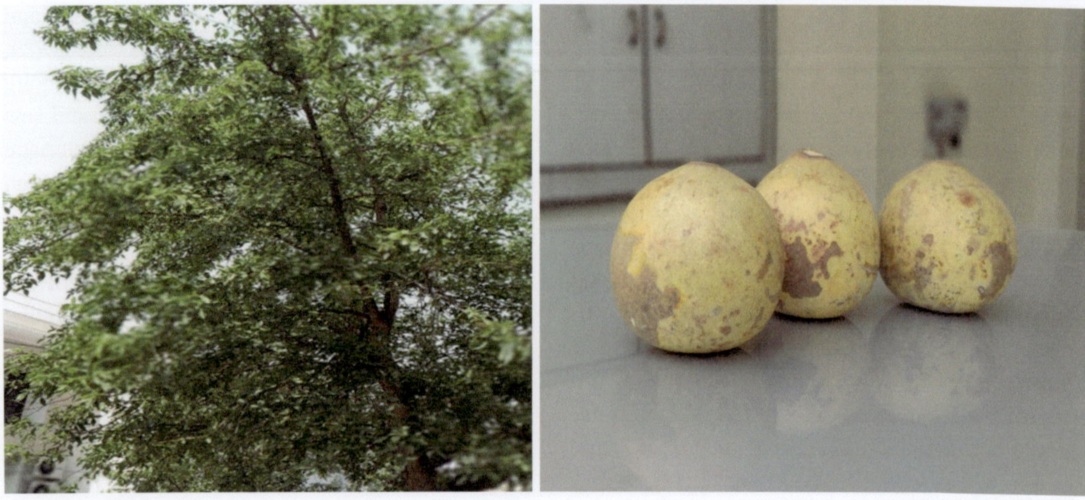

Fig. 28.4 Bel fruits on the tree, and when fully ripe (Photo source: Dr. Satpal Mehra, Ludhiana)

28.4.2 Medicinal Properties

Bel fruit and leaves have been reported to show a wide range of therapeutic effects, such as antidiarrheal, antibacterial, cardioprotective, antioxidant, inhibition of lipid peroxidation, anti-ulcerative colitis, antidiabetic, antiviral, antifungal, radiation- and gastro-protective properties. Various compounds extracted from bel were found to be biologically active against many diseases, such as cancer, diabetes, and cardiovascular diseases. The crude extract of bel fruit can be used in the treatment of many microbial diseases, diabetes, and gastric ulcer. Maity et al. (2009) have produced an exhaustive review of all the above medicinal benefits of bel bark, leaves, and fruits, including the biological activities of some isolated chemical constituents as well as preclinical studies on some crude extracts as well as pure compounds from *Aegle marmelos* for therapeutic applications. The potential use of bark, leaves, and fruits of *Aegle marmelos* as an antidiarrheal, antibacterial, and antifungal agent in the traditional system of medicine in India have also been reviewed by Sharma et al. (2011) and Akram et al. (2012). Synthesis, physicochemical properties, and biomedical applications of sulfated *Aegle marmelos* gum for modulating drug release dosages have been investigated by Jindal et al. (2017). The modified gum showed higher viscosity, shear force, firmness, consistency, cohesiveness, and index of viscosity when compared to unmodified gum or sodium alginate and was also superior in terms of antimicrobial and anticoagulant activities.

The use of radiotherapy in cancer cure as well as in palliative care had many side effects due to the radiosensitivity of adjoining normal tissues of the tumor. Under such circumstances, radioprotective compounds are needed to minimize the cytotoxic effects of ionizing radiations, which are mainly due to the generation of free radicals. *Aegle marmelos* fruit being a rich source of antioxidants has been suggested to relieve this oxidative stress. The plausible reasons for the use of bel fruit having radioprotective effects have been reviewed by Baliga et al. (2010).

The anti-inflammatory activities of the young roots of *Aegle marmelos* have been made use of in Ayurveda for the treatment of many inflammatory disorders in different parts of India. Rajaram et al. (2018) have recently investigated the anti-inflammatory activities of bel tree roots and found that the region in which this tree is grown as well as the age of the plant plays an important role in exhibiting anti-inflammatory effect. An exhaustive review on the importance of using *Aegle marmelos* bark, leaves, and fruits in the traditional Indian system of medicine for curing various disease conditions, its radioprotective and chemoprotective properties, and treatment of cancer has been published by Baliga et al. (2013). The hepatoprotective effect of bel leave extract can be augmented with piperine co-administered in a paracetamol model of Wistar rats (Rathee et al. 2018). Their results showed that bel leaf extract exerts hepatoprotective activity through its antioxidant and anti-inflammatory properties, and this effect was enhanced by piperine. The whole extract of bel fruit being rich in phytochemicals has been shown to exhibit protective effects against isoproterenol-induced myocardial infarction in rats (Krushna et al. 2017). Using molecular docking studies, they confirmed their results of cardioprotection offered by bel are mainly due to the presence of various bioactive compounds in this fruit.

Removal of man-made chemicals such as pesticides and herbicides from the aqueous system is becoming more important because of their adverse effects on the aquatic and native microbes. One of the selective herbicides, atrazine, used as a weed killer in agriculture, forests, and homes, leaches into the ground, thus contaminating our water supplies. Sivarajasekar et al. (2017) have modelled the use of microwave-irradiated bel fruit shell in a fixed-bed column for sorptive removal of atrazine from the aqueous solution. According to their results, the use of a dose-response model was the best-suited model for the removal of atrazine from aqueous solutions using the fixed-bed column. In another study, the removal of fluorine from aqueous solution by using bel shell activated carbon to well below the permissible limit has successfully been achieved by Singh et al. (2017). This variety of diverse uses and medicinal benefits make the *Aegle marmelos* a highly useful fruit tree for mankind.

28.5 Custard Apple or Sitaphal (*Annona squamosa*)

Custard apple is a small branched tree or shrub, belonging to the family Annonaceae, which bears edible fruits known as sitaphal, custard apple sweet sops, or sugar apple. This family contains 129 genera and more than 2000 species (Awachare et al. 2018). The tree grows to a height of 3–8 m and bears fruits with white yellow-tinged edible sweet aromatic pulp, with one oblong shiny brown to black seed in each carpel. Although this tree is native to subtropical Americas and West Indies, it has now spread to Asian countries such as India, Indonesia, Thailand, Taiwan, and many South American countries like Brazil and Argentina. It was introduced to Florida in the USA (Fig. 28.5).

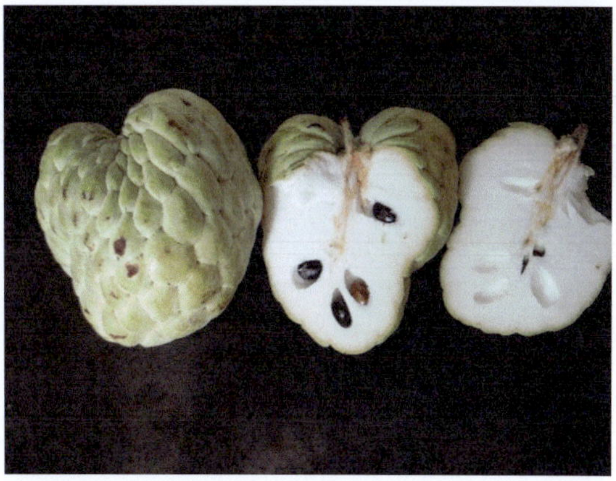

Fig. 28.5 Custard apple fruit (Photo source: Prof. Jiwan S. Sidhu)

28.5.1 Chemical Composition

Custard apple fruit has a wide range of phytochemicals like alkaloids, terpenoids and phenolics, such as quercetin with proven activities. In one earlier publication, Morton (1987b) has listed the use of sweet apple crushed leaves in traditional Indian, Thai, and American medicine for treating dysentery, urinary tract infection, and healing of wounds, and for cleaning floors and repelling lice from hens. Satish Kumar et al. (2011) have reviewed extensively the chemical constituents present in custard apple and the medicinal values of different parts of this tree, such as coolant, sedative, antiemetic, cough suppressant, antitumor activity, for strengthening muscles, seeds for destroying lice in hair, bark as a tonic, crushed leaves applied to ulcers and wounds, and as a decoction for curing dysentery.

In another review article, Gajalakshmi et al. (2011) have combined various studies covering the traditional, phytochemical, and pharmacological aspects of this medicinal plant. The fruit possesses analgesic, anti-inflammatory, antimicrobial, antioxidant, antilipidemic, anti-ulcer, mollusticidal, genotoxic, vasorelaxant, antitumor, hepatoprotective, larvicidal, insecticidal, anthelmintic activities, whereas the roots, leaves and seeds also offer several medicinal properties. Recently, Ma et al. (2017) have reviewed the phytochemicals and biological activities of custard apple. The fruit finds application in the preparation of many products, such as candies, ice cream, and beverages. Different parts of this tree exhibit anticancer, antioxidant, antidiabetic, antihypertensive, hepatoprotective, antiparasitic, antimalarial, insecticidal, antimicrobial, and mollusticidal activities. The major phytochemicals reported by them were acetogenins, diterpenes, alkaloids, and cyclopeptides.

28.5.2 Medicinal Properties

Custard apple fruit is only second to the Indian gooseberry (*Phyllanthus emblica* L.) in its antioxidant capacity but has higher antioxidant properties than starfruit (*Averrhoa carambola*) as reported by Silva and Sirasa (2018). Seeds from custard apple are generally discarded as waste material but have been shown to be more effective than that of propyl thiouracil, a standard antithyroidic drug (Panda and Kar 2007a). They suggested the presence of a phytochemical, quercetin, in custard apple seed extract may be responsible for the mediation of antithyroidal activity. Although custard apple is a very sweet fruit, a structural polysaccharide (M.W. 2.28×10^6 Da) consisting of rhamnose, arabinose, xylose, mannose, glucose, galactose, glucuronic acid, and galacturonic acid has been shown to exhibit α-glucosidase activity which prevents the sudden rise of blood glucose levels (Ren et al. 2017). Custard apple leaves show antidiabetic effects due to quercetin-3-O-glucoside, possibly mediated through the insulin stimulating and/or free-radical scavenging properties (Panda and Kar 2007b). In case of streptozotocin-induced diabetic rats, Kaleem et al. (2006) have reported that the custard apple leaf extract, when administered orally, reduced the blood glucose level, lipids, and lipid peroxidation but increased the activities of plasma insulin and antioxidant enzymes such as catalase, superoxide dismutase, reduced glutathione, and glutathione peroxidase. They suggested that *Annona squamosa* leaf extract may be useful for the prevention or early treatment of diabetes mellitus. Similar results on the antioxidant and antilipidemic potential of custard apple leaf extract in Type-2 diabetic models have also been reported by Gupta et al. (2008).

The bark from custard apple tree has been used by Yadav et al. (2011b) to treat ulcer. In a similar study, Chen et al. (2012) have used custard apple seed extract to treat malignant sores (cancer). Using FT-IR and HPLC, they identified the presence of two acetogenins compounds in the seed extract: 12,15-cis-squamostatin-A and bullatacin. These compounds exhibited significant antitumor activities against human hepatoma cells *in vitro* as well as *in vivo*, thus offering a potential for developing anti-liver cancer drugs from custard apple seed extract. Tundis et al. (2017) have recently reviewed various studies published from 2009 to 2016 exploring the potential of Annona species as a rich source of potential antitumor agents.

Emergence of drug-resistant strains is becoming a serious problem the world over. Natural products from herbal plants are becoming the favoured material of choice for developing antimicrobial chemicals. Leaves, bark, and seeds of custard apple offer an interesting alternative to chemical antimicrobials. Dholvitayakhun et al. (2017) have tested the custard apple leaf extract for its inhibitory action against Gram-positive *Bacillus cereus* and Gram-negative *Campylobacter jejuni* using scanning and transmission microscopy to study the antibacterial mechanism of action. Their results suggested that *Annona squamosa* leaf extract inhibits bacterial growth by disrupting the synthesis of peptidoglycans in the cell walls, thus leading to cell death due to osmotic lysis. Silver nanoparticles were synthesized with *Annona squamosa* plant extract and tested against third-stage larvae from mosquitoes by Khader et al. (2018). They observed effective larvicidal activity with custard apple plant extract against larvae even at very low concentrations and suggested that the extract and nanoparticles may be a better control measure against mosquitoes. *Annona squamosa* leaf extract has been reported to exhibit a broad spectrum but heat-labile activity against many common foodborne pathogens, such as *Bacillus cereus*, *Listeria monocytogenes*, and *Staphylococcus aureus* (Dholvitayakhun et al. 2012).

For the removal of aquatic pollution coming from colored effluents from fabric, paint, paper and leather industries, a number of approaches have been suggested. For the removal of methyl red, a dye, Khan et al. (2018a, b) have employed activated carbon derived from custard apple fruit shell. They performed equilibrium isotherm and kinetic studies, and according to their findings, methyl red adsorption followed a pseudo-first order and pseudo-second order rate equation for potassium carbonate and phosphoric acid activated carbons, respectively. A note of caution on the consumption of custard apple fruit has been sounded by Bonneau et al. (2017) because of the presence of annonaceous acetogenins, which are neurotoxins possibly responsible for atypical Parkinsonism/dementia clusters.

28.6 Jackfruit (*Artocarpus heterophyllus*)

Consumption of fruits and vegetables as a source of phenolics, carotenoids, vitamin E, and vitamin C are known to reduce the risk of various chronic diseases such as diabetes, cancer, atherosclerosis, inflammation, and cardiovascular diseases, mainly because of their ability to scavenge free radicals (Chen et al. 2017; Kabir et al. 2017; Kabir and Sidhu 2011; Sidhu 2012; Sidhu and Zafar 2012; Zafar and Sidhu 2017). Jackfruit tree is native to Southwest Asia and belongs to the family Moraceae; its fruit is the largest tree-borne fruit weighing up to 35 Kg. The flesh of the fruit has the aroma of apple, pineapple, mango, and banana; both the fruit and seeds are eaten. The flesh of jackfruit is rich in starch, sugars, and dietary fiber (Fig. 28.6).

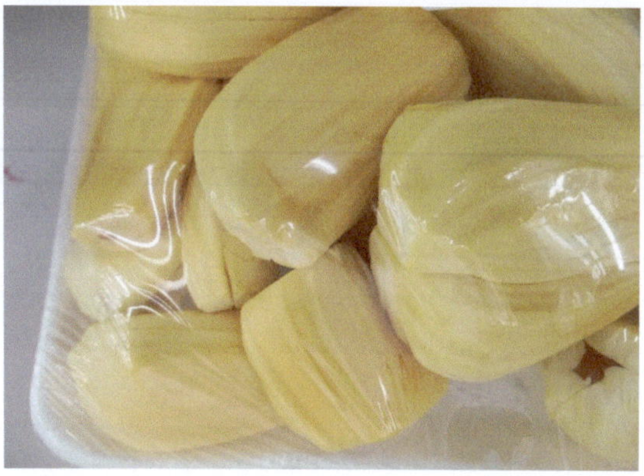

Fig. 28.6 Jackfruit cut pieces (Photo source: Prof. Jiwan S. Sidhu)

28.6.1 Chemical Composition

The jackfruit is reported to be a good source of carbohydrates, protein, fat, flavonoids, phytosterols, prenylflavones, vitamins, and minerals. Baliga et al. (2011a) have reviewed extensively the phytochemistry, nutritional, and pharmacological properties of jackfruit. A water-soluble polysaccharide isolated from jackfruit pulp has been reported to exhibit strong antioxidant properties and relatively lower reducing power and thus can be used as an effective natural antioxidant application in medical and food industries (Zhu et al. 2017). Wen et al. (2017) have identified a flavonoid C-glycoside having good antioxidant but low cytotoxicity properties from jackfruit pulp. The bioactivity of a stable nanoemulsion prepared from jackfruit pulp by high-pressure homogenization (twice at 800 bars) has been optimized by using 5% miglyol plus 0.5% sucrose monostearate (Ruiz-Montanez et al. 2017). Starch granules extracted from the seeds of jackfruit were reported to be similar in diameter to that from rice and potato starch but were larger than that of maize and waxy rice (Zhang et al. 2018a, b). The jackfruit seeds are reported to accumulate primary and secondary metabolites which have a capacity to scavenge reactive nitrogen species (Fernandes et al. 2017).

A protein isolate prepared from jackfruit seeds by high-intensity ultrasound application has been found to meet the techno-functional properties of food industry (Resendiz-Vazquez et al. 2017). A high-amylose starch (26.56–38.34%) extracted from jackfruit seeds has been found to serve as a functional food rich in resistant starch (Zhang et al. 2018a, b). Based on particle size these starch samples were divided into three grades (5.53–14.46 μm), the smallest size suitable as a thickening or gelling agent, the second group used in glutinous foods, and the third group for filling in confectionery or weaning foods.

After removing the pulp from the jackfruit, its peel (rind) and rachis are discarded as waste material. Daud et al. (2017) have found these waste materials to be highly rich in many phenolic compounds and thus can be used as a source of natural antioxidants in new product development. Moorthy et al. (2017) have optimized the yield of pectin from jackfruit peel using ultrasound-assisted extraction techniques. Later, Xu et al. (2018) have also extracted pectin from jackfruit peel using ultrasonic-microwave-assisted extraction technique and have characterized its biological activity. They found the pectin extracted from jackfruit to be rich in galactose, rhamnose, arabinose, glucose, and galacturonic acid with high degree of methyl-esterification and can be used as natural antioxidants in the food industry. Starch extracted from jackfruit seed has been used to prepare microencapsulated vanilla oil using an ultrasound method by Zhu et al. (2018). Their results showed that jackfruit seed starch has tremendous potential for microencapsulation of food flavors for industrial applications. Some of the phenolic compounds reported in jackfruit leaf extract are tabulated in Table 28.2.

Table 28.2 Main phenolic compounds and their contents in jackfruit leaf extract (Ref Chen et al. 2017)

Sl no	Phenolic fractions	Detected phenolics and their quantities (μg/g DW)
1	Free	Gallic acid (27.51 ± 0.37), (+)-catechin (49.36 ± 1.08), epicatechin (698.50 ± 27.02), ferulic acid (22.95 ± 1.41), rutin (36.01 ± 0.89), isoquercitrin (42.29 ± 0.91), quercitrin (52.75 ± 2.85)
2	Esterified	Gallic acid (76.24 ± 2.67), (+)-catechin (34.72 ± 1.37), epicatechin (254.99 ± 9.61), ferulic acid (38.22 ± 0.60), rutin (43.29 ± 1.33), isoquercitrin (22.53 ± 2.44), quercitrin (28.44 ± 1.44).
3	Insoluble bound	Gallic acid (144.92 ± 2.5), (+)-catechin (202.22 ± 2.88), epicatechin (427.78 ± 5.87), ferulic acid (117.73 ± 1.31), rutin (272.99 ± 11.33), isoquercitrin (202.63 ± 4.90), quercitrin (286.47 ± 18.29).

28.6.2 Medicinal Properties

Jackfruit is reported to possess antioxidant, anti-inflammatory, antibacterial, antifungal, anticarcinogenic, antineoplastic, hypoglycemic, and wound-healing properties. The decoction of leaves possesses hypoglycemic effects both in healthy individuals as well as in noninsulin-dependent diabetic patients (Baliga et al. 2011a). Wang et al. (2016b) have isolated new phenolic compounds from the leaves of jackfruit showing moderate to weak inhibitory activity against the proliferation of PC-3, NCI-H460, and A549 cancer cell lines. Anti-angiogenic effect of the jackfruit seed methanolic extract has shown potential as a candidate for future anticancer therapy (Oktavia et al. 2017). Antiviral activity of the dichloromethane extract of jackfruit leaves against hepatitis C virus has been reported by Hafid et al. (2017). In a recent study, Burci et al. (2018) have also shown the potential anticancer effects of Brazilian jackfruit seed extract. From jackfruit peel, a waste product from the processing industry, Govindaraj et al. (2018) have developed pectin/apatite bionanocomposites for bone-healing applications. These bionanocomposites having good biocompatibility may find applications as bone graft materials. Flavonoids extracted from the roots of jackfruit have been found to be natural inhibitors for cathepsins κ (Catκ) and thus can find use in preventing osteoporosis (Yuan et al. 2017). Suryadevara et al. (2017) have prepared from jackfruit starch, a novel natural super-disintegrant, a fast-dissolving

Table 28.3 Total phenolics, flavonoids, and free radical scavenging activity of jackfruit leaf extract

Method of analysis	Free phenolic fractions	Esterified phenolic fractions	Insoluble bound phenolic fractions	Total
DPPH radical scavenging activity[a]	27.74 ± 0.97	70.70 ± 1.34	135.81 ± 1.08	234.25 ± 1.10
ABTS radical cation scavenging activity[a]	44.49 ± 0.87	57.35 ± 0.87	34.22 ± 1.01	136.05 ± 2.70
Ferric reducing antioxidant power[a]	23.87 ± 0.18	38.58 ± 1.02	179.67 ± 0.78	242.12 ± 0.16
Total flavonoid contents[a]	3.73 ± 0.15	5.50 ± 0.18	26.72 ± 0.76	36.00 ± 0.86
Total phenolic contents[b]	2.76 ± 0.04	5.09 ± 0.03	20.81 ± 0.15	28.67 ± 0.13

[a]Determined as (μmol Trolox/g, DW)
[b]Determined as (mg GAE/g DW) (Reference: Chen et al. 2017)

tablet formulation for Irbesartan medicine. Chen et al. (2017) investigated and reported significant antioxidant activity of jackfruit leaf extract and total phenolics, and flavonoid content in the extract (Table 28.3).

With the evolution of industrialization, a number of aromatic dyes, phenols, agrochemicals, and many other pollutants having carcinogenic effects have entered our food and water resources. Effluents from textile, paper, dye manufacturing, food packaging, and leather tanning industries are rich in chemicals having cancer risk and are a threat to our aquatic and human life. Scientists are always on the lookout for developing various treatments to eliminate these harmful chemicals from our food and water supplies. Vidya et al. (2017) have used hazard-free green synthesis of zinc oxide nano-photo-catalyst using jackfruit leaf extract for the degradation of Congo red dye in water treatment applications. Nava et al. (2017) have used jackfruit peel extract-mediated green synthesis of zinc oxide nanoparticles for the absorption of methylene blue dye. Lim et al. (2017) have prepared a highly effective low-cost biosorbent from *Artocarpus camansi* fruit peel for methylene blue dye.

28.7 Ber or Indian Plum (*Zizyphus mauritiana* Lam)

Zizyphus mauritiana, also known as ber, Indian jujube, Indian plum, or Chinese apple, belongs to the Rhamnaceae, is a native fruit of South Asia and East Africa. The tree can be an evergreen shrub or grows tall up to 15 m high. It can grow in a wide range of soils and under wide climatic and soil conditions, ranging from sandy soil to black soil, and in deserts with scanty rain. A few cultivars have been shown to offer good resistance to an important insect (fruit fly, *Carpomyia vesuviana*) infesting the fruit (Haldhar et al. 2018). An extensive review about the role of *Zizyphus mauritiana* in alleviating household food insecurity and illnesses in the arid and semiarid regions of the world has been published recently, as this has multiple uses such as culinary, fodder, and medicinal uses (Maruza et al. 2017). Another cultivar, *Zizyphus jujube* Mill, has also been reviewed for its chemical composition, including bioactive compounds for human consumption (Ji et al. 2017). They reported the fruit to have immunomodulatory, antioxidant, antitumor, hepatoprotective and hypoglycemic activities, and gastrointestinal-protective effects. The best point of harvesting superior quality fruit in Brazil is suggested to be 56 days after anthesis (Bastos et al. 2016) (Fig. 28.7).

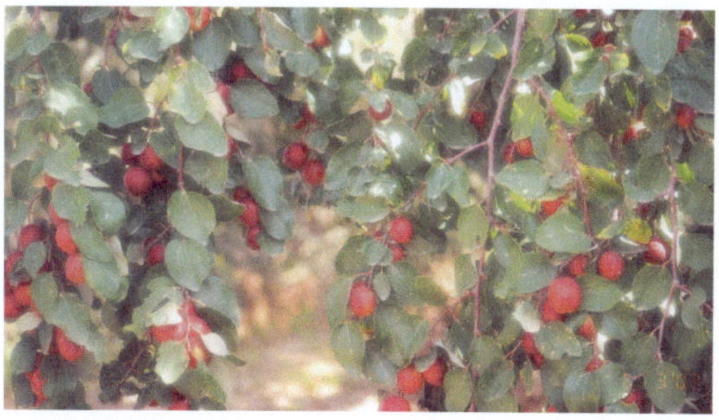

Fig. 28.7 Zizyphus tree bearing fruits (Photo source: Dr. Narayanan Bhat, Kuwait)

28.7.1 Chemical Composition

Interest in Zizyphus fruit is growing because the fruit is a rich source of many valuable nutrients and phytochemicals required for maintaining good health. The fruit has been shown to be rich in phenolics and ascorbic acid, and has a good antioxidant capacity (Wojdylo et al. 2016). Changes in antioxidant activity and phenolic compounds have been reported in several publications. Un-colored jujube has natural antioxidants, mostly proanthocyanidins, but the half-red ripening stage is proper for picking fruits for table purposes (Wu et al. 2012).

The sugar content and types of sugars change with the stage of ripening. As the fruit ripens to change from green to a fully ripe stage, the sucrose content decreases, but glucose and fructose contents gradually keep on increasing with ripening (Zozio et al. 2014a). The phenolic profiles of fruits are affected by the stage of development, but the antioxidant capacity is more impacted by the flavonols and condensed tannins (Zozio et al. 2014b). Wang et al. (2016a) have followed the changes in phenolic compounds in three stages of fruit maturity. The white maturity stage (WM) had the highest levels of total phenolic content, total flavonoid content, and individual phenolic compound content. The phenolic content and their antioxidant activities decreased with the increasing maturity stage from half-red maturity stage (HM) to the red maturity stage (RM). Caffeic acid was the predominant phenolic during the WM stage but rutin at the HM and RM stages. Catechin and rutin have also been earlier reported in the ripe fruits by San and Yildirim (2010). The cultivars also differed in phenolic contents and β-carotenes, α-tocopherols, and fatty acids. Wide variation in the nutritive value of Zizyphus fruits from Zambezi valley in Zimbabwe has been reported by Nyanga et al. (2013). The antioxidant activity and phenolic content of 12 commercial cultivars of Zizyphus fruits have been reported by Koley et al. (2016). Physicochemical and antioxidant activity of different fruits of the Zizyphus genotype are tabulated in Table 28.4. Indian jujube is a good source of vitamin C and total phenolics which ranged from 19.54 to 99.49 mg/100 g and 172 to 328.6 mg GAE/100 g, respectively.

28.7.2 Medicinal Properties

The genus *Zizyphus* has about 170 species, most of which are important economic plants with edible fruits having nutritional and medicinal value. The seeds have been used to treat insomnia and the bark and roots as anti-inflammatory and anti-infection agents for burns and diarrhea (Ji et al. 2012). They have isolated three novel nortriterpenes from the roots of *Zizyphus mauritiana*, which have shown anticancer as well as antimicrobial activities. Shanmugavasan et al. (2011) have designed a pyrolyser to extract medicinal oil from the stem of *Zizyphus jujube* plant and found the oil to contain various degradation products of cyclopeptide alkaloids present in the stem. They reported these phytochemicals to have sedative property and may be responsible for the curative nature of this oil. Iqbal et al. (2017a) have reviewed literature on the plant-derived anticancer agents and have explored the vast avenues for research in this area. According to their review, phytochemicals present in plants are considered suitable candidates for the development of anticancer drugs without having any side effects.

The exposure of *Zizyphus mauritiana* leaves to gamma radiations at a dosage of 12.5 kGy has been shown to enhance the levels of certain phytochemicals and have augmented their biological activities (Khattak and Rahman 2016). The methanolic extract of *Zizyphus mauritiana* roots has been shown to have the maximum zone of inhibition for *E. coli* but the least against *Klebsiella pneumoniae*. These extracts showed a broad spectrum of antimicrobial activity (Priyanka et al. 2015). Panseeta et al. (2011) have isolated cyclopeptide alkaloids from the roots of *Zizyphus mauritiana* grown in Thailand, which exhibited potent antiplasmodial activity against the parasite *Plasmodium falciparum*. These compounds also exhibited antimycobacterial activity against *Mycobacterium tuberculosis*. Deshpande et al. (2013) have obtained

Table 28.4 Content of antioxidant molecules, antioxidant activity, and physicochemical composition of some Zizyphus genotypes (Ref: Koley et al. 2016)

Sl No	Cultivar	Antioxidant component (content)	Antioxidant activity (Trolox/g.)	Physicochemical composition
1	Chuhara	Total phenolics: 258.06 ± 37.99[a] Total flavonoids: 8.36 ± 1.47[b] Ascorbic acid: 99.49 ± 1.53[c]	FRAP: 9.96 ± 1.6 CUPRAC: 13.57 ± 2.7 DPPH: 15.42 ± 3.2 TEAC: 15.76 ± 2.7	TA: 0.22 ± 0.005 TSS: 15 ± 0.58 TSS/TA: 66.96 pH: 4.58 ± 0.06
2	Gola	Total phenolics: 252.23 ± 18.29[a] Total flavonoids: 21.97 ± 2.09[b] Ascorbic acid: 57.65 ± 4.59[c]	FRAP: 8.58 ± 2.5 CUPRAC: 12.56 ± 1.3 DPPH: 23.19 ± 2.5 TEAC: 22.94 ± 1.3	TA: 0.25 ± 0.005 TSS: 15 ± 0.29 TSS/TA: 58.59 pH: 4.35 ± 0.06
3	Umran	Total phenolics: 172.08 ± 31.77a Total flavonoids: 10.76 ± 0.85[b] Ascorbic acid: 19.54 ± 1.85[c]	FRAP: 7.41 ± 1 CUPRAC: 8.01 ± 1.2 DPPH: 14.56 ± 1 TEAC: 12.74 ± 1.2	TA: 0.22 ± 0.005 TSS: 15 ± 0.58 TSS/TA: 66.9 pH: 5.37 ± 0.12
4	ZG-3	Total phenolics: 328.65 ± 13.98[a] Total flavonoids: 14.58 ± 0.59[b] Ascorbic acid: 83.16 ± 0.51[c]	FRAP: 11.65 ± 3.7 CUPRAC: 15.1 ± 1.7 DPPH: 39.64 ± 3.7 TEAC: 29.45 ± 1.7	TA: 0.32 ± 0.002 TSS: 15 ± 0.00 TSS/TA: 46.87 pH: 4.72 ± 0.12
5	Elaichi	Total phenolics: 267.28 ± 18.39[a] Total flavonoids: 16.07 ± 2.58[b] Ascorbic acid: 71.56 ± 1.15[c]	FRAP: 11.95 ± 2.9 CUPRAC: 12.21 ± 1.8 DPPH: 21.82 ± 2.9 TEAC: 21.1 ± 1.8	TA: 0.28 ± 0.001 TSS: 10 ± 0.00 TSS/TA: 34.72 pH: 4.99 ± 0.12

[a]Total phenolics expressed as mg GAE/100 g
[b]Total flavonoids expressed as mg CAE/100 g
[c]Ascorbic acid expressed as mg/100 g
FRAP ferric reducing antioxidant power, *CUPRAC* cupric ion antioxidant reducing capacity, *DPPH* 2,2-diphenyl-1-picrylhydrazyl, *TEAC* trolox equivalent antioxidant capacity, *TA* total acidity, *TSS* total soluble solids

chloroform, ethanol, and aqueous extracts of Z. mauritiana bark and evaluated them for antioxidant, anti-inflammatory, and adipocyte differentiation inhibitory potential. The chloroform, ethanol, and aqueous extracts showed good antioxidant activity, but the anti-inflammatory potential was shown only by the chloroform extract. However, the aqueous extract showed adipocyte inhibition and induced glucose uptake in CHO-HIRC-mycGLUT4e GFP cells. The polyphenols extracted from the jujube peel have been shown to provide protective effects against isoproterenol-induced myocardial ischemia and aluminum-induced oxidative damage in rats (Cheng et al. 2012).

28.8 *Lasura* or Assyrian Plum (*Cordia myxa*)

Lasura is a flowering tree belonging to the Boraginaceae, bearing broad leaves, and deciduous in nature, found mainly in Asia from Myanmar to Afghanistan but grows in many other countries, including the State of Kuwait. The tree matures in 50–60 years and grows to a height of 10–15 m. The tree bears fruits in the months of July–August, and the fruits are pale yellow to light brown or sometimes pink in color. The fruit is full of a glue-like mucilage with a somewhat translucent appearance. Pulp from half-ripe fruits is used as paper glue. The fully ripe fruit is quite sweet and enjoyed by children. The fruit, bark, and roots have been used in traditional medicine in Asian countries (Fig. 28.8).

28.8.1 Chemical Composition

The fruits of *Cordia myxa* contain moisture 6 g, crude protein 35 g, crude fat 37, and carbohydrate 18 g per 100 g. A maximum yield of hydrocolloid (0.5%) from *Cordia myxa* leaf has been obtained by Samavati et al. (2014). According to them, the leaf extract hydrocolloid had moisture, crude protein, water-soluble and water-insoluble

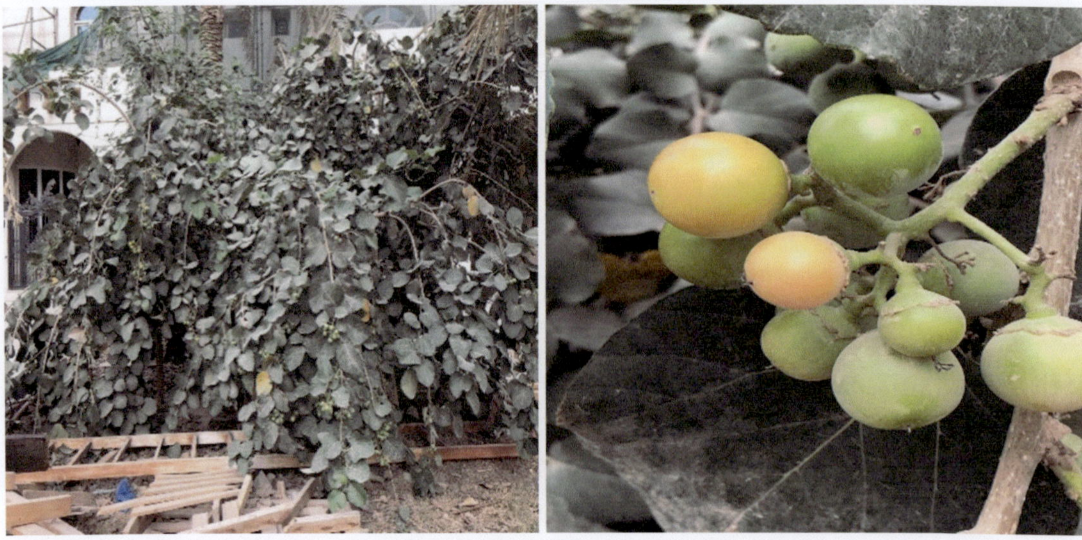

Fig. 28.8 Lasura tree bearing fruits. (Photo source: Mr. Abdul Aziz Al-Naqi, Kuwait)

ash, and total phenolics in the following quantities: 21.63 ± 0.94%, 14.27 ± 0.55%, 3.07 ± 0.16%, and 2.61 ± 0.19 mg gallic acid/g, respectively. An anionic polysaccharide rich in uronic acid with good adhering properties extracted from the ripe fruits of *Cordia myxa* when used as coating on Chilgoza (*Pinus gerardiana*) nuts extended its shelf life by about 95% as compared to carboxymethyl cellulose (60% extension) (Haq et al. 2013). Haq et al. (2014) have prepared an edible film using *Cordia myxa* gum for use in low-cost packaging of food materials and drugs. Steady shear flow properties of Cordia myxa leaf gum as a function of concentration and temperature have been investigated by Chaharlang and Samavati (2015), who observed a non-Newtonian shear-thinning behavior of this gum.

28.8.2 Medicinal Properties

The fruit, leaves, bark, and seed of Cordia myxa have been reported to possess antidiabetic, antiulcer, anti-inflammatory, immune-modulating, and analgesic activity in a review by Jamkhande et al. (2013). In another review, Matias et al. (2015) have discussed the principal botanical aspects, ethnopharmacological information, and evaluation of Cordia species' bioactive compounds. Later, Al-Snafi (2016) has reviewed the pharmacological and therapeutic importance of *Cordia myxa* and reported the plant to be rich in many phytochemicals such as, glycosides, flavonoids, oil, sterols, terpenoids, alkaloids, phenolic acids, coumarins, tannins, resins, saponins, gums, and mucilage. Pharmacological studies revealed this tree to possess analgesic, anti-inflammatory, immunomodulatory, antimicrobial, antiparasitic, insecticidal, cardiovascular, respiratory, and gastrointestinal-protective effects.

The *Cordia myxa* fruit mucilage has been utilized as a tablet binder and emulsifier as it is nontoxic, biodegradable, cheap, economic, and an easily available option in the list of pharmaceutical excipients (Dinda and Mukharjee 2009; Pawar and Jadhav 2015). In another study by applying response surface methodology, metformin-loaded gum Cordia/gellan beads have been prepared using an ionic-gelation technique by Ahuja et al. (2010). Their mathematical model was found to be robust and accurate for optimization of controlled release of metformin hydrochloride.

The *Cordia myxa* fruit has been studied for its effects on experimentally induced colitis in rats by Al-Awadi et al. (2001). Histological observations showed in colitis rats a significant decrease in glutathione peroxidase and superoxide dismutase and lower concentrations of trace elements, which was reversed with Cordia fruit ingestion. Their results suggested that the anti-inflammatory effects of *Cordia myxa* fruit may partly be due to its antioxidant properties and restoring the levels of trace minerals in the inflamed colon, liver, and plasma. The methanolic extract of *Cordia dichotoma* tree bark was reported to contain a phytochemical, apigenin, which significantly reduced the inflammatory enzymes and this extract can be used for the treatment of ulcerative colitis (Ganjare et al. 2011). The leaf extract from *Cordia dichotoma* has been evaluated for its reversible contraceptive potential in rats after withdrawal (Bhattacharya and Saha 2013).Two major phytonutrients, apigenin and luteolin, were found to exhibit no toxicity but were useful as an antifertility drug with reversible contraceptive potential in rats. In a later study, Sharma et al. (2015) have assessed the antifertility activity of hydro-alcoholic extract of *Cordia dichotoma* leaves being used by Meena community women in Rajasthan state of India. Their results showed that the hydro-alcoholic extract of *C. dichotoma* leaves possesses significant antifertility activity.

28.9 *Phalsa* or Falsa (*Grewia asiatica* L.)

Phalsa is native to Southeast Asia, from India, Pakistan, to Cambodia, but now it is widely cultivated in other tropical countries also. It has now spread from Philippines to Australia and got established. It is a shrub or small tree growing only up to 8 m tall, with broad rounded leaves and yellow flowers. The fruits when ripe have sweet and sour taste and attain purple to black in color. It is available in the market usually during summer months, and by using sugar it is suitable for the preparation of squash or jam. The genus *Grewia* belongs to family Malvaceae and has about 150 species which bear edible fruits having nutritional and therapeutic attributes (Wani et al. 2015). Apart from nutritional value, the stem, roots and leaves also are used for medicinal purposes (Fig. 28.9).

28.9.1 Chemical Composition

Most fruits are known to be rich sources of many phytochemicals exhibiting antioxidant, antielastase, anticollagenase, antityrosinase, and anti-inflammatory activities. These polyphenolic compounds are known to scavenge free radicals, inhibit enzymes causing skin-aging and skin-darkening and can, therefore, be utilized to formulate products for general health maintenance as well as anti-aging and skin-whitening creams (Singh et al. 2016). In another study, Adebiyi et al. (2017) have studied the *in vitro* antioxidant activity and total phenolic and flavonoid contents for ethanolic extracts of stem and leaf of *Grewia*

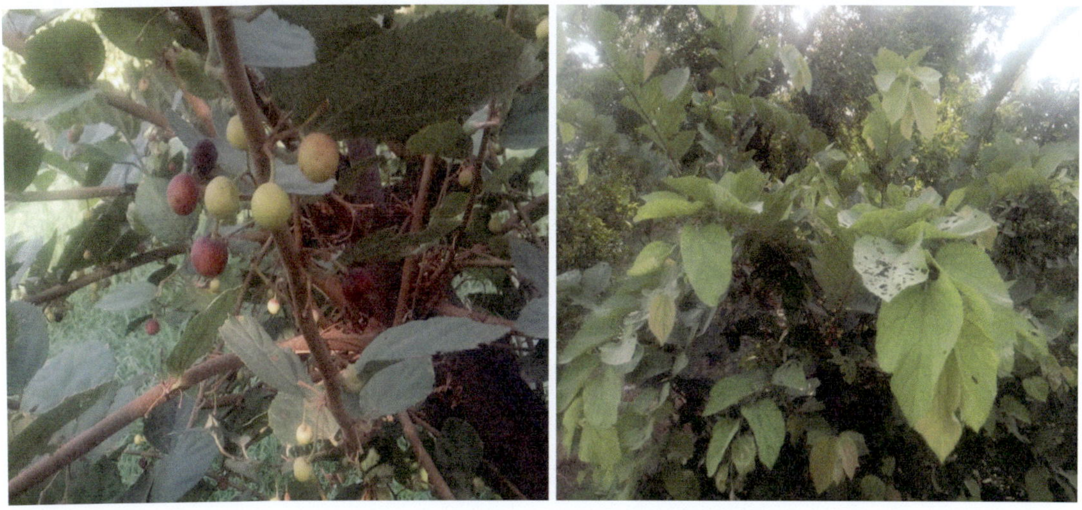

Fig. 28.9 Phalsa tree bearing fruits. (Photo source: Dr. Ramesh Batta, New Delhi)

carpinifolia, and they attributed the high antioxidant activity to the presence of high levels of flavonoids and phenolics in these plant parts. Phalsa fruit is known to be a rich source of triterpenoids and flavonoids having various putative health benefits, but its full commercialization is impeded due to a short shelf life and presence of large seed in relation to its pulp component. Wani and Latto (2017) have investigated the auxin response factor (GaARF) cloning and expression in relation to reproductive maturation in *Grewia asiatica* L. with the objective of reducing the seed volume in the fruit. Their results suggested that targeting GaARF is a prospective means for elucidation of maturation and fruit set without fertilization.

28.9.2 Medicinal Benefits

Different parts of *Grewia* species are being used as folk medicine in different parts of the world. Goyal (2012) has reviewed the phytochemical and pharmacological properties of the genus *Grewia*. According to the review, a high concentration of tannins, saponins, flavonoids, glycosides, phenols, and steroids in the bark and roots, and absence of alkaloids in the leaves and bark were observed. Different parts of this plant have been used in folk medicine for antidiabetic, antihypertensive, antifertility activities; for the alleviation of inflammation, respiratory, cardiac, and blood disorders; as a demulcent and febrifuge; for the treatment of diarrhea and skin lesions; as a tranquilizer; for antibacterial activity; for the treatment for headache, eye complaints, sores, cholera, spleen enlargement, piles, rheumatism, joint pain, indigestion, eczema, typhoid fever, dysentery, syphilis ulceration in the mouth, throat complaints; and for apoptosis of cancer cells. Chandiran et al. (2013a) have reported that extracts from aerial parts of *Grewia serrulata* DC were found to be rich in flavonoids, saponins, glycosides, terpenoids, steroids, phenols, and were nontoxic in tested dosages up to 800 mg/kg body wt/per day in rats. Histopathological evaluation showed no abnormalities with the test drug treatment.

Nanoparticles do show a considerably changed physical, chemical, and biological behavior compared with their macroscale counterparts. Sana et al. (2015) achieved eco-friendly synthesis of silver nanoparticles using *Grewia flaviscences* leaves which showed antibacterial activity against Gram-positive *Bacillus species* and Gram-negative *Pseudomonas aeruginosa*. Ahamed et al. (2010) have investigated the *in vitro* antioxidant and *in vivo* prophylactic effects of two γ-lactones isolated from *Grewia tiliaefolia* against hepatotoxicity in carbon tetrachloride-intoxicated rats. Their results showed that the bark extract and the γ-lactones had significant free radical scavenging activity as well as protected the hepatocytes from carbon tetrachloride-induced liver damage in rats, possibly due to their antioxidant effects by eliminating the deleterious effects of toxic metabolites from carbon tetrachloride.

The physicochemical characterization of seed oil obtained from *Grewia bicolor* for its putative pharmaceutical, cosmetic, and industrial uses have been investigated by Nyakudya et al. (2015). Although *Grewia bicolor* yielded a low amount of seed oil, it was rich in palmitic, stearic, oleic, and linoleic acids, and can be used as an industrial ingredient for the manufacture of soaps, cosmetics, and pharmaceutical products. The ethanolic extract of *Grewia bicolor* roots given by intraperitoneal administration to rats during early pregnancy (1–4 days) did not affect the number of conception sites but did increase resorption significantly (Mohamed et al. 1990). They found the active compound to be a peptide which exhibited serotonin-like rise in blood pressure. Mulholland et al. (2002) have investigated the uterogenic effect of compounds extracted from the stem of *Grewia occidentalis* and identified the active compounds in this wood extract as oleanonic acid and coniferaldehyde ((E)-4-hydroxy-3-methoxycinnamaldehyde). The aqueous and supercritical fluid extracts from the wood caused uterine muscle contraction in guinea pigs. Chandiran et al. (2013b) have studied the antioxidant and hypoglycemic properties of aqueous and ethanolic extracts of aerial parts of *Grewia serrulate* DC on normal and hyperglycemic rats. The ethanolic extract was found to possess strong free radical scavenging activity and showed reduction in blood glucose levels both in normal and glucose-loaded hyperglycemic rats.

28.10 Future Research Needs

Mother Earth is filled with an enormous population of diverse plant species which are known to be a rich source of many phytochemicals having not only health-promoting properties but also an immense source of medicinal compounds. Looking at the functional features, the health benefits of bioactive compounds like phenolics, flavonoids, carotenoids, glycosides, steroids, alkaloids, terpenoids, lignans, mucopolysaccharides, many vitamins and minerals, and their incorporation into functional foods have attracted more attention of food scientists and health professional across the globe. Most of these plant parts have shown numerous medicinal properties like antioxidative, anti-inflammatory, antidiabetic, hypoglycemic, anti-hypercholesterolemic, cardioprotective, hepatoprotective, immunomodulatory, antipyretic, analgesic, antitussive, anticancer, antifertility, gastroprotective, and snake venom-neutralizing activities, but their mechanism of action is still not fully understood. The list of these beneficial properties of these plant parts, such as roots, bark, wood, leaves, fruits and seeds, seems to be incomplete and needs further investigation. Well-planned clinical trials on the role of these bioactive compounds in promoting good human health as well as their toxic effects, if any, need to be undertaken in the future.

References

Abid M, Yaich H, Hidouri H, Attia H, Ayadi MA. Effect of substituted gelling agents from pomegranate peel on color, textural and sensory properties of pomegranate jam. Food Chem. 2018;39:1047–54.

Adaramoye O, Erguen B, Nitzsche B, Hopfner M, Jung K, Rabien A. Punicalagin, a polyphenol from pomegranate fruit, induces growth inhibition and apoptosis in human PC-3 and LNCaP cells. Chem Biol Interact. 2017;274:100–6.

Adebiyi OE, Olayemi FO, Ning-Hua T, Guang-Zhi Z. *In vitro* antioxidant activity, total phenolic and flavonoid contents of ethanol extract of stem and leaf of *Grewia carpinifolia*. Beni-Seuf Univ J Appl Sci. 2017;6:10–4.

Ahad S, Tanveer S, Malik TA, Nawchoo IA. Anticoccidial activity of fruit peel of *Punica granatum* L. Microb Pathog. 2018;116:78–83.

Ahamed MBK, Krishna V, Dandin CJ. *In vitro* antioxidant and *in vivo* prophylactic effects of two -lactones isolated from *Grewia tiliaefolia* against hepatotoxicity in carbon tetrachloride intoxicated rats. Eur J Pharmacol. 2010;631:42–52.

Ahmed HH, El-Abhar HS, Hassanin EAK, Abdelkader NF, Shalaby MB. *Punica granatum* suppresses colon cancer through downregulation of Wnt/β-Catenin in rat model. Braz J Pharmacol. 2017;27:627–35.

Ahuja M, Yadav M, Kumar S. Application of response surface methodology to formulation of ionotropically gelled gum cordia/gellan beads. Carbohydr Polym. 2010;80:161–7.

Akram M, Hamid A, Asif HM. *Aegle marmelos*: a potential of phytomedicine. Wudpacker J Med Plant. 2012;1(1):8–10.

Al-Awadi FM, Srikumar TS, Anim JT, Khan I. Antiinflammatory effects of *Cordia myxa* fruit on experimentally induced colitis in rats. Nutrition. 2001;17(5):391–6.

Al-Snafi AE. The pharmacological and therapeutic importance of *Cordia myxa*- A review. IOSR J Pharm. 2016;6(6):47–57.

Ambarwati D, Fatmawati F, Nooryanto M, Santoso S, Baktiyani SCW, Nurdiana N. *Punica granatum* fruit extract inhibits the production of pro-inflammatory cytokines and angiogenic factors of HUVEC cells induced by plasma from patients with pre-eclampsia. Clin Nutr Exp. 2017;15:9–14.

Ambigaipalan P, de Camargo AC, Shahidi F. Identification of phenolic antioxidants and bioactives of pomegranate seeds following juice extraction using HPLC-DAD-ESI-MS. Food Chem. 2017;221:1883–94.

Anon. 2018. Pomegranate. http://en.wikipedia.org/wiki/pomegranate. Accessed 17 Mar 2018.

Awachare CM, Kurian RM, Upreti KK, Laxman RH. Morpho-physiological diversity in *Annona* species. Sci Hortic. 2018;234:58–62.

Ayyanar M, Subash-Babu P, Ignacimuthu S. *Syzygium cumini* (L.) Skeels., a novel therapeutic agent for diabetes: folk medicinal and pharmacological evidences. Complement Ther Med. 2013;21:232–43.

Aziz ARA, AbouLaila MR, Aziz M, Omar MA, Khaled S. *In vitro* and *in vivo* anthelmintic activity of pumpkin seeds and pomegranate peels extracts against *Ascaridia galli*. Beni-Seuf Univ J Appl Sci. 2018;7:231–4.

Bag A, Bhattacharyya SK, Pal NK, Chattopadhyay RR. *In vitro* antibacterial potential of *Eugenia jambolana* seed extract against multidrug resistant human bacterial pathogens. Microbiol Res. 2012;167:352–7.

Baliga MS, Bhat HP, Pereira MM, Mathias N, Venkatesh P. Radioprotective effects of *Aegle marmelos* (L.)

Correa (Bael): a concise review. J Altern Complement Med. 2010;16(10):1109–16.

Baliga MS, Shivashankara AR, Haniadka R, Dsouza J, Bhat HP. Phytochemistry, nutritional and pharmacological properties of *Artocarpus heterophyllus* Lam (jackfruit): a review. Food Res Int. 2011a;44:1800–11.

Baliga MS, Bhat H, Baliga BRV, Wilson R, Palatty PL. Phytochemistry, traditional uses and pharmacology of *Eugenia jambolana* Lam. (black plum): a review. Food Res Int. 2011b;44:1776–89.

Baliga MS, Thilakchand KR, Rai MP, Rao S, Venkatesh P. *Aegle marmelos* (L.) Correa (Bael) and its phytochemicals in the treatment and prevention of cancer. Integr Cancer Ther. 2013;12(3):187–96.

Balyan U, Sarkar B. Integrated membrane process for purification and concentration of aqueous *Syzygium cumini* (L.) seed extract. Food Bioprod Process. 2016;98:29–43.

Bastos VJ, Neves LC, da Silva PMC, Shahab M, Colombo RC, Roberto SR. Harvest point determination of Indian jejube fruit (*Zizyphus mauritiana* L.) based on physicochemical and functional parameters. Sci Hortic. 2016;213:392–402.

Bera K, Ray S, Raja W, Ray B. Structural insight of an antioxidative arabinogalactan protein of *Aegle marmelos* fruit gum and its interaction with -lactoglobulin. Int J Biol Macromol. 2017;99:300–7.

Bezerra M, Araujo A, Santos K, Correia R. Caprine frozen yoghurt produced with fresh and spray dried jambolan fruit pulp (*Eugenia jambolana* Larn) and *Bifidobacterium animalis* subsp. *lactis* BI-07. LWT-Food Sci Technol. 2015;62:1099–104.

Bhatt ID, Rawat S, Badhani A, Rawal RS. Nutraceutical potential of selected wild edible fruits of the Indian Himalayan region. Food Chem. 2017;215:84–91.

Bhattacharya P, Saha A. Evaluation of reversible contraceptive potential of *Cordia dichotoma* leaves extract. Braz J Pharmacogn. 2013;23(2):342–50.

Biswas TK, Chakrawarti S, Pandit S, Jana U, Dey SK. Pilot study evaluating the use of *Emblica officinalis* standardized fruit extract in cardio-respiratory improvement and antioxidant status of volunteers with smoking history. J Herb Med. 2014;4:188–94.

Bonneau N, Baloul L, ba Ndob IB, Senejoux F, Champy P. The fruit of *Annona squamosa* L. as a source of environmental neurotoxins: from quantification of squamocin to annotation of Annonaceous acetogenins by LC-MS/MS analysis. Food Chem. 2017;226:32–40.

Branco IG, Moraes ICF, Argandona EJS, Madrona GS, Santos C, Ruiz ALTG, Carvalho JE, Haminiuk CWI. Influence of pasteurization on antioxidant and in vitro anti-proliferative effects of jambolan (*Syzygium cumini* L. Skeels) fruit pulp. Indus Crops Prod. 2016;89:225–30.

Burci LM, da Silva CB, Rondon JN, et al. Cute and subacute (28 days) toxicity, hemolytic and cytotoxic effect of *Artocarpus heterophyllus* seed extracts. Toxicol Rep. 2018. https://doi.org/10.1016/j.toxrep.2018.02.006

Carvalho TIM, Nogueira TYK, Mauro MA, Gomez-Alonso S, Gomes E, Da-Silva R, et al. Dehydration of jambolan (*Syzygium cumini* L.) juice during foam mat drying: quantitative and qualitative changes of the phenolic compounds. Food Res Int. 2017;102:32–42.

Castro-Lopez C, Ventura-Sobrevilla JM, Gonzalez-Hernandez MD, Rojas R, Ascacio-Valdes JA, Aguilar CN, Martinez-Avila GCG. Impact of extraction techniques on antioxidant capacities and phytochemical composition of polyphenol-rich extracts. Food Chem. 2017;237:1139–48.

Chaharlang M, Samavati V. Steady shear flow properties of *Cordia myxa* leaf gum as a function of concentration and temperature. Int J Biol Macromol. 2015;79:56–62.

Chandiran IS, Jayaveera KN, Karimulla S. Preliminary phytochemical and preclinical toxicity studies of *Grewia serrulata* DC. Drug Invent Today. 2013a;5:267–74.

Chandiran IS, Jayaveera KN, Karimulla S. Antioxidant property of *Grewia serrulate* DC and its hypoglycemic effect on normal and hyperglycemic rats. J Pharm Res. 2013b;6:813–7.

Chansriniyom C, Bunwatcharaphansakun P, Eaknai W, Nalinratana N, Ratnawong A, Khongkow M, et al. A synergistic combination of *Phyllanthus emblica* and *Alpinia galangal* against H_2O_2-induced oxidative stress and lipid peroxidation in human ECV304 cells. J Func Food. 2018;43:44–54.

Charoensiddhi S, Anprung P. Bioactive compounds and volatile compounds of Thai bael fruits (*Aegle marmelos* (L.) Correa) as a valuable source for functional food ingredients. Int Food Res J. 2008;15(3):287–95.

Chen Y, Xu SS, Chen JW, Wang Y, Xu HQ, Fan NB, Li X. Anti-tumor activity of *Annona squamosa* seeds extract containing annonaceous acetogenin compounds. J Ethnopharmacol. 2012;142(2):462–6.

Chen GL, Zhang X, Chen SG, Han MD, Gao YQ. Antioxidant activities and contents of free, esterified and insoluble-bound phenolics in 14 subtropical fruit leaves collected from the south of China. J Funct Food. 2017;30:290–302.

Cheng D, Zhu C, Cao J, Jiang W. The protective effects of polyphenols from jujube peel (*Zizyphus jejube* Mill) on isoproterenol-induced myocardial ischemia and aluminum-induced damage in rats. Food Chem Toxicol. 2012;50:1302–8.

Chinprahast N, Siripatrawan U, Leerahawong A, Triananwuttikul K. Effects of blanching and vacuum impregnation on physicochemical and sensory properties of Indian gooseberry (*Phyllanthus emblica* L.). J Food Process Preserv. 2013;37:57–65.

Czieczor L, Bentkamp C, Damerow L, Blanke M. Non-invasive determination of the quality of pomegranate fruit. Postharvest Biol Technol. 2018;136:74–9.

Daud MNH, Fatanah DN, Abdullah N, Ahmad R. Evaluation of antioxidant potential of *Artocarpus heterophyllus* L. J33 variety fruit waste from different extraction methods and identification of phenolic constituents by LCMS. Food Chem. 2017;232:621–32.

Deng Y, Li Y, Yang F, Zeng A, Yang S, Luo Y, et al. The extract of *Punica granatum* (pomegranate) peel induces apoptosis and impairs metastasis in prostate cancer cells. Biomed Pharmacother. 2017;93:976–84.

Derakhshan Z, Ferrante M, Tadi M, Ansari F, Heydari A, Hosseini MS, et al. Antioxidant activity and total phenolic content of ethanolic extract of pomegranate peels, juice and seeds. Food Chem Toxicol. 2018;114:108–11.

Deshpande M, Tondare PR, Paygude SV, Apte KG, Parab PB. Evaluation of antioxidant, anti-inflammatory and adipocyte differentiation inhibitory potential of *Zizyphus mauritiana* bark extract. Pharmacogn J. 2013;5(5):205–10.

Dholvitayakhun A, Trachoo N, Sakee U, Tim Cushnie TP. Potential applications for *Annona squamosa* leaf extract in the treatment and prevention of food borne bacterial disease. Nat Prod Commun. 2012;7:1–2.

Dholvitayakhun A, Trachoo N, Narkkong NA, Tim Cushnie TP. Using scanning and transmission electron microscopy to investigate the antibacterial mechanism of action of the medicinal plant *Annona squamosa* L. J Herbal Med. 2017;7:31–6.

Diamanti AC, Igoumenidis PE, Mourtzinos I, Yannakopoulou K, Karathanos VT. Green extraction of polyphenols from whole pomegranate fruit using cyclodextrins. Food Chem. 2017;214:61–6.

Dinda SC, Mukharjee B. Gum cordia- A new tablet binder and emulsifier. Acta Pharm Sci. 2009;51:189–98.

Dureante M, Montefusco A, Marrese PP, Soccio M, Pastore D, Piro G, Mita G, Lenucci MS. Seeds of pomegranate, tomato and grapes: an underestimated source of natural bioactive molecules and antioxidants from agri-food by-products. J Food Compos Anal. 2017;63:65–72.

Elzayat EM, Auda SH, Alanazi KH, Al-Agamy MH. Evaluation of wound healing activity of henna, pomegranate and myrrh herbal ointment blend. Saud Pharmaceut J. 2018;26:733. https://doi.org/10.1016/j.jsps.2018.02.016.

Ender P, Vural G, Nevzat A. Organic acids and phenolic compounds in pomegranates (*Punica granatum* L.) grown in Turkey. J Food Compos Anal. 2002;15:567–75.

Ezhilarasi AA, Vijaya JJ, Kaviyarasu K, Kennedy LJ, Ramalingam RJ, Al-Lohedan HA. Green synthesis of NiO nanoparticles using *Aegle marmelos* leaf extract for the evaluation of *in-vitro* cytotoxicity, antibacterial and photocatalytic properties. J Photochem Photobiol B Biol. 2018;180:39–50.

Faria AF, Marques MC, Mercadante AZ. Identification of bioactive compounds from jambolan (*Syzygium cumini*) and antioxidant capacity evaluation in different pH conditions. Food Chem. 2011;126:1571–8.

Fatima N, Pingali U, Muralidhar N. Study of pharmacodynamic interaction of *Phyllanthus emblica* extract with clopidogrel and ecosprin in patients with type II *diabetes mellitus*. Phytomedicine. 2014;21:579–85.

Fernandes F, Ferreres F, Gil-Izquierdo A, Oliveira AP, Valentao P, Andrade PB. Accumulation of primary and secondary metabolites in edible jackfruit seed tissue and scavenging of reactive nitrogen species. Food Chem. 2017;233:85–95.

Gajalakshmi S, Divya R, Deepika VD, Mythili S, Sathiavelu A. Pharmacological activities of *Annona squamosa*: a review. Int J Pharmaceut Sci Res. 2011;10(2):24–9.

Gajera HP, Gevariya SN, Patel SV. Nutritional profile and molecular fingerprints of indigenous black jamun (*Syzygium cumini* L.) landraces. J Food Sci Technol. 2018;55(2):730–9.

Ganjare AB, Nirmal SA, Patil AN, Golakiya BA. Use of apigenin from Cordia dichotoma in the treatment of colitis. Fitoterapia. 2011;82:1052–6.

Govindaraj D, Rajan M, Hatamleh AA, Munusamy MA. From waste to high-value product: jackfruit peel derived pectin/apatite bionanocomposites for bone healing applications. Int J Biol Macromol. 2018;106:293–301.

Goyal PK. Phytochemical and pharmacological properties of the genus Grewia: a review. Int J Pharm Pharm Sci. 2012;4(4):72–8.

Gulube Z, Patel M. Effect of Punica granatum on the virulence factors of cariogenic bacteria Streptococcus mutans. Microb Pathog. 2016;98:45–9.

Gupta RK, Kesari AN, Diwakar S, Tyagi A, Tandon V, Chandra R, Watal G. In vivo evaluation of anti-oxidant and anti-lipidemic potential of Annona squamosa aqueous extract in Type-2 diabetic models. J Ethnopharmacol. 2008;118(1):21–5.

Hafid AF, Aoki-Utsubo C, Permanasari AA, et al. Antiviral activity of the dichloromethane extracts from *Artocarpus heterophyllus* leaves against hepatitis C virus. Asian Pac J Trop Biomed. 2017;7:633–9.

Haldhar SM, Bhargava R, Krishna H, Berwal MK, Saroj PL. Bottom-up effects of different host plant resistance cultivars on ber (Zizyphus mauritiana) fruit fly (Carpomyia vesuviana) interactions. Crop Protect. 2018;106:117–24.

Haq MA, Alam MJ, Hasnain A. Gum Cordia: a novel edible coating to increase the shelf life of *Chilgoza* (*Pinus gerardiana*). LWT-Food Sci Technol. 2013;50:306–11.

Haq MA, Hasnain A, Azam M. Characterization of edible gum cordia film: effects of plasticizers. LWT-Food Sci Technol. 2014;55:163–9.

Iqbal J, Ababsi BA, Mahmood T, Kanwal S, Ali B, Shah SA, Khalil AT. Plant-derived anticancer agents: a green anticancer approach. Asian Pac J Trop Biomed. 2017a;7(12):1129–50.

Iqbal Z, Asif M, Aslam N, Akhtar N, Asmawi MZ, Fei YM, Jabeen Q. Clinical investigations on gastroprotective effects of ethanolic extract of *Phyllanthus emblica* L. fruits. J Herb Med. 2017b;7:11–7.

Jafari SM, Ghalenoel MG, Dehnad D. Influence of spray drying on water solubility index, apparent density, and anthocyanin content of pomegranate juice powder. Powder Technol. 2017;311:59–65.

Jamkhande PG, Barde SR, Patwekar SL, Tidke PS. Plant profile, phytochemistry and pharmacology of *Cordia dichotoma* (Indian cherry): a review. Asian Pac J Trop Biomed. 2013;3(12):1009–12.

Jana K, Bera TK, Ghosh D. Antidiabetic effects of Eugenia jambolana in the streptozotocin diabetic male albino rat. Biomar Genom Med. 2015;7:116–24.

Jang H, Srichayet P, Park WJ, Heo HJ, Kim DO, Tongchitpakadee S, et al. *Phyllanthus emblica* L. (Indian gooseberry) extracts protect against retinal degeneration in a mouse model of amyloid beta-induced Alzheimer's disease. J Funct Food. 2017;17:330–8.

Ji CJ, Zeng GZ, Han J, He WJ, Zhang YM, Tan NH. Zizimauritic acids A-C, three novel nortriterpenes from *Zizyphus mauritiana*. Bioorg Med Chem Lett. 2012;22:6377–80.

Ji X, Peng Q, Yuan Y, Shen J, Xie X, Wang M. Isolation, structures and bioactivities of the polysaccharides from jujube fruit (*Zizyphus mauritiana* mill): a review. Food Chem. 2017;227:349–57.

Jindal M, Rana V, Kumr V, Sapra B, Tiwary AK. Synthesis, physico-chemical and biomedical applications of sulfated *Aegle marmelos* gum: green chemistry approach. Arab J Chem. 2017;10:S2151–9.

Kabir Y, Sidhu JS. Antioxidative functional factors in nuts. In: Shi J, Ho CT, Shahidi F, editors. Functional foods of the east. New York: Taylor and Francis; 2011. p. 343–97.

Kabir Y, Shekhar HU, Sidhu JS. Phytochemical Compounds and Functional properties of mangoes. In: Siddiq M, Brecht JK, Sidhu JS, editors. Handbook of mango fruit: production, postharvest science, processing technology and nutrition. 1st ed. New York: Wiley-Blackwell Publishing Co; 2017. p. 237–54.

Kachkoul R, Houssaini TS, Miyah Y, Mohim M, ElHabbani R, Lahrichi A. The study of the inhibitory effect of calcium oxalate monohydrate crystallization by two medicinal and aromatic plants: *Ammi visnaga* and *Punica granatum*. Prog Urol. 2018;28(3):156–65.

Kaleem M, Asif M, Ahmed QU, Bano B. Antidiabetic and antioxidant activity of *Annona squamosa* extract in streptozotocin-induced diabetic rats. Singapore Med J. 2006;47(8):670–5.

Karimi M, Sadeghi R, Kokini J. Pomegranate as a promising opportunity in medicine and nanotechnology. Trends Food Sci Technol. 2017;69:59–73.

Khader SZA, Ahmed SSZ, Sathyan J, Mahboob MR, Venkatesh KP, Ramesh K. A comparative study on larvicidal potential of selected medicinal plants over green synthesized silver nanoparticles. Egypt J Basic Appl Sci. 2018;5:54–62.

Khan EA, Shahjahan, Khan TA. Adsorption of methyl red on activated carbon derived from custard apple (*Annona squamosa*) fruit shell: equilibrium isotherm and kinetic studies. J Mol Liquid. 2018a;249:1195–211.

Khan A, Ahmed T, Rizwan M, Khan N. Comparative therapeutic efficacy of *Phyllanthus emblica* (*amla*) fruit extract and procaine penicillin in the treatment of subclinical mastitis in dairy buffaloes. Microb Pathog. 2018b;115:8–11.

Khattak K, Rahman TU. Effect of gamma radiations on the vitamins, phytochemicals, antimicrobials and antioxidant properties of *Zizyphus mauritiana* Lam. leaves. Rad Phys Chem. 2016;127:243–8.

Kho YL, Jung W, Kwon D, Kim JH. Identification of estrone in pomegranate (*Punica granatum*) extracts by liquid chromatography-tandem mass spectrometry. Food Sci Biotechnol. 2010;19(3):809–13.

Kim ND, Mehta R, Yu WP, Neeman I, Livney T, Amichay TA. Chemopreventive and adjuvant therapeutic potential of pomegranate (*Punica granatum*) for human breast cancer. Breast Cancer Res Treatment. 2002;71:203–17.

Koley TK, Kaur C, Nagal S, Walia S, Jaggi S, Sarika. Antioxidant activity and phenolic content in genotypes of Indian jujube (*Zizyphus mauritiana* Lamk). Arab J Chem. 2016;9:S1044–52.

Kotsampasi B, Christodoulou C, Tsiplakou E, Mavrommatis A, Mitsiopoulou C, Karaiskou C, et al. Effects of dietary pomegranate pulp silage supplementation on milk yield and composition, milk fatty acid profile and blood plasma antioxidant status of lactating dairy cows. Anim Feed Sci Technol. 2017;234:228–36.

Krushna GS, Shivaranjani VL, Umamaheshwari J, Srinivasulu C, Hussain SA, Karren MA, et al. *In vivo* and molecular docking studies using whole extract and phytocompounds of *Aegle marmelos* fruit protective effects against isoproterenol-induced Myocardial infarction in rats. Biomed Pharmacol. 2017;91:880–9.

Kumar S, Singh A, Kumar B. Identification and characterization of phenolics and terpenoids from ethanolic extracts of *Phyllanthus* species by HPLC-ESI-QTOF-MS/MS. J Phrmaceut Anal. 2017;7:214–22.

Lan Y, Wu J, Wang X, Sun X, Hackman RM, Li Z, Feng X. Evaluation of antioxidant capacity and flavor profile change of pomegranate wine during fermentation and aging process. Food Chem. 2017;232:777–87.

Lansky EP, Newman RA. *Punica granatum* (pomegranate) and its potential for prevention and treatment of inflammation and cancer. J Ethnopharmacol. 2007;109:177–206.

Lee CJ, Chen LG, Liang WL, Hseih MS, Wang CC. Inhibitory effects of punicalagin from *Punica granatum* against type II collagenase-induced osteoarthritis. J Funct Food. 2018;41:216–22.

Les F, Carpene C, Arbones-Mainar JM, Decaunes P, Valero MS, Lopez V. Pomegranate juice and its main polyphenols exhibit direct effects on amine oxidases from human adipose tissue and inhibit lipid metabolism in adipocytes. J Funct Food. 2017;33:323–31.

Li X, Liu L, Pischetsrieder M. Pomegranate (*Punica granatum* L.) wine polyphenols affect Nrf2 activation and antioxidant enzyme expression in human neuroblastoma cells (SH-SY5Y). J Funct Food. 2017a;38:140–10.

Li Y, Xu J, Yuan C, Ma H, Liu T, Liu F, et al. Chemical composition and anti-hyperglycemic effects of triterpenoid enriched *Eugenia jambolana* Lam. berry extract. J Funct Food. 2017b;28:1–10.

Lim LBL, Priyantha N, Tennakoon DTB, et al. Breadnut peel as a highly effective low-cost biosorbent for methylene blue: equilibrium, thermodynamic and kinetic studies. Arab J Chem. 2017;10:S3216–28.

Lu CC, Yang SH, Hsia SM, Wu CH, Yen GC. Inhibitory effects of *Phyllanthus emblica* L. on hepatic steatosis and liver fibrosis in vitro. J Funct Food. 2016;20:20–30.

Ma C, Chen Y, Li X, Chen Y. A review on *Annona squamosa* L.: phytochemicals and biological activities. Am J Chin Med. 2017;45(5):933–64.

Maity P, Hansda D, Bandyopadhyay U, Mishra DK. Biological activities of crude extracts and chemical constituents of bael, *Aegle marmelos* (L.) Corr. Ind J Exptl Biol. 2009;47:849–61.

Maruza IM, Musemwa L, Mapurazi S, Matsika P, Munyati VT, Ndhieve S. Future prospects of *Zizyphus mauritiana* in alleviating household food insecurity and illnesses in arid and semi-arid areas: a review. World Develop Perspect. 2017;5:1–6.

Matias EFF, Alves EF, do Nascimento Silva MK, Carvalho VRA, Coutinho HDM, da Costa JGM. The genus *Cordia*: botanists, etho, chemical and pharmacological aspects. Braz J Pharmacogn. 2015;25:542–52.

Mirdehghan SH, Rahemi M. Seasonal changes of mineral nutrients and phenolics in pomegranate (*Punica granatum L.*). Sci Hortic Fruit. 2007;111:120–7.

Mishra T, Pal M, Kumar A, Rai D, Tewari SR. Termiticidal activity of *Punica granatum* fruit rind fractions and its compounds against *Microcerotermes beesoni*. Indus Crops Prod. 2017;107:320–5.

Mohamed AH, Karrar MA, Salih AM, Bashir AK, Ali MB, Khalid SA. Pharmacological activities of *Grewia bicolor* roots. J Ethnopharmacol. 1990;28(3):285–92.

Moorthy IG, Prakash Maran J, Ilakya S, Anitha SL, Pooja Sabarima S, Priya B. Ultrasound assisted extraction of pectin from waste *Artocarpus heterophyllus* fruit peel. Ultrason Sonochem. 2017;34:525–30.

Morsy MK, Mekawi E, Elsabash R. Impact of pomegranate peel nanoparticles on quality attributes of meatballs during refrigerated storage. LWT-Food Sci Technol. 2018;89:489–95.

Morton J. Pomegranate (*Punica granatum* L.). In: Morton JF, editor. Fruits of warm climates. Miami, FL: ECHO; 1987a. p. 352–5.

Morton J. Sugar apple. In: Morton JF, editor. Fruits of warm climates. Miami, FL: ECHO; 1987b. p. 69–72.

Mulholland DA, Sewram V, Raynor M, Thornell K, Raidoo DM. Coupling SFE to uterotonic bioassay: an online investigation of the uterotonic activity of compounds from *Grewia occidentalis* (Tiliaceae). South Afr J Bot. 2002;68:68–71.

Murhekar S, Wright MH, Greene AC, Brownlie JC, Cock IE. Inhibition of *Shewanella* spp. Growth by *Syzygium australe* and *Syzygium luehmannii* extracts: natural methods for the prevention of fish spoilage. J Food Sci Technol. 2017;54(10):3314–26.

Mustafa E, Dogan A. Pomegranate/Roma- *Punica granatum*. In: Exotic fruits. New York: Academic Press; 2018. p. 355–61.

Nahid S, Mazumdar K, Rahman Z, Islam S, Rashid MH, Kerr PG. Cardio- and hepato-protective potential of methanolic extract of *Syzygium cumini* (L.) Skeels seeds: a diabetic rat model study. Asian Pac J Trop Biomed. 2017;7(2):126–33.

Nasifah I, Soeharto S, Nooryanto M. Effects of anti-lipid peroxidation of *Punica granatum* fruit extract in endothelial cells induced by plasma of severe pre-eclamptic patients. J Ayurveda Integr Med. 2017;8:215–7.

Nava OJ, Soto-Robles CA, Gómez-Gutiérrez CM, et al. Fruit peel extract mediated green synthesis of zinc oxide nanoparticles. J Mol Struct. 2017;1147:1–6.

Nyakudya TT, Nosenga N, Chivandi E, Erlwanger KH, Gundidza M, Gundidza E, Magwa ML, Muredzi P. *Grewia bicolor* seed oil: putative pharmaceutical, cosmetic and industrial uses. South Afr J Bot. 2015;97:154–8.

Nyanga L, Gadaga TH, Nout MJR, Smid EJ, Boekhout T, Zwietering MH. Nutritive value of masau (*Zizyphus mauritiana*) fruits from Zambezi Valley in Zimbabwe. Food Chem. 2013;138:168–72.

Oktavia S, Wijayanti N, Retnoaji B. Anti-angiogenic effect of *Artocarpus heterophyllus* seed methanolic extract in *ex ovo* chicken chorioallantoic membrane. Asian Pac J Trop Biomed. 2017;7:240–4.

Panda S, Kar A. *Annona squamosa* seed extract in the regulation of hyperthyroidism and lipid-peroxidation in mice: possible involvement of quercetin. Phytomedicine. 2007a;14(12):799–805.

Panda S, Kar A. Antidiabetic and antioxidative effects of *Annona squamosa* leaves are possibly mediated through quercetin-3-O-glucoside. Biofactors. 2007b;31(3–4):201–10.

Panseeta P, Lomchoey K, Prabpai S, Kongsaeree P, Suksamrarn A, Ruchirawat S, Suksamrarn S. Antiplasmodial and antimycobacterial cyclopeptide alkaloids from the root of *Zizyphus mauritiana*. Phytochemistry. 2011;72:909–15.

Pawar HA, Jadhav P. Isolation, characterization and investigation of *Cordia dichotoma* fruit polysaccharide as a herbal excipient. Int J Biol Macromol. 2015;72:1228–36.

Peixoto MPG, Freitas LAP. Spray-dried extracts from *Syzygium cumini* seeds: physicochemical and biological evaluation. Braz J Pharmacogn. 2012;23(1):145–52.

Prabhu DL, Chandrasekar S, Ambashankar K, Dayal JS, Ebeneezar S, Ramachandran K, et al. Effect of dietary *Syzygium cumini* leaf powder on growth and non-specific immunity of *Litopenaeus vannamei* (Boone 1931) and defense against virulent strain of *Vibrio parahaemolyticus*. Aquaculture. 2018;489:9–20.

Priyanka C, Kumar P, Bankar SP, Karthik L. In vitro antibacterial activity and gas chromatography- mas spectroscopy analysis of *Acacia karoo* and *Zizyphus mauritiana* extracts. J Taibah Univ Sci. 2015;9:13–9.

Purena R, Seth R, Bhatt R. Protective role of *Emblica officinalis* hydro-ethanolic leaf extract in cisplatin induced nephrotoxicity in rats. Toxicol Rep. 2018;5:270–7.

Raghu V, Patel K, Srinivasan K. Comparison of ascorbic acid content of *Emblica officinalis* fruits determined by different analytical methods. J Food Comp Anal. 2007;20:529–33.

Rajaram A, Vanaja GR, Vyakaranam P, Rachamallu A, Reddy GV, et al. Anti-inflammatory profile of *Aegle marmelos* (L.) Correa (Bilva) with special reference to young roots grown in different parts of India. J Ayurveda Integr Med. 2018;9:90–8.

Ramlagan P, Rondeau P, Planesse C, Neergheen-Bhujun VS, Fawdar S, Bourdon E, Bahorun T. Punica granatum L. mesocarp suppresses advanced glycation end products (AGEs)- and H2O2-induced oxidative stress and pro-inflammatory biomarkers. J Funct Food. 2017;29:115–26.

Rathee D, Kamboj A, Sachdev R, Sidhu S. Hepatoprotective effect of *Aegle marmelos* augmented with piperine co-administration in paracetamol model. Braz J Pharmacogn. 2018;28:65–72.

Raza A, Butt MS, Ul-Haq I, Suleria HAR. Jamun (*Syzygium cumini*) seed and fruit extract attenuates hyperglycemia in diabetic rats. Asian Pac J Trop Biomed. 2017;7(8):750–4.

Ren YY, Zhu ZY, Sun HQ, Chen LJ. Structural characterization and inhibition on α-glucosidase activity of acidic polysaccharide from *Annona squamosa*. Carbohydr Polym. 2017;174:1–12.

Resendiz-Vazquez JA, Ulloa JA, Urias-Silvas JE, Bautista-Rosales PU, Ramirez-Ramirez JC, Rosas-Ulloa P, et al. Effect of high-intensity ultrasound on the technofunctional properties and structure of jackfruit (*Artocarpus heterophyllus*) seed protein isolate. Ultrason Sonochem. 2017;37:436–44.

Rodriguez KAF, Amorim LV, Dias CN, Moraes DFC, Carneiro SMP, Carvalho FAA. *Syzygium cumini* (L.) Skeels essential oil and its major constituent -pinene exhibit anti-*Leishmania* activity through immunomodulation in vitro. J Ethnopharmacol. 2015;160:32–40.

Ruiz-Montanez G, Ragazzo-Sanchez JA, Picart-Palmade L, Calderon-Santoyo M, Chevalier-Lucia D. Optimization of nanoemulsions processed by high pressure homogenization to protect a bioactive extract of jackfruit (*Artocarpus heterophyllus* lam). Innov Food Sci Emerg Technol. 2017;40:35–41.

Sahebhar A, Ferri C, Giorgini P, Bo S, Nachtigal P, Grassi D. Effects of pomegranate juice on blood pressure: a systematic review and meta-analysis of randomized controlled trials. Pharmacol Res. 2017;115:149–61.

Samavati V, Lorestani M, Joolazadeh S. Identification and characterization of hydrocolloid from *Cordia myxa* leaf. Int J Biol Macromol. 2014;65:215–21.

San B, Yildirim AN. Phenolic, alpha-tocopherol, beta-carotene and fatty acid composition of four promising jejube (*Zizyphus jejube* Miller) selections. J Food Comp Anal. 2010;23:706–10.

Sana SS, Badineni VR, Arla SK, Boya VKN. Eco-friendly synthesis of silver nanoparticles using leaf extract of *Grewia flaviscences* and study of their antimicrobial activity. Mater Lett. 2015;145:347–50.

Sandeep NC, Raghavendra Rao H, Hemachandra Reddy K. Extraction and characterization of physico-chemical and tensile properties of *Aegle marmelos* fiber. Mater Today Proc. 2017;4:3158–65.

Sankhari JM, Jadeja RN, Thounaojam MC, Devkar RV, Ramachandran AV. Safety evaluation of *Eugenia jambolana* seed extract. Asian Pac J Trop Med. 2010;1(1):982–7.

Santhalakshmy S, Bosco SJD, Francis S, Sabeena M. Effect of inlet temperature on physicochemical properties of spray-dried jamun fruit juice powder. Powd Technol. 2015;274:37–43.

Sathyanarayanan S, Chandran R, Thankarajan S, Abrahamse H, Thangaraj P. Phytochemical composition, antioxidant and anti-bacterial activity of *Syzygium calophyllifolium* Walp. Fruit. J Food Sci Technol. 2018;55(1):341–50.

Satish Kumar BN, Behera GM, Baidya M. Pharmacognosy, phytochemistry and pharmacology of *Annona squamosa* L.: a review. Res J Pharmacogn Phytochem. 2011;3(3):93–102.

Savikin K, Zivkovic J, Alimpic A, Zdunic G, Jankovic T, Duletc-Lausevic S, Menkovic N. Activity guided fractionation of pomegranate extract and its antioxidant, antidiabetic and antineurodegenerative properties. Indus Crops Products. 2018;113:142–9.

Shanmugavasan A, Vaitheeswaran KSR, Ramachandran T. Design and development of pyrolyser to extract medicinal oil from the stem of *Zizyphus jujuba*. J Anal App Pyrol. 2011;92:176–83.

Sharma GN, Dubey SK, Sharma P, Sati N. Medicinal value of Bael (*Aegle marmelos*) (L.) Corr: a review. Int J Curr Pharm Rev Res. 2011;1(3):12–22.

Sharma B, Siddiqui MS, Kumar SS, Ram G, Chaudhary M. Liver protective effects of aqueous extract of *Syzygium cumini* in Swiss albino mice on alloxan induced diabetes mellitus. J Pharm Res. 2013;6:853–8.

Sharma P, Manjusha RS, Malhotra H, Nitesh DS, Singh S. Antifertility potential of hydro-alcoholic extract of *Cordia dichotoma* G. Forsh. leaves: a folklore medicine used by Meena community in Rajasthan state of India. Asian Pac J Reprod. 2015;4(2):100–5.

Sharma RJ, Gupta RC, Singh S, Bansal AK, Singh IP. Stability of anthocyanins-enriched extracts, and formation of fruit pulp of *Eugenia jambolana* (*jamun*). Food Chem. 2016;190:808–17.

Sidhu JS. Tropical fruits II: production, processing and quality of guava, lychee and papaya. In: Sinha N, editor. Handbook of fruits and fruit processing. 2nd ed. New York: Wiley-Blackwell Publishing Co; 2012. p. 591–628.

Sidhu JS, Zafar TA. Super fruits: pomegranate, wolfberry, Aronia (chokeberry), acai, noni, amla. In: Sinha N, editor. Handbook of fruits and fruit processing. 2nd ed. New York: Wiley-Blackwell Publishing Co.; 2012. p. 653–79.

Silva KDRR, Sirasa MSF. Antioxidant properties of selected fruit cultivars grown in Sri Lanka. Food Chem. 2018;238:203–8.

da Silva PM, de Moura MC, Gomes FS, da Silva Trentin D, de Oliveira APS, de Mello GSV, et al. PgTel, the lectin found in *Punica granatum* juice, is an antifungal agent against *Candida albicans* and *Candida krusei*. Int J Biol Macromol. 2018;108:391–400.

Singh JP, Kaur A, Singh N, Nim L, Shevkani K, Kaur H, Arora DS. *In vitro* antioxidants and antimicrobial properties of *jambolan* (*Syzygium cumini*) fruit polyphenols. LWT-Food Sci Technol. 2016;65:1025–30.

Singh K, Lataye DH, Wasewat KL. Removal of fluorine from aqueous solution by using bael (*Aegle marmelos*) shell activated carbon: kinetic, equilibrium and thermodynamic study. J Fluor Chem. 2017;194:23–32.

Sivarajasekar N, Balasubramani K, Mohanraj N, Prakash Maran J, Sivamani S, Ajmal Koya P, Karthik V. Fixed-bed adsorption of atrazine onto microwave irradiated *Aegle marmelos* Correa fruit shell: statistical optimization, process design and breakthrough modeling. J Mol Liquids. 2017;241:823–30.

Srinivasan P, Subramaniyan V, Kothandaraman S, Palani M. Anti-diabetic activity of quercetin extracted from *Phyllanthus emblica* L. fruits: in silica and in vivo approaches. J Pharma Anal. 2018;8:109. https://doi.org/10.1016/j.jpha.2017.10.005.

Suppakul P, Boonlert R, Buaphet W, Sonkaew P, Luckaqnatinvong V. Efficacy of superior antioxidant Indian gooseberry extract-incorporated edible Indian gooseberry puree/methylcellulose composite films on enhancing the shelf life of roasted cashew nut. Food Control. 2016;69:51–60.

Suryadevara V, Lankapalli SR, Danda LH, Pendyala V, Katta V. Studies on jackfruit seed starch as a novel natural superdisintegrant for the design and evaluation of irbesartan fast dissolving tablets. Integr Med Res. 2017;6(3):280–91.

Tsai CC, Chou CH, Liu YC, Hsieh CW. Ultrasound-assisted extraction of phenolic compounds from *Phyllanthus emblica* L. and evaluation of antioxidant activities. Int J Cosmetic Sci. 2014;36:471–6.

Tundis R, Xiao J, Loizzo MR. *Annona* species (*Annonaceae*): a rich source of potential anti-tumor agents? Ann N Y Acad Sci. 2017;1398(1):30–6.

Tung YT, Huang CZ, Lin JH, Yen GC. Effect of *Phyllanthus emblica* L. fruit on methionine and choline-deficiency diet-induced nonalcoholic steatohepatitis. J Food Drug Anal. 2018;26:1245. https://doi.org/10.1016/j.jfda.2017.12.005.

Vadde R, Radhakrishnan S, Kurundu HEK, Reddivari L, Vanamala JKP. Indian gooseberry (*Emblica officinalis* Gaertn.) suppresses cell proliferation and induces apoptosis in human colon cancer stem cells independent of p53 status vie suppression of c-Myc and cyclin d1. J Funct Food. 2016;25:267–78.

Vaithiyanathan V, Mirunalini S. Chemo preventive potential of fruit juice of *Phyllanthus emblica* L. (amla) against mammary cancer by altering oxidant/antioxidant status, lipid profile levels and estrogen/progesterone receptor status in female Sprague-Dawley rats. Biomed Prevent Nutr. 2013;3:357–66.

Varghese S, Joseph MM, Aravind SR, Unnikrishnan BS, Sreelekha TT. The inhibitory effect of anti-tumor polysaccharide from *Punica granatum* on metastasis. Int J Biol Macromol. 2017;103:1000–10.

Vidya C, Manjunatha C, Chandraprabha MN, Rajshekar M, Mal AR. Hazard free green synthesis of ZnO nano-photo-catalyst using Artocarpus heterophyllus leaf extract for the degradation of Congo red dye in water treatment applications. J Environ Chem Eng. 2017;5:3172–80.

Wafa BA, Makni M, Ammar S, Khannous L, Hassana AB, Bouaziz M, et al. Antimicrobial effect of the Tunisian Nan variety *Punica granatum* L. extract against *Salmonella enterica* (Serovar Kentucky and Enteritidis) isolated from chicken meat and phenolic composition of its peel extract. Int J Food Microbiol. 2017;241:123–31.

Wang B, Huang Q, Venkitasamy C, Chai H, Gao H, Cheng N, et al. Changes in phenolic compounds and their antioxidant capacities in jejube (*Zizyphus jujube* Miller) during three maturity stages. LWT-Food Sci Technol. 2016a;66:56–62.

Wang X, Di X, Shen T, Wang S, Wang X. New phenolic compounds from the leaves of *Artocarpus heterophyllus*. Chin Chem Lett. 2016b;28:37–40.

Wang ST, Chou CT, Su NW. A food-grade self-nanoemulsifying delivery system for enhancing oral bioavailability of ellagic acid. J Funct Food. 2017;34:207–15.

Wani TA, Pandith SA, Rana S, Bhat WW, Dhar N, Razdan S, Chandra S, Kitchlu S, Sharma N. Promiscuous breeding behavior in relation to reproductive success in Grewia asiatica L. (Malvaceae). Flora. 2015;211:62–71.

Wani TA, Latto SK. Auxin response factor (GaARF) cloning and expression in relation to reproductive maturation in *Grewia asiatica* L. Plant Gene. 2017;12:123–30.

Wen L, Zhao Y, Jiang Y, Yu L, Zeng X, Yang J, Tian M, Liu H, Yang B. Identification of a flavonoid C-glycoside as potent antioxidant. Free Rad Biol Med. 2017;110:92–101.

Wojdylo A, Carbonell-Barrachina AA, Legua P, Hernanandez F. Phenolic composition, ascorbic acid content, and antioxidant capacity of Spanish jejube (*Zizyphus jejube* Mill.) fruits. Food Chem. 2016;201:307–14.

Wu CS, Gao QH, Guo XD, Yu JG, Wang M. Effect of ripening stage on physicochemical properties and antioxidant profiles of a promising table fruit 'pear jejube' (*Zizyphus jujube* Mill.). Sci Hortic. 2012;148:177–84.

Xi J, He L, Yan L. Continuous extraction of phenolic compounds from pomegranate peel using high voltage electrical discharge. Food Chem. 2017;230:354–61.

Xu SY, Liu JP, Huang X, Du LP, Shi FL, Dong R, Huang XT, Zheng K, Liu Y, Cheong KL. Ultrasonic-microwave assisted extraction, characterization and biological activity of pectin from jackfruit peel. LWT-Food Sci Technol. 2018;90:577–82.

Yadav SS, Meshram GA, Shinde D, Path RC, Manohar SM, Upadhye MV. Antibacterial and anticancer activity of bioactive fractions of *Syzygium cumini* L. seeds. HAYATI J Biosci. 2011a;18(3):118–22.

Yadav DK, Singh N, Dev K, Sharma R, Sahai M, Palit G, Maurya R. Anti-ulcer constituents of *Annona squamosa* twigs. Fitoterapia-Milano. 2011b;82(4):666–75.

Yuan WJ, Yuan JB, Peng JB, Ding YQ, Zhu JX, Ren G. Flavonoids from the roots of *Artocarpus heterophyllus*. Filoterpia. 2017;117:133–7.

Zafar TA, Sidhu JS. Composition and nutritional properties of mangoes. In: Siddiq M, Brecht JK, Sidhu JS, editors. Handbook of mango fruit: production, postharvest science, processing technology and nutrition. 1st ed. New York: Wiley-Blackwell Publishing Co; 2017. p. 217–36.

Zhang Y, Zhang Y, Xu F, Li S, Tan L. Structural characterization of starches from Chinese jackfruit seeds (*Artocarpus heterophyllus* Lam). Food Hydrocoll. 2018a;80:141–8.

Zhang Y, Hu M, Zhu R, Wu G, Tan L. Functional properties and utilization of *Artocarpus heterophyllus* Lam. seed starch from new species in China. Int J Biol Macromol. 2018b;107:1395–405.

Zhu K, Zhang Y, Nie S, Xu F, He S, Gong D, Wu G, Tan L. Physicochemical properties and in vitro antioxidant activities of polysaccharide from *Artocarpus heterophyllus* Lam. pulp. Carb Polymers. 2017;155:354–61.

Zhu H, Zhang Y, Tian J, Chu Z. Effect of a new shell material- jackfruit seed starch on novel flavor microcapsules containing vanilla oil. Indus Crops Prod. 2018;112:47–52.

Zivkovic J, Savikin K, Jankovic T, Cujic N, Menkovic N. Optimization of ultrasound-assisted extraction of polyphenolic compounds from pomegranate peel using response surface methodology. Sep Purific Technol. 2018;194:40–7.

Zozio S, Servent A, Hubert G, Hiol A, Pallet D, Mbeguie-A-Mbegguie D. Physicochemical and biochemical characteristics of ripening in jujube (*Zizyphus mauritiana* Lamk) fruits from to accessions grown in Guadeloupe. Sci Hortic. 2014a;175:290–7.

Zozio S, Servent A, Cazal G, Mbeguie-A-Mbegguie D, Ravion S, Pallet D, Abel H. Changes in antioxidant activity during the ripening of jejube (*Zizyphus mauritiana* Lamk). Food Chem. 2014b; 150:448–56.

Emerging Roles of Nutraceuticals from Selected Fermented Foods in Lifestyle-Related Disease Prevention

29

Jahidul Islam, Hitoshi Shirakawa, and Yearul Kabir

Contents

29.1 Introduction

In the present world, lifestyle-related diseases are a major public health problem. People are prone to suffer with this type of diseases depending on their daily lifestyle behavior. Intake of high- or low-fiber diet, smoking, alcohol consumption, and physical inactivity are the major factors responsible for the occurrence of diseases like diabetes, cancer, cardiovascular diseases, and neurodegeneration diseases. Lifestyle diseases not only reduced people's quality of life and life expectancy but also create a burden on health systems and economics, and on society. In 2013, 382 million people were diagnosed to have diabetes around the world and this incidence is expected to be 592 million by 2035 (Guariguata et al. 2014; Prabu et al. 2012).

Over the last two decades, the food industry has advanced and started sophisticated research in the development of healthier, more physiological benefits, which may reduce chronic disease risk. Thus, foods are often titled as "functional"

J. Islam · H. Shirakawa
Laboratory of Nutrition, Graduate School of Agricultural Science, Tohoku University, Sendai, Japan

Y. Kabir (✉)
Department of Biochemistry and Molecular Biology, University of Dhaka, Dhaka, Bangladesh

S. Sen, R. Chakraborty (eds.), *Herbal Medicine in India*, https://doi.org/10.1007/978-981-13-7248-3_29

when they have nutritional components vital for healthy living or "nutraceuticals" when considered to ameliorate or prevent disease or disorders through a variety of mode of actions (Perez-Gregorio and Simal-Gandara 2017). Generally, nutraceuticals are food or part of food which play an important role in modifying and maintaining normal physiological function and help in eliminating numerous lifestyle-related diseases like obesity, cardiovascular diseases, cancer, osteoporosis, arthritis, inflammation, and nonalcoholic fatty liver diseases (NAFLD) (Ramaa et al. 2006; Prabu et al. 2012; Khan et al. 2011). Although limited clinical studies on fermented foods have been done, there is confirmation that fermented foods deliver health benefits over the starting food materials. Study revealed that high nutraceuticals containing fermented foods provide many health benefits by acting as antioxidant as well as antimicrobial and anti-inflammatory agents (Selhub et al. 2014). Thus, this chapter will elucidate the relevance, and potentially the necessity, of certain fermented foods in the human diet and describes their health benefits especially in lifestyle-related disease prevention.

29.2 Nutraceuticals and Fermented Foods

The nutraceutical industries have primarily been categorized into three major parts, notably herbal products, dietary supplements, and functional foods. Among these, herbal/natural products and the dietary supplements are fast growing. The top most countries having nutraceutical markets include the United States, the United Kingdom, and Japan (Das et al. 2012). It is estimated that demand for nutraceutical ingredients has increased 5.8% annually and in 2010, the total nutraceutical market was found to be $ 15.5 billion globally (Prabu et al. 2012). On the other hand, China and India are the fastest growing nutraceutical markets (Prabu et al. 2012). The food components used as nutraceuticals are all natural and can be classified as dietary fiber, prebiotics, probiotics, vitamins, polyunsaturated fatty acids, polyphenols, and spices (Das et al. 2012).

In the fermentation process, functional microorganisms enzymatically transform the chemical constituents of raw materials of foods thereby enhancing the bioavailability of nutrients, enriching tastes and smells of the food, making the biopreservative process, removing toxic components, and finally producing antioxidant, antimicrobial, and probiotic functions with stimulating health-promoting bioactive compounds (Marco et al. 2017; Tamang et al. 2009). Nutraceuticals, for example, phenolic compounds in foods, have attracted great interest due to their beneficial effects on human health. Fermentation process can modulate phenolic compounds content in different foods. *Lactobacillus*-mediated fermented mottled cowpea had the highest soluble total phenolic content (TPC) (about 750 mg GAE/100 g DW) among the edible legumes compared to nonfermented samples (Gan et al. 2016). Soybeans incubated with *Aspergillus oryzae* at 30 °C for 48 h resulted in 23 times elevated genistein aglycones content when compared to unfermented soybean flour (da Silva et al. 2011). Barley fermented by *Lactobacillus johnsonii*, *L. reuteri*, and *L. acidophilus* showed a 20 times elevated total free phenolic acid compared to the unfermented sample (Hole et al. 2012). Cheonggukjang fermented by *Bacillus pumilus* for 60 h generates 2.8-fold, 7.6-fold, and 4.5-fold increases in gallic acid, catechin, and epicatechin, respectively (Cho et al. 2009).

29.2.1 Role of Nutraceuticals from Fermented Foods in Cancer Prevention

Cancer is a complicated disease with different phenotypes and origins. About 5–10% of all cancer cases can occur due to genetic defects, whereas the remaining 90–95% have been observed for environment and lifestyle factors (Anand et al. 2008). Fermented soybean products are one of the richest sources of isoflavones, which act as a phytoestrogen in humans (Klejdus et al. 2005). The isoflavone content has been reported as follows: genistein 8 mg daidzein 0.5 mg and glycitein 7.2 mg per 100 g in fermented soybean (Nakajima et al. 2005). Genistein is widely known for its anticancer effects (Cui et al. 2017). Chui et al. demonstrated that genistein significantly inhibited B16F10 cell proliferation and induced apoptosis in a time- and concentration-dependent manner. Genistein (100 μM) decreased the p-FAK, p-paxillin, tensin-2, vinculin, and α-actinin expression level, which finally regulates the FAK/paxillin and MAPK signaling pathways and regulates cancer progression (Cui et al. 2017). Genistein inhibited both the invasion of breast carcinoma cells and tumor growth in nude mice carrying MCF-7 and MDA-MB-231 xenografts by downregulating the matrixmettaloproteinase-9 (MMP-9), a gene involved in tumor cell migration (Shao et al. 1998). In a large, meta-analysis study, it is observed that soy intake was linked to lower incidence and mortality rate due to breast cancer (Chi et al. 2013). In another prospective cohort study of postmenopausal women, increasing amounts of daidzein consumption are responsible for reduced breast cancer recurrence (Guha et al. 2009).

Flavonols such as kaempferol and quercetin are abundantly found in Mulberry leaf extract which was fermented by *L. plantarum*, and these bioactive compounds have been involved in cancer prevention and progression (Lee et al. 2015a). The COX-2-catalyzed synthesis of prostaglandin E2 plays a key role in inflammation and its associated diseases and cancer (O'Leary et al. 2004). Quercetin and quercetin conjugates reduce COX-2 mRNA expression and activity in both unstimulated and Il-1β-stimulated $CaCO_2$ cells (O'Leary et al. 2004). Supplementing a diet containing quercetin (0–4.5 g/kg) suppresses the formation of early preneoplastic lesions in colon carcinogenesis by decreasing proliferation and increasing apoptosis (Warren et al. 2009). Besides, serum interleukin-6 (IL-6), a proinflammatory cytokine, is considered a sign of inflammation as well as colorectal carcinogenesis, which was found lower in participants taking flavonols, especially kaempferol and quercetin (Bobe et al. 2010). Kaempferol decreased cell viability and induced a G2/M phase cell cycle arrest in a concentration-dependent manner in SK-HEP-1 human hepatic cancer cells, which implies that kaempferol may be useful for long-term cancer prevention (Huang et al. 2013). Indole-3-carbinol (I3C) is another nutraceutical found in fermented cabbage (Tolonen et al. 2002). In C33A cervical cancer cells, I3C reduced Bcl-2 protein in a time- and dose-dependent manner (Chen et al. 2001).

Besides, cancer also develops through exposure to carcinogens. It is found that probiotics reduced the consumed carcinogens by several different practices, including emphasizing detoxification, improving apoptosis (programmed death of damaged cells), and inhibiting tumor growth (Aso and Akazan 1992). *Bifidobacterium breve* and *L. casei*, found in fermented foods like sauerkraut and kefir, both reduce intestinal absorption of toxicants such as bisphenol A. (Oishi et al. 2008). Bisphenol A has been shown to play a role in the pathogenesis of several endocrine disorders as well as hormone-dependent tumors such as breast and prostate cancer (Konieczna et al. 2015). Kimchi, a fermented cabbage dish, comprises probiotic strains that breaks down the organophosphorus pesticides by that toxin as food and breaks down sodium nitrate, a cancer-causing food preservative (Cho et al. 2009). Previously, fermented mung bean and soybean have been separately reported to have antioxidant, cytotoxic, and immunomodulatory effects (Ali et al. 2016). Nutraceuticals, for example, free amino acids and soluble phenolic acids (especially protocatechuic acid), were found in fermented mung bean. Both fermented mung bean and soybean products possessed cytotoxicity activities against breast cancer MCF-7 cells by arresting the G0/G1 phase followed by apoptosis. Moreover, they also induced splenocyte proliferation and enhanced serum interleukin-2 and interferon-γ to limit breast cancer cell proliferation (Ali et al. 2016).

29.2.2 Role of Nutraceuticals from Fermented Food for Metabolic Syndrome Prevention

Metabolic syndrome (MetS) characterizes a group of disorder including obesity, elevated blood pressure, and impaired glucose metabolism, dyslipidemia, and cardiometabolic risk. The prevalence of metabolic syndrome is currently reaching epidemic proportions throughout the world (Wu et al. 2010). The treatment of MetS is basically dependent on an improvement of lifestyle, physical exercise, and a balanced low-energy diet.

Rice bran is a by-product of the rice milling process and a rich source of dietary fiber and numerous bioactive molecules like indole compounds (Islam et al. 2017). Fermented rice bran (FRB) prepared by dual fermentation of rice bran using *Aspergillus kawachii* and *Lactobacillus sp.* is effective against MetS observed in an animal model (Alauddin et al. 2016). Alauddin et al. (2016) showed that long-term supplementation of 5% FRB significantly reduced both systolic and diastolic blood pressure and improved leptin impairment and increased serum adiponectin levels and angiotensin-converting enzyme (ACE) inhibitory activity as well as insulin sensitivity. Besides, chronic FRB supplementation downregulated the gluconeogenesis and lipogenesis in the liver and alleviate MetS (Alauddin et al. 2016).

Monacolin K (lovastatin), a metabolite generated by Monascus, has been described as a 3-hydroxy-3-methylglutaryl-coenzyme A (HMG-CoA) reductase inhibitor (statins) with cholesterol-lowering action which is found in red mold rice (RMR). RMR is produced through the fermentation of ordinary rice with *Monascus* species. Water extracts of RMR suppress the glycerol-3-phosphate dehydrogenase (GPDH) activity and lipid accumulation, a marker of adipogenesis, in a dose-dependent manner in 3T3-L1 preadipocytes (Jeon et al. 2004). Animal study revealed that RMR (0.4 or 2%) doses for 6 weeks had lower weight gain and less fat pads mass accompanied with smaller fat cells compare to HF diet. Besides, RMR supplement considerably reduced serum total cholesterol and low-density lipoprotein (LDL) cholesterol and successfully prevented metabolic disorder in even providing high-fat diet (Chen et al. 2008).

Kimchi, another popular fermented food, contains beneficiary probiotic strain, notably lactic acid bacteria (Park et al. 2012). Park et al. demonstrated that 12 weeks of dietary intervention of HF-KCO (high-fat diet containing 3% kimchi manufactured with the starter culture *W. koreensis* OK1-6) on C57BL/6J mice significantly lowers the obesity by decreasing leptin and the mRNA expression level of liver X receptor α (LXRα), SREBP2, stearoyl-CoA desaturase-1 (SCD1), peroxisome proliferator-activated receptor γ (PPARγ), and CPT1 along with body and epididymal fat weight in the HF-KCO group compared to other control and HF diet group (Park et al. 2012). Red ginseng roots have bioactive compounds like saponins (ginsenosides) and nonsaponins (Oh et al. 2014). Both compounds have been recognized as potential compounds in maintaining blood glucose and insulin levels (Oh et al. 2014). Besides fermented ginseng roots (FGR) have elevated amount of saponins compared to nonfermented red ginseng (Oh et al. 2014). Study revealed that consuming 2.7 g/day of FGR for 4 weeks had reduced fasting and postprandial glucose, and increased fasting and postprandial insulin levels in human subjects (Oh et al. 2014). Kho et al. demonstrated that FRG 250 mg/kg/day for 8 weeks supplementation significantly reduced body weight, epididymal fat weight, and adipocyte size and prevented high-fructose-diet-induced hyperlipidemia and hypertension (Kho et al. 2016). FRG prevented endothelial dysfunction by downregulating endothelin-1 (ET-1) and adhesion molecules in the aorta as well as markedly upregulating the insulin receptor substrate 1 (IRS-1) and glucose transporter type 4 (Glut4) in the muscle and finally ameliorated MetS (Kho et al. 2016).

In addition, another Korean traditional fermented soybean pastes, called Doenjang, has investigated its protective effect against obesity and type 2 diabetes, where flavonoids and *Bacillus* probiotic strains are the major nutraceuticals (Kim et al. 2018). Long-term fermented soybean pastes (LFSPs) protects high-fat-diet (HFD)-induced nonalcohol fatty liver disease (NAFLD) and insulin resistance in obese mice. LFSPs improved glucose tolerance and increased adiponectin levels and attenuated HFD-induced gut permeability and lowered serum lipopolysaccharide (LPS) level to protect against NAFLD and insulin resistance (Kim et al. 2018).

Probiotics are also used as biotherapies during prevention of metabolic disorders (Mallappa et al. 2012). In a study, Kaddoka et al. (2010) revealed that probiotic LG2055 strain significantly reduced the abdominal adiposity and body weight in a study conducted with 87 high body mass index subjects who were randomly divided into two groups receiving either *L. gasseri* SBT 2055 (LG2055) or placebo and thus playing a role in obesity prevention.

Diabetes mellitus (DM) is another major health problem in the world. Type 2 diabetes is a complex metabolic disorder caused by insulin resistance, impaired insulin signaling and β-cell dysfunction, and abnormal glucose and lipid metabolism (Bahadoran et al. 2013). Elevated oxidative stress plays an important role in the occurrence and development of diabetes mellitus. Quercetin is well known for its antioxidative properties, abundantly present in the fermented onion (*Allium cepa*), when *Aspergillus kawachii* is used for fermentation (Yang et al. 2012). It has been reported that intraperitoneal-injected quercetin (15 mg/kg/day) reduced the oxidative stress and NO production and increased the antioxidant activity as well as maintain the pancreatic β-cell integrity in streptozotocin (STZ)-induced diabetes in rats (Coskun et al. 2005; Kim et al. 2007). Berries are considered as a rich source of bioactive phenolic compounds that can bind and prevent the enzyme dipeptidyl peptidase-IV (DPP-IV), a current target for type 2 diabetes therapy (Johnson and de Mejia 2016). Johnson and de Mejia extracted phenolic compounds like anthocyanins, predominantly delphinidin-3-arabinoside from fermented berry beverages which increased the insulin secretion from pancreatic β-cells *in vitro* by modulating DPP-IV and its substrate GLP-1 action (Johnson and de Mejia 2016).

29.2.3 Role of Nutraceuticals from Fermented Foods in Neurodegeneration and Anti-Aging

Aging is one of the key factors responsible for neurological disorder and enhanced neuroinflammation due to decrease antioxidant activity in the body. There is a growing interest toward the nutritional supplements like fermented food products or herbal medicines for the prevention and treatment of neurodegenerative diseases (Rehman et al. 2017). Anthocyanins are the major polyphenolic compounds found in fermented strawberry (Hornedo-Ortega et al. 2017), which prevented D-galactose (D-gal)-induced oxidative stress and elevated inflammatory response causing memory and synaptic dysfunction. Supplemented anthocyanins significantly improved behavioral performance by inhibiting activated astrocytes and neuroinflammation by suppressing inflammatory markers including p-NF- KB, inducible nitric oxide synthase (iNOS), and TNF-α in the hippocampus and cortex regions of D-gal-treated rats' brain (Rehman et al. 2017). Thus, anthocyanins could be an excellent nutraceutical for prevention of age-related neurodegenerative diseases such as Alzheimer's disease (AD) (Rehman et al. 2017). Monacolin k and gamma-aminobutyric acid (GABA) are the major active functional compounds that are isolated from red mold rice (RMR), which is being fermented by *Monascus purpureus* (Kim et al. 2016). GABA is the main inhibitory neurotransmitter in the central nervous system. Oral supplementation of GABA is an effective approach for memory performance and neurochemical profile in hippocampus of rats and can be used for the treatment of AD (Tabassum et al. 2017). Monacolin K also prevented amyloid beta peptide–induced neurotoxicity via repressing small G-protein-mediated inflammation, a potent synergism of anti-inflammatory and antioxidative effect in PC12 cell (Lee et al. 2008). Further, probiotics in fermented foods may also influence brain function via gut microbiota. Probiotic bacteria like *Lactobacillus* and *Bifidobacterium* strains are capable of producing GABA from glutamate (Barrett et al. 2012). Desbonnet et al. demonstrated that 14-day treatment of probiotics containing *Bifidobacteria infantis* on Sprague-Dawley rats significantly reduced the IFN-γ, TNF-α, and IL-6 cytokines and increased the plasma concentrations of tryptophan compared to control following mitogen stimulation (Desbonnet et al. 2008). Thus, *Bifidobacteria* treatment opens an encouraging evidence that this probiotic may possess antidepressant properties. Therefore, it is hypothesized that fermented foods containing nutraceuticals might improve cognitive function by modulating the release of neurotransmitters (Desbonnet et al. 2008).

Isoflavone (genistein and daidzein) and β-glucan content were found elevated in fermented barley and soybean formula (BS) by yeast fermentation (Lee et al. 2015b). In a clinical study with BS-containing drink (3 g/day) for 8 weeks significantly improved the hyaluronan (HA) and skin barrier function *in vitro* and reduced Hyal2 expression in human dermal fibroblasts (HDF). BS also recovered ultraviolet (UV) B-induced downregulation of HA in HaCaT cells. Thus, BS has promising potential for development as a health functional food to enhance skin health (Lee et al. 2015b).

29.2.4 Role of Nutraceuticals from Fermented Food in Cardiovascular Disease Prevention

Cardiovascular disease (CVD) is the key cause of mortality and morbidity in the world (Micha et al. 2012). Major risk factors for CVD include presence of type 2 diabetes, dyslipidemia, obesity, and inflammation. Dietary components lessen CVD risk by attenuating associated risk factors, notably legumes. Diets containing fermented legumes are considered as a cardioprotective diet as they are associated with better weight management and glycemic control, reduced blood pressure, and a better plasma lipid profile (Bouchenak and Lamri-Senhadji 2013).

Nutraceuticals such as isoflavones, phytosterols, and lecithins are abundantly found in soybeans, which may act collectively or independently for cardioprotection (Ramdath et al. 2017). Dietary soy isoflavones increase arterial vasodilatation, improve endothelial function, and decrease blood pressure (BP), perhaps by nitric oxide (NO)-dependent mechanism in animal experiments (Mahn et al. 2005). Besides, this soy isoflavones also increase renal blood flow and sodium excretion, and interact with estrogen receptors to inhibit ACE activity in the renin–angiotensin–aldosterone system (Nagata et al. 2016). In an epidemiological study, it has been shown that there is an inverse association between consuming whole soy foods/products and CVD risk (Gil-Izquierdo et al. 2012). Same results were observed in dietary intakes of natto (fermented soy beans) and CVD mortality in Japanese adults, especially reductions in mortality from stroke by taking soy protein and natto (Nagata et al. 2016).

Isoflavones also decreased hypertension via endothelial vasodilation. In a study on postmenopausal women, isoflavone supplementation for 6 months increased endothelial vasodilation by significantly reducing cellular adhesion molecules (Colacurci et al. 2005). A reduction in SBP was found in pre- or hypertensive, mildly hyperglycemic postmenopausal women after taking isoflavones (100 mg), along with soy protein, for 6 months (Liu et al. 2013), although several studies found no effect on BP after intake of soy isoflavones (81–100 mg/day) for 6 weeks (Wong et al. 2012) or 1 year on menopausal women (Curtis et al. 2013).

Pigeon pea (*Cajanus cajan* L.) is another well-known grain legume crop in tropical and subtropical countries and contains high levels of phytosterol. Water extracts of *Bacillus subtilis*-mediated fermented pigeon pea has been shown to possess antidyslipidemic activity (Lee et al. 2015c). In an animal model, 100 mg/kg body weight of fermented pigeon pea significantly maintained both systolic and diastolic blood pressure (30 mmHg) in spontaneously hypertensive rats compared to nonfermented ones. Thus, *Bacillus*-fermented pigeon pea containing bioactive molecules is beneficial for cardiovascular disease prevention and can be used as a new source of nutraceuticals (Lee et al. 2015c).

29.2.5 Role of Nutraceuticals from Fermented Food in Ulcerative Colitis Disease Prevention

The occurrence and prevalence of inflammatory bowel diseases (IBDs) including ulcerative colitis (UC) and Crohn's disease are rapidly grow-

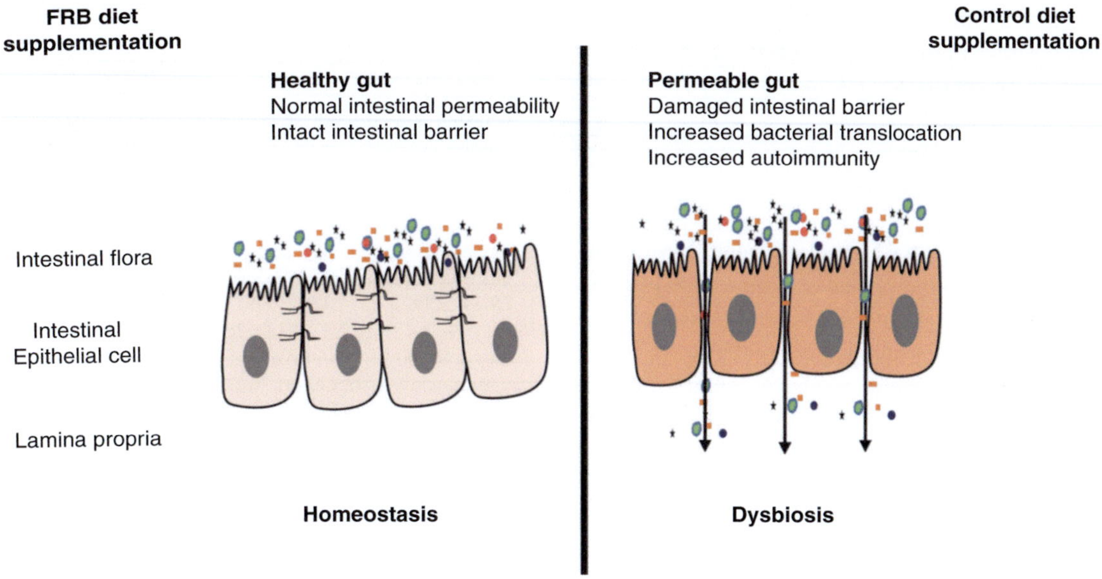

Fig. 29.1 Role of fermented rice bran in tight junctions (TJs) barrier integrity

ing in Western countries and in developed Asian countries (Kanai et al. 2014). It is a chronic immune disorder of unclear etiology (Islam et al. 2017). Environmental factors, especially lifestyle patterns for prolong intake of westernized diet (low fiber) resulting in the dysregulated composition of intestinal microbiota or dysbiosis, is responsible for its occurrence (Islam et al. 2017). Drugs that are used for suppressing the immune system have been effective in patients with IBD but termination of these drugs leads to relapse in the majority of patients (Kanai et al. 2014).

Fermented rice bran (FRB) is an excellent source of nutraceuticals like high fiber (Alauddin et al. 2016) and gut microbiome-induced short chain fatty acids (SCFAs) (Islam et al. 2017). Islam et al. explored the anti-colitis effect of FRB supplementation in a murine model of UC by 3% dextran sodium sulfate (DSS) and reported that the FRB-supplemented group significantly reduced the myeloperoxidase (MPO) and thiobarbituric acid-reactive substance levels and proinflammatory cytokine transcript (Tnf-a, Il-1b, Il-6, and Il-17) levels in the colon compared to the nonfermented group. Dietary FRB alleviated colitis via elevated production of SCFAs and tryptophan, which might regulate tight junction (TJ) barrier integrity and intestinal homeostasis (Fig. 29.1). Therefore, FRB could be a possible preventive dietary supplementation for UC (Islam et al. 2017). Hahm et al. demonstrated that fermented kimchi can significantly prevent DSS-induced colitis-associated cancer (CAC) in 12 weeks. Probiotics, *L. plantarum*, contained in the fermented kimchi, showed significantly inhibitory actions of IL-6, STAT3, and NF-κB, while in nonfermented kimchi, the involvement of probiotics and cancer prevention was highlighted (Hahm et al. 2018). Soy isoflavones such as genistein, daidzein, and its metabolite equol exhibit estrogen-like activity in the colon and enhance tight junctions (TJ) proteins and decrease proinflammatory cytokines production in experimental colitis (Verdu et al. 2002; Suzuki and Hara 2011). Woo et al. (2016) demonstrated the anti-colitis effects of fermented barley and soybean mixture (BS) on intestinal inflammation using a murine model of IBD. Orally administrated BS (100 and 200 mg/kg/day) for 3 days alleviated the severity of colitis by decreasing proinflammatory cytokines and epithelial barrier dysfunction, inducing an increase of TJ protein levels in colonic tissues. Supplementation of BS increased the levels of *Lactobacilli* and *Bacteroides* in the gut, protecting against inflammatory bowel disease (Woo et al. 2016).

29.3 Conclusion

Fermented foods have excellent health-promoting benefits due to the presence of functional microorganisms and optimistic source of nutraceuticals. Fermented foods are treated globally as health foods and therapeutic foods, although sophisticated research is still needed to validate the health claims of fermented foods by clinical trials and animal model experiments. Consequently, there is a need to provide consumers with more information to effectively guide them in making wider choices of fermented foods that contain optimal levels of health-promoting nutraceuticals.

References

Alauddin M, Shirakawa H, Koseki T, Kijima N, Ardiansyah, Budijanto S, Islam J, Goto T, Komai M. Fermented rice bran supplementation mitigates metabolic syndrome in stroke-prone spontaneously hypertensive rats. BMC Complement Altern Med. 2016;16(1):442.

Ali NM, Yeap SK, Yusof HM, Beh BK, Ho WY, Koh SP, Abdullah MP, Alitheen NB, Long K. Comparison of free amino acids, antioxidants, soluble phenolic acids, cytotoxicity and immunomodulation of fermented mung bean and soybean. J Sci Food Agric. 2016;96(5):1648–58.

Anand P, Kunnumakkara AB, Sundaram C, Harikumar KB, Tharakan ST, Lai OS, Sung B, Aggarwal BB. Cancer is a preventable disease that requires major lifestyle changes. Pharm Res. 2008;25(9):2097–116.

Aso Y, Akazan H. Prophylactic effect of a Lactobacillus casei preparation on the recurrence of superficial bladder cancer. Urol Int. 1992;49(1):125–9.

Bahadoran Z, Mirmiran P, Azizi F. Dietary polyphenols as potential nutraceuticals in management of diabetes: a review. J Diabetes Metab Disord. 2013;12:43.

Barrett E, Ross RP, O'Toole PW, Fitzgerald GF, Stanton C. γ-Aminobutyric acid production by culturable bacteria from the human intestine. J Appl Microbiol. 2012;113:411–7.

Bobe G, Albert PS, Sansbury LB, Lanza E, Schatzkin A, Colburn NH, Cross AJ. Interleukin-6 as a potential indicator for prevention of high-risk adenoma recurrence by dietary flavonols in the polyp prevention trial. Cancer Prev Res (Phila). 2010;3(6):764–75.

Bouchenak M, Lamri-Senhadji M. Nutritional quality of legumes, and their role in cardiometabolic risk prevention: a review. J Med Food. 2013;16:185–98.

Chen DZ, Qi M, Auborn KJ, Carter TH. Indole-3-carbinol and diindolylmethane induce apoptosis of human cervical cancer cells and in murine HPV16-transgenic preneoplastic cervical epithelium. J Nutr. 2001;131(12):3294–302.

Chen WP, Ho BY, Lee CL, Lee CH, Pan TM. Red mold rice prevents the development of obesity, dyslipidemia and hyperinsulinemia induced by high-fat diet. Int J Obes. 2008;32(11):1694–704.

Chi F, Wu R, Zeng YC, Xing R, Liu Y, Xu ZG. Post-diagnosis soy food intake and breast cancer survival: a meta-analysis of cohort studies. Asian Pac J Cancer Prev. 2013;14:2407–12.

Cho K, Math R, Islam S, Lim W, Hong S, Kim J, Yun M, Cho J, Yun H. Biodegradation of chlorpyrifos by lactic acid bacteria during kimchi fermentation. J Agri Food Chem. 2009;57(5):1882–9.

Colacurci N, Chiantera A, Fornaro F, de Novellis V, Manzella D, Arciello A, Chiantera V, Improta L, Paolisso G. Effects of soy isoflavones on endothelial function in healthy postmenopausal women. Menopause. 2005;12:299–307.

Coskun O, Kanter M, Korkmaz A, Oter S. Quercetin, a flavonoid antioxidant, prevents and protects streptozotocin-induced oxidative stress and beta-cell damage in rat pancreas. Pharmacol Res. 2005;51(2):117–23.

Cui S, Wang J, Wu Q, Qian J, Yang C, Bo P. Genistein inhibits the growth and regulates the migration and invasion abilities of melanoma cells via the FAK/paxillin and MAPK pathways. Oncotarget. 2017;8(13):21674–91.

Curtis PJ, Potter J, Kroon PA, Wilson P, Dhatariya K, Sampson M, Cassidy A. Vascular function and atherosclerosis progression after 1 y of flavonoid intake in statin-treated postmenopausal women with type 2 diabetes: a double-blind randomized controlled trial. Am J Clin Nutr. 2013;97:936–42.

Das L, Bhaumik E, Raychaudhuri U, Chakraborty R. Role of nutraceuticals in human health. J Food Sci Technol. 2012;49(2):173–83.

da Silva LH, Celeghini RMS, Chang YK. Effect of the fermentation of whole soybean flour on the conversion of isoflavones from glycosides to aglycones. Food Chem. 2011;128:640–4.

Desbonnet L, Garrett L, Clarke G, Bienenstock J, Dinan TG. The probiotic Bifidobacteriainfantis: an assessment of potential antidepressant properties in the rat. J Psychiatr Res. 2008;43(2):164–74.

Gan RY, Shah NP, Wang MF, Lui WY, Corke H. Fermentation alters antioxidant capacity and polyphenol distribution in selected edible legumes. Int J Food Sci Technol. 2016;51(4):875–84.

Gil-Izquierdo A, Penalvo JL, Gil JI, Medina S, Horcajada MN, Lafay S, Silberberg M, Llorach R, Zafrilla P, Garcia-Mora P, Ferreres F. Soy isoflavones and cardiovascular disease epidemiological, clinical and -omics perspectives. Curr Pharm Biotechnol. 2012;13(5):624–31.

Guariguata L, Whiting DR, Hambleton I, Beagley J, Linnenkamp U, Shaw JE. Global estimates of diabetes prevalence for 2013 and projections for 2035. Diabetes Res Clin Pract. 2014;103:137–49.

Guha N, Kwan ML, Quesenberry CP, Weltzien EK, Castillo AL, Caan BJ. Soy isoflavones and risk of cancer recurrence in a cohort of breast cancer survivors: the life after cancer epidemiology study. Breast Cancer Res Treat. 2009;118:395–405.

Hahm KB, Han YM, Park JM. P061 probiotic kimchi prevented colitis-associated cancer. J Crohns Colitis. 2018;12(1):S123–4.

Hole AS, Rud I, Grimmer S, Sigl S, Narvhus J, Sahlstrøm S. Improved bioavailability of dietary phenolic acids in whole grain barley and oat groat following fermentation with probiotic Lactobacillus acidophilus, Lactobacillus johnsonii, and Lactobacillus reuteri. J Agric Food Chem. 2012;60:6369–2 75.

Hornedo-Ortega R, Álvarez-Fernández MA, Cerezo AB, Garcia-Garcia I, Troncoso AM, Garcia-Parrilla MC. Influence of fermentation process on the anthocyanin composition of wine and vinegar elaborated from strawberry. J Food Sci. 2017;82(2):364–72.

Huang WW, Tsai SC, Peng SF, Lin MW, Chiang JH, Chiu YJ, Fushiya S, Tseng MT, Yang JS. Kaempferol induces autophagy through AMPK and AKT signaling molecules and causes G2/M arrest via downregulation of CDK1/cyclin B in SK-HEP-1 human hepatic cancer cells. Int J Oncol. 2013;42(6):2069–77.

Islam J, Koseki T, Watanabe K, Ardiansyah BS, Oikawa A, Alauddin M, Goto T, Aso H, Komai M, Shirakawa H. Dietary supplementation of fermented rice bran effectively alleviates dextran sodium sulfate-induced colitis in mice. Nutrients. 2017;9(7):E747.

Jeon T, Hwang SG, Hirai S, Matsui T, Yano H, Kawada T, Lim BO, Park DK. Red yeast rice extracts suppress adipogenesis by down-regulating adipogenic transcription factors and gene expression in 3T3-L1 cells. Life Sci. 2004;75:3195–203.

Johnson MH, de Mejia EG. Phenolic compounds from fermented berry beverages modulated gene and protein expression to increase insulin secretion from pancreaticβ-cells in vitro. J Agric Food Chem. 2016;64:2569–81.

Kadooka Y, Sato M, Imaizumi K, Ogawa A, Ikuyama K, Akai Y, et al. Regulation of abdominal adiposity by probiotics (Lactobacillus gasseri SBT2055) in adults with obese tendencies in a randomized controlled trial. Eur J Clin Nutr. 2010;64:636–43.

Kanai T, Matsuoka K, Naganuma M, Hayashi A, Hisamatsu T. Diet, microbiota, and inflammatory bowel disease: lessons from Japanese foods. Korean J Intern Med. 2014;29(4):409–15.

Khan TM, Hassali MA, Al-Haddad MSM. Nutraceuticals use among the inhabitants of Penang, Malaysia. Int J Collab Res Intern Med Public Health. 2011;3(5):402–14.

Kho MC, Lee YJ, Park JH, Kim HY, Yoon JJ, Ahn YM, et al. Fermented red ginseng potentiates improvement of metabolic dysfunction in metabolic syndrome rat models. Nutrients. 2016;8(6):E369.

Kim EK, Kwon KB, Song MY, Han MJ, Lee JH, Lee YR, et al. Flavonoids protect against cytokine-induced pancreatic beta-cell damage through suppression of nuclear factor kappaB activation. Pancreas. 2007;35(4):e1–9.

Kim B, Hong VM, Yang J, Hyun H, Im JJ, Hwang J, Yoon S, Kim JE. A review of fermented foods with beneficial effects on brain and cognitive function. Prev Nutr Food Sci. 2016;21(4):297–309.

Kim MS, Kim B, Park H, Ji Y, Holzapfel W, Kim DY, Hyun CK. Long-term fermented soybean paste improves metabolic parameters associated with non-alcoholic fatty liver disease and insulin resistance in high-fat diet-induced obese mice. Biochem Biophys Res Commun. 2018;495(2):1744–51.

Klejdus B, Mikelová R, Petrlová J, Potesil D, Adam V, Stiborová M, et al. Evaluation of isoflavone aglycon and glycoside distribution in soy plants and soybeans by fast column high-performance liquid chromatography coupled with a diode-array detector. J Agric Food Chem. 2005;27:5848–52.

Konieczna A, Rutkowska A, Rachoń D. Health risk of exposure to Bisphenol a (BPA). Rocz Panstw Zakl Hig. 2015;66(1):5–11.

Lee CL, Wang JJ, Pan TM. Red mold rice extract represses amyloid beta peptide-induced neurotoxicity via potent synergism of anti-inflammatory and antioxidative effect. Appl Microbiol Biotechnol. 2008;79(5):829–41.

Lee NK, Jeong JH, Oh J, Kim Y, Ha HS, Jeong YS. Conversion of flavonols Kaempferol and Quercetin in mulberry (Morus Alba L.) leaf using plant-fermenting lactobacillus Plantarum. J Food Biochem. 2015a;39(6):765–70.

Lee S, Kim JE, Suk S, Kwon OW, Park G, Lim TG, Seo SG, Kim JR, Kim DE, Lee M, Chung DK, Jeon JE, Cho DW, Hurh BS, Kim SY, Lee KW. A fermented barley and soybean formula enhances skin hydration. J Clin Biochem Nutr. 2015b;57(2):156–63.

Lee BH, Lai YS, Wu SC. Antioxidation, angiotensin converting enzyme inhibition activity, nattokinase, and antihypertension of Bacillus subtilis (natto)-fermented pigeon pea. J Food Drug Anal. 2015c;23(4):750–7.

Liu ZM, Ho SC, Chen YM, Woo J. Effect of soy protein and isoflavones on blood pressure and endothelial cytokines: a 6-month randomized controlled trial among postmenopausal women. J Hypertens. 2013;31:384–92.

Mahn K, Borras C, Knock GA, Taylor P, Khan IY, Sugden D, et al. Dietary soy Isoflavone induced increases in antioxidant and eNOS gene expression lead to improved endothelial function and reduced blood pressure in vivo. FASEB J. 2005;19:1755e7.

Mallappa RH, Rokana N, Duary RK, Panwar H, Batish VK, Grover S. Management of metabolic syndrome through probiotic and prebiotic interventions. Indian J Endocrinol Metab. 2012;16(1):20–7.

Marco ML, Heeney D, Binda S, Cifelli CJ, Cotter PD, Foligné B, Gänzle M, et al. Health benefits of fermented foods: microbiota and beyond. Curr Opin Biotechnol. 2017;44:94–102.

Micha R, Kalantarian S, Wirojratana P, Byers T, Danaei G, Elmadfa I, et al. Estimating the global and regional burden of suboptimal nutrition on chronic disease: methods and inputs to the analysis. Eur J Clin Nutr. 2012;66(1):119–29.

Nagata C, Wada K, Tamur T, Konishi K, Goto Y, Koda S, Kawachi T, Tsuji M, Nakamura K. Dietary soy and natto intake and cardiovascular disease mortality in Japanese adults: the Takayama study. Am J Clin Nutr. 2016;105:426–31.

Nakajima N, Nozaki N, Ishihara K, Ishikawa A, Tsuji H. Analysis of isoflavone content in tempeh, a fermented soybean, and preparation of a new isoflavone-enriched tempeh. J Biosci Bioeng. 2005;100(6):685–7.

Oh MR, Park SH, Kim SY, Back HI, Kim MG, Jeon JY, et al. Postprandial glucose-lowering effects of fermented red ginseng in subjects with impaired fasting glucose or type 2 diabetes: a randomized, double blind, placebo-controlled clinical trial. BMC Complement Altern Med. 2014;14:237.

Oishi K, Sato T, Yokoi W, Yoshida Y, Ito M, Sawada H. Effect of probiotics, Bifidobacterium breve and lactobacillus casei, on Bisphenol a exposure in rats. Biosci Biotechnol Biochem. 2008;72(6):1409–15.

O'Leary KA, de Pascual-Teresa S, Needs PW, Bao YP, O'Brien NM, Williamson G. Effect of flavonoids and vitamin E on cyclooxygenase-2 (COX-2) transcription. Mutat Res. 2004;551(1–2):245–54.

Park JA, TirupathiPichiah PB, Yu JJ, Oh SH, Daily JW 3rd, Cha YS. Anti-obesity effect of kimchi fermented with Weissellakoreensis OK1-6 as starter in high-fat diet-induced obese C57BL/6J mice. J Appl Microbiol. 2012;113(6):1507–16.

Perez-Gregorio R, Simal-Gandara J. A critical review of bioactive food components, and of their functional mechanisms, biological effects and health outcomes. Curr Pharm Des. 2017;23(19):2731–41.

Prabu SL, Prakash TNKS, Kumar CD, Kumar SS, Ragavendran T. Nutraceuticals: a review. Elixir Pharm. 2012;46:8372–7.

Ramaa CS, Shirode AR, Mundada AS, Kadam VJ. Nutraceuticals-an emerging era in the treatment and prevention of cardiovascular diseases. Curr Pharm Biotech. 2006;7:15–23.

Ramdath DD, Padhi EM, Sarfaraz S, Renwick S, Duncan AM. Beyond the cholesterol-lowering effect of soy protein: a review of the effects of dietary soy and its constituents on risk factors for cardiovascular disease. Nutrients. 2017;9(4):E324.

Rehman SU, Shah SA, Ali T, Chung JI, Kim MO. Anthocyanins reversed D-Galactose-induced oxidative stress and neuroinflammation mediated cognitive impairment in adult rats. Mol Neurobiol. 2017;54(1):255–71.

Selhub EM, Logan AC, Bested AC. Fermented foods, microbiota, and mental health: ancient practice meets nutritional psychiatry. J Physiol Anthropol. 2014;33:2.

Shao ZM, Wu J, Shen ZZ, Barsky SH. Genistein exerts multiple suppressive effects on human breast carcinoma cells. Cancer Res. 1998;58:4851–7.

Suzuki T, Hara H. Role of flavonoids in intestinal tight junction regulation. J Nutr Biochem. 2011;22:401–8.

Tabassum S, Ahmad S, Madiha S, Khaliq S, Shahzad S, Batool Z, Haider S. Impact of oral supplementation of glutamate and GABA on memory performance and neurochemical profile in hippocampus of rats. Pak J Pharm Sci. 2017;30(3):1013–21.

Tamang JP, Tamang B, Schillinger U, Guigas C, Holzapfel WH. Functional properties of lactic acid bacteria isolated from ethnic fermented vegetables of the Himalayas. Int J Food Microbiol. 2009;135:28–33.

Tolonen M, Taipale M, Viander B, Pihlava JM, Korhonen H, Ryhänen EL. Plant-derived biomolecules in fermented cabbage. J Agric Food Chem. 2002;50(23):6798–803.

Verdu EF, Deng Y, Bercik P, Collins SM. Modulatory effects of estrogen in two murine models of experimental colitis. Am J Physiol Gastrointest Liver Physiol. 2002;283:G27–36.

Warren CA, Paulhill KJ, Davidson LA, Lupton JR, Taddeo SS, Hong MY, et al. Quercetin may suppress rat aberrant crypt foci formation by suppressing inflammatory mediators that influence proliferation and apoptosis. J Nutr. 2009;139(1):101–5.

Wong WW, Taylor AA, Smith EO, Barnes S, Hachey DL. Effect of soy isoflavone supplementation on nitric oxide metabolism and blood pressure in menopausal women. Am J Clin Nutr. 2012;95:1487–94.

Woo JK, Choi S, Kang JH, Kim DE, Hurh BS, Jeon JE, et al. Fermented barley and soybean (BS) mixture enhances intestinal barrier function in dextran sulfate sodium (DSS)-induced colitis mouse model. BMC Complement Altern Med. 2016;16(1):498.

Wu SH, Liu Z, Ho S, Wu SH. Metabolic syndrome and all-cause mortality: a meta-analysis of prospective cohort studies. Eur J Epidemiol. 2010;25(6):375–84.

Yang EJ, Kim SI, Park SY, Bang HY, Jeong JH, So JH, Rhee IK, Song KS. Fermentation enhances the in vitro antioxidative effect of onion (*Allium cepa*) via an increase in quercetin content. Food Chem Toxicol. 2012;50(6):2042–8.

Food Grains of India: A Brief Note on Their Therapeutic Potential

30

Saikat Sen

Contents

30.1 Introduction

Food or dietary constituents that afford a health beneficial and health-promoting effect beyond the basic nutritional value are considered as functional food. Cereals are produced in more than 73% of the world harvested area, which accounts for 60% food production in the world (Das et al. 2012). Cereals such as rice, wheat, barley, oat, psyllium, flaxseed, and maize are accepted as important functional food and nutraceuticals as these foods are an important source of dietary fiber, energy, minerals, proteins, vitamins, and antioxidants essential for human health. Cereal and food products based on cereal component provide opportunities to incorporate prebiotics, probiotics, and a large amount of fibers in human diet. Evidence from preclinical research, clinical trial, and epidemiological study has clearly indicated the beneficial effect of whole-grain cereals and their bioactive mole-

S. Sen (✉)
Faculty of Pharmaceutical Science, Assam Down Town University, Guwahati, Assam, India

S. Sen, R. Chakraborty (eds.), *Herbal Medicine in India*,
https://doi.org/10.1007/978-981-13-7248-3_30

cule against metabolic diseases such as diabetes and obesity, cardiovascular diseases, and cancer (Das et al. 2012).

Agriculture is one of the key areas for economic development of India. More than1.2 billion people of India depend on agriculture, and the sectors also provide employment for 54.6% of the country's population (Khatkar et al. 2016). India accounts to only 2.4% of the world's geographical area, but needs to support nearly 17% of the world's population and 15% of livestock. Moreover, India consists of 179.9 million hectares of agricultural land and considered as a nation with the second-largest agricultural land. Food grain is produced from foremost part of the cropped area of Indian agriculture (65%). Additionally, India is considered the world's highest producer of millets and second highest producer of rice, wheat, and pulses (Khatkar et al. 2016). This chapter highlights the therapeutic potential and bioactive molecule of wheat, rice, and millets besides their nutritive value.

30.2 Food Grains in India

30.2.1 Wheat

Wheat is an annual plant belongs to the genus Triticum (family *Gramineae*) family. Some of the common species of wheat are *Triticum dicoccum* Schuh L. (Emmer wheat), *Triticum durum* Desf. (Macaroni wheat), *T. vulgare Hist* (common bread wheat), *Triticum spherococcum* Mihi (Indian dwarf wheat), and *Triticum aestivum* (Mexican dwarf wheat). In India, Uttar Pradesh, Punjab, Madhya Pradesh, Haryana, Rajasthan, Bihar, and Gujarat are the key Indian states that produce wheat. Worldwide demand for wheat from India is increasing. Export of India's wheat is more in Nepal, Afghanistan UAE, Bangladesh, and Somalia (Anonymous 2018a).

30.2.2 Rice

Rice (*Oryza sativa*) is very important staple food and cereal that sustains two-thirds of the world population. Rice belongs to genus *Oryza* (family Poaceae) that comprises 24 species. Among these species, only two of them (*Oryza sativa* and *Oryza glaberrima*) are cultivated, and the remaining species are wild. *Oryza sativa* is further subgrouped as *indica*, *japonica*, and *javanica* subspecies. In India subspecies, *indica* is cultivated mainly (Mahajan et al. 2017). Rice can be grouped in various categories depending on their size, smell, color, etc. Aromatic rice such as Basmati and Joha are very popular in India. Moreover, India offers a wide variety of rice. Furthermore, black rice of Manipur is believed to have several therapeutic activities.

30.2.3 Millets

Millets, a small seeded crop, is considered a super grain and one of the oldest foods recognized by humans. Common millet varieties that grow in India include pearl millet or bajra (*Pennisetum typhoides/Pennisetum glaucum*), sorghum or great millet or jowar (*Sorghum vulgare*), finger millet or ragi (*Eleusine coracana*), proso/common millet or barri (*Panicum miliaceum*), barnyard millet or jhangora (*Echinochloa frumentacea*), foxtail/Italian millet or kangni (*Setaria italica*), kodo millet or kodra (*Paspalum scrobiculatum*), and little millet or moraiyo (*Panicum sumatrense*). Some other different varieties of millets found worldwide are *Coix lacryma* jobi, *Hygroryza aristata*, *Eragrostis tef, Digitaria exilis,* and *Brachiaria deflexa* (Anonymous 2018b; Morya et al. 2017; Shahidi and Chandrasekar 2013).

30.3 Bioactive Molecules in Food Grains

30.3.1 Wheat

The presence of fatty acids (i.e., linoleic, linolenic, palmitic, oleic, and stearic acid) and phytosterols (i.e., β-sitosterol, campesterol, and stigmasterol) was observed in hulled, durum, and soft wheat (Veronika and Magdalena 2017).

Different varieties of wheat are investigated, and wheat kernels are identified as major source of phytosterol. Sitosterol, campesterol, stigmasterol, avenasterols, and stanols are found in wheat. Cyanidine-3-glucoside and peonidine-3-glucoside are detected as main anthocyanins found in pericarp in purple wheat seeds. Furthermore, cyanidine-3-galactoside, peonidine-3-glucoside, delphinidine-3-glucoside, and delphinidine-3-rutinoside are also detected in blue/purple wheat seed. Also, cyanidine-3-galactoside, peonidin-3-glucoside, pelargonidin-3-glucoside, and ferulic acid were found in wheat cultivar Hedong Wumai (Havrlentova et al. 2014). Vitamin E (tocopherols and tocotrienols) and carotenoids (i.e., lutein, β-cryptoxanthin, zeaxanthin, and β-carotene) were detected in wheat flour and bran. Bran of wheat is a major source of different phenolic compounds. Wheat phenolics include ferulic, sinapic, caffeic, vanillic, protocatechuic, p-coumaric, p-hydroxybenzoic, and syringic acid. These bioactive molecules possess strong antioxidant activity (Havrlentova et al. 2014). Cyanidin 3-rutinoside, apigenin glycosides, and tricin are also reported in wheat (Sen and Chakraborty 2017). Phytic acid, alkylresorcinols (ARs), betaine, choline, niacin, pantothenic acid, riboflavin, biotin, thiamine, pyridoxine, folate, lutein, and minerals (iron, manganese, magnesium, phosphorus, zinc, and selenium) are some other bioactive compounds available in wheat grain and wheat bran. Lignans are also considered as key biomolecule available in wheat bran (Mateo Anson et al. 2012; Onipe et al. 2015. Wheat grass juice (WGJ) is found to possess various beneficial effects on health. Chemical analysis revealed that juice is rich in minerals (i.e., magnesium, zinc, selenium, iron, potassium, boron, and molybdenum.), vitamins (i.e., vitamin E, vitamin C, vitamin B12, folic acid, and pyridoxine), and antioxidant molecules such as β-carotene, apigenin, quercetin, and luteolin (Chauhan 2014).

30.3.2 Rice

Rice is loaded with diverse compounds such as vitamin, minerals, flavonoids, phenolic cods, coumarins, among others. Moreover, rice bran is one of the most vital part which contains health promotive compounds. Table 30.1 included the list of compounds isolated from rice parts.

30.3.3 Millets

Millets are loaded with different biomolecules which are responsible for diverse biological activities. Millets consist of different essential amino acids such as arginine, histidine, lysine, tryptophan, phenylalanine, tyrosine, methionine, cystine, threonine, leucine, isoleucine, and valine (Chandra et al. 2016). Millets are also found to contain diverse phytomolecules (Table 30.2).

30.4 Therapeutic Potential

Oxidative stress became a key underlying factor for a number of diseases such as cardiovascular diseases, CNS-related disorders, metabolic disorders, cancer, and ageing. Foods such as different food grains are good sources of nutrients, minerals (zinc, selenium, iron, etc.), vitamins (vitamin C and vitamin E), amino acids, and phytoconstituents especially phenolic compounds (phenolic acid, coumarins, flavonoid, tannin, etc.) which act in synergy and confer health promotive, curative, and preventive effect. Antioxidant activity confers by food grains is a key mechanism by which they are immerging as a therapeutic substance beside their nutritive value (Sen and Chakraborty 2017). Phenolics are well-known antioxidant substance, and different *in vitro* and *in vivo* studies confirmed the therapeutic effectiveness in treatment of diabetes, cancer, hyperlipidemia, CNS disorders, cardiovascular diseases, etc. Wheat, rice, and millets are the very good source of phenolic compounds. Bran of food grain contains large amount and diverse phenolic acid, coumarins, flavonoid, tannins etc., and antioxidant activity exerted by this compound is responsible for their therapeutic efficacy may be in apart.

Table 30.1 Compounds isolated from rice grain parts

Group of molecule	Compounds
Vitamin	Vitamin E (α-tocopherol, β-tocopherol, γ-tocopherol, δ-tocopherol, α-tocotrienol, β-tocotrienol, γ-tocotrienol, δ-tocotrienol), thiamine, riboflavin, niacin, vitamin B6
Minerals	Na, Mg, Zn, Fe, Cu, K
Amino acid	Alanine, aspartic acid, arginine, cysteine, glycine, histidine, glutamic acid, isoleucine, leucine, methionine, phenylalanine, lysine, proline, serine, threonine, tyrosine, valine, tryptophan (Ravichanthiran et al. 2018)
Phenolic acids (hydroxycinnamic and hydroxybenzoic acid)	1-O-caffeoylquinic acid; 3-O-p-coumaroylquinic acid; tricaffeoyl-hydroxyferulic acid; caffeoyl-coumaroyl-quinic acid; 5-O-feruloyl quinic acid; Z-ferulic acid; 4-O-caffeoylquinic acid; coumaroylquinic acid; caffeic acid; gallic acid; dihydro gallic acid derivative; protocatechuic acid; p-hydroxybenzoic acid; vanillic acid; syringic acid; p-coumaric acid; ferulic acid; caffeic acid; caffeic acid hexoside; carnosic acid; sinapic acid; chlorogenic acid; cinnamic acid; ethyl-3,4-dihydroxybenzoic acid; 3,4-dihydroxybenzoic acid; 4-hydroxy-3-methoxyphenylacetic acid; 4-hydroxy-3-methoxy cinnamic acid; 3,4-dihydroxy methyl benzoic acid; 4-hydroxy-3-methoxy methyl benzoic acid; p-methoxyphenol; hydroxybenzoic acid-O-hexoside; o-cresol; guaiacol; 3,5-xylene; 6′-O-(E)-sinapoylsucrose; tricaffeoyl-hydroxyferulic acid; 6′-O-(E)-feruloylsucrose; feruloyl quinic acid; rutinoside; sinapoyl; sinapoyl tartrate; dihydroxybenzoic acid-O-pentoside (Goufo and Trindade 2014; Bhat and Riar 2017)
Flavonoids (other than anthocyanin and proanthocyanidin)	Luteolin; quercetin; apigenin; kaempferol; isorhamnetin; myricetin; isovitexin; hesperidin; naringenin; rutin; tricin; tricin 4′O-(threo-b-guaiacylglyceryl) ether; tricin 4′-O-(erythro-b-guaiacylglyceryl) ether; apigenin-7-O-glucoside; luteolin-7-O-glucoside; quercetin-3-O-rutinoside; quercetin-3-O-glucoside; isorhamnetin-3-O-glucoside; isorhamnetin-7-O-rutinoside; myricetin-7-O-glucoside; isorhamnetin-3-O-acetylglucoside; taxifolin-7-O-glucoside; 5,6,3′,4′,5′-pentahydroxyflavone-7-O-glucoside; 5,3′,4′,5′-tetrahydroxyflavanone-7-O-glucoside; apigenin-6-C-glucoside-8-C-arabinoside; (+)-3′-O-methyltaxifolin; 3′-O-methyltaxifolin-5-O-glucoside; brassicin; isorhamnetin-4′-O-glucoside; 3′-O-methyltaxifolin-7-O-glucoside; 3′-O-methyltaxifolin-4′-O-glucoside; brassicin-4′-O-glucoside; isorhamnetin-7-O-cellobioside; quercetin-3-O-rhamnoside; quercetin hexoside; quercetin-uronic acid (Goufo and Trindade 2014; Bhat and Riar 2017) 3′-O-methyltaxifolin; tricinin; brassicin; isorhamnetin-4′-O-β-D-glucopyranoside; 3′-O-methyltaxifolin-7-O-β-D-glucosyranoside; 3-O-methyltaxifolin-5-O-β-D-glucosyranoside; 3′-O-methyltaxifolin-4′-O-β-D-glucosyranoside; brassicin-4′-O-β-D-glucosyranoside; isorhamnetin-7-O-β-D-cellobioside; taxifolin-O-hexoside; quercetin-3-O-glucoside; quercetin-3-O-rutinoside; diosmedin-8-hexoside; isorhamnetin-3-O-glucoside; luteolin 6/8-C-pentoside-6/8-C-hexoside; apigenin 6/8-C-pentoside-8/6-C-hexoside (Caro et al. 2013; Cho et al. 2013)
Anthocyanin and proanthocyanidin	peonidin-3-O-glucoside, catechin, epicatechin, cyanidin-3-O-glucoside, cyanidin-3-O-galactoside, cyanidin-3-O-rutinoside, cyanidin-3-O-arabidoside, petunidin-3-glucoside, pelargonidin-3-O-glucoside, delphinidin, malvidin, cyanidin-3-O-(6″-O-p-coumaryl) glucoside, peonidin-3-O-(6″-O-p-coumaryl) glucoside (Caro et al. 2013, Goufo and Trindade 2014)
Carotenoids	Lutein, zeaxanthin, lycopene, and β-carotene (Cho et al. 2013)
Phytosterol	Stigmasterol, β-sitosterol, stigmastanol, campesterol, δ7-avenasterol, and δ5-avenasterol (Ravichanthiran et al. 2018)
Others	Dietary fiber, γ-oryzanol, phytic acid, syringaldehyde, procyanidin B1, ellagic acid, ellagic acid deoxyhexoside hydroxybenzoylhexsose, and (E)-coniferaldehyde (Bhat and Riar 2017; Ravichanthiran et al. 2018) arachidic acid, behenic acid, and gamma amino butyric acid (Das et al. 2014) Nonstarch (triglycerides, phospholipids, glycolipids, monoglycosyl glycerides, diglycosyl diglycerides, sterol glycosides, acyl sterol glycosides) and starch lipids (phosphatidylcholine, phosphatidylethanolamine, lysophosphatidyl ethanolamine, and free fatty acids) (Choudhury and Juliano 1980)

Table 30.2 Phytocompounds present in different millets

Millets	Phytochemicals present
Pennisetum typhoides/P. glaucum (Pearl millet, Bajra)	p-Hydroxybenzoic acid, vanillic acid, syringic acid, protocatechuic acids, gentisic acid, coumaric acid, caffeic acid, ferulic acid, cinnamic acid, cis/trans p-coumaric acid. Undecane, naphthalene, nitroisobutylglycerol, n-hexadecanoic acid, linoleic acid, oleic acid amide, β-tocopherol, β-sitosterol, omega 3-fatty acid, lutein, zeaxanthin, β-carotene (Shuhua et al. 2015; Sen and Chakraborty 2017; Khan et al. 2017; Dykes and Rooney 2006; Shahidi and Chandrasekar 2013)
Sorghum vulgare (Sorghum, great millet, Jowar)	Gallic acid; p-hydroxybenzoic acid; vanillic acid; syringic acid; salicylic acid; protocatechuic acid; gentisic acid; *p*-coumaric acid; *o*-coumaric acid; caffeic acid; ferulic acid; cinnamic acid; sinapic acid; apigeninidin; apigeninidin-5-glucoside; luteolinidin; luteolinidin-5-glucoside; 5-methoxyluteolinidin; 5-methoxyluteolinidin 7-glucoside; 7-methoxyapigeninidin; 7-methoxyapigeninidin 5-glucoside; luteolinidin 5-glucoside; 5-methoxyapigeninidin; 7-methoxyluteolinidin; luteoforol; apiforol; apigenin; luteolin; eriodictyol; eriodictyol 5-glucoside; naringenin; kaempferol 3-rutinoside-7-glucuronide; taxifolin; taxifolin 7-glucoside; catechin; procyanidin B-1; epicatechin-(epicatechin)$_n$-catechin; prodelphinidin; proapigeninidin; proluteolinidin; malvidin; tricin; quercetin 3,4′-dimethyl ether; *trans*-resveratrol; *trans*-piceid; peonidin; pelargonidin; pelargonidin-3,5-diglucoside; cyaniding; cyanidin-3-glucoside; cyanidin-3,5-diglucoside; cyanidin-3-rutinoside (Dykes and Rooney 2006; Awika et al. 2004; Vanamal et al. 2017). Epicatechin gallate; polyflavon 3-ol; proluteolinidin; proapigeninidin; procyanidin; prodelphinidin; heteropolyflavan-3-ol; quercetin-3,4′-O-di-beta-glucopyranoside; 2-O-caffeoylglycerol-O-glucoside; 1-O-caffeoylglycerol-O-glucoside; taxifolin and its derivatives; epicat-(4beta → 6)-epicatechin-(2beta → 7,4beta → 8)-epicatechin; robinetinidol-(4alpha → 6)-catechin-(6 → 4alpha)-robinetinidol; luteolin-7-oglucside; [epicatechin-(4beta → 8)]5-epicatechin; [epicatechin-(4beta → 8)]5-epicatechin, eriodictyol-5-O-galactoside; N′.n′-dicafferoylspermidine, robinetinidol-(4alpha → 6)-catechin-(6 → 4alpha)-robinetinidol; 6-C-glucosyl-8-C-arabinosyl-apigenin; N1-caffeoyl-N 10-feruloyl spermidine; pentahydroxyflavanone-(3 → 4)-catechin-7-*O*-glucoside; luteolin-3′,7-di-O-glucoside; pentahydroxyflavanone-(3 → 4)-catechin-7-O-glucoside; pyrano-eriodictyol-(3 → 4)-catechin-7-O-glucoside and its isomer; procyanidin; eriodictyol-7-o-galactoside; eriodictyol deoxyhexoside; luteolin and its isomer; 7-o-methly-luteolinidin; campesterol; stigmasterol; caffeoylglycolic acid methyl ester (Awika and Rooney 2004; Rao et al. 2018; Choo et al. 2015)
Eleusine coracana (Finger millet, Ragi)	Arabinoxylan, p-hydroxybenzoic acid, vanillic acid, syringic acid, protocatechuic acid, gentisic acid, sinapic acid, caffeic acid, *trans*-ferulic acid, *trans*-cinnamic acid, *p*-coumaric acid, chlorogenic acid, salicylic acid, gallic acid, quercetin, catechin, gallocatechin, epicatechin, epigallocatechin, taxifolin, vitexin, tricin, luteolin, myricetin, apigenin, kaempferol, naringenin, daidzein, procyanidin B1 and B2, orientin, isoorientin, isovitexin, saponarin, violanthin, lucenin-1, saponarin, violanthin, proanthocyanidins, 4-O-methyl gallic acid, phloroglucinol, trans-feruloyl-malic acid, dimer of prodelphinidin, daidzein, catechin gallates, trimmers of catechin, tetramers of catechin, oleic acid, linoleic acid, palmitic acid, 6″-O-3-hydroxy-3-methylglutaroyvitexin, 4″-O-3-hydroxy-3-methylglutaroyvitexin, 6″-O-malonylvitexin, lutein, zeaxanthin, and β-carotene (Shan et al. 2015; Udeh et al. 2017; Devi et al. 2014; Oseghale et al. 2017; Sen and Chakraborty 2017; Taylor 2017)
Panicum miliaceum (Proso, common millet, Barri)	Gallic acid; p-hydroxybenzoic acid; vanillic acid; syringic acid; protocatechuic acid; gentisic acid; *p*-coumaric acid; caffeic acid; *trans*-ferulic acid; cinnamic acid; sinapic acid; chlorogenic acid; glycosylvitexin, glycolsylorientin, vixetin, tannin; zeaxanthin; lutein; kaempferol; apigenin; myricetin (Shan et al. 2015; Taylor 2017; Shahidi and Chandrasekar 2013; Jana 2007; Dias-Martins et al. 2018)
Echinochloa frumentacea (Barnyard millet, Jhangora)	N-p-coumaroyl serotonin; feruloyl serotonin; tricin and its methyl ester; luteolin; luteolin-7-glucoside; 3,4-dihydroxy benzoic acid; 4-hydroxybenzoic acid; kaempferol; biochanin A; formononetin; echinochlorins A-C; 5,7-dihydroxy-3′,4′,5′-trimethoxy flavones; quercetin; flavones; apigenin-8-C-sophoroside; 2-methoxy-4-hydroxycinnamic acid; p-coumaric acid; quercetin-3-O-glucoside; ferulic acid; vanillic acid; sinapic acid; naringenin; and apigenin (Taylor 2017; Molla et al. 2016; Woo et al. 2015; Seo et al. 2015; Lee et al. 2014)

(continued)

Table 30.2 (continued)

Millets	Phytochemicals present
Setaria italic (Foxtail millet, Kangni)	Gallic acid, p-hydroxybenzoic acid, vanillic acid, syringic acid, protocatechuic acid, gentisic acid, *p*-coumaric acid, caffeic acid, *trans*-ferulic acid, cinnamic acid, sinapic acid, chlorogenic acid, ferulic acid, sinapic acid, kaempferol, catechin, myricetin, daidzein, luteolin, quercetin, apigenin, naringenin, lutein, zeaxanthin, and β-carotene (Shahidi and Chandrasekar 2013; Shan et al. 2015; Pradeep and Sreerama 2018; Dykes and Rooney 2006)
Paspalum scrobiculatum (Kodo millet, Kodra)	Gallic acid; p-hydroxybenzoic acid; vanillic acid; syringic acid; protocatechuic acid; gentisic acid; *p*-coumaric acid; caffeic acid; *trans*-ferulic acid; cinnamic acid; sinapic acid; kaempferol; apigenin; vitexin; isovitexin; luteolin; quercetin; chlorogenic acid; arachidonic amide; pterin-6-carboxylic acid; N-(3,5-dinitropyridin-2-yl) l-aspartic acid ester; 9-octadecenoic acid; methyl-10-trans, 12,cisoctadecadienoate; stigmasterol; C-sitosterol; pregnenolone; campesterol; N, Propyl 9,12,15-octadecatrienoate; pregan-20-one, 2-hydroxy-5,6-epoxy-15-methyl; hexadecanoic acid; butyl-6,9,12,15-octadecatetraenoate; quercetin; cinnamic acid (Taylor 2017; Shahidi and Chandrasekar 2013; Woo et al. 2015; Sharma et al. 2017; Ramasamy et al. 2017)
Panicum sumatrense (Little millet, Moraiyo)	Gallic acid, p-hydroxybenzoic acid, vanillic acid, syringic acid, protocatechuic acid, gentisic acid, *p*-coumaric acid, caffeic acid, *trans*-ferulic acid, cinnamic acid, sinapic acid, chlorogenic acid, ferulic acid, kaempferol, catechin, myricetin, daidzein, luteolin, quercetin, apigenin, and naringenin (Shahidi and Chandrasekar 2013; Pradeep and Sreerama 2018)

30.4.1 Wheat

Wheat is considered as important functional food. Wheat seed, bran, and even wheatgrass are loaded with diverse biomolecule importantly with different antioxidant molecule. Whole wheat, bran, and seed possess strong antioxidant activity (Merike et al. 2010) and found useful in different treatment of different oxidative stress-related disorder. Some of the possible therapeutic benefits of wheat are discussed in this study.

30.4.1.1 Inflammatory Potential

5-*n*-ARs isolated from different wheat bran produced anti-inflammatory activity. Moreover, AR significantly inhibit the expression of TNF-α, IL-1β, and IL-6 in LPS-activated Raw264.7 macrophage cells. Reduction in NF-κB p65 nuclear translocation, κB (IκBα) kinase, and JNK phosphorylation was observed with ARs treatment (Liu et al. 2018). Ethanol extract of whole wheat flour exhibited significant anti-inflammatory activity evaluated by measuring inhibition of interleukin-1β (IL-1β) mRNA expression (Whent et al. 2012). Antioxidant and anti-inflammatory activities of different wheat fractions are observed during gastrointestinal (GI) transit. Ferulic acid is the major component responsible for such activity (Anson et al. 2008).

30.4.1.2 Anticancer Activity

Phytochemicals present in wheat such as phytosterol, vitamin E, selenium, and phenolics are investigated for anticancer activity. Lunasin, BiP-peptide isolated from wheat seed, exhibited anticancer activity in preclinical studies (Poudel and Bhatta 2017). Lipophilic extracts of wheat bran exerted potent cytotoxic activity. Fractions containing phytosteroids, unsaturated free fatty acid, and ARs found to inhibit the growth of human prostate adenocarcinoma (PC3) cells significantly (Liu et al. 2012). Extract of wheat germ has been investigated for their potent *in vitro* cytotoxic effect against different human cell line including MCF-7 breast cancer, H9 human lymphoid cell, and gastric cancer cells, etc. (Poudel and Bhatta 2017). Immature and mature wheat kernels were investigated for anticancer activity. Immature wheat kernels showed significant antiproliferative activities tested against HT-29 and Caco-2 (colon cancer cells) and HeLa (cervical cancer cells) (Kim and Kim 2016). Antiproliferative activity of whole wheat flour was investigated using HT-29 adenocarcinoma cells, and the result was impressive. Presence of phenolics, carotenoids, and α-tocopherol was observed in wheat flour (Whent et al. 2012).

30.4.1.3 Immunomodulatory Effect

Wheat bran-derived polysaccharides (WBP) exhibited immunomodulatory activity. WBP found to enhance intracellular nitric oxide, prostaglandin E2, and tumor necrosis factor-α (TNF-α) in RAW 264.7 cells. It also increases enhanced inducible nitric oxide synthase, TNF-α, and cyclooxygenase-2 (COX-2) expression. Phosphorylated p38 mitogen-activated protein kinase (MAPK), activator protein-1 (AP-1) activity, and nuclear factor (NF)-κB are also activated by WBP. In *in vivo* assay, it increases serum cytokines IL-2 and IFN-γ production in immunosuppressed mice (Shen et al. 2017). Wheat extract can produce an immunomodulatory effect through induction of IL-10 (Yamazaki et al. 2008). Arabinoxylans (AR) isolated from wheat found to have immunomodulatory activity. It found to produce pro-inflammatory response *in vitro*, *in vivo*, and in humans (Fadel et al. 2018)

30.4.1.4 Antidiabetic Potential

Extracts of wheat bran are found to be processed *in vitro* antidiabetic activity. Ethanol extracts significantly inhibit baker's yeast and rat intestinal enzymes, whereas petroleum ether fraction of ethanolic extract significantly inhibits rat intestinal α-glucosidase. ARs are major bioactive molecules responsible for such activity (Tu et al. 2013). Feruloyl oligosaccharides from wheat bran exerted antioxidant and hypoglycemic effect in alloxan-induced diabetic rats (Ou et al. 2007). Insoluble fibers of wheat (*Triticum aestivum*) exhibited *in vitro* hypoglycemic effect tested through *glucose adsorption capacity study, glucose diffusion and glucose dialysis retardation index estimation, starch digestibility activity,* and *estimation of residual amylase activity* (Bisoi et al. 2012). Water extractable arabinoxylan extracts from wheat aleurone and bran found to possess strong α-glucosidase inhibitory activity (Malunga et al. 2017).

30.4.1.5 Cardiovascular Effect

Cholesterol and LDL are found to decrease in serum after consumption of whole wheat. A study reported that phytoestrogen (also available in wheat) protects blood vessels from atherosclerosis after it binds to specific receptor located intracellularly. It also protects blood vessels from arterial spasm (Saleh et al. 2017). Ethanolic extract of wheat bran administration is found to control atherosclerosis in hyperlipidemic rabbits (Rashi and Ashok 2018.

30.4.1.6 Effect on GUT Health

Arabinoxylan and cellulose are scantily fermented in the gut and thus help to maintain or improve gut health. Whole-grain consumption increases butyrate-producing bacteria. Wheat contains a large amount of fibers especially in bran and thus act as laxative, and several studies indicated dietary fibers are helpful in controlling body weight and lipid profile and maintaining healthy gut (Kumar et al. 2011; Poudel and Bhatta 2017). Wheat bran is found to promote healthy digestive tract in pig. Wheat bran enhanced water retention capacity and the concentration of butyric acid and increased microbial fermentation in intestinal digesta. Wheat bran in pig also decreased the level of intestinal enterobacteria and coliform bacteria especially *E.coli* attachment to ileum (Liu et al. 2018). Arabinoxylan oligosaccharides derived from wheat bran alter gut microbiota composition positively, blunted *Clostridium* and *Turicibacter*, and enhanced and *Butyricicoccus* strongly. Arabinoxylan oligosaccharides found to reduce adiposity efficiently. Crude fraction of wheat bran enhances fat excretion and increases *Akkermansia* genus and also counteract gut overexpression of IL1β (Francesco et al. 2017).

Besides the antioxidant molecule, wheat is enriched with protein, minerals, and vitamins especially thiamine, riboflavin, and niacin, which boost the internal rejuvenation and maintain internal harmony. Wheat is useful in prevention and treatment of pyorrhea. Other beneficial uses of wheat include treatment of acne, pimples, tonsil pain, chest pain, scars, etc. (Kumar et al. 2011). Bioactive molecules of wheat such as ferulic acid also boost the immunity. Ferulic acid improving γδ T-cell proliferation and thereby promote immunity (Poudel and Bhatta 2017). Additionally, wheat bran also produced significant antimicrobial activity against *Escherichia coli, Pseudomonas aeruginosa, Bacillus subtilis, Staphylococcus aureus, Candida albicans, and Aspergillus niger* (Elhassan et al. 2017).

Further, WGJ is investigated for different biological activity, and its beneficial activity was well reported. Supplement of WGJ is also available commercially. Intake of WGJ causes increased number of RBC and blood oxygen level. A clinical study reported the beneficial effect of WGJ on thalassemic patients by reducing the transfusion rate and increasing mean time interval between transfusions. General well-being along with improved appetite and decreased musculoskeletal aches and pains was observed in patients under investigation. Preclinical and several investigation studies also reported possible therapeutic activity/beneficial effect of WGJ in cancer, arthritis, tooth disorder, ulcer, kidney swelling, constipation, skin disorder, digestive system disorders, circulatory disorder, diabetes, inflammatory condition, anemia, eczema, common colds, etc. (Chauhan 2014; Sareen et al. 2014).

30.4.2 Rice

Rice grain, rice bran, and rice hull bioactive molecule of rice (i.e., phenolic compounds, γ-oryzanol, and vitamin E) showed remarkable therapeutic potency when tested through preclinical or clinical studies. Therapeutic potential of rice includes the following:

- Antioxidant activity
- Hypolipidemic activity
- Antidiabetic activity
- Anti-inflammatory activity
- Anticancer activity
- Immunomodulatory activity
- Hepatoprotective activity
- Nephroprotective activity
- Protective effect against reproductive disorder
- Neuroprotective potential
- Probiotic activity
- Antidiarrheal activity
- Laxative effect
- Anti-allergic activity

Antioxidant activity of rice grain part and phytochemicals against *in vitro* free radical scavenging assay methods include DPPH radical, ABTS radical, nitric oxide radical, superoxide radical, hydroxyl radical, hydrogen peroxide scavenging assay, and reducing power ability assay (Goufo and Trindade 2014). Bran extract and isolated anthocyanin and proanthocyanidins from rice had the significant inhibitory effect of xanthin oxidase, NO, MDA, through which extracts or compounds provide protection against oxidative stress related to $KBrO_3$-induced kidney injury (Hao et al. 2015). Moreover, rice was found to enhance superoxide dismutase (SOD) and glutathione peroxidase (GSH-Px) level in CCl_4-induced hepatotoxic animals (Hou et al. 2013). Black rice and rice extract found to prevent human LDL oxidation and DNA nicking (Hu et al. 2003). Thai red rice extract was found to increase GSH and maintain the level of hepatic transaminases, thus conferring liver protection in paracetamol-treated mice (Sinthorn et al. 2016). Seven different pigmented whole rice cultivars of Kashmir, India, was analyzed, and six flavonoids, six phenolics, eleven hydroxycinnamic acid derivatives, three anthocyanins, seven hydroxybenzoic acid derivatives, and seven flavonoid glucosides of different flavonoid compounds were identified. Extract and fractions of different cultivars produced significantly *in vitro* radical scavenging effect and lipid peroxidation inhibition (Bhat and Riar 2017).

Brown, black, Joha rice, and cold press rice bran oil demonstrated activity against prostaglandin 2 (PGE-2), nitric acid (NO), tumor necrosis factor-α (TNF-α), inducible NOS, and endothelial NOS in LPS-stimulated murine macrophage cell line (Debnath et al. 2013; Settharaksa et al. 2014). Indian Njavara rice extract exhibited anti-inflammatory activity in carrageenan-induced paw edema in rats, and rice extract also restrained COX, LOX, NOS, and myeloperoxidase tested through *in vitro* models (Nair et al. 2011). Parboiled germinated brown rice was found to be effective against liver fibrosis in rat, and its action may relate to the inhibitory effect on transforming growth factor β-1 (TGF-β1) and platelet-derived growth factor (PDGF), (TNF-α, IL-1β,

IL-6 (Wunjuntuk et al. 2016a, b). Rice from Sri Lanka showed inhibitory effect on methylglyoxal-mediated protein glycation, acetyl, and butyryl-cholinesterase activity. *In vivo* hypoglycemic effect of bran extract was also examined by the authors (Abeysekera et al. 2015). Black rice bran and rice hull smoke extract were evaluated for hypoglycemic activity and found that blood glucose level was reduced through stimulation of insulin level, inhibitory effect on α-glucosidase, enhanced glucose metabolism, and pancreatic β-cells regeneration in experimental diabetic rodents (Wunjuntuk et al. 2016a, b). A number of studies confirmed hypolipidemic activity of rice, particularly rice bran or rice bran oil in animals and human. Rice bran oil demonstrated antioxidant and antilipidemic activities in human volunteers (Rajnarayana et al. 2001). A double-blind, randomized, placebo-controlled study on human volunteers with mild to moderate hypercholesterolemia confirmed cholesterol-lowering effects of yellow yeast rice (Sewon et al. 2018)

A number of studies and their phytochemicals such as phenolic acids, γ-oryzanol, GABA, vitamin E, and their derivatives exerted *in vivo* antioxidant activity, protect protein and DNA from oxidation, and confer protective effect on hepatic cytochrome P450 enzymes and its members such as CYP2E1 in CCl_4-induced hepatotoxic animals (Wunjuntuk et al. 2016a). The extract of germinated brown rice produced hepatoprotective activity in hypercholesterolemic rabbits (Esa et al. 2013). Traditionally, rice was also used during painful urination and other urinary system-related dysfunctions (Cabanting and Perez 2016). Rice extract was found useful in vaginal atrophy, pain in time of urination, and dryness of the vaginal wall (Muhammad et al. 2013). Melatonin and tryptophan are considered as neuroprotective agents, and the presence of these compounds were noted in brown, white, and black glutinous rice, which inhibit the production of ROS and sustain cell viability and gene expression of brain-derived neurotrophic factor (BDNF) in hippocampal neuronal HT22 cells of mouse against neurotoxicity-induced by H_2O_2 (Chumpiya et al. 2016). GABA in pre-germinated brown rice exerted protective effect against oxidative stress-induced neuronal cell (SK-N-SH) damage (Soiampornkul et al. 2012).

Anticancer/antiproliferative activity of rice grain, rice bran, and biomolecule of rice was successfully evaluated on different *in vitro* studies carried out using HL-60, MCF-7, caco-2, marmoset B-lymphoblastoid B95-98, V-79 lung cells, cervical, liver, and stomach cancer cell lines (Nam et al. 2005; Miyoshi et al. 2001). Fermented/non-fermented rice extract and rice bran produced anticancer activity through a number of mechanisms such as fragmentation of DNA, oncogene damage, inhibition of CYT_{450}s and initiation and post termination phases, AMP-protein kinase activation, and NK cell activation (Kuno et al. 2006, 2016). Immunoactivatory activity of glycoprotein, feruloylated oligosaccharides, and polysaccharides from rice in murine macrophages cells (RAW 264.7) was observed, and the activity may be related to the release of NO, PGE_2, IL-1β, IL-6, IL-10, and TNF-α to equip immune response macrophages cells without any cytotoxicity (Park et al. 2013; Fang et al. 2012). Korean rice exhibited potent anti-allergic activity by reducing histamine level *in vivo* and murine model (Kim et al. 1999).

Rice bran was found to confer protection against rotavirus diarrhea induced in gnotobiotic pigs. Moreover, rice bran promotes the growth of probiotics such as *Lactobacillus rhamnosus* (Yang et al. 2015). Laxative effect of rice bran fiber was well documented which enhance fecal production and stool rates (Sohail et al. 2017)

30.4.3 Millets

Millets are rich source of minerals such as iron, calcium, magnesium, potassium, zinc, phosphorous, vitamins (i.e., B-complex vitamins, niacin, vitamin B6, folic acid), dietary fiber, antioxidant molecules including phenolic compounds, protein, and essential amino acid (i.e. methionine and cysteine). Millets are gluten-free, thus considered as an alternative for the gluten-intolerant peoples. Additionally, millets are easily digestible and contain a large amount of lecithin which found to restore function of nerve cell, regenerate myelin fiber, and strengthen brain cell metabolism, thus promoting better nervous system function. Higher fat content was reported in millets (Habiyaremye et al. 2017). Millet possesses strong antioxidant activity (Dykes and Rooney 2006). Furthermore, millet is a loaded with a good amount of phosphorus that is considered as a vital component of ATP and required to uphold cell structure and formation of mineral matrix of the bone (Habiyaremye et al. 2017). It is a source of high level of calcium millets, and their products can be helpful in the prevention of osteoporosis and other bone-related ailments (Kumar et al. 2016). Millets contain different biomolecules which act synergy and produce preventive and curative effects. They can retard the ageing process and may exert preventive effect on age-onset degenerative diseases (Habiyaremye et al. 2017).

30.4.3.1 Pearl Millet (Bajra)

Lipid and phenolic compounds isolated from pearl millet reduced proliferation of mitogen-induced T cell. Compared with lipids exerted, phenolic compounds produced strong effects on phosphorylation of ERK-1/ERK2 and C^{a2+} signaling in mitogen-activated T cells (Nani et al. 2015). Bran of pearl millet was found effective in the treatment of hyperlipidemia in experimental rats (Javed et al. 2012). The extract of pearl millet was found to possess antimicrobial activity against *Serratia marcescens, Salmonella typhi, Proteus vulgaris, and Staphylococcus epidermidis* (Ndiku and Ngule 2015). Methanol, ethyl acetate, and petroleum ether extract of pearl millet inhibited the growth of *E. coli*, *Bacillus cereus*, and *Serratia liquefaciens*, respectively (Ndiku et al. 2016). Antiradical and other bioactivities such as inhibition of DNA scission and proliferation of HT-29 adenocarcinoma cells of pearl millets were successfully investigated. Pearl millets also found to restrain oxidation of LDL cholesterol and liposome (Chandrasekara and Shahidi 2011).

As a rich source of fiber, pearl millets are not only an important source of prebiotics but also useful to develop functional food containing probiotic microbial cultures, as researchers isolated one probiotic actinomycete based on the properties from pearl millet grain (Kunchala et al. 2017). In addition, pearl millet was also found beneficial in inflammatory bowel disease, inflammation, hypertension, atherosclerosis, and other cardiac diseases (Dias-Martins et al. 2018). Grains of pearl millet are gluten-free in nature and thus can be considered as an alternative of wheat (wheat contain gluten protein) which may provide an advantage in metabolic disorders in individuals allergic to gluten protein (Dias-Martins et al. 2018).

30.4.3.2 Sorghum (Jowar)

A number of studies have been carried out to find effect of sorghum-based test meal on different disease conditions or on healthy human. Majority of the studies indicated toward the beneficial effect of sorghum or its component on energy balance, redox balance, maintain lipid profile, glycemic control, gut health and gut microbiota, and cell-mediated immune system (Stefoska-Needham et al. 2015). A systemic study which includes 6 observational and 19 interventional studies concluded that intake of sorghum attenuated blood glucose responses and reduced the expression of oxidative stress markers. It was also observed that sorghum is a right component for the formulation of oral rehydration solutions and also helpful as medical adjunct to enhance immune responses in HIV-positive patients (Simnadis et al. 2016).

Preclinical studies found the beneficial effect of sorghum in hyperlipidemic condition. Proposed hypolipidemic mechanism of sorghum includes decrease in absorption of cholesterol absorption with increase in excretion of fecal sterol excretion, sterols present sorghum decline absorption of cholesterol, and level of liver cholesterol (Stefoska-Needham et al. 2015). The beneficial effect of sorghum on cardiovascular disease evaluated successfully. Low-tannin sorghum grain was found effective to reduce cholesterol level in guinea pig. Rat liver microsomal HMG-CoA reductase was found to inhibit by sorghum extract. Sorghum potently improved blood thinning and integrity of erythrocyte membrane of fish blood (Awika and Rooney 2004).

In vivo study was found the antidiabetic potential of sorghum which may be linked to the regulation of PPAR-γ-mediated metabolism in mice (Park et al. 2012). Another study showed that sorghum extract reduced blood glucose level and hyperlipidemia in streptozotocin-induced diabetic rats. The extract also decreased phosphoenolpyruvate carboxykinase expression and the phosphor-p38/p38 ratio, while enhancing phosphor adenosine monophosphate-activated protein kinase (AMPK)/AMPK ratio. These results indicated that the extract has a significant effect on hepatic gluconeogenesis (Kim and Park 2012).

Anticancer effect of sorghum extract or phytochemicals on human epithelial larynx carcinoma cell line (Hep-2), human colon carcinoma cells, breast cancer cell lines, etc., was evaluated successfully (Stefoska-Needham et al. 2015). Anti-inflammatory effects of sorghum may be linked with their ability to inhibit lipopolysaccharide-mediated production of nitric oxide, TNF-α, and interleukin-6 (Stefoska-Needham et al. 2015). Proanthocyanidins-rich bran of different varieties of sorghum showed *in vitro* antioxidant and anticancer activities in HepG2 cells lines. Upregulation of phosphorylated 5′AMP-activated protein kinase α level and downregulation of phosphorylated extracellular signal-regulated kinase 1/2 (ERK1/2) and p38 may be linked with anticancer activity of extract (Zhu et al. 2017).

Golden gelatinous sorghum found to possess anti-inflammatory activity in 12-O-tetradecanoylphorbol-13-acetate-induced ear inflammation in mice. Extract reduced expression of inflammatory mediators, that is, COX-2, inducible nitric oxide synthase. *In vitro* study using lipopolysaccharide-induced Raw264.7 cells also confirms the anti-inflammatory effect of sorghum (Shim et al. 2013). Caffeoylglycolic acid methyl ester, a key phytomolecule of sorghum grain, produced anti-inflammatory activity tested on Raw264.7 cells. The extract is a strong inducer of heme oxygenase-1 (HO-1) expression through Nrf2/HO-1 pathway (Choo et al. 2015).

30.4.3.3 Finger Millet (Ragi)

Antimicrobial activities of finger millets were investigated by different researchers. Phenolic extract of seed cote was found active against *Bacillus cereus*, *Aspergillus niger*, while extract of fermented millet inhibits the growth of *Escherichia coli*, *Salmonella sp*. Finger millet also showed antimicrobial activity against *Bacillus cereus*, *Yersinia enterocolitica*, *Staphylococcus aureus*, *Listeria monocytogenes*, *Escherichia coli*, *Pseudomonas aeruginosa*, *Streptococcus pyogenes*, *Klebsiella pneumonia Chethan*, *Serratia marcescens*, *and Malleshi* (Devi et al. 2014).

The phenolic compound of finger millet was found to produce antidiabetic activity which is evident by the inhibition of malt amylase, α glucosidase, and pancreatic amylase. *In vivo* studies on experimental animals also support antidiabetic potential of finger millet. Finger millet phenolic compound also decreased the risk of diabetic cataract, complication of diabetes, and ageing and enhanced dermal wound healing in diabetic rats (Devi et al. 2014; Shahidi and Chandrasekar 2013). Polyphenols of seed coat of finger millet effectively inhibit albumin glycation induced by fructose (Chandra et al. 2016).

Whole grain and bran of finger millet supplementation were found to retain body weight, improve lipid profile and anti-inflammatory status, reduce oxidative stress, regulate several obesity-related gene expressions, and enhance beneficial gut bacteria such as *Bifidobacteria*, *Lactobacillus*, *and Roseburia*, while suppressing the *Enterobacter* abundance in cecal contents. Results suggested that bran produced better activity in the prevention of high-fat diet-induced changes (Murtaza et al. 2014). A study on diabetic patients showed the beneficial effect of finger millet toward wound healing by improving the synthesis of nerve growth factor (NGF) and antioxidant status (Chandra et al. 2017). Diet-included finger millet prevented mucosal ulceration and thus indicated toward antiulcer activity of finger millet. Finger millet supplementation also reduced the elevated cholesterol level in animals. Statins (i.e., pravastatin, monacolin J, lovastatin, pravastatin, mevastatin) produced for fermentation of finger millets were found to inhibit hydroxymethylglutarate to mevalonate enzymatic conversion by HMG-CoA reductase (Chandra et al. 2017).

A number of studies have confirmed the anticancer/antiproliferative effect of finger millet or isolated bioactive component on HepG2 liver cancer cell line, K562 cancer cell, and human chorionic myeloid leukemia cell (Oseghale et al. 2017). Purified AR isolated from finger millet produced mitogenic activity and causes of macrophages (including phagocytosis) activation. It was also found that observed immunostimulatory activity of AR is directly related to the content of ferulic acid (Prashanth et al. 2015). Finger millets contain high level of iron. Betterment in hemoglobin status was observed after intake of germinated finger millet-based food. The product of fermented millet in young children acts as probiotic to cure diarrhea (Chandra et al. 2017). A research carried out on the extract of finger millets revealed that extract averted carbon tetrachloride-induced hepatotoxicity in experimental animals (Singh et al. 2015). Another study concluded that aqueous and ethanol fractions of finger millet inhibited the crystal growth formation and improved kidney function. Finger millet also found to ameliorate pathology related with kidney positively (Oseghale et al. 2017).

The beneficial effect of finger millets on the prevention of gastrointestinal disorders and malnutrition was also evaluated. Finger millet can serve as an alternative to wheat. Moreover, finger millet contains a large amount of dietary fibers (mixture of soluble and insoluble) or roughage that are not easily undergoing breakdown during digestion and assist to avert gastrointestinal disorders, coronary heart disease, colon cancer, and diabetes. High level of cellulose and insoluble fiber in finger millet acts as laxative and also prevents constipation. Soluble fibers of millets help in lubrication and regulate inflamed digestive tract (Kumar et al. 2016).

30.4.3.4 Proso/Common Millet (Barri)

Nine varieties of Chinese proso millet were examined for their antioxidant, antiproliferative activities. Chinese proso millets showed significant *in vitro* antioxidant and antiproliferative effects tested on MDA-MB-231-breast cell lines (Shen et al. 2018). *In vitro* study against MDA breast cancer and HepG2 liver cancer cells established the antiproliferative activities of proso millet (Zhang et al. 2014). Butanol fraction of 80% ethanol extract of grain of proso millet exerted cytotoxic activity on 3T3-L1 preadipocytes. Fraction induced apoptotic cell death that may be related to mitochondria-dependent activation of caspase-3 and successive PARP cleavage. Fraction also reduced terminal differentiation of 3T3-L1 preadipocytes into mature adipocytes without exerting a significant cytotoxic effect, through reduced expression of transcription factors (i.e., PPARγ1 and C/EBPα) (Jun et al. 2014). Linoleic acid isolated from proso millet exhibited histone deacetylase inhibitory activity and cytotoxic effect against human leukemia K562 and prostate cancer LNcaP cell line (Aburai et al. 2007).

Intake of proso and other millets decreased the risk of type 2 diabetes. Millets contain a large amount of magnesium, which may control glucose and insulin level in the body though their regulating effect on various enzymatic reactions (Habiyaremye et al. 2017). A preliminary study showed the beneficial effect of diet supplementation containing dietary protein from proso millet on plasma cholesterol level in rats (Nishizawa et al. 1990). Supplementation of diet based on proso millet to hyperlipidemic rats positively ameliorates plasma HDL cholesterol, LDL cholesterol, total cholesterol, and triglycerides level (Bora et al. 2018). Enhanced neuronal density in different parts of hippocampus was observed in rat treated with alcoholic extract of proso millet seed compared to the control animals. Results suggested that proso millet causes neurogenesis in the mouse hippocampus (Bornarodi et al. 2017).

30.4.3.5 Barnyard Millet (Jhangora)

Hydroalcoholic extract of grains of barnyard millet showed significant hypoglycemic and hypolipidemic activity in alloxan-induced diabetic rat (Ravirala et al. 2013). Ethyl acetate extract grains of barnyard millet and eight isolated compounds

(N-p-coumaroyl serotonin, feruloyl serotonin, tricin and its methyl ester, luteolin, luteolin-7-glucoside, 3,4-dihydroxy benzoic acid, 4-hydroxybenzoic acid) from extract showed significantly inhabited α-glucosidase obtained from *Saccharomyces cerevisiae*. Compounds such as N-p-coumaroyl serotonin, feruloylserotonin, and luteolin produced potent activity (Seo et al. 2015). Due to the promising biological activity, barnyard millet was considered as alternative of rice for *khichdi* preparation for diabetic people and also to prepare biscuit with low glycemic index (Anju and Sarita 2010; Joshi and Srivastava 2016). Ethanol (80%) extract of grains of barnyard millet and its fractions showed more potent anti-inflammatory activity. Fractions particularly methylene chloride fraction causes downregulation of expression of iNOS, COX-2, IL-1β, IL-6, and TNF-α transcripts in LPS-stimulated Raw264.7 cells and also induced the activation of MAPKs, such as ERK, JNK, and p38MAPK. Kaempferol and biochanin present in fraction may be responsible for anti-inflammatory effect exerted by the millet (Lee et al. 2014). Alcoholic extract, fractions (n-hexane, chloroform, ethyl acetate, and n-butanol), and isolated compounds (5,7-dihydroxy-3′,4′,5′-trimethoxy flavones; tricin; quercetin; flavones; apigenin-8-C-sophoroside; 2-methoxy-4-hydroxycinnamic acid; p-coumaric acid; quercetin-3-O-glucoside) of barnyard millet were found to possess potent cytotoxic activity tested using the colon (HCT-116), cervical (HELA), liver (HEPG-2), and breast (MCF-7) adenocarcinoma cell (Molla et al. 2016).

Hypolipidemic and anti-obesity effects of barnyard millet were examined. Hydroalcoholic extracts significantly change the lipid profile toward normal value and reduced atherogenic index (MB18). Methanol extract of barnyard millet caryopses produced strong *in vitro* antioxidant and *in vivo* hepatoprotective and anti-hepatotoxic activity against paracetamol, and D-Galactosamine induced hepatic damage in experimental animal, respectively (Vanapatla et al. 2017). Antibacterial and antifungal potency of barnyard millet were successfully examined against *Staphylococcus aureus, Bacillus megaterium, Escherichia coli, Pseudomonas aeruginosa, Aspergillus niger, Fusarium oxysporum, Fusarium solani, Fusarium oxysporum*, etc. EcAMP1, an antifungal peptide isolated from barnyard millet grain kernels, was found effective against *F. graminearum* and *F. solani, A. alternata*, A. *solani, B. Sorokiniana, P. infestans, P. debaryanum*, and *P. ultimum* (Al-Snafi 2017).

30.4.3.6 Foxtail Millet (Kangni)

A study examined anti-inflammatory activity of bound polyphenols of inner shell of foxtail millet bran on LPS-induced HT-29 cells and in nude mice. Bound polyphenols found to restrain pro-inflammatory cytokine (IL-1β, IL-6, IL-8) levels and increased IL-10 (an anti-inflammatory cytokine) expression through inhibition of nuclear factor-kappaB (NF- κB)-p65 nuclear translocation. It was also observed that bound polyphenols exerted anti-inflammatory activity via the signaling cascade of ROS/miR-149/Akt/NF-κB axis (Shi et al. 2017). FMBP, a secretory peroxidase of class III from bran of foxtail millet bran, showed significant growth inhibitory effect on human colon cancer cell, but not against normal colon cell. Moreover, FMBP causes accumulation of reactive oxygen species in the cancer cell which in part is responsible for the downregulation of expression of Nrf2 expression and decrease of catalase activities and glutathione level. Accumulation of ROS may block the STAT3 signaling pathway, which is responsible for anticancer effects on colon cancer cells (Shan et al. 2015). Foxtail millet extract reduced viability of androgen-sensitive lymph node metastasis type of prostate cancer (LNCaP) cells (Kim et al. 2016). Another study concluded that isolated phenolic acid compounds of foxtail millet produced antiproliferative activity on MDA human breast cancer cells and human HepG2 liver cancer cells (Sharma and Niranjan 2018).

Ethanolic extract of foxtail millet and its fractions showed a number of pharmacological activities which include antioxidant, analgesic, anti-inflammatory, hypoglycemic, cytotoxic, and CNS depressant (only against certain model) activities (Dasgupta et al. 2012, 2016a, b). *In vivo* and *in vitro* studies confirmed the antidiabetic potential of foxtail millet. Insoluble dietary fibers of foxtail millet could hold up the glucose diffusion, enhance glucose absorption in GIT, inhibit α-amylase activity, and slow down the digestion of carbohydrates. Bioactive components of foxtail millet produced *in vivo* hypoglycemic and hypolipidemic activity. Foxtail millet reduced atherogenic index and reduced LDL peroxidation and triglyceride and CRP levels (Sharma and Niranjan 2018). Intake of foxtail millet biscuits and burfi (with low glycemic index) was found effective in type 2 diabetic individuals. It reduced serum glucose, cholesterol, triglyceride, and VLDL levels (Thathola et al. 2011).

Different extracts of foxtail millet seed exerted antimicrobial activity against *Bacillus cereus, B. Megaterium, B. Subtilis, Sarcina lutea, Staphylococcus aureus, E. coli, Pseudomonas aeruginosa, Salmonella paratyphi, S. Typhi, Shigella boydii, S. Dysenteriae, Vibrio mimicus, V. parahaemolyticus, Aspergillus niger, Candida albicans, and Saccharomyces cerevisiae.* However, crude extract did not produce significant antidiarrheal effect (Dasgupta et al. 2016a, b).

30.4.3.7 Kodo Millet (Kodra)

A study examined the bioactivity of phenolic extract of pearl and kodo millet dehulled grains, hull, and whole grain. Kodo millet extract showed strong inhibitory effect against LDL cholesterol and liposome oxidation; pearl millet exhibited lesser potent activity compared to kodo millet. All extracts showed inhibition of DNA scission. Hull of millets found to contain three times more total phenolic content than the whole grain. Antioxidant activity exerted by hull is found more followed by whole grain and dehulled grain. Extracts were found to inhibit cell proliferation of HT-29 adenocarcinoma cell (Chandrasekara and Shahidi 2011). Polyphenol-rich extract of kodo millet inhibited the growth of human cervical cancer line (HeLa). Membrane blebbing, loss of potential of mitochondrial membrane, enhanced generation of ROS, DNA damage, activation of caspase-9, reduced expression of Bcl-2, and cleavage of poly ADP-ribosome polymerase are responsible for anticancer activity of extract (Ramasamy et al. 2017).

Dermal wound healing activity of kodo and finger millets was accessed on rats. Water paste of both millet grains were found effective. Significant enhancement in protein, collagen content, rate of wound contraction, and reduction in lipid peroxidation and period of epithelialization was observed after 2 weeks of treatment (Hegde et al. 2005). Ethanol and water extracts of kodo millet showed antidiabetic activity on alloxan-induced diabetic rats. Treatment with extract found to enhance liver glycogen and reduced glycated hemoglobin level (Jain et al. 2010). A randomized crossover study found that a daily diet of kodo millet-based food (idli and sewai upma) could help a better control of blood glucose in diabetic individuals (Yadav et al. 2013). The beneficial effect of kodo millet was examined in high fat diet-induced hyperlipidemic rats. Millet was found to reduce elevated LDL, VLDL, triglyceride, and cholesterol levels, while HDL level increased significantly (Narra et al. 2013).

30.4.3.8 Little Millet (Moraiyo)

Insoluble fibers of kodo millet, proso millet, barnyard millet, finger millet, and great millet showed significant hypoglycemic activity when examined through several *in vitro* assay methods such as glucose adsorption capacity study, glucose diffusion and glucose dialysis retardation index estimation, starch digestibility activity, and estimation of residual amylase activity (Bisoi et al. 2012). Anti-adipogenic activities such as foxtail, sorghum, and proso millet was evaluated using mouse 3T3-L1 fibroblast cells. Results showed that water extract millets inhibited adipocyte differentiation. Proso millet exhibited maximum anti-adipogenic activity, which is related to downregulation of PPAR-γ, sterol regulatory element-binding protein 1, and CCAAT/enhancer binding protein-α gene. Extracts also alter the ratio of monounsaturated fatty acids to saturated fatty acids in adipocytes (Park et al. 2011). Bran extracts of foxtail, barnyard, and proso millet were examined for immunomodulating effect using mouse macrophage cell line (Raw264.7 cells). Methanol extract of bran of millets suppressed the production of NO, TNF-α, and IL-6 in

LPS-stimulated macrophages. Phenolic component present in extract may be responsible for the above activities. Proso millet extract showed better immunosuppressing effect compared to other extracts (Hosoda et al. 2012). Millet-enriched diets found to attenuate hypertension induced by high salt intake and myocardial damage in experimental male rat (Wei et al. 2018).

30.5 Scope and Things to Remember

This review mainly concentrates on the therapeutic benefit of wheat, rice, and millets. Therapeutic benefit confirmed by the wheat, rice, and millets is well documented, and several further researches are going on using new varieties/cultivar to find mechanism of action and isolate bioactive molecules. In the twenty-first century, we are going through a time where a large number of people are living an unhealthy lifestyle with stress and in polluted environment which contribute for a number of disorders. Therefore, research toward the food grain is beneficial for the future. Preclinical studies and epidemiological studies/randomized trial on healthy human/patients also showed the beneficial effect exerted by these food grains. Whole grains consist of the entire grain including bran and germ, which are rich in phenolic components, fibers, minerals, vitamins, etc. Higher consumption of whole grains is found to reduce the risk of cardiovascular disease, cancer, and all-cause and disease-specific mortality. Food grains were also found as preventive or curative agents in case of diabetes and other associated disorders (Singhal and Kaushik 2016; Aune et al. 2016). Oxidative stress is considered as a major underlying cause involved in the pathogenesis of cancer, metabolic diseases, CNS-related diseases, cardiovascular diseases, cancer, and ageing. Wheat, rice, and millets are found to contain a large number of antioxidant molecules such as phenolic compounds, carotenoids, vitamin E, minerals (e.g., zinc, selenium), etc., which may produce added health benefits, by virtue of antioxidant property of those phytochemicals. However, at the same time, interaction between numerous phytoconstituent is complex. A healthy diet which includes whole food grains is essential for physical and mental well-being. Oftentimes, in preclinical studies, the therapeutic benefit of isolated phytomolecules is almost consistent. However, the results of randomized controlled trials (RCTs) to find the effect of isolated molecule/antioxidant are not consistent. Positive, negative, or null effect of such antioxidant supplements are observed through RCTs (Sen and Chakraborty 2017). These observations clearly direct toward the complex beneficial synergism of constitutes when present as a part of whole grain. Consumption of whole grain was found to confer health-promotive and disease-preventive effect.

In recent time, research is ongoing in almost all parts of the world to find therapeutic efficacy of food grains. However, certain issues need to be documented properly, such as variety/cultivar of food grain used, location, and systemic research to find the molecular mechanism and phytochemical responsible for such effect. It is well noted that the quality of soil, environment, and related factors are key factors which may be responsible for variation in phytoconstituents. Work on developing products based on whole grain and bran along with developing processing techniques is essential. Multidisciplinary collaborative researches are essential to make sure this observation and results can be used in a sustainable, appropriate, and economically sound way. Wheat, rice, and millets are not only good sources of nutrients and fibers but also contain antioxidants and other bioactive molecules. Bran of wheat, rice, and millets are loaded with diverse phytochemicals that are important therapeutically. Wheat, rice, and millets are truly wonderful food grains that could protect us from diverse health-related issues. Current evidence suggested that incorporation of wheat, rice, and millets in regular diet could be useful. Research on these food grains and phytochemicals present on wheat, rice, and millets could pave the way for new therapeutic approach to cure cardiovascular, antimicrobial, and metabolic disorders, hepatic problems, diabetes mellitus, neurodegenerative diseases, cancer, etc.

References

Abeysekera WKSM, Arachchige SPG, Ratnasooriya WD, Choudhary MI, Dalvandi K, Chandrasekharan NV. Anti-diabetic related health food properties of traditional rice (Oryza sativa L.) in Sri Lanka. J Coast Life Med. 2015;3(10):815–20.

Aburai N, Esumi Y, Koshino H, Nishizawa N, Kimura K. Inhibitory activity if linoleic acid isolated from proso and Japanese millet toward histone deacetylase. Biosci Biotechnol Biochem. 2007;71(8):20161–4. MPO 18

Al-Snafi AE. Pharmacology of *Echinochloa crus-galli* – a review. Indo Am J P Sci. 2017;4(01):117–22.

Anju T, Sarita S. Suitability of foxtail millet (Setaria italica) and barnyard millet (Echinochloa frumentacea) for development of low glycemic index biscuits. Malays J Nutr. 2010;16(3):361–8.

Anonymous. Exports from India of wheat. 2018a. http://agriexchange.apeda.gov.in/product_profile/exp_f_india.aspx?categorycode=0603. Accessed 24 Aug 2018.

Anonymous. About millets. 2018b. http://millets.res.in/millets.php. Accessed 24 Aug 2018.

Anson NM, Berg RVD, Havenaar R, Haenen G, Bast A. Antioxidant and anti-inflammatory potency of different wheat varieties and fractions. Proc Nutr Soc. 2008;67(OCE1):E56. https://doi.org/10.1017/S0029665108006654.

Aune D, Keum N, Giovannucci E, Fadnes LT, Boffetta P, Greenwood DC, et al. Whole grain consumption and risk of cardiovascular disease, cancer, and all cause and cause specific mortality: systematic review and dose-response meta-analysis of prospective studies. BMJ. 2016;353:i2716. https://doi.org/10.1136/bmj.i2716.

Awika JM, Rooney LW. Sorghum phytochemicals and their potential impact on human health. Phytochemistry. 2004;65:1199–221.

Awika J, Rooney LW, Waniska RD. Properties of 3-Deoxyanthocyanins from Sorghum. J Agric Food Chem. 2004;52:4388–94.

Bhat FM, Riar CS. Characterizing the pigmented traditional rice cultivars grown in temperate regions of Kashmir (India) for free and bound phenolics compounds and in vitro antioxidant properties. J Cereal Sci. 2017;76:253–62.

Bisoi PC, Sahoo G, Mishra SK, Das C, Das KL. Hypoglycemic effects of insoluble fiber rich fraction of different cereals and millets. J Food Process Technol. 2012;3:191.

Bora P, Das P, Mohan P, Barthakur A. Evaluation of hypolipidemic property of proso millet (*Panicum miliaceum* L.) in high fat diet induced hyperlipidemia in rats. J Entomol Zool Stud. 2018;6(3):691–5.

Bornarodi A, Tehranipour M, Mahdavi-Shahri N. The effect of alcoholic extract of *Panicum miliaceum* L. seed on hippocampus neuronal density in male mouse. Feyz. 2017;21(4):335–44.

Cabanting RMF, Perez LM. An ethnobotanical study of traditional rice landraces (*Oryza sativa* L.) used for medical treatment in selected local communities of the Philippines. J Ethnopharmacol. 2016;194:767–73.

Caro GP, Cros G, Yokota T, Crozier A. Phytochemical profiles of black, red, brown, and white rice from the Camargue region of France. J Agric Food Chem. 2013;61:7976–86.

Chandra D, Chandra S, Pallavi, Sharma AK. Review of finger millet (*Eleusine coracana* (L.) Gaertn): a power house of health benefiting nutrients. Food Sci Human Wellness. 2016;5:149–55.

Chandrasekara A, Shahidi F. Bioactivities and antiradical properties of millet grains and hulls. J Agric Food Chem. 2011;59:9563–71.

Chauhan M. A pilot study on wheat grass juice for its phytochemical, nutritional and therapeutic potential on chronic diseases. Int J Chem Stud. 2014;2(4):27–34.

Cho JG, Song NY, Nam TG, et al. Flavonoids from the grains of C1/R-S transgenic rice, the transgenic *Oryza sativa* spp. japonica, and their radical scavenging activities. J Agric Food Chem. 2013;61:10354–9.

Choo Y-Y, Lee S, Nguyen P-H, et al. Caffeoylglycolic acid methyl ester, a major constituent of sorghum, exhibits anti-inflammatory activity via the Nrf2/heme oxygenase-1 pathway. RSC Adv. 2015;5:17786.

Choudhury NH, Juliano BO. Effect of amylose content on the lipids of mature rice grain. Phytochemistry. 1980;19:1385–9.

Chumpiya S, Plaingarm W, Tencomnao T. Neuroprotective effect of rice and corn extracts against H_2O_2 -induced neurotoxicity in HT22 murine hippocampal neuronal cells. Med Health. 2016;11(2):151–70.

Das A, Raychaudhuri U, Chakraborty R. Cereal based functional food of Indian subcontinent: a review. J Food Sci Technol. 2012;49(6):665–72.

Das KR, Medhabati K, Nongalleima K, Devi HS. The potential of dark purple scented rice- from staple food to nutraceutical. Curr World Environ. 2014;9(3):867–76.

Dasgupta T, Asaduzzaman M, Qais N. Pharmacological potential investigation of setaria italic (Poaceae). Germany: LAMBERT Academic Publishing; 2012.

Dasgupta T, Ganguly A, Asaduzzaman M, Qais N. Evaluation of anti-microbial, hypoglycemic and anti-diarrheal activities of Setaria italica seeds. Dhaka Univ J Pharm Sci. 2016a;15(1):31–5.

Dasgupta T, Poddar SK, Ganguly A, Qais N. Anti-inflammatory and Neuropharmacological activities of the seed extract of Setaria italic. J App Pharm Sci. 2016b;6(5):193–7.

Debnath T, Park SR, Kim DH, et al. Anti-oxidant and anti-inflammatory activities of *Inonotus obliquus* and germinated brown rice extracts. Molecules. 2013;18:9293–304.

Devi PB, Vijayabharathi R, Sathyabama S, Malleshi NG, Priyadarisini VB. Health benefits of finger millet (Eleusine coracana L.) polyphenols and dietary fiber: a review. J Food Sci Technol. 2014;51(6):1021–40.

Dias-Martins AM, Pessanha KLF, Pacheco S, Rodrigues JAS, Carvalho CWP. Potential use of pearl millet (Pennisetum glaucum (L.) R. Br.) in Brazil: food security, processing, health benefits and nutritional products. Food Res Int. 2018;109:175–86.

Dykes L, Rooney LW. Review sorghum and millet phenols and antioxidants. J Cereal Sci. 2006;44:236–51.

Elhassan FA, Suad AGHO, Dahawi FAA. Antimicrobial activities of six types of wheat bran. IOSR J Appl Chem. 2017;10(3):61–9.

Esa NM, Kadir KA, Amom Z, Azlan A. Antioxidant activity of white rice, brown rice and germinated brown rice (*in vivo* and *in vitro*) and the effects on lipid peroxidation and liver enzymes in hyperlipidaemic rabbits. Food Chem. 2013;141:1306–12.

Fadel A, Plunkett A, Li W, et al. Arabinoxylans from rice bran and wheat immunomodulatory potentials: a review article. Nutr Food Sci. 2018;48:97–110.

Fang H, Chen Y, Chen H, Lin S, Fang Y. Immunomodulatory effects of feruloylated oligosaccharides from rice bran. Food Chem. 2012;134:836–40.

Francesco S, Laure BB, Joran V, Christophe MC, Kristin V, Patrice DC, Audrey MN, Nathalie MD. Fat binding capacity and modulation of the gut microbiota both determine the effect of wheat bran fractions on adiposity. Sci Rep. 2017;7:5621.

Goufo P, Trindade H. Rice antioxidants: phenolic acids, flavonoids, anthocyanins, proanthocyanidins, tocopherols, tocotrienols, c-oryzanol, and phytic acid. Food Sci Nutr. 2014;2(2):75–104.

Habiyaremye C, Matanguihan JB, D'Alpoim GJ, et al. Proso Millet (*Panicum miliaceum* L.) and its potential for cultivation in the pacific northwest, US: a review. Front Plant Sci. 2017;7:1961. https://doi.org/10.3389/fpls.2016.01961.

Hao J, Zhu H, Zhang Z, Yang S, Li H. Identification of anthocyanins in black rice (Oryza sativa L.) by UPLC/QTOF-MS and their in vitro and in vivo antioxidant activities. J Cereal Sci. 2015;64:92–9.

Havrlentova M, Pšenáková I, Žofajová A, Rückschloss L, Kraic J. Anthocyanins in wheat seed–a mini review. Nova Biotechnologica et Chimica. 2014;13(1):1. https://doi.org/10.2478/nbec-2014-0001.

Hegde PS, Anitha B, Chandra TS. *In vivo* effect of whole grain flour of finger millet (Eleusine coracana) and kodo millet (Paspalum scrobiculatum) on rat dermal wound healing. Indian Exp Biol. 2005;43:254–8.

Hosoda A, Okai Y, Kasahara E, et al. Potent immunomodulating effects of bran extracts of traditional japanese millets on nitric oxide and cytokine production of macrophages (raw264.7) induced by lipopolysaccharide. J UOEH. 2012;34(4):285–96.

Hou F, Zhanga R, Zhanga M, et al. Hepatoprotective and antioxidant activity of anthocyanins in black rice bran on carbon tetrachloride-induced liver injury in mice. J Funct Food. 2013;5:1705–13.

Hu C, Zawistowski J, Ling W, Kitts DD. Black Rice (*Oryza sativa* L. *indica*) pigmented fraction suppresses both reactive oxygen species and nitric oxide in chemical and biological model systems. J Agric Food Chem. 2003;51:5271–7.

Jain S, Bhatiaa G, Barika R, et al. Antidiabetic activity of *Paspalum scrobiculatum* Linn. in alloxan induced diabetic rats. J Ethnopharmacol. 2010;127:325–8.

Jana K. Nutritionally important components of proso millet (*Panicum miliaceum* L.). FoodReview. 2007;1(1):91–100.

Javed I, Aslam B, Khan MZ, Rahman ZU, Muhammad F, Saleemi MK. Lipid lowering efficacy of *Pennisetum glaucum* bran in hyperlipidemic albino rats. Pak Vet J. 2012;32(2):201–5.

Joshi S, Srivastava S. Barnyard millet as a substitute of rice in preparation of khichdi for diabetics. Int J Sci Res. 2016;5(6):1798–802.

Jun DY, Lee JY, Han CR, et al. Pro-apoptotic and anti-adipogenic effects of proso millet (Panicum miliaceum) grains on 3t3-l1 preadipocytes. J Life Sci. 2014;24(5):505–14.

Khan IU, Meena RC, Raiger PR, Rathore BS, Satyavathi CT, Singh B. Evaluation and identification of volatile bio active compounds in methanol extract of pearl millet genotypes by gas chromatography-mass spectroscopy. Int J Pure App Biosci. 2017;5(2):526–31.

Khatkar BS, Chaudhary N, Dangi P. Production and consumption of grains: India. In: Wrigley C, Corke H, Seetharaman K, Faubion J, editors. Encyclopedia of food grains. 2nd ed. Oxford: Academic Press; 2016. p. 367–73.

Kim MJ, Kim SS. Antioxidant and antiproliferative activities in immature and mature wheat kernels. Food Chem. 2016;196:638–45.

Kim J, Park Y. Anti-diabetic effect of sorghum extract on hepatic gluconeogenesis of streptozotocin-induced diabetic rats. Nutr Metab. 2012;9:106.

Kim HM, Yi D, Shin HY. The evaluation of antianaphylactic effect of *Oryza sativa* L. in rats. Am J Chin Med 1999:63–71, 27.

Kim J-H, Cho H-D, Hong S-M, et al. Antioxidant and antiproliferating effects of Setaria italica, Panicum miliaceum and Sorghum bicolor extracts on prostate cancer cell lines. Korean J Food Preserv. 2016;23(7):1033–41.

Kumar P, Yadava RK, Gollen B, Kumar S, Verma RK, Yadav S. Nutritional contents and medicinal properties of wheat: a review. Life Sci Med Res. 2011;22:1–10.

Kumar A, Metwal M, Kaur S, et al. Nutraceutical value of finger millet [Eleusine coracana (L.) Gaertn.], and their improvement using omics approaches. Front Plant Sci. 2016;7:934. https://doi.org/10.3389/fpls.2016.00934.

Kunchala R, Durgalla P, Banerjee R, et al. Probiotic potential *Streptomyces* species from the grains of pearl millet (*Pennisetum glaucum*). Afr J Microbiol Res. 2017;11(14):553–9.

Kuno T, Hirose Y, Yamada Y, et al. Chemoprevention of mouse urinary bladder carcinogenesis by fermented brown rice and rice bran. Oncol Rep. 2006;15:533–8.

Kuno T, Nagano A, Mori Y, et al. Preventive effects of fermented brown rice and rice bran against prostate carcinogenesis in TRAP rats. Nutrients. 2016;8:421.

Lee JY, Jun DY, Yoon YH, Ko JY, Woo KS, Woo MH, Kim YH. Anti-inflammatory effect of flavonoids kaempferol and biochanin a-enriched extract of barnyard millet (Echinochloa crus-galli var. frumentacea) grains in LPS-stimulated RAW264.7 cells. J Life Sci. 2014;24(11):1157–67.

Liu L, Winter KM, Stevenson L, Morris C, Leach DN. Wheat bran lipophilic compounds with *in vitro* anticancer effects. Food Chem. 2012;130:156–64.

Liu J, Hao Y, Wang Z, et al. Identification, quantification and anti-inflammatory activity of 5-n-alkylresorcinols from 21 different wheat varieties. J Agric Food Chem. 2018;66:9241–7.

Mahajan G, Kumar V, Chauhan BS. Rice production in India. In: Chauhan B, Jabran K, Mahajan G, editors. Rice production worldwide. Cham: Springer; 2017. p. 53–91.

Malunga LN, Izydorczyk M, Beta T. Antiglycemic effect of water extractable arabinoxylan from wheat aleurone and bran. J Nutr Metab. 2017;2017:1. https://doi.org/10.1155/2017/5784759.

Mateo Anson N, Hemery YM, Bast A, Haenen GR. Optimizing the bioactive potential of wheat bran by processing. Food Funct. 2012;3:362–75.

Merike V, Kersti M, Tuuli L, Kati H, Mihkel K. Phenolic compounds and the antioxidant activity of the bran, flour and whole grain of different wheat varieties. Procedia Chem. 2010;2:76–82.

Miyoshi N, Koyama Y, Katsuno Y, et al. Apoptosis induction associated with cell cycle dysregulation by rice bran agglutinin. J Biochem. 2001;130(6):799–805.

Molla SGE, Motaal AA, Hefnawy HE, Fishawy AE. Cytotoxic activity of phenolic constituents from Echinochloa crus-galli against four human cancer cell lines. Rev Bras Farmacogn. 2016;26:62–7.

Morya GGK, Vinita, Mishra HS, Shakya S, Bahadur R, Yadav KN. The indigenous food grains. Int J Adv Ayurveda Yoga Unani Siddha Homeopathy. 2017;6:447–52.

Muhammad SI, Ismail M, Mahmud RB, Salisu AM, Zakaria ZA. Germinated brown rice and its bioactives modulate the activity of uterine cells in oophorectomised rats as evidenced by gross cytohistological and immunohistochemical changes. BMC Complement Altern Med. 2013;13(198):1–9.

Murtaza N, Baboota RK, Jagtap S, et al. Finger millet bran supplementation alleviates obesity-induced oxidative stress, inflammation and gut microbial derangements in high-fat diet-fed mice. Br J Nutr. 2014;1:12.

Nair SV, Bhaskar S, Helen A. Anti-inflammatory activity of *Oryza sativa* L. (Njavara). J Nat Remedies. 2011;11(1):24–30.

Nam SH, Choi SP, Kang MY, Koh HJ, Kozukue N, Friedman M. Bran extracts from pigmented rice seeds inhibit tumor promotion in lymphoblastoid B cells by phorbol ester. Food Chem Toxicol. 2005;43:741–5.

Nani A, Belarbi M, Ksouri-Megdiche W, et al. Effects of polyphenols and lipids from Pennisetum glaucum grains on T-cell activation: modulation of Ca^{2+} and ERK1/ERK2 signaling. BMC Complement Altern Med. 2015;15:426.

Narra S, Ramadurg B, Saraswathi CD. Antihyperlipidemic activity of *Paspalum scrobiculatum* L. grains extract in albino rats. Res J Pharmacol Pharmacodynamics. 2013;5:362–70.

Ndiku HM, Ngule MC. Comparative study on the antibacterial and chemical constituents of Pennisetum glaucum (pearl millet) and Zea mays (maize). Int J Nutr Metab. 2015;7(4):46–51.

Ndiku HM, Mwitari PG, Irungu B, Ngule CM, Hellen MN, Peter GM, Beatrice I, Chrispus MN. Antibacterial activity of P*ennisetum glaucum* crude extracts and prepurified fractions against selected pathogenic microorganisms. Br J Pharm Res. 2016;14(1):1–9.

Nishizawa N, Oikawa M, Hareyama S. Effect of dietary protein from proso millet on the plasma cholesterol metabolism in rats. Agric Biol Chem. 1990;54(1):229–30.

Onipe OO, Jideani AIO, Beswa D. Composition and functionality of wheat bran and its application in some cereal food products. Int J Food Sci Technol. 2015;50:2509–18.

Oseghale IO, Imieje VO, Erharuyi O, Iheanacho C, Falodun A. A review of the phytochemistry and pharmacology of eleusine coracana Linn (poaceae): a popular Nigerian edible grain. Trop J Nat Prod Res. 2017;1(6):227–35.

Ou S-Y, Jackson GM, Jiao X, et al. Protection against oxidative stress in diabetic rats by wheat bran feruloyl oligosaccharides. J Agric Food Chem. 2007;55(8):3191–5.

Park M-Y, Seo D-W, Lee J-Y, et al. Effects of *Panicum miliaceum* L. extract on adipogenic transcription factors and fatty acid accumulation in 3T3-L1 adipocytes. Nutr Res Pract. 2011;5(3):192–7.

Park JH, Lee SH, Chung I-M, Park Y. Sorghum extract exerts an anti-diabetic effect by improving insulin sensitivity via PPAR-γ in mice fed a high-fat diet. Nutr Res Pract. 2012;6(4):322–7.

Park H, Yu A, Choi I, et al. Immunostimulatory effects and characterization of a glycoprotein fraction from rice bran. Int Immunopharmacol. 2013;17:191–7.

Poudel R, Bhatta M. Review of nutraceuticals and functional properties of whole wheat. J Nutr Food Sci. 2017;7:571.

Pradeep PM, Sreerama YN. Phenolic antioxidants of foxtail and little millet cultivars and their inhibitory effects on α-amylase and α-glucosidase activities. Food Chem. 2018;247:46–55.

Prashanth MRS, Shruthi RR, Muralikrishna G. Immunomodulatory activity of purified arabinoxylans from finger millet (Eleusine coracana, v. Indaf 15) bran. J Food Sci Technol. 2015;52(9):6049–54.

Rajnarayana K, Prabhakar MC, Krishna DR. Influence of rice bran oil on serum lipid peroxides and lipids in human subjects. Indian J Physiol Pharmacol. 2001;45(4):442–4.

Ramasamy S, Anupam K, Ratnavathi CV, Karunagaran D, Chandra TS. Paspalum scrobiculatum polyphenol rich extracts inhibit human cervical cancer cell proliferation and induce apoptosis in vitro. Biochem Mol Biol. 2017;31:1. https://doi.org/10.1096/fasebj.31.1_supplement.lb162.

Rao S, Santhakumar AB, Chinkwo KA, Wu G, Johnson SK, Blanchard CL. Characterization of phenolic compounds and antioxidant activity in sorghum grains. J Cereal Sci. 2018;84:103. https://doi.org/10.1016/j.jcs.2018.07.013.

Rashi C, Ashok P. Wheat bran extract mimics statin like action in hyperlipidemic rabbits: an experimental study. Asian J Pharm Clin Res. 2018;11(3):402–5.

Ravichanthiran K, Ma ZF, Zhang H, et al. Phytochemical profile of brown rice and its nutrigenomic implications. Antioxidants. 2018;7:71. https://doi.org/10.3390/antiox7060071.

Ravirala R, Kotagiri S, Vrushabendra SBM, Archana Swamy P, Vishwanath Swamy KM. Hypoglycemic and hypolipidemic activities of hydro-alcoholic extract of *Mchinochloa frumentacea* link grains in alloxan induced diabetic rats. J Pharmacol Toxicol Studies. 2013;1(2):38–51.

Saleh ASM, Wang P, Wang N, Yang S, Xiao Z, Ahmed SS, Peng W, Na W, Shu Y, Zhigang X. Technologies for enhancement of bioactive components and potential health benefits of cereal and cereal-based foods: research advances and application challenges. Crit Rev Food Sci Nutr. 2017;59:1–21. https://doi.org/10.1080/10408398.2017.1363711.

Sareen M, Baghla P, Dhaka P, Mathur E, Sobti P, Khajuria S. Wheat grass-a wonder herb. Sys Rev Pharm. 2014;5(1):4–5.

Sen S, Chakraborty R. Food in health preservation and promotion: A special focus on the interplay between oxidative stress and pro-oxidant/antioxidant. In: Shekhar HU, Howlader ZH, Kabir Y, editors. Exploring the nutrition and health benefits of functional. Hershey: IGI Global; 2017. p. 265–300.

Seo KH, Ra JE, Lee SJ, et al. Anti-hyperglycemic activity of polyphenols isolated from barnyard millet (*Echinochloa utilis* L.) and their role inhibiting a-glucosidase. J Korean Soc Appl Biol Chem. 2015;58:571–9.

Settharaksa S, Madaksa F, Charkree K, Charoenchai L. The study of anti-inflammatory and antioxidant activity in cold press rice bran oil from rice in Thailand. Int J Pharm Pharm Sci. 2014;6(7):428–31.

Sewon J, Jaekyung L, Oran K, Won KJ, Bumjo O. A randomized, double-blind, placebo-controlled trial investigating cholesterol-lowering effects and safety of yellow yeast rice in adults with mild to moderate hypercholesterolemia: a study protocol. Medicine. 2018;97:e11634.

Shahidi F, Chandrasekar A. Millet grain phenolics and their role in disease risk reduction and health promotion: a review. J Funct Foods. 2013;5:570–81.

Shan S, Shi J, Li Z, et al. Targeted anti-colon cancer activities of a millet bran-derived peroxidase were mediated by elevated ROS generation. Food Funct. 2015;6:2331.

Sharma N, Niranjan K. Foxtail millet: properties, processing, health benefits and uses. Food Rev Int. 2018;34:329–63.

Sharma S, Saxena DC, Riar SC. Using combined optimization, GC–MS and analytical technique to analyze the germination effect on phenolics, dietary fibers, minerals and GABA contents of Kodo millet (Paspalum scrobiculatum). Food Chem. 2017;233:20–8.

Shen T, Wang G, You L, et al. Polysaccharide from wheat bran induces cytokine expression via the toll-like receptor 4-mediated p38 MAPK signaling pathway and prevents cyclophosphamide-induced immunosuppression in mice. Food Nutr Res. 2017;61:1344523. https://doi.org/10.1080/16546628.2017.1344523.4.

Shen R, Ma Y, Jiang L, Dong J, Zhu Y, Ren G. Chemical composition, antioxidant, and antiproliferative activities of nine Chinese proso millet varieties. Food Agric Immunol. 2018. (online published;29:625. https://doi.org/10.1080/09540105.2018.1428283.

Shi J, Shan S, Li H, Song G, Li Z. Anti-inflammatory effects of millet bran derived-bound polyphenols in LPS-induced HT-29 cell via ROS/miR-149/Akt/NF-κB signaling pathway. Oncotarget. 2017;8(43):74582–94.

Shim T-J, Kim TM, Jang KC, Ko J-Y, Kim DJ. Toxicological evaluation and anti-inflammatory activity of a golden gelatinous sorghum bran extract. Biosci Biotechnol Biochem. 2013;77:697–705.

Shuhua S, Jiangying S, Zhen L, Huixian G, Tonglin S, Zongwei L, Zhuoyu L. Targeted anti-colon cancer activities of a millet bran-derived peroxidase were mediated by elevated ROS generation. Food Funct. 2015;6:2331.

Simnadis TG, Tapsell LC, Beck EJ. Effect of sorghum consumption on health outcomes: a systematic review. Nutr Rev. 2016;0(0):1–18.

Singh N, Meenu G, Sekhar A, Abraham J. Evaluation of antimicrobial and anticancer properties of finger millet (*Eleusine coracana*) and pearl millet (*Pennisetum glaucum*) extracts. Pharma Innov J. 2015;3(11):82–6.

Singhal P, Kaushik G. Therapeutic effect of cereal grains: A review. Crit Rev Food Sci Nutr. 2016:56748–59.

Sinthorn W, Chatuphonprasert W, Chulasiri M, Jarukamjorn K. Thai red rice extract provides liver protection in paracetamol-treated mice by restoring the glutathione system. Pharm Biol. 2016;54:5770–9.

Sohail M, Rakha A, Butt MS, Iqbal MJ, Rashid S. Rice bran nutraceutics: a comprehensive review. Criti Rev Food Sci Nutr. 2017;57:3771–80.

Soi-ampornkul R, Junnu S, Kanyok S, et al. Antioxidative and neuroprotective activities of the pre-germinated brown rice extract. Food Nutr Sci. 2012;3:135–40.

Stefoska-Needham A, Beck EJ, Johnson SK, Tapsell LC. Sorghum: an underutilized cereal whole grain with the potential to assist in the prevention of chronic disease. Food Rev Int. 2015;31(4):401–37.

Taylor JRN. Millets: their unique nutritional and health-promoting attributes. In: Taylor JRN, Awika JM, editors. Gluten-free ancient grains, Woodhead Publishing series in food science, technology and nutrition. Duxford: Woodhead Publishing; 2017. p. 55–103.

Thathola A, Srivastava S, Singh G. Effect of foxtail millet (Setaria italica) supplementation on serum glucose, serum lipids and glycosylated hemoglobin in type 2 diabetics. Diabetol Croat. 2011;40:23–8.

Tu J, Chen J, Zhu S, et al. Inhibition of wheat bran and it's active compoments on α-glucosidase *in vitro*. Pharmacogn Mag. 2013;9(36):309–14.

Udeh HO, Duodu KG, Jideani AIO. Finger millet bioactive compounds, bioaccessibility, and potential health effects – a review. Czech J Food Sci. 2017;35(1):7–17.

Vanamal JKP, Massey AR, Pinnamaneni SR, Reddivari L, Reardon KF. Grain and sweet sorghum (*Sorghum bicolour* L. Moench) serves as a novel source of bioactive compounds for human health. Crit Rev Food Sci Nutr. 2017;58:2867. https://doi.org/10.1080/10408398.2017.1344186.

Vanapatla SR, Syed S, Pallerla P, Bobbala RK. Antioxidant and hepatoprotective studies on methanolic extract of caryopses of Echinochloa frumentacea link. Int J Pharmacog Phytochem Res. 2017;9(10):1386–91.

Veronika C, Magdalena L. Chemical composition and nutritional value of emmer wheat (T*riticum dicoccon* schrank): a review. J Cent Eur Agric. 2017;18(1):117–34.

Wei S, Cheng D, Yu H, Wang X, Song S, Wang C. Millet-enriched diets attenuate high salt-induced hypertension and myocardial damage in male rats. J Funct Foods. 2018;44:304–12.

Whent M, Huang H, Xie Z, et al. Phytochemical composition, anti-inflammatory, and antiproliferative activity of whole wheat flour. J Agric Food Chem. 2012;60:2129–35.

Woo MH, Nguyen DH, Zhao BT, Seo UM, Nguyen TT, Jun DY, Kim YH. Echinochlorins A˜C from the grains of Echinochloa utilis (Barnyard Millet) and their anti-inflammatory activity. Planta Med. 2015;81:81–PX66. https://doi.org/10.1055/s-0035-1556510.

Wunjuntuk K, Kettawan A, Charoenkiatkul S, Rungruang T. Parboiled germinated brown rice protects against CCl_4-induced oxidative stress and liver injury in rats. J Med Food. 2016a;19(1):15–23.

Wunjuntuk K, Kettawan A, Rungruang T, Charoenkiatkul S. Anti-fibrotic and anti-inflammatory effects of parboiled germinated brown rice (Oryza sativa 'KDML 105') in rats with induced liver fibrosis. J Funct Foods. 2016b;26:363–72.

Yadav N, Chaudhary K, Singh A, Gupta A. Evaluation of hypoglycemic properties of kodo millet based food products in healthy subjects. IOSR J Pharm. 2013;3:14–20.

Yamazaki K, Murray JA, Kita H. Innate immunomodulatory effects of cereal grains through induction of IL-10. J Allergy Clin Immunol. 2008;121(1):172–8.

Yang X, Twitchell E, Li G, et al. High protective efficacy of rice bran against human rotavirus diarrhea via enhancing probiotic growth, gut barrier function, and innate immunity. Sci Rep. 2015;5:15004, 1–12. https://doi.org/10.1038/srep15004.

Zhang L, Liu R, Niu W. Phytochemical and antiproliferative activity of proso millet. PLoS One. 2014;9(8):e104058. https://doi.org/10.1371/journal.pone.0104058.

Zhu Y, Shi Z, Yao Y, Hao Y, Ren G. Antioxidant and anticancer activities of proanthocyanidins-rich extracts from three varieties of sorghum (*Sorghum bicolor*) bran. Food Agric Immunol. 2017;28:1530. https://doi.org/10.1080/09540105.2017.1351526.

Medicinal Aspect of Mushrooms: A View Point

31

Banani Das, Biplab De, Rishiraj Chetree, and Subhash C. Mandal

Contents

31.1 Introduction

Nature has served as a resource for an array of substances with health benefits and many of the modern-day drugs are actually derived from natural origin (Kinsalin et al. 2014). Huge number of species of diversified categories of mushrooms has always attracted mankind both as source of food and for medicine. An estimate suggests that there are about 140,000 species of which 22,000 species are only known. If it is now assumed that only 5% of the unknown species are useful, then it would count that about 7000 of the unknown species will be of beneficial use for mankind (Hawksworth 2001).

B. Das
Government Degree College, Dharmanagar, Tripura, India

B. De (✉) · R. Chetree
Regional Institute of Pharmaceutical Science and Technology (RIPSAT), Agartala, Tripura, India

S. C. Mandal
Division of Pharmacognosy, Department of Pharmaceutical Technology, Jadavpur University, Kolkata, West Bengal, India

S. Sen, R. Chakraborty (eds.), *Herbal Medicine in India*,
https://doi.org/10.1007/978-981-13-7248-3_31

The association of human with mushroom is older than any recorded history. Before the evolvement of modern medicine, humans were dependent on the nature of the treatment of their illness as well as for variety of their healthcare needs. In this regard the use of medicinal plants is well established, and mushrooms were not an exception from these needs (Molitoris 1994). Medicinal uses of mushroom have been suggested in the early records of Materia Medica (Abugri et al. 2016). The health benefits of mushrooms find their place in the ancient texts of Greek and Roman writers as well as in traditional Chinese medicine and even in Ayurveda. "Father of Medicine" the famous Greek philosopher Hippocrates had also mentioned about the usefulness of mushrooms (Adhikari 1981). In China, Japan, and some Southeastern countries, cultivation of medicinal mushrooms is a tradition (Molitoris 1994). R.G. Wasson claimed that the Soma plant was used in the preparation of the vedic juice "Soma Rasa" and was actually obtained from the juice of the mushroom *Amanita muscaria* (Wasson 1969). Ayurveda categorizes Mushrooms as *Tamsika* food and considers them as a medicine for enhancing vigor and vitality (Adhikari 1981).

Exploration and validation of the history and ethnic knowledge of the use of mushrooms have been a basis for a number of novel bioactive agents which may serve as leads for drug discovery (Aly et al. 2011; Valverde et al. 2015). Mushrooms are significantly nutritious since they are low in fat and calories, whereas they are rich in protein including essential amino acids and dietary fiber. They are also a good source of various vitamins and trace elements (Aida et al. 2009; Aly et al. 2011; Valverde et al. 2015).

A variety of medicinal properties of the mushrooms have been reported like antioxidant, antidiabetic, anticancer, immunomodulating, anti-allergic, anticholesterolemic, cardiovascular protector, and hepatoprotective effects and antimicrobial benefits such as antibacterial, antiviral, antifungal, and antiparasitic (Valverde et al. 2015). The varied medicinal properties of mushrooms are attributed to the presence of bioactive compounds like glycosides, polysaccharides, alkaloids, terpenoids, volatile oils, phenolics, flavonoids, ergosterols, carotenoids, tocopherols, folates, lectins, enzymes, ascorbic acid, organic acids, etc. (Aida et al. 2009; Valverde et al. 2015).

31.2 Cultivation of Mushrooms

Collection and cultivation of mushrooms for medicinal purpose are a common practice in some Asian countries like China and Japan. In India ethnic groups consume nearly 283 species of wild mushrooms out of 2000 species recorded world over (Purkayastha and Chandra 1985; Sachan et al. 2013; Sarma et al. 2010). Wild mushrooms are an important non-timber source that is sold in traditional markets as food or medicines (Pilz et al. 1999). East Asian countries artificially cultivate more than 60 species of mushrooms on a commercial scale, out of which more than 30 species are cultivated in China. Considering the facts it needs to be mentioned that China has now become the biggest mushroom producer, consumer, and exporter country in the world (Chang 2006).

31.2.1 Mushroom Cultivation in India

The inception of commercial cultivation of mushroom is recorded way back from the year 1960 to 1961 with the cultivation of button mushroom in Himachal Pradesh. However, the cultivation of button mushroom attained pace from the year 1990 onwards with some other North Indian States like Haryana, Punjab, Uttar Pradesh, and Uttaranchal following the footsteps of Himachal Pradesh (Chang 2006). In recent years India has witnessed a major upliftment with respect to the cultivation of various types and strain of mushrooms (Chang 2006; Gaze 2005).

31.2.2 Popularly Cultivated Mushrooms in India

Button mushrooms (*Agaricus sp.*) are one of the most extensive and popular variety cultivated in the North Indian states of Jammu and Kashmir,

Himachal Pradesh, Punjab, Haryana, Uttaranchal, and Bihar (Singh et al. 2011).

Oyster mushroom (*Pleurotus sp.*), because of its low substrate specificity and its adaptive ability to grow in varying agroclimatic condition, is a popular commercially grown species. In spite of this, its cultivation is limited to a few places with a temperature range of 25–40 °C (Tewari 2004).

The milky mushroom, an Indian origin variety, is a new entrant into the world of edible mushrooms, with huge prospects in commercial cultivation. A temperature range of 30–35 °C is ideal for its growth. Its hassle-free production techniques, sustainable yield, increased shelf life, attractive color, and shape have attracted many Indian mushroom cultivators toward commercial cultivation of milky mushrooms (Krishnamoorthy and Muthusankaranarayanan 1998).

31.2.3 Medicinal Mushroom Cultivation in India

The first mushroom which acquired a lot of importance in India is *Ganoderma lucidum* (Mahajna et al. 2010). Various reports suggest that this bitter-tasting exclusive mushroom has been successfully cultivated on sawdust, wheat straw plus rice, and wheat bran. Another mushroom of medicinal importance *shiitake* mushroom has been cultivated on wood logs, saw dust, wheat straw, rice bran, and calcium carbonate mixture. Domestic cultivation of few other mushrooms like *Flammulina velutipes* (Sharma et al. 2005), *Auricularia polytricha* (Sharma 1989), *Trametes versicolor* (Veena and Pandey 2007), *Pycnoporus cinnabarinus* (Veena and Pandey 2007) has been also reported.

31.3 Medicinal Significance Mushrooms

Traditional uses of the Mushrooms have been recorded since Neolithic and Paleolithic eras. Greek physician Dioscorides included *Laricifomes officinalis* (Villars: Fr.) in his De Materia medica for treatment of a disease now known as tuberculosis (Samorini 2001). China has a long history of the use of mushrooms as medicine but their health-promoting basic active principles were investigated by scientists in the 1960s (Gunde-Cimmerman 1999).

Mushrooms have been used in the treatment of a number of simple to complex diseases. Many workers have discussed and reported the medicinal use of mushrooms, viz. reported the use of *Pleurotus sajor-caju* in renal failure, antitumor effects were reported by Ikekawa et al. (1969), whereas Bahl in 1983 reported their use in epilepsy, wounds, skin diseases, heart ailments, rheumatoid arthritis, cholera, diaphoretic, diarrhea, dysentery, cold, anaesthesia, liver disease, gall bladder diseases, and also as vermicides (Bahl 1983; Chihara et al. 1969).

Ganoderma lucidum a basidiomycete white rot fungus is considered as one of the important variety of medicinal mushrooms, popularly known as "Lingzhi" in Chinese and "Reishi" in Japanese. Its medicinal properties are documented in Chinese literature of the Shen Nong Materia Medica in 102–200 AD and in the Chinese Pharmacopoeia. The use of this fungus is common in East Asian countries for various health benefits including longevity and remedy for illness (Sudheesh et al. 2009; Xin-Cun et al. 2012). Use of the fungus by certain Indian tribal groups for treatment of joint pain has also been reported (Harsh et al. 1993; Pala et al. 2013; Panda and Tayung 2015). Various pharmacological effects attributed to *Ganoderma lucidum* include hepatoprotective, antidiabetic, antihypertensive, cardioprotective, immune modulatory, antioxidant, anticancer, cholesterol lowering, anti-inflammatory, sleep induction, stress reduction, etc. (Chang et al. 2015; Sanodiya et al. 2009; Wachtel-Galor et al. 2011).

Mushrooms like *Cordyceps*, enoki, maitake, lion's mane, and splitgill also find their place in cancer treatment. Shiitake, blazei, enoki, cordyceps, maitake, mesima, and oyster exhibit cholesterol lowering properties (Hobbs 1995). *Cordyceps*, shiitake, and maitake have proven their credentials in stress reduction. *Cordyceps* find their use in improvement of sexual pleasure and physical stamina (Sharma 2008). Liver protecting attributes of shiitake, cordyceps, chaga, and Turkey have also been reported. Turkey tail and shiitake show antidiabetic property activity (Hobbs 1995).

31.3.1 Antioxidant Activity

Free radicals are highly reactive atoms or molecules containing unpaired electrons. Excessive production of free radicals can cause oxidative damage to different parts of cells such as lipids, proteins, and DNA, hampering normal functioning of the cell and can result in loss of enzyme activity, mutagenesis, and carcinogenesis (Halliwell and Gutteridge 1997). Antioxidants are compounds that play a protective role against the free radical damage (Mau et al. 2004; Oyetayo 2007; Sanodiya et al. 2009). Intake of antioxidants in the form of supplements and foods may be helpful in maintaining the balance between free radicals and antioxidants, and mushrooms serve as a very good source of antioxidants (Ferreira et al. 2009; Khatua et al. 2013). Many researchers have reported the antioxidant properties of several mushrooms like *A. bisporus*, *P. sajor-caju*, *G. lucidum*, *Cordyceps sinensis, Inonotus obliquus, Lentinula edodes,* etc. (Kozarski et al. 2015; Lakshmi et al. 2008; Oyetayo 2007; Sharma 2008; Wachtel-Galor et al. 2011; Zhou et al. 2007). Presence of antioxidant compounds of various parts of mushrooms is recorded as flavonoids, phenolics, polysaccharides, glycosides, tocopherols, carotenoids, ergothioneine, and ascorbic acid (Kozarski et al. 2015; Valverde et al. 2015).

31.3.2 Anticancer Potential

Cancer is one of the deadliest diseases of the world in recent years. Nonspecificity of target and severe side effects are some of the major disadvantages of the majority of available anticancer drugs, which has stressed on the need for effective yet less toxic variants. Mushrooms with proven anticancer properties are of much interest to the scientific fraternity (Patel and Goyal 2012).

Mushrooms have been known to be used in China, Korea, Japan, Russia, United States, and Canada in cancer therapy (Mizuno 1999). There are several thousand species of mushrooms on earth (both *Basidiomycetes* and *Ascomycetes*) and reports suggest that about 200 species of higher *Basidiomycetes* show antitumor activity (Lucas et al. 1957). Antitumor activity of mushrooms is mainly attributed to the presence of polysaccharides or polysaccharide-protein complexes such as β-glucan (Ganeshpurkar et al. 2010). They exert anticancer properties through immunomodulation and strengthen immune system of the host. Many of such polysaccharide-related compounds are clinically used like Lentinan from *Lentinula edodes*, Schizophyllan from *Schizophyllum commune*, Grifolan from *Grifola frondosa* and protein-bound polysaccharide Krestin/PSK, and polysaccharide peptides/PSP derived from different strains of *Trametes versicolor* as adjuvant to major anticancer therapies (Chihara et al. 1969, 1970a, b; Ganeshpurkar et al. 2010; Patel and Goyal 2012).

31.3.3 Management of Metabolic Disorders

A variety of mushrooms and associated products like their extracts, polysaccharide fraction, and isolated compounds are known to be beneficial in the management of obesity, hyperglycemia, hypercholesterolemia, and hypertension. Apart for the most active compounds like β-glucans and lectines, small compounds such as eritadenine, triterpenes, sterols, and phenolic compounds also exhibit hypoglycemic, hypotensive, hypocholesterolemic, and anti-obesity activity (Kundakovic and Kolundzic 2013).

31.3.3.1 In Obesity and Hyperlipidemia

Anti-obesity and antihyperlipidemic effects of mushrooms have been investigated in several studies. In a study *Lentinula edodes* has been associated with antihyperlipidemic activity and prevention of body weight gain where rats on high fat diet enriched with *L. edodes* have significantly lowered plasma triacylglycerol (TAG) and fat deposition in comparison to rats fed with high fat diet without the *L. edodes* (Handayani et al. 2011).

Studies revealed *Ganoderma lucidum* mushrooms reduce obesity in mice by modulating the composition of the gut microbiota (Chang et al. 2015; Friedman 2016). A polysaccharide from edible mushroom *Tremella fuciformis* had shown to inhibit the differentiation of 3T3-L1 adipocytes by reducing the mRNA expression suggesting the possible significance of the polysaccharide as an anti-obesity prebiotic (Jeong et al. 2008b). *Pleurotus tuber-regium* polysaccharides attenuate hyperglycemia and oxidative stress in experimental diabetic rats (Huang et al. 2012; Friedman 2016).

31.3.3.2 In Hypercholesterolemia

Mushrooms along with their extracts are rich sources of ergosterol, eritadenine, β-glucans, and inhibitors of the enzyme HMG-CoA reductase, the chief enzyme involved in biosynthesis of endogenous cholesterol (Gil-Ramírez et al. 2016). Research reports suggest that water extract of *L. edodes* shows cholesterol-lowering activity through inhibition of HMG-CoA reductase and modulation of transcriptional profile of some genes involved in the cholesterol metabolism (Yang et al. 2013; Gil-Ramírez et al. 2014, 2016; Caz et al. 2015). Beneficial effects of *Agaricus bisporus* on hypercholesterolemia have also been reported (Jeong et al. 2010). Significant reduction of serum cholesterol was observed on supplementation of hypercholesterolemic diet with *A. brasiliensis* (de Miranda et al. 2017).

31.3.3.3 In Diabetes

Antidiabetic properties of derived polysaccharides from mushrooms were reported from the following: *Agaricus brasiliensis* (Yu et al. 2013), *Agrocybe chaxingu* (Lee et al. 2010), *Catathelasma ventricosum, Phellinus linteus, Pleurotus abalonus* (Friedman 2016), *Grifola frondosa* (Lei et al. 2012), *Pleurotus eryngii* (Li et al. 2014), *Pleurotus florida, Pleurotus sajor-caju*, *Tremella fuciformis*, *Ganoderma lucidum, Tremella aurantialba* (Friedman 2016), *Lentinus strigosus* (Yamac et al. 2008), and *Pleurotustuber-regium* (Kwon et al. 2009).

Reduction of blood glycated hemoglobin and serum glucose levels was observed in alloxan-induced hyperglycemic mice on oral administration of *Pleurotus eryngii* extracts (Li et al. 2014). Aqueous extracts of *Pleurotus pulmonarius* (Badole et al. 2008) and *Hericium erinaceus* have exhibited antidiabetic effect (Liang et al. 2013). Water-soluble polysaccharide from fermented broth of *Pleurotus citrinopileatus* (Hu et al. 2006b) helped to reduce fasting blood glucose. Dietary intake of *Agaricus bisporus* has shown both hypoglycemic and hypocholesterolemic effects in streptozotocin-induced diabetic male Sprague-Dawley rats (Jeong et al. 2010). Antidiabetic effects of *A. sylvaticus* (Mascaro et al. 2014) and *A. blazei* (Friedman 2016) have also been investigated.

31.3.4 As Antihypertensive

Researchers have been in the quest for anti-hypertensive properties of mushrooms since long. Research shows antihypertensive property of *Marasmius androsaceus* is credited to the presence of a bioactive compound 3,3,5,5-tetram ethyl-4-piperidone (TMP) in it (Zhang et al. 2009). Vasodilatory potential of lentinan obtained from *Lentinula edodes* helps in maintaining low blood pressure (Bisen et al. 2010). Various researches from time to time have revealed the antihypertensive potential of the hot water extract of *Tricholoma giganteum*, *Grifola frondosa* Talpur et al. 2002), *Pholiota ostreatus*, *Pleurotus cornucopiae* (Jang et al. 2011), *Pholiota nebrodensis*, and *Pholiota cystidiosus* (Hagiwara et al. 2005); methanolic extract of *Ganoderma lucidum* and *Hypsizygus marmoreus*; and hot water extract of *Hypsizygus marmoreus* (Kang et al. 2013), *Sarcodon aspratus* (Kiyoto et al.

2008), *and Agaricus bisporus* (Lau et al. 2012) through ACE inhibition.

31.3.5 In Neurodegenerative Disease

Mushrooms have proven to be beneficial in the management of neurodegenerative diseases. The role of *Hericium erinaceus* in neuro health is well established through various preclinical and clinical studies (Sabaratnam et al. 2013). Bioactive compounds from Hericenones (A-H) and Erinacines (A-K and P-Q) from *Hericium erinaceus* induce nerve growth factor synthesis (Phan et al. 2015; Sabaratnam et al. 2013). Another bioactive compound dilinoleoyl-phosphatidylethanolamine from the same mushroom exhibits its neuroproactive potential through reducing oxidative stress in endoplasmic reticulum of neuro-2a cells (Nagai et al. 2006).

Termitomycesphins A, B, C, D, G, and H extracted from *Termitomyces albuminosus* along with Termitomycamides B and E from the same mushroom show neuroprotective roles (Qi et al. 2000; Qu et al. 2012). A number of bioactive compounds from *Ganoderma lucidum* help to prolong the lifespan of yeast and exert neuroprotective role via an increase in neurotrophin such as nerve growth factor and brain-derived neurotrophic factor (Weng et al. 2010; Zhang et al. 2011). Dictyophorines A and B, isolated from the mushroom *Dictyophora indusiata*, stimulate NGF-synthesis (Kawagishi et al. 1997). Apart from the abovementioned ones other neuroprotective compounds from *Dictyophora indusiata* are Dictyoquinazols A, B, and C (Lee et al. 2002b).

Some bioactive compounds isolated from *Mycoleptodonoides aitchisonii* have played protective role against endoplasmic reticulum stress-induced cell death (Choi et al. 2009) –neuronal death. Cordycepin from Cordyceps militaris plays a protective role on the impairment of neural growth and development induced by microglia overactivation of hippocampal cultured neurons (Peng et al. 2015). Cordyceps militaris promotes neuritogenesis of neuro2A cell lines *in vitro*, whereas *in vivo* studies revealed its beneficial effect on reversal of scopolamine-induced memory impairment in rats (Lee et al. 2011). Methanolic extracts of *Cordyceps ophioglossoides* mycelium prevent neuronal death and improvement of β-amyloid peptide-induced memory insufficiency in rats (Jin et al. 2004). Uridine from *Pleurotus giganteus* stimulates neurite outgrowth in neuro2A cells (Phan et al. 2015). Oral ingestion of ergothioneine derived from *Pleurotus cornucopiae* is helpful in the promotion of neuronal differentiation and attenuate symptoms of depression in mice (Nakamichi et al. 2016).

31.3.6 Other Medicinal Uses

Data from a clinical trial revealed the effectiveness of *Cordyceps sinensis* on asthma patients (Wang et al. 2016). Mycelial extract and culture filtrate of *Cordyceps sphecocephala* J201 showed anti-asthmatic activities in ovalbumin-induced mice animal model of asthma (Heo et al. 2010). *Ganoderma lucidum* has shown hepatoprotective activity in both *in vitro* and *in vivo* studies (Gao et al. 2002; Zhang et al. 2002b; Wachtel-Galor et al. 2011). Ganopoly, the polysaccharide-containing preparation of *Ganoderma lucidum*, has proven its potential against hepatitis B in phase I/II study (Gao et al. 2002).

Oral administration of proteoglycan isolated from *Phellinus linteus* showed to reduce collagen-induced arthritis in mice whereas their ethanol extract showed an anti-inflammatory effect against croton oil-induced ear edemas test in mice. At the same time, ethanol extract has also exhibited anti-angiogenic and antinociceptive activity (Kim et al. 2003, 2004). Ganoderic acids A, B, G, H and compound C6 isolated from *Ganoderma lucidum* showed an antinociceptive effect in writhing test (Koyama et al. 1997). Methanol extract of *Pleurotus pufmonanus* was able to reduce carrageenan and formalin-induced paw edema (Jose et al. 2002).

Bioassay-guided isolation followed by purification of fatty acid fraction and three compounds, ergosterol, ergostra-4, 6, 8(14), 22-tetraen-3-one (2), and 1-oleoyl-2-linoleoyl-3-palmitoylglycerol from hexane extract of the cultured mycelia of *Grifola frondosa*, was able to inhibit cyclooxygenases 1 and 2 (Zhang et al. 2002a). Acetone and methanol extracts of the mushrooms *Amanita rubescens*, *Cantharellus cibarius*, *Lactarius piperatus*, *Russula cyanoxantha*, *Boletus aestivalis*, *Boletus edulis, and Leccinum carpini* have demonstrated strong antioxidant and antimicrobial activity (Kosanic et al. 2013). Methanolic extracts of *Lycoperdon perlatum*, *Clavaria vermicularis*, *Marasmius oreades*, and *Pleurotus pulmonarius* showed significant antioxidant and antimicrobial efficacy (Ramesh and Manohar 2010).

Researchers have also suggested the antioxidant potential of *Lepista nuda*, *Lentinus edodes*, *Agrocybe cylindracea*, *Cantharellus lutescens*, and *Hydnum repandum* (Murcia et al. 2002). Applanoxidic acid A, isolated from *Ganoderma annulare* (Fr.) Gilbn., showed weak antifungal activity (Smania et al. 2003). Steroids 5a-ergosta7,22-dien-3b-ol or 5,8-epidioxy-5a,8a-ergosta-6,22-dien-3b-ol, isolated from *Ganoderma applanatum* (Pers.) Pat., showed weak antimicrobial activity against certain number of both gram-positive and gram-negative microorganisms (Smania et al. 1999). Oxalic acid from *Lentinula edodes* (Berk.) Pegler showed antimicrobial effect (Bender et al. 2003). Ethanolic mycelial extracts from *L. edodes* possess antiprotozoal activity (Badalyan 2004). Epicorazines A, B, and C isolated from *Podaxis pistillaris* exhibited antibacterial activity against certain bacteria (Al-Fatimi et al. 2006).

Ganodermadiol isolated from *Ganoderma pfeifferi* possessed antiviral activity against influenza virus type A and herpes simplex virus type 1, whereas lucidadiol and applanoxidic acid G isolated from the same mushroom showed antiviral activity against influenza virus type A (Mothana et al. 2003). Mycelia extracts of *Kuehneromyces mutabilis* (Mentel et al. 1994), ethanolic extracts, and two isolated phenolic compounds hispolon and hispidin from *Inonotus hispidus* (Awadh et al. 2003) and ergosterol peroxide present in several mushrooms had demonstrated antiviral activity against influenza viruses type A and B (Lindequist et al. 1989).

Intake of *Tricholoma populinum* was able to reduce symptoms of allergy in a patient with thromboangiitis obliterans and in another patient with urticaria (Kreisel et al. 1990). Hispolon and hispidin isolated from *Inonotus hispidus* inhibited chemiluminescence response of human mononuclear blood cells and suppression of mitogen-induced proliferation of spleen lymphocytes of mice (Ali et al. 1996).

31.4 Conclusion

Mushrooms used as food and also as the sources of medicine around the globe and India are also not left behind. India, because of its diverse habitats and varied ecological condition, houses a wide variety of mushrooms. Many ethnic groups from various parts of India rely on different wild mushrooms that are available locally for their day-to-day needs, that is, as food or for any medicinal use. The scientific validation of the ethno use of the mushrooms has been one of the top priorities of the scientific world, and as a result of which, many bioactive substances have been isolated from them, out of which some are already in the market while some are in the pipeline. Considering all aspects, cultivation and promotion of medicinal mushrooms in India is the need of the hour to make mushrooms as food for medicine. However, more research and development on medicinal mushrooms should be fortified to attain the goal (Tables 31.1 and 31.2).

Table 31.1 Ethno-medicinal use of mushrooms

Sl no.	Name of mushroom species	Claimed ethno uses	References
1	*Volvariella* sp.	Used in rheumatism and lowering high blood pressure	Panda and Tayung (2015)
2	*Astraeus hygrometricus* (Pers.) Morgan	Spore mass is blended with mustard seed oil and used as a salve against burns. Acts as a hemostatic agent	Panda and Tayung (2015); Kumar et al. (2017)
3	*Geastrum* sp.	Used to reduce staunch bleeding and reduce swelling	Panda and Tayung (2015)
4	*Termitomyces reticulates*	Lowering high blood pressure	Panda and Tayung (2015)
5	*Lactarius* sp.	Used to reduce high blood pressure	Panda and Tayung (2015)
6	*Lycoperdon sp.*	Used to cure wound	Panda and Tayung (2015)
7	*Tuber* sp.	Used to cure wound	Panda and Tayung (2015)
8	*Russula sp.*	Used in malnutrition and weakness	Panda and Tayung (2015); Dutta and Acharya (2014)
9	*Daldinia concentrica* (Bolton) Ces. and De Not	Getting relief from burning, itching, and healing minor skin infections	Dutta and Acharya (2014)
10	*Schizophyllum. commune* Fr.	Used as tonic	Dutta and Acharya (2014)
11	*Termitomyces clypeatus* R. Heim	Treatment of pox	Dutta and Acharya (2014)
12	*Cordyceps sinensis* (Berk.) Sacc.	Used as aphrodisiac, invigorative, revitalizer, and antiaging	Dutta and Acharya (2014)
13	*Pisolithus arhizus* (Scop.) Rauschert	Getting relief from burning, itching, and healing minor skin infections	Dutta and Acharya (2014)
14	*Calocybe gambosa*	Used to increase immunity	Vishwakarma et al. (2016)
15	*Calocybe indica*	Used to get relief from stomach pain	Vishwakarma et al. (2016)
16	*Macrolepiota procera*	Used in diabetes and high blood pressure	Vishwakarma et al. (2016)
17	*Tuber aestivum*	Commonly used in healthcare	Vishwakarma et al. (2016)
18	*Agaricus bisporus* (Lange) Imbach	Powder form of this mushroom is mixed with butter and used for the treatment of leucoderma. Used as tonic for patients with CVD. Enhances insulin secretion	Pala et al. (2013), Venkatachalapathi and Paulsamy (2016).
19	*Agaricus campestris* L.: Fr	Fresh fruiting body is crushed and applied to scalds and burns	Pala et al. (2013)
20	*Amanita muscaria* var. *formosa* Pers.	Preparations from dry powder are used for rheumatoid arthritis	Pala et al. (2013)
21	*Auricularia auricula-judae* (Bull.) J. Schröt.	Used to cure cold, sore throats, sore eyes, jaundice, and as an astringent. It is traditionally recommended as food for patients with hypertension, CVD, and diabetes	Pala et al. (2013), Venkatachalapathi and Paulsamy (2016), Kumar et al. (2017)
22	*Bovista plumbea* Pers.	Used for the treatment of frost bite and to heal wounds	Pala et al. (2013)
23	*Coprinopsis atramentaria* (Bull.) Redhead	Its acid formulations are used to cure kidney problems, pus cells in urine, and removal of gall stones	Pala et al. (2013)
24	*Coprinus comatus* (O.F. Mull.: Fr.). Pers.	Consumed as food. Its preparations are recommended for the treatment of respiratory disorders	Pala et al. (2013)
25	*Coprinellus micaceus* (Bull.: Fr.)	Used to treat skin infections and is consumed as food prior the deliquescence of gills	Pala et al. (2013)
26	*Flammulina velutipes* (Curt.) Singer	Recommended for diabetes	Pala et al. (2013)

Table 31.1 (continued)

Sl no.	Name of mushroom species	Claimed ethno uses	References
27	*Fomes fomentarius* (L.) Fr.	Used as a disinfectant for wounds and as an anti-inflammatory agent. Its extract is used to cure arthritis	Pala et al. (2013)
28	*Fomitopsis pinicola* (Sw.: Fr.) P. Karst.	Used to stop bleeding during minor injuries. Extract is used in rheumatoid arthritis	Pala et al. (2013)
29	*Ganoderma applanatum* (Pers.) Pat.	Powder obtained from the dry fruiting body is added to vegetables in very small quantities during cooking with the belief that it reduces the chances of disease	Pala et al. (2013)
30	*Gomphus floccosus* (Schwn.) Singer	Paste obtained from the sporocarp is applied externally for eczema. Its extract also is used for washing the feet in case of athlete's foot	Pala et al. (2013)
31	*Gyromitra sphaerospora* (Peck) Sacc.	Used for the treatment of goiter	Pala et al. (2013)
32	*Helvella lacunose* Afzl.: Fr.	Known to cure piles	Pala et al. (2013)
33	*Helvella macropus* (Pers.) P. Karst.	Used for the treatment of asthma by the tribal people	Pala et al. (2013)
34	*Hericium coralloides* (Scop.) Pers.	Consumed with the belief that it lowers the risk of cancer and heart disease. It also used as food. Recommend for patients with hypertension	Pala et al. (2013)
35	*Humaria hemisphaerica* (Wigg.) Fuckel	Used in combination with mustard oil for the treatment of blisters on skin	Pala et al. (2013)
36	*Inonotus hispidus* (Bull.) P. Karst.	Extract obtained from the fruiting body is used externally as a disinfectant and to cure boils	Pala et al. (2013)
37	*Langarmania gigantia* (Batsch ex Pers.) Rostk.	Used to cure stomach ulcers	Pala et al. (2013)
38	*Lactarius deliciosus* (L.: Fr.) Gray	Its powder is used for the treatment of frostbite	Pala et al. (2013)
39	*Lentinus tigrinus* (Bull.) Fr.	Recommended for diabetic patients by local Hakims	Pala et al. (2013)
40	*Lycoperdon perlatum* Pers.	Locally used to dress wounds for quick healing and by bee keepers to intoxicate the honey bees. Spores are sprinkled on wounds to stop bleeding	Pala et al. (2013)
41	*Lycoperdon pyriforme* Schaeff.	Tribal people use it for treatment of frostbite and sprinkle spores on wounds to stop bleeding. Spore mass used as burn remedy	Pala et al. (2013), Kumar et al. (2017)
42	*Morchella esculenta* Fr.	Paste of the dried fruiting body is blended with a glass of lukewarm milk and given to men with sexual weakness (aphrodisiac)	Pala et al. (2013)
43	*Morchella vulgaris* (Pers.) Boud.	Tribal people also use it for treatment of respiratory problems and as an aphrodisiac	Pala et al. (2013)
44	*Panaeolus sphinctrinus* (Fr.) Quél.	Paste of the sporocarp is blended with a tea in small concentrations and is used as an aesthetic agent	Pala et al. (2013)
45	*Peziza repanda* Pers.	Used against diabetes, constipation, and eczema	Pala et al. (2013)
46	*Phallus impudicus* L.	Gelatinous material inside the egg covering is used for healing wounds and burns	Pala et al. (2013)

(continued)

Table 31.1 (continued)

Sl no.	Name of mushroom species	Claimed ethno uses	References
47	*Pleurotus ostreatus* (Jacq.: Fr.) P. Kumm.	Locally used for the treatment of hypertension, diabetes, jaundice, and asthma. It is also believed to reduce the chances of tumor	Pala et al. (2013), Venkatachalapathi and Paulsamy (2016), Sachan et al. (2013)
48	*Ramaria formosa* (Pers.) Quél.	Recommended for cardiac and diabetic patients by local herbalists	Pala et al. (2013)
49	*Trametes versicolor* (L.) Lloyd	Paste obtained from the sporocarp is used against dermatitis	Pala et al. (2013)
50	*Verpa bohemica* (Krombh.) J. Schrot.	Used for the treatment of urinary disorders	Pala et al. (2013)
51	*Russula delia*	Used in malnutrition, weakness, and nutritional disorder	Sachan et al. (2013)
52	*Termitomyces eurrhizus*	Used to cure rheumatism, diarrhea, hypertension	Sachan et al. (2013)
53	*Agaricus silvaticus*	Used to cure rheumatism, diarrhea, high blood pressure	Sachan et al. (2013)
54	*Lentinus sajor-caju*	Used in high fever	Sachan et al. (2013)
56	*Ophiocordyceps sinensis*	Increase longevity and as female aphrodisiac. Treatment of erectile dysfunction, infertility, general weakness, tuberculosis, bronchitis, malignant tumor, cough and cold, rheumatism, arthritis, jaundice, prostate enlargement, liver and kidney diseases, coronary heart disease, chronic pain, sciatica and backache, hypertension, dizziness, diabetics, and alcoholic hepatitis	Gupta and Karkala (2017), Panda and Swainl (2011)
57	*Agaricus augustus* Fr.	Used to cure high cholesterol, problem in the arteries, and ulcer	Venkatachalapathi and Paulsamy (2016)
58	*Agaricus campestris* L.	Diabetes and ulcer	Venkatachalapathi and Paulsamy (2016)
59	*Agaricus heterocystis* Heinem.	Used as antitumor. To cure cholesterol and kidney problem	Venkatachalapathi and Paulsamy (2016)
60	*Bovista nigrescens* Pers.	Used in the treatment of broken skin or wound and to stop bleeding	Venkatachalapathi and Paulsamy (2016)
61	*Calocybe indica* Kuhner ex Donk.	Used in the management of diabetes	Venkatachalapathi and Paulsamy (2016)
62	*Clavulina rugosa* (Fr.) Schroet.	Used to cure skin diseases	Venkatachalapathi and Paulsamy (2016)
63	*Clitocybe nuda* (Bull.) H.E.	Used to cure cardiovascular problem	Venkatachalapathi and Paulsamy (2016)
64	*Coprinus sp.*	Used to cure diabetes, circulatory disease, digestive disorders, piles	Venkatachalapathi and Paulsamy (2016)
65	*Daedaleopsis confragosa* (Bolton) J.	Used to cure skin diseases	Venkatachalapathi and Paulsamy (2016)
66	*Ganoderma lucidum* (Curtis) P.	Improves immune system, protects the liver, lowers blood pressure, and inhibits cholesterol synthesis	Venkatachalapathi and Paulsamy (2016)
67	*Hygrocybe psittacina* (Schaeff.) P.	Used to cure skin diseases	Venkatachalapathi and Paulsamy (2016)

Table 31.1 (continued)

Sl no.	Name of mushroom species	Claimed ethno uses	References
68	*Lentinus sajor–caju* (Fries) Fries.	Used to decrease lower cholesterol and as anticancer agent	Venkatachalapathi and Paulsamy (2016)
69	*Lentinus squarrosulus* Mont.	As antiulcer	Venkatachalapathi and Paulsamy (2016)
70	*Pleurotus tuber-regium* (Rumph. Ex Fr.)	Used to cure cough, indigestion, and dysentery	Venkatachalapathi and Paulsamy (2016)
71	*Lycoperdon echinatum* Pers.	Used to cure wound healing	Venkatachalapathi and Paulsamy (2016)
72	*Marasmius androsaceus* (L.) Fr.	In blood purification, nerve problems, rheumatism, and as anti-inflammatory agent	Venkatachalapathi and Paulsamy (2016)
73	*Melanoleuca grammopodia* Bull.	Used to cure skin diseases	Venkatachalapathi and Paulsamy (2016)
74	*Mycena galericulata* (Scop.) Gray	Used to cure skin diseases	Venkatachalapathi and Paulsamy (2016)
75	*Pisolithus arhizus* (Scop.) Rauschert.	Used to cure skin diseases and heal wound	Venkatachalapathi and Paulsamy (2016)
76	*Pleurotus sajor-caju* (Fr.) Singer	Used to reduce cholesterol	Venkatachalapathi and Paulsamy (2016)
77	*Pleurotus sapidus* Schulzer and Kalchbr.	Used to cure skin diseases and to heal wound	Venkatachalapathi and Paulsamy (2016)
78	*Russula delica* (Pers.) Fr.	Used to cure skin diseases and to heal wound	Venkatachalapathi and Paulsamy (2016)
79	*Scleroderma citrinum* Pers.	Used to cure skin diseases and to heal wound	Venkatachalapathi and Paulsamy (2016)
80	*Termitomyces heimii*	Wound healing	Venkatachalapathi and Paulsamy (2016)
81	*Termitomyces microcarpus* (Berk. and Broome) R.	Skin diseases and wound healing	Venkatachalapathi and Paulsamy (2016)
82	*Trametes versicolor* (L.) Lloyd.	Increase immune system and depression	Venkatachalapathi and Paulsamy (2016)
83	*Volvariella speciosa* (Fr.) Singer.	Antitumor	Venkatachalapathi and Paulsamy (2016)
84	*Ganoderma lucidum* (Curtis) P. Karst.	Used for enhancing milk secretion	Kumar et al. (2017)
85	*Geastrum triplex*	Spore mass used as burn remedy	Kumar et al. (2017)
86	*Lycoperdon perlatum* Pers.	Spore mass used as burn remedy	Kumar et al. (2017)
87	*Phallus sp.*	As aphrodisiac	Kumar et al. (2017)
88	*Stereum* sp.	As burn remedy	Kumar et al. (2017)
89	*Truffle*	As mouth freshener	Kumar et al. (2017)

Table 31.2 Medicinal significance mushrooms—reported activity and/or as a source of therapeutic agent

Sl no.	Name of the mushroom	Medicinal uses	References
1	*Penicillium notatum*	Antibacterial	Fleming (1929)
2	*Cephalosporium acremonium (Acremonium chrysogenum)*	Antibacterial	Newton and Abraham (1955), Demain et al. (1988)
3	*Penicillium griseofulvum*	Antifungal	Desai (1960), Oxford et al. (1939)
4	*Fuszdzum coccneui*	Antibiotic	Godtfredsen et al. (1962).
5	*Penicillium citrinum*	Antilipidemic, inhibits melanoma cell growth and proliferation	Endo et al. (1976), Hanjani et al. (2001)
6	*Aspergillus niger*	Hypocholesterolemic	Javed et al. (2014)
		Inhibit pancreatic cancer cell proliferation	Muller et al. (1998)
7	*Zalerion arboricola*	Antifungal	Robert et al. (1992)
8	*Pleurotus tuber-regium*	Hepatoprotective, anti-breast cancer	Dandapat et al. (2015), Zhang et al. (2006)
		Antihyperglycemic	Huang et al. (2012)
9	*Ganoderma lucidum*	Hypoglycemic, immunomodulating, antitumor, antioxidative, anti-decrepitude	Miyazaki and Nishijima (1981), Zhu et al. (2007), Wachtel-Galor et al. (2011)
		Antiviral	El-Mekkawy et al. (1998)
		Anti-allergic	Tasaka et al. (1988)
		Anti-inflammatory	Koyama et al. (1997)
		Inhibits the biosynthesis of cholesterol	Komoda et al. (1989), Wachtel-Galor et al. (2011)
		Reduces obesity	Chang et al. (2015)
		Antitumor activity	Yoshiaki et al. (1985).
10	*Auricularia auricula*	Reduces LDL cholesterol and serum total cholesterol	Cheung (1996)
11	*Schizophyllum commune*	Immunomodulatory, antitumor	Ooi and Liu (2000)
12	*Hericium erinaceus*	Amelioration of expression of TNF-α, IL-1β, IL-12, and other cytokinin	Diling et al. (2017)
		Advantageous effect in treatment of Alzheimer's disease	Mori et al. (2009)
		Neuroprotective activities	Kuo et al. (2016)
13	*Lentinus edodes*	Reduce plasma cholesterol and phospholipids, modification of hepatic phospholipid metabolism, anti-atherosclerotic (as nutritional supplement), hyperhomocysteinemic effect, antihypertensive, hypoglycemic	Byung et al. (2002), Chibata et al. (1969), Kabir et al. (1987), Kaneda and Tokuda (1966), Yamada et al. (2002), Yang et al. (2013)
		Induces nonspecific cytotoxicity in macrophage, enhances cytokine production, and	Bisen et al. (2010)
		antitumor	Chihara (1969), Chihara et al. (1970b)
14	*Coriolus versicolor*	Immunomodulating, antitumor, anti-radiative, antihyperglycemic, and anti-inflammatory	Cui and Chisti (2003)
15	*Grifola frondosa*	Macrophage activation, induction of IL-1, IL-6, TNF-α secretion	Yang et al. (2007)
		Hypocholesterolemic, antitumor, Hypoglycemic, anticancer	Fukushima et al. (2001), Cun et al. (1994), Horio and Ohtsuru (2001), Konno et al. (2002)
		Anti-inflammatory activity	Zhang et al. (2002a)
		Antihypertension	Preuss et al. (2010)

Table 31.2 (continued)

Sl no.	Name of the mushroom	Medicinal uses	References
16	*Inonotus obliquus*	Antitumor	Lee et al. (2009)
		Immunomodulating	Kim (2005)
		Enhances expression of IL-1β, IL- 6, TNF-α, iNOS in macrophages	Won et al. (2011)
		Anti-inflammation Hypoglycemic	Young-Mi et al. (2005), Ho-Gyoung et al. (2007), Lu et al. (2010)
17	*Agaricus blazei*	Antitumor	Mizuno (1999)
		Induction of TNF, IFN-γ, and IL-8 production	Sorimachi et al. (2001)
		Reduction of atherosclerotic lesions	Sijun et al. (2011)
18	*Flammulina velutipes*	Antitumor, anti-inflammatory, antiviral, immunomodulatory effect. Increases NO, IL-1 production, and TNF-α secretion	Leung et al. (1997), Wu et al. (2010b), Yin et al. (2010)
		Hypocholesterolemic, anti-allergic	Fukushima et al. (2001), Sano et al. (2002)
19	*Ganoderma applanatum*	Antitumor, immunomodulation Enhances TNF-α, IL-1β, and NO production	Jeong et al. (2008a), Ren et al. (2012), Zhang et al. (2007), Gao et al. (2004)
20	*Polyporus umbellatus*	Antitumor	Zhao et al. (2010)
21	*Clitopilus caespitosus*	Antitumor	Zhang et al. (2007)
22	*Pleurotus citrinopileatus*	Immunomodulating, antihyperglycemic, antihyperlipidemic, hepatoprotective, anticancer	Hu et al. (2006a, b), Zhang et al. (2007)
23	*Trametes robiniophila*	Antitumor, anticancer, immunomodulatory effect	Jia et al. (2009)
24	*Tremella fuciformis*	Immunomodulating, hyperglycemia	Friedman (2016), Han et al. (2015)
25	*Tremella aurantialba*	Enhances mouse spleen lymphocyte proliferation	Du et al. (2010)
		Antitumor, hyperglycemia, antioxidant, immunomodulatory	Zhang et al. (2004), Deng et al. (2016), Du et al. (2011)
26	*Pleurotus ostreatus*	Hyperglycemia, antitumor	Patel and Goyal (2012), Friedman (2016)
		Macrophage activation, activates NF-kB	Kong et al. (2014)
27	*Morchella esculenta*	Anti-inflammatory, immunomodulating	Cui et al. (2011), Ajmal et al. (2015)
28	*Omphalia lapidescens*	Antitumor	Ohno et al. (1992)
29	*Phellinus linteus*	Murine B-cell activation, induces IL-12, IFN-γ production. Blocks NF-kB, TNF-α, IL-1α, IL-1β, and IL-4 production. Antidiabetic and anticancer effect	Wu et al. (2013), Kim et al. (2004), Wang et al. (2012), Ho et al. (2007)
30	*Armillaria tabescens*	Anti-inflammation, antigastric	Lee et al. (2018)
		Antitumor	Kiho et al. (1992)
31	*Dictyophora Indusiata*	Antitumor	Hara et al. (1991)
32	*Peziza vesiculosa*	Immunomodulatory antitumor	Mimura et al. (1985), Suzuki et al. (1982)
33	*Tricholoma mongolium*	Increase in IL-5 induction with decrease in IL-4 and IL-17	Wang et al. (1996)
34	*Cordyceps sinensis*	Anti-inflammation	Zhenquan et al. (2010)
35	*Agaricus bisporus*	Reduces LDL cholesterol, serum total cholesterol. Increases hepatic LDL receptor mRNA. Reduces serum adipocytokine/fat deposition/triglycerides in the liver	Fukushima et al. (2000), Neyrinck et al. (2009)
		Hypoglycemic	Ahmad et al. (1984)
		Antibacterial property	Tambekar et al. (2006)

(continued)

Table 31.2 (continued)

Sl no.	Name of the mushroom	Medicinal uses	References
36	*Pleurotus cornucopiae*	Reduced adhesion of monocytes	Keith (2010)
		Antihypertensive	Hagiwara et al. (2005)
		Anti-inflammatory and antitumor	Wang et al. (2013)
		Hepatoprotective	Ei et al. (2009)
37	*Pleurotus florida*	Antitumor, antidiabetic	Nayana and Janadharan (2000), Friedman (2016)
		Immunoenhancing	Roy et al. (2009)
38	*Pleurotus ostreatus*	Cholesterol lowering effect, immunomodulatory, hepatoprotective	Bobek et al. (1991, 1993), Refale et al. (2009), Lakshmi et al. (2004)
39	*Antrodia camphorata*	Anti-hepatitis, anticancer	Lee et al. (2002a), Hsu et al. (2005)
		Immunomodulatory Anti-inflammatory	Shen et al. (2003, 2004)
40	*Cryptoporus volvatus*	Inhibits influenza virus replication Anticancer	Gao et al. (2014), Narisawa et al. (1992)
41	*Morchella conica*	Increases the release of TNF-α and NO in macrophage	Pfab et al. (2008)
42	*Polystictus versicolor*	Antiviral and immunopotentiating activity	Chen et al. (1986)
43	*Sarcodon aspratus*	Stimulates proliferation of lymphocyte, increases TNF-α release	Mizuno et al. (2000)
44	*Sclerotinia sclerotiorum*	Effect of Peyer's patch cell	Hashimoto et al. (1991)
45	*Sparassis crispa*	Antitumor Hypoglycemic	Ren et al. (2012), Friedman (2016)
46	*Xylaria nigripes*	Immunomodulatory	Ko et al. (2011)
47	*Agrocybe cylindracea* (DC.) Maire	Hypoglycemic	Kiho et al. (1994)
48	*Agrocybe aegerita*	Hypocholesterolemic	Ng (2005)
49	*Agaricus campestris*	Hyperglycemic	Gray and Flatt (1998).
45	*Boletus edulis*	Antitumor	Ren et al. (2012)
46	*Calvatia gigantea*	Antitumor	Lucas et al. (1958)
47	*Collybia maculata*	Antiviral	Leonhardt et al. (1987)
48	*Ganoderma pfeifferi*	Antimicrobial	Mothana et al. (2003)
49	*Ganoderma annulare*	Antifungal	Smania et al. (2003)
50	*Ganoderma applanatum*	Anti-allergic, antibacterial	Smania et al. (1999), Sano et al. (2002)
51	*Hypsizygus marmoreus*	Antifungal, antiplatelet activity	Suzuki et al. (2011), Park et al. (2011)
52	*Hericium coralloides*	Antinociceptive, antiviral activity	Saito et al. (1998).
53	*Inonotus hispidus*	Anti-allergic, antiviral activity	Ali et al. (1996), Awadh et al. (2003)
54	*Kuehneromyces mutabilis*	Antiviral	Mentel et al. (1994)
55	*Lentinula edodes*	Antitumor, immunomodulation, antiviral, antibacterial, antifungal, hypolipidemic, hepatoprotective	Chihara et al. (1969), Patel and Goyal (2012), Yap and Ng (2005), Bisen et al. (2010)
56	*Fomitopsis officinalis*	Anti-TB activity	Hwang et al. (2013)
57	*Agaricus brasiliensis*	Anti-ischemia/reperfusion	Song et al. (2010)
58	*Agaricus sylvaticus*	Hypocholesterolemic	Percario et al. (2008)
		Antidiabetic	Mascaro et al. (2014)
		Immunomodulatory	Fortes et al. (2009)
59	*Cordyceps militaris*	Anti-inflammatory	So and Eun (2005)

Table 31.2 (continued)

Sl no.	Name of the mushroom	Medicinal uses	References
61	*Pholiota nameko*	Hypolipidemic	Li et al. (2010)
62	*Pleurotus nebrodensis*	Antihypertensive, antitumoral, anti-HIV-1, immunostimulating activity	Miyazawa et al. (2008), Lv et al. (2009), Cui et al. (2015)
63	*Polyporus confluens*	Cardioprotective	Yan et al. (2015)
64	*Tricholoma giganteum*	Hypocholesterolemic	Sugiyama et al. (1992)
65	*Pleurotus pulmonarius*	Antihypertension, anti-inflammatory, anti-cholinesterase	Dae et al. (2004), Nguyen et al. (2016)
66	*Pleurotus cystidiosus*	Antifungal	Menikpurage et al. (2009)
67	*Pleurotus djamor*	Antiproliferative activity	Wu et al. (2010a)
68	*Pleurotus sajor-caju*	Antineoplasic, anti-inflammatory	Dalonso et al. (2010), Silveira et al. (2014)
69	*Pleurotus eous*	Antibacterial Antitumor	Suseem and Saral (2013)
70	*Pleurotus eryngii*	Antibacterial activity	Li and Shah (2014)
71	*Pleurotus abalonus*	Antitumor	Ren et al. (2015)
72	*Inonotus obliquus*	Antibacterial and antiproliferative	Nagajyothi et al. (2014)
73	*Volvariella volvacea*	Antibacterial	Ayodele and Idoko (2011)
74	*Cheimonophyllum candissimum*	Antibacterial	Stadler and Anke (1994).
75	*Clitocybe cyathiformis*	Antimicrobial	Arnone et al. (1993)
76	*Clitocybe diatreta*	Antifungal	Arnone et al. (1996)
77	*Crepidotus fulvotomentosus*	Antibacterial and antifungal	Weber et al. (1989)
78	*Flagelloscypha pilatii*	Antifungal	Heim et al. (1988)
79	*Oudemansiella radicata*	Antifungal	Anke et al. (1990)

References

Abugri D, McElhenney WH, Willian KR. Fatty acid profiling in selected cultivated edible and wild medicinal mushrooms in the Southern United States. J Exp Food Chem. 2016;2:1–7.

Adhikari MK. Chyau: Ayurvediya vishleshan ek vivechana (Mushrooms: an Ayurvedic concepts). J Nep Pharm Assoc. 1981;9:17–21.

Ahmad N, Bansal AK, Kidwai JR. Effect of PHA-B fraction of *Agaricus bisporus* lectin on insulin release and 45Ca2C uptake by islet of Langerhans *in vitro*. Acta Diabetol. 1984;21:63–70.

Aida FMNA, Shuhaimi M, Yazid M, Maaruf AG. Mushroomas a potential source of prebiotics: a review. Trends Food Sci Technol. 2009;20(11–12):567–75.

Ajmal M, Akram A, Ara A, Akhund S, Nayyar BG. *Morchella Esculenta*: an edible and health beneficial mushroom. Pak J Food Sci. 2015;25(2):71–8.

Al-Fatimi MAA, Jülich WD, Jansen R, Lindequist U. Bioactive components of the traditionally used mushroom *Podaxis pistillaris*. Evid Based Complement Alternat Med. 2006;3(1):87–92.

Ali NAA, Pilgrim H, Ludke J, Lindequist U. Inhibition of chemiluminescence response of human mononuclear cells and suppression of mitogeninduced proliferation of spleen lymphocytes of mice by hispolon and hispidin. Pharmazie. 1996;51:667–70.

Aly AH, Debbab A, Proksch P. Fifty years of drug discovery from fungi review. Fungal Divers. 2011;50:3–19.

Anke T, Werle A, Bross M, Steglich W. XXXXIII Oudemansin X, a new antifungal *e*-β-methoxyacrylate from *Oudemansiella radicata* (Relhan ex Fr.) Sing. J Antibiot. 1990;43(8):1010–1.

Arnone A, Cardillo R, Nasini G, Pava OVD. Cyathiformines A-D, new chorismate derived metabolites from fungus *Clitocybe cyathiformis*. Tetrahedron. 1993;49:7251–8.

Arnone A, Capelli S, Nasini G, Meille SV, Pava OVD. Secondary mould metabolites II structure elucidation of diatretol- A new Diketopiperazine metabolite from the fungus *Clitocybe diatreata*. Liebigs Ann. 1996;11:1875–7.

Awadh AAN, Mothana RAA, Lesnau A, Pilgrim H, Lindequist U. Antiviral activity of extracts and compounds from *Inonotus hispidus*. Fitotherapia. 2003;74(5):483–5.

Ayodele SM, Idoko ME. Antimicrobial activities of four wild edible mushrooms in Nigeria. Int J Sci Nat. 2011;2(1):55–8.

Badalyan SM. Antiprotozoal activity and mitogenic effect of mycelium of culinary-medicinal shiitake mushroom

Lentinus edodes (Berk.) Singer (Agaricomycetidae). Int J Med Mushrooms. 2004;6:131–8.

Badole SL, Patel NM, Thakurdesai PA, Bodhankar SL. Interaction of aqueous extract of *Pleurotus pulmonarius* (Fr.) Quel-Champ with glyburide in alloxan induced diabetic mice. Evid Based Complement Alternat Med. 2008;5(2):159–64.

Bahl N. Medicinal value of edible fungi. In: Proceeding of the International Conference on Science and Cultivation Technology of Edible Fungi. Indian Mushroom Science II. 1983. pp. 203–9.

Bender S, Dumitrache CN, Backhaus J, Christie G, Cross RF, Lonergan GT. A case for caution in assessing the antibiotic activity of extracts of culinary-medicinal Shiitake mushroom [*Lentinus edodes* (Berk.) Singer] (Agaricomycetidae). Int J Med Mushrooms. 2003;5:31–5.

Bisen PS, Baghel RK, Sanodiya BS, Thakur GS, Prasad GB. *Lentinus edodes*: a macrofungus with pharmacological activities. Curr Med Chem. 2010;17(22):2419–30.

Bobek P, Ginter E, Jurcovicova M, Ozdin D, Mekinova D. Cholesterol lowering effect of the mushroom *Pleurotus ostreatus* in hereditary hypercholesterolemic rats. Ann Nutr Metab. 1991;35:191–5.

Bobek P, Kuniak L, Ozdin L. The mushroom *Pleurotus ostreatus* reduces secretion and accelerates the fractional turnover rate of very low density lipoproteins in the rat. Ann Nutr Metabol. 1993;37(3):142–5.

Byung KY, Dong HK, Sang CJ, Surajit D, Young SC, Joon SS, Sang CL, Chi HS. Hypoglycemic effect of a *Lentinus edodes* exopolymer produced from a submerged mycelia culture. Biosci Biotechnol Biochem. 2002;66:937–42.

Caz V, Gil-Ramírez A, Largo C, Tabernero M, Santamaría M, Martín-Hernández R, et al. Modulation of cholesterol-related gene expression by dietary fiber fractions from edible mushrooms. J Agric Food Chem. 2015;63(33):7371–80.

Chang ST. Development of culinary medicinal mushrooms industry in China: past, present and future. Int J Med Mushrooms. 2006;8:1–17.

Chang CJ, Lin CS, Lu CC, Martel J, et al. *Ganoderma lucidum* reduces obesity in mice by modulating the composition of the gut microbiota. Nat Commun. 2015;6:7489.

Chen H, Li Z, Jiang J, Li G, Xue Y, Zhen Y. The antiviral and immunopotentiating activities of polysaccharide from *Polystictus versicolor* (L.) Fr. In mice. Kangshengsu. 1986;11(5):390–5.

Cheung PCK. The hypocholesterolemic effect of two edible mushrooms: Auricularia auricula (tree-ear) and Tremella fuciformis (white jelly-leaf) in hypercholesterolemic rats. Nutr Res. 1996; 16:1721–5.

Chibata I, Okumura K, Takeyama S, Kotera K. Lentinacin: a new hypocholesterolemic substance in *Lentinus edodes*. Experientia. 1969;25:1237–8.

Chihara G, Maeda Y, Hamuro J, Sasaki T, Fukuoka F. Inhibition of mouse sarcoma 180 by polysaccharides from *Lentinus edodes* (Berk.) Sing. Nature. 1969;222:687–8.

Chihara G, Hamuro J, Maeda Y, Arai Y, Fukuoka F. Antitumor polysaccharide derived chemically from natural glucan (pachyman). Nature. 1970a;225:943–4.

Chihara G, Hamuro J, Maeda YY, Arai Y, Fukuoka F. Fractionation and purification of the polysaccharides with marked antitumor activity, especially lentinan, from Lentinus edodes. Cancer Res. 1970b;30:2776–81.

Choi JH, Horikawa M, Okumura H, Kodani S, Nagai K, Hashizume D, Koshino H, Kawagish H. Endoplasmic reticulum (ER) stress protecting compounds from the mushroom *Mycoleptodonoides aitchisonii*. Tetrahedron. 2009;65(1):221–4.

Cui J, Chisti Y. Polysaccharopeptides of *Coriolus versicolor*: physiological activity, uses, and production. Biotechnol Adv. 2003;21:109–22.

Cui HL, Chen Y, Wang SS, Kai GQ, Fang YM. Isolation, partial characterization and immunomodulatory activities of polysaccharide from *Morchella esculenta*. J Sci Food Agric. 2011;91:2180–5.

Cui HY, Wang CL, Wang YR, Li ZJ, Zhang YN. The polysaccharide isolated from *Pleurotus nebrodensis* (PN-S) shows immune-stimulating activity in RAW264.7 macrophages. Chin J Nat Med. 2015;13:355–60.

Cun Z, Mizuno T, Ito H, Shimura K, Sumiya T, Kawade M. Antitumor activity and immunological property of polysaccharides from the mycelium of liquid-cultured *Grifola frondosa*. J Jpn Soc Food Sci Technol. 1994;41:724–33.

Dae HL, Jae HK, Jeong SP, Young JC, Jong SL. Isolation and characterization of a novel angiotensin I-converting enzyme inhibitory peptide derived from the edible mushroom *Tricholoma giganteum*. Peptides. 2004;25:621–7.

Dalonso N, Souza R, Silveira ML, Ruzza AA, Wagner TM, Wisbeck E, Furlan SA. Characterization and antineoplasic effect of extracts obtained from *Pleurotus sajor-caju* fruiting bodies. Appl Biochem Biotechnol. 2010;160:2265–74.

Dandapat S, Sinha MP, Kumar M, Jaggi Y. Hepatoprotective efficacy of medicinal mushroom *Pleurotus tuber-regium*. Envir Exp Biol. 2015;13:103–8.

Demain AL, Zhang J, Cephalosporin C. Production by *Cephalosporium acremonium*: the methionine story. Critical Rev Biotechnol. 1988;18(4):283–94.

de Miranda AM, Rossoni Júnior JV, Souza E, Silva L, Dos Santos RC, Silva ME, Pedrosa ML. *Agaricus brasiliensis* (sun mushroom) affects the expression of genes related to cholesterol homeostasis. Eur J Nutr. 2017;56(4):1707–17.

Deng C, Sun Y, Fu H, Zhang S, Chen J, Xu X. Antioxidant and immunomodulatory activities of polysaccharides extracted from *Tremella aurantialba* mycelia. Mol Med Rep. 2016;14(5):4857–64.

Desai SC. Effect of griseofulvin on *Trichophyton rubrum* and *T. violaceum* infections. Arch Dermatol. 1960;81:849.

Diling C, Xin Y, Chaoqun Z, Jian Y, Xiaocui T, Jun C, et al. Extracts from *Hericium erinaceus* relieve inflammatory bowel disease by regulating immunity and gut microbiota. Oncotarget. 2017;8(49):85838–57.

Du XJ, Zhang JS, Yang Y, Tang Q, Pan YJ. Purification, chemical modification and immunostimulating activity of polysaccharides from *Tremella aurantialba* fruit bodies. J Zhejiang Univ Sci B. 2010;1:437–42.

Du XJ, Zhang JS, Jia W. Antitumor and immunomodulating activities of the extracts from *Tremella aurantialba* fruiting bodies in vitro. Nat Prod Res Dev. 2011;23(2):351–5.

Dutta AK, Acharya K. Traditional and ethno-medicinal knowledge of mushrooms in West Bengal, India. Asian J Pharm Clin Res. 2014;7(4):36–41.

Ei BK, Hasimoto Y, Muzandu K, Ikenaka Y, Ibrahim ZS, Kazusaka A, Fuzita S, ishizuka M. Protective effect of *Pleurotus cornupiae* mushroom extract on carbo tetrachloride induced hepatotoxicity. Jpn J Vet Res. 2009;57(2):109–18.

El-Mekkawy S, Meselhy MR, Nakamura N, Tezuka Y, Hattori M, Kakiuchi N. Anti-HIV-1 and anti- HIV-1-protease substances from *Ganoderma lucidum*. Phytochemistry. 1998;49:1651–7.

Endo A, Kuroda M, Tsujita Y. ML-236A, ML-236B, and ML-236C, new inhibitors of cholesterogenesis produced by *Penicillium citrinum*. J Antibiot. 1976;2(12):1346–8.

Ferreira ICFR, Barros L, Abreu RMV. Antioxidants in wild mushrooms. Curr Med Chem. 2009;16(12):1543–60.

Fleming A. Classics in infectious diseases: on the antibacterial action of cultures of a Penicillium, with special reference to their use in the isolation of B. influenza. Br J Exp Pathol. 1929;10(3):226–36.

Fortes RC, Novaes MRCG, Recova VL, Melo AL. Immunological, hematological and glycemia effects of dietary supplementation with *Agaricus sylvaticus* on patients' colorectal cancer. Exp Biol Med. 2009;234:53–62.

Friedman M. Mushroom polysaccharides: chemistry and antiobesity, antidiabetes, anticancer, and antibiotic properties in cells, rodents, and humans. Foods. 2016;5(4):80.

Fukushima M, Nakano M, Morii Y, Ohashi T, Fujiwara Y, Sonoyama K. Hepatic LDL receptor mRNA in rats is increased by dietary mushroom (*Agaricus bisporus*) fiber and sugar beet fiber. J Nutr. 2000;130:2151–6.

Fukushima M, Ohashi T, Fujiwara Y, Sonoyama K, Nakano M. Cholesterol-lowering effects of maitake (*Grifola frondosa*) fiber, shiitake (*Lentinus edodes*) fiber, and enokitake (*Flammulina velutipes*) fiber in rats. Exp Biol Med. 2001;226:758–65.

Ganeshpurkar A, Rai G, Jain AP. Medicinal mushrooms: towards a new horizon. Pharmacog Rev. 2010;4(8):127–35.

Gao Y, Zhou S, Chen G, Dai X, Ye J, Gao H. A phase I/II study of a *Ganoderma lucidum* (Curt.:Fr.) P.Karst. (Ling Zhi, Reishi mushroom) extract in patients with chronic hepatitis B. Int J Med Mushrooms. 2002;4(4):2321–7.

Gao Y, Chan E, Zhou S. Immunomodulating activities of Ganoderma, a mushroom with medicinal properties. Food Rev Int. 2004;20:123–61.

Gao L, Sun Y, Si J, Liu J, Sun G, Sun X, Cao L. *Cryptoporus volvatus* extract inhibits influenza virus replication *in vitro* and *in vivo*. PLoS One. 2014;9(12):e113604.

Gaze R. The larger world of global mushrooms. Mushroom J. 2005;670:11–3.

Gil-Ramírez A, Ruiz-Rodríguez A, Marín FR, Reglero G, Soler-Rivas C. Effect of ergosterol-enriched extracts obtained from *Agaricus bisporus* on cholesterol absorption using an in vitro digestion model. J Funct Foods. 2014;11:589–97.

Gil-Ramírez A, Caz V, Smiderle FR, Martin-Hernandez R, Largo C, Tabernero M, Marín FR, Iacomini M, Reglero G, Soler-Rivas C. Water-soluble compounds from *Lentinula edodes* influencing the HMG-CoA reductase activity and the expression of genes involved in the cholesterol metabolism. J Agric Food Chem. 2016;6(9):1910–20.

Godtfredsen WO, Jahnsen S, Lorck H, Roholt K, Tybring L. Fusidic acid: a new antibiotic. Nature. 1962;193:987.

Gray AM, Flatt PR. Insulin-releasing and insulinlike activity of *Agaricus campestris* (mushroom). J Endocrinol. 1998;157:259–66.

Gunde-Cimmerman N. Medicinal value of the genus *Pleurotus* (fr). P Karst (Agaricales s.l. Basidiomycetes). Int J Med Mushrooms. 1999;1:69–80.

Gupta G, Karkala M. Yarsagumba: a miracle mushroom its history, cultivation, phytopharmacology and medicinal uses. Int J Herb Med. 2017;5(2):69–72.

Hagiwara S, Takahashi M, Shen Y, Kaihou S, Tomiyama T, Yazawa M, et al. A phytochemical in the edible tamogitake mushroom (*Pleurotus cornucopiae*), D-Mannitol, inhibits ACE activity and lowers the blood pressure of spontaneously hypertensive rats. Biosci Biotechnol Biochem. 2005;69(8):1603–5.

Halliwell B, Gutteridge JMC. Free radicals in biology and medicine. Oxford: Oxford University Press; 1997.

Han CK, Chiang HC, Lin CY, Tang CH, Lee H, Huang DD, et al. Comparison of immunomodulatory and anticancer activities in different strains of *Tremella fuciformis* Berk. Am J Chin Med. 2015;43(8):1637–55.

Handayani D, Chen J, Meyer BJ, Huang XF. Dietary Shiitake mushroom (*Lentinus edodes*) prevents fat deposition and lowers triglyceride in rats fed a high-fat diet. J Obes. 2011;2011:258051. https://doi.org/10.1155/2011/258051.

Hanjani AS, Stagliano NE, Yamada M, Huang PL, Liao JK, Moskowitz MA. Mevastatin, an HMG-CoA reductase inhibitor, reduces stroke damage and upregulates endothelial nitric oxide synthase in mice. Stroke. 2001;32(4):980–6.

Hara C, Kumazawa Y, Inagaki K, Kaneko M, Kiho T, Ukai S. Mitogenic and colony-stimulating factor-inducing activities of polysaccharide fractions from the fruit bodies of *Dictyophora indusiata* Fisch. Chem Pharml Bull. 1991;39:1615–6.

Harsh NSK, Rai BK, Tiwari DP. Use of Ganoderma lucidum in folk medicine. J Trop Biodivers. 1993;1:324–6.

Hashimoto K, Suzuki I, yadomae T. Oral administration of SSG,a beta glucan obtained from *Sclerotinia sclerotiorum* affects the function of Peyer's patch cells. Int J Immnopharmacol. 1991;176:5513–8.

Hawksworth DL. Mushrooms: the extent of the unexplored potential. Int J Med Mushrooms. 2001;3:333–7.

Heim J, Anke T, Mocek U, Steffan B, Steglich W. Antibiotics from basidiomycetes. XXIX: Pilatin, a new antibiotically active marasmane derivative from cultures of *Flagelloscypha pilatii* agerer, J Antibiot (Tokyo) 1988; 41(12):1752-1757.

Heo JC, Nam SH, Nam DY, Kim JG, Lee KG, Yeo JH, Yoon CS, Park CH, Lee SH. Anti-asthmatic activities in mycelial extract and culture filtrate of *Cordyceps sphecocephala* J201. Int J Mol Med. 2010;26(3):351–6.

Ho GK, Deok HY, Won HL, Sang KH, Bhushan S, Chun HK, et al. *Phellinus linteus* inhibits inflammatory mediators by suppressing redox-based NF- B and MAPKs activation in lipopolysaccharide-induced RAW 264.7 macrophage. J Ethnopharmacol. 2007;114:307–15.

Hobbs C. Medicinal mushrooms. An exploration of tradition, healing and culture. Santa Cruz: Botanica Press; 1995.

Ho-Gyoung K, Deok HY, Chun HK, Bhushan S, Woo-chul C, So-yeon L, et al. Ethanol extract of *Inonotus obliquus* inhibits lipopolysaccharide-induced inflammation in RAW 264.7 macrophage cells. J Med Food. 2007;10:80–9.

Horio H, Ohtsuru M. Maitake (*Grifola frondosa*) improve glucose tolerance of experimental diabetic rats. J Nutr Sci Vitaminol. 2001;47:57–63.

Hsu YL, Kuo YC, Pl K, Ng LT, Kuo YH, Lin CC. Apoptotic effects of extract from *Antrodia camphorata* fruiting bodies in human hepatocellular carcinoma cell lines. Cancer Lett. 2005;221(1):77–89.

Hu SH, Wang JC, Lien JL, Liaw ET, Lee MY. Antihyperglycemic effect of polysaccharide from fermented broth of *Pleurotus citrinopileatus*. Appl Microbiol Biotechnol. 2006a;70(1):107–3.

Hu SH, Liang ZC, Chia YC, Lien JL, Chen KS, et al. Antihyperlipidemic and antioxidant effects of extracts from *Pleurotus citrinopileatus*. J Agric Food Chem. 2006b;54(6):2103–10.

Huang HY, Korivi M, Chaing YY, Chien TY, Tsai YC. *Pleurotus tuber-regium* polysaccharides attenuate hyperglycemia and oxidative stress in experimental diabetic rats. Evid Based Complement Alt Med. 2012;2012(7):856381. https://doi.org/10.1155/2012/856381.

Hwang CH, Jaki BU, Klein LL, Lankin DC, McAlpine JB, Napolitano JG, Fryling NA, Franzblau SG, Cho SH, Stamets PE, Wang Y, Pauli GF. Chlorinated coumarins from the polypore mushroom, *Fomitopsis officinalis*, and their activity against *Mycobacterium tuberculosis*. J Nat Prod. 2013;76(10):1916–22.

Ikekawa T, Uehara N, Maeda Y, Nakanishi M, Fukuoka F. Antitumor activity of aqueous extracts of edible mushrooms. Cancer Res. 1969;29:734–75.

Jang JH, Jeong SC, Kim JH, Lee YH, Ju YC, Lee JS. Characterisation of a new antihypertensive angiotensin I converting enzyme inhibitory peptide *from Pleurotus cornucopiae*. Food Chem. 2011;127(2):412–8.

Javed S, Bukhari SA, Zovia I, Meraj M. Screening of indigenously isolated fungi for lovastatin production and its in vivo evaluation. Curr Pharm Biotechnol. 2014;15(4):422–7.

Jeong YT, Yang BK, Jeong SC, Kim SM, Song CH. *Ganoderma applanatum*: a promising mushroom for antitumor and immunomodulating activity. Phytother Res. 2008a;22(5):614–9.

Jeong HJ, Yoon SJ, Pyun YR. Polysaccharides from edible mushroom Hinmogi (*Tremella fuciformis*) inhibit differentiation of 3T3-L1 adipocytes by reducing mRNA expression of PPARγ, C/EBPα, and leptin. Food Sci Biotechnol. 2008b;17:267–73.

Jeong SC, Yang BK, Islam R, Koyyalamudi SR, Pang G, Cho KY, Song CH. White button mushroom (*Agaricus bisporus*) lowers blood glucose and cholesterol levels in diabetic and hypercholesterolemic rats. Nutr Res. 2010;30(1):49–56.

Jia XN, Dong W, Lu WD, Guo LZ, Wei YX. *In vivo* imuunomodulatory and tumor inhibitory activities of polysaccharides isolated from solid state cultured *Trametes robinophila* Murrill. World J Microbiol Biotechnol. 2009;25:2057–63.

Jin D, Park B, Lee J, Choi H, Lee Y, Yang J. Mycelial extract of *Cordyceps ophioglossoides* prevents neuronal cell death and ameliorates β-amyloid peptide-induced memory deficits in rats. Biol Pharm Bull. 2004;27(7):1126–9.

Jose N, Ajith TA, Jananrdhanan KK. Antioxidant, anti-inflammatory and antitumor activities of culinary-medicinal mushroom *Pleurotus pulmonarius* (Fr.) Quel. (Agaricomycetidae). Int J Med Mushrooms. 2002;4(4):329–35.

Kabir Y, Yamaguchi M, Kimura S. Effect of shiitake (*Lentinus edodes*) and maitake (*Grifola frondosa*) mushrooms on blood pressure and plasma lipids of spontaneously hypertensive rats. J Nutr Sci Vitaminol. 1987;33:341–6.

Kaneda T, Tokuda S. Effect of various mushroom preparations on cholesterol levels in rats. J Nutr. 1966;90:371–6.

Kang MG, Kim YH, Zanabaatar B, Kim MK, Seo GS, Lee JS. Characterization of an antihypertensive angiotensin I-converting enzyme inhibitory peptide from the edible mushroom *Hypsizygus marmoreus*. BioMed Res Int. 2013;2013:283964. https://doi.org/10.1155/2013/283964.

Kawagishi H, Ishiyama D, Mori H, Sakamoto H, Ishiguro Y, Furukawa S, Li J. Dictyophorines A and B, two stimulators of NGF-synthesis from the mushroom Dictyophora indusiata. Phytochemistry. 1997;45(6):1203–5.

Keith RM. Both common and specialty mushrooms inhibit adhesion molecule expression and *in vitro* binding of monocytes to human aortic endothelial cells in a pro-inflammatory environment. J Nutr. 2010;9:29.

Khatua S, Paul S, Acharya K. Mushroom as the potential source of new generation of antioxidant: a review. Res J Pharm Technol. 2013;6(5):496–505.

Kiho T, Shiose Y, Nagai K, Ukai S. Polysaccharides in fungi. XXX. Antitumor and immunomodulating activities of two polysaccharides from the fruiting bodies of *Armillariella tabescens*. Chem Pharm Bull. 1992;40:2110–4.

Kiho T, Sobue S, Ukai S. Structural features and hypoglycemic activities of two polysaccharides from a hot-water extract of *Agrocybe cylindracea*. Carbohydr Res. 1994;251:81–7.

Kim YR. Immunomodulatory activity of the water extract from medicinal mushroom *Inonotus obliquus*. Mycobiology. 2005;33(3):158–62.

Kim GY, Kim SH, Hwang SY, Kim HY, Park YM, Park SK. Oral administration of proteoglycan isolated from *Phellinus linteus* in the prevention and treatment of collagen-induced arthritis in mice. Biol Pharm Bull. 2003;26(6):823–31.

Kim SH, Song YS, Kim SK, Kim BC, Lim CJ, Park EH. Anti-inflammatory and related pharmacological activities of the n-BuOH subfraction of mushroom *Phellinus linteus*. J Ethnopharmacol. 2004;93(1):141–6.

Kinsalin VA, Kumar PS, Duraipandiyan V, Ignacimuthu S, Al-Dhabi NA. Antimicrobial activity of methanol extracts of some traditional medicinal plants from Tamil Nadu, India. Asian J Pharm Clin Res. 2014;7(1):36–40.

Kiyoto M, Saito S, Hattori K, Cho NS, Hara T, Yagi Y, Aoyama M. Inhibitory effects of L-pipecolic acid from the edible mushroom, *Sarcodon aspratus* on angiotensin-I-converting enzyme. J Wood Sci. 2008;54(2):179–81.

Ko HJ, Song A, Lai MN, Ng L. Immunomodulatory properties of *Xylaria nigripes* in peritoneal macrophage cells of Balb/c mice. J Ethnopharmacol. 2011;138(3):762–8.

Komoda Y, Shimizu M, Sonoda Y, Sato Y. Ganoderic acid and its derivatives as cholesterol synthesis inhibitors. Chem Pharm Bull. 1989;37:531–3.

Kong F, Li FE, He Z, Jiang Y, Hao R, Sun X, Tong H. Antitumor and macrophage activation induced by alkali extracted polysaccharide from *Pleurotus ostreatus*. Int J Biol Biol Macromol. 2014;69:561–6.

Konno S, Aynehchi S, Dolin DJ, Schwartz AM, Choudhury MS, Tazakin HN. Anticancer and hypoglycemic effects of polysaccharides in edible and medicinal Maitake mushroom [*Grifola frondosa* (Dicks.:Fr.) S.F.Gray]. Int J Med Mushrooms. 2002;4:185–95.

Kosanic M, Rankovi B, Dasic M. Antioxidant and antimicrobial properties of mushrooms. Bulg J Agric Sci. 2013;19(5):1040–6.

Koyama K, Imaizumi T, Akiba M, Kinoshita K, Takahashi L, Suzuki A. Antinociceptive components of *Ganoderma lucidum*. Planta Med. 1997;63(3):224–7.

Kozarski M, Klaus A, Jakovljevic D, Todorovic N, Vunduk J, Petrović P, et al. Antioxidants of edible mushrooms. Molecules. 2015;20:19489–525.

Kreisel H, Lindequist U, Horak M. Distribution, ecology and immunosuppressive properties of *Tricholoma populinum* (Basidiomycetes). Zentralbl Mikrobiol. 1990;145(5):393–6.

Krishnamoorthy AS, Muthusankaranarayanan A. Indian farmers Digest. XXXI. 1998. pp. 7–8, 43–44.

Kumar M, Harsh NSK, Prasad R, Pandey VV. An Ethnomycological survey of Jaunsar, Chakrata, Dehradun, India. J Threatened Taxa. 2017;9(9):10717–25.

Kundakovic T, Kolundzic M. Therapeutic properties of mushrooms in managing adverse effects in the metabolic syndrome. Curr Top Med Chem. 2013;13(21):2734–44.

Kuo HC, Lu CC, Shen CH, Tung SY, Hsieh MC, Lee KC, et al. *Hericium erinaceus mycelium* and its isolated erinacine A protection from MPTP-induced neurotoxicity through the ER stress, triggering an apoptosis cascade. J Transl Med. 2016;14:78.

Kwon AH, Qiu Z, Hashimoto M, Yamamoto K, Kimura T. Effects of medicinal mushroom (*Sparassis crispa*) on wound healing in streptozotocin-induced diabetic rats. Am J Surg. 2009;197(4):503–9.

Lakshmi B, Jose N, Ajith TA, Janadharan KK. Antimutagenic activity of methanolic extract of culinary medicinal oyster mushroom, *Pleurotus ostreatus* (Jacq.: Fr.) Kumm. (strain floric Eger nom. Nud.) and its protective effect against benzo(á) pyrene induced heptic damages. Int J Med Mushrooms. 2004;6:139–49.

Lakshmi B, Tilak JC, Adhikari S, Devasagayan TPA, Janardhanan KK. Evaluation of antioxidant activity of selected Indian mushrooms. Pharm Biol. 2008;42(3):179–85.

Lau CC, Abdullah N, Shuib AS, Aminudin N. Proteomic analysis of antihypertensive proteins in edible mushrooms. J Agric Food Chem. 2012;60(50):12341–8.

Lee IH, Huang RL, Chen CT, Chen HC, Hsu WC, Lu MK. *Antrodia camphorate* polysaccharides exhibit antihepatitis B virus effects. FEMS Microbil Lett. 2002a;209(1):63–7.

Lee IK, Yun BS, Han G, Cho DH, Kim YH, Yoo ID. Dictyoquinazols A, B, and C, new neuroprotective compounds from the mushroom *Dictyophora indusiata*. J Nat Prod. 2002b;65(12):1769–72.

Lee SH, Hwang HS, Yun JW. Antitumor activity of water extract of a mushroom, *Inonotus obliquus*, against HT-29 human colon cancer cells. Pytother Res. 2009;23(12):1784–9.

Lee BR, Lee YP, Kim DW, Song HY, Yoo KY, Won MH, et al. Amelioration of streptozotocin-induced diabetes by *Agrocybe chaxingu* polysaccharide. Mol Cells. 2010;29(4):349–54.

Lee B, Park J, Park J, Jinhee P, Hyun-Jae S, Sunoh K, et al. *Cordyceps militaris* improves neurite outgrowth in Neuro2a cells and reverses memory impairment in rats. Food Sci Biotechnol. 2011;20(6):1599–608.

Lee S, Lee D, Park JY, Seok S, Jang TS, Park HB, et al. Antigastritis effects of *Armillariella tabescens* (Scop.) Sing. and the identification of its anti-inflammatory metabolites. J Pharm Pharmacol. 2018;70:404–12.

Lei H, Guo S, Han J, Wang Q, Zhang X, Wu W. Hypoglycemic and hypolipidemic activities of MT-α-glucan and its effect on immune function of diabetic mice. Carbohydr Polym. 2012;89(1):245–50.

Leonhardt K, Anke T, Hillen-Maske E, Steglich W. 6-Methylpurine, 6-methyl-9-β-D-ribofuranosylpurine, and 6-hydroxymethyl-9-β-D-ribofuranosylpurin as antiviral metabolites of *Collybia maculate* (basidiomycetes). Z Naturforsch C. 1987;42:420–4.

Leung MKY, Fung KP, Choy YM. The isolation and characterization of an immunomodulatory and anti-tumor polysaccharide preparation from *Flammulina velutipes*. Immunopharmacology. 1997;35:255–63.

Li JP, Lei YL, Zhan H. The effects of the king oyster mushroom *Pleurotus eryngii* (higher Basidiomycetes) on glycemic control in alloxan-induced diabetic mice. Int J Med Mushrooms. 2014;16(3):219–25.

Li S, Shah NP. Antioxidant and antibacterial activities of sulphated polysaccharides from *Pleurotus eryngii* and *Streptococcus thermophilus* ASCC 1275. Food Chem. 2014;165:262–70.

Li H, Zhang M, Ma G. Hypolipidemic effect of the polysaccharide from *Pholiota nameko*. Nutrition. 2010;26:556–62.

Liang B, Guo Z, Xie F, Zhao A. Antihyperglycemic and antihyperlipidemic activities of aqueous extract of *Hericium erinaceus* in experimental diabetic rats. BMC Complement Altern Med. 2013;13:253.

Lindequist U, Lesnau A, Teuscher E, Pilgrim H. Untersuchungen zur antiviralen Wirksamkeit von Ergosterolperoxid. Pharmazie. 1989;44:579–80.

Lu X, Chen H, Dong P, Fu L, Zhang X. Phytochemical characteristics and hypoglycaemic activityof fraction from mushroom *Inonotus obliquus*. J Sci Food Agric. 2010;90:276–80.

Lucas EH, Byerrum M, Clarke DA, Reilly HC, Stevens JA, Stock CC. Production of oncostatic principles in vivo and in vitro by species of the genus Calvatia. Antibiot Annu. 1958;6:493–6.

Lucas EH, Montesano R, Pepper MS, Hafner M, Sablon E. Tumor inhibitors in *Boletus edulis* and other holobasidiomycetes. Antibiot Chemother. 1957;7:1–4.

Lv H, Kong Y, Yao Q, Zhang B, Leng FW, Bian HJ, et al. Nebrodeolysin, a novel hemolytic protein from mushroom *Pleurotus nebrodensis* with apoptosis-inducing and anti-HIV-1 effects. Phytomedicine. 2009;16(2–3):198–205.

Mahajna J, Dotan N, Zaidman BZ, Petrova RD, Wasser SP. Pharmacological values of medicinal mushrooms for prostate cancer therapy: the case of *Ganoderma lucidum*. Nutr Cancer. 2010;61:16–26.

Mascaro MB, Franca CM, Esquerdo KF, Lara MAN, Wadt NSY, Bach EE. Effects of dietary supplementation with *Agaricus sylvaticus* Schaeffer on glycemia and cholesterol after streptozotocin induced diabetes in rats. Evid Complement Altern Med. 2014;2014:107629. https://doi.org/10.1155/2014/107629.

Mau CN, Huang SJ, Chen CC. Antioxidant properties of methanolic extracts from *Grifola frondosa, Morchella esculenta* and *Termitomyces albuminosus* mycelia. Food Chem. 2004;87:111–8.

Menikpurage IP, Abeytunga DT, Jacobsen NE, Wijesundara RL. An oxidized ergosterol from *Pleurotus cystidiosus* active against anthracnose causing Colletotrichum gloeosporioides. Mycopathologia. 2009;167(3):155–62.

Mentel R, Meinsen D, Pilgrim H, Herrman B, Lindequist U. *In vitro* antiviral effect of extracts of *Kuehneromyces mutabilis* on influenza virus. Die Parmazie. 1994;49(11):859–60.

Mimura H, Ohno N, Suzuki I, Yadomae T. Purification, antitumor activity, and structural characterization of b-1,3-glucan from *Peziza vesiculosa*. Chem Pharm Bull. 1985;33:5096–9.

Miyazaki T, Nishijima M. Studies on fungal polysaccharides.XXVII. Structural examination of a water-soluble, antitumor polysaccharide of *Ganoderma lucidum*. Chem Pharm Bull. 1981;29:3611–25.

Miyazawa N, Okazaki M, Ohga S. Antihypertensive effect of *Pleurotus nebrodensis* in spontaneously hypertensive rats. J Oleo Sci. 2008;57:675–81.

Mizuno T. Extraction and development of antitumor-active polysaccharides from medicinal mushrooms in Japan. Int J Med Mushrooms. 1999;1(1):9–29.

Mizuno M, Shiomi Y, Minato K, Kawakami S, Ashida H, Tsuchida H. Flucogalactan isolated from *Sarcodon aspratus* elicits release of tumor necrosis factor alpha and nitric oxide from murine macrophages. Immunopharmacology. 2000;46(2):113–21.

Molitoris HP. Mushrooms in medicine. Folia Microbiol. 1994;39(2):91–8.

Mori K, Inatomi S, Ouchi K, Azumi Y, Tuchida T. Improving effects of the mushroom Yamabushitake (*Hericium erinaceus*) on mid cognitive impairment: a double-blind placebo-controlled clinical trial. Phytother Res. 2009;23:367–72.

Mothana RAA, Awadh NAA, Jansen R, Wegner U, Mentel R, Lindequist U. Antiviral lanostanoid triterpenes from the fungus *Ganoderma pfeifferi* BRES. Fitoterapia. 2003;74(1–2):177–80.

Muller C, Bockhorn AG, Klusmeier S, Kiehl M, Roeder C, Kalthoff H, et al. Lovastatin inhibits proliferation of pancreatic cancer cell lines with mutant as well as with wild type K-ras oncogene but has different effects o protein phosphorylation and induction of apoptosis. Int J Oncol. 1998;12:717–23.

Murcia MA, Martínez-Tomé M, Jiménez AM, Vera AM, Honrubia M, Parras P. Antioxidant activity of edible fungi (truffles and mushrooms): losses during industrial processing. J Food Protect. 2002;65(10):1614–22.

Nagai K, Chiba A, Nishino T, Kubota T, Kawagishi H. Dilinoleoyl- phosphatidylethanolamine from Hericium erinaceum protects against ER stress-dependent Neuro-2a cell death via protein kinase C pathway. J Nutr Biochem. 2006;17(8):525–30.

Nagajyothi PC, Sreekanth TV, Lee JI, Lee KD. Mycisynthesis: antibacterial, antioxidant and antiproliferative activities of silver nanoparticles synthesized from *Inonoyus obliqus* (chaga mushroom) extract. J Photochem Photobiol. 2014;130:299–304.

Nakamichi N, Nakayama K, Ishimoto T, Masuo Y, Wakayama T, Sekiguchi H, et al. Food-derived hydrophilic antioxidant ergothioneine is distributed to the brain and exerts antidepressant effect in mice. Brain Behav. 2016;6(6):e00477. https://doi.org/10.1002/brb3.477.

Narisawa T, Fukaura Y, Kotanagi H, Asakawa Y. Inhibitory effect of cryptoporic acid E, a product from fungus *Cryptoporus volvatus* on colon carcinogenesis induced with N-methyl-N-Nitrosourea in rats and with 1,2-Dimethylhydrazine in mice. Jpn J Cancer Res. 1992;83:830–4.

Nayana J, Janadharan KK. Antioxidant and antitumor activity of *Pleurotus florida*. Curr Sci. 2000;79(7):941–3.

Newton GGF, Abraham EP. Cephalosporin C, a new antibiotic containing sulphur and D-α-aminoadipic acid. Nature. 1955;175:548.

Neyrinck AM, Bindels LB, De Backer F, Pachikian D. Dietry supplementation with chitosan derieved from mushrooms changes adipocytokine profile in diet induced obese mice, a phenomenon linked to its lipid lowering action. Int Immunopharmacol. 2009;9(6):767–73.

Ng YF. In vitro and in vivo antioxidant activity and hypocholesterolemic effect in extracts of *Agrocybe aegerita*. M.Phil. thesis. Hong Kong: The Chinese University of Hong. 2005.

Nguyen TK, Im KH, Choi J, Shin PG, Lee TS. Evaluation of antioxidant, anti-cholinesterase, and anti-inflammatory effects of culinary mushroom *Pleurotus pulmonarius*. Mycobiology. 2016;44(4):291–301.

Ohno N, Miura T, Saito K, Nishijima M, Miyazaki T, Yadomae T. Physicochemical characteristics and antitumor activities of a highly branched fungal (1----3)-beta-D-glucan, OL-2, isolated from *Omphalia lapidescens*. Chem Pharm Bull (Tokyo). 1992;40(8):2215–8.

Ooi VEC, Liu F. Immunomodulation and anti-cancer activity of polysaccharide-protein complexes. Curr Med Chem. 2000;7:715–29.

Oxford AE, Raistrick H, Simonart P. Studies in the biochemistry of micro-organisms: Griseofulvin, C(17) H(17)O(6)Cl, a metabolic product of Penicillium griseo-fulvum Dierckx. Biochem J. 1939;33(2):240–8.

Oyetayo FL. Potential antioxidant properties of Nigerian edible mushrooms. Agro Food Industry Hi-tech. 2007;18(4):44–5.

Pala SA, Wani AH, Bhat MY. Ethnomycological studies of some wild medicinal and edible mushrooms in the Kashmir Himalayas (India). Int J Med Mushrooms. 2013;15(2):211–20.

Panda AK, Swainl KC. Traditional uses and medicinal potential of *Cordyceps sinensis* of Sikkim. J Ayurveda Integr Med. 2011;2(1):2–9.

Panda MK, Tayung K. Documentation and ethnomedicinal knowledge on wild edible mushrooms among ethnic tribes of Northern Odisha, India. Asian J Pharm Clin Res. 2015;8(4):139–43.

Park JY, Oh WJ, Kwak DM, Kim MG, Seo GS, Hong SB, Rhee MH. The antiplatelet activity of *Hypsizygus marmoreus* extract is involved in the suppression of intracellular calcium mobilization and integrin $\alpha_{IIb}\beta_3$ activation. J Med Plant Res. 2011;5(11):2369–77.

Patel S, Goyal A. Recent Developments in mushrooms as anticancer therapeutics: a review. 3 Biotech. 2012;2(1):1–15.

Peng J, Wang P, Ge H, Qu X, Jin X. Effects of cordycepin on the impairments of growth and development of hippocampal cultured neurons. PLoS One. 2015;10(5):e0125902. https://doi.org/10.1371/journal.pone.0125902.

Percario S, Odorizzi VF, Souza DR, Pinhel MA, Gennari JL, Gennari MS, Godoy MF. Edible mushroom *Agaricus sylvaticus* can prevent the onset of atheroma plaques in hipercholesterolemic rabbits. Cell Mol Boil (Noisy-le-Grand, France). 2008;54(Suppl):OL 1055–61.

Pfab R, Haberl B, Kleber J, Zilker T. Cerebellar effects after consumption of edible morels (*Morchella conica, Morchella esculenta*). Clin Toxicol. 2008;46(3):256–60.

Phan CW, David P, Wong KH, Naidu M, Sabaratnam V. Uridine from Pleurotus giganteus and its neurite outgrowth stimulatory effects with underlying mechanism. PLoS One. 2015;10(11):e0143004. https://doi.org/10.1371/journal.pone.0143004.

Pilz D, Smith J, Amaranthus MP, Alexander S, Molina R, Louma D. Mushrooms and timber: managing commercial harvesting in the Oregon Cascades. J For. 1999;97:4–11.

Preuss HG, Echard B, Bagchi D, Perricone NV. Maitake mushroom extracts ameliorate progressive hypertension and other chronic metabolic perturbations in aging female rats. Int J Med Sci. 2010;7(4):169–80.

Purkayastha RP, Chandra A. Manual of Indian edible mushrooms. New Delhi: Today and Tomorrow's Printers and Publishers; 1985.

Qi J, Ojika M, Sakagami Y. Termitomycesphins A–D, novel neuritogenic cerebrosides from the edible Chinese mushroom *Termitomyces albuminosus*. Tetrahedron. 2000;56(32):5835–41.

Qu Y, Sun K, Gao L, Sakagami Y, Kawagishi H, Ojika M, Qi J. Termitomycesphins G and H, additional cerebrosides from the edible Chinese mushroom *Termitomyces albuminosus*. Biosci Biotechnol Biochem. 2012;76(4):791–3.

Ramesh C, Manohar GP. Antimicrobial properties, antioxidant activity and bioactive compounds from six wild edible mushrooms of Western Ghats of Karnataka, India. Pharmacog Res. 2010;2(2):107–12.

Refale FM, Esmat AY, Daba AS, Taha SM. Characterization of polysaccharides from *Pleurotus ostreatus* mycelium: assessment of toxicity and immunomodulation in vivo. Micol App Int. 2009;21:61–7.

Ren D, Jiao Y, Yang X, Yuan L, Guo L, Zhao Y. Antioxidant and antitumor effects of polysaccharides from the fungus *Pleurotus abalonus*. Chem Biol Interact. 2015;237:166–74.

Ren L, Perera C, Hemar Y. Antitumor activity of mushroom polysaccharides: a review. Food Funct. 2012;3:1118.

Robert ES, David FS, Henry J, Kenneth EW, August JK, Kent AG, et al. Pneumocandins from *Zalerion arboricola*. I. Discovery and isolation. J Antibiot. 1992;45(12):1853–66.

Roy SK, Das D, Mondal S, Maiti D, Bhunia B, Maiti T, Islam SS. Structural studies of an immunoenhancing water soluble glucan isolated from hot water extract of an edible mushroom, *Pleurotus florida*, cultivar Assam lorida. Carbohydr Res. 2009;344(18):2596–601.

Sabaratnam V, Kah-Hui W, Naidu M, David PR. Neuronal health – can culinary and medicinal mushrooms help? J Tradit Complement Med. 2013;3(1):62–8.

Sachan SKS, Patra JK, Thatoi HN. Indigenous knowledge of ethnic tribes for utilization of wild mushrooms as food and medicine in similipal biosphere reserve, Odisha, India. J Agric Technol. 2013;9(2):403–16.

Saito T, Aoki F, Hirai H, Inagaki T, Matsunaga Y, Sakakibara T. Erinacine E as a kappa opioid receptor agonist and its new analogs from a basidiomycete, *Hericium ramosum*. J Antibiot. 1998;51:983–90.

Samorini G. Fungi Hallucinogeni. In: Guo J, Cheng HY, Wei X, editors. Studi etnomicologici. Dozza, Bologna, Italy, Shen: Telesterion; 2001. p. 250.

Sano M, Yoshino K, Matsuzawa T, Ikekawa T. Inhibitory effects of edible higher basidiomycetes mushroom extracts on mouse type IV allergy. Int J Med Mushrooms. 2002;4:37–41.

Sanodiya BS, Thakur GS, Baghel RK, Prasad GB, Bisen PS. *Ganoderma lucidum:* a potent pharmacological macrofungus. Curr Pharm Biotechnol. 2009;10(8):717–42.

Sarma TC, Sarma I, Patiri BN. Wild edible mushrooms used by some ethnic tribes of Western Assam. The Bioscan. 2010;3:613–25.

Sharma VP. Recycling of wastes from mushroom industry for cultivation of some edible fungi, PhD. Thesis. Dr. Y. S. Parmar University of Horticulture and Forestry, Solan. 1989.

Sharma TK. Vegetable caterpillar, Science Reporter. National Institute of Science Communication and Information Resources (NISCAIR), CSIR. 2008. pp. 33–5.

Sharma VP, Sharma SR, Kumar S. Nutritional requirements for mycelial growth and cultivationof Flammulina velutipes. Mushrooms Res. 2005;14:13–8.

Shen YC, Chen CF, Wang YH, Chang TT, Chou CJ. Evaluation of the immunomodulatory activity of some active principles isolated from the fruiting bodies of *Antrodia camphorata*. Chinese Pharm J. 2003;55(50):313–8.

Shen YC, Wang YH, Chou YC, Chen CF, Lin LC, Chang TT, Ten JH, Chou CJ. Evaluation of the anti-inflammatory activity of Zhankuic acids isolated from the fruiting bodies *Antrodia camphorata*. Planta Med. 2004;70(4):310–4.

Sijun D, Yoshiyuki F, Yumiko S, Michiko F, Yun Z, Makoto Y, et al. Estrogen-like activity and dual roles in cell signaling of an *Agaricus blazei* Murrill mycelia-dikaryon extract. Microbiol Res. 2011;167(4):231–7.

Silveira MLL, Smiderle FR, Moraes CP, Borato DG, Baggio CH, Ruthes AC, et al. Structural characterization and anti-inflammatory activity of a linear β-D-glucan isolated from *Pleurotus sajor-caju*. Carbohydr Polym. 2014;113:588–96.

Singh M, Bhuvnesh V, Kamal S, Wakchaure GC. Mushrooms: cultivation, marketing and consumption. Solan, Himachal Pradesh: Directorate of Mushroom Research (ICAR; 2011. p. 1–2.

Smania EF, Delle Monache F, Smania A Jr, Yunes RA, Cuneo RS. Antifungal activity of sterols and triterpenes isolated from *Ganoderma annulare*. Fitoterapia. 2003;74(4):375–7.

Smania A Jr, Delle Monache F, Smania EFA, Cuneo RS. Antibacterial activity of steroidal compounds isolated from *Ganoderma applanatum* (Pers.) Pat. (Aphyllophoromycetideae) fruit body. Int J Med Mushrooms. 1999;1(4):325–30.

So YW, Eun HP. Anti-inflammatory and related pharmacological activities of cultured mycelia and fruiting bodies of *Cordyceps militaris*. J Ethnopharmacol. 2005;96:555–61.

Song Z, Ben H, Junbo G, Changlin Z, Xin L, Pingang L. Characterization of chemical composition of *Agaricus brasiliensis* polysaccharides and its effect on myocardial SOD activity, MDA and caspase-3 level in ischemia-reperfusion rats. Int J Biol Macromol. 2010;46(3):363–6.

Sorimachi K, Akimoto K, Inafuku K, Okubo A, Yamazaki S. Secretion of TNF-γ, IL-8 and nitric oxide by macrophages activated with *Agaricus blazei* Murrill fractions *in vitro*. Cell Struct Funct. 2001;26:103–8.

Stadler M, Anke H. New nematicidal and antimicrobial compounds from the basidiomycete *Cheimonophyllum candissimum* (Berk & Curt.) sing. I. Producing organism, fermentation, isolation, and biological activities. J Antibiot (Tokyo). 1994;47(11):1284–9.

Sudheesh NP, Ajith TA, Janardhanan KK. Ganoderma lucidum (Fr.) P. Karst enhances activities of heart mitochondrial enzymes and respiratory chain complexes in the aged rat. Biogerontology. 2009;10:627–36.

Sugiyama K, Kawagishi H, Tanaka A, Saeki S, Yoshida S, Sakamoto H, Ishiguro Y. Isolation of plasma cholesterol-lowering components from ningyotake (*Polyporus confluens*) mushroom. J Nutr Sci Vitaminol (Tokyo). 1992;38:335–42.

Suseem SR, Saral AM. Analysis on essential fatty acid esters of mushroom *Pleurotus eous* and its antibacterial activity. Asian J Pharm Clin Res. 2013;6:188–91.

Suzuki T, Umehara K, Tashiro A, Kobayashi Y, Dohra H, Hirai H, Kawagishi H. An antifungal protein from the culinary medicinal beech mushroom, *Hypsizygus marmoreus* (Peck) Bigel. (Agaricomycetideae). Int J Med Mushroom. 2011;13(1):27–31.

Suzuki I, Yadomae T, Yonekubo H, Nishijima M, Miyazaki T. Antitumor activity of an immunomodulating material extracted from a fungus, *Peziza vesiculosa*. Chem Pharm Bull (Tokyo). 1982;30(3):1066–8.

Talpur NA, Echard BW, Fan AY, Jaffari O, Bagchi D, Preuss HG. Antihypertensive and metabolic effects of whole maitake mushroom powder and its fractions in two rat strains. Mol Cell Biochem. 2002;237(1-2):129–36.

Tambekar DH, Sonar TP, Khodje MV, Khante BS. The novel antibacterial from two edible mushrooms *Agaricus bisporus* and *Pleurotus sajor* caju. Int J Pharm. 2006;2:584–7.

Tasaka K, Mio M, Izushi K, Akagi M, Makino T. Anti-allergic constituents in the culture medium of Ganoderma lucidum. (II). The inhibitory effect of cyclooctasulfur on histamine release. Agents Actions. 1988;23:157–60.

Tewari RP. Now in the limelight; Mushroom. The Hindu Survey of Indian Agriculture. 2004; pp. 132–3.

Valverde ME, Hernández-Pérez T, Octavio Paredes-López O. Edible mushrooms: improving human health and promoting quality life. Int J Microbiol. 2015;2015:376387.

Veena SS, Pandey M. Tramete sp, a potential species for diversification of Indian Mushroom Ind. In: Proceedings International Conference on Mushroom Biology and Biotechnology. Solan: NRCM; 2007. p. 125.

Venkatachalapathi A, Paulsamy S. Exploration of wild medicinal mushroom species in Walayar valley, the Southern Western Ghats of Coimbatore District Tamil Nadu. Mycosphere. 2016;7(2):118–30.

Vishwakarma P, Singh P, Tripathi NN. Nutritional and antioxidant properties of wild edible macrofungi from North-Eastern Uttar Pradesh, India. Indian J Trad Knowl. 2016;15(1):143–8.

Wachtel-Galor S, Yuen J, Buswell JA, et al. *Ganoderma lucidum* (Lingzhi or Reishi): a medicinal mushroom. In: Benzie IFF, Wachtel-Galor S, editors. Herbal medicine: biomolecular and clinical aspects. 2nd ed. Boca Raton, FL: CRC Press/Taylor & Francis; 2011. p. 175–200.

Wang S, Bao L, Zhao F, Wang Q, Li S, Ren J, Li L, Wen H, Guo L, Liu H. Isolation, identification, and bioactivity of monoterpenoids and sesquiterpenoids from the mycelia of edible mushroom *Pleurotus cornucopiae*. J Agric Food Chem. 2013;61:5122–9.

Wang G, Dong L, Zhang Y, Ji Y, Xiang W, Zhao M. Polysaccharides from *Phellinus linteus* inhibit cell growth and invasion and induce apoptosis in Hep G2 human hepatocellular carcinoma cells. Biologia. 2012;67(1):247–54.

Wang N, Li J, Huang X, Chen W, Chen Y. Herbal medicine *Cordyceps sinensis* improves health-related quality of life in moderate-to-severe asthma. Evid Based Complement Alternat Med. 2016;2016:6134593. https://doi.org/10.1155/2016/6134593.

Wang H, Ooi V, Ng T, Chiu K, Chang S. Hypotensive and vasorelaxing activities of a lectin from the edible mushroom *Tricholoma mongolicum*. Pharmacol Toxicol. 1996;79:318–23.

Wasson RG. Soma: divine mushroom of immortality. Harcourt, brace & world. New York: New York Press; 1969. p. 3–4.

Weber W, Anke T, Steffan B, Steglich W. Antibiotics from basidiomycetes XXXII strobilurin E: a new cytostatic and antifungal (E)- methoxyacrylate antibiotic from *Crepidotus fulvotomentosus* Peck. J Antibiot (Tokyo). 1989;43:207–12.

Weng Y, Xiang L, Matsuura A, Zhang Y, Huang Q, Qi J. Ganodermasides A and B, two novel anti-aging ergosterols from spores of a medicinal mushroom *Ganoderma lucidum* on yeast via UTH1 gene. Bioorg Med Chem. 2010;18(3):999–1002.

Won DP, Lee JS, Kwon DS, Lee E, Shin WC, Hong WK. Immunostimulating activity by polysaccharides isolated from fruiting body of *Inonotus obliquus*. Mol Cells. 2011;31:165–73.

Wu DM, Duan WQ, Liu Y, Cen Y. Anti-inflammatory effect of the polysaccharides of golden needle mushroom in burned rats. Int J Biol Macromoles. 2010b;46(1):100–3.

Wu SJ, Liaw CC, Pan SZ, Yang HC, Ng LT. *Phellinus linteus* polysaccharides and their immunomodulatory properties in human monocytic cells. J Funct Food. 2013;5:679–88.

Wu X, Zheng S, Cui L, Wang H, Ng TB. Isolation and characterization of a novel ribonuclease from the pink oyster mushroom *Pleurotus djamor*. J Gen Appl Microbiol. 2010a;56(3):231–9.

Xin-Cun W, Rui-Jiao X, Yi L, Dong-Mei W, Yi-Jian Y. The species identity of the widely cultivated Ganoderma, '*G. lucidum*' (Ling-zhi), in China. PLoS One. 2012;7(7):e40857.

Yamac M, Kanbak G, Zeytinoglu M, Bayramoglu G, Senturk H, Uyanoglu M. Hypoglycemic effect of *Lentinus strigosus* (Schwein.) Fr. crude exopolysaccharide in streptozotocin-induced diabetic rats. J Med Food. 2008;11(3):513–7.

Yamada T, Oinuma T, Niihashi M, Mitsumata M, Fujioka T, Hasegawa K, Nagaoka H, Itakura H. Effects of *Lentinus edodes* mycelia on dietaryinduced atherosclerotic involvement in rabbit aorta. J Atheroscler Thromb. 2002;9:149–56.

Yan B, Jing L, Wang J. A polysaccharide (PNPA) from *Pleurotus nebrodensis* offers cardiac protection against ischemia–reperfusion injury in rats. Carbohydr Polymers. 2015;133:1–7.

Yang H, Hwang I, Kim S, Hong E, Jeung E. *Lentinus edodes* promotes fat removal in hypercholesterolemic mice. Exp Ther Med. 2013;6(6):1409–13.

Yang BK, Jeong YT, Jeong H, Song CH. Chemical characteristics and immune-modulating activities of exobiopolymers produced by *Grifola frondosa* during submerged fermentation process. Int J Biol Macromol. 2007;41:327–33.

Yap AT, Ng ML. The medicinal benefits of lentinan (β-i, 3-D glucan) from *Lentinus edodes* (Berk.) Singer (shiitake Mushroom) through oral administration. Int J Med Mushrooms. 2005;7:175–91.

Yin H, Wang Y, Wang Y, Chen T, Tang H, Wang M. Purification, characterization and immune- modulating properties of polysaccharide isolated from *Flammulina velutipes* mycelium. Am J Chin Med. 2010;38(1):191–204.

Yoshiaki S, Reiko O, Noriko W, Etsu K, Akira M. Structures and antitumor activities of the polysaccharides isolated from fruiting body and the growing culture of mycelium of *Ganoderma lucidum*. Agric Biol Chem. 1985;49(9):2641–53.

Young-Mi P, Jong-Heon W, Yang-Hee K, Jong-Won C, Hee-Juhn P, Kyung-Tae L. *In vivo* and *in vitro* anti-inflammatory and anti-nociceptive effects of the methanol extract of *Inonotus obliquus*. J Ethnopharmacol. 2005;101:120–8.

Yu H, Han C, Sun Y, Qi X, Shi Y, Gao X, Zhang C. The agaricoglyceride of royal sun medicinal mushroom, Agaricus brasiliensis (higher Basidiomycetes) is anti-inflammatory and reverses diabetic glycemia in the liver of mice. Int J Med Mushrooms. 2013;15(4):357–64.

Zhang M, Cheung PCK, Chiu LCM, Wong EYL, Ooi VEC. Cell-cycle arrest and apoptosis induction in human breast carcinoma MCF-7 cells by carboxymethylated β-glucan from the mushroom sclerotia of *Pleurotus tuber-regium*. Carbohydr Polym. 2006;66:455–62.

Zhang M, Cui SW, Cheung PCK, Wang Q. Antitumor polysaccharides from mushrooms: a review on their isolation process, structural characteristics and antitumor activity. Trend Food Sci Technol. 2007;18:4–19.

Zhang XQ, Ip FC, Zhang DM, Ip NY, Ye WC. Triterpenoids with neurotrophic activity from Ganoderma lucidum. Nat Prod Res. 2011;25(17):1607–13.

Zhang Y, Mills G, Nair MG. Cyclooxygenase inhibitory and antioxidant compounds from the mycelia of the edible mushroom *Grifola frondosa*. J Agr Food Chem. 2002a;50(26):7581–5.

Zhang W, Qu W, Zhang X. The anti hyperglycemic activity of polysaccharides from *Tremella aurantialba* mycelium. Acta Nutrimenta Sinica. 2004;26(4):300–3.

Zhang G, Wang Y, Ni W, Teng H, Lin Z. Hepatoprotective role of *Ganoderma lucidum* polysaccharide against BCG-induced immune liver injury in mice. World J Gastroenterol. 2002b;8(4):728–33.

Zhang L, Yang M, Song Y, Sun Z, Peng Y, Qu K, Zhu H. Antihypertensive effect of 3,3,5,5-tetramethyl-4-piperidone, a new compound extracted from *Marasmius androsaceus*. J Ethnopharmacol. 2009;123(1):34–9.

Zhao YY, Chao X, Zhang Y, Lin RC, Sun WJ. Cytotoxic steroids from *Polyporus umbellatus*. Planta Med. 2010;76(15):1755–8.

Zhenquan L, Pengtao L, Dan Z, Huiling T, Jianyou G. Anti-inflammation effects of *Cordyceps sinensis* mycelium in focal cerebral ischemic injury rats. Inflammation. 2010;34:639–44.

Zhou X, Lin J, Yin Y, Zhao J, Sun X, Tang K. Ganodermataceae: Natural products and their related pharmacological functions. Am J Chin Med. 2007;35(4):559–74.

Zhu XL, Chen AF, Lin ZB. *Ganoderma lucidum* polysaccharides enhance the function of immunological effector cells in immunosuppressed mice. J Ethnopharmacol. 2007;111:219–26.

32 Study on Nutraceuticals of a Certain Ethnomedicinal Plants of Arunachal Pradesh, India

Chandan Tamuly

Contents

32.1 Introduction

In today's changing times, there is an urgent need to address the challenge of greater food production with regard to the technological enhancement and easy access to latest developments in the agricultural sector amidst ever-growing population. An immediate and single solution is not possible instantly. Knowledge of various food resources and their nutritive value will be of most help for devising alternate food resources. For this, a systematic, planned and thorough analysis of the sources is necessary. The deterioration of food situation in many of the developing countries may be attributed to the increase of populations, changing scenarios of the agricultural practices and the high price of essential staple food (Ezeagu et al. 1996). It has estimated that almost 50% of children and an equal number of women suffer from protein calorie malnutrition as adjudged by the anthropometric parameter. Deficiency in micronutrients (vitamins and minerals), particularly iron deficiency anaemia, is the main reason for the death of women in childbearing age and undermines the productivity of the country (Bamji 2007). Recently throughout the world, every measure is being taken to boost food production by conventional agriculture; and also a great emphasis is being given to the alternative foods and dietary supplements (Radimer et al. 2004).

In India, various supplementary nutrition programmes are running in different sectors in its National Plan of Action on Nutrition to combat the malnutrition. However, 80% of the Indian populations is living in rural and semi-urban areas, where a considerable population is still undernourished (Sundriyal and Sundriyal 2001). People living in the rural areas either do not produce sufficient

C. Tamuly (✉)
Natural Product Chemistry Section, CSIR-North East Institute of Science and Technology Branch Itanagar, Naharlagun, Arunachal Pradesh, India
e-mail: ctamuly@neist.res.in

S. Sen, R. Chakraborty (eds.), *Herbal Medicine in India*,
https://doi.org/10.1007/978-981-13-7248-3_32

food or could not afford various supplementary diets. Survey reports from the National Nutrition Monitoring Bureau show that Indian diets are qualitative deficient in micronutrient due to inadequate intake of vegetables, fruits, pulses and millets (Anonymous 2001). Wild edible plants particularly leafy vegetables play an important role in fulfilling the nutritional requirements of the rural population by an unconventional means (Singh and Arora 1978), as these are easily available and can be found throughout the year. These wild edible plants not only enhance the food quality but also make a significant contribution in generation of the income (Sundriyal and Sundriyal 2004; Duke and Atchley 1986). Many of such plant has been identified, but lack of the data on their chemical nutrition composition has limited the prospectus for their utilization (Vijayakumari et al. 1994). The contribution of the ethnomedicinal plant which is used as a wild vegetable in diet and economy of the ethnic people of Arunachal Pradesh is quite emerging and therefore there is an urgent need of evaluation in terms of quantitative and qualitative. During the recent years there has been growing interest in evaluation of nutritional value of the various wild edible plants (Anonymous 1970–1988; Duke and Atchley 1986; Dhyani and Khali 1993; Maikhuri et al. 1994; Negi et al. 1993; Akpanyung et al. 1995; Arora and Pandey 1996; Samant and Dhar 1997; Bhardwaj et al. 2007). From the literature survey, it was found that there are large numbers of edible plants which are commonly available in the local market or in the forest area (Angami et al. 2006). So there is a promising scope for the study of nutraceuticals of the edible plants.

32.2 Study Area

The state of Arunachal Pradesh is the largest North-East states of India situated in the easternmost flank of Himalaya and lies in between 26°28″ to 29°39 N and 91°30′ to 97°30′E. This encompasses an area of 83,743 sq. km, and 82% of the area is under forest cover. The state has been the traditional habitat of tribal people of Paleo-Mongoloid stock, speaking mostly the Tibeto-Burman group of Sino-Tibetan language. The total population of the state spreading over 22 districts is about 16.01 lakh in 2017 with density of 13 persons per sq. km (census 2011). It has 25 tribes and 125 subtribes with varied composition and cultural diversity. The state is also very rich in biotic as well as ethnic diversity and inhibited the tribes including the aboriginal people *Nyishi, Adi, Apatani, Mompas, Idu Mishmis, Golos,* etc. The people living in this state have been leading an intricate life and depended on the forest plants. The area is bounded by Bhutan in the West, the Indian states of Assam in the South, Tibet in the North and Myanmar in the East. A wide range of topography, varied climatic condition and high annual precipitation makes the state of Arunachal Pradesh, one of the richest phytogeographic regions of the world. It is estimated that more than 26% of the flowering plants are found in this state and covering 2.5% of the total geographic region of the country (Baishya 1999). All about 4117 flowering plants belonging to 1295 genera and 192 families (Chowdhery 1996) and 452 pteridophytes (Baishya 1999) are accounted from the state.

The field study was carried out in the Papum Pare district of the state situated in the capital city Itanagar. The terrain is characterized by steep hill slopes or valleys, and the households are scattered and consisting of hamlets. The climate of the area is tropical to subtropical climate, warm in winter, hot and humid in summer and prolonged rain. Papum Pare district of Arunachal Pradesh is having an area of 2875 sq. km. with population of 1,383,727 (2011 census). Nyishi tribe is a predominant tribe in this district and having rich knowledge about the wild edible plants. Many of these plants are nonconventional and lesser known to people of other parts of the country. It is urgently required to document this information and start R&D before it is too late. The economy of the area depends on hill cultivation and the majority of forest produces. The plants come into their life as food, medicine, fodder fuel, poison, etc. Literature survey shows that about 153 types of plants or plant parts are being used in the food systems (Angami et al. 2006; Haridasan et al. 1990; Arora and Pandey 1996; Maikhuri 1991; Baishya et al. 2001; Bhardwaj et al. 2007; Deka et al. 2013; Chaudhuri et al. 2018; Ghosh et al. 2014; Payum et al. 2013a, b, 2014; Seal 2011; Seal and Chaudhuri 2015; Seal et al. 2017; Tamuly et al. 2013; Tag and Tsering 2012; Tag et al. 2014).

Table 32.1 represents the nutritive value of important wild edible species found in Arunachal Pradesh. It is clear that in the table few nutritive parameters have been reported and need to cover more species with a diverse parameter for upgradation of the data bank. The nutritional value of 40 species is reported in Table 32.1. Table 32.2 represents wild edible plants available in Arunachal Pradesh. From the table, it was found that recorded 153 species are used as wild edible plants by tribal people of the state. But indigenous communities continuously include wild edible plants to their daily food intake, and sales from the surplus add to their income. Out of total 153 species, 76 species are used as vegetable, 41 plant species are used as ethnomedicine and 60 species are used as fruits. It is important to note that sometimes, same species are used in different purposes like as vegetable, medicine and spices. Out of 76 vegetable species, 31 species are used as ethnomedicine, and out of 41 species, 8 fruits species are used as ethnomedicine.

32.3 Discussion

Arunachal Pradesh has a vast geographical area and is rich in forest resources. However, there is a great scope for the improvement of the scientific management of the resources for the sustainable utilization. Use of a large number of wild species by the tribal to meet their diverse requirements is largely due to the prevalence of diversity of vegetation in the area. The tribal communities draw their sustenance mainly from the forests, which provide them food, plants and other material requirement. Their lives are much dependent on forest or natural plant wealth. The biological wealth is so intrinsically important to the lifestyle and systems of the indigenous communities that wild plants make an important contribution for the sustenance of local communities.

The rich natural resource contributes lots for nutrition, health and socio-economy upliftment of the tribal people. Traditionally they are getting good sources of protein, carbohydrate, vitamins, minerals, etc. to a greater extent (Dhyani and Khali 1993; Maikhuri et al. 1994; Negi and Gaur 1994). In the remote area, the people mainly depends upon the variety of the plant species for survival. The medicine, foods, house construction, fuel, woods and other items are obtained from the forest.

A total 153 plant species have been recorded from the Arunachal Pradesh (Table 32.2). These wild edible plants can be used as one of the best sources of protein, sugar, crude fibre and mineral especially Ca, P and Mg. It is interesting to note that most of the plants are available throughout the year. One of the advantages of these wild edible plants is that these plant species have some additional medicinal properties. For example, *Spilanthes acmella* is used as a remedy for cough and mouth freshener. The leaves are used as a condiment or eaten raw or boiled to remove constipation. The chemical constituent purified from the root of *Piper pedicellatum* exhibited an antituberculosis activity (Rukachaisirikul et al. 2004), and *Adhatoda vasica* is used for the treatment of cough and as a bronchodilator (Joshi et al. 1994). There are lots of unexplored wild edible plant species which may be utilized as a source of nutritious food items for the society. It may help to upliftment of socioeconomic as well as the cultural development of tribal people of the region. So it is suggested that these wild edible plant with rich nutritional value may be cultivated with systematic manner. The consumption of these plants will help to meet the nutritional requirement of the local inhabitants of Arunachal Pradesh. Furthermore it will help to conserve the various species of wild edible plant in the forest area and enrichment of national database system of nutritional food items.

Table 32.1 Nutritional value of wild edible plant of Arunachal Pradesh

Plant species	Part used	Moisture (%)	Protein (%)	Fat (%)	Carbohydrate (%)	Fibre (%)	Vit. C (mg/100 g)	K (%)	P (%)	Ca (%)	Na (%)	Fe (%)
Adhatoda vasica	Leaves	79.5	2.44	2.64	–	11.65	17.5	1.50	0.479	1.19	0.19	0.023
Albizia procera Benth	Leaves	78	1.61	–	18.46	–	–	–	–	–	–	–
Artocarpus lakoocha M Beib	Fruits	–	0.70	1.10	13.30	2.00	20.6	–	–	–	–	–
Baccaurea sapida Muell-Arg	Fruits	35.6	5.58	0.73	51.90	20.4	273	0.73	0.132	0.16	0.035	0.75
Bambusa balcooa Roxb.	Tender shoot	90	2.4	0.05	1.48	1.0	5.24	0.603	0.060	0.017	0.006	0.0002
Basella rubra	Leaves	88	5.15	0.86	–	–	23.4	0.402	–	0.378	0.043	0.021
Clerodendrum colebrookianum	Leaves	70.5	5.50	1.96	–	10.15	30.1	2.56	0.75	1.54	0.014	0.019
Colocasia esculenta (L.) Schott	L, Stem		0.30	0.30	4.10	0.60	–	–	0.02	0.06	–	0.050
Dendrocalamus hamiltonii Nees & Arn.	Tender shoot	88	3.90	0.50	5.70	–	–	0.057	0.065	1.12	0.039	–
Diplazium esculentum Sw.	Tender leaves	86	–	8.00	–	–	–	2.37	0.500	1.020	0.079	0.560
Elaeagnus umbellata	Fruits	14	15.13	4.36	62.45	21.80		0.29	0.10	0.81	0.47	–
Emblica officinales Gaertn.	Fruits	81	0.50	0.10	14.10	3.60	–	–	–	–	–	–
Euphorbia hirta L.	Tender plant (Lv.)	78	4.65	–	–	–	–	–	–	–	–	–
Fagopyrum esculentum Moench.	Tender leaves (S)	81	10.30	2.40	65.00	8.60	–	0.50	0.36	0.12	–	0.0649
Ficus glomerata Roxb.	Fruits	14	7.40	5.60	49.00	17.90	–	–	1.05	–	–	–
Glochidion multiloculari	Leaves	70	3.30	3.56	–	–	15.5	0.565	–	0.603	0.095	0.0008
Maianthemum purpureum	Shoot	13	27.17	5.54	42.45	10.16	–	0.73	0.07	1.09	0.53	–
Mangifera sylvatica Roxb.	Fruits	78	2.32	0.56	80.81	8.53	12.00	–	–	–	–	–
Mussaenda incana	Leaves	78.2	2.96	5.96	–	16.15	20.1	1.20	0.451	0.575	0.017	0.029
Mussaenda roxburghii	Leaves	81	2.80	1.46	–	–	12.1	0.426	–	0.367	0.032	0.012
Oenanthe javanica (Bl.) DC.	Leaves	76	17.13	2.56	–	12.20	–	4.96	0.22	–	–	0.013
Panax bipinnatifidus	Tender shoot Tuber	25										
Phoebe cooperians	Fruits	72	2.95	7.01	–	–	160.0	0.248	–	0.468	0.035	0.0023
Pouzolzia bennettiana	Leaves	87	3.96	2.14	–	12.75	29.41	3.11	1.28	4.00	0.014	0.43
Pouzolzia viminea	Leaves	90	2.46	1.48	–	15.3	19.6	1.90	1.13	0.50	0.02	0.039
Pyrus pashia	Leaves	26	1.79	0.89	66.61	21.22	–	0.80	0.13	0.65	0.09	–
Rhynchotechum ellipticum	Leaves	82	7.76	1.52	46.49	11.31		2.066		3.51	0.048	0.0047
Rubus ellipticus Smith	Fruits	80	8.10	9.50	72.70	7.90	11.00	1.50	0.16	–	–	0.509
Rubus niveus Thunb.	Fruits	85	1.23	–	5.24	–	17.70	0.002	0.028	0.04	0.002	0.0012
Solanum khasianum	Fruits	89	4.82	2.45	–	–	20.0	0.437	–	0.078	0.065	0.0010

Solanum nigrum L.	Fruits, leaves, tender shoots	–	17.50	21.50	20.00	–	11.00	–	0.07	0.41	–	0.0205
Solanum torvum	Leaves	76	0.56	0.95	–	–	17.6	0.415	–	0.03	0.058	0.0007
Spondias pinnata (L.f.) Kurz	Fruits	90	0.70	3.00	4.50	1.00	216.50	–	0.11	0.37	–	0.040
Syzigium cuminii (L.) Skeels	Fruits	84	0.70	0.30	14.00	0.90	442.30	0.34	0.075	0.046	0.05	0.0113
Terminalia chebula Retz.	Fruits	53	1.25	3.90	80.61	7.10	–	1.27	0.041	0.811	0.078	0.031
Vernonia anthelmintica	Leaves	85	3.55	2.29		13.65	35.29	5.20	1.10	0.41	0.021	0.005
Zanthoxylum rhetsa	Leaves	82	5.31	1.68	–	–	14.7	0.396	–	0.208	0.051	0.0028
Zingiber pardochlamys	Rhizome	89	2.8	2.26	–	–	21.4	0.258	–	0.027	0.051	0.0027
Ziziphus mauritiana Lam. {(Linn.) Gaertn.}	Fruits	82	0.80	0.30	17.00	–	50.60	1.50	0.05	0.021	–	0.430

(Ref: Anonymous 1970–1988; Duke and Atchley 1986; Kapur and Sarin 1990; Dhyani and Khali 1993; Maikhuri et al. 1994; Negi and Gaur 1994; Bokhary and Parvez 1995; Akpanyung et al. 1995; Arora and Pandey 1996; Samant and Dhar 1997; Bhardwaj et al. 2007; Deka et al. 2013; Chaudhuri et al. 2018; Ghosh et al. 2014; Payum et al. 2013a, b, 2014; Seal 2011; Seal and Chaudhuri 2015; Seal et al. 2017, Tamuly et al. 2013; Ali 2009; Pareek and Sharma 1993; Rawat and Choudhery 1998; Sundriyal and Sundriyal 2003; Tag and Tsering 2012; Tag et al. 2014).

Table 32.2 Wild edible plant of Arunachal Pradesh

Scientific name	Family	Vernacular name	Parts used	Uses
Adhatoda vasica	Acanthaceae	Ogik (Adi)	Leave	Vegetable, medicinal
Albizia procera Benth.	Mimosaceae	–	Leaves	Vegetable
Allium hookeri	Liliaceae	Losun (A)	Leaves, bulb	Vegetable, medicinal
Allium reballum M Beib.	Liliaceae	Alomana (I)	Leaves	Vegetable
Allium sativum (var) L	Liliaceae	Losun (Nishi)	Leaves, bulb	Vegetable, medicinal
Allium sativum (var) L	Liliaceae	Losun(Nishi)	Leaves	Vegetable, medicinal
Alocasia macrorrhiza (L.) Schott	Araceae	Enge (Adi)	Leaves	Vegetable, medicinal
Alternanthera sessilis R.Br.	Amaranthaceae	–	Leaves	Vegetable
Amaranthus spinosus L.	Amaranthaceae	Mora sag (N), Khotuka (Ak)	Leaves	Vegetable, medicinal
Amaranthus viridis Linn.	Amaranthaceae	Nyipak O (N)	Leaves	Vegetable, medicinal
Amomum aromaticum Roxb.	Zingiberaceae	Papia (A)	Seed	Spices
Amomum dealbatum Roxb.	Zingiberaceae	Papia (A)	Seed	Spices
Amomum subulatum roxb	Zingiberaceae	Taje (Adi)	Seed	Spices
Artocarpus chaplasha Roxb.	Moraceae	Chamin gulo (N)	Fruits	Pickle
Artocarpus heterophyllus	Moraceae	Bellang (Adi)	Fruits	Medicinal
Artocarpus lakoocha Roxb.	Moraceae	Belang (A)	Fruits	Pickle
Baccaurea sapida Muell-Arg.	Euphorbiaceae	Lateku (As)	Fruit	Taken raw
Bambusa balcooa Roxb.	Poaceae	Erbu (A)	Tender shoot	Vegetable
Bambusa tulda Roxb.	Poaceae	Bah (As)	Tender shoot	Vegetable
Basella rubra		Poi(A)	Leaves	Vegetable
Bauhinia ÿirsuteÿe L.	Caesalpiniaceae	Bah (As)	Flowers	Vegetable
Begonia josephi A.DC.	Begoniaceae	Gumbolopang (A)	Tender shoot	Taken raw
Begonia ÿirsute D. Don	Begoniaceae	Donpolapang (A), Bayia (N)	Tender shoot	Vegetable, medicinal
Begonia roxburghii A. DC.	Begoniaceae	Bayia (N), Lukhu (Ap)	Leaves, Stem	Vegetable, medicinal
Begonia chinensis (L) Willd.	Asteraceae	–	Tender leaves	Vegetable, medicinal
Bischofia javanica Blume		Sitir (Adi)	Leaves	Medicinal
Bombax ceiba L.	Bombacaceae	Semi phul (C)	Flowers	Vegetable
Calamus acanthospathus	Arecaceae	Tasar (Nishi)	Fruits	Vegetable
Calamus erectus Roxb.	Arecaceae	Tarea (N), Uhdum bizi (C)	Stem, fruits	Vegetable
Calamus flagellum Griff.	Arecaceae	Golar/Raiding (A)	Stem, fruits	Vegetable
Calamus latifolius Roxb.	Arecaceae	Golar/Raiding (A)	Stem, fruits	Taken raw
Callicarpa arborea Roxb.	Verbenaceae	Tato (N), Yaohorin (A), Poirek (C)	Bark	Mouth freshener, medicinal
Canarium strictum Roxb.	Burseraceae	Poirek gulo (C), Dhuna (Ap), Singlu (N)	Fruits	Taken raw
Cardamine ÿirsute L.	Brassicaceae	Serampeti (N)	Whole plant	Vegetable
Caryota urens L.	Arecaceae	Rani sengor (C)	Tender stem	Vegetable

Table 32.2 (continued)

Scientific name	Family	Vernacular name	Parts used	Uses
Castanopsis hystrix A. DC. (=*C. rufescens* Hk. f & Thoms.)	Fagaceae	Kora (N)	Fruits	Taken raw
Castanopsis indica A. DC	Fagaceae	Kora (N), Bazana gulo (C)	Fruits	Taken raw
Centella asiatica L.	Apiaceae	Mengoni (C), Narang (N), Glankhako (Ap)	Leaves, shoot	Vegetable, medicinal
Chenopodium album. L.	Chenopodiaceae	Machiosak (A)	Leaves, tender shoot	Vegetable
Cinnamomum tamala Nees & Ebrm.	Lauraceae	Tejpat (C)	Leaves	Spices
Citrus medica L.	Rutaceae	Jamir (C), Narang (N), Pinchi (A)	Fruits	Taken raw, medicinal
Clerodendrum colebrookianum Walp.	Verbenaceae	Poto (N), Ongin/Oin (A), Heliasak (C), Khamo (T)	Leaves	Vegetable, medicinal
Clerodendrum viscosum Vent.		Ongin/Oin/Heliasak (C)	Leaves	Vegetable, medicinal
Colocasia esculenta (L.) Schott	Araceae	Teu (T), Annyi (A), Kochu (As), Thoks (Ak)	Leaves, stem	Vegetable
Cordia myxa L.	Boraginaceae	–	Fruits	Pickle
Crassocephalum crepidioides (Benth.) S. Moore	Asteraceae	Tong phul, Thung nam (T)	Leaves, tender shoot	Vegetable, medicinal
Curcuma aromatica Salisb.	Zingiberaceae	Jangali haladhi (A)	Flower	Vegetable
Curcuma sps.	Zingiberaceae	Teeta haladhi	Flower	Vegetable
Dendrocalamus hamiltonii Nees & Arn.	Poaceae		Tender shoot	Vegetable
Dendrocalamus strictus (Roxb.) Nees.	Poaceae	Eeng	Tender shoot	Vegetable, medicinal
Dillenia indica L.	Dilleniaceae	Olu gulo (C), Champak (A)	Fruits	Taken raw, vegetable, medicinal
Dioscorea alata L.	Dioscoreaceae	Ogit (A)	Tubers	Vegetable
Dioscorea bulbifera L.	Dioscoreaceae	Uli (Adi)		Medicinal
Diospyros kaki L. f	Ebenaceae	Kesdu goch (As)	Fruits	Taken raw
Diplazium esculentum Sw.	Athyriaceae	Rukja/Horon (T), Lochanch (Ak)	Tender leaves	Vegetable
Docynia indica. Decne.	Rosaceae	–	Fruits	Taken raw
Duabanga grandiflora (Roxb. Ex DC.) Walp.	Sonneratiaceae	Hojo Gulo (C)	Fruit	Taken raw
Elaeagnus pyriformis Hk. f.	Elaeagnaceae	Maza sok bizi (C)	Fruits	Taken raw
Elaeagnus latifolia L.	Elaeagnaceae	Gamyamrap (M), Makhachi (S)	Fruits	Taken raw
Elaeocarpus floribundus Bl.	Elaeocarpaceae	Jalpai (As), Goroshi (I)	Fruits	Taken raw
Elatostema sessile Forst.	Urticaceae	–	Leaves, tender shoot	Vegetable
Emblica officinales Gaertn.	Euphorbiaceae	Amolodi (C)	Fruits	Taken raw, medicinal
Ensete superbum Cheesman	Musaceae	Colon/Kopak (A), Namninyah (S), Napkhoi (T)	Fruits, stem	Vegetable,\
Eryngium foetidum L.	Apiaceae	Ori-ritak (Adi)		Taken raw

(continued)

Table 32.2 (continued)

Scientific name	Family	Vernacular name	Parts used	Uses
Erythrina stricta Roxb.	Fabaceae	Chemroy (T)	Flowers	Vegetable
Euphorbia hirta L.	Euphorbiaceae	–	Tender plant	Vegetable
Fagopyrum esculentum Moench.	Polygonaceae	Papor (C), Hukuna (N)	Tender leaves	Vegetable, medicinal
Ficus cordata Thunberg.	Moraceae	Takuk (Adi)	Leaves	Medicinal/ vegetable
Ficus glomerata Roxb.	Moraceae	Jagana Gulo (C)	Fruits	Taken raw
Ficus hispida L. f	Moraceae	Kukto Belo (A)	Fruits	Taken raw
F. roxburghii Wall.	Moraceae	Tatuk (A)	Fruits	Taken raw
F. cunia Buch.-Ham.	Moraceae	Sorbek gulo (C)	Fruits	Taken raw
Fissistigma polyanthum Merr.	Annonaceae	Lisu gulo(C), Dardo (N)	Fruits	Taken raw
Fragaria indica Andr.	Rosaceae	–	Fruits	Taken raw
Giradina pedunculata Roxb.	Clusiaceae	Prejang bizi (A)	Fruits	Taken raw, medicinal
Girardinia zeylanica Decne.	Urticaceae	Oguma (Ak)	Leaves	Vegetable
Glochidion multiloculari		Gaam oying(A)	Leaves	Vegetable
Gnaphalium pensylvanicum Willd (=*G. purpureum* L.)	Asteraceae	Tap (N)	Leaves	Vegetable
Gynocardia odorata R.Br.	Flacourtiaceae	Toko (A)	Fruits	Vegetable
Gynura cusimbua (D. Don) S. Moore.	Asteraceae	Nakling (A) Buli/Yogin (N)	Leaves	Vegetable, medicinal
Houttuynia cordata Thunb.	Saururaceae	Amuli (I), Thingnaluk (T)	Leaves	Vegetable
Hydrocotyle sibthorpioides Lam.	Apiaceae	Killing-kiro (Adi)	Leaves	Vegetable
Ipomoea cymosa Roem. & Schult.	Convolvulaceae	Kalmau (As)	Tuber	Vegetable
Laportea crenulata Gaud	Urticaceae	Peji (Adi)	Tender leaves	Vegetable, medicinal
Ipomoea batatas	Convolvulaceae	E-phen pher	Tuber	Vegetable
Lasia spinosa Thw.	Araceae	–	Tender shoot	Vegetable
Litsea cubeba	Lauraceae	Rajil ∗Adi)	Fruits, leaves	Spice, medicinal
Livistona jenkinsiana Griff.	Arecaceae	Toko (As)	Fruits	Taken raw
Maesa indica Wall.	Myrsinaceae	Chonium (N)	Fruits	Taken raw
Mahonia napaulensis DC.	Berberidaceae	Taming (Ap)	Bark, stem, fruits	Taken raw, medicinal
Mangifera sylvatica Roxb.	Anacardiaceae	Tagol (N), Jharbuo aam (C)	Fruits	Taken raw
Melastoma malabathricum L.	Melastomaceae	Daidassa (N)	Fruits, leaves	Taken raw, medicinal
Mentha arvensis L.	Lamiaceae	Pudina (As)	Leaves	Pickle
Mesua ferrea L.	Clusiaceae	–	Fruits	Taken raw
Mimusops elengi L.	Sapotaceae	Bokul (As)	Fruits	Taken raw
Morus indica L.	Moraceae	Ashihushi (I)	Fruits	Taken raw
Morus alba L	Moraceae	Hinskai	Fruits	Vegetable, medicinal
Murraya koenigii (L.) Spreng	Rutaceae	–	Leaves	Spices
Musa balbisiana Colla	Musaceae	Kopak/Colon (A), Wegoin (Ak)	Inflorescence	Vegetable

Table 32.2 (continued)

Scientific name	Family	Vernacular name	Parts used	Uses
Musa sapientum L.	Musaceae	Kolung (Adi)	Inflorescence	Taken raw
Musa sp	Musaceae	Jharbuo kala (C)	Fruits, stem	Vegetable
Mussaendaglabra Vahl	Rubiaceae	Takshap (Adi)	Leave	Taken raw, vegetable
Mussaenda roxburghii Hk. f.	Rubiaceae	Dongkorio/Taksap (As)	Tender leaf	Vegetable
Mussaenda incana	Rubiaceae	Takshap(Adi, Nishi)	Leaves	Vegetable, medicinal
Myrica esculenta Buch.-Ham.	Myricaceae	–	Fruits	Taken raw
Oenanthe javanica (Bl.) DC.	Apiaceae	Kebunamul/Babon (N)	Leaves, tender shoot	Vegetable, medicinal
Oxalis corniculata L.	Oxalidaceae	Bangal amelia (C), Sajang Habo (N), Okhui hamang (Ap)	Leaves, stem	Vegetable, medicinal
Paederia scandens (Lour.) Merr. (=*P. foetida* L.)	Rubiaceae	Phadobas lodi (C), Tapin Rimin (N), Paritaro (Ap)	Leaves, stem, fruits	Vegetable, medicinal
Passiflora edulis Sim.	Passifloraceae	Bel (A)	Fruits, leaves	Taken raw, vegetable, medicinal
Passiflora nepalensis Wall.	Passifloraceae	Meya (As)	Fruits	Vegetable
Phlogacanthus tubiflorus Nees	Acanthaceae	Basak patta (C)	Inflorescence, leaves	Vegetable, medicinal
Phoebe cooperiana U.N Kanjilal ex A. Das	Lauraceae	Tambor (A)	Fruits	Taken raw
Pinanga gracilis (Roxb.) Blume	Arecaceae	Morizya (C), Tachar (N)	Fruits	Taken raw
Piper betleoides C. DC.	Piperaceae	Jangali pan (A)	Leaves, stem	Mouth freshener, medicinal
Piper pedicellatum C. DC.	Piperaceae	Namar (A)	Leaves, stem	Vegetable
Piper sylvaticum Roxb.	Piperaceae	–	Leaves	Vegetable
Plantago major L.	Plantaginaceae	Arisapana (I)	Leaves, stem	Vegetable, medicinal
Polygonum alatum Buch.-Ham. ex Spreng.	Polygonaceae	Mejia daro aga (C), Uyushayan (A), Ahopi (I)	Leaves, tender shoot	Vegetable
Polygonum chinense L.	Polygonaceae	Okung (A)	Leaves	Vegetable
Pouzolzia bennettiana	Urticaceae	Osik (Nishi, Adi)	Leaves	Vegetable, medicinal
Pouzolzia viminea	Urticaceae	Oyik (Apa, Nishi)	Leaves	Vegetable, medicinal
Prunus persica Batsch	Rosaceae	Amuchi (I), Kompe (A)	Fruits	Taken raw
Pyrus pashia Buch.-Ham. ex D.Don	Rosaceae	Semo (Ap)	Fruits	Taken raw
Rhus semialata Murr. (=*R. javanica* Linn.)	Anacardiaceae	Amashi (I), Tamo (Ap)	Fruits	Spices, medicinal
Rhynchotechum ellipticum	Gesneriaceae	Jooke (N)	Leaves	Vegetable
Rubus ellipticus Sm.	Rosaceae	Aingkushi (I), Nintcho (N), Komrupsiang (M)	Fruits	Taken raw
Rubus lineatus Reinw.	Rosaceae	Kada aphal (C), Chichi nintch (N), Achin barin (A)	Fruits	Taken raw

(continued)

Table 32.2 (continued)

Scientific name	Family	Vernacular name	Parts used	Uses
Rubus niveus Thunb.	Rosaceae	–	Fruits	Taken raw
Saurauia napaulensis DC.	Actinidiaceae	–	Fruits	Taken raw
Solanum indicum L.	Solanaceae	Bake (N), Fisook (Ak)	Fruits	Vegetable, medicinal
Solanum khasianum	Solanaceae	Kopir (Adi)	Leaves	Vegetable
Solanum kurzii	Solanaceae	Kopir (Adi)	Fruits	Vegetable
Solanum nigrum L.	Solanaceae	Bhul potting (C), Hor (N)	Fruits, leaves, tender shoot	Vegetable, medicinal
Solanum spirale Roxb	Solanaceae	Bangko	Fruits	Medicinal
Solanum torvum Sw.	Solanaceae	Bor bagulo (C), Akapu (Ak)	Fruits	Vegetable
Spilanthes paniculata Wall ex DC.	Asteraceae	Namlang marchang Vajungnam (T), Marcha (N) Paynson (Ak)	Tender plants	Vegetable, medicinal
Spondias axillaris Roxb.	Anacardiaceae	Ban gulo/Separisi gulo (C), Balam (N)	Fruits	Taken raw
Spondias pinnata (L.f.) Kurz	Anacardiaceae	Amara gulo (C)	Fruits	Taken raw
Syzygium cuminii (L.) Skeels	Myrtaceae	Aamun (As)	Fruits	Taken raw, medicinal
Terminalia bellirica Roxb.	Combretaceae	Bahid (N)	Fruits	Taken raw
Terminalia chebula Retz.	Combretaceae	Ohtyal gulo (C)	Fruits	Taken raw, medicinal
Trevesia palmata Vis.	Araliaceae	Togo (N)	Leaves	Vegetable
Vangueria spinosa Hook. f.	Rubiaceae	Pobon gulo (C)	Fruits	Taken raw
Vernonia anthelmintica	Asteraceae	Yugin (Nishi)	Leaves	Vegetable, medicinal
Vitis sp	Vitaceae	Tapsi gulo (C)	Fruits	Taken raw
Zanthoxylum armatum DC.	Rutaceae	Onier (N), Khagi (M), Tsogok (T), Machang (S)	Fruits	Spices, medicinal
Zanthoxylum hamiltonian Wall. Ex Hook	Rutaceae	Ombeng (Adi)	Fruits, leaves	Medicinal
Zanthoxylum oxyphyllum	Rutaceae	Honyor (N)	Leaves	Vegetable, medicinal
Zanthoxylum rhetsa	Rutaceae	Honyor(N, A)	Leaves	Vegetable, medicinal
Zingiber pardochlamys	Zingiberaceae	Red ginger(A)	Flower	Vegetable
Ziziphus mauritiana Lam.	Rhamnaceae	Makhachi (S), Tehanghat (T)	Fruits	Taken raw

Abbreviation used: *A* Adi, *As* Assamese, *Ak* Aka, *Ap* Apatani, *C* Chakma, *I* Idu Mishimi, *M* Monpa, *N* Nyshi, *S* Sinpho, *T* Tangsa

32.4 Conclusion

These wild edible plants form a good source of protein, fat, vitamins, carbohydrate and minerals and are available in the different season in a year. These species provide ecological security as they are disease resistant and grow in diverse climatic condition. Such species may be promoted for large-scale cultivation for benefit of socioeconomic condition of the tribal people. Some species like *Clerodendrum colebrookianum*, *Solanum nigrum*, *Piper pedicellatum*, *Pouzolzia bennettiana*, *Spilanthes acmella*, *Vernonia anthelmintica* and *Zanthoxylum armatum* are sold extensively in the local market of the state. For example, in the market survey, it was found that around 4.0–5.0 lakhs rupees *Piper pedicellatum* are sold in five markets of capital complex in a month in the winter season. It also needs to start research in genetic improvement, plant breeding and tissue culture on wild edible plant species. Since the nutritional value of the plant may be changed, it is also necessary to study the nutritional value in the different growth stage of the wild edible plant.

In the developing countries, 789 million people are still suffering from malnutrition especially infants and children in rural areas. Unfortunately, a large number of children in the remote area untouched by the govt. scheme launched low-cost nutritious food for school children. This type of edible plant definitely will help to overcome such type of problems. So by cultivating these plants in large scale, the plant species may be conserved as well.

Acknowledgements Thanks to Director Jorhat Assam, North East Institute of Science and Technology, for providing facilities and valuable advice.

References

Akpanyung EO, Udoh AP, Akpan EJ. Chemical composition of the edible leaves of *Pterocarpus mildbraedii*. Plant Foods Hum Nutr. 1995;48:209–15.

Ali A. Nutritional evaluation of edible *Portulaca oleracia* as plant food. Food Anal Methods. 2009;2:204–7.

Angami A, Gajurel PR, Rethy P, Singh B, Kalita SK. Status and potential of wild edible plants of Arunachal Pradesh. Ind J Tradit Knowl. 2006;5(4):541–50.

Anonymous. Wealth of India. New Delhi: CSIR; 1970–1988.

Anonymous. National Nutrition Monitoring Bureau, Report, National Institute of Nutrition. Hyderabad: Indian Council of Medical Research; 2001.

Arora RK, Pandey A. Wild edible plants of India conservation and use ICAR. New Delhi: National Bureau of Plant Genetics Resources; 1996.

Baishya AK. Studies on Ferns and Fern-allies of Arunachal Pradesh, PhD thesis. Guwahati University, Guwahati, India. 1999.

Baishya AK, Hoque S, Bora PJ, Kalita N. Flora of Arunachal Pradesh, on overview. Arunachal Forest News. 2001;19(1&2):1–25.

Bamji MS. Nutrition secure India – how do we get there? Nutrition conclave discusses the forward. Curr Sci. 2007;93(11):1473–5.

Bhardwaj R, Rai AK, Wangchu L, Sureja AK Singh D, Singh RK, Tag H. Biodiversity of edible wild plant and use in maintaining health and nutrition 7th International food data conference on Food Composition and Biodiversity at Sao Paulo, Brazil on October 21–24, 2007. http://www.fcf.usp.br/7ifdc/pdf/session02/7ifdc_session02_06_rakesh_bhardwaj.pdf.

Bokhary HA, Parvez S. Fungi inhabiting household environments in Riyadh, Saudi Arabia. Mycopathologia. 1995;130:79–87.

Chaudhuri K, Nurul Hasan SK, Barai AC, Das S, Seal T, Bag BG. Nutraceutical evaluation of *Rhynchotechum ellipticum*, a potent wild edible plant consumed by the tribal of North-Eastern region in India and green synthesis of gold nanoparticles using its leaf extract. J Pharmacog Phytochem. 2018;7(3):1434–42.

Chowdhery HJ. Arunachal Pradesh. In: Mudgal V, Hajra PK, editors. Floristic diversity and conservation strategies in India. Calcutta: BSI Publication; 1996.

Deka DC, Kumar V, Prasad C, Kumar K, Gogoi BJ, Singh L, Srivastava RB. Oroxylum indicum– a medicinal plant of North East India: an overview of its nutritional, remedial, and prophylactic properties. J Appl Pharm Sci. 2013;3(Suppl 1):S104–12.

Dhyani PP, Khali MP. Fruit yield and economics of jelly and jam production from fruits of some promising *Ficus* (fig) tree crops. Ecol Food Nutr. 1993;30:169–78.

Duke JA, Atchley A. Handbook of Proximate analysis tables of higher plants. Boca Raton, FL: CRC Press, Inc.; 1986.

Ezeagu IE, Metges CC, Proll J, Petzke KJ, Akinsoyinu AO. Chemical composition and nutritive value of some wild gathered tropical plant seeds. Food Nutr Bull. 1996;17:275–8.

Ghosh G, Gosh GC, Melkania U, Majumdar U. Traditional medicinal plants used by the Adi, Idu and Khamba tribes of Dehang-Debang biosphere Reserve in Arunachal Pradesh. Int J Agric Environ Biotechnol. 2014;7(1):165–71.

Haridasan K, Bhuyan LR, Deori ML. Wild edible plants of Arunachal Pradesh. Arunachal Forest News. 1990;8(1&2):1–8.

Joshi BS, Yili B, Puar MS. Dubose KK Pelletier SW H^1 and C^{13} NMR assignment for some pyrrolo [2,1b] Quinazoline alkaloids of *Adhatoda vasica*. J Nat Prod. 1994;57(7):953–62.

Kapur SK, Sarin YK. Flora of Trikuta Hills (Shri Vaishno Devi Shrine). Dehradun: Bishen Singh Mahendra Pal Singh; 1990.

Maikhuri RK. Nutritional value of some lesser known wild food plants and their role in tribal nutrition: a case study in Northeast India. Trop Sci. 1991;31:397–405.

Maikhuri RK, Semwal RL, Singh A. Nautiyal Wild fruits as a contribution to sustainable rural development: a case study from the Garhwal Himalaya. Int J Sust Dev World Eco. 1994;1:56–68.

Negi KS, Gaur RD. Principal wild edible plants of Western Himalaya, Uttar Pradesh, India. In: Gupta BK, editor. Higher Plants of Indian Subcontinent, vol. III. Dehradun: Bishen Singh Mahendra Pal Singh; 1994. p. 1–78.

Negi KS, Tiwari JK, Gaur RD, Pant KC. Notes on ethnobotany of five districts of Garhwal Himalaya, Uttar Pradesh, India. Ethnobotany. 1993;5:73–81.

Pareek OP, Sharma S. Under-utilized fruits. Indian Hortic. 1993;38:47–56.

Payum T, Das AK, Shankar R, Tamuly C, Hazarika M. Ethnobotany and antioxidant determination of *Phoebe cooperiana* fruit- a highly utilized wild fruit in Arunachal Pradesh, India. Int J Pharm Sci Res. 2013a;4(8):3196–201.

Payum T, Das AK, Tamuly C, Shankar R, Hazarika M. Antioxidant potential of *Solanum kurzii* Br. berry: a folk medicinal food berry used in Arunachal Pradesh, North East India. Global J Med Res. 2013b;13(6):1–6.

Payum T, Das AK, Shankar R. Nutraceutical folk food plants used among indigenous people of east Siang district of Arunachal Pradesh, India. Am J Pharm Tech Res. 2014;4(4):696–704.

Radimer K, Bindwald B, Hughes J, Ervin SC, Picciano MF. Dietary supplement use by US adults- date from the National Health & Nutritional examination survey 1999–2000. Am J Epidermiol. 2004;260(4):339–49.

Rawat RS, Choudhery S. Ethno Medico Botany of Arunachal Pradesh (Nishi and Apatani Tribes). Dehradun: Bishen Singh Mahendra Pal Singh; 1998.

Rukachaisirikul T, Prabpal S, Kongsaeree P, Suksamran A. (+)- Bornyl Piperate, a New Monoterpene Ester from *Piper* aff. *Pedicellatum* Roots. Chem Pharm Bull. 2004;52(6):760–1.

Samant SS, Dhar U. Diversity, endemism and economic potential of wild edible plants of Indian Himalaya. Int J Sust Develop World Eco. 1997;4:179–91.

Seal T. Determination of nutritive value, mineral contents and antioxidant activity of some wild edible plants from Meghalaya State, India. Asian J Appl Sci. 2011;4(3):238–46.

Seal T, Chaudhuri K. Antioxidant activities of five wild edible fruits of Meghalaya State in India and effect of solvent extraction system. Int J Pharma Sci Res. 2015;6(12):5134–40.

Seal T, Pillai B, Chaudhuri K. Evaluation of nutritional potential of five unexplored wild edible plants consumed by the tribal people of Arunachal Pradesh state in India. J Food Nutr Res. 2017;5(1):1–5.

Singh HB, Arora RK. Wild edible plants of India. 1st ed. New Delhi: ICAR Publication; 1978.

Sundriyal RC, Sundriyal M. Wild edible of the Sikkim Himalaya: nutritive values of selected species. Econ Bot. 2001;55(3):377–99.

Sundriyal M, Sundriyal RC. Underutilized edible plant of Sikkim Himalaya: need for domestication. Curr Sci. 2003;85(6):731–6.

Sundriyal M, Sundriyal RC. Wild edible plant of Sikkim Himalaya: marketing, value addition and implication for management. Econ Bot. 2004;58(2):300–15.

Tag H, Tsering J. Ethnobotanical Study and Nutritional Analysis on Middle and High Altitude Wild Edible flora of West Kameng and Tawang Sector of Arunachal Pradesh for defence Food Security. Technical Report, DRL, Defence Research Laboratory, Defence R&D Organization, Ministry of Defence, Post Bag No. 2, Tezpur-Assam 784001 (India). 2012. p. 3–98.

Tag H, Tsering J, Hui PK, Gogoi BJ, Veer V. Nutritional potential and traditional uses of high altitude wild edible plants in eastern Himalayas, India. Int J Nutr Food Eng. 2014;8(3):238–43.

Tamuly C, Saikia B, Hazarika M, Bora J, Bordoloi MJ, Sahu OP. Correlation between phenolic, flavonoid, and mineral contents with antioxidant activity of underutilized vegetables. Int J Veg Sci. 2013;19:34–44.

Vijayakumari K, Siddhuraja P, Janardhanan K. Nutritional assessment and chemical composition of the lesser known tree legumes, *Acacia leucophloea*. Food Chem. 1994;50:285–8.

Part V

Herbal Medicine—Validation, Quality Control & IPR Issues

Herb-Drug Interactions: Focus on Adverse Drug Reactions and Pharmacovigilance of Herbal Medicines

33

Kuppusamy Asokkumar
and Subramaniam Ramachandran

Contents

Asokkumar Kuppusamy and Ramachandran Subramaniam contributed equally to this work.

K. Asokkumar (✉)
Department of Pharmacology, College of Pharmacy, Sri Ramakrishna Institute of Paramedical Sciences, Coimbatore, Tamil Nadu, India

S. Ramachandran
Pharmacology Section, Pharmacopoeia Commission for Indian Medicine & Homoeopathy, PLIM Campus, Post Kavi Nagar, Ghaziabad, Uttar Pradesh, India

S. Sen, R. Chakraborty (eds.), *Herbal Medicine in India*,
https://doi.org/10.1007/978-981-13-7248-3_33

33.1 Introduction

The consumption of medicinal herbs and herbal product(s) or medicine(s) is increasing in developing and developed countries (Bodeker 1995; Shaw et al. 2012). Centuries ago, medicinal plants or herbs were used to prevent and treat the diseases before emergence of modern medicine (Sheeja et al. 2006). Industrialisation and urbanisation in the last century decreased the use of medicinal plants or herbs. But in last two decades, the medicinal plants consumption has increased significantly for various ailments. World Health Organization (WHO) stated that about 70% of the world population currently uses medicinal herbs as complementary or alternative medicine (Wills et al. 2000). Consumption rate of herbal products is increasing consistently in United States of America, Canada and Europe. The highest sale of herbal products has been reported in France and Germany. Herbal medicines (HM) are used in the treatment of various diseases or indication by different age groups. Studies revealed that 45% of parents give herbal medicines to children and 45 and 67% of women use herbs in pregnancy and for premenopausal symptoms, respectively (Fasinu et al. 2012).

According to WHO, herbal medicines include herbs, herbal materials, herbal preparations and finished herbal products. Herbs include crude plant material and all parts of herbs, fresh juices, oils, resin, gums and dry powder of herbs. The powdered herbal materials, tinctures, extracts and fatty oils of herbal materials are basis of herbal preparations. Finished herbal products consist of herbal preparations made from one or more herbs, and the mixture herbal products in addition to the active ingredients may also contain excipients. The traditional use of herbal medicines refers to the extensive historical use and is generally recognised to be safe and effective, and national authorities may have accepted its use (WHO 2004a).

Although consumer's common belief of "natural" always means "safe" and medicines obtained from natural source are harmless, the toxic in nature of few medicinal plants are too. The herbal medicines may produce side effects which might be adverse in nature. Most commonly, adverse events/effects are reported on herbal products/medicines due to quality issues. It may occur due to adulteration of herbal medicines with various drug substances like corticosteroids, cardiac tonics, antihistaminic and nonsteroidal anti-inflammatory drugs. The reasons for the adverse events are use of wrong species of medicinal plants, doses, medication errors at the time of dispensing by healthcare professionals and use of consumers, drug interaction, presence of heavy metals, microorganism and residues of pesticide (WHO 2004b).

HM use in the prevention and treatment of diseases as an alternative and/or together with conventional therapies is observed as common practice, and it is a one of the important areas of interest in research field to ensure the safety during concomitant use. In the developing countries, a significant proportion of the people depends on herbs or herbal medicine for primary healthcare need. For example, alternative medicines used in some parts of Africa was estimated as 80%, and concomitant use of herbs with conventional medicines in the United States was estimated at 20–30%. The survey in Nigeria reveals that conventional medicines are used along with herbs by 46% of diabetes mellitus patients, 39.1% of hypertensive patients and 65% of cancer patients. The regulations are not stringent to prove the safety, efficacy or quality of herbal remedies or medicines in many countries due to false belief that natural herbs are harmless. But it is reported in regular practice that herbs are not free from side, toxic or adverse effects and interaction with herbs or conventional drug (Ondieki et al. 2017).

Polypharmacy is a major complex issue for the inappropriate prescribing of drugs and adverse reactions/adverse drug reactions (ADR) and adverse events or experience or adverse drug event (ADE). The drug-drug interaction (DDI) or herb-drug interaction (HDI) occurs due to polypharmacy and poor awareness or a lack of coordination of patients and healthcare providers. Studies reported that 19.2% of Turkish elderly, 16% of US population and 14.1% of Taiwanese take herbal medicines and supplements along with prescription drug. About 14–16% of

American adults and 49.4% of Israeli population are reported to be habitual in concomitant use of herbal and conventional medicine (Giveon et al. 2004). About less than 40% of patients disclose use of herbal medicines or supplement to healthcare professionals, but unawareness of potential risks of HDIs is noticed with physicians. Although the awareness of the potential of HDIs is increased, healthcare providers and consumers are finding difficulties to take rational decisions for the safe use of herbal and conventional medicines due to absence of significant wide clinical data in different population (Fasinu et al. 2012).

33.2 Adverse Drug Reactions

WHO defines ADR is a response to a drug that is noxious and unintended, and that occurs at doses normally used in humans for the prophylaxis, diagnosis or therapy of disease or for the modification of physiological function. An unexpected adverse reaction is an adverse reaction, the nature or severity of which is not consistent with domestic labelling or market authorisation or expected from the characteristics of the drug. The adverse event/experience (AE) is defined as any untoward medical occurrence that may present during treatment with a pharmaceutical product but that does not necessarily have a causal relationship with this treatment. The serious adverse event (SAE) is any untoward medical occurrence that at any dose results in death, requires inpatient hospitalisation or prolongation of existing hospitalisation and results in persistent or significant disability/incapacity and life-threatening condition. But the side effect is defined as any unintended effect of a pharmaceutical product occurring at doses normally used in humans that is related to the pharmacological properties of the drug. ADR classified as Type A (acute/augmented), Type B (bizarre/idiosyncratic), Type C (chronic/cumulative) and Type D (delayed onset) are classified well in conventional medicine usage, and same may also be applied to herbal medicines (WHO 2004b; Shaw et al. 2012).

The safety and efficacy of herbs or herbal medicines is mostly based on practical experience, and immediate or acute toxicity of herbal medicines may be identified effectively within hours or days due to faster onset of toxic symptoms. But traditional knowledge or experience is not sufficient to effectively identify the herbs or herbal medicines' mediated idiosyncratic, chronic, cumulative or delayed life-threatening ADR and drug interaction with concomitant administered herbs or herbal medicines or conventional medicines. Specifically, administration of herbal medicines to elder and children needs more attention to identify the ADR. Since it is commonly believed that herbs or herbal medicines are safe, the first signs of the ADR may not be recognised properly after the intake or stopping its use. A good example for chronic toxicity (Type C) is nephropathy induced by aristolochic acid and its cumulative and delayed renal symptoms noticed after 2 years of withdrawal of the intake of herbs (Zhang et al. 2012; Gujjarlamudi 2016).

The countries such as Germany, UK, USA, Australia and Canada have banned the species of *Aristolochia* since the phytoconstituent present in it causes aristolochic acid nephropathy and high incidence for the occurrence of upper urinary tract cancer. It was initially reported in a Belgian cohort study which was carried out on 100 patients after the consumption of slimming tablets containing *Aristolochia fangchi* (Chinese herb) as one of the herb. The exposure to species of *Aristolochia* in traditional Chinese medicines and its use revealed a significant incidence of upper urothelial cancer in Taiwan. *Aristolochia indica* L. is commonly used in India and Bangladesh, and its possible association between chronic interstitial and upper urothelial cancer fibrosis in both country populations is undiagnosed. Similar to *Aristolochia* species, ADRs of many of the plant species or herbal medicines is required to monitor continuously with proper documentation to ensure the safety and have to make it as an integral part of the worldwide regulation of herbal medicines (Michl et al. 2013).

33.3 Pharmacovigilance and Herbal Medicine

WHO stated that pharmacovigilance (PV) is the science and activities relating to the detection, assessment, understanding and prevention of adverse effects of drugs or any other possible drug-related problems. An important goal of PV is the safe and proper use of effective medicines of all types (WHO 2004b). PV focuses on following areas:

1. Herbals
2. Traditional and complementary medicines
3. Blood products
4. Biologicals
5. Medical devices
6. Vaccines

Apart from above areas, PV looks at the issues which are important to science as follows:

1. Substandard medicines
2. Medication errors
3. Lack of efficacy reports
4. Use of medicines for indications that are not approved and for which there is inadequate scientific basis
5. Case reports of acute and chronic poisoning
6. Assessment of drug-related mortality
7. Abuse and misuse of medicines
8. Adverse interactions of medicines with chemicals, other medicines and food

PV specifically aims to:

1. Improve patient care and safety in relation to the use of medicines and all medical and paramedical interventions
2. Improve public health and safety in relation to the use of medicines
3. Contribute to the assessment of benefit, harm, effectiveness and risk of medicines, encouraging their safe, rational and more effective (including cost-effective) use
4. Promote understanding, education and clinical training in pharmacovigilance and its effective communication to the public

The above aims of PV may be achieved by:

1. Early detection of previously unknown adverse reactions and interactions
2. Detection of increases in frequency of (known) adverse reactions
3. Identification of risk factors and possible mechanisms underlying adverse reactions
4. Estimation of the quantitative aspects of benefit/risk and analysis and dissemination of the information needed to improve the prescription, dispensing, provision and regulation of medicines

33.3.1 Pharmacovigilance Systems and Safety Monitoring of Herbal Medicines

Safety of drugs in any form for herbal medicines and herbal products is a fundamental principle of use and quality control. The regulatory and ethnic differences in the preparation and use of various types of medicines may vary, but it is equally important to monitor safety of medicines including herbal medicines and products. Pharmacovigilance on herbal medicines is important due to its wide use and acceptance throughout the world. The worldwide consumption of herbal medicines is enormous so that in terms of population exposure alone, it is essential. The monitoring of the safety of herbal medicines is important for the benefit of public health and to identify the risks associated with their use. Herbal medicines are concomitantly taken with other medicines, and hence it is important to assess and understand the problems of any adverse effects arising. WHO guidelines for setting up and running pharmacovigilance centre provide practical technical guidance on safety monitoring of herbal medicines within PV systems (WHO 2002, 2004b).

33.3.2 Sources of Adverse Drug Reports of Herbal Medicine

The source of reports for the ADR and AE is important in the view of quality of report but not on its source according to the recommendation of Council for International Organizations of Medical Sciences (CIOMS) Working Group V. The basis for the quality reports are systematic preparation, documentation, recording of data, follow-up and justified and analysed data. The clinical trials (CT) and voluntary/spontaneous reports are utmost common sources for the information of ADR and AE of the medicines. In the case of herbal medicine, according to national circumstances, it is essential to encourage the prescribers, dispensers, consumers and others to report the ADR, AE and SAE (WHO 2004b).

Globally, ADR reporting system in post-marketing surveillance set-up is based on the voluntary report through healthcare professionals who have direct relationship with the care of the patient/consumer. The considerable quantity of herbal medicines is sold directly as non-prescription medicines without previous documented post-marketing safety data unlike conventional/allopathic medicines. In this scenario, the community pharmacists and nurses may play a predominant role as source for the report of safety of non-prescription medicines including herbal medicines. The positive value needs to provide for the concern of consumers about the possible ADR/AE/SAE of herbal medicines and herbal products. It is essential to accept the adverse reaction report submitted by consumer as serious source of information, and it may be first useful signal for the unknown effects of herbal medicines (WHO 2004b).

The adverse reaction is also obtained from manufacturers of herbal medicines, and it is an important source of reporting points. The manufacturers can collect the ADR/SE/SAE information of the HM from consumer and healthcare professionals through their representative as well as conducting of various industry and educational programmes. It may be helpful to identify the new signal or signals not reported through voluntary reporting system. The national poisons centre, drug information centres and consumer organisations are other important source of report for the adverse reactions of herbal medicines (WHO 2004b).

33.3.3 Specific Area for Safety Monitoring of Herbal Products

The safety monitoring of herbal product may be divided in the following categories for the complete coverage:

1. According to their regulatory status
   (a) Herbal medicines in the prescription medicines category
   (b) Herbal medicines in the non-prescription medicines category
   (c) Other herbal products intended for use in healthcare
2. According to their registration/marketing status
   (a) Herbal medicines undergoing the new drug development process: in clinical trials prior to national drug regulatory approval
   (b) Herbal medicines undergoing the new drug development process: under post-marketing safety surveillance
   (c) Herbal medicines undergoing re-evaluation under the current protocol: in clinical trials
   (d) Herbal medicines undergoing re-evaluation under the current protocol: under post-marketing safety surveillance
   (e) Herbal medicines on the market: under post-marketing safety surveillance
   (f) Other herbal products marketed for healthcare, such as dietary supplements

The report of adverse events occurring in CT is explained in national guidelines on good clinical practice for trials on pharmaceutical products (WHO 1995, 2004b).

33.3.4 Reporting of Herbal Medicine-Suspected Adverse Reactions

The details of reporting of herbal medicine mediated suspected adverse reactions such as network of various PV centres, status of person identifying the adverse reaction and their reporting centre and elements required to document in the case report form including model reporting form for suspected adverse reactions, how to report and mode of report. It also covers coding of adverse events or adverse reactions and therapeutic classification proposed by Uppsala Monitoring Centre (UMC), data links for the herbal substances and other reporting issues related to PV activities are available in "WHO Guideline on Safety Monitoring of Herbal Medicines in Pharmacovigilance System" (http://apps.who.int/medicinedocs/en/m/abstract/Js7148e/).

33.3.5 Evaluation of Case Report and Data Management of Adverse Reaction of Herbal Medicine

The details of method and basis for the assessment of individual case report, standard approach for causality assessment, detection of signals at national and international level, role of advisory committee, methods for the analysis of basis of suspected adverse reactions, use of technical expertise and data management of adverse reactions of herbal medicines are available in "WHO Guideline on Safety Monitoring of Herbal Medicines in Pharmacovigilance System" (http://apps.who.int/medicinedocs/en/m/abstract/Js7148e/).

33.4 Mechanism of HDIs

The biotransformation is an important action of physiological system of human to convert the drug from one form to another form. The HDI may be occurring due to overlapping of herbal medicines or allopathic drugs or its metabolites to bind to the receptors or enzymes. The two major mechanism of HDI is pharmacokinetic and pharmacodynamic nature. These effects lead to changes in the efficacy (pharmacodynamic) of the herbal medicines. Similarly, intrusion in the absorption (A), distribution (D) and competition in the metabolism (M) and elimination (E) pathways may lead to change in the ADME (pharmacokinetic) of herbs or herbal medicines (Fasinu et al. 2012; Marchetti et al. 2007; Izzo 2005). Both aspects of HDI are explained in following section.

33.4.1 Pharmacokinetic and HDI

The induction or inhibition of cytochrome P450 (CYP) metabolic enzymes of hepatic and intestine is a main underlying mechanism of pharmacokinetic HDI. The efflux proteins and drug transporters like P-glycoprotein are also reported in many cases of HDI. The bioavailability of drugs affected by P-glycoprotein (P-gp) and presystemic effect of CYP also influence co-administered herbal medicine effects and lead to lower or higher levels of affected drugs in blood. The low molecular substrates transport wide range of substance via organic anion transporters (OATs) which are member of the solute carrier family SLC22A (Fasinu et al. 2012). The drugs such as antibiotics, angiotensin-converting enzyme (ACE) inhibitors, diuretics and antivirals are excreted via OAT1 and OAT3 which are almost completely expressed in the kidney and accountable for the renal secretion (Burckhardt 2012). OAT3 is essential for the replication of influenza A virus, and its inhibitor is effective in limiting influenza A virus infection. Therefore, OAT1 and OAT3 are considered as therapeutic targets for hypertension and influenza A infection. The compounds obtained from herbal medicine, *Salviae miltiorrhizae Radix et Rhizoma,* such as lithospermic acid, rosmarinic acid, salvianolic acid A, salvianolic acid B, tanshinol and anthraquinones in rhubarb, inhibiting human OAT1 and OAT3, are good examples for HDI on transporters (Wang and Sweet 2012; Ma et al. 2014).

33.4.1.1 Phase I Metabolising Enzymes and HDI

The enzyme CYP1A2 is responsible for the metabolism of almost 20% of the available therapeutic drug and is mainly found in the liver (15%). The commonly used drugs such as acetaminophen (analgesic), propranolol (antihypertension), clomipramine (antidepressant) and warfarin (anticoagulant), which are substrates of CYP1A2 phase I enzyme, showed pharmacokinetic interaction with herbal drugs. For example, paracetamol (acetaminophen) is metabolised via CYP1A2, CYP3A4 and CYP2E1 and produce toxic compound N-acetyl-*p*-benzoquinone (NAPQI). It is detoxified by conjugation with glutathione in normal conditions, and intake of overdose of paracetamol increases this metabolic route and it becomes saturated. Hence, increased production of NAPQI allows it to bind to proteins resulting in damage of liver and finally produces cell death. The induction of CYP1A2 occurs after the intake of *Allium sativum* and *Curcuma longa* with paracetamol due to the accumulation of NAPQI which leads to increased toxicity. At the same time the intake of *Phyllantus amarus*, *Mormodica charantia*, *Eucalyptus globulus*, *Glycine max*, *Harpagophytum procumbens*, *Mentha piperita*, *Trifolium pratense* and *Punica granatum* with paracetamol may reduce the NAPQI levels due to inhibition of CYP1A2 enzyme (Wang and Zhou 2009; Lee et al. 2001).

The CYP2C9 is isoform CYP2C, and approximately 15% of drug is metabolised by this enzyme. For example, drugs such as ibuprofen (nonsteroidal anti-inflammatory drugs), losartan (antihypertensive), fluoxetine (antidepressant), phenytoin (antiepileptic) and fluvastatin (antihypercholesterolemic drug) are metabolised by CYP2C9. The CYP2C9 also metabolise the endogenous bioactive substances like steroids, melatonin, retinoids and arachidonic acid. Ibuprofen is commonly used to treat pain and inflammation, and it is metabolised by CYP2C9 to active metabolite (*S*)-ibuprofen. Herbal species such as *Allium sativum*, *Eucalyptus globulus*, *Harpagophytum procumbens*, *Mentha piperita*, *Punica granatum*, *Trifolium pratense* and *Zingiber officinale* are substrates for CYP2C9 may inhibit the (*S*)-ibuprofen formation and it leads to therapeutic failure. Similarly, the metabolism of losartan, fluoxetine, phenytoin and fluvastatin is also affected by concomitant use of above-mentioned plants by inhibition of biotransformation of drugs (Berka et al. 2011; Baxter and Stockley 2008; Mo et al. 2009).

The commonly used drugs such as omeprazole (antiulcer), amitriptyline and fluoxetine (antidepressant), diazepam and phenobarbital (sedative and hypnotic) and almost 10% of the clinical drugs are metabolised by CYP2C19. The concomitant intake of *Allium sativum*, *Eucalyptus globulus*, *Mentha piperita* and *Trifolium pratense* with above drugs noticed to inhibit CYP2C19 enzyme. The CYP2D6 metabolises about 25% of clinical drugs such as timolol and propafenone (beta blocker), amitriptyline (antidepressant), chlorpheniramine (antihistamine) and haloperidol and risperidone (antipsychotic). The polymorphism on CY2D6 is commonly reported, and it may influence the metabolism of drugs. Likewise, concomitant intake of *Eucalyptus globulus*, *Harpagophytum procumbens, Mentha piperita*, *Phyllanthus amarus*, *Punica granatum* and *Trifolium pratense* has shown inhibition of CYP2C19 enzyme in preclinical studies. The enzyme CYP2E1 is involved in the metabolism of ethanol and activation of some carcinogens, procarcinogens and toxicants to low molecular weight compounds. The use of *Allium sativum*, *Momordica charantia*, *Phyllanthus amarus*, *Phyllanthus urinaria* and *Punica granatum* reduces the CYP2E1 levels and activity in the liver, and hence concomitant intake of medicine would alter its therapeutic effect (Zhou et al. 2009; Mazzari and Prieto 2015).

The enzyme CYP3A metabolises greater than 50% of clinical drugs which exists in isoform CYP3A4, CYP3A5 and CYP3A7. This family of CYP3A is involved in the metabolism of macrolide antibiotics, antiarrhythmics, benzodiazepines, immunomodulators, HIV antivirals, antihistamines, calcium channel blockers and HMG-CoA reductase inhibitors. It was reported that *Uncaria tomentosa* inhibits CYP3A4 which leads to increase in the minimum effective concentration (C_{min}) values of antiretroviral agents and increased the risk of toxicity of anti-HIV drugs. The preclinical pharmacokinetic study revealed that *Allium sativum* increases the half-life of atorvastatin (HMG-CoA reductase inhibitor) in rats by inhibition of CYP3A4 (Zhou et al.

Table 33.1 Pharmacokinetic interaction of herbal/herbal medicine with phase 1 drug metabolic enzymes

		Phase I enzymes					
S. no	Herbal/herbal medicine	CYP1A2	CYP2C9	CYP2C19	CYP2D6	CYP2E1	CYP3A
1.	*Allium sativum*	+	–, +	–	NE	–	NE, – (CYP3A4,5,7)
2.	*Curcuma longa*	+	–	NR		NE	NE (CYP3A4)
3.	*Eucalyptus globulus*	–	NR	–	–	NR	– (CYP3A4)
4.	*Glycine max*	–	NR	NR		NE	NR
5.	*Harpagophytum procumbens*	NE, –	NE, –	NE	NE, –	NR	NE, – (CYP3A4)
6.	*Mentha piperita*	–	–	–	–	–	– (CYP3A4)
7.	*Phyllanthus amarus*	–	NR	NR	–	–	– (CYP3A4,5,7)
8.	*Punica granatum*	–	–	NR	–	–	– (CYP3A4,5,7)
9.	*Trifolium pratense*	–	–	–	–	–	– (CYP3A4)
10.	*Zingiber officinale*	NR	–	NR	NR	–	CYP3A4
11.	*Phyllanthus urinaria*	NR	NR	NR	NR	–	NR
12.	*Chamomilla recutita*	NR	NR	NR	NR	NR	– (CYP3A4)
13.	*Foeniculum vulgare*	NR	NR	NR	NR	NR	– (CYP3A4)
14.	*Mormodica charantia*	NR	NR	NR	NR	NR	– (CYP3A4)
15.	*Uncaria tomentosa*	NR	NR	NR	NR	NR	– (CYP3A4)

(+) indicates enzyme induction; (–) indicates enzyme inhibition; *NE* no effect, *NR* no report

2009; Mazzari and Prieto 2015).The pharmacokinetic interaction of herbal medicine on induction and/or inhibition of phase 1 metabolic enzymes has been given in Table 33.1.

33.4.1.2 Phase II Drug-Metabolising Enzymes and HDI

The conjugation or phase II biotransformation occurs when metabolites (active/inactive drug) formed during phase 1 metabolism interact with functional groups of phase II metabolic enzymes. Generally, the metabolite (active/inactive drug) will be converted to water-soluble form to facilitate the elimination process of drug. The glutathione conjugation and glucuronidation are major pathways, and sulfonation, methylation and acetylation are other relevant phase 2 metabolism pathways for drugs which include plant medicines. The formation of toxic metabolite, N-acetyl–*p*–benzoquinone (NAPQI), occurs due to action of phase I enzymes in liver during biotransformation of acetaminophen. As happened with phase I, the conjugation of glutathione with NAPQI occurs in normal conditions to detoxify, and overdose of acetaminophen augments this metabolic route and it becomes saturated. The excess formation of NAPQI leads to binding to proteins and damage liver cells. The plants mentioned in Table 33.3 either inhibit or increase the glutathione levels when in concomitant administration with acetaminophen (Mazzari and Prieto 2015).

The uridine diphosphate glucuronosyltransferases (UGTs) are vital enzymes in phase 2 reactions which catalyses the drug or metabolite of phase 1 reaction during glucuronidation in the liver. The drugs containing chemical groups such as alcohols, hydroxyl amines, phenols, amines, sulphonamides, carboxylic acids and thiols would undergo conjugation reaction. For example, phase 1 metabolite of ibuprofen predominantly undergoes glucuronidation pathway. The *Allium sativum* induced the UGTs expression and *Curcuma longa* inhibited the UGTs expression in liver which leads to alteration of the pharmacokinetic profile of this class of drugs apart from glucuronidation (Mazzari and Prieto 2015).The pharmacokinetic interaction of herbal medicine on induction and/or inhibition of phase 2 enzyme (UGTs) and interference is given in Table 33.2.

33.4.1.3 Transporter and HDI

The oral bioavailability of drugs is affected by human drug efflux transporters acting alone or together with drug-metabolising enzymes. The transporters ATP binding cassette (ABC) are found in kidney, intestinal epithelium, liver and endothelium of blood capillaries of brain which

Table 33.2 Pharmacokinetic interaction of herbal/herbal medicine with phase 2 enzymes

S. no	Herbal/herbal medicine	Phase 2 enzymes	
		Glutathione levels	Glucuronidation (UGT level)
1.	*Achillea millefolium*	–	NR
2.	*Aloe vera/Aloe barbadensis*	–, +	NR
3.	*Allium sativum*	+	+
4.	*Anacardium occidentale*	+	NR
5.	*Baccharis trimera*	–	NR
6.	*Bauhinia forficate*	–	NR
7.	*Bauhinia variegate*	+	NR
8.	*Calendula officinalis*	+	NR
9.	*Chamomilla recutita*	+	NR
10.	*Croton cajucara*	+	NR
11.	*Cynara scolymus*	+, NE	NR
12.	*Curcuma longa*	+	–
13.	*Foeniculum vulgare*	+	NR
14.	*Glycine max*	+	NR
15.	*Mentha piperita*	+	NR
16.	*Mentha pulegium*	+	NR
17.	*Mikania glomerata*	NE	NR
18.	*Mormodica charantia*	+	NR
19.	*Phyllanthus amarus*	+	NR
20.	*Phyllanthus niruri*	+	NR
21.	*Punica granatum*	–, +	NR
22.	*Psidium guajava*	+	NR
23.	*Ruta graveolens*	+	NR
24.	*Zingiber officinale*	+, NE	NR

(+) indicates enzyme induction; (–) indicates enzyme inhibition; *NE* no effect, *NR* no report

affect efflux of drug and change the concentration gradient of it. A significant alteration of absorption of drugs administered by oral route occurred due to drug's return back to gastrointestinal tract lumen by utilisation of ATP as an energy source through P-glycoprotein (P-gp) and repeated exposure to enterocyte metabolism producing decreased bioavailability of drugs. Thus, P-gp plays crucial role in the regulation of ADME of clinically important therapeutic substance. The herbal drug or its constituents may modulate P-gp and can cause induction of efflux of drugs either by competitive or non-competitive inhibition. The herbal drugs or its phytoconstituents mediated inhibition of ATP binding and coupling or hydrolysis of ATP-hydrolysed molecules leading to depletion of energy needs for the P-gp-bound substrate drugs translocation (Mamindla et al. 2016).

The xenobiotics crosses biological membrane through drug transporter proteins like P-gp, and its action results in alteration of pharmacokinetic property of drugs. The *Achillea millefolium* inhibits P-gp and *Allium sativum* activates P-gp, and this may affect the concomitantly administered drug's bioavailability and action. The drug saquinavir (HIV-protease inhibitor) is a substrate of CYP3A4 and absorbed in the intestine through P-gp. The induction of P-gp activity by garlic extracts can reduce the bioavailability of concomitantly administered vital drugs (Williamson et al. 2009).

The natural products such as paclitaxel, vinca alkaloids (vincristine), anthracyclines (doxorubicin), camptothecins (topotecan) and epipodophyllotoxins (teniposide) possess high levels of resistance to P-gp. The Alisol B23-acetate of *Alisma orientalis* increased vinblastine, doxorubicin and rhodamine-123 anticancer action via reduction of efflux activity of P-gp confirmed by *in vitro* studies in MDR cell lines. Grapefruit juice (*Citrus paradisi*) inhibited P-gp rhodamine-123 efflux *in vitro* in Caco-2 cells and in healthy volunteers. It also increased nifedipine bioavailability in rats and talinolol in Caco-2 cells. The catechins of green tea (*Camellia sinensis*) modulate P-gp transport through either inhibition or activation by heterotopic allosteric mechanism. The daunorubicin and rhodamine-123 inhibited 6-gingerol through P-gp-mediated efflux of KB-C2 cells. The *Ginkgo biloba* (ginkgo) extract significantly reduced P-gp activity was noticed in *in vitro* or *in vivo* studies (Mamindla et al. 2016).

The other transporters such as multi-drug resistance-associated protein-2 (MRP2) and breast cancer resistance protein (BCRP) are ABC subfamily members. The MRP2 is located in the bile canalicular membrane of hepatocytes, and BCRP, ABC gene, is recognised as placenta-specific. But little data is available on these transporters for HDI than P-gp. The grape juice also modulates MRCP2 and BRCP apart from P-gp. The *in vitro* assay using MCF-7, M-X100 cells showed genistein, biochanin A, pigenin and kaempferol from *Silybum marianum* increase the BCRP substrate mitoxantrone accumulation by inhibition of BCRP. At the same time, BCRP does not confer resistance to vinca alkaloids, epipodophyllotoxins, paclitaxel or cisplatin (Mamindla et al. 2016).

Apart from above transport proteins, the solute carrier transporters such as OATs, organic anion-transporting polypeptides (OATPs) and organic cation transporters (OCTs) mediate the substrates uptake in cells and influence oral bioavailability of concomitantly administered drugs and hepatobiliary, intestinal and renal excretion of drugs. The furanocoumarin phytoconstituents, naringin, from *Citrus paradisi* inhibited the influx or uptake active transporter OATP1A2 *in vitro*, and it may affect the bioavailability of drugs. The *in vitro* studies reveal that catechin and epigallocatechin inhibiting OATPB might inhibit the bioavailability of concomitantly administered drug (Kalliokoski and Niemi 2009).

The effect of 172 extracts (hexane, dichloromethane, n-butanol and aqueous) prepared from 37 medicinal plants was studied on OATP1 and OATP3 by *in vitro* using HEK293 cells. The effect of 172 extracts on transporters with 6-carboxylfluorescein (6-CF) uptake in HEK-OAT1 and HEK-OAT3 cells has been reported. The three hexane extracts (*Achillea biebersteinii, Chaerophyllum bulbosum, Symphytum asperum*), 17 dichloromethane extracts (*Anchusa azurea, Camphorosmalessingii, Chaerophyllum bulbosum, Echium russicum, Elaeagnus orientalis, Glycyrrhiza glabra, Hypericum scabrum, Juncus effusus, Juniperus oblonga*, *Melandrium album, Polygonum hydropiper, Primula macrocalyx, Solanum dulcamara, Stachys lavandulifolia, Symphytum asperum, Zygophyllum fabago*), 12 n-butanol extracts (*Anchusa azurea, Artocarpus altilis, Chaerophyllum bulbosum, Echium russicum, Glycyrrhiza glabra, Hypericum scabrum, Juniperus oblonga, Mentha longifolia, Scutellaria orientalis, Symphytum asperum, Thymus kotschyanus, Zygophyllum fabago*) and 1 aqueous extract (*Thymus kotschyanus*) showed inhibitory effects on both OAT1 and OAT3. Therefore, clinical use of conventional drugs with above said plants may cause HDI, and it may affect pharmacokinetic of either conventional drug or herbal drug (Lu et al. 2017).

As of now, no much clinical data is available on herb-drug interactions via transporter, but significant *in vivo* and *in vitro* studies to support the possibility of HDI via transporters were reported. These data may be useful to initiate the pharmacovigilance on transporters which may influence in HDI and to document clinical data.

33.4.2 Pharmacodynamic and HDI

The synergistic, inhibitory and/or additive effect of herbal products during concomitant administration of conventional medications can occur due to interaction with common binding sites of receptor and may serve as the basis of HDI. The pharmacodynamic (PD) interactions are those herbal medicine and conventional drug interactions leading to cause changes in pharmacological responses of drugs (Ma et al. 2009). Clinical data (Zhang et al. 2017) on PD-HDI has given in Table 33.3 and Table 33.4.

Table 33.3 Clinical data of pharmacodynamic interaction of herbal medicine with conventional drug

S. no.	Herbal medicine	Conventional drug	Effect
1.	Free and easy wanderer plus (Chinese herbal medicine)	Carbamazepine	Combination of both can improve the tolerability of carbamazepine (i.e., significantly lower discontinuation rate, fewer side effects, and low level of serum carbamazepine) in the 26-week treatment of mood disorders.
2.	Shakuyaku-kanzo-to (traditional Japanese herbal medicine)	Antipsychotic	Combination of both during two-week treatment decreased the extrapyramidal symptoms of antipsychotic drugs.

Table 33.3 (continued)

S. no.	Herbal medicine	Conventional drug	Effect
3.	Aqueous extract of saffron	Olanzapine	Administration of aqueous extract of saffron for 12 weeks can prevent metabolic syndrome and increases in blood glucose in schizophrenia patients on olanzapine treatment.
		Fluoxetine	Treatment of saffron (15 mg, b.i.d.) for 4 weeks can improve fluoxetine-related sexual dysfunction among the patients with major depressive disorder.
4.	*Ginkgo biloba* extract 360 mg daily	Haloperidol	*Ginkgo biloba* extract (360 mg OD) administration for 12 weeks significantly enhanced the efficiency of haloperidol (0.25 mg/kg/day) in schizophrenia patients on their positive symptoms.
5.	Cranberry juice	Warfarin	A significant increase in sensitivity of healthy subjects to warfarin noticed with administration of cranberry juice concentrate capsule for 2 weeks (1000 mg t.i.d.) without influencing the pharmacokinetics of warfarin enantiomers. So careful monitoring of warfarin blood level is important, if both administered together.
6.	*Ginkgo biloba* extract	Iodine-131	Treatment of *Ginkgo biloba* extract (120 mg OD) for 1 month can protect from possible oxidative and genotoxic damage associated with iodine-131 therapy reported in 10 patients with thyroid cancer, without any adverse modification of the clinical outcome. But further large study is required.
7.	*Rhizoma notoginseng* extract	Aspirin	Synergistic action was noticed by combined intake of aspirin (50 mg/day) with *Rhizoma notoginseng* extract (sanchi tong shu capsule 200 mg t.i.d.) in patients with light and moderate ischemic stroke in acute and subacute stages.
8.	Bergamot polyphenolic fraction	Rosuvastatin	An enhanced rosuvastatin effect on low-density lipoprotein cholesterol (LDL-C), lipoxygenase-1 expression and protein kinase B phosphorylation was noticed in patients with hyperlipidaemia with administration of oral bergamot polyphenolic fraction (1000 mg OD) for 30 days. It reduced daily dose of rosuvastatin for achieving the target levels of cholesterol.
9.	Total ginsenosides	Ulinastatin	Total ginsenosides are major components of Shenmai injection which contains red ginseng and *Radix ophiopogonis*. It is widely used for treating coronary heart disease, organ protection and adjunct therapy to tumour chemotherapy. Co-administration of Shenmai injection (100 ml b.i.d. for 7 days) can effectively synergise with intravenous ulinastatin (100,000 units t.i.d.) against septic acute lung injury and acute respiratory distress syndrome.
10.	Fuzheng Yiliu decoction	Chemotherapy	Oral administration of Fuzheng Yiliu decoction 3 days before chemotherapy and lasting to the end of 2 cycles of chemotherapy enhanced therapeutic effects on malignant gastrointestinal tumour of chemotherapy and reduce the toxic and side effects on bone marrow and digestive tract.
11.	St. John's wort	Oral contraceptive	The co-administration of *Hypericum perforatum* increased intra-cyclic bleeding episodes, adversely affected compliance to oral contraceptives and decreased 3-keto-desogestrel concentration in serum. It may possibly increase the risk of unintended pregnancies. But no evidence for the effect of *Hypericum perforatum* and oral contraceptive on health female. A caution is required when combined use of above plants with oral contraceptives.
		Atorvastatin or simvastatin	A significant increase of LDL-C serum level and total cholesterol was noticed in hypercholesterolemic patients receiving atorvastatin or simvastatin compared with control during co-administration of St. John's wort product b.i.d. for 4 weeks at least 3 months. The efficacy of both drugs was reduced, and it may not administer with *Hypericum perforatum*.

33.5 Monitoring the Safety of Herbal Medicines and Its Challenges

The challenges associated with monitoring the safety of herbal medicines in regulatory aspects, quality assurance and control procedures [Good manufacturing practices (GMP) and good agricultural and good collection practices (GACP)] as well as standards for herbal materials mentioned in the national or regional pharmacopoeias are available in "WHO Guideline on Safety Monitoring of Herbal Medicines in Pharmacovigilance System" (http://apps.who.int/medicinedocs/en/m/abstract/Js7148e/). It also covers the role of herbal drugs providers in monitoring the safety of herbal medicines, lack of proper knowledge about herbal medicine and its concomitant use with other system of medicine and conventional medicines, attitudes of the patient or consumer about herbal medicine (i.e. natural means safe) and self-medication with other food or health products.

33.5.1 Other Practical Key Issues of Herbal Medicines

The ecological origin (soil, climate, photoperiod), genotype, various plant parts (stems, leaves, root bark and root), harvesting time (time of day, season and year), storage conditions, processing and extraction of herbs, combinations of herbs and/or its processing as medicines can influence and arise safety or lack of efficacy issues due to variation of quality and quantity of phytoconstituents in the herbs. An intrinsic variability of single herbal ingredient can result in product that may be relatively altered and may not be essentially bioequivalent. A careful assessment on variation or resemblance of the chemistry or biological activity may be needed at the time of combining reports of ADR or efficacy (Shaw et al. 2012).

Major changes may be adopted in various aspects of procedures followed in herbal drug manufacture to enhance the pharmacological action and to produce quick onset of drug action, and this could limit time factor and pave way to practice of herbal medicines. The effect of use of herbal drugs followed by ancient eternities has to be further strengthened, and this may change patient attitude towards quick relief from diseases and would enhance the traditional treatment procedure. The pesticides are commonly used in the cultivation of medicinal plants for the commercial purpose, and analysis of pesticide content is important during the selection of raw material to avoid safety issues. The substitution and adulteration of medicinal plants with view of equal potency and non-availability of medicinal plants will affect the quality, safety and efficacy of herbal medicines. The safety issues of herbal medicines are also reported due to presence of heavy metal, and it needs special attention to identify and detect excess amount of these metals to avoid/reduce ADR and have to be documented. The safety issues of herbal medicines arise due to the open market availability of combinations of herbs through over the counter (OTC) and prescription of herbal medicines by non-registered vaidya or experienced persons. The above factors have considerable role in the ADR of herbal medicines which is not well documented due to absence or stringent non-implementation of regulation in many countries.

33.6 Clinical Data on Herb-Drug Interactions

Herbal medicines involved in drug interactions with conventional drugs during consumption or studied in pharmacokinetic trials are given in Table 33.4 according to the therapeutic category of conventional drugs. There are many interactions reported with limited clinical significance, and a few herbs, especially St. John's wort (*Hypericum perforatum*), may aggravate AE from serious to life-threatening condition. Therefore pharmacovigilance (safety monitoring) on herbal medicines or drugs is vital to prevent the potential interactions with conventional drugs; specifically, narrow therapeutic index conventional drugs are prescribed to the patients.

Table 33.4 Clinical data on herbal-drug interactions

S. no	Herbal/herbal medicine name	Prescribed/conventional drug	Reported HDI[a]	Mechanism/scientific reason[a]	Reference
Anticoagulant					
1.	*Peumus boldus*	Warfarin	Increased anticoagulant effect	Anticoagulant action due to coumarins from *Peumus boldus*	Lambert and Cormier (2001)
2.	*Matricaria recutita*	Warfarin	Bleeding	Anticoagulant action due to coumarins from *Matricaria recutita*	Segal and Pilote (2006)
3.	*Chlorella pyrenoidosa*	Warfarin	Decreased anticoagulant effect	Vitamin K present in *Chlorella pyrenoidosa* may inhibit warfarin effect	Ohkawa et al. (1995)
4.	*Vaccinium macrocarpon*	Warfarin	Enhanced anticoagulant effect and fatal haemorrhage	Yet to be established	Griffiths et al. (2008)
5.	*Salvia miltiorrhiza*	Warfarin	Increased anticoagulant effect	Additive effect, but need to be established	Chan (2001)
6.	*Angelica sinensis*	Warfarin	Increased anticoagulant effect	Anticoagulant action due to coumarins from *Angelica sinensis*	Page and Lawrence (1999)
7.	*Trigonella foenum-graecum*	Warfarin	Increased anticoagulant effect	Anticoagulant action due to coumarins from *Trigonella foenum-graecum*	Lambert and Cormier (2001)
8.	*Panax quinquefolius* (American ginseng)	Warfarin	Decreased anticoagulant effect	Yet to be established	Yuan et al. (2004)
9.	*Lycium barbarum* (Chinese wolfberry)	Warfarin	Increased anticoagulant effect	Yet to be established	Leung et al. (2008); Lam et al. (2001)
10.	*Camellia sinensis*	Warfarin	Decreased anticoagulant effect	Vitamin K present in *Camellia sinensis* may inhibit warfarin effect	Taylor and Wilt (1999)
11.	*Grifola frondosa*	Warfarin	Increased anticoagulant effect	Yet to be established	Hanselin et al. (2010)
12.	*Glycine max*	Warfarin	Decreased anticoagulant effect	Yet to be established	Cambria-Kiely (2002)
13.	*Hypericum perforatum*	Warfarin	Increased clearance of warfarin and decreased anticoagulant effect	PKI	Jiang et al. (2004)
14.	*Allium sativum*	Fluindione	Decreased anticoagulant effect of fluindione	Yet to be established	Pathak et al. (2003)
Anti-HIV drugs					
15.	*Uncaria tomentosa*	Atazanavir, ritonavir, saquinavir	Increased blood concentration of the drugs	Yet to be established	López Galera et al. (2008)
16.	*Allium sativum*	Ritonavir	Severe gastrointestinal toxicity	Yet to be established	Laroche et al. (1998)
		Saquinavir	Decreased blood concentration of saquinavir	Reduction of saquinavir absorption due to induction of P-glycoprotein in the gut (PKI)	Piscitelli et al. (2002)

(continued)

Table 33.4 (continued)

S. no	Herbal/herbal medicine name	Prescribed/conventional drug	Reported HDI[a]	Mechanism/scientific reason[a]	Reference
17.	*Ginkgo biloba*	Efavirenz	Virologic failure due to reduction of blood concentration of efavirenz	Yet to be established	Wiegman et al. (2009)
18.	*Hypericum perforatum*	Lamivudine	Enhanced HIV RNA viral load	Yet to be established	Zhou et al. (2007)
		Nevirapine	Decreased blood concentration of nevirapine	Induction of intestinal CYP3A (PKI)	de Maat et al. (2001)
		Indinavir	Decreased blood concentration of indinavir	Induction of CYP34A by St. John's wort may be a reason for interaction (PKI)	Piscitelli et al. (2000)
Anaesthetic					
20.	*Aloe vera*	Sevoflurane	Blood loss in surgery	Additive effect on platelet function and its mechanism yet to be established (PKI)	Lee et al. (2004)
21.	*Hypericum perforatum*	Anaesthetics	Delayed emergence	Use of *Hypericum perforatum* needs to be discontinued before the 2 or 3 weeks surgery	Irefin and Sprung (2000)
Anticholinergic					
22.	*Areca catechu*	Procyclidine	Bradykinesia, rigidity, jaw tremors	Antagonistic action due to arecoline from *Areca catechu* (PDI)	Deahl (1989)
Sedative and hypnotics					
23.	*Salvia miltiorrhiza*	Midazolam	Higher blood concentration of midazolam	Induction of CYP3A4 (PKI)	Qiu et al. (2010)
24.	*Hydrastis canadensis*	Midazolam	Increased blood concentration of midazolam	Induction of CYP3A4 (PKI)	Gurley et al. (2005b)
25.	*Piper methysticum*	Alprazolam	Lethargic and disoriented state	Yet to be established	Almeida and Grimsley (1996)
26.	*Passiflora incarnata*	Lorazepam	Dizziness, hand tremor, throbbing and muscular fatigue	Additive CNS-depressant effect, but yet to be established (PKI)	Carrasco et al. (2009)
27.	*Schisandra sphenanthera*	Midazolam	Midazolam concentration increased in blood	Augmented oral bioavailability of midazolam (PKI)	Xin et al. (2009)
28.	*Hypericum perforatum*	Alprazolam	Decreased blood concentration of alprazolam	Yet to be established	Markowitz et al. (2003)
		Midazolam	Increased blood concentration of midazolam	Induction of intestinal and possibly hepatic CYP3A4(PKI)	Gurley et al. (2005b)
		Zolpidem	Decreased zolpidem concentration in blood	Increased CYP3A4 activity (PKI)	Hojo et al. (2011)
29.	*Valeriana officinalis*	Lorazepam	Dizziness, hand tremor, throbbing and muscular fatigue	Additive CNS-depressant effect (PDI)	Carrasco et al. (2009)

Antipsychotic, antidepressant and anxiolytic drugs					
30.	*Oenothera biennis*	Fluphenazine	Seizure	Seizure threshold lowered due to gamolenic acid present in *Oenothera biennis* (PKI)	Holman and Bell (1983)
31.	*Ginkgo biloba*	Risperidone	Priapism	Priapism is a serious adverse effect of antipsychotic medications and both drugs possess vasodilating action (PDI)	Lin et al. (2007)
		Trazodone	Coma	Yet to be established	Galluzzi et al. (2000)
32.	*Panax ginseng*	Phenelzine	Sleeplessness, tremor and headaches	Yet to be established	Shader and Greenblatt (1988); Jones and Runikis (1987)
33.	*Piper methysticum*	Paroxetine	Lethargic state	Yet to be established	Rubin et al. (2006)
34.	*Hypericum perforatum*	Amitriptyline	Decreased blood concentration of amitriptyline	Interaction due to induction of CYP3A4 and/or induction of P-gp, but yet to be established (PKI)	Johne et al. (2002)
		Bupropion	Orofacial dystonia	Both inhibit dopamine reuptake due to additive effects on dopaminergic transmission (PDI)	Milton and Abdulla (2007)
		Bupropion	Decreased blood concentration of bupropion	PKI	Lei et al. (2010)
		Buspirone	Serotonin syndrome, hypomanic episode	Additive action on 5-HT uptake (PDI)	Dannawi (2002)
		Paroxetine	Serotonin syndrome	Additive action on 5-HT uptake (PDI)	Gordon (1998)
		Venlafaxine	Serotonin syndrome	Additive action on 5-HT uptake (PDI)	Borrelli and Izzo (2009)
		Sertraline	Serotonin syndrome	Additive action on 5-HT uptake (PDI)	Barbenel et al. (2000)
		Nefazodone	Serotonin syndrome	Additive action on 5-HT uptake (PDI)	Lantz et al. (1999)
CNS stimulants					
35.	*Curcuma longa*	Caffeine	Synergism of CYP2A6 action/ antagonism of CYP1A2 action	PKI	Chen et al. (2010)
Antidiarrhoeal agents					
36.	*Valeriana officinalis*	Loperamide	Acute delirium	Yet to be established	Khawaja et al. (1999)
Analgesic, anti-inflammatory and antipyretic agents					
37.	*Allium sativum*	Paracetamol	Changes in paracetamol pharmacokinetic variables	No clinical significance	Gwilt et al. (1994)

(continued)

Table 33.4 (continued)

S. no	Herbal/herbal medicine name	Prescribed/conventional drug	Reported HDI[a]	Mechanism/scientific reason[a]	Reference
38.	*Ginkgo biloba*	Aspirin	Spontaneous hyphema	No clinical significance	Rosenblatt and Mindel (1997)
		Ibuprofen	Fatal intracerebral haemorrhage	No clinical significance	Meisel et al. (2003)
39.	*Hibiscus sabdariffa*	Paracetamol	Alteration in pharmacokinetic parameters of acetaminophen	Clinical significance is uncertain	Kolawole and Maduenyi (2004)
Antihypertensive drugs					
40.	*Ginkgo biloba*	Talinolol	Increased blood concentration of talinolol	Talinolol is a P-glycoprotein probe, yet to be established (PKI)	Fan et al. (2009a)
41.	*Mentha piperita*	Felodipine	Increased blood concentration of felodipine	May be CYP3A4 inhibition (PKI)	Dresser et al. (2002)
42.	*Schisandra chinensis*	Talinolol	Increased blood concentration of talinolol	Inhibition of P-gp in humans (PKI)	Fan et al. (2009a)
43.	*Hypericum perforatum*	Ephedrine, phenylephrine	Decreased responsiveness to vasopressor	Yet to be established	Irefin and Sprung (2000)
		Talinolol	Decreased blood concentration of talinolol	Talinolol is a P-gp probe, yet to be established (PKI)	Schwarz et al. (2007)
		Verapamil	Decreased blood concentration of verapamil	Induction of intestinal CYP3A4 (PKI)	Borrelli and Izzo (2009)
		Nifedipine	Decreased blood concentration of nifedipine	Induction of intestinal CYP3A4 (PKI)	Tannergren et al. (2004)
44.	*Hydrastis canadensis*	Debrisoquine	Decreased debrisoquine urinary recovery ratio	Inhibition of CYP2D6 (PKI)	Gurley et al. (2005a, b)
45.	*Commiphora wightii*	Diltiazem, propranolol	Decreased diltiazem and propranolol area under the curve and peak plasma concentration	Yet to be established	Dalvi et al. (1994)
Antihyperlipidaemic drugs					
46.	*Camellia sinensis*	Simvastatin	Increased simvastatin levels in blood associated with statin intolerance	Minor effects of green tea on simvastatin metabolising CYP3A4 (PKI)	Werba et al. (2008)
47.	*Hypericum perforatum*	Atorvastatin	Reduction of atorvastatin efficacy	Induction of CYP3A4 and/or P-gp (PKI)	Andrén et al. (2007)
		Rosuvastatin	Reduced efficacy of rosuvastatin	Reduction of blood levels of rosuvastatin (PKI)	Gordon et al. (2009)
		Simvastatin	Decreased blood concentration of simvastatin	Induction of CYP3A4 and/or P-gp by *Hypericum perforatum* (PKI)	Sugimoto et al. (2001)

Antiulcer drugs					
48.	*Ginkgo biloba*	Omeprazole	Reduction of omeprazole and omeprazole sulphone in blood concentrations	Omeprazole is a CYP2C19 probe, but mechanism is yet to be established (PKI)	Yin et al. (2004)
49.	*Hypericum perforatum*	Omeprazole	Decreased blood concentration of omeprazole	Induction of CYP2C19 by *Hypericum perforatum* (PKI)	Wang et al. (2004a, b)
50.	*Glycyrrhiza glabra*	Omeprazole	Reduction of plasma concentration of omeprazole	Glycyrrhizin of *Glycyrrhiza glabra* induces CYP3A4 and catalysed sulfoxidation of omeprazole	Tu et al. (2010)
Antidiabetic agents					
51.	*Allium sativum*	Chlorpropamide	Hypoglycaemia	Intake of karela may be responsible of the interaction	Aslam and Stockley (1979)
52.	*Ginkgo biloba*	Tolbutamide	Possible decreased blood concentration of tolbutamide	Tolbutamide is a substrate of CYP2C9 and its interaction is uncertain	Uchida et al. (2006)
53.	*Opuntia polyacantha*	Glipizide and metformin	Hypoglycaemic effect	Additive hypoglycaemic effect, but yet to established (PDI)	Sobieraj and Freyer (2010)
54.	*Hypericum perforatum*	Gliclazide	Decreased blood concentration of gliclazide	Yet to be established	Xie et al. (2005)
55.	*Momordica charantia*	Metformin, glibenclamide	Hypoglycaemic effect	Synergism with oral hypoglycaemics and potentiates their hypoglycaemia in type 2 diabetes	Tongia et al. (2004)
56.	Trigonella foenum-graecum	Sulfonylurea	Hypoglycaemic effect	Combined therapy with sulfonylureas drug lower the blood glucose level and reason yet to be established	Lu et al. (2008)
Anticonvulsants					
57.	*Hypericum perforatum*	Mephenytoin	Levels of mephenytoin metabolites increased in urinary excretion	CYP2C19 induction by *Hypericum perforatum* (PKI)	Wang et al. (2004a, b)
58.	*Ginkgo biloba*	Phenytoin and valproic acid	Fatal seizure	Yet to be established	Kupiec and Raj (2005)
Muscle relaxants					
59.	*Allium sativum*	Chlorzoxazone	Reduction of serum ratio of 6-hydroxychlorzoxazone/ chlorzoxazone	Inhibition of CYP2E1 by *Allium sativum* (PKI)	Gurley et al. (2002)
60.	*Piper methysticum*	Chlorzoxazone	Reduction of serum ratio of 6-hydroxychlorzoxazone/ chlorzoxazone	Inhibition of CYP2E1 by *Piper methysticum* (PKI)	Gurley et al. (2005a, b)

(continued)

Table 33.4 (continued)

S. no	Herbal/herbal medicine name	Prescribed/conventional drug	Reported HDI[a]	Mechanism/scientific reason[a]	Reference
61.	*Hypericum perforatum*	Chlorzoxazone	Increased serum hydroxychlorzoxazone/ chlorzoxazone ratios	Induction of CYP2E1 by *Hypericum perforatum* and induction high in younger than elder patients (PKI)	Gurley et al. (2005a, b)
Immunosuppressants					
62.	*Hypericum perforatum*	Tacrolimus	Decreased blood concentration of tacrolimus	CYP3A4 and/or P-gp induction by *Hypericum perforatum* (PKI)	Dresser et al. (2003)
		Prednisone	Manic episode	Concomitant drugs may influence, but no clinical significance in PKI both together administration	Saraga and Zullino (2005)
		Cyclosporine	Reduction of cyclosporine concentration in blood	Serious and potentially fatal interactions and well documented. Induction of CYP3A4 and/or P-glycoprotein by *Hypericum perforatum* (PKI)	Breidenbach et al. (2000)
63.	*Schisandra sphenanthera*	Tacrolimus	Increased tacrolimus concentration in blood	Inhibition of CYP3A4 (PKI)	Jiang et al. (2010)
64.	Red yeast rice (produced by fermentation process)	Cyclosporine	Rhabdomyolysis	Red yeast rice contains natural statins (CYP3A4 substrates) and its blood concentration may be theoretically increased by cyclosporine (inhibitor of CYP3A4)	Prasad et al. (2002)
65.	*Berberis aristata*	Cyclopsorine A	Combined administration of berberine elevated cyclosporine A concentration in the blood of renal transplant recipients	Combined administration of berberine may permit reduction of cyclosporine A dosage possibly due to inhibition of CYP3A4 in liver and/or small intestine by berberine (PKI)	Wu et al. (2005)
Anticancer drugs					
66.	*Hypericum perforatum*	Imatinib	Decreased blood concentration of imatinib	Induction of CYP3A4 by *Hypericum perforatum* may be responsible for interaction (PKI)	Frye et al. (2004)
		Irinotecan	Decreased levels of active metabolite (SN-38) of irinotecan in blood	Induction of CYP3A4 by *Hypericum perforatum* may be responsible for interaction (PKI)	Mathijssen et al. (2002)
67.	*Viscum album*	Busulfan	Organ fibrosis and death	Yet to be established	Gutsch (1982)
68.	*Panax ginseng*	Imatinib	Hepatotoxicity	Both drugs elevated liver enzymes levels and mechanism yet to be established	Bilgi et al. (2010)

Vitamins					
69.	*Camellia sinensis*	Folic acid	Decreased blood concentration of folate	Reduction of C_{max} and AUC of folate by green and black tea (PKI)	Alemdaroglu et al. (2008)
Antimalarial drugs					
70.	*Hibiscus sabdariffa*	Chloroquine	Reduction of chloroquine concentration in blood	Reduction of AUC and C_{max} of chloroquine. Mechanism yet to be established (PKI)	Mahmoud et al. (1994)
Antiparkinsonian agents					
71.	*Piper methysticum*	Levodopa	Reduced efficacy of levodopa	Dopamine antagonism (PDI), but yet to be established	Schelosky et al. (1995)
Antiprotozoals					
72.	*Silybum marianum*	Metronidazole	Decreased blood concentration of metronidazole	Yet to be established (PKI)	Rajnarayana et al. (2004)
Cardiotonic drugs and other cardiac drugs					
73.	*Hypericum perforatum*	Digoxin	Decreased blood concentration of digoxin	Digoxin is a P-gp substrate, but pharmacokinetics of digoxin not altered with extracts contains low hyperforin (PKI)	Mueller et al. (2004)
		Ivabradine	Decreased blood concentration of ivabradine	Induction of CYP3A4 by *Hypericum perforatum*	Portolés et al. (2006)
Antimigraine drugs					
74.	*Hypericum perforatum*	Eletriptan	Serotonin syndrome	Concomitant use of *Hypericum perforatum*, eletriptan and fluoxetine may inhibit 5-HT reuptake and development of serotonin syndrome possibly due to eletriptan which binds to $5\text{-HT}1_D$ and $5\text{-HT}1_B$ receptors (PDI)	Bonetto et al. (2007)
Antihistaminic					
75.	*Hypericum perforatum*	Fexofenadine	Decreased blood concentration of fexofenadine	Fexofenadine is a P-gp substrate; exact mechanism need to be established	Bonetto et al. (2007)
76.	*Hypericum perforatum*	Methadone	Decreased blood concentration of methadone	*Hypericum perforatum* mediated induction of CYP3A4 and/or P-gp (PKI)	Eich-Höchli et al. (2003)

(continued)

Table 33.4 (continued)

S. no	Herbal/herbal medicine name	Prescribed/conventional drug	Reported HDI[a]	Mechanism/scientific reason[a]	Reference
Oral contraceptive and steroid drugs					
77.	*Hypericum perforatum*	Oral contraceptive	Reduction of efficacy due to altered PK of oral pill leads to increased bleeding	CYP3A4 induction by *Hypericum perforatum* (PKI) may be a reason for interaction. No PKI was observed in clinical trial with low hyperforin extract and oral contraceptive	Pfrunder et al. (2003); Murphy et al. (2005)
		Tibolone	Acute hepatitis	Yet to be established	Etogo-Asse et al. (2008)
Antifungal drugs					
78.	*Hypericum perforatum*	Voriconazole	Transient increase followed by a decreased blood concentration	PKI (CYP2C19 substrate)	Rengelshausen et al. (2005)
Antitubercular drugs					
79	*Carum carvi*	Fixed dose combination containing rifampicin, isoniazid and pyrazinamide	Increase in plasma levels of rifampicin, isoniazid and pyrazinamide	Possible due to *Carum carvi* influence on the P-glycoprotein	Choudhary et al. (2014); Sachin et al. (2009)

[a]Details of other drug or herbal medicine or food administered with conventional drug may influence the reported HDI or/and possible scientific reason/mechanism of HDI can be obtained from given reference. *PKI* pharmacokinetic interaction, *PDI* pharmacodynamic interaction, *CT* clinical trial

References

Alemdaroglu NC, Dietz U, Wolffram S, Spahn-Langguth H, Langguth P. Influence of green and black tea on folic acid pharmacokinetics in healthy volunteers: potential risk of diminished folic acid bioavailability. Biopharm Drug Dispos. 2008;29:335–48.

Almeida JC, Grimsley EW. Coma from the health food store: interaction between kava and alprazolam. Ann Intern Med. 1996;125:940–1.

Andrén L, Andreasson A, Eggertsen R. Interaction between a commercially available St John's Wort product (Movina) and atorvastatin in patients with hypercholesterolemia. Eur J Clin Pharmacol. 2007;63:913–6.

Aslam M, Stockley IH. Interaction between curry ingredient (karela) and drug (chlorpropamide). Lancet. 1979;1:607.

Barbenel DM, Yusufi B, O'Shea D, Bench CJ. Mania in a patient receiving testosterone replacement post orchidectomy taking St John's Wort and sertraline. J Psychopharmacol. 2000;14:84–6.

Baxter K, Stockley IH. Stockley's drug interactions: a source book of interactions, their mechanisms, clinical importance, and management. Chicago: Pharmaceutical Press; 2008.

Berka K, Hendrychova T, Anzenbacher P, Otyepka M. Membrane position of ibuprofen agrees with suggested access path entrance to cytochrome P450 2C9 active site. J Phys Chem A. 2011;115:11248–55.

Bilgi N, Bell K, Ananthakrishnan AN, Atallah E. Imatinib and *Panax ginseng:* a potential interaction resulting in liver toxicity. Ann Pharmacother. 2010;44:926–8.

Bodeker G. Traditional health systems: policy, biodiversity, and global interdependence. J Altern Complement Med. 1995;1:231–43.

Bonetto N, Santelli L, Battistin L, Cagnin A. Serotonin syndrome and rhabdomyolysis induced by concomitant use of triptans, fluoxetine and hypericum. Cephalalgia. 2007;27:1421–3.

Borrelli F, Izzo AA. Herb-drug interactions with St John's Wort *(Hypericum perforatum):* an update on clinical observations. AAPS J. 2009;11:710–27.

Breidenbach T, Hoffmann MW, Becker T, Schlitt H, Klempnauer J. Drug interaction of St John's Wort with cyclosporin. Lancet. 2000;355:1912.

Burckhardt G. Drug transport by Organic Anion Transporters (OATs). Pharmacol Ther. 2012;136: 106–30.

Cambria-Kiely JA. Effect of soy milk on warfarin efficacy. Ann Pharmacother. 2002;36:1893–6.

Carrasco MC, Vallejo JR, Pardo-de-Santayana M, Peral D, Martín MA, Altimiras J. Interactions of *Valeriana officinalis* L. and *Passiflora incarnata* L. in a patient treated with lorazepam. Phytother Res. 2009;23:1795–6.

Chan TY. Interaction between warfarin and danshen *(Salvia miltiorrhiza).* Ann Pharmacother. 2001;35:501–4.

Chen Y, Liu WH, Chen BL, Fan L, Han Y, Wang G, Hu DL, Tan ZR, Zhou G, Cao S, Zhou HH. Plant polyphenol curcumin significantly affects CYP1A2 and CYP2A6 activity in healthy, male Chinese volunteers. Ann Pharmacother. 2010;44:1038–45.

Choudhary N, Khajuria V, Gillani ZH, Tandon AR, Arora E. Effect of *Carum carvi*, a herbal bioenhancer on pharmacokinetics of antitubercular drugs: a study in healthy human volunteers. Perspect Clin Res. 2014;5:80–4.

Dalvi SS, Nayak VK, Pohujani SM, Desai NK, Kshirsagar NA, Gupta KC. Effect of gugulipid on bioavailability of diltiazem and propranolol. J Assoc Physicians India. 1994;42:454–5.

Dannawi M. Possible serotonin syndrome after combination of buspirone and St John's Wort. J Psychopharmacol. 2002;16:401.

Deahl M. Betel nut-induced extrapyramidal syndrome: an unusual drug interaction. Mov Disord. 1989;4:330–2.

Dresser GK, Wacher V, Wong S, Wong HT, Bailey DG. Evaluation of peppermint oil and ascorbyl palmitate as inhibitors of cytochrome P4503A4 activity *in vitro* and *in vivo*. Clin Pharmacol Ther. 2002;72:247–55.

Dresser GK, Schwarz UI, Wilkinson GR, Kim RB. Coordinate induction of both cytochrome P4503A and MDR1 by St John's Wort in healthy subjects. Clin Pharmacol Ther. 2003;73:41–50.

Eich-Höchli D, Oppliger R, Golay KP, Baumann P, Eap CB. Methadone maintenance treatment and St John's Wort-a case report. Pharmacopsychiatry. 2003;36:35–7.

Etogo-Asse F, Boemer F, Sempoux C, Geubel A. Acute hepatitis with prolonged cholestasis and disappearance of interlobular bile ducts following tibolone and *Hypericum perforatum* (St John's Wort). Case of drug interaction? Acta Gastroenterol Belg. 2008;71:36–8.

Fan L, Mao XQ, Tao GY, Wang G, Jiang F, Chen Y, Li Q, Zhang W, Lei HP, Hu DL, Huang YF, Wang D, Zhou HH. Effect of *Schisandra chinensis* extract and *Ginkgo biloba* extract on the pharmacokinetics of talinolol in healthy volunteers. Xenobiotica. 2009a;39:249–54.

Fan L, Tao GY, Wang G, Chen Y, Zhang W, He YJ, Li Q, Lei HP, Jiang F, Hu DL, Huang YF, Zhou HH. Effects of *Ginkgo biloba* extract ingestion on the pharmacokinetics of talinolol in healthy Chinese volunteers. Ann Pharmacother. 2009b;43:944–9.

Fasinu PS, Bouic PJ, Rosenkranz B. An overview of the evidence and mechanisms of herb-drug interactions. Front Pharmacol. 2012;3:69. https://doi.org/10.3389/fphar.2012.00069.

Frye RF, Fitzgerald SM, Lagattuta TF, Hruska MW, Egorin MJ. Effect of St John's Wort on imatinib mesylate pharmacokinetics. Clin Pharmacol Ther. 2004;76:323–9.

Galluzzi S, Zanetti O, Binetti G, Trabucchi M, Frisoni GB. Coma in a patient with Alzheimer's disease taking low dose trazodone and *Gingko biloba*. J Neurol Neurosurg Psychiatry. 2000;68:679–80.

Giveon SM, Liberman N, Klang S, Kahan E. Are people who use "natural drugs" aware of their potentially harmful side effects and reporting to family physician? Patient Educ Couns. 2004;53:5–11.

Gordon JB. SSRIs and St John's Wort: possible toxicity? Am Fam Physician. 1998;57:950.

Gordon RY, Becker DJ, Rader DJ. Reduced efficacy of rosuvastatin by St John's Wort. Am J Med. 2009;122:e1–2.

Griffiths AP, Beddall A, Pegler S. Fatal haemopericardium and gastrointestinal haemorrhage due to possible interaction of cranberry juice with warfarin. J R Soc Promot Heal. 2008;128:324–6.

Gujjarlamudi HB. Polytherapy and drug interactions in elderly. J Midlife Health. 2016;7(3):105–7.

Gurley BJ, Gardner SF, Hubbard MA, Williams DK, Gentry WB, Cui Y, Ang CY. Cytochrome P450 phenotypic ratios for predicting herb-drug interactions in humans. Clin Pharmacol Ther. 2002;72:276–87.

Gurley BJ, Gardner SF, Hubbard MA, Williams DK, Gentry WB, Cui Y, Ang CY. Clinical assessment of effects of botanical supplementation on cytochrome P450 phenotypes in the elderly: St John's Wort, garlic oil, *Panax ginseng* and *Ginkgo biloba*. Drugs Aging. 2005a;22:525–39.

Gurley BJ, Gardner SF, Hubbard MA, Williams DK, Gentry WB, Khan IA, Shah A. *In vivo* effects of goldenseal, kava kava, black cohosh, and valerian on human cytochrome P450 1A2, 2D6, 2E1, and 3A4/5 phenotypes. Clin Pharmacol Ther. 2005b;77:415–26.

Gutsch J. On the state of therapy of chronic myeloid leukemia in adults with the mistletoe preparation Helixor. Ärztezeitschrift für Naturheilverfahren. 1982;23:523–44.

Gwilt PR, Lear CL, Tempero MA, Birt DD, Grandjean AC, Ruddon RW, Nagel DL. The effect of garlic extract on human metabolism of acetaminophen. Cancer Epidemiol Biomark Prev. 1994;3:155–60.

Hanselin MR, Vande Griend JP, Linnebur SA. INR elevation with maitake extract in combination with warfarin. Ann Pharmacother. 2010;44:223–4.

Hojo Y, Echizenya M, Ohkubo T, Shimizu T. Drug interaction between St John's Wort and zolpidem in healthy subjects. J Clin Pharm Ther. 2011;36:711–5.

Holman CP, Bell AFJ. A trial of evening primrose oil in the treatment of chronic schizophrenia. J Orthomol Psychiatry. 1983;12:302–4.

Irefin S, Sprung J. A possible cause of cardiovascular collapse during anesthesia: long-term use of St John's Wort. J Clin Anesth. 2000;12:498–9.

Izzo AA. Herb-drug interactions: an overview of the clinical evidence. Fundam Clin Pharmacol. 2005;19:1–16.

Jiang X, Williams KM, Liauw WS, Ammit AJ, Roufogalis BD, Duke CC, Day RO, McLachlan AJ. Effect of St John's Wort and ginseng on the pharmacokinetics and pharmacodynamics of warfarin in healthy subjects. Br J Clin Pharmacol. 2004;57:592–9.

Jiang W, Wang X, Xu X, Kong L. Effect of *Schisandra sphenanthera* extract on the concentration of tacrolimus in the blood of liver transplant patients. Int J Clin Pharmacol Ther. 2010;48:224–9.

Johne A, Schmider J, Brockmöller J, Stadelmann AM, Störmer E, Bauer S, Scholler G, Langheinrich M, Roots I. Decreased plasma levels of amitriptyline and its metabolites on comedication with an extract from St. John's Wort *(Hypericum perforatum)*. J Clin Psychopharmacol. 2002;22:46–54.

Jones BD, Runikis AM. Interaction of ginseng with phenelzine. J Clin Psychopharmacol. 1987;7:201–2.

Kalliokoski A, Niemi M. Impact of OATP transporters on pharmacokinetics. Br J Pharmacol. 2009;158:693–705.

Khawaja IS, Marotta RF, Lippmann S. Herbal medicines as a factor in delirium. Psychiatr Serv. 1999;50:969–70.

Kolawole JA, Maduenyi A. Effect of zobo drink (*Hibiscus sabdariffa* water extract) on the pharmacokinetics of acetaminophen in human volunteers. Eur J Drug Metab Pharmacokinet. 2004;29:25–9.

Kupiec T, Raj V. Fatal seizures due to potential herb-drug interactions with *Ginkgo biloba*. J Anal Toxicol. 2005;29:755–8.

Lam AY, Elmer GW, Mohutsky MA. Possible interaction between warfarin and *Lycium barbarum* L. Ann Pharmacother. 2001;35:1199–201.

Lambert JP, Cormier J. Potential interaction between warfarin and boldo-fenugreek. Pharmacotherapy. 2001;21:509–12.

Lantz MS, Buchalter E, Giambanco V. St John's Wort and antidepressant drug interactions in the elderly. J Geriatr Psychiatry Neurol. 1999;12:7–10.

Laroche M, Choudhuri S, Gallicano K, Foster B. Severe gastrointestinal toxicity with concomitant ingestion of ritonavir and garlic. Can J Infect Dis. 1998;9:471P.

Lee KJ, You HJ, Park SJ, Kim YS, Chung YC, Jeong TC, Jeong HG. Hepatoprotective effects of *Platycodon grandiflorum* on acetaminophen-induced liver damage in mice. Cancer Lett. 2001;174:73–81.

Lee A, Chui PT, Aun CS, Gin T, Lau AS. Possible interaction between sevoflurane and *Aloe vera*. Ann Pharmacother. 2004;38:1651–4.

Lei HP, Yu XY, Xie HT, Li HH, Fan L, Dai LL, Chen Y, Zhou HH. Effect of St John's Wort supplementation on the pharmacokinetics of bupropion in healthy male Chinese volunteers. Xenobiotica. 2010;40:275–81.

Leung H, Hung A, Hui AC, Chan TY. Warfarin overdose due to the possible effects of *Lycium barbarum* L. Food Chem Toxicol. 2008;46:1860–2.

Lin YY, Chu SJ, Tsai SH. Association between priapism and concurrent use of risperidone and *Ginkgo biloba*. Mayo Clin Proc. 2007;82:1289–90.

López Galera RM, Ribera Pascuet E, Esteban Mur JI, Montoro Ronsano JB, Juárez Giménez JC. Interaction between cat's claw and protease inhibitors atazanavir, ritonavir and saquinavir. Eur J Clin Pharmacol. 2008;64:1235–6.

Lu FR, Shen L, Qin Y, Gao L, Li H, Dai Y. Clinical observation on *Trigonella foenum-graecum* L. total saponins in combination with sulfonylureas in the treatment of type 2 diabetes mellitus. Chin J Integr Med. 2008;14:56–60.

Lu H, Lu Z, Li X, Li G, Qiao Y, Borris RP, Zhang Y. Interactions of 172 plant extracts with human organic anion transporter 1 (SLC22A6) and 3 (SLC22A8): a study on herb-drug interactions. Peer J. 2017;5:e3333. https://doi.org/10.7717/peerj.3333.

Ma XH, Zheng CJ, Han LY, Xie B, Jia J, Cao ZW, Li YX, Chen YZ. Synergistic therapeutic actions of herbal ingredients and their mechanisms from molecular interaction and network perspectives. Drug Discov Today. 2009;14:579–88.

Ma L, Zhao L, Hu H, Qin Y, Bian Y, Jiang H, Zhou H, Yu L, Zeng S. Interaction of five anthraquinones from rhubarb with human organic anion transporter 1(SLC22A6) and 3 (SLC22A8) and drug-drug interaction in rats. J Ethnopharmacol. 2014;153:864–71.

de Maat MM, Hoetelmans RM, Math t RA, van Gorp EC, Meenhorst PL, Mulder JW, Beijnen JH. Drug interaction between St. John's Wort and nevirapine. AIDS. 2001;15:420–1.

Mahmoud BM, Ali HM, Homeida MM, Bennett JL. Significant reduction in chloroquine bioavailability following co-administration with the Sudanese beverages Aradaib, Karkadi and Lemon. J Antimicrob Chemother. 1994;33:1005–9.

Mamindla S, Prasad KVSRG, Koganti B. Herb-drug interactions: an overview of mechanisms and clinical aspects. Int J Pharm Sci Res. 2016;7:3576–86.

Marchetti S, Mazzanti R, Beijnen JH, Schellens JH. Concise review: clinical relevance of drug-drug and herb-drug interactions mediated by the ABC transporter ABCB1 (MDR1, P-glycoprotein). Oncologist. 2007;12:927–41.

Markowitz JS, Donovan JL, DeVane CL, Taylor RM, Ruan Y, Wang JS, Chavin KD. Effect of St John's Wort on drug metabolism by induction of cytochrome P4503A4 enzyme. JAMA. 2003;290:1500–4.

Mathijssen RH, Verweij J, de Bruijn P, Loos WJ, Sparreboom A. Effects of St John's Wort on irinotecan metabolism. J Natl Cancer Inst. 2002;94:1247–9.

Mazzari AL, Prieto JM. Corrigendum: herbal medicines in Brazil: pharmacokinetic profile and potential herb-drug interactions. Front Pharmacol. 2015;6:23. https://doi.org/10.3389/fphar.2015.00023.

Meisel C, Johne A, Roots I. Fatal intracerebral mass bleeding associated with *Ginkgo biloba* and ibuprofen. Atherosclerosis. 2003;167:367.

Michl J, Jennings HM, Kite GC, Ingrouille MJ, Simmonds MS, Heinrich M. Is aristolochic acid nephropathy a widespread problem in developing countries? A case study of *Aristolochia indica* L. in Bangladesh using an ethnobotanical-phytochemical approach. J Ethnopharmacol. 2013;149:235–44.

Milton JC, Abdulla A. Prolonged oro-facial dystonia in a 58-year-old female following therapy with bupropion and St John's Wort. Br J Clin Pharmacol. 2007;64:717–8.

Mo SL, Zhou ZW, Yang LP, Wei MQ, Zhou SF. New insights into the structural features and functional relevance of human cytochrome P4502C9. Part I. Curr Drug Metab. 2009;10:1075–126.

Mueller SC, Uehleke B, Woehling H, Petzsch M, Majcher-Peszynska J, Hehl EM, Sievers H, Frank B, Riethling AK, Drewelow B. Effect of St John's Wort dose and preparations on the pharmacokinetics of digoxin. Clin Pharmacol Ther. 2004;75:546–57.

Murphy PA, Kern SE, Stanczyk FZ, Westhoff CL. Interaction of St John's Wort with oral contraceptives: effects on the pharmacokinetics of norethindrone and ethinyl estradiol, ovarian activity and breakthrough bleeding. Contraception. 2005;71:402–8.

Ohkawa S, Yoneda Y, Ohsumi Y, Tabuchi M. Warfarin therapy and chlorella. (in Japanese. Rinsho Shinkeigaku. 1995;35:806–7.

Ondieki G, Nyagblordzro M, Kikete S, Liang R, Wang L, He X. Cytochrome P450 and P-Glycoprotein-mediated interactions involving African herbs indicated for common noncommunicable diseases. Evid Based Complement Alternat Med. 2017;2017:2582463. https://doi.org/10.1155/2017/2582463.

Page RL, Lawrence JD. Potentiation of warfarin by dong quai. Pharmacotherapy. 1999;319:870–6.

Pathak A, Léger P, Bagheri H, Senard JM, Boccalon H, Montastruc JL. Garlic interaction with fluindione: a case report. Therapie. 2003;58:380–1.

Pfrunder A, Schiesser M, Gerber S, Haschke M, Bitzer J, Drewe J. Interaction of St John's Wort with low-dose oral contraceptive therapy: a randomized controlled trial. Br J Clin Pharmacol. 2003;56:683–90.

Piscitelli SC, Burstein AH, Chaitt D, Alfaro RM, Falloon J. Indinavir concentrations and St John's Wort. Lancet. 2000;355:547–8.

Piscitelli SC, Burstein AH, Welden N, Gallicano KD, Falloon J. The effect of garlic supplements on the pharmacokinetics of saquinavir. Clin Infect Dis. 2002;34:234–8.

Portolés A, Terleira A, Calvo A, Martínez I, Resplandy G. Effects of *Hypericum perforatum* on ivabradine pharmacokinetics in healthy volunteers: an open-label, pharmacokinetic interaction clinical trial. J Clin Pharmacol. 2006;46:1188–94.

Prasad GV, Wong T, Meliton G, Bhaloo S. Rhabdomyolysis due to red yeast rice *(Monascus purpureus)* in a renal transplant recipient. Transplantation. 2002;74:1200–1.

Qiu F, Wang G, Zhang R, Sun J, Jiang J, Ma Y. Effect of danshen extract on the activity of CYP3A4 in healthy volunteers. Br J Clin Pharmacol. 2010;69:656–62.

Rajnarayana K, Reddy MS, Vidyasagar J, Krishna DR. Study on the influence of silymarin pre-treatment on metabolism and disposition of metronidazole. Arzneimittelforschung. 2004;54:109–13.

Rengelshausen J, Banfield M, Riedel KD, Burhenne J, Weiss J, Thomsen T, Walter-Sack I, Haefeli WE, Mikus G. Opposite effects of short-term and long-term St John's Wort intake on voriconazole pharmacokinetics. Clin Pharmacol Ther. 2005;78:25–33.

Rosenblatt M, Mindel J. Spontaneous hyphema associated with ingestion of *Ginkgo biloba* extract. N Engl J Med. 1997;336:1108.

Rubin D, McGovern B, Kopelman RI. Back to basics. Am J Med. 2006;119:482–3.

Sachin BS, Monica P, Sharma SC, Satti NK, Tikoo MK, Tikoo AK, Suri KA, Gupta BD, Johri RK. Pharmacokinetic interaction of some antitubercular drugs with caraway: implications in the enhancement of drug bioavailability. Hum Exp Toxicol. 2009;28:175–84.

Saraga M, Zullino DF. St John's Wort, corticosteroids, cocaine, alcohol … and a first manic episode (in French). Praxis (Bern 1994). 2005;94:987–9.

Schelosky L, Raffauf C, Jendroska K, Poewe W. Kava and dopamine antagonism. J Neurol Neurosurg Psychiatry. 1995;58:639–40.

Schwarz UI, Hanso H, Oertel R, Miehlke S, Kuhlisch E, Glaeser H, Hitzl M, Dresser GK, Kim RB, Kirch W. Induction of intestinal P-glycoprotein by St John's Wort reduces the oral bioavailability of talinolol. Clin Pharmacol Ther. 2007;81:669–78.

Segal R, Pilote L. Warfarin interaction with *Matricaria chamomilla*. CMAJ. 2006;174:1281–2.

Shader RI, Greenblatt DJ. Bees, ginseng and MAOIs revisited. J Clin Psychopharmacol. 1988;8:235.

Shaw D, Graeme L, Pierre D, Elizabeth W, Kelvin C. Pharmacovigilance of herbal medicine. J Ethnopharmacol. 2012;140:513–8.

Sheeja K, Shihab PK, Kuttan G. Antioxidant and anti-inflammatory activities of the plant *Andrographis paniculata* Nees. Immunopharmacol Immunotoxicol. 2006;28:129–40.

Sobieraj DM, Freyer CW. Probable hypoglycemic adverse drug reaction associated with prickly pear cactus, glipizide, and metformin in a patient with type 2 diabetes mellitus. Ann Pharmacother. 2010;44:1334–7.

Sugimoto K, Ohmori M, Tsuruoka S, Nishiki K, Kawaguchi A, Harada K, Arakawa M, Sakamoto K, Masada M, Miyamori I, Fujimura A. Different effects of St John's Wort on the pharmacokinetics of simvastatin and pravastatin. Clin Pharmacol Ther. 2001;70:518–24.

Tannergren C, Engman H, Knutson L, Hedeland M, Bondesson U, Lennernäs H. St John's Wort decreases the bioavailability of R- and S-verapamil through induction of the first-pass metabolism. Clin Pharmacol Ther. 2004;75:298–309.

Taylor JR, Wilt VM. Probable antagonism of warfarin by green tea. Ann Pharmacother. 1999;33:426–8.

Tongia A, Tongia SK, Dave M. Phytochemical determination and extraction of *Momordica charantia* fruit and its hypoglycemic potentiation of oral hypoglycemic drugs in diabetes mellitus (NIDDM). Indian J Physiol Pharmacol. 2004;48:241–4.

Tu JH, Hu DL, Dai LL, Sun Y, Fan L, Zhang M, Tan ZR, Chen Y, Li Z, Zhou HH. Effect of glycyrrhizin on CYP2C19 and CYP3A4 activity in healthy volunteers with different CYP2C19 genotypes. Xenobiotica. 2010;40:393–9.

Uchida S, Yamada H, Li XD, Maruyama S, Ohmori Y, Oki T, Watanabe H, Umegaki K, Ohashi K, Yamada S. Effects of *Ginkgo biloba* extract on pharmacokinetics and pharmacodynamics of tolbutamide and midazolam in healthy volunteers. J Clin Pharmacol. 2006;46:1290–8.

Wang L, Sweet DH. Active hydrophilic components of the medicinal herb *Salvia miltiorrhiza* (Danshen) potently inhibit organic anion transporters 1 (Slc22a6) and 3 (Slc22a8). Evid Based Complement Alternat Med. 2012;2012:872458. https://doi.org/10.1155/2012/872458.

Wang B, Zhou SF. Synthetic and natural compounds that interact with human cytochromeP4501A2 and implications in drug development. Curr Med Chem. 2009;16:4066–218.

Wang LS, Zhou G, Zhu B, Wu J, Wang JG, Abd El-Aty AM, Li T, Liu J, Yang TL, Wang D, Zhong XY, Zhou HH. St John's Wort induces both cytochrome P450 3A4-catalyzed sulfoxidation and 2C19-dependent hydroxylation of omeprazole. Clin Pharmacol Ther. 2004a;75:191–7.

Wang LS, Zhu B, Abd El-Aty AM, Zhou G, Li Z, Wu J, Chen GL, Liu J, Tang ZR, An W, Li Q, Wang D, Zhou HH. The influence of St John's Wort on CYP2C19 activity with respect to genotype. J Clin Pharmacol. 2004b;44:577–81.

Werba JP, Giroli M, Cavalca V, Nava MC, Tremoli E, Dal Bo L. The effect of green tea on simvastatin tolerability. Ann Intern Med. 2008;149:286–7.

WHO. Guidelines for good clinical practice (GCP) for trials on pharmaceutical products. In: The use of essential drugs, Sixth report of the WHO Expert Committee. Geneva: WHO; 1995. Annex 3 (WHO Technical Report Series, No. 850).

WHO. Guidelines for assessing quality of herbal medicines with reference to contaminants and residues. Geneva: WHO; 2004a. http://apps.who.int/medicinedocs/en/d/Js14878e/. Accessed Dec 2018

WHO. Guideline on safety monitoring of herbal medicines in pharmacovigilance system. Geneva: WHO; 2004b. http://apps.who.int/medicinedocs/en/m/abstract/Js7148e/. Accessed 24 Dec 2018

Wiegman DJ, Brinkman K, Franssen EJ. Interaction of *Ginkgo biloba* with efavirenz. AIDS. 2009;23:1184–5.

Williamson EM, Driver S, Baxter K. Stockley's herbal medicines interactions: a guide to the interactions of herbal medicines, dietary supplements and nutraceuticals with conventional medicines. Chicago: Pharmaceutical Press; 2009.

Wills RB, Bone K, Morgan M. Herbal products: active constituents, modes of action and quality control. Nutr Res Rev. 2000;13:47–77.

World Health Organization (WHO). The importance of pharmacovigilance: safety monitoring of medicinal products. Geneva: World Health Organization; 2002.

Wu X, Li Q, Xin H, Yu A, Zhong M. Effects of berberine on the blood concentration of cyclosporin A in renal transplanted recipients: clinical and pharmacokinetic study. Eur J Clin Pharmacol. 2005;61:567–72.

Xie R, Tan LH, Polasek EC, Hong C, Teillol-Foo M, Gordi T, Sharma A, Nickens DJ, Arakawa T, Knuth DW, Antal EJ. CYP3A and P-glycoprotein activity induction with St John's Wort in healthy volunteers from 6 ethnic populations. J Clin Pharmacol. 2005;45:352–6.

Xin HW, Wu XC, Li Q, Yu AR, Xiong L. Effects of *Schisandra sphenanthera* extract on the pharmacokinetics of midazolam in healthy volunteers. Br J Clin Pharmacol. 2009;67:541–6.

Yin OQ, Tomlinson B, Waye MM, Chow AH, Chow MS. Pharmacogenetics and herb-drug interactions: experience with *Ginkgo biloba* and omeprazole. Pharmacogenetics. 2004;14:841–50.

Yuan CS, Wei G, Dey L, Karrison T, Nahlik L, Maleckar S, Kasza K, Ang-Lee M, Moss J. Brief communication: American ginseng reduces warfarin's effect in healthy patients: a randomized, controlled trial. Ann Intern Med. 2004;141:23–7.

Zhang L, Yan J, Liu X, Ye Z, Yang X, Meyboom R, Chan K, Shaw D, Duez P. Pharmacovigilance practice and risk control of traditional Chinese medicine drugs in China: current status and future perspective. J Ethnopharmacol. 2012;140:519–25.

Zhang XL, Chen M, Zhu LL, Zhou Q. Therapeutic risk and benefits of concomitantly using herbal medicines and conventional medicines: from the perspectives of evidence based on randomized controlled trials and clinical risk management. Evid Based Complement Alternat Med. 2017;2017:9296404. doi: https://doi.org/10.1155/2017/9296404.

Zhou SF, Zhou ZW, Li CG, Chen X, Yu X, Xue CC, Herington A. Identification of drugs that interact with herbs in drug development. Drug Discov Today. 2007;12:664–73.

Zhou SF, Liu JP, Chowbay B. Polymorphism of human cytochrome P450 enzymes and its clinical impact. Drug Metab Rev. 2009;41:289–95.

Scientific Validation of Herbal Medicine

34

Vivek V. Bhosale and Dibyendu Banerjee

Contents

34.1 Introduction

Herbal medicines also known as traditional medicines are either the mainstay of healthcare delivery in some countries or serves as a complement to it in some other countries. The opportune use of herbal medicine is supported by the World Health Organization (WHO) which also encourages the use of remedies which have been proven to be harmless and effective. The WHO definition for herbal medicine defines it to be an extract or preparation from one or more plants that have therapeutic as well as other human health benefits. In some traditional practices, herbal medicines also contain some materials of inorganic or animal origin (WHO 1993).

A series of technical guidelines has been developed by WHO which includes guidelines on good manufacturing practices (GMP) for herbal medicines. These guidelines encompass the criteria such as quality assurance of medicinal plants and herbal materials, assessment of herbal medicines, assessment of quality of herbal medicines with reference to contaminants and residues, guidelines on good agricultural and collection practices (GACP) for medicinal plants and quality control methods for medicinal plant materials (WHO 2007a, b; Anonymous 1997).

V. V. Bhosale (✉)
CSIR- Central Drug Research Institute,
CDRI communication number: 9854,
Lucknow, Uttar Pradesh, India
e-mail: drvivekbhosale@cdri.res.in

D. Banerjee
CSIR- Central Drug Research Institute,
Lucknow, Uttar Pradesh, India

S. Sen, R. Chakraborty (eds.), *Herbal Medicine in India*,
https://doi.org/10.1007/978-981-13-7248-3_34

The guidelines aim to elucidate the basic criteria for the evaluation of quality, safety and efficacy of herbal medicines, thus assisting national regulatory authorities, scientific organizations and manufacturers for product development and dossier submission. The US FDA guidelines, European agency guidelines and Indian guidelines are based on the same principles derived from WHO guidelines.

34.2 European Union Guidelines (Anonymous 2004)

The European Medicines Agency has laid down two ways of registration of herbal medicinal products:

(a) Directive 2001/83/EC (4) requires that applications for authorization to place a medicinal product on the market have to be accompanied by a dossier containing particulars and documents relating in particular to the results of physicochemical, biological or microbiological tests as well as pharmacological and toxicological tests and clinical trials carried out on the product and thus proving its quality, safety and efficacy (Official Journal of European Union 2004).
(b) Some herbal medicinal products are prepared traditionally, and do not require doctors' supervision. If evidence of long traditional use of medicinal products already exists, directive 2004/24/EC can process it (Sharma 2015).

The evidence of traditional use is accepted as evidence of efficacy of the product. However, authorities may still ask for evidence to support safety. Physicochemical and microbiological tests as quality control are to be included in the product specifications. The product should meet the standards of quality listed in the authentic pharmacopoeias of the member state or European Pharmacopoeia. Moreover, the scientific publication evidences should support the medical use of the herbal medicine for at least 30 years, including its 15 years of use within the European community. The Committee on Herbal Medicinal Products reviews the traditional use registration of the product. The application states that the product has been in use within the European community for less than 15 years for simplified registration procedure under the directive (Sharma 2015).

34.3 US FDA Botanical Guidelines (Food and Drug Administration 2016)

The US FDA botanical guidelines define botanicals as

1. the products in which animal or animal parts as well as minerals have been used as a minor ingredient. The Chinese or Ayurvedic traditional botanical products are prepared traditionally in this way.
2. The derivatives of botanical species in which genes were modified with techniques like recombinant DNA technology or cloning for production of a single molecular entity.
3. The products which gives single molecular entity such as antibiotics, amino acids, and vitamins after fermentation processes by yeast, bacteria, plant cells, or other microorganisms, including plants used as substrates.
4. Paclitaxel like highly purified substances which are derived from a naturally occurring source. The estrogen synthesized from yam extracts which are modified chemically can also be considered as botanical product.

In the USA a botanical product produced to diagnose, cure, mitigate or treat disease can meet the definition of a drug under section 201 (g) (1) (B) of the FD&C Act. The regulations will be applied to it. Botanical drugs may differ in some characteristics like chemical composition due to possibilities of changes in agricultural practices and collection of botanical raw material(s). The conditions during manufacture and process of optimization also make lot of differences. US FDA requires bridging studies to justify these differences. Currently, two botanical products have been approved for marketing as prescription drugs. For example, sinecatechins (Veregen®) is a topical ointment commercialized for the treatment of external genital and perianal warts. Another drug is crofelemer (Mytesi™) for the treatment of diarrhea associated with anti-HIV drugs. These have fulfilled the criteria under the Botanical Guidance definition of a botanical drug product.

34.4 Indian Phytopharmaceutical Guidelines for Herbal Medicine

In Indian regulations, the major class of drugs included under Ayurveda, Siddha, or Unani (ASU) system is (Department of AYUSH 2013):

1. Classical ASU drugs should be mentioned in the authoritative books of ASU system drugs. The list of text book is given in Drugs and Cosmetics Act, 1940 and Rules, 1945. The manufacturing and nomenclature and formulations are similar as described in the authoritative texts. The issue of license to manufacture of these categories of drugs is based on citation in authoritative books and published literature. If the drug is meant for a new indication then proof of effectiveness is essential.
2. Patent or proprietary products containing traditional or new ingredients which are different from the classical medicine. This category of drugs requires proof of effectiveness based on the pilot study as relevant for ASU drugs. The Department of Ayurveda, Unani, Siddha, and Homeopathy (AYUSH) introduced Rule 158(B) in 2010 in this regard. (Central Council for Research in Ayurvedic Sciences 2018).

The GCP guidelines which allowed researchers to voluntarily use ASU medicine while taking up clinical trials were introduced by Ministry of AYUSH (Department of AYUSH 2013).

In India, the Department of AYUSH and regulatory authorities approves the use of ASU drugs as per the requirements given in Table 34.1. The phytopharmaceuticals which are well characterized as per phytopharma guidelines are under the purview of the Central Drugs Standard Control Organization (CDSCO) (Ministry of Health and Family Welfare, Govt. of India 2015). The gazette notification has been issued for phytopharmaceuticals. It states the requirements needed for submission of scientific data relating to quality, safety, and efficacy for evaluation of a herbal drug. It also describes the procedure for obtaining permission for marketing on similar to synthetic drugs. Phytochemical drug refers to purified and standard fraction consisting of at least four bioactive or phytochemical compound extracted from a medicinal plant or its part that has been qualitatively and quantitatively assessed to be used internally or externally by human beings or animals. These drugs are useful for diagnosis, treatment, mitigation or prevention of diseases or disorders. They cannot be used for administration through parenteral route. This provision is laid down by Rule 2 (eb) of the Drugs and Cosmetics (D&C) Rules, 1945.

The clinical trial permission of phytopharmaceuticals requires data as per clinical trial rules 2019 by Drug Controller General of India. The new rules 2019, part B states that the data has to be submitted along with an application to seek permission for conducting clinical trials or for import or manufacturing a phytochemical drug in the country (NewDrugs_CTRules_2019 2019). The regulatory requirements for NDA for the phytopharmaceutical drug need standard requirements for a new drug safety and pharmacological information, human studies, and confirmatory clinical trials. The part I of new rules 2019 deals with required data already available such as botanical name of the plant (including vernacular or scriptural name, wherever applicable), product monograph, claims to be made for the phytopharmaceutical product, published literature including clinical studies if available, contraindications, etc. The extent of exposure on human population and number of years for which the product is being sold is also important to take any decision. (NewDrugs_CTRules_2019 2019).

The part II of the new rules deals with identification, authentication of the source of the plant used for extraction and fractionation purpose, formulations, safety, marketing information, etc. The plant identification involves description about the taxonomical identity of the plant that has been used as a source for the phytopharmaceutical drug describing the botanical name including genus, species, and family, followed by

Table 34.1 Research criteria for evaluating the safety/toxicity of ASU drugs

S. no.	Category	Ingredient(s)	Indication(s)	Requirement of nonclinical safety data	Requirement of nonclinical efficacy data
Classical ASU drugs as defined under Section 3 (a) of the Drugs and Cosmetics Act, 1940					
1.1	Ayurvedic, Siddha and Unani drugs given in 158B as referred in Section 3(a) of Drugs and Cosmetics Act, 1940	As given in the text	As per text	No requirement	No requirement
1.2	Any change in dosage form of ASU drugs as described in Section 3(a) of Drugs and Cosmetics Act, 1940	As given in the text	As per text	No requirement	No requirement
1.3	ASU drugs referred in Section 3(a) of Drugs and Cosmetics Act, 1940 to be used for new indication*	As given in the text	New	Not Required	Required
2.1.	Patent or proprietary drugs as defined under Section 3(h) of Drugs and Cosmetics Act, 1940 containing crude drugs /aqueous axtract(s) /hydro-alcoholic extracts)	As given in the text	Textual rationale	No requirement	No requirement
2.2	Patent or proprietary drugs as defined under Section 3(h) containing other than aqueous and hydro-alcoholic extract(s)/ any other solvent-based extract(s)	As specified	As specified/ claimed	Requirement as follows: *For oral preparations*:* 1. Single-dose toxicity test (acute toxicity) in mice and rats 2. Repeated-dose systemic toxicity studies (long-term toxicity studies in rats 3. Reproductive and developmental toxicity studies 4. Genotoxicity 5. Carcinogenicity *metal-associated toxicity in case of any metal/mineral as one of the ingredients *For topical preparations:* 1. Dermal toxicity study 2. Photo-allergy or dermal photo-toxicity 3. Allergenicity/hypersensitivity in guinea pigs	Required
	2.4 Patent or proprietary drugs as defined under Section 3(h) containing any of the ingredients of Schedule E (1) of the D&C Act, 1940	As given in the text	Indication as claimed/ specified	*For oral preparations:* 1. Single-dose toxicity test (acute toxicity) in mice and rats 2. Repeated-dose systemic toxicity studies (long-term toxicity studies) in two species: one rodent (rat) and one nonrodent rabbit/dog. 3. Reproductive and developmental toxicity studies 4. Genotoxicity 5. Carcinogenicity *metal-associated toxicity in case of any metal/mineral as one of the ingredient *For topical preparations:* 1. Dermal toxicity study 2. Photo-allergy or dermal photo-toxicity 3. Allergenicity/hypersensitivity in guinea pigs	Required

Adopted from CCRS guidelines from Ministry of AYUSH, Government of India (2018)

the authority citation which means the name of the taxonomist who named the species and the variety of the cultivar, if any. It should also accompany the description about the natural habitat and geographical distribution and location of the plant, the time, and season of collection. The categories of the species description are (a) endangered or threatened under the Endangered Species Act or the Convention on International Trade in Endangered Species of Wild Fauna and Flora (CITES), (b) requiring special protection under the Biological Diversity Act, 2002 (18 of 2003), and (c) any known genotypic, chemotypic, and ecotypic variability of species. (NewDrugs_CTRules_2019 2019).

The data about phytopharmaceutical drugs should be generated for specifications regarding the quality, namely: (a) foreign matter, (b) total ash content, (c) acid insoluble ash, (d) pesticide residue, (e) heavy metal contamination, (f) microbial load, (g) chromatographic fingerprint profile with phytochemical reference marker, (h) assay for bioactive or phytochemical compounds, and (i) chromatographic fingerprint of a sample as per test method mentioned for the quality control of the phytopharmaceutical drug with pictographical documents. The purification, fractionation, and extraction procedures of the plant-based drug should be described in detail. The formulation details about markers, vehicles, and stabilizers should be mentioned. The stability studies should be performed as Drugs and Cosmetics Act. There is no difference for toxicity studies between new drugs and phytopharmaceutical drugs (NewDrugs_CTRules_2019 2019).

The details for requirements of phytopharmaceutical drug can be found in the phytopharmaceutical guidelines available at Indian regulatory authority CDSCO website (Ministry of Health and Family Welfare, Govt. of India. Gazette Notification G.S.R. 918(E) dated 30.1.2015 and NewDrugs_CTRules_2019 2019). Once the CDSCO approves a new phytopharmaceutical drug, its marketing status will be like that of a new chemical entity-based drug. The new regulation for phytopharmaceutical is in line with regulations in the USA, China, and other countries (Narayana and Katiyar 2013). It is expected that this new regulations will promote innovations and scientific development of new phytopharmaceutical drugs and will enhance the acceptance of the use of herbal products by modern doctors in the community. This would further encourage researchers to increase the research in phytopharmaceutical drug development area (Bhatt 2016).

34.5 Issues in Scientific Validation of Herbal Medicine

Herbal medicines can be defined as natural products originating from plants or their parts with varying chemical composition depending upon several factors like chemotype, botanical species used, and part of plant such as root, leaves, flowers, etc. used. The extrinsic factors like storage conditions, sunlight, humid environment, type of soil, land, harvesting time, and geographic area also affects quality of raw medicinal plant materials. It is because of these changing factors that marketed products containing the same ingredients vary in their contents and concentrations and quality from batch to batch. The standardization and maintaining quality changes with time. This variability may lead to significant differences in pharmacological activity at both pharmacodynamics and pharmacokinetic level (Bhatt 2016). The good manufacturing practices (GMP) are expected to enhance the quality results for herbal medicines. Another issue with phytopharmaceutical drug is about its pharmacokinetic properties which are difficult to establish. The validity of Ayurvedic herbal drugs can be tested using radiotracer technology which involves the labeling of the molecule designed for therapeutics with C-14 to study its absorption, biodistribution, and excretion in small animals. Similarly herbal drugs can be studied by tritium labeling. Arjun bark has been studied in this manner already. Radioisotope techniques of C-14 urea can be a new approach for study of plant parts. The C-14 radiolabeled plant parts can be fed to small animals. The whole-body autoradiography maybe performed to study the biodistribution of the plant-based drugs (Lele 2010). The action of herbal drugs is difficult to study, but the screening of Ayurvedic drugs based on mechanism is a novel approach. The enzymes and ligands are particularly possible targets. This can be illustrated by the example of study on Triphala using I-125 cholecystokinin (CCK) as ligand and mouse pancreatic membrane as receptor. The researchers group in collaboration with USA showed that the "Triphala" constituents act on CCK receptors (Lele 2010).

The clinical trials of herbal medicine have to face challenges like the adversity and side effects it may cause in patients (Firenzuoli and Gori 2007). Also, the inclusion criteria for enrollment of patients in clinical trial should be based on both modern and traditional medicine (Parveen et al. 2015). To eliminate biasness and isolate placebo effects, blinding is used as a gold standard in randomized clinical trials (RCT). Generally, double-blind clinical trials are carried out which means that neither the investigator nor the subject knows about the treatment allotment. As far as herbal medicines are considered, carrying out double-blind clinical trials might be difficult. The herbal treatment involves multidimensional treatment approach which involves counseling, listening, explaining as well as lifestyle and dietary advice while prescribing herbal medicines. For example, it gets difficult to maintain double blindness for certain natural products such as ginger, which has a peculiar odor. Therefore for such products single blinding is done where the investigator but not the patient is aware of the treatment allocation (Leung 2004). The challenge of protocol violations also occurs frequently. It is because the practitioners may feel uncomfortable with the protocol, and they may like to provide best therapeutic practice. To reduce this therapist variability treatment manuals detailing the precise procedures to be followed should be provided to the practitioner (Walker and Anderson 1999).

34.6 Conclusion

Scientific validation of herbal medicine should not be based only on regulatory bodies and good manufacturing practices (GMP) requirements. The academic institutions, research institutes, hospitals, industry, and pharmacy faculties should work together to increase the quality of herbal products and robust data generation regarding safety and efficacy. Efforts should also be made to validate scientific evidence with double-blind placebo controlled trials which will increase the faith of people in herbal medicines.

References

Anonymous. Quality assurance of pharmaceuticals - a compendium of guidelines and related materials, Vol. 1. 1997. http://apps.who.int/medicinedocs/pdf/h1813e/h1813e.pdf. Accessed 29 Apr 2019.

Anonymous. Directive 2004/24/EC of the European Parliament and of The Council of 31 March 2004. Official Journal of the European Union. 2004. https://eurlex.europa.eu/LexUriServ/LexUriServ.do?uri=OJ:L:2004:136:0085:0090:en:PDF. Accessed 29 Apr 2019.

Bhatt A. Phytopharmaceuticals: a new drug class regulated in India. Perspect Clin Res. 2016;7(2):59–61.

Central Council for Research in Ayurvedic Sciences, Ministry of AYUSH – Govt. of India. General guidelines for safety/toxicity evaluation of ayurvedic formulations. 2018. http://www.ccras.nic.in/sites/default/files/viewpdf/Publication/CCRAS_Guideline%20of%20Safety_Toxicity.pdf. Accessed 29 Apr 2019.

Department of AYUSH, Govt. of India. Good Clinical Practice Guidelines for Clinical Trials of ASU medicine. 2013. http://ayush.gov.in/sites/default/files/5110899178-Final%20Book%2028-03-13_0.pdf. Accessed 29 Apr 2019

Drugs and Cosmetics (Eighth Amendment) Rules, 2015, Ministry of Health and Family Welfare, Govt. of India. Gazette Notification G.S.R. 918(E). 2015. http://www.cdsco.nic.in/writereaddata/GSR%20918-E-dated-30-11-2015.pdf. Accessed 29 Apr 2019.

Firenzuoli F, Gori L. Herbal medicine today: clinical and research issues. Evid Based Complement Alternat Med. 2007;4(Suppl 1):37–40.

Food and Drug Administration, US. Botanical Drug Development Guidance for Industry. 2016. https://www.fda.gov/media/93113/download. Accessed 29 Apr 2019

Lele RD. Four new approaches for validation of Ayurvedic herbal drugs. Int J Ayurveda Res. 2010;1(3):136–7.

Leung PC. Complementary medicine. In: Machin D, Day S, Green S, editors. Textbook of clinical trials. 1st ed. Chichester: John Wiley & Sons; 2004. p. 63–84.

Narayana DA, Katiyar C. Draft amendment to drugs and cosmetics rules to license science based botanicals phytopharmaceuticals as drugs in India. J Ayurveda Integr Med. 2013;4:245–6.

NewDrugs_CTRules_2019. New Drugs and Clinical Trials Rules 2019 G.S.R. 227(E), Ministry of health and family welfare, New Delhi, the 19th March, 2019. 2019. https://cdsco.gov.in/opencms/opencms/system/modules/CDSCO.WEB/elements/download_file_division.jsp?num_id=NDI2MQ==2019. Accessed 30 Apr 2019.

Official Journal of the European Union. 2004. https://eur-lex.europa.eu/LexUriServ/LexUriServ.do?uri=OJ:L:2004:136:0085:0090:EN:PDF

Parveen A, Parveen B, Parveen R, Ahmad S. Challenges and guidelines for clinical trial of herbal drugs. J Pharm Bioallied Sci. 2015;7(4):329–33.

Sharma S. Current status of herbal product: regulatory overview. J Pharm Bioallied Sci. 2015;7(4):293–6.

Walker LG, Anderson J. Testing complementary and alternative therapies within a research protocol. Eur J Cancer. 1999;35:1614–8.

WHO. Research Guidelines for Evaluating the Safety and Efficacy of Herbal Medicines. 1993. http://apps.who.int/medicinedocs/en/d/Jh2946e/

WHO, guidelines for assessing quality of herbal medicines with reference to contaminants and residues. 2007a. http://apps.who.int/medicinedocs/documents/s14215e/s14215e.pdf

WHO. Guidelines on Good Manufacturing Practices (GMP) for herbal medicines. 2007b. http://apps.who.int/medicinedocs/documents/s14215e/s14215e.pdf

Scientific Validation of Aristas 35

Vidhu Aeri and Shikha Mishra

Contents

35.1 Introduction

Arista is a self-fermented Ayurvedic formulation. Fermentation is prescribed as a scientific method of preparing herbal formulations like Aristas and Asvas in classical texts of Ayurveda (Shrivastava 1998; Valiathan 2003, 2007, 2009). This technology has not been used in any other system of medicine as explained in Ayurveda. Susruta (Susruta, 44th Chapter) reads, "arishta has better properties and functions than any other mode of

V. Aeri (✉) · S. Mishra
Department of Pharmacognosy and Phytochemistry, School of Pharmaceutical Education and Research, Jamia Hamdard, New Delhi, India
e-mail: vaeri@jamiahamdard.ac.in

S. Sen, R. Chakraborty (eds.), *Herbal Medicine in India*,
https://doi.org/10.1007/978-981-13-7248-3_35

drug preparation because of the combination of different types of medical materials and their transformation."

Fermentation increases the nutritional value. It removes major fraction of sugars, making the components more bio-available. It can extract a wider range of active ingredients as the ratio of solvent changes with time from aqueous to aqueous- alcoholic. Also increased extraction rate occurs due to rupture of cells, active transport and enzyme-based action. Fermentation actively breaks the cells of biomass and exposes it to the solvent further assisting in the extraction process. However, no theoretical basis is provided with reference to fermentation technology in any of the Ayurvedic classics (Valiathan 2003, 2007, 2009).

In Ayurvedic Formulary of India (AFI), the traditional method of preparation of Aristas has been given. With reference to analysis, out of 24 Asava/Arista mentioned in API, 14 are either identified or assayed on the basis of gallic acid. In current scenario of strict quality control and for increasing the worldwide acceptability of traditional Indian medicine, the method of preparation and analysis needs to be standardized.

Asokarista, a classical herbal Ayurvedic formulation, is for gynaecological disorders. It contains *Saraca asoca* (bark), *Woodfordia fruticosa* (flower), *Cuminum cyminum* (fruit), *Cyperus rotundus* (rhizome), *Zingiber officinale* (rhizome), *Berberis aristata* (stem), *Nymphaea stellata* (flower), *Terminalia chebula* (fruit pericarp), *Terminalia belerica* (fruit pericarp), *Phyllanthus emblica* (fruit pericarp), *Mangifera indica* (endosperm), *Adhatoda vasica* (root) and *Santalum album* (heartwood) along with jaggery. The quantity of Ashoka bark is 100 times than other herbal ingredients. It has been indicated for dysmenorrhoea and menorragia in Ayurvedic treatises (Anonymous 2008).

The traditional medicinal preparations are marketed as polycomponent products' post-proper standardization and safety data. The plant-based search for new chemical entities (NCEs) indicated in conventional areas of cancer, antidiabetic, hepatoprotective, immunomodulatory and metabolic diseases are receiving attention for the development of traditional medicine-based formulations. These drugs in general are single plant extracts, or their standardized fractions.

The fingerprint profile and marker-based compound analyses are techniques useful for standardization of traditional medicinal formulations. However, this type of standardization does not ensure consistent biological activity or stability. Hence production of quality botanical medicines has become a challenge to regulatory authorities and scientific groups. This calls for optimization of extraction process and fermentation parameters in addition to evaluation of biotransformed products.

The research on scientific validation of Aristas encompassed the prospects as discussed in the chapter.

35.2 Methods

The research on scientific validation of Aristas encompassed the prospects as follows.

35.2.1 Evaluation of Pre- and Post-fermented Aqueous Decoction of *Saraca asoca* by High-Performance Thin-Layer Chromatography (Aeri and Mishra 2015)

Standardization of plant-based drugs is not just an analytical operation for identification and assay of active compounds with reference to markers. In fact it should comprise of entire information and thereby checkpoints right from its inception to ensure consistent composition of the herbal formulation. The principle of synergy is to be understood. It is now recognized that it is not a pure compound but a group of compounds which are responsible for the biological activity of a specific botanical. The very basis of the Ayurvedic drugs is to administer drugs as whole or processed extracts, which calls for measure of group of compounds rather than one single compound.

The present investigation explored the changes brought in by fermentation during the preparation of Ayurvedic formulation Arista with respect to physicochemical parameters based on correlation approach. The bark material was extracted with boiling water and fermented with *Woodfordia fruticosa* flowers after addition of jaggery. The fermentation broth was analyzed each day for14 days with reference to physicochemical parameters, and high-performance thin-layer chromatography (HPTLC) profile based on marker compounds (gallic acid and kaempferol) suggested by API.

The physicochemical properties of the formulation improved with the progress in days. The pH, specific gravity, solid content and sugar content decreased whereas phenolic content increased. Fermentation initiated on third day, resulting in generation of alcohol producing a quantifiable amount of alcohol by the fourth day. Marker compounds (gallic acid and kaempferol) were quantified in the fermented product, and quantity of gallic acid was found to be 3.24 times higher than the decoction. Kaempferol was identified in the fermented product but not in decoction, thereby indicating hydrolysis of flavonol glycosides during the process of fermentation.

An important finding was the presence of high amount of iron and calcium in the fermented product. The time required for the relevant fermentation study was 7–8 days. Thereafter, alcohol content exceeds the permissible level; however, it remains within +5% of higher limit till the completion of study. Traditional fermentation method improved the quality of formulation in terms of organoleptic and phytochemical properties.

35.2.2 Standardization Based on Specific Markers

It is an erroneous and difficult task to identify a specific marker compound for each traditional formulation because of the presence of number of plants. Asavas and Aristhas contain more than 20 plants in equal quantity. Hence, it is difficult to identify a quantitative marker for standardization of the formulation.

35.2.2.1 A Comparative Study of Prepared and Marketed Asokarista with Respect to Physicochemical Parameters and Phytochemical Markers (Mishra and Aeri 2015)

Arista is self-fermented Ayurvedic formulation, and fermentation helps in improving the quality of preparation. However fermentation being a vital process, there is a vital need to control its composition. Present work documents the physicochemical changes during processing of Ayurvedic formulation, Asokarista, and establishes its chemical marker.

The formulation was initiated by preparing a decoction of the bark with water, followed by fermenting it with *Woodfordia fruticosa* flowers. It was analyzed during processing (decoction), at beginning of storage and then at 30, 60 and 90 days at ambient conditions. The physicochemical parameters specified in API were evaluated, and assay was carried out based on phytochemical markers (lyoniside and lyoniresinol) of *Saraca asoca* using validated HPLC method. The formulation was completed in 8 days and complied with pharmacopoeial limits. The physicochemical properties of the formulation improved with the time span. Lyoniside was qualitatively and quantitatively assessed in decoction. However, its content decreased during fermentation. On the contrary, the content of lyoniresinol increased on storage.

The quality control parameters specified in API were also evaluated for two reputed commercial brands in comparison to laboratory-formulated preparation. All the formulations were evaluated for lyoniside and lyoniresinol content at various time intervals. The physical appearance of prepared formulation (PF-A) was similar to commercial formulations (CF-1 and CF-2). The odor (alcoholic-acidic) and taste (sour-sweet) were identical. The pH of decoction was 4.1 which became 3.3 when formulation is completed as various acids liberated during fermentation. Specific gravity of the decoction (1.12) was higher than finished formulation (1.07). The solid content decreased from 18.7 to 11.2% due to fermentation. Phenolic content increased by four times, from 0.025 to 0.082%. *Saraca asoca* bark has been reported to contain tannins and other phenolic compounds, which may be hydrolyzed during fermentation to release more quantity of phenolic compounds (Chaudhary et al. 2006; Arai et al. 2004).

Phenolic compounds are antioxidants, and their increased content indicated the increased antioxidant potential of arista. Apart from antioxidant, *Saraca asoca* bark has also been reported to contain, DNA-binding property, menstrual cycle regulatory activity, and DNA topoisomerase inhibitory property (Mukherjee et al. 2012).

Arista is an alcoholic preparation and has a specified limit of ethanol. The alcohol content was 8% in prepared formulation which is within limit. The prepared formulation was evaluated for iron and calcium content since the presence of organic iron and calcium compound in *Saraca asoca* was suggested in earlier literature. Prepared formulation contained 3767 mg calcium and 61 mg elemental iron in 100 ml dosage. Increase in the content of elemental calcium and iron after fermentation also highlights the role of fermentation in overall quality of studied gynaecological formulation. It was concluded that the use of incubator produced identical formulation in lesser duration. During the duration of processing, chemical marker of main component, *Saraca asoca*, is converted to its aglycone, lyoniresinol. Moreover, substantial quantity of elemental iron and calcium was detected in the formulation.

35.2.3 Quantitation of Lyoniside and Lyoniresinol

Besides the basic objective to record the various features of identification of single crude drug, the follow-up objective should be the developing of fingerprinting of marker compounds of the botanicals being used traditionally for therapeutic use in different parts of the country. The chemical profiling of the secondary metabolites may be utilized for the identification of plant material. Based on sophisticated analytical techniques the chemical compounds can be evaluated qualitatively and quantitatively. The very basis of the traditional drugs is to administer crude drugs as whole or their processed extracts, indicating that for a better evaluation of the plant material, a set of compounds need to be quantified than a single compound.

Sadhu et al. (2007) reported the presence of lignan glycosides in *Saraca asoca* bark. Lyoniside is the major component of *S. asoca* bark so it was estimated in decoction and different formulations (PF-A, CF-1 and CF-2). It is reported that microbes from Woodfordia flowers contain β-glucosidase enzyme which might be responsible for conversion of lyoniside into lyoniresinol. Lyoniside is a glycoside which yields lyoniresinol on deglycosylation, so the content of lyoniresinol was also evaluated. In all the formulations, lyoniresinol was present in good quantity which means that major portion of lyoniside was converted to lyoniresinol during fermentation. It has been reported that *Woodfordia fruticosa* flowers contain microorganisms which produce glycosidase, so it can be postulated that the conversion of lyoniside to lyoniresinol is deglycosylation rather that hydrolysis. Bhondave reported that mobilization of active phytoconstituents was independent of alcohol generation and perhaps microbial biotransformation plays an important role (Bhondave et al. 2013).

The developed HPLC procedure was validated in terms of specificity, sensitivity, accuracy and precision. The authors want to report here that traditional fermentation takes almost 30–37 days for similar changes to take place, but in our study it has been done in 8 days. This study establishes the presence of calcium and iron in a traditional gynaecological formulation. The chemical marker for main component, *Saraca asoca*, gets modified during fermentation, and its aglycone represents the chemical milieu of traditional formulation. On storage, the chemical composition was not modified significantly, and it retains its original character.

35.2.4 Modern Methods of Extraction to Enhance the Yield of Bioactive Marker

The protocols for production of fermented Ayurvedic drugs have been enriched by adding to the prescriptions available in the classics

(Valiathan 2003). Consequence to this, the other texts enriched the medicinal literature of Asvas and Aristas (Valiathan 2007, 2009; Shrivastava 1998). The protocols for the production of such medicines were flexible to allow physicians to innovate the medicines. However, the basic philosophy is followed to keep the basic ingredients constant.

35.2.4.1 Optimization of Microwave-Assisted Extraction Conditions for Preparing Lignan-Rich Extract from *Saraca asoca* Bark Using Box–Behnken Design (Mishra and Aeri 2016c)

The main bioactive constituents of *S. asoca* are lignans, flavonoids, catechin and anthocyanidin. Sadhu et al. (2007) reported five lignan glycosides (lyoniside, nudiposide, 5-methoxy-9 -b-D-xylopyranosyl-(-)-isolariciresinol, icariside E3 and schizandriside) from *S. asoca* stem bark. Further, Mukherjee et al. (2012) isolated another lignan glycoside, saracoside, from *S. asoca* bark. Mittal et al. (2013) have identified 34 catechin derivatives, 34 flavonoids and 17 other compounds in various parts of *S. asoca* plant. Ahmad et al. (2016) have isolated 30,5-dimethoxy epicatechin, 30-deoxyepicatechin-3-O-b-D-glucopyranoside, 30-deoxycatechin-3-O-a-L-rhamnopyranoside and epigallocatechin from *S. asoca* bark. Swamy et al. (2013) showed the cardioprotective activity of alcoholic extract of *S. indica* bark against cyclophosphamide-induced cardiotoxicity, whereas Arora et al. (2015) have shown significant hepatoprotection against CCl4-induced hepatotoxicity. Yadav et al. (2015) have shown the anti-breast cancer activity of *S. indica* bark extract along with its safe nature. Recently, Asokan et al. (2015) have studied the *in vitro* antioxidant activity of *S. asoca* bark in various assays. Lyoniside is a xyloside of lyoniresinol, an arylnaphathalene type of lignan, which has a structural similarity to secoisolariciresinol, and a precursor of mammalian lignans, enterodiol and enterolactone. Lignans are polyphenolic compounds structurally described by 8–80 coupling of two phenylpropanoid units (Moss 2000). They occur either in free form or glycosidically linked to a wide variety of different carbohydrates. Some of the plant lignans are metabolized by the colon microflora to the "enterolignans" (enterolactone and enterodiol). These enterolignans, also called mammalian lignans, have been reported to possess antiestrogenic, weakly estrogenic, anticarcinogenic, antioxidant and antimicrobial effects (Sicilia et al. 2003; Smeds et al. 2007). Recently, several new techniques have been described for efficient extraction of secondary metabolites from complex herbal matrices, i.e. supercritical fluid extraction (Ghoreishi et al. 2012), ultrasonic-assisted extraction (Gu et al. 2005), accelerated solvent extraction (Cicchetti and Chaintreau 2009), pressurized hot water extraction (Li-Chun et al. 2012) and microwave-assisted extraction (Delazar et al. 2012; Gallo et al. 2010; Tomaniová et al. 1998). Among all of them, microwave-assisted extraction is quite suitable for extraction of polar metabolites, since it requires a solvent with high dielectric constant. Further, the variables to be used for extraction of lyoniside were optimized using Box–Behnken method combined with response surface methodology. Box and Wilson introduced response surface methodology (RSM) in 1951, and Montgomery further evolved it (Myers et al. 2004). It consists of processing the process optimization work. Originally, it was defined as a statistical technique for multiple regression analysis, which uses data acquired from prior designed experiments for solving multivariate equations. Response surfaces are graphical representations of these equations, which are used to explain the individual and collective effect of the independent variables on the dependent variable (response) and to find out the mutual interactions between the independent variables and their subsequent effect on the dependent variable (response) (Mudahar et al. 1989; Wei et al. 2012). RSM employs design of experiments (DOE) techniques, e.g. central composite design (CCD), Box–Behnken design (BBD), full and fractional factorial designs and regression analysis methods. Design of experiments technique is employed before, during and after the regression analysis to estimate the accuracy of the model. The most desirable condition for the use of experimental design is the smallest number of factor levels. The Box–Behnken design is one such method. It is formed by merging two factorials with balanced incomplete block designs, which considerably decreases the number of experiments. In this system, only 15 experiments are required for a three-factor, three-level study. It consists of replicated center points, and the area of interest is a set of points located at the midpoints of edges of the multidimensional cube. It is also suitable for the exploration of quadratic response surfaces and creating a second-order polynomial model (Gaur et al. 2014). In the present work, an efficient method has been developed for enhanced extraction of lyoniside from *S. asoca* stem bark, and its process variables have been optimized using the Box–Behnken design.

Lyoniside is the chief constituent of *Saraca asoca* Linn. (Caesalpiniaceae) bark. Hence, there is an immediate need to develop an efficient method to isolate Lyoniside. A rapid extraction method for lyoniside based on microwave-assisted extraction of *S. asoca* bark was developed and optimized using response surface methodology (RSM). Lyoniside was analyzed and quantified by high-performance liquid chromatography coupled with ultraviolet detection (HPLC-UV). The extraction solvent ratio (%), material solvent ratio (g/ml) and extraction time (min) were optimized using Box–Behnken design (BBD) to obtain the highest extraction efficiency. The optimal conditions were the use of 1:30 material solvent ratio with 70:30 mixture of methanol/water for 10 min duration. The optimized microwave-assisted extraction yielded 9.4 mg/g of lyoniside content in comparison to reflux extraction under identical conditions which yielded 4.2 mg/g of lyoniside content. The experimental values agreed closely with the predicted values under optimum conditions. The analysis of variance (ANOVA) indicated a high goodness-of-fit model and the RSM method for optimizing lyoniside extraction from the bark of *S. asoca*. The three variables significantly affected the lyoniside content. Increased polarity of solvent medium enhances the lyoniside yield. The present study shows the applicability of microwave-assisted extraction in extraction of lyoniside from *S. asoca* bark.

Present work indicates the superiority of microwave-assisted extraction over conventional extraction for isolation of lignan, in particular, lyoniside. The use of experimental design further enhances the quality of the process by decreasing the number of trials and effectively utilizing the resources and extraction time.

35.3 Application of Modern Methods: Biotechnological Aspect

35.3.1 Fermentation Process of Traditional Asokarista Using *Wickerhamomyces anomala* and Its Optimization Using Three-Factor, Three-Level Box–Behnken Design (Mishra and Aeri 2016a)

The effects of selected variables on fermentation of decoction of *Saraca asoca* bark were evaluated to develop a suitable method for preparing its polyherbal formulation. *Saraca asoca* bark was fermented using *Wickerhamomyces anomalus* (non-*Saccharomyces* yeast), and the method was optimized using response surface methodology (RSM). The independent variables, substrate volume (ml), temperature (°C) and time (hours),were optimized using three-factor, three-level Box–Behnken design to obtain the good content of secoisolariciresinol, lyoniresinol and 5-methoxy isolariciresinol. Secoisolariciresinol and 5-methoxy isolariciresinol were first isolated from *S. asoca* bark. The method yielded a quadratic polynomial equation to predict the effect of independent variables on selected responses (<0.0001). All three variables significantly (p-value <0.0001–0.0068) affected the selected responses. The experimental values agreed closely with the predicted values, and the analysis of variance signified a good model fit. The optimum conditions were 67.03 ml substrate volume, 30.95 °C and 64.86 h resulting in 23.24,

21.20, 25.06 μg of secoisolariciresinol, lyoniresinol and 5-methoxy Isolariciresinol content. This is the first report of biotechnological production of Asokarista using *Wickerhamomyces anomalus* in 48 h rather than 35 days mentioned in traditional method. Also, secoisolariciresinol has been found in fermented *Saraca asoca* bark for the first time. It has been ascertained that *Wickerhamomyces anomalus* causes deglycosylation in traditional Ayurvedic formulations during fermentation. Present study proved the possibility of using pure strain, *Wickerhamomyces anomalus*, for formulating traditional formulation.

35.3.2 Biotechnological Changes Observed and Looking for New Pharmacophores

Research has been carried out on Asvas and Aristhas related to fermentation (Valiathan 2007; Katiyar 2008; Sekar and Mariappan 2008; Mulay and Khale 2011; Sayyad et al. 2012; Kadam et al. 2012). The literature indicates that no research has been carried out on the chemical and functional changes in the starting materials brought about by fermentation.

35.3.3 Biotransformation of Lignan Glycoside to Its Aglycone by *Woodfordia fruticosa* Flowers: Quantification of Compounds Using a Validated HPTLC Method (Mishra and Aeri 2016b)

Saraca asoca Linn. (Caesalpiniaceae) is an important traditional remedy for gynaecological disorders, and it contains lyoniside, an aryl tetra linlignan glycoside. The aglycone of lyoniside, lyoniresinol possesses structural similarity to enterolignan precursors which are established phytoestrogens. The present work illustrated the biotransformation of lyoniside to lyoniresinol using *Woodfordia fruticosa* Kurz. (Lythraceae) flowers. The simultaneous quantification of lyoniside and lyoniresinol using a validated HPTLC method was also carried out.

The decoction (aqueous extract) was of *S. asoca* bark was fermented using *W. fruticosa* flowers. The substrate and fermented products were simultaneously analyzed using solvent system/toluene/ethyl acetate/formic acid (4:3:0.4) at 254 nm. The method was validated for specificity, accuracy, precision, linearity, sensitivity and robustness as per ICH guidelines.

The substrate showed the presence of lyoniside; however, it decreased as the fermentation proceeded. On third day, lyoniresinol reappeared in the medium. In 8 days most of the lyoniside was converted to lyoniresinol. The developed method was specific for lyoniside and lyoniresinol. Lyoniside and lyoniresinol showed linearity in the range of 250–3000 and 500–2500 ng. The method was accurate as resulted in 99.84% and 99.83% recovery, respectively, for lyoniside and lyoniresinol. Aryl tetralin lignan glycoside, lyoniside, was successfully transformed into lyoniresinol using *W. fruticosa* flowers and their contents were simultaneously analysed using developed validated HPTLC method.

The principal crude drug *Saraca asoca* contains lyoniside as a major chemical constituent, As per literature survey, this compound has not been reported for any gynaecological activity. The formulation being a fermented product, it was hypothesized that lyoniside gets converted to some other compound during fermentation which might have gynaecological properties. Biotransformation is a process which can be defined as the use of biological system to induce chemical changes in compounds that are not their natural substrates. The present work was carried out to estimate the content of lyoniside and lyoniresinol in aqueous extract and fermented extract over the duration of fermentation (8 days).

The present work indicates the change in chemical constituent of extract during fermentation using *W. fruticosa*. Lignan glycoside, lyoniside, successfully transformed into lyoniresinol during this process. A new HPTLC method was developed and validated for their quantification. The developed method was unique as it simultaneously quantifies glycoside and aglycone.

35.4 Conclusion

A scientific validation of arishtas will help to understand the basis of philosophy behind the preparation of said formulations, change in chemistry after fermentation, the role of microbial biotransformation and the selection of relevant markers for the quality control and standardization of aristhas. Moreover, it will also help to introduce biotechnological techniques so as to enhance the production of pharmacophores, which may lead to the development of new formulations.

References

Aeri V, Mishra S. Evaluation of pre- and postfermented aqueous decoction of *Saraca asoca* by high-performance thin-Layer Chromatography. J Planar Chromat. 2015;28:36. https://doi.org/10.1556/JPC.28.2015.1.6.

Ahmad F, Misra L, Tewari R, et al. Anti-inflammatory flavanolglycosides from *Saraca asoca* bark. Nat Prod Res. 2016;30(4):489–92.

Anonymous. Ayurvedic Pharmacopoeia of India, Monographs-API, Part II, Vol. II. 2008.

Arai MA, Masada A, Ohtsuka T, Kageyama R, Ishibashi M. The first Hes1 dimer inhibitors from natural products. Bioorg Med Chem Lett. 2004;19:5778–81.

Arora B, Choudhary M, Arya P. Hepatoprotective potential of *Saraca ashoka* (Roxb.) De Wilde bark by carbon tetrachloride induced liver damage in rats. Bull Fac Pharm – Cairo University. 2015;53:23–8.

Asokan A, Thangavel M, Nisha P. In vitro antioxidant activity of *Saraca indica* methanolic bark extract. Int J Curr Microbiol Appl Sci. 2015;4:515–20.

Bhondave P, Burase R, Takale S, Paradkar A, Patil S, Mahadik K, Harsulkar A. Yeast consortium isolated from Woodfordia fruticosa flowers proved to be instrumental for traditional Ayurvedic fermentation. Int J Pharmaceut Biomed Res. 2013;4:37–45.

Chaudhary S, Kohli KR, Sharma G. An open clinical trial to evaluate the efficacy of a herbal preparation for menstrual irregularities. J Endrocrinol Rep. 2006;10:43–7.

Cicchetti E, Chaintreau A. Comparison of extraction techniques and modeling of accelerated solvent extraction for the authentication of natural vanilla flavors. J Sep Sci. 2009;32:1957–64.

Delazar A, Nahar L, Hamedeyazdan S. Microwave-assisted extraction in natural products isolation. Methods Mol Biol. 2012;864:89–115.

Gallo M, Ferracane R, Graziani G. Microwave assisted extraction of phenolic compounds from four different spices. Molecules. 2010;15:6365–74.

Gaur PK, Mishra S, Kumar A. Development and optimization of gastroretentive mucoadhesive microspheres of gabapentin by box–Behnken design. Artif Cells Nanomed Biotechnol. 2014;42:167–77.

Ghoreishi SM, Kamali H, Ghaziaskar HS. Optimization of supercritical extraction of linalyl acetate from lavender via box– Behnken design. Chem Eng Technol. 2012;35:1641–8.

Gu X, Cai J, Zhu X. Dynamic ultrasound-assisted extraction of polyphenols in tobacco. J Sep Sci. 2005;28:2477–81.

Kadam PV, Yadav KN, Patel AN, Navsare VS, Narappanawar NS, Patil MJ. Comparative account of traditionally fermented biomedicine from Ayurveda: Mustakarishta. Int J Res Ayurveda Pharm. 2012;3(3):429–32.

Katiyar CK. Aqueous alcoholic extraction of medicinal and aromatic plants by fermentation. In: Handa SS, Khanuja SS, Longo G, Rakesh DD, editors. Extraction technologies for medicinal and aromatic plants. Trieste: International Centre for Science and High Technology; 2008. p. 107–12.

Li-Chun ZH, Ying D, Xin X. Ultrasound-assisted extraction of syringin from the bark of Ilex rotunda thumb using response surface methodology. Int J Mol Sci. 2012;13:7607–16.

Mishra S, Aeri V. A comparative study of prepared and marketed asokarista with respect to physicochemical parameters and phytochemical markers. Int J Pharmacog Phytochem Res. 2015;7(1):144–9.

Mishra S, Aeri V. Fermentation process of traditional Asokarista using Wickerhamomyces anomala and its optimization using 3 factor, 3 level box-behnken design. Separat Sci Technol. 2016a;51(9):1579–88.

Mishra S, Aeri V. Biotransformation of lignan glycoside to its aglycone by *Woodfordia fruticosa* flowers: quantification of compounds using a validated HPTLC method. Pharm Biol. 2016b;55(1):360–6.

Mishra S, Aeri V. Optimization of microwave-assisted extraction conditions for preparing lignan-rich extract from *Saraca asoca* bark using box-Behnken design. Pharm Biol. 2016c;54:1255–62.

Mittal A, Kadyan P, Gahlaut A. Nontargeted identification of the phenolic and other compounds of *Saraca asoca* by high performance liquid chromatography – positive electro-spray ionization and quadrupole time-of-flight mass spectrometry. ISRN Pharmaceutics. 2013;2013:293935. https://doi.org/10.1155/2013/293935.

Moss GP. Nomenclature of lignans and neolignans (IUPAC recommendations 2000). Pure Appl Chem. 2000;72:1493–523.

Mudahar GS, Toledo RT, Floros JD. Optimization of carrot dehydration process using response surface methodology. J Food Sci. 1989;54:714–9.

Mukherjee T, Chowdhury S, Kumar A, Majumder HK, Jaisankar P, Mukhopadhyay S. Saracoside: a new lignan glycoside from *Saraca indica*, a potential inhibitor of DNA topoisomerase IB. Nat Prod Commun. 2012;7:767–9.

Mulay S, Khale A. Asavarishtas through improved fermentation technology. Int J Pharm Sci Res. 2011;2(6):1421–5.

Myers RH, Montgomery DC, Vining GG. Response surface methodology: a retrospective and literature survey. J Qual Technol. 2004;36:53–77.

Sadhu SK, Khatun A, Phattanawasin P, Ohtsuki T, Ishibashi M. Lignan glycosides and flavonoids from *Saraca asoca* with antioxidant activity. J Nat Med. 2007;61:480–2.

Sayyad SF, Randive DS, Jagtap SM, Chaudhari SR, Panda BP. Preparation and evaluation of fermented Ayurvedic formulation: Arjunarishta. J Appl Pharma Sci. 2012;5:122–4.

Sekar S, Mariappan S. Traditionally fermented biomedicines, aristas and asavas from ayurveda. Indian J Tradit Knowl. 2008;7(4):548–56.

Shrivastava S. Sarangadhara Samhita. Varanasi: Chaukhamba Orientalia; 1998.

Sicilia T, Niemeyer HB, Honig DM. Identification and stereochemical characterization of lignans in flaxseed and pumpkin seeds. Agric Food Chem. 2003;51:1181–8.

Smeds AI, Eklund PC, Sjoholm RE. Quantification of a broad spectrum of lignans in cereals, oilseeds, and nuts. Agric Food Chem. 2007;55:1337–46.

Swamy AV, Patel UM, Koti B. Cardioprotective effect of *Saraca indica* against cyclophosphamide induced cardiotoxicity in rats: a biochemical, electrocardiographic and histopathological study. Indian J Pharmacol. 2013;45:44–8.

Tomaniova´ M, Hajšlova J, Pavelka J Jr. Microwave assisted solvent extraction – a new method for isolation of polynuclear aromatic hydrocarbons from plants. J Chromatogr. 1998;A827:21–9.

Valiathan MS. The legacy of Caraka. Hyderabad: Orient Longman Pvt. Ltd; 2003.

Valiathan MS. The legacy of Susruta. Hyderabad: Orient Longman Pvt. Ltd; 2007.

Valiathan MS. The legacy of Vagbhata. Hyderabad: Universities Press (India) Pvt. Ltd; 2009.

Wei LZ, Li-Chun S, Yin-Shi L. Optimization of pressurized liquid extraction of three major acetophenones from Cynanchum bungei using a box–Behnken design. Int J Mol Sci. 2012;13:14533–44.

Yadav NK, Saini KS, Hossain Z. *Saraca indica* bark extract shows in vitro antioxidant, antibreast cancer activity and does not exhibit toxicological effects. Oxidative Med Cell Longev. 2015;2015:1. https://doi.org/10.1155/2015/205360.

Challenges and Opportunities in Standardization of Homeopathic Drugs and Dilutions

Arun K. Sharma, Bitasta Mandal, Swati Madan, and Satyendra K. Rajput

36

Contents

A. K. Sharma
Centre for Pharmacology and Toxicology, Amity Institute of Pharmacy, Amity University, Noida, India

B. Mandal
Centre for Pharmacognosy and Phytomedicine, Amity Institute of Pharmacy, Amity University, Noida, India

S. Madan
Centre for Pharmacognosy and Phytomedicine, Amity Institute of Pharmacy, Amity University, Noida, India

Amity Institute of Indian System of Medicine, Amity University, Noida, India

S. K. Rajput (✉)
Centre for Pharmacology and Toxicology, Amity Institute of Pharmacy, Amity University, Noida, India

Amity Institute of Indian System of Medicine, Amity University, Noida, India
e-mail: skrajput95@amity.edu

S. Sen, R. Chakraborty (eds.), *Herbal Medicine in India*,
https://doi.org/10.1007/978-981-13-7248-3_36

36.1 Introduction

Homeopathy is the longest originated complementary and alternative medicine which came into being in Europe more than 200 years ago. The demand of homeopathic remedies are on an unprecedented rise which has attracted the attention of researchers as well as sceptics towards the safety, quality and efficacy of homeopathic medicines and has led to an uprise in the experimental and clinical studies on homeopathic drugs.

The homeopathic system of medicine was introduced by Samuel Hahnemann who presumed that an ailment could be treated by administering a medicine which would exhibit similar symptoms of the particular illness when provided to a healthy person but to a slighter extent

(Loudon 2006). Therefore, the principle of homeopathy is based on 'similia' or 'simile' which implies 'let likes be cured by likes' (Bellavite et al. 2005). Another principle on which homeopathy is based is that the therapies employed in homeopathic system will continue to exhibit their efficacy following repeated dilutions and succussion even when the dilutions reach beyond Avogadro's number (Ernst 2002). Homeopathic medicines are prepared from a variety of natural and synthetic sources including plants, minerals, microorganisms, insects, animal tissues, and body secretions from animals and even from patients which are administered in the form of hydroalcoholic extracts called as mother tinctures and high dilutions. Treatment method in homeopathic system involves administration of drugs prepared by potentization which includes serial dilution and succussion (vigorous shaking).

Hahnemann suggested the use of dilutions of astronomical scale and up to a degree where not even a single molecule of source material could exist in the suggested final formulation which led to a huge controversy during that time (Handley 1997). In order to find out which therapy is efficacious as per the situation and for employing the law of similars, homeopaths examine their medications on healthy volunteers and explicitly record the symptoms caused which is called 'proving' (Ernst 2008). However, when these provings were reviewed in detail, it was concluded that the ambiguity on whether the high dilutions used for treatment can actually aggravate effects in healthy volunteers has not yet been made clear (Dantas et al. 2007). In the current practice of homoeopathy ultrahigh dilutions are used. Many experimental and clinical studies have reported such ultrahigh dilutions to exert detectable biological effects and to be better than placebos. However, a comprehensive review of all these studies is indispensable in assessing the reliability of the same. Improvement in a patient can be due any factor irrespective of any treatment that the person is undergoing, and hence, the conflict between the trials and observational data remains controversial (Ernst 2007). Nevertheless, use of high dilutions is not the only mode of drug administration. For certain drugs, even lower dilutions like mother tinctures are directly administered.

Since its origin, the system of homoeopathy has been criticized particularly regarding the use of high dilutions as medicines because medicines in high potencies such as 30 and 200C are made by incorporating extremely large dilution factors (10^{60} and 10^{400}, respectively) with many orders of magnitude greater than Avogadro's number which rules out the probability of the presence of any measurable remains of the starting materials. There exists no rationale for detection of the retention of characteristics of the starting materials and neither any evidence for existence of any physical entity in these high-potency medications (Kaur 2013). Homoeopathy has been in practice since a long time which suggests that these drugs affect biological processes at least in some or the other way. Therefore, clinical studies relating to success of homeopathic drugs may serve as a vital source of information pertaining to the probable efficacy of certain drugs. Reports on the efficacy of high dilutions mandate a systematic proving of efficacy of these drugs. However, in order to ensure the effectiveness of high dilutions administered there arises a necessity for standardization of diluted drugs which implies the extent to which it can be diluted without compromising its therapeutic benefits (Satti 2005) and the dilutions should be prepared according to the definitions finalized by the World Health Organization (WHO).

36.2 Homeopathic Drug Standardization

Standardization is the method of establishing a set of standards or inherent features, constant parameters, and definitive qualitative and quantitative values that are representative of quality, efficacy, safety, and reproducibility (Kumari 2016). To ensure a satisfactory product quality it is imperative to detect the validity and origin of the source materials and describe the manufacturing process. Evaluation of identity and purity is carried out with the source material and with the least diluted source used for potentization.

The process is carried out as per the homeopathic pharmacopoeias and other official guidelines and certified as per GMP. The source material should be characterized to detect its origin, history, and nature:

- Botanical origin characterized by the scientific name—genus, species, subspecies/variety, authority, and name of family; other information like ecotype, chemotype, and phenotype; part used; the state of material; probable pharmacologically active or toxic constituents; and macroscopic and microscopic details;
- Biological origin characterized by the physical, anatomical, and histological state;
- Mineral or chemical origin characterized by the physical form, structural formula and relative molecular mass (WHO 2009).

Mainly three methods of drug standardization are there—physical, chemical, and biological (Fig. 36.1). However, methods of standardization vary as per the source material used for preparing the finished product. For plant-derived material a description of the macroscopic and microscopic features, identity tests, limit tests for pesticides, heavy metals, pathogenic microbes, purity tests, and complementary tests such as foreign matter, total ash, water content, bitterness value, loss on drying, and radioactive contamination are imperative. For animal sources a brief description of the source, part used including its anatomical and histological details, identity tests, purity tests, moisture content, toxic content assessment, and method of preparation should be indicated. For human-derived material source, identification, material used, anatomical and histological features, identity and purity determination, water content and procedure of preparation should be specified. For sources derived from minerals and chemicals a detailed method of preparation, description and features, identity, and purity tests, and quantification of toxic components are a must. Likewise, for mother tinctures the procedure for preparation, appearance and description,

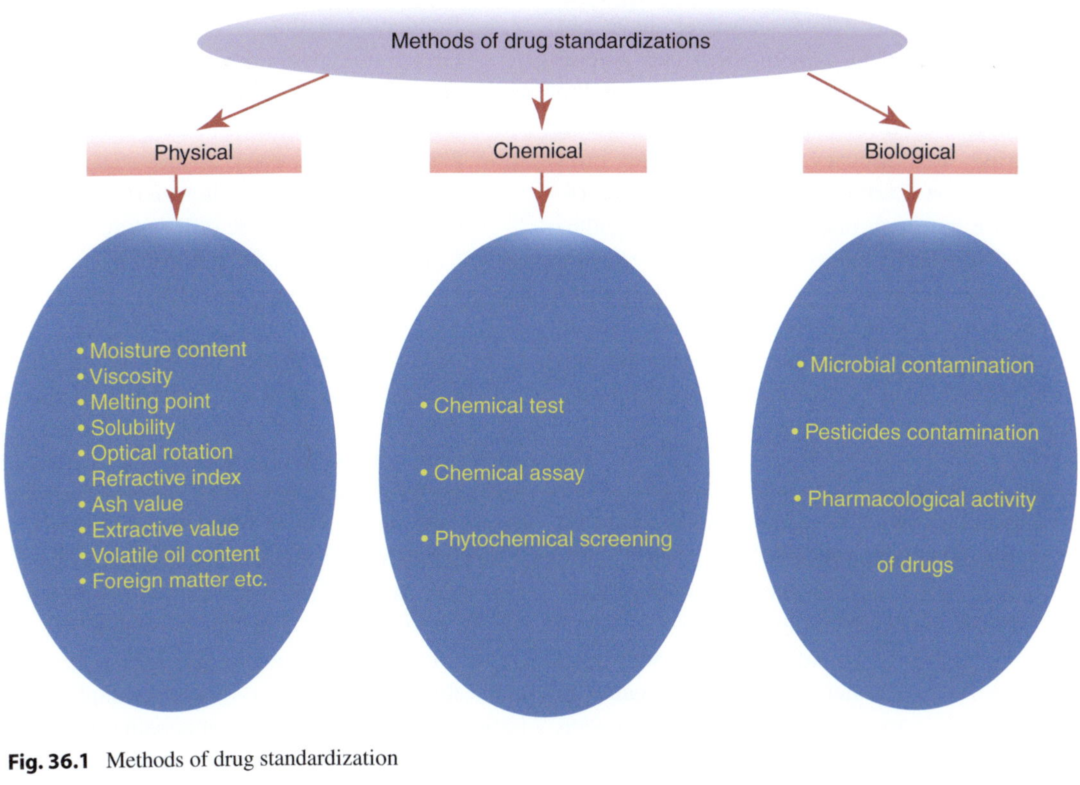

Fig. 36.1 Methods of drug standardization

identity and purity evaluation, method for stability tests, and detection of toxic constituents are mandatory. Similarly, finished products should be evaluated for identity and content, quality of dosage form, any chances of contamination with impurities due to manufacturing, and stability (Jadhav et al. 2016; Rao et al. 2014; WHO 2009).

36.3 Biological Standardization of Homeopathic Medicines

When we follow the protocols in a precise and organized way then a concise and brief conclusion regarding the purity and efficacy of the drug is reached. In case of drugs for the treatment of different ailments, the biological standardization gives rise to the curiosity related to the degree of dilution that leads to the desired observations, and hence, the target should be on the methods followed and the ways to lessen the possible errors in biological standardizations. Literature highlights a large number of validated *in vitro* and *in vivo* biological assays for a variety of homeopathic drugs and their dilutions that have displayed reproducible results which, however, have not been implemented in a methodical and precise manner till now for the standardization of the same. Moreover, these assessments give stress on displaying their efficacy rather than the brief mode of action. Current improvements in technology and a thorough understanding of the pathogenesis of the majority of diseases provide remarkable opportunities to standardize homeopathic drugs including high dilutions. As an example, some of the *in vitro* and *in vivo* antioxidant methods used for standardization of homeopathic medicines are reported below:

- *In vitro* methods:
  - 1,1-diphenyl-2-picrylhydrazyl (DPPH) radical scavenging activity
  - Hydrogen peroxide scavenging (H_2O_2) assay
  - Nitric oxide scavenging activity
  - Peroxynitrite radical scavenging activity
  - Trolox equivalent antioxidant capacity (TEAC) method/ABTS radical cation decolorization assay
  - Total radical-trapping antioxidant parameter (TRAP) method
  - Ferric reducing-antioxidant power (FRAP) assay
  - Superoxide radical scavenging activity
  - Hydroxyl radical scavenging activity
  - Hydroxyl radical averting capacity (HORAC) assay
  - Oxygen radical absorbance capacity (ORAC) method
  - Reducing power assay
  - Phosphomolybdenum method
  - Ferric thiocyanate (FTC) method
  - Thiobarbituric acid (TBA) method
  - N,N-dimethyl-p-phenylenediamine (DMPD) method
  - β-carotene linoleic acid method/conjugated diene assay
  - Xanthine oxidase assay
  - Cupric ion reducing antioxidant capacity (CUPRAC) assay
  - Metal chelating assay
- *In vivo* models:
  - Ferric reducing ability of plasma (FRAP) assay
  - Reduced glutathione (GSH) assay
  - Glutathione peroxidase (GPx) assay
  - Glutathione S-transferase (GST) assay
  - Superoxide dismutase (SOD) assay
  - Catalase (CAT) assay
  - Gamma-glutamyl transferase (GGT) assay
  - Glutathione reductase (GR) assay
  - Lipid hydroperoxide (LPO) assay
  - Low-density lipoprotein (LDL) activity

In addition, the biological assays together with the chromatographic fingerprinting methods can reveal the association of the molecular fingerprint with the biological efficacy of mother tinctures (Kardile et al. 2015). Several research papers on biological activity of high dilutions pose a challenge to the pharmacologists to either reproduce such results and confirm the efficacy of the homeopathic drugs or to systematically refute such claims through a series of controlled and validated experiments. As an example, biological standardization of homeopathic preparations having anti-inflammatory properties have been mentioned here according to the type of source material.

- Plant origin
- Various chemicals such as glucocorticoids (GCs) and mometasone furoate (MF); endogenous factors such as tumour necrosis factor alpha (TNF-α); enzymes and proteins such as copper and zinc superoxide dismutase (SOD), proinflammatory peptide substance (PPS), RGD peptides, interleukin-4 (IL-4), IL-10, interferon-ɣ (IFN- α), cyclooxygenase (COX), lipoxygenase (LOX), and cytokines such as interleukin-1 (IL-1); reactive oxygen species (ROS), nitric oxide (NO) and prostaglandin E2; and pro-inflammatory cells such as T and natural killer (NK) cells are well known to play a vital role in the development of inflammatory events. When any of these methods are followed for mother tinctures or diluted preparations and concise results are exhibited then these drugs are regarded as the standard ones.
- Animal origin
- *Apis mellifera*, cartilage from *Sus scrofa* and *Lachesis muta* are currently used as anti-inflammatory homeopathic remedies. Honey possesses antioxidant benefits, but the therapeutic findings obtained are not standardized with regard to its antioxidant properties. This is because the literature does not support any systematized approach taking into account the different markers of antioxidant activity and making the proper correlations to furnish a detailed observation of the antioxidant capacity of honey sample. The lack of standardization relies also on the fact that honey is a highly complex mixture of at least 200 phytoconstituents whose composition is strictly dependent on floral and geographical origin. A combination of different antioxidant assays such as Folin-Ciocalteu assay for total phenolic content (PC), ferric reducing antioxidant power (FRAP) assay for total antioxidant activity, 1,1-diphenyl-2-picrylhydrazyl (DPPH) assay to evaluate antiradical capacity, and oxygen radical absorbance capacity (ORAC) assay for antilipoperoxidant activity may lead to reliable results.
- Mineral origin
- Studies focusing on standardization of homeopathic preparations with respect to determination of active ingredients along with evaluation of their purity, mainly the presence of toxic metals such as cadmium and lead, are a must owing to their widespread therapeutic use (Opoka et al. 2004). For mineral sources different methods of standardization exist such as determination of the concentration of various metals such as zinc, iron and copper by atomic absorption spectrophotometer, determination of calcium and magnesium by complexometric titration, phosphorus determination by titration method after precipitation with ammonium molybdate reagent, and determination of sodium and potassium using flame photometer. However, the biological standardization of the same is lacking.

There are reports available on various active principles in medicinal plants used in the formulation of anti-inflammatory homeopathic medicines and molecular mechanisms of their anti-inflammatory activity (Kardile et al. 2015). If it is assumed that the active ingredient is responsible for the anti-inflammatory activity, then projected maximum dilution which will contain at least a few molecules of this active ingredient can be determined. Depending upon the reported concentrations of such active ingredients in the source material, the maximum homeopathic dilution that may contain at least a few molecules of the active ingredient has been determined. The estimated maximum dilution containing at least a few molecules of the active ingredient may provide a rough estimate of the maximum homeopathic dilution of the particular drug which may be considered to exhibit its effect through interaction with a definite biological target. There are scientific reports highlighting the effects of such active principles on the process of inflammation. This is an effort to suggest that if the specified active ingredient contributes to the anti-inflammatory property of the specific homeopathic drug, then what maximum dilution may be used so that at least a few molecules of the active ingredient will be present in the administered dose.

36.4 Obstacles in the Quality Control and Standardization of Homeopathic Preparations

36.4.1 Standardization of Homeopathic Dilutions

The foremost matter of dispute which revolves around the field of homeopathy making it a controversial one is the extremely diluted preparations employed where the chances of occurrence of the molecules of the starting material is scarce. Homeopathic dilutions beyond 12C (or 24×) levels can still possess active atoms or molecules of the therapeutic material though with less probability, and this is mainly by virtue of random distribution of drug particles in the dilution vehicle such as water, alcohol, or lactose. It is unscientific to claim that probability drops down from 100 to 0 while moving in a single step from 12 to 13C dilution. It is only that the chances of the presence of an atom or a molecule drop down in any level of dilution no matter how small it is. Theoretically this probability will grow extremely small but never zero as long as the serial dilution is maintained throughout the dilution process (Milgrom and Chatfield 2011). Nevertheless, the specific parameters for standardization of the diluted homeopathic preparations are lacking. The matter that raises doubt is regarding the biological activity observed even when the dilution is beyond the limit. This complication renders the efficacy of homeopathic drugs to a highly controversial state.

Majority of the homeopathic drugs occur in chemical forms such as molecules and atoms which further arises the curiosity regarding whether the effectiveness is originating due to the chemical presence of the drug at atomic or molecular level which was used during its proving or due to some secret force emerging from the drug. Since, this form of energy is unknown to us hence, it cannot be modelled for research. The key problem related to Avogadro is the drug's capacity either to pass or to fail the standard with certainty when assessed with active ingredients at extreme levels of dilution, which assists in reproducing the outcomes in a very explicit way. This will pave the way to develop the base for quality control in the homeopathic drug industry (Satti 2005).

36.4.2 Other Complications Associated with Homeopathic Drug Standardization

Standardization of homeopathic medicines is an arduous task due to the wide variety of source materials used to prepare high dilutions, variations in composition of the source material, and problems related to identity, stability of the active constituents and the possibility of contamination during manufacturing. Lack of advanced chemical and analytical assays for standardization of high dilutions and less attention given to detailed mechanism of action of drugs subjected to biological testing makes the standardization process more complicated. For standardization of high dilutions, identification and quantification of the active components is a must which is, however, not feasible in such extreme degrees of dilutions, and hence, there is a demand for prudent experimentation to confirm the reproducibility of the results (Kardile et al. 2015). Further there are inconsistencies in pharmacopoeial compendias of different countries which suggest different methods of attaining dilutions. For example, the mother tincture is regarded as 1x dilution in The Homeopathic Pharmacopoeia of India, whereas the same is considered in German and France homeopathic pharmacopoeias as 1:4 and 1:9 dilution of mother tincture. Therefore, WHO has taken steps to mitigate such disparities to lessen the complexity of homeopathic standardization.

Safety aspects of homeopathic medicines should be given prime importance as they also include lower dilutions (apart from highly diluted ones) that may contain starting material that may be harmful. Safety issues include safety pertaining to the source material as well as the method of preparation of the final product. Homeopathic preparations include sources from microbes, animals and humans which may contain hazardous pathogenic agents as well as plants which may be loaded with pesticide residues and heavy metals. Implementation of appropriate GMP guidelines related to manufacturing process, premises, personnel, packaging and labeling will help in ensuring the desired quality and safety of the final product (WHO 2009).

Moreover, the content of starting material present in homeopathic medicines may depend on the method of preparation which may lead to safety issues due to negligence of the disparities in the method of preparation. For example, significant deviations are observed from a comparison of the 'identically' entitled pharmacopoeial monographs on *Aconitum napellus* in different pharmacopoeias, e.g. the Pharmacopoeia française (Phf), the German Homeopathic Pharmacopoeia (GHP), the Homoeopathic Pharmacopoeia of the United States (HPUS) and the Homoeopathic Pharmacopoeia of India (HPI) which reveals considerable differences. *Aconitum napellus* 1× = 1DH made according to the German Homeopathic Pharmacopoeia is closer to *Aconitum napellus* mother tincture than to the 1× = 1DH, both made according to the Pharmacopoeia française. In case of India, there are no specifications for the alkaloidal content due to the belief that the action of the therapeutic agent will be seldom affected by minor variations in the quantity of physiologically active alkaloids in the end product. It is assumed that the action is exhibited qualitatively and not quantitatively (WHO 2009).

There occurs an alteration in the quality of material obtained from natural origin on account of the differences in the natural, biological and geographical features of the source material (Baker et al. 2002). Materials obtained from plant origin often fail to exhibit persistent chemical composition and reproducible pharmacological action mainly due to the hindrances pertaining to their identification, fluctuations in genetic features and environmental conditions, harvesting methods and deviations in the preparation and processing of extracts as well as insufficient scientifically established information regarding active constituents. Additionally, age of the plant, environmental conditions and geographical distribution, methods adopted for collection and storage also lead to disparities in the chemical composition of the plant material (Marcus and Grollman 2002). There is an urgent requirement to validate the correlation between the content of biochemical marker with the biological efficacy of the particular plant material which may serve as a boon to standardization of homeopathic preparations.

There is also an issue regarding the true identity of the plant drugs used in manufacture of homeopathic medicines. Certain medicines like *Toxicodendron pubescens* is generally described as *Rhus toxicodendron* in homeopathic literature. However, as per the current practice of nomenclature, this name is not used by botanists. Such disagreements need to be removed from the identity of plants. As the content of active constituents vary with changes in soil composition and environmental factors, therefore, it is necessary to specify which part of the plant is to be used in preparation of mother tincture. There are huge variations in the chemical composition of different parts like roots, bark, leaves, etc. Even inclusion of unwanted part or exclusion of the specified part may lead to deviation in the medicinal properties.

Herbal medicines and other folk remedies are gaining the attention of the general population for improving health condition as well as preventing and curing various ailments. During the past two decades, they have attracted the attention to a greater extent in Western countries due to their high pharmacological activities with low toxicity and rare complications. Despite this, herbal medicines have not been officially recognized worldwide because the quantity and quality of their safety and efficacy data are far from sufficient to meet the criteria required to support their use everywhere. Therefore, WHO provides guidelines for the evaluation of the quality of herbal medicines (WHO 2000).

36.5 Conclusion

Homeopathy is considered by many scientists and physicians throughout the world as questionable and ineffective. At the most it is considered that homeopathy is effective but only because of consultation (Satti 2004, 2005). The lack of faith on homeopathic medicines is because of non-existence of convenient and systematic standardized methods to prove the exact therapeutic interpretation. Majorly, standardized parameters are followed for the mother tinctures. But when the mother tincture gets diluted, standardized parameters similar to those followed for mother tinctures are not executed. When *in vitro* studies exhibit best results for specific therapeutic interventions then *in vivo* studies are performed and specific assays for specific dilutions are finalized. No justified methods exist for the standardization of homeopathic drugs except the guidelines for the preparation of high dilutions. Validated biological assays are a must for the quality control of homeopathic preparations and their dilutions. The key concept is to develop and advance the field of homeopathic medicines on the basis of validated experimental evidences rather than theoretical assumptions.

References

Baker C, Borneman J, Abecassis J. The Homoeopathic Pharmacopoeia of the United States. In: Homeopathic Pharmacopoeia Convention of the United States. 2002.

Bellavite P, Conforti A, Piasere V, Ortolani R. Immunology and homeopathy. 1. Historical background. Evid Based Complement Alternat Med. 2005;2(4):441–52.

Dantas F, Fisher P, Walach H, Wieland F, Rastogi DP, Teixeira H, Koster D, Jansen JP, Eizayaga J, Alvarez ME, Marim M, Belon P, Weckx LL. A systematic review of the quality of homeopathic pathogenetic trials published from 1945 to 1995. Homeopathy. 2007;96(1):4–16.

Ernst E. A systematic review of systematic reviews of homeopathy. Br J Clin Pharmacol. 2002;54(6):577–82.

Ernst E. The 'dirty tricks' experience can play on us. Postgrad Med J. 2007;83(978):287–8.

Ernst E. The truth about homeopathy. Br J Clin Pharmacol. 2008;65(2):163–4.

Handley R. Search of the later Hahnemann. 1st ed. New Delhi: Elsevier; 1997.

Jadhav HP, Chaudhari GG, Patil DD, Jadhav RB, Reddy NM, Shirkhedkar AA, Goyal SN, Patil CR. Standardization of homeopathic mother tincture of *Toxicodendron pubescens* and correlation of its flavonoid markers with the biological activity. Homeopathy. 2016;105(1):48–54.

Kardile MV, Patil C, Haidar A, Mahajan UB, Goyal S. Homeopathic drug standardization through biological evaluations: an untrodden avenue. Int J High Dilution Res. 2015;14(4):16–37.

Kaur H. Homeopathic research-understanding the challenges. J Homeop Ayurv Med. 2013;2(1):1–4.

Kumari R. A review on the standardization of herbal medicines. Int J Pharm Sci Res. 2016;7(2):97–106.

Loudon I. A brief history of homeopathy. J R Soc Med. 2006;99(12):607–10.

Marcus DM, Grollman AP. Botanical medicines--the need for new regulations. N Engl J Med. 2002;347(25):2073–6.

Milgrom LR, Chatfield K. "It's the consultation, stupid!". Isn't it? J Altern Complement Med. 2011;17:573e575.

Opoka W, Krzek J, Kierszniewska A, Rzeszutko W. Direct determination of Pb(II) and Cd(II) ions as impurities in some homeopathic drugs by using stripping voltammetry. Acta Pol Pharm. 2004;61(1):3–7.

Rao PP, Subramanian P, Sudhakar P. Standardisation of homoeopathic drug: *Plectranthus fruticosus*. Indian J Res Homeopathy. 2014;8(4):194–9.

Satti JA. Complementary nano-scale therapeutic approach through frequency base bio-synchronization. Proceedings of the 3rd International Conference on Non-Linear Dose-Response Relationship in Biology, Toxicology and Medicine, June 8–10, 2004, University of Massachusetts, Amherst, MA. Nonlinearity Biol Toxicol Med. 2004;2:381–2.

Satti J. Homeopathic drug standardization. Semin Integr Med. 2005;3(4):113–22.

World Health Organization. General guidelines for methodologies on research and evaluation of traditional medicines. 2000.

World Health Organization. Safety issues in the preparation of homeopathic medicines. 2009.

Translation of Traditional Knowledge from Lab to Layman from Herbal Sources

37

M. Kannan, P. Sathiyarajeswaran, and M. S. Shree Devi

Contents

M. Kannan (✉)
LR&DD and Department of Clinical Research, Siddha Central Research Institute (Central Council for Research in Siddha, Ministry of AYUSH, Govt. of India), Chennai, Tamil Nadu, India
e-mail: m.kannan77@gov.in

P. Sathiyarajeswaran
Siddha Central Research Institute (Central Council for Research in Siddha, Ministry of AYUSH, Govt. of India), Chennai, Tamil Nadu, India

M. S. Shree Devi
Department of Pharmacy, Siddha Central Research Institute (Central Council for Research in Siddha, Ministry of AYUSH, Govt. of India), Chennai, Tamil Nadu, India

S. Sen, R. Chakraborty (eds.), *Herbal Medicine in India*,
https://doi.org/10.1007/978-981-13-7248-3_37

37.1 Introduction

Translational medicine/research is rising, the new order that intends and that aims to fill the gap between bench and bedside, to comprise a close linkage across the whole pipeline of developing a new idea/hypothesis to the final clinical practice (Fitzgerald 2005; Lauer and Skarlatos 2010; Wang et al. 2009). The projections of translational research on the new drug development and the clinical therapy of various diseases have been extensively discussed (Paterson 2011; Simon 2010; Von Herrath and Chan 2009).

The WHO evaluates that around three-quarters of the total populace at present utilize herbs and different types of customary MEDs to treat their diseases. The formulations, which are sold as over-the-counter (OTC) items, have an alternate convention with respect to planning, getting permission, and advertising. The dynamic standards of natural arrangements are not frequently very much characterized. Likewise, the directions with respect to wellbeing and viability are not known to researchers or customers.

A medication is characterized as being safe, if it causes no known or potential damage to clients. There are three classifications of safety that should be considered, as these would manage the idea of the wellbeing prerequisites that should be guaranteed. The three classes are as per the following:

1. Category 1: Safety established by use over a long time
2. Category 2: Safe under specific conditions of use (such herbal medicines should preferably be covered by well-established documentation)
3. Category 3: Herbal medicines of uncertain safety (the safety data required for this class of drugs will be identical to that of any new substance) (WHO 2003)

As indicated by the WHO (1996a, b), standardization and quality control of drugs is the procedure associated with the physicochemical assessment of raw drug-covering perspectives, for example, choice and treatment of raw material, safety, efficacy, and reliability evaluation of completed item, documentation of wellbeing and hazard in light of involvement, arrangement of item data to buyer, and item promotion (Folashade et al. 2012). Experimentally approved and innovatively standardized herbal medicine might be inferred utilizing a protected way of turnaround pharmacology approach in light of customary information database. This may assume an imperative job in sedate revelation, advancement, and therapeutics, notwithstanding managing a run of the mill Western predisposition against herbal medicine (Joshi et al. 2004). The WHO has set certain measures for home-grown medications, which include the different parameters.

37.2 Standardization

Standardization of drug means validation of its identity, quality and purity throughout all phases of its cycle, i.e. shelf life, storage, distribution, and use by various parameters. As we all together know in our Siddha system of medicines, drug standardization of Siddha formulation is a big task. Strong cut guidelines have not been developed so far. So, it is necessary to encourage ISM manufacturing industry people for drug standardization work. The Ministry of AYUSH, Govt. of India established Pharmacopoeial Commission of Indian medicines and Homoeopathy (PCIM and H) for setting up drug standard of ASU and H medicines. To understand drug standardization the following aspects need to be learnt and implemented in our existing system.

37.2.1 Method of Standardization

There are different techniques involved in standardization of crude/finished compound drugs such as:

1. Macroscopic methods
2. Microscopic method
3. Physical methods
4. Chemical methods
5. Biological methods

37.2.2 Crude Drug Standardization

Crude ASU drug testing involves the following testing protocol for drug standardization:

1. Medico-botanical survey/identification, habitat, synonyms, regional names, etc.
2. Collection and preservation of raw material
3. Testing of drugs as per approved pharmacopoeial testing protocol
   (a) Identity by pharmacognosy profile, chemical identification, and TLC/HPTLC fingerprint profile
   (b) Purity by physicochemical profile
   (c) Strength by active marker/assay estimation
   (d) Safety by heavy metal profiling, microbiological limit test analysis, aflatoxin analysis and pesticide residue analysis
   (e) Siddha properties and action—*Gunam* (character), *Veeriyam* (potency), and *Vipakam* (post-digestive transformation)
   (f) Dose and *Anupanam* (vehicle)

37.2.3 Pharmacognostic Drug Analysis (Dept. of AYUSH 2016)

1. Macroscopic examination
2. Visual examination as size, colour, surface, characteristics, texture, and other examination like odour and taste
3. Macroscopic examination involves various steps as preparation of sample, inspection by microscopy, inspection by colour filter of ground glass, histochemical detection, and section study (T.S./L.S.)
4. TLC (Pharmacopoeia Commission For Indian Medicine and Homoeopathy 2016)/HPTLC fingerprinting
5. Identification/marking for phytochemicals

37.2.4 Compound Drug Standardization

Compound ASU drug testing involves the following testing protocol (Ayurvedic Pharmacopoeia of India 2008, 2016; Unani Pharmacopoeia of India 2016) for drug standardization:

1. Literature survey/drug reference
2. Collection and preservation of raw material
3. Testing of raw material by above testing protocol
4. Definition
5. Formulation composition
6. Method of preparation (manufacturing SOPs)
7. Testing of compound formulation on undermentioned pharmacognostic and physicochemical testing protocol (compound drug testing protocol) such as:
   (a) Identity by description, microscopic profile if any, chemical identification if any, and TLC/HPTLC fingerprinting profile
   (b) Purity-physicochemical profile
   (c) Strength-active marker/assay if any
   (d) Safety by heavy metal profiling, microbiological limit test analysis, aflatoxin analysis, and pesticide residue analysis
   (e) Storage
   (f) Therapeutic use
   (g) Dose and *Anupanam* (vehicle)
   (h) Self-life of drug by stability study

There is various physicochemical testing employed for drug profiling which depend on the specific characteristics of drug as per method given in Ayurvedic Pharmacopoeia of India (API) and Siddha Pharmacopoeia of India (SPI) (Ayurvedic Pharmacopoeia of India 1999, 2001a, b, 2004, 2006, 2009; Siddha Pharmacopoeia of India 2008, 2016).

USP (United States Pharmacopoeia), IP (Indian Pharmacopoeia), etc. such as:

1. Determination of foreign matter
2. Determination of ash value (at 500–8000 °C).
3. Determination of extractable matter.
4. Determination of water and volatile matter.
5. Determination of moisture content (L.O.D. at 110 °C).
6. Determination of bitterness value.
7. Determination of haemodynamic activity.
8. Determination of tannins.
9. Determination of swelling index.
10. Determination of foaming index.
11. Determination of pesticide residue.
12. Determination of total chlorine, phosphorous, and phosphates
13. Determination of arsenic and heavy metal.
14. Determination of bulk density.
15. Determination of radioactive contamination.
16. Comparative TLC/HPLC/HPTLC/GC-MS.
17. Determination of inorganic content by ICP, etc. Various test may be carried out for drug standardization.

In drug standardization chemist/technical person must know the state-of-the-art instrumentation technique, having knowledge of OQ (operation qualification), IQ (installation qualification), DQ (design qualification), PQ (performance qualification), instrument manual and SOPs (standard operating procedures) for instrument handling and maintenance, STP (standard testing procedures) and WI (work instruction for various common instrument used in the drug standardization or quality control process as pH meter, single distillation unit, double distillation unit, Soxhlet assembly, water bath, viscometer, tintometer, bulk density apparatus, polarimeter, refractometer, microscope, titration unit, hot air oven, magnetic stirrer, filtration unit, infrared spectroscopy, moisture balance, Karl fischer titrator, muffle furnace, vacuum evaporator, dissolution apparatus, friability apparatus, hardness tester, top loading balance, autoclave, B.O.D., incubator, laminar flow, microbiological colony counter, and antibiotic zone reader. In drug standardization work so many sophisticated instruments are also used frequently as and when they are in need for application as paper chromatography setups, column chromatography apparatus, double beam spectrophotometer, HPTLC unit, HPLC unit, LCMS,

G.C./M.S. unit, and ICP unit. Microbiological testing is also carried out for estimation of:

1. Total aerobic bacterial count
2. Total yeast and mould count
3. Presence of pathogens like *Salmonella*, *P. aeruginosa*, *E. coli*, and *S. aureus*. Stability study should also be carried out for drug standardization work for real-time stability studies (to see the changes in the quality standards at various intervals is found suitable for ascertaining the shelf life of the ASU medicines) in standard storage condition – Temp.1/6/12/18/24/30/36 months as per stability study testing protocol.

37.2.5 Drug Standardization Needs and Challenges

Drug standardization is required for the development of Indian system of medicines (viz. Siddha) for the following reasons (Kataria et al. 2011):

1. For Siddha physician, to cure disease, drug is one among the choice; medicine would be of good quality with highest efficacy and safety.
2. Identification of drug.
3. Purity of drug.
4. Safety of drug.
5. Strength of drug.
6. Efficacy of drug.
7. To follow GMP and GLP standards given by WHO.

37.3 Huge Cry for Metallic Drugs: Safety and Efficacy

The quality, safety and efficacy of the metallic preparations of Siddha system have to be assessed and brought to the public in order to maintain the authenticity of the age-old medicines. In Tamil Nadu, where the system was originated, a quantity of about 50,000 kg of metallic preparations of Siddha are prepared every year; if there is any iota of truth in the cry that these metal contents are toxic, it would have resulted in chaos already in the healthcare system of the state. Siddha medicine is being used in India, especially in Tamil Nadu, for "thousands of years".

Siddhar's concepts on purification of metals, grinding, heat application, compound formulation, adjuvant, antidote, diet regimen, etc. are astonishing facts which are to be verified and tuned using modern parameters and instrumentation. The present generation of Siddha practitioners, scientists and scholars should be duty bound to shoulder any challenge and conduct advanced researches to prove before the modern scientists that the benefits of metallic preparations outweigh the occasional and mild side effects.

37.4 Genotoxicity

Genotoxic substances are fit for causing hereditary transformation and of adding to the improvement of tumours. Genotoxicants incorporate the both-certain substance mixes and certain kinds of radiations. Normal genotoxins like fragrant amines are accepted to cause changes since they are nucleophilic and frame solid covalent bonds with DNA coming about with development of fragrant amine DNA adducts avoiding exact replication. Genotoxicity or on the other hand hereditary toxicology has advanced from the underlying investigations of quality changeability illustrated by Muller utilizing X-beam radiation, trailed by (Auerbach 1947). Hereditary toxicology evaluates the impacts of concoction and physical specialists on the inherited material, DNA and hereditary procedures of living cells (Prestone and Hoffmann 2001). It likewise incorporates mutagenicity, and cancer-causing nature considers and in addition thinks about on results of the DNA. There are numerous substances which cause or deliver genotoxicity, for instance, different synthetic compounds such as bug sprays and pesticides. A few medications may likewise cause genotoxic impacts like allopathic and Ayurvedic drugs. Ayurvedic solution has been utilized in India for a large number of years and is progressively been utilized worldwide amid the most recent couple of decades as proved by quickly becoming worldwide and national markets of Ayurvedic drugs. In India, around 25,000 successful plant-based definitions are utilized in customary and people drug. In excess of 1.5 million specialists are utilizing the conventional restorative framework for medicinal services in India (Kochhar 1981).

37.5 Preclinical Trial

Preclinical trial is a laboratory test of a new drug or a new medical device, usually done on animal subjects, to see if the hoped-for treatment really works and if it is safe to test on humans. There are two types of research: basic and applied basic research. Basic research means discovering new facts about how things work, how they are made, or what causes a biological event to occur, and applied basic research means taking the information discovered in basic research and investigating how to use it to treat and prevent sicknesses.

Determining whether a drug is ready for clinical trials (the so-called move from bench to bedside) involves extensive preclinical studies that yield preliminary efficacy, toxicity, pharmacokinetic and safety information. Wide doses of the drug are tested using *in vitro* (test tube or cell culture) and *in vivo* (animal) experiments which are guided by good number of guidelines such as OECD, WHO and AYUSH guidelines. However, there are too many complications in adopting this; exclusively in

AYUSH drugs many of the drugs traditionally are given with adjuvants such as honey/ghee/milk, etc. Complexity of herbo-mineral drugs is also a greater risk. Many of the external therapies mentioned under AYUSH stream lack testing model; hence it is the need of the hour to develop a guideline for testing AYUSH drugs having in mind all the complexities and scope for proving fundamental theories and laws. It is also possible to perform in silico profiling using computer models of the drug–target interactions.

37.6 Good Clinical Practice Guidelines for ASU Medicines (Anonyms 2013)

The Department of AYUSH has issued good clinical practice (GCP) guideline in March 2013 for clinical trial in Ayurveda, Siddha and Unani (ASU) medicines which will facilitate the researcher and institutions in adopting a standard way of good practice while conducting the ASU clinical trials. The GCP is a set of guidelines which encompasses the design, conduct, termination, audit, analysis, reporting and documentation of the studies involving human subjects. These guidelines are formulated based on CDSCO Document on GCP Guidelines (2001) for Clinical Trials on Pharmaceutical Products. The guidelines seek to establish two cardinal principles: protection of the rights of human subjects and authenticity of ASU medicine clinical trial data generated.

37.7 Regulatory Laws in India for Herbal Drugs

There are various regulatory laws in India for the regulation of herbal drugs. Some of these are Drugs and Cosmetics Act, 1940, Indian Medicine Central Council Act, 1970, Drugs and Magic Remedies Act (Objectionable Act), 1954, Biological Diversity Act 2002, Wild Life Protection Act, 1972, and Indian Forests Act, 1865 (Sharma 2006).

37.7.1 Indian Drugs and Cosmetics Act, 1940 (for Herbal Drug Regulation)

All traditional medicines such as Ayurveda, Unani, and Siddha products containing primarily one or more medicinal plant ingredients are governed under Chapter IVA of Drugs and Cosmetics Act, which was introduced in 1969. Before this amendment, definition of products containing herbs or herbal ingredients was non-existent in the Indian Drug Laws (Verma 2006). A recent amendment of the Drugs and Cosmetics Act 1940 has made some of its provisions applicable to the Ayurvedic drugs, which are defined to include medicines for internal or external use in human beings for diagnosis, prevention, mitigation, or treatment of diseases and which are mentioned in and manufactured exclusively in accordance with the formulae described in literature listed in Schedule I of the act (Mittal 2007).

37.7.2 Wild Life Protection Act, 1972

The Government of India enacted Wild Life (Protection) Act (1972), with the objective of effectively protecting the wild life of this country and to control poaching, smuggling, and illegal trade in wildlife and its derivatives. The ministry has proposed further amendments in the law by introducing more rigid measures to strengthen the act. The objective is to provide protection to the listed endangered flora and fauna and ecologically important protected areas (Wildlife (Protection) Act 2011). The act provides the establishment of Wildlife Advisory Board and appointment of wildlife wardens and other staff to implement the act. In the year 1991, the wildlife act was further modified. This amendment was based on the recommendations of Indian Wildlife Board and Ministry of Environment and Forests (Moef 2011). The Chief Wildlife Warden may, on application, grant to any persona permission to enter or reside in a sanctuary for all or any of the following purposes, namely: (a) investigation or study of wildlife and purposes, ancillary or incidental thereof, (b) photography, (c) scientific research, (d) tourism and (e) transaction of lawful business with any person residing in the sanctuary (Wildlife (Protection) Act 1972).

37.7.3 Biodiversity Act, 2002

The act aims at the conservation of biological resources and associated knowledge as well as facilitating access to them in a sustainable manner and through a process. For the purposes of implementing the objectives of the act, it establishes the National Biodiversity Authority in Chennai (Biodiversity Act 2011). The National Biodiversity Authority may appoint such officers and other employees as it considers necessary for the efficient discharge of its functions under this act (The Biological Diversity Act 2002).

37.8 Manufacture of Siddha Drugs

Ayurvedic, Siddha, and Unani drugs are required to be manufactured according to the formulae prescribed in the first schedule of the act. A license is necessary for the manufacture of these drugs and is required to be manufactured from genuine and properly identified raw materials (D&C Act 2011). The manufacture of drugs should be carried out under the directions and supervision of competent technical staff, and one of whom should have at least one of the following qualifications:

- A degree or diploma in Siddha or Siddha Pharmacy or Siddha system of medicines recognized by the central or the state government
- A degree or diploma in pharmaceutical chemistry with at least 1 year experience or a degree in chemistry or botany with at least 2 years of experience in the manufacture of the Siddha drugs
- A Vaid or Hakim registered in a State Register of Practitioners of indigenous systems of medicines having experience of at least 4 years in the manufacture of Ayurvedic or Siddha or Unani drugs
- Qualified pharmacist in Ayurveda, Siddha, or Unani system of medicine with at least 8-year experience in the manufacture of Siddha drugs

37.8.1 Manufacture on More than One Set of Premises

If Siddha (including Ayurvedic) or Unani drugs are required to be manufactured on more than one set of premises, a separate application shall be made and a separate license shall be obtained with regard to each such set of premises.

37.9 Indian Drugs and Cosmetics Act: Spurious Drugs

Person who manufactures any spurious drugs shall be liable to imprisonment for 1–3 years and a fine of not < ₹ 5000 on first conviction and an imprisonment for 2–6 years and a minimum fine of ₹ 10,000 on subsequent convictions. For the manufacture of adulterated drugs or manufacture without a valid license, imprisonment up to 2 years and a fine of at least ₹ 2000 for any subsequent conviction are prescribed.

37.10 Sale of Siddha, Ayurveda and Unani Drugs

No license is necessary for effective sale of Siddha, Ayurveda and Unani drugs, but dealers in such drugs can sell only products manufactured by a person licensed to manufacture drugs under the act. Some of the largest OTC brands in India are registered as "Siddha Medicines" because of their plant-based natural active ingredients.

37.11 Administrative Agencies Regarding the Regulation of Herbal Drugs

The central government and state government appoint some administrative bodies for efficient running of the act. These bodies are divided into three parts: advisory, analytical, and executive. Advisory body includes Drug Consultative Committee and Drug Technical Advisory Board; the analytical body involves Central Drugs Laboratory, Drug Control Laboratories in States, and Government Analyst; and the executive body comprises Licensing Authorities, Drug Inspectors, and Custom Collectors. The board is required to be constituted of the director general of health services, drug controller of India, director of Central Drugs Laboratory, a principal officer dealing with indigenous system of medicines in the Ministry of Health, a government analyst for Ayurvedic and Unani drugs, a pharmacognosist, a phytochemist and in addition, four persons, two from among the members of the Ayurveda Pharmacopoeia Committee and each from the members of the Siddha/Unani Pharmacopoeia Committee, one person, who is a teacher in Dravyaguna and Bhaishajya, Kalpana, one teacher in pharmacology and pharmacy, and one person each to represent Ayurvedic and Unani systems of medicine.

37.12 Labeling Provisions (Rule-161) of Herbal Drugs

Label must have the following:

1. Name of the formulation.
2. True list of ingredients used in the formulation together with the quantity of each ingredient.
3. If the list is long, a separate list has to be enclosed with the packing and references to be made on the label.
4. If ingredients are from Schedule E (I) the word "Caution: To be taken under medical supervision" should be printed both in English and Hindi languages.
5. Correct statements of weights and measures
6. Name and address of the manufacturers
7. Manufacturing license number
8. Batch number
9. Date of manufacturing and expiry date
10. The words, "for external use only," if the medicine is meant for external application,
11. Testing for heavy metals limits for export is mandatory with effect from January 1, 2006.

37.13 Mass Production

The Government of India appointed the Chopra Committee on Indigenous System of Medicine in 1948 which became a landmark. It accepted all the above proposals and recommended the establishment of the Drugs Enquiry Committee in 1946.The Drugs Enquiry Committee recommended mass production. But the situation prevailing was not indicative for the industry as such. The manufacturers were aware of only small-scale production laid down in the classical texts. The present system did not link the possibility of linking technology with production. The recommendations of the committee were primarily focused on the commercialization and standardization of the industry. It was well realized that mass production was possible only through mechanization. The mechanized production was resorted by majority of the companies, and this prevented the preparation of medicines by hand by vaidhyars. This was a serious handicap for the sector. But the lack of standardization was still a problem. Different texts followed different methods and included different ingredients. We may delineate a second phase of commercialization of the Ayurvedic medical sector in the end of the twentieth century, marked by a move from bulk to mass industrialized production. In this later phase, the process was not necessarily under the control of the vaidyas, but with the manufacturing firms. This phase was governed by the dynamics of the market and state regulations on drug development; and at this juncture, clinical testing and usage of scientific methods became a necessity. Today there are hypermodern factories of Ayurvedic medicine and the production process is completely mechanized, where the phases of traditional medicine production are no longer visible, though this is not true in the case of numerous small manufacturers.

37.14 Import of Herbal Drugs

There is no provision for import of Siddha, Ayurveda, and Unani drugs. The drugs being indigenous to the country are not manufactured outside India and as such no provisions for their import have been made.

37.15 Export

In India, about 80% of the rural population uses medicinal herbs or indigenous systems of medicine (WHO 2012). It is estimated that nearly 960 plant species are used by the Indian herbal industry, and the turnover of the industry is more than ₹ 80 billion. Herbal exports include medicines of AYUSH (Ayurveda, Unani, Siddha, and homoeopathy) products, which occupy a share of 3% of total Indian pharmaceutical export. Seventy percent of export from the herbal sector consists largely of raw materials and is estimated to be ₹ 10 billion per annum. Thirty percent of the export consists of finished products, including herbal extracts (Working Group on Access to Health Systems including AYUSH 2012). However, India's share in the global herbal export market is less than 1% (Singh 2006). Although the AYUSH industry represents one of the oldest traditional forms of medicine in India, it has not been able to exploit the opportunities of the emerging market (Wakdikar 2004; Vaidya and Devasagayam 2007).

37.16 On the Platter

Last decade recorded developments of health-related products, especially for NCD by various scientific organizations in India. In the year 1987 clinical trial carried out for psoriasis in Siddha Central Research Institute, Chennai, with a plant-based oil has been patented and commercialized as 777 oil through Dr. JRK's Research Pharmaceuticals Private Ltd. DRDO developed a drug for vitiligo and commercialized through AIMIL Pharmaceuticals. AIMIL pharmaceuticals also commercialized BGR-34 of CSIR parallelly CCRAS have commercialized AYUSH 82 antidiabetic compound as IME-9. Central Council for Research in Siddha has published a patent for Diabetic named as D5 *Chooranam* in which commercialization is under way.

These are also some of the drugs which have taken their right path using the existing guidelines and legal pathways from a lab translating to the benefit to the layman.

References

Anonyms. Good Clinical Practice Guidelines for Clinical Trials in Ayurveda, Siddha and Unani Medicine (GCP – ASU). New Delhi: Department of AYUSH, Ministry of Health and Family Welfare, Government of India; 2013.

Auerbach. Bioaccumulation of polyacrylamide aromatic compounds: 2. Modelling bioaccumulation in marine organisms chronically exposed to dispersed oil. Environ Toxicol Chem. 1947;20:1185–95.

Ayurvedic Pharmacopoeia of India Part-I, V-II, V-I. Ministry of AYUSH, Govt of India. 1st ed. 1999.

Ayurvedic pharmacopoeia of India Part-I, Ministry of AYUSH, Govt of India. 2001a.

Ayurvedic Pharmacopoeia of India Part-II, V-III. Ministry of AYUSH, Govt of India. 1st ed. 2001b.

Ayurvedic Pharmacopoeia of India Part-I, V-IV. Ministry of AYUSH, Govt of India. 1st ed. 2004.

Ayurvedic Pharmacopoeia of India Part-I, V-V. Ministry of AYUSH, Govt of India. 1st ed. 2006.

Ayurvedic Pharmacopoeia of India Part-II, V-III. (Form.), Ministry of AYUSH, Govt of India. 1st ed. 2008.

Ayurvedic Pharmacopoeia of India Part-I, V-VI. Ministry of AYUSH, Govt of India. 1st ed. 2009.

Ayurvedic Pharmacopoeia of India Part-II, V-I. Ministry of AYUSH, Govt of India. 1st ed. 2016.

Biodiversity Act. 2011. http://www.moef.nic.in/modules/rules-and-regulation/bio-diversity/. Accessed 03 Oct 2011.

Dept. of AYUSH. Macroscopic and microscopic atlas of Pharmacopoeial drugs part- I, V-V. Ministry of Health and Family Welfare, Govt of India. 2016.

Fitzgerald GA. Opinion, anticipating change in drug development, the emerging era of translational medicine and therapeutics. Nat Rev Drug Discov. 2005;4(10):815–8.

Folashade KO, Omoregie HE, Ochogu AP. Standardization of herbal medicines – a review. Int J Biodivers Conserv. 2012;4:101–12.

Joshi K, Chavan P, Warde D, Patwardhan B. Molecular markers in herbal drug technology. Curr Sci. 2004;87:159.

Kataria S, Bhardwaj S, Middha A. Standardization of medicinal plant material. Int J Res Ayurveda Pharm. 2011;2(4):1100–9.

Kochhar SL. Tropical crops: a textbook of economy botany. London: Macmillan Pub Ltd; 1981.

Lauer MS, Skarlatos S. Translational research for cardiovascular diseases at the National Heart, Lung, and Blood Institute, moving from bench to bedside and from bedside to community. Circulation. 2010;121(7):929–33.

Mittal BM. A textbook of forensic pharmacy. Delhi: Vallabh Prakashan; 2007. p. 73–143.

Moef. 2011. http://www.moef.nic.in/modules/rules-and-regulation/wildlife/. Accessed 02 Oct 2011.

Paterson NE. Translational research in addiction, toward a framework for the development of novel therapeutics. Biochem Pharmacol. 2011;81:1388–407.

Pharmacopoeia Commission for Indian Medicine & Homoeopathy. TLC Atlas Part-I, V-I, Ministry of AYUSH, Govt of India. 2016.

Prestone RJ, Hoffmann GR. Genetic toxicology. In: Klaassen CD, editor. Casarette and Doull's toxicology, the basic science of poison. 6th ed. New York: McGraw- Hill Medical Publishing Division; 2001.. https://accesspharmacy.mhmedical.com/content.aspx?sectionid=53483730&bookid=958.

Sharma SK. Infrastructure status, regulation & quality control of Indian medicine. Department of Ayurveda, Yoga & Naturopathy, Unani, Siddha, Homoeopath (AYUSH). New Delhi: Ministry of Health & Family Welfare, Government of India; 2006.

Simon R. Translational research in oncology, key bottlenecks and new paradigms. Expert Rev Mol Med. 2010;12:e32.

Singh H. Prospects and challenges for harnessing opportunities in medicinal plants sector in India. LEAD J. 2006;2:198–211.

The Biological Diversity Act. 2002. http://www.genecampaign.org/home/Biological%20Diversity%20Act%20 2002.pdf. Accessed 01 Oct 2011.

The Drugs and Cosmetics Act and Rules, Government of India Ministry of Health and Family Welfare. 2011. http://www.cdsco.nic.in/html/copy%20of%201.%20 dandcact121.pdf. Accessed 01 Oct 2011.

The Siddha Pharmacopoeia of India Part-1, V-I. Ministry of AYUSH, Govt of India. 1st ed. 2008.

The Wildlife (Protection) Act, Part- I 1972 with the Wildlife (protection) Amendment Act. 1972. http://www.westbengalforest.gov.in/pdf/the_wildlife_p_act_1972.pdf. Accessed 05 Jan 2012.

Unani Pharmacopoeia of India Part-II, V-I. Ministry of AYUSH, Govt of India. 2016.

Vaidya ADB, Devasagayam TPA. Current status of herbal drugs in India: an overview. J Clin Biochem Nutr. 2007;4:1–11.

Verma R. Drug regulations and plant-based pharmaceuticals in post. Izatnagar: Indian Veterinary Research Institute; 2006.

Von Herrath M, Chan A. How can we improve the translational landscape for a faster cure of type 1 diabetes? J Clin Invest. 2009;119(5):1061–5.

Wakdikar S. Global health care challenge: Indian experiences and new prescriptions. Electron J Biotechnol. 2004;7:214–20.

Wang PS, Heinssen R, Oliveri M, Wagner A, Goodman W. Bridging bench and practice, translational research for schizophrenia and other psychotic disorders. Neuropsychopharmacology. 2009;34(1):204–12.

WHO. Quality assurance of pharmaceuticals: a compendium of guidelines and related materials, good manufacturing practices and inspection. Geneva: World Health Organization; 1996a.

WHO. Guidelines for the Assessment of Herbal Medicines. In: WHO Technical Report Series. Geneva: World Health Organization; 1996b.

WHO. WHO Guidelines for the Regulation of Herbal Medicines in the South East Asia Region. 2003. http://apps.who.int/medicinedocs/en/m/abstract/Js22299en/.

Wildlife (Protection) Act. 2011. http://www.legalserviceindia.com/articles/wild.htm. Accessed 11 Oct 2011.

Working Group on "Access to Health Systems including AYUSH," Government of India Planning Commission. Eleventh Five-year Plan (2007–2012) [homepage on the Internet]. 2012. http://planningcommission.nic.in/plans/planrel/11thf.htm. Accessed 20 Mar 2012.

World Health Organization. Traditional medicine, fact sheet no. 134 [homepage on the Internet]. 2012. http://www.who.int/mediacentre/factsheets/fs134/en/. Accessed 20 Mar 2012.

Role of Traditional Knowledge Digital Library (TKDL) in Preservation and Protection of Indigenous Medicinal Knowledge of India

38

Mohd Shoaib Ansari

Contents

38.1 Introduction

Traditional or indigenous knowledge generally refers to the local knowledge that is unique to a culture and society. It naturally involves a profound understanding of environmental processes and the ability to extract useful products from the local habitat in a sustainable manner. It is an integral part of the practices, institutions, relations and rituals of the community. Traditional knowledge also includes the knowledge, teaching and wisdom of these communities. Traditional knowledge passes from person to person for generations, mainly through stories, legends, folklore, rituals, songs and laws (Bardi et al. 2011).

Over the past two decades, traditional knowledge has received a great attention on the international level. There are many reasons for recognizing its importance in people's lives and

M. S. Ansari (✉)
Government Kaktiya Post-Graduate College, Jagdalpur, India

S. Sen, R. Chakraborty (eds.), *Herbal Medicine in India*,
https://doi.org/10.1007/978-981-13-7248-3_38

in biodiversity conservation, concerns about the rapid loss of TK and global cultural diversity, and concerns about unauthorized and inappropriate patenting and use without sharing the benefits with the original owners. Many countries and communities around the world take this issue into account at national and international level. For the continued survival of indigenous and rural people, the conservation of species, habitat and biodiversity is essential. By protecting indigenous people's customs and habitat, we are simultaneously reducing emissions from deforestation and ecosystem degradation. Furthermore, the opportunity for cultural survival is a basic human right. Traditional knowledge is facing major biopiracy problems (Conforto 2004).

38.1.1 Importance of Traditional Knowledge in Medicine

Medical science has made considerable progress in human healthcare. In this achievement, scientific innovation and the rapid development of new medicines play an important role. Despite these achievements, however, more than one-third of the world's population lacks affordable essential medicines. Modern medicine and advanced treatment for a large part of the world's population are not available. Traditional medicine, therefore, plays an important role in healthcare because it is widely available throughout the world, even in remote areas. Because of its local availability and low costs, it is affordable for most people living in developing countries. Herbal medicines and acupuncture are the most commonly used traditional medicines and alternative therapies (Carlos 2002; World Health Organization 2002).

Traditional medicine and alternative medicine today play an increasingly important role in the health sector reform in many countries. The 40% population of China, 71% of Chile, 40% of Colombia, and 65% population of India use traditional medicine to meet its primary needs in healthcare. In developed countries, traditional, supplementary and alternative medicines are increasingly popular. For example, the population that used these medicines at least once is 31% in Belgium, 48% in Australia, 49% in France, 70% in Canada and 42% in the United States (Hasan 2010; WHO Traditional medicine Secretariat 2003).

38.1.2 Challenges Involved in Protecting Knowledge of Traditional Medicine

The effectiveness of traditional medicine has been extensively studied and discussed. For example, *Artemisia annua* has been one of the traditional Chinese medicines for malaria management since ancient times. *Artemisinin* and its derivatives have recently been developed as antimalaria drugs by modern scientific research. These findings have led to further research into new medicines based on traditional medicines (Apte 2006).

There is a modern mechanism required for protection and preservation of traditional medicinal practices. There are three major issues involved in designing a protection mechanism, and they are as follows (Brush 2007):

- Which technique is suitable for preservation and sharing benefits of traditional medicine and how it would be effective?
- The knowledge of traditional medicine mostly originates from community practice. This knowledge is adapted, utilized and patented by scientists and firms from developed countries, without taking consent of the people of the belonging communities. So, how would the intellectual property rights of the holders of TK be protected when it is used by the scientist to create modern drugs?
- Herbal pharmaceutical production requires a large number of medicinal plants. These plants can be planted by researchers on their farms, and it will affect the right of knowledge belonging people. So, how can we stop the loss of biodiversity caused by the rapid expansion of the international market for herbal products? (Vadi 2007).

38.1.3 The Gaps Between Traditional Medicine Areas and Existing Modern Patent Law

In order to protect traditional knowledge and biodiversity, protection under international patent law and most national patent laws is not sufficient. For example, traditional medical practices differed from those in modern practice and no records of who invented them are available. Similarly, it is very difficult to protect other traditional non-medicinal therapies using current patent protection rules because these therapies have not been developed by a single person or organization. These have been developed by traditional community practices over a long period (Finetti 2011).

The intellectual property standards set out in the Agreement on Trade-Related Aspects of Intellectual Property Rights (TRIPS Agreement) protect innovation by patenting the discovery of new chemical components and innovative know-how in the manufacture of products, trademarks and trade secrets. Due to their intrinsic characteristics, this patenting approach is hard to apply to herbal medicines. They fail to comply with all modern patent law requirements (Martin 2010). There are reasons why herbal products and medicines are not properly protected by IPRs or patents:

- Traditional medicines are raw materials of plants, such as leaves, flowers, fruits, seeds, stems, wood, bark, roots, rhizomes or other parts of plants that can be used in whole or fragmented or powdered form. Therefore, existing patent law protection for herbal medicinal products cannot be sought by claiming the discovery of new chemical entities or by developing an inventive step.
- Many traditional medicines are powdered plant materials, extracts, tinctures or fatty oils prepared in alcohol, honey or other liquids by steeping or heating these materials. The production process is usually simple and involves no sophisticated process and which cannot be protected under current patent laws. (Zhang 2004).

38.2 India and Traditional Knowledge

India has a long tradition of civilization and has a wealth of traditional knowledge in ancient scriptures which consist of the *Vedas*, *Puranas*, *Upanishads*, *Brahma sutras*, two *epics*, *Bhagavad-Gita*, *Arthashastra*, *Shastra*s, *Smritis*, *Manusmriti* and scriptures in various regional languages. India is one of the world's most biodiverse countries. It only covers 2.4% of the world's land area but holds 7–8% of the world's recognized species. There are 26 agro-climate zones in the world and 16 agro-climate zones in India alone. Its diverse agro-climate zones range from the trans-Himalayan region to Kerala, Andaman and Nicobar coastal areas. India is home to a wide variety of herbs, shrubs, tubers, mangroves and rhizomes (Dubey et al. 2004). The Botanical Survey of India and the Zoological Survey of India reported more than 47,000 plant species and 81,000 animal species. This natural wealth has created a rich collection of traditional medicine systems, including Ayurveda, Yoga, Unani, Homeopathy and Siddha (Vaidya and Devasagayam 2007).

38.2.1 Defining Biopiracy and Biopiracy of Indian Traditional Knowledge

The term piracy is defined as an unauthorized publication or reproduction of another person's work or material. It is the stealing of someone's work illegally or without taking any permission. Biopiracy can be defined as the stealing of biomedical knowledge from communities and individuals without their consent (Mooney 2000). There is not a well-accepted definition of biopiracy. Even though the Action Group on Erosion, Technology and Concentration (ETC Group 2017) defines it as:

> '...the appropriation of the knowledge and genetic resources of farming and indigenous communities by individuals or institutions seeking exclusive monopoly control (usually patents or plant breeders' rights) over these resources and knowledge'.

The main problem with biopiracy is the exploitation of biological resources and the knowledge of indigenous tribes and traditional communities by professional organizations and multinational companies. The innovations and the discovery of pharmaceutical and agricultural research are not new as they are inventive because they are based on centuries of traditional societies' knowledge (Mgbeoji 2006).

Traditional knowledge has always been a treasure that is easily accessible and therefore susceptible to misuse. Traditional knowledge, especially concerning the treatment of different diseases, has led to the development of biologically active molecules in technology-rich countries. Traditional knowledge is often misappropriated because it is easily assumed that since it is in the public domain, communities have abandoned all their claims.

CSIR found that nearly 80% of the 4,896 references to individual plant-based medicinal patents in the US Patent Office in 2000 related to only seven Indian medicinal plants. Three years later, nearly 15,000 patents spread over the United States, United Kingdom and other registers of patent offices on such medicines. This number increased to 35,000 in 2005, clearly demonstrating the interest of the developed world in developing countries' traditional knowledge. There is no patent examiners from developing countries, who can examine the claims and cross-check it from traditional practices of indigenous communities (National Knowledge Commission 2005). Some major biopiracy cases regarding Indian products are discussed below.

38.2.1.1 Neem

The neem plant is very useful for controlling the attack of fungal diseases on food crops and pests. It can be used to cure a cold and flu using its seed oil. It also relieves malaria, skin problems and even meningitis. In 1994 the US Department of Agriculture and the W.R. Grace Company received a patent (EPO patent No.436257) for a method to control fungi in plants with the help of neem oil extracted from hydrophobic from the European Patent Office (EPO). In 1995, a group of international NGOs and Indian farmer's representatives lodged a legal objection to this patent. They submitted evidence that the fungicidal effect of neem seed extracts was known and used in Indian agriculture to protect crops for centuries and that it is not patentable. The EPO revoked the patent in May 2000 (Goyal and Arora 2009).

38.2.1.2 Turmeric

The turmeric is used as a spice for flavouring Indian dishes. It has traditionally been used as a medicine for healing wounds and rashes for centuries. In 1995, a US patent (No.5, 401504) for the use of turmeric in wound healing was granted to two expatriate Indians at the University of Mississippi Medical Centre. The Council of Scientific and Industrial Research (CSIR), India, filed a case for re-examination with the US Patent Office in which the patent was challenged on the grounds of prior art. CSIR argued that turmeric had been used for the cure of wounds and rashes for thousands of years, and its medicinal use was therefore not a new invention. They show traditional knowledge in ancient Sanskrit manuscripts and a paper published in the Indian Medical Association journal in 1953. In 1997, the US Patent Office revoked this patent.

38.2.1.3 Basmati Rice

RiceTec. Inc., an American company, applied before the UK Trade Mark Registry Office for the registration of the trademark 'Texmati'. Agricultural and Processed Food Export Development Authority (APEDA), India, opposed and argued that basmati varieties already have been cultivated in India that RiceTec claims to be unique. This US utility patent was unique in claiming the rice plant that had similar characteristics to the traditional Indian basmati rice. It was dismissed in 2001.

38.2.1.4 Rice Biopiracy

Syngenta is a biotech company that has attempted to collect the precious collections of 22,972 rice varieties from rice bowl of India, Chhattisgarh. Syngenta has signed a memorandum of understanding with the Indira Gandhi Agricultural University (IGAU) for Dr. Richharia's priceless rice diversity collection. Dr. Richharia is the former director of the Central Rice Research

Institute (CRRI), Cuttack, and is known as India's rice sage who has pioneered the field.

38.2.1.5 Pharmaceuticals

Indigenous knowledge in the field of pharmaceutical research contributes to the identification of the material in the development of the drugs. It often provides information on its uses in the treatment of certain diseases, preparation methods and dosage. Some of the other recent examples of patents granted on the basis of biological resources that relate to 'inventions' are:

- *Phyllanthus* has been used for the treatment of jaundice traditionally.
- Treatment of diabetes by using composition of Jamun, Gurmar, bitter gourd and eggplant.
- Using neem tree for production of various products.
- Basmati rice varieties that grow in a temperate climate in the absence of sunlight.
- Using methi as a tonic to bring down blood glucose levels.
- Kala jeera or Kalonji compositions to increase immune functions and treat diabetes, hepatitis and asthma.

38.3 Traditional Knowledge Digital Library (TKDL)

It was a matter of concern to protect and preserve traditional knowledge for the developing countries. India has started protection of its traditional knowledge from patent biopiracy very late after above-mentioned cases. The Department of Ayurveda, Yoga and Naturopathy, Unani, Siddha and Homoeopathy (AYUSH) formed an interdisciplinary task force to create an approach paper on the establishment of a Traditional Knowledge Digital library in 1999. (Menon 2009).

TKDL is aimed at Indian medicine systems i.e. Ayurveda, Unani, Siddha, Homeopathy and Yoga to make them available in public domain. This knowledge is documented by collecting and sifting in five international languages, *English*, *Spanish*, *German*, *French* and *Japanese* from existing literature available in *Sanskrit*, *Arabic*, *Persian*, *Urdu* and *Tamil* (Hirwade 2010). The information containing two lakh formulations was transcribed in order to achieve the TKDL project objective. Each *Sloka* is read and translated into a structured language by subject experts using the classification of traditional knowledge resources (TKRC). The *Slokas* are categorized in the database. The abstraction is carried out by the subject experts and all the codes are translated using TKRC and stored into the database. The codes once stored in the metadata directory are converted to different languages using Unicode Technology. It can be noted that the software does not transliterate, but rather a knowledge-based conversion, in which data is converted into these languages using Unicode and Metadata methodology. The software also converts traditional terminology to modern terminology, e.g. turmeric to *Curcuma longa*, Jwar to fever, Mussoric to small pox, etc. Figure 38.1 shows the home page of the TKDL (Ansari 2016; Gupta 2005).

38.3.1 Traditional Knowledge Resource Classification (TKRC)

The TKDL expert group estimated that approximately 200 numbers of incorrect patents concerning Indian medical systems were granted at the international level every year. The main reason is that traditional medical knowledge exists in Indian languages and patent examiners at the international patent office did not understand it because of language and format barriers. The TKDL breaks these barriers and translated the information into five international languages and structured scientifically into the database. The use of IT tools and a new classification system, Traditional Knowledge Resource Classification (TKRC), enable the conversion of available information into 34 million A4 pages.

TKRC is an innovative structured system of classification based on the International Patent Classification (IPC). It has approximately 27,000 Ayurveda, Unani, Siddha and Yoga subgroups. The aim of the creation of TKRC is not only to provide Indian traditional medicine a structured classification but also to use as an abstracting and retrieval tool Fig. 38.2 represents the hierarchy of the TKRC scheme.

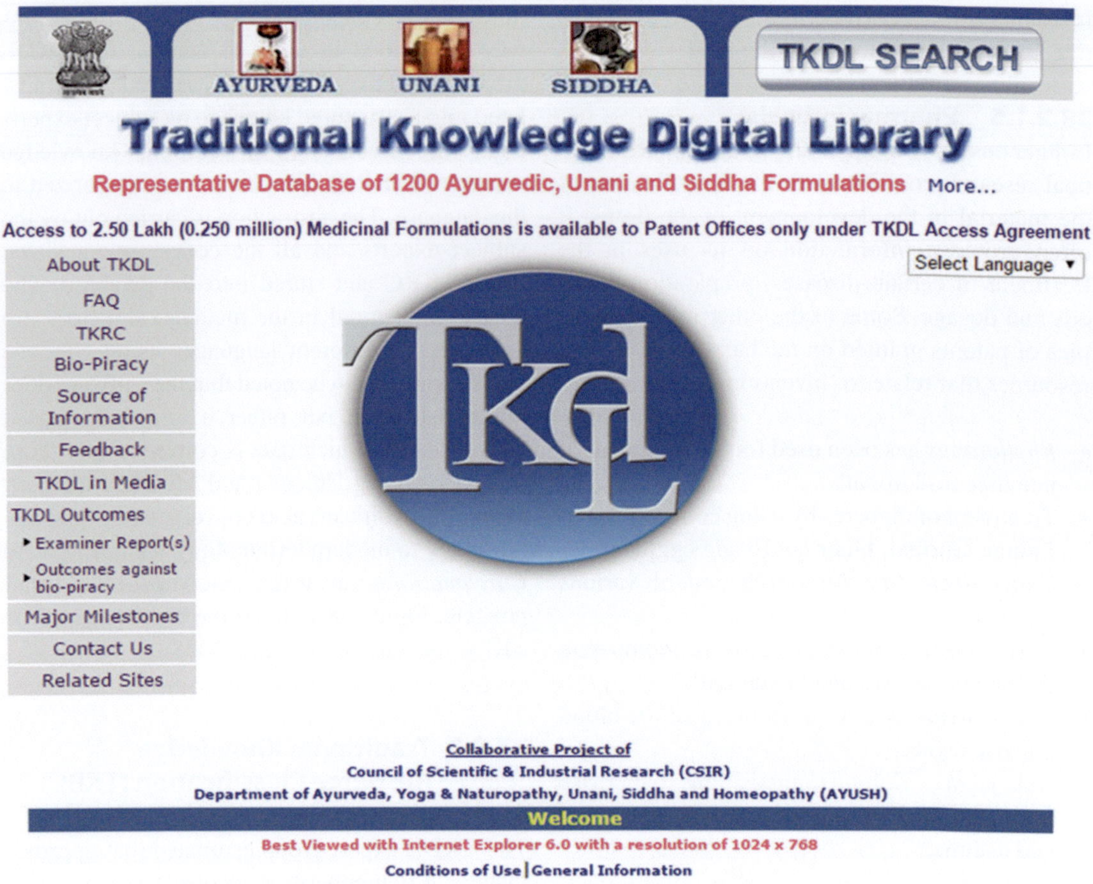

Fig. 38.1 Traditional Knowledge Digital Library (TKDL) Homepage (www.tkdl.res.in/)

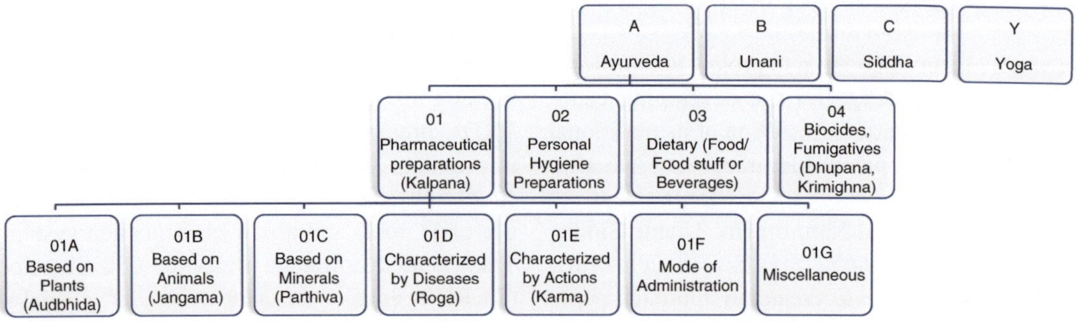

Fig. 38.2 Structure of classification in TKRC (http://www.tkdl.res.in/tkdl/langdefault/common/Section.asp)

The TKRC is mainly divided into the following sections:

- A—Ayurveda
- B—Unani
- C—Siddha
- Y—Yoga

Section A (Ayurveda) is divided into the following classes:

- 01—Pharmaceutical preparations (Kalpana)
- 02—Personal hygiene preparations
- 03—Dietary (food/foodstuff or beverages)
- 04—Biocides, fumigations (Dhupana, Krimighna)

The sub-section 01 (pharmaceutical preparations) are divided into following subclasses based on the material used:

- 01A—Based on plants (Audbhida)
- 01B—Based on animals (Jangama)
- 01C—Based on minerals (Parthiva)
- 01D—Characterized by diseases (Roga)
- 01E—Characterized by actions (Karma)
- 01F—Mode of administration
- 01G—Miscellaneous

For example, the subclass A01A represents pharmaceutical preparations based on plants, which is described as:

A—Ayurveda
01—Pharmaceutical preparations (Kalpana)
A—Based on plants (Audbhida)

38.3.2 Breaking Down Barriers Between TK Holders and Patent Examiners

The TKDL is a unique, proprietary database that integrates a variety of knowledge systems—Ayurveda, Unani, Siddha, modern science and medicine, classic languages—and Sanskrit, Arabic, Urdu, Persian, Tamil and international languages, English, Japanese, French and German. It is based on 148 state-of-the-art books relating to Indian medical systems, available at a cost of around US$ 1,000. The TKDL links patent examiners worldwide to these knowledge books. The TKDL is available to all patent offices which have signed a non-disclosure access agreement with TKDL. Patent examiners may only use the TKDL database for search and examination purposes under this agreement. The TKDL content can only be disclosed to third parties for citation purposes. The TKDL Access Agreement has integrated non-disclosure mechanisms to protect the interests of India and to counter any possible misuse. India has signed TKDL Access Agreements with the EPO and patent offices in Australia, Germany, Japan, New Zealand, Canada, the United States and the United Kingdom (Twarog and Kapoor 2004).

38.3.3 TKDL Database: Current Status

The TKDL database is a tool for understanding the existing codified knowledge of the Indian medical systems as a prior art. It is not a user or diagnostic database. TKDL contains scanned images of the original scriptural medical formulations. It covers two lakh formulations taken from different ancient manuscripts. It is important to note that TKDL does not contain all the information available in the Indian medical systems rather than comprehensive. TKDL is a dynamic database in which formulations are continually added and updated according to the inputs of database user. The complete database was made available to all IPR offices around the world to facilitate the search for prior art and to prevent biopiracy.

The representative database having 1200 formulations can be accessed from the official TKDL website. The current transcription status of the traditional medicine formula in TKDL is shown in Table 38.1.

38.3.4 Content Analysis of Representative Database of TKDL

The detailed content analysis of the representative database of TKDL reveals that the database has 41.66% formulation from Ayurveda, 41.66% formulations from Unani and 16.66% formulations from Siddha. The database still has to add formulations in Yoga. These formulations use approximately 308 plants as ingredients

Table 38.1 Present status of TKDL (http://www.tkdl.res.in/tkdl/langdefault/common/SourceInfo.asp?GL=Eng accessed on 3 October 2017)

Sr. no.	Discipline	No. of text (including volumes) used for transcription	Transcribed
1	Ayurveda	75	97,337
2	Unani	10	1,75,150
3	Siddha	50	23,016
4	Yoga	15	1,680
Total		150	2,97,183

other than animal or mineral origin ingredients. They are used in turn to treat 214 diseases (Table 38.2).

38.3.5 Search Types and Search Options in TKDL

The TKDL has a search interface that provides full-text search and retrieval of traditional IPC knowledge and multi-language keywords. The search functionality includes single or multiple word searches, proximity searches, complex Boolean searches, phrase searches, field searches, etc. Simple search allows the user to search for a combination of keywords. This is a searchable database that can be started by clicking on the Homepage icons of Ayurveda, Unani or Siddha. The following is the screenshot of its search interface (Fig. 38.3).

Table 38.2 Contents of representative TKDL database (http://www.tkdl.res.in/tkdl/langdefault/Common/More.asp?GL=Eng accessed on 3 October 2017)

Sr. no.	Subjects	No. of formulations	Percentage
1	Ayurveda	500	41.66
2	Unani	500	41.66
3	Siddha	200	16.66
4	Yoga	–	–
Total		1200	100

38.3.5.1 Simple Search

Various search terms, including keywords, diseases and IPC codes can be used with the 'OR' operator (the use of the 'AND' operator is not accepted). The corresponding menu lists all available search terms in this database and can be used to select the corresponding search term.

Features of Simple Search

- Terms to be searched may be selected from corresponding help menus or entered.
- Ultimately, you can enter single or multiple search terms.
- Using the operator OR, multiple search terms can be searched.
- Tick the checkbox labelled 'with local name' to search using local names.

38.3.5.2 Advanced Search

This option allows a combination of multiple search terms, such as keywords, IPC code, disease, title and bibliography, to be searched individually also. All these terms can be chosen from suitable help menus.

Features of Advanced Search

- The search terms can be entered or selected from the corresponding help menu in the text box provided.

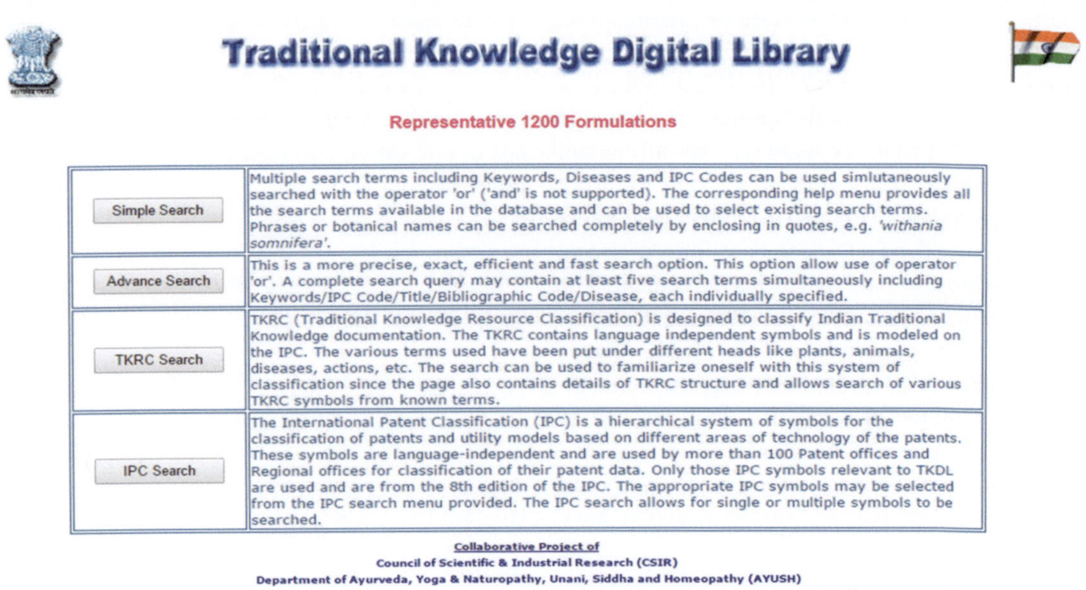

Fig. 38.3 Traditional Knowledge Digital Library (TKDL) Search Window (http://www.tkdl.res.in/tkdl/langdefault/common/Global_Search.asp?GL=Eng)

- You can search for a single term, but the text box at the top should not be left empty.
- The keyword help can be used to find appropriate keywords. It provides a comprehensive list of the keywords used in the database, including plant ingredients, animal or mineral. Traditional names and Sanskrit, Tamil or Urdu terms can be used directly (in diacritical terms).
- A list of all diseases which can be cured by formulations in the database is provided in the Disease Help menu.
- Formulations can be also searched by given title by select Title option in the search window.
- The 'with local name' checkbox can be used to search by local names.
- The OR can be used to get results that contain both search terms including standard and common language. For example, Curcuma OR cough gives all formulations that either contain Curcuma or cough.
- The 'Knowledge is known' drop-down menu can be used to view the formulations on the basis of the time period. For example, selecting 200 years will show all types of formulations that is 200 years old.
- The options 'along with a summary' and 'without a summary' can be selected to view result accordingly.

It also has also two additional search options.

38.3.5.3 TKRC Search

The TKRC is designed to classify document on traditional Indian knowledge. The TKRC has independent language symbols and is modelled on the IPC. The different terms used were put under different heads, such as animals, plants, diseases, actions and so on. The search can be used to familiarize people with this classification system, as the page also contains TKRC structure details and allows to search for different TKRC symbols from known terms.

38.3.5.4 IPC Search

The International Patent Classification (IPC) is a system of symbols for the classification of patents and utility models based on various fields of patent technology. These symbols are language independent and are used for the classification of their patent data by more than 100 national patent and regional offices. The TKDL used only those IPC symbols from the eighth IPC edition which are relevant to them. The appropriate IPC symbols can be selected from the provided IPC search menu. The IPC search allows you to search for single or multiple symbols.

38.4 Success of TKDL Against Biopiracy

TKDL team identified 1155 applications for patents at the International Patent Offices, such as the European Patent Office (EPO), US Patent and Trademark Office (USPTO), the Canadian Intellectual Property Office (CIPO), the UK Patent and Trademark Office (UKPTO), the German Patent and Trade Mark Office (DPMA), IP Australia and the Controller General for Patents, Designs and Trademarks (CGPDTM) for patents related to Indian medicine systems. The most significant success has been achieved in 220 cases where the patent applications have either been cancelled/withdrawn/terminated/declared dead or the claims have been amended by the applicants or have been rejected by the examiner on the basis of TKDL proposals (Tables 38.3 and 38.4).

Table 38.3 Patent office-wise number of cases withdrawn/cancelled/declared dead/terminated (http://www.tkdl.res.in/tkdl/langdefault/Common/outcomemain.asp?GL=Eng)

Sl. no	Patent office	No. of cases
1	European Patent Office (EPO)	129
2	The US Patent and Trademark Office (USPTO)	25
3	Controller General of Patents, Designs and Trademarks (CGPDTM)	24
4	Canadian Intellectual Property Office (CIPO)	37
5	IP Australia (AIPO)	4
6	UK Patent and Trademark Office (UKPTO)	1
	Total	220

38.4.1 TKDL Success Against MNC

Many multinational companies tried to take patent of traditional Indian medicinal knowledge, but they failed. On the basis of TKDL submissions, the examiners have refused their patent applications. Some famous successes against MNCs are given in Table 38.5.

Table 38.4 Year-wise number of cases withdrawn/cancelled/declared dead/terminated (http://www.tkdl.res.in/tkdl/langdefault/Common/outcomemain.asp?GL=Eng)

Sl. no.	Year	No. of cases
1	2017	1
2	2016	4
3	2015	15
4	2014	28
5	2013	45
6	2012	53
7	2011	44
8	2010	22
9	2009	8
	Total	220

38.5 Conclusion

The protection of indigenous traditional knowledge raises many issues. The issues concerning the protection of such knowledge in accordance with existing IPR laws are very complex. Most of developing countries are mostly unaware of the protection of traditional knowledge, and this cause biopiracy. Another important issue is the extent to which TK can be protected and preserved. The identification of TK and codification in standard level is a very tough task.

Indian government started the preservation and protection of their indigenous knowledge under the TKDL project. The traditional knowledge recorded in TKDL becomes knowledge of the public domain and cannot be regarded for a patent. The database is easily accessible to patent offices worldwide, and nobody can obtain a recorded patent. If a person requests for a patent, the examiner can easily check the database and reject the application, which could be a mere copy of traditional Indian knowledge.

Table 38.5 Successful cases defended by TKDL

Country	Patent application no.	Name of Company	Description of claim which was denied or withdraw
USA	EP1906980	Natreon Inc.	Treatment of a range of illnesses including diabetes, depression, insomnia, convulsions and gastritis using ashwagandha
	EP1825845	Jan Marini Skin Research, Inc.	Use of brahmi, ashwagandha, tea leaves and turmeric as anti-ageing and anti-inflammatory medicine
	EP2116253	Phytrix JV, LLC	Treatment of HIV-associated diseases using Phyllanthus/Bhumi Aamla
	EP1942917	Juice Beauty	Treatment of acne, freckles and skin marks Using grapes, lemon, apple and aloe vera
	EP1709995	Al-Jassim, Rawaa	Treatment of conjunctivitis and allergic disorders using Black seeds
	EP1959977	Jaffe, Russell M.	Treatment of indigestion, constipation and diabetes using Babool
Korea	EP1971354	Seoul National University Industry Foundation	Treatment of liver-related diseases using licorice/mulaithi
	EP1781309	PuriMed Co. Ltd.	Use of Indian lotus for the treatment of heart diseases
Italy	EP1520585	Data Medica Padova S.p.A	Using Pista as an anti-cancer medicine
	EP2133089	Indena S.p.A	Use of Abuqanus to treat asthma and breathlessness
	EP2070545	Bios Line S.p.a.	Use of olive, turmeric and mint for the treatment of dysentery
	EP2014295	Velleja Research SRL	Use of licorice/mulaithi, turmeric and chamomile as anti-inflammatory and anti-infective medicine in the genital area

Table 38.5 (continued)

Country	Patent application no.	Name of Company	Description of claim which was denied or withdraw
Japan	EP1949889	Mercian Corporation	Treatment of skin marks and acne using grapes
Germany	EP2218455	Cognis IP Management GmbH	Use of horse gram/kulattha as an antioxidant for wound healing medicine
	EP1967197	Cognis IP Management GmbH	Treatment of obesity using Gheekawaar
	EP2065031	Evonik Goldschmidt GmbH	Use of Arjuna as an anti-wrinkle and anti-ageing agent
	EP1759706	PRIEBE INGRID	Treatment of skin, renal and urinary disorders using yellow gentian
China	EP1849473	Livzon Pharmaceutical	The use of mint and kalamegha for avian influenza treatment
	EP1889638	Jumpsun Bio-Medicine Co., Ltd.	Obesity and diabetes treatment with Bengal gram/chana
Switzerland	EP2263481	NESTEC SA	Green tea extracts of improved bioavailability
	EP2133080	Haelan Schweiz	Use of pomegranate/anaar and alsi for the treatment of heart, skin and diabetes diseases
Australia	EP1729593	Natbio Pty Ltd.	Use of ginger to treat malabsorption and inflammation
India	EP1660106	Avesthagen Limited	Use of arjuna as a cardiotonic and diabetes and obesity treatment
Britain	EP1937231	GW Pharma Limited	Use of Bhaang to treat bronchitis and cough
	EP2090315	Kapur MBBS, B., Dr.	Using opium, fenugreek and spinach as immunomodulators
Netherlands	EP1607006	Unilever N.V	Using apple juice and grape juice as a cardiotonic
Brazil	EP2101800	Ache Laboratories	Treatment of diabetes, hypertension and obesity using grape
Canada	EP2089505	Herbal Infusion Corporation	Use of turmeric for reducing alcoholic hangover
Cyprus	EP1958641	Bionature	Treatment of inflammation using *Pistacia lentiscus*/Mastgee
Israel	EP2015761	Naveh Pharma	Treatment of diseases of throat using rose and sweet violet/Banafshah
Spain	EP1747786	Perdix Eurogroup SL	Using watery extract of muskmelon as an anti-vitilgo cream
Kenya	EP1807098	Amcod Limited	Use of Gheekawaar, Daal Chini and neem for the treatment of diabetes
Denmark	EP2044850	Clara's ApS	Use of turmeric, cumin, ginger and onion as a slimming agent
	EP2094287	Ocumedic ApS	Treatment of eye disease using Naarangi
Argentina	EP2008661	Spannagel Lucia Antonia	Treating wound using aloe vera, Marigold and Brahmi as a healing agent
Norway	EP2091353	Biorigin Scandinavia AS	Treatment of worm infestation and external parasites using rice, wheat, sunflower and barley
New Zealand	EP 1750809	Industrial Research Limited and Otago Innovation Limited	Citrus fruit skin extract for angiogenesis promotion

The increasing impact of the TKDL has already being felt at internationally. The TKDL team of the EPO has identified 220 applications for patents concerning Indian medicinal systems submitted by third parties since July 2009. The applications were refused or withdrawn by the applicant after TKDL had submitted the evidence. A recent study by a TKDL expert team at the EPO shows a sharp decline (44%) in the number of patent applications for Indian medical systems submitted. The results show that TKDL is clearly an effective dissuasive agent against biopiracy.

References

Ansari MS. Evaluation of role of traditional knowledge digital library and traditional Chinese medicine database in preservation of traditional medicinal knowledge. DESIDOC J Lib Inform Technol. 2016;36(2):73–8.

Apte T. A simple guide to intellectual property rights, biodiversity and traditional knowledge. Pune, New Delhi: Kalpavriksh-Grain-IIED; 2006.

Bardi M, Guti errez-Oppe E, Politano R. Traditional knowledge products in Latin America and their misappropriation. J Intellect Prop Law Prac. 2011;6:34–42.

Brush S. Whose knowledge; whose genes; whose rights? In: Brush S, Stabinsky D, editors. Indigenous people and intellectual property rights. Washington, DC: Island Press; 2007. p. 1–24.

Carlos M. Protection and promotion of traditional medicine-implications for public health in developing countries. 2002. http://www.southcentre.org/publications/traditionalmedicine/toc.htm. Accessed 21 Aug 2016.

Conforto D. Traditional and modern-day biopiracy: redefining the biopiracy debate. J Environ Law Litig. 2004;19:357–96.

Dubey NK, Kumar R, Tripathi P. Global promotion of herbal medicine: India's opportunity. Curr Sci. 2004:37–41.

ETC Group. Biopiracy. Montoring power, Tracking technology, Strenghening diversity. 2017. http://www.etcgroup.org/content/biopiracy. Accessed 12 Jan 2017.

Finetti C. Traditional knowledge and the patent system: two worlds apart? World Pat Inform. 2011;33:58–66.

Goyal AK, Arora S. India's fourth National Report to the convention on biological diversity. New Delhi: Ministry of Environment and Forests, Government of India; 2009.

Gupta VK. Traditional knowledge digital library. Subregional experts meeting in Asia on intangible cultural heritage. Bangkok. 2005.

Hasan I. Alternative medicine. Articleworld.org. 2010. http://www.articleworld.org/Alternative_medicine#axzz1PbHzzkAZ. Accessed 19 Sept 2017.

Hirwade MA. Protecting traditional knowledge digitally: a case study of TKDL. In: National Workshop on Digitization Initiatives & Applications in Indian Context, DNC, Nagpur. 2010. http://eprints.rclis.org/14020/1/TKDL_paper.pdf. Accessed 20 Aug 2016.

Martin VA. Biopiracy: the need for a protective solution? 2010. http://www.jur.lu.se/Internet/Utbildning/kurser/JCA803.nsf/43e828219552/. Accessed 20 Aug 2016.

Menon R. Traditional knowledge receives a boost from the government. India together. 2009. http://www.indiatogether.org/. Accessed 25 Jul 2015.

Mgbeoji S. Global Biopiracy: patents, plants and indigenous knowledge. Vancouver, BC: University of British Columbia Press; 2006.

Mooney P. Why we call it biopiracy. In: Svarstad H, Dhillion S, editors. Responding to bio-prospecting: from biodiversity in the south to medicines in the north. Oslo: Spartacus Forlag; 2000. p. 37–44.

National Knowledge Commission. Traditional knowledge. 2005. http://knowledgecommissionarchive.nic.in/focus/traditional.asp. Accessed 25 Aug 2016.

Twarog S, Kapoor P. Protecting and promoting traditional knowledge: systems, national experiences and international dimensions. In: United Nations Conference on Trade and Development. New York and Geneva: United Nations; 2004.. http://unctad.org/en/docs/ditcted10_en.pdf. Accessed 21 Aug 2016.

Vadi V. Intangible heritage: traditional medicine and knowledge governance. J Intellect Prop Law Pract. 2007;2:682–91.

Vaidya AD, Devasagayam TP. Current status of herbal drugs in India: an overview. J Clin Biochem Nutr. 2007;41:1–11.

WHO Traditional medicine. Secretariat. World Health Organization Fifty-Sixth World Health Assembly A56/18. Geneva: World Health Organization; 2003.. http://apps.who.int/gb/archive/pdf_files/WHA56/ea5618.pdf. Accessed 6 May 2016

World Health Organization. Traditional medicine – growing needs and potential. 2002. http://whqlibdoc.who.int/hq/2002/WHO_EDM_2002.4.pdf. Accessed 13 Jun 2017.

Zhang X. Traditional medicine: its importance and protection. Protecting and promoting traditional knowledge: systems, national experiences and international dimensions. New York: United Nations; 2004.. http://unctad.org/en/docs/ditcted10_en.pdf. Accessed 8 Jul 2017

Further Readings

Traditional Knowledge Resource Classification. http://www.tkdl.res.in/tkdl/langdefault/common/TKRC.asp

TKDL-Traditional Knowledge Digital Library. www.tkdl.res.in

Correction to: Preclinical and Clinical Trials of Indian Medicinal Plants in Disease Control

Md. Harun Al Rashid, Anindita Kundu, Vivekananda Mandal, Phurpa Wangchuk, and Subhash C. Mandal

Correction to:
S. Sen, R. Chakraborty (eds.), *Herbal Medicine in India*, https://doi.org/10.1007/978-981-13-7248-3_9

The original version of Chapter 9 was inadvertently published with incorrect author name "Harun Al Rashid" instead of "Md. Harun Al Rashid". The chapter has been updated.

The updated online version of this chapter can be found at
https://doi.org/10.1007/978-981-13-7248-3_9

S. Sen, R. Chakraborty (eds.), *Herbal Medicine in India*,
https://doi.org/10.1007/978-981-13-7248-3_39